Leadership
and
Nursing Care Management

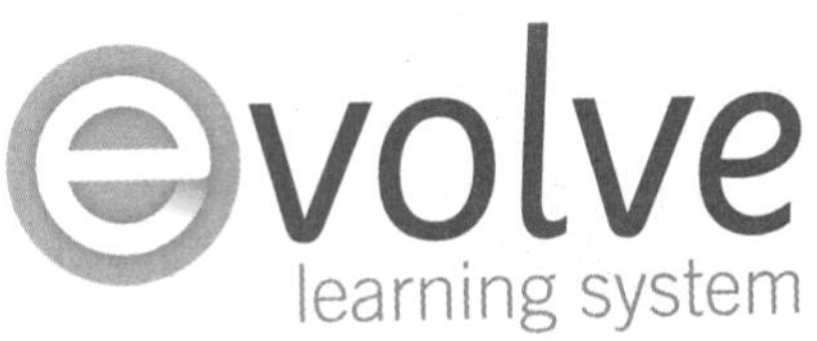

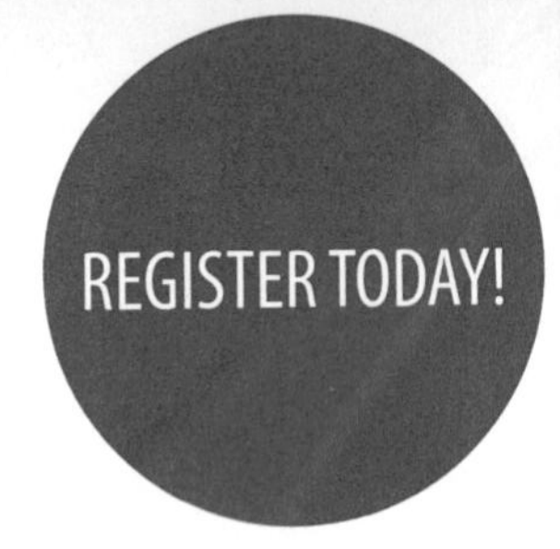

To access your Student Resources, visit the web address below:

http://evolve.elsevier.com/Huber/leadership/

Evolve Student Learning Resources for Huber: Leadership and Nursing Care Management, Fourth Edition, offers the following features:

- **Case Studies**
  Case scenarios with accompanying questions and answer guidelines apply chapter content to real-life nursing practice.
- **Glossary**
  A comprehensive alphabetical listing gives readers access to a compilation of all key terms within the text.
- **Research Notes**
  Additional summaries of current research studies complement the recent literature studies in the text.
- **Short-Answer Study Questions**
  Essay questions promote critical thinking related to important concepts.
- **Study Questions**
  Matching and true-or-false questions reinforce the key content covered in the text.
- **WebLinks**
  Links to hundreds of websites supplement the textbook content.

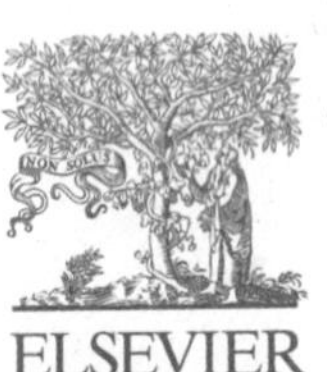

Leadership and Nursing Care Management

Fourth Edition

Diane L. Huber, PhD, RN, FAAN, NEA-BC
Professor
College of Nursing and College of Public Health
The University of Iowa
Iowa City, Iowa

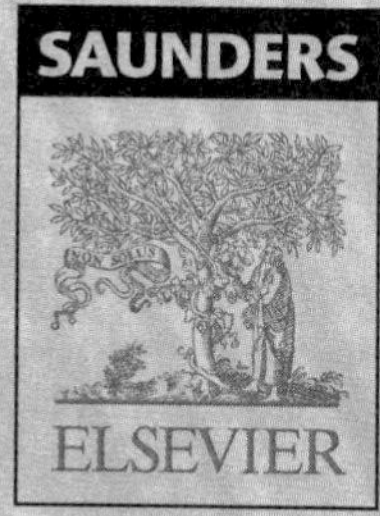

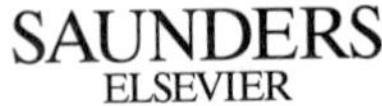

3251 Riverport Lane
Maryland Heights, Missouri 63043

LEADERSHIP AND NURSING CARE MANAGEMENT ISBN: 978-1-4160-5984-4

Library of Congress Cataloging-in-Publication Data

Leadership and nursing care management / [edited by] Diane L. Huber. – 4th ed.
p.; cm.
Includes bibliographical references and index.
ISBN 978-1-4160-5984-4 (pbk.: alk. paper) 1. Nursing services—Administration. 2. Leadership. 3. Nurse administrators. I. Huber, Diane.
[DNLM: 1. Nursing Services–organization & administration. 2. Leadership. 3. Nursing, Supervisory. WY 105 L4327 2010]
RT89.H83 2010
362.17'3068–dc22

2009016322

Managing Editor: Nancy O'Brien
Senior Acquisitions Editor: Kristin Geen
Associate Developmental Editor: Angela Perdue
Developmental Editor: Jamie Horn
Editorial Assistant: Jennifer Palada
Publishing Services Manager: Deborah L. Vogel
Senior Project Manager: Jodi M. Willard
Book Designer: Charles Seibel

Printed in United States of America

Last digit is the print number: 9 8 7 6 5 4 3 2 1

Contributors

Lecia A. Albright, BS, CPHQ, FNAHQ
Principal and Owner
LARA Consulting, LLC
Spotsylvania, Virginia

G. Rumay Alexander, EdD, MSN, BSN
Associate Clinical Professor
Director, Office of Multicultural Affairs
School of Nursing
University of North Carolina at Chapel Hill
Chapel Hill, North Carolina

Mary K. Anthony, PhD, RN, CS
Associate Dean for Research
Associate Professor
Kent State University
Kent, Ohio

Bonnie Weaver Battey, PhD, RN
Nursing Education Consultant
Antioch, California

Sharon A. Eck Birmingham, DNSc, MA, BSN, RN
Chief Nursing Executive
AtStaff, Inc.;
Adjunct Faculty
University of North Carolina, School of Nursing
Durham, North Carolina

Karen W. Budd, PhD, RN
Director, Graduate Programs
College of Nursing
Kent State University
Kent, Ohio

Thomas R. Clancy, PhD, MBA, RN
Clinical Professor
School of Nursing
University of Minnesota
Minneapolis, Minnesota

Sean P. Clarke, RN, PhD, FAAN
RBC Chair in Cardiovascular Nursing Research
Lawrence S. Bloomberg Faculty of Nursing, University of Toronto, and University Health Network
Toronto, Ontario, Canada

Robert W. Cooper, PhD
Employers Mutual Distinguished Professor of Insurance, College of Business and Public Administration
Drake University
Des Moines, Iowa

Karen S. Cox, RN, PhD, FAAN
Executive Vice President/Co-Chief Operating Officer
The Children's Mercy Hospital
Kansas City, Missouri

Kathleen B. Cox, PhD, RN
Assistant Professor
University of Virginia School of Nursing
Charlottesville, Virginia

Kathy Craig, MS, RN, CCM
Craig Research Continuum, LLC
Founder and President
Davidsonville, Maryland, and Kingston, Ontario, Canada

Laura Cullen, MA, RN, FAAN
Evidence-Based Practice Coordinator
Research Quality and Outcomes Manager
Nursing Services and Patient Care
University of Iowa Hospitals and Clinics
Iowa City, Iowa

Cindy Jean Dawson, RN, MSN, CORLN
Nurse Manager
Otolaryngology Head and Neck Surgery Clinic
Oral Surgery Clinic
University of Iowa Hospitals and Clinics
Iowa City, Iowa

Amy London Deutschendorf, MS, RN, APRN, BC
Senior Director, Clinical Resource Management
The Johns Hopkins Hospital
Baltimore, Maryland

Karen N. Drenkard, RN, PhD, CNAA, BC
Senior Vice President/Chief Nurse Executive
Inova Health System
Falls Church, Virginia

Therese A. Fitzpatrick, RN, PhD
Clinical Instructor
University of Illinois at Chicago, College of Nursing
Chicago, Illinois;
Executive Vice President and Healthcare Practice Leader
The Optimé Group
Evanston, Illinois

Betsy Frank, RN, PhD, ANEF
Professor
Indiana State University
Terre Haute, Indiana

Maryanne Garon, DNSc, MSN, RN
Associate Professor and Graduate Program Coordinator
Department of Nursing
California State University
Fullerton, California

Gregory O. Ginn, BA, MEd, MBA, PhD, CPA
Associate Professor of Health Care Administration and Policy
University of Nevada
Las Vegas, Nevada

L. Jean Henry, PhD
Assistant Professor
Health Science, Kinesiology, Recreation, and Dance
University of Arkansas
Fayetteville, Arkansas

Katherine R. Jones, PhD, RN, FAAN
Sarah Cole Hirsh Professor
Associate Dean for Evidence-Based Practice
Frances Payne Bolton School of Nursing
Case Western Reserve University
Cleveland, Ohio

Susan R. Lacey, RN, PhD, FAAN
Director, Bi-State Nursing Workforce Innovation Center
Director of Nursing Workforce & Systems Analysis
Children's Mercy Hospitals and Clinics
Kansas City, Missouri

Jo Manion, PhD, RN, NEA-BC, FAAN
Founder and Consultant
Manion and Associates
Oviedo, Florida

Maureen T. Marthaler, RN, MS
Associate Professor
Purdue University—Calumet
Hammond, Indiana

Amelia Sanchez McCutcheon, RN, PhD
Chief Nurse Officer and Executive Lead, Professional Practice
Vancouver Coastal Health Authority
Vancouver, British Columbia, Canada

Matthew D. McHugh, PhD, JD, MPH, CRNP, RN
Assistant Professor of Nursing
Center for Health Outcomes and Policy Research
University of Pennsylvania School of Nursing
Philadelphia, Pennsylvania

Raquel Meyer, RN, PhD(c)
Canadian Institutes of Health Research Doctoral Fellow
Lawrence S. Bloomberg Faculty of Nursing
University of Toronto
Toronto, Ontario, Canada

Jacqueline Moss, PhD, RN
Associate Professor and Assistant Dean for Clinical Simulation and Technology
University of Alabama at Birmingham, School of Nursing
Birmingham, Alabama

Mary Ellen Murray, PhD, RN
Associate Dean for Academic Affairs
Associate Professor
University of Wisconsin—Madison, School of Nursing
Madison, Wisconsin

Lynne S. Nemeth, PhD, RN, MS
Associate Professor
College of Nursing
Medical University of South Carolina
Charleston, South Carolina

Heidi Nobiling, RN, MA, MBA, NEA-BC
Senior Assistant Director
University of Iowa Hospitals and Clinics
Iowa City, Iowa

Luc R. Pelletier, MSN, APRN, PMHCNS-BC, FAAN, FNAHQ
Clinical Nurse Specialist
Sharp Mesa Vista Hospital;
Core Adjunct Faculty
National University
San Diego, California

Beth Pickard, BSN
President and CEO
AtStaff, Inc.
Durham, North Carolina

Belinda E. Puetz, PhD, RN
Principal, Puetz Consulting Services, Inc.;
Editor-in-Chief, Journal for Nurses in Staff Development
Cantonment, Florida

Richard W. Redman, PhD, RN
Professor
Director, Doctoral and Post-Doctoral Programs
University of Michigan School of Nursing
Ann Arbor, Michigan

Gene S. Rigotti, RN, MSN, CCNA, BCC
Director, Professional Practice
Inova Health System
Falls Church, Virginia

Claudia DiSabatino Smith, RN, PhD(c), NE-BC
Director, Nursing Research
St. Luke's Episcopal Hospital
Houston, Texas

Judith Lloyd Storfjell, PhD, RN, FAAN
Associate Professor and Associate Dean
Executive Director, Institute for Healthcare Innovation
University of Illinois at Chicago, College of Nursing
Chicago, Illinois

Kathleen Williams, RN, BSN, CORLN
Assistant Nurse Manager, Department of Nursing
University of Iowa Hospitals and Clinics
Iowa City, Iowa

Dana Woods, MBA, BA
Director of Marketing and Strategy Integration
American Association of Critical-Care Nurses
Aliso Viejo, California

Linda L. Workman, RN, PhD
VP Center of Professional Excellence
Patient Services, Cincinnati Children's Hospital Medical Center;
Associate Professor
University of Cincinnati College of Nursing
Cincinnati, Ohio

EVOLVE RESOURCES

Case Studies, Study Questions, Instructor's Manual, and PowerPoint Lecture Slides

Jean Nagelkerk, PhD, FNP-BC
Vice Provost for Health
Grand Valley State University
Grand Rapids, Michigan

TEST BANK

Susan Turner, RN, BSN, MSN, FNP
Lead Instructor, RN Program
Gavilan College
Gilroy, California

Reviewers

Jeanne Campbell Brock, MSN, RNC, WHNP
Curriculum Coordinator
Indiana University/Methodist Family Medicine Residency
Indianapolis, Indiana

Gloria Fowler, MN, RN, CNAA
Clinical Assistant Professor and Director of Student Affairs
University of South Carolina
College of Nursing
Columbia, South Carolina

Jaynelle F. Stichler, DNSc, RN, FACHE
Associate Professor
School of Nursing
Chair—Nursing Leadership in Health Systems
San Diego State University
San Diego, California

Preface

The time is now for strong leadership and care management in nursing. Highlighted by a series of reports from the prestigious Institute of Medicine (IOM), it is clear that nurses matter to health care delivery systems. Yet the United States is in the midst of a severe and continuing nurse shortage. Strong nurse leaders and administrators are important for clients (and their safety), for delivery systems (and their viability), and for payers (and their solvency). Some have called this the Age of the Nurse, but pressures remain to balance cost and quality considerations in a complex, chaotic, and turbulent health care environment. Although society's need for excellent nursing care remains the nurse's constant underlying reason for existence, nursing is in reality much more than that. It is the Age of the Nurse precisely because nurses offer cost-effective expertise in solving problems related to the coordination and delivery of health care to individuals and populations in society. Nurses are well prepared to lead clinical change strategies and to effectively manage the coordination and integration of interdisciplinary teams, population needs, and systems of care across the continuum.

It can be argued that nursing is a unique profession in which the primary focus is caring—giving and managing the care that clients need. Thus nurses are both health care providers and health care coordinators; that is, they have both clinical and managerial role components. Beginning with the first edition of *Leadership and Nursing Care Management*, it has been this text's philosophy that these two components can be discussed separately but in fact overlap. Because all nurses are involved in coordinating client care, leadership and management principles are a part of the core competencies they need to function in a complex health care environment.

The turbulent swirl of change in this country's health care industry has provided both challenges and opportunities for nursing. Nurses have needed a stronger background in nursing leadership and client care management to be prepared for contemporary and future nursing practice. As nurses mature in advanced practice roles and as the health care delivery system restructures, nurses will become increasingly pivotal to cost-effective health care delivery. Leadership and management are crucial skills and abilities for complex and integrated community and regional networks that employ and deploy nurses to provide health care services to clients and communities.

Today nurses are expected to be able to lead and manage care across the health care continuum—a radically different approach to nursing than has been the norm for hospital staff nursing practice. In all settings, including both nurse-run and interdisciplinary clinics, nursing leadership and management are complementary skills that add value to solid clinical care and client-oriented practice. Thus there is an urgent need to advance nurses' knowledge and skills in leadership and management. In addition, nurses who are expected to make and implement day-to-day management decisions need to know how these precepts can be practically applied to the organization and delivery of nursing care in a way that conserves scarce resources, reduces costs, and maintains or improves quality of care.

The primary modality for health care in the United States has moved away from acute care hospitalization. As prevention, wellness, and alternative sites for care delivery become more important, nursing's already rich experiential tradition of practice in these settings is emerging. This text reflects this contemporary trend by blending the hospital and nonhospital perspectives when examining and analyzing nursing care, leadership, and management. The reader will notice examples from the wide spectrum of nursing practice settings in the specific applications of nursing leadership and care management principles.

PURPOSE AND AUDIENCE

The intent of this text is to provide both a comprehensive introduction to the field and a synthesis of the knowledge base and skills related to both nursing leadership and nursing management. It is an evidence-based blend of practice and theory. It breaks new ground by explaining the intersection of nursing care with leading people and managing organizations and systems. It highlights the evidence base for care management. It combines traditional management perspectives and theory with contemporary health care trends and issues and consistently integrates leadership and management concepts. These concepts are illustrated and made relevant by practice-based examples.

The impetus for writing this text comes from teaching both undergraduate and graduate students in nursing leadership and management and from perceiving the need for a comprehensive, practice-based textbook that blends and integrates leadership and management into an understandable and applicable whole.

Therefore the main goal of *Leadership and Nursing Care Management* is twofold: (1) to clearly differentiate traditional leadership and management perspectives, and (2) to relate them in an integrated way with contemporary nursing trends and practice applications. This textbook is designed to serve the needs of nurses and nursing students who seek a foundation in the principles of coordinating nursing services. It will serve the need for these principles in relation to client care, peers, superiors, and subordinates.

ORGANIZATION AND COVERAGE

This fourth edition continues the format first used with the third edition. The first two editions were Dr. Huber's single-authored texts. The edited book approach draws together the best thinking of experts in the field—both nurses and nonnurses—to enrich and deepen the presentation of core essential knowledge and skills. Beginning with the first edition, a hallmark of *Leadership and Nursing Care Management* has been its depth of coverage, its comprehensiveness, and its strong evidence-based foundation. This fourth edition continues the emphasis on explaining theory in an easily understandable way to enhance comprehension. A "Practical Tips" feature has been added to augment the existing features of previous editions.

In addition, the content of this fourth edition has been reorganized and refreshed to integrate leadership and care management topics with the nurse executive leadership competencies of the 2005 American Organization of Nurse Executives (AONE). As the professional organization that speaks for nurse leaders, managers, and executives, AONE has identified the evidence-based core competencies in the field, and the content of this book has been aligned accordingly to reflect the knowledge underlying quality management of nursing services. This will help the reader develop the crucial skills and knowledge needed for core competencies. In addition, this new organizational schema can serve as a guidepost for building curricula and continuing educational offerings.

The organizational framework of this book groups the 38 chapters into the following five parts:

- **Part I: Leadership** aligns with the AONE competency category of the same name and provides an orientation to the basic principles of both leadership and management. Part I contains chapters on leadership, management, change, and organizational climate and culture.
- **Part II: Professionalism** aligns with the AONE competency category of the same name and addresses the nurse's role and career

development. The reader is prompted to examine the role of the nurse leader and manager. Part II discusses the three core content areas of critical thinking and decision making, managing time and stress, and legal and ethical issues, which form the foundation for leadership and care management skills.

- **Part III: Communication and Relationship Building** aligns with the AONE competency category of the same name. Part III focuses on communication techniques, motivation, team building, delegation, power and conflict, and workplace diversity. These are essential knowledge and skills areas for nurse leaders and managers as they work with and through others in care delivery.
- **Part IV: Knowledge of the Health Care Environment** covers the AONE competency category of the same name and features a broad array of chapters. Part IV starts with an overview of the health care delivery system and health policy and then covers evidence-based practice, organizational structure aspects, models of care delivery, case and population management, patient acuity, quality, and outcomes. This discussion highlights the importance of understanding the health care system and the organizational structures within which nursing care delivery must operate. This section includes information on traditional organizational theory, such as mission statements, policies and procedures; and the dynamics of decentralized and shared governance.
- **Part V: Business Skills** aligns with the AONE competency category on business skills and principles and contains an extensive grouping of chapters related to human resource management, health care financing, workplace violence, and all-hazards disaster preparedness. These chapters discuss the opportunities and challenges for the nurse manager-leader when dealing with the health care workforce. The wide range of human resource responsibilities of nurse managers is reviewed, and resources for further study are provided. The significant share of scarce organization budgets consumed by the human resources of an institution makes this area of management a key challenge that requires intricate skills in leadership and management. This section examines some of the important factors that nurse leader-managers must consider in the nursing and health care environment. Also in this section are chapters that build on organizational theory and demonstrate the importance of integrating organizations and systems with the current technology and theory applications, including data management and informatics, strategic management, and marketing.

Each of the 38 chapters in this text is organized into a consistent format that highlights the following features:

- Concept definitions
- Study questions
- Theoretical and research background
- Leadership and management implications
- Current issues and trends
- Practical tips for practice leadership

This format is designed to bridge the gap between theory and practice and to increase the relevance of nursing leadership and management by demonstrating the way in which theory translates into behaviors appropriate to contemporary leadership and nursing care management.

TEXT FEATURES

In addition to the traditional text features—chapter objectives, chapter summary, and references—this book contains other interesting and effective aids to readers' comprehension, critical thinking, and application.

Leading & Managing Defined

A definition box near the beginning of each chapter provides a quick summary of the key terms and accompanying definitions needed to master each chapter's content. Key terms within this box are boldfaced within the text to give the reader quick access to a more detailed contextual discussion of each word or phrase.

Leadership & Management Behaviors

In every chapter, this box summarizes applicable behaviors that fall under either leadership or management and also identifies the behaviors that overlap these areas. This box is designed to help readers reflect on the chapter content in a way that distinguishes leadership from management and also demonstrates how the two concepts are integrated.

Critical Thinking Exercises

Found at the end of each chapter, this feature challenges readers to inquire and reflect, to analyze critically the knowledge they have absorbed, and to apply it to the situation.

Research Notes

These summaries of current research studies are highlighted in every chapter and introduce the reader to the liveliness and applicability of the available literature in nursing leadership and management.

Case Studies

Found at the end of each chapter, these vignettes introduce the reader to the "real world" of nursing leadership and management and demonstrate the ways in which the chapter concepts operate in specific situations. These vignettes show the creativity and energy that characterize expert nurse administrators as they tackle issues in practice.

Practical Tips for Practice Leadership

This new feature provides the reader with a few helpful hints about applying the knowledge being gained in the daily practice of nursing.

TEACHING AND LEARNING AIDS

evolve Resources for Students

Case Studies. With accompanying questions and answer guidelines, these case scenarios encourage critical thinking and apply the text content to real-life nursing practice.

Glossary. A comprehensive alphabetical listing gives readers access to a compilation of all key terms within the text.

Study Questions. Short-answer, matching, true-or-false, and fill-in-the-blank questions reinforce content learned in the text.

Research Notes. Additional summaries of current research studies compliment the recent literature studies provided in the text.

WebLinks. These links to hundreds of websites supplement textbook content.

evolve Resources for Faculty

Instructor's Manual. Includes a chapter focus, key terms, learning objectives, teaching strategies (**NEW!**), chapter outline, critical thinking activities, learning activities (featuring both class discussions and essay questions), a case study with analysis questions to facilitate classroom discussion, and other additional resources.

PowerPoint Lecture Slides. Each chapter includes between 15 and 30 slides to guide classroom lectures.

Test Bank. Includes 400 NCLEX-style questions. The test bank has been revised to incorporate text page references and a greater number of application-based questions.

evolve eBooks

Make the most of your time with Evolve eBooks. With easy access from your computer or any Internet browser, you and your students can:

- Search across an entire library of Elsevier e-textbooks simultaneously
- Create focused, customized study documents
- Make and share notes, highlights, and more

Evolve eBooks revolutionize the way your students study and learn. Please contact your Elsevier sales representative for more information, or visit **http://evolve.elsevier.com/ebooks.**

Diane L. Huber

Acknowledgments

This book is dedicated to my husband, Bob Huber. He made this book a reality and was the text and graphics support behind it. For his love, caring, and support I am eternally grateful. To my children, Brad Gardner and Lisa Witte, and their spouses, Nonalee Gardner and John Witte, for their enthusiasm and love. I am forever privileged that they are in my life. I thank them for the gifts of Kathryn Anne Gardner (the Princess), Anthony James Gardner (A.J.), and Logan Witte. I love being Grandma to these wonderful people. Also special are Chris Huber; Beth and Brad Nau and grandchildren Brandon, Danielle, Creighton, and the late Cameron Nau; and Von and Kirk Danielson and Kory, Ryan, and Sean Danielson.

To my professional colleagues who inspired me and served as examples of excellence in nursing, I am grateful. To my nursing students, past and future, my thanks for being a source of continual intellectual stimulation and challenge.

This book's first two editions evolved under the tender care of Thomas Eoyang, former Editorial Manager at W.B. Saunders Company, whose guidance, support, and caring were invaluable. To the editors in the Elsevier Nursing Division, including Kristin Geen, Senior Acquisitions Editor; Jamie Horn, Developmental Editor; and Jennifer Palada, Editorial Assistant, who worked so hard to facilitate everything related to the 4th edition, and to the excellent staff at Elsevier, a sincere thank you.

Diane L. Huber

CONTRIBUTOR ACKNOWLEDGMENTS

Chapter 8

The author of Chapter 8 gratefully acknowledges the editorial review of the manuscript by James R. Acree, PhD, MSN, MS, BSNA, BSN, CRNA, RN.

Chapter 28

The authors gratefully acknowledge the assistance of Dr. Cheryl Jones for an insightful chapter review, Kraig McKinley for manuscript editing, and Sherry Turner for reference documentation.

Chapter 35

The authors would like to thank their colleagues Fran Vasaly, RN, Infection Control Practitioner, Inova Health System; Dan Hanfling, MD, FACEP, Director of Emergency Management and Disaster Medicine, Inova Health System/Inova Fairfax Hospital; Allan Morrison, MD, FACP, FIDSA, Medical Chief of Infection Control, Inova Health System/Inova Fairfax Hospital; and Greg Brison, Director of Safety and Security, Inova Alexandria Hospital.

Contents

PART IV
KNOWLEDGE OF THE HEALTH CARE ENVIRONMENT

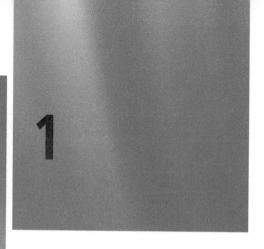

1 Leadership Principles

Diane L. Huber

PART I

CHAPTER OBJECTIVES

- Define and describe leadership
- Formulate the process of leadership
- Critique the qualities of leadership
- Analyze leadership styles
- Distinguish among theories of leadership
- Specify the linkage between followership and leadership
- Apply leadership to nursing practice
- Exercise critical thinking to conceptualize and analyze possible solutions to a practice exercise

"The nurse leader plays a critical role in the business of the healthcare organization and the quality and safety of the services provided" (O'Connor, 2008, p. 21). Strong evidence for the nurse leader's critical role both in the business of a health care organization and in the quality and safety of service delivery has been laid out by the Institute of Medicine (IOM) (Institute of Medicine [IOM], 2004), the American Nurses Credentialing Center's (ANCC) Magnet Recognition Program® (American Nurses Credentialing Center [ANCC], 2008), and the American Organization of Nurse Executives (American Organization of Nurse Executives [AONE], 2005). The IOM focus is on five areas of management practice:

- Implementing evidence-based management
- Balancing tensions between efficiency and reliability
- Creating and sustaining trust
- Actively managing the change process through communication, feedback, training, sustained effort and attention, and worker involvement
- Creating a learning environment

The ANCC's Magnet™ program acknowledges excellence in nursing services and leadership based on 14 Forces of Magnetism. The AONE 2005 nurse executive competencies are described in five domains of skill:

- Communication and relationship management
- Leadership
- Business skills and principles
- Knowledge of the health care environment
- Professionalism

Taken together, these source documents overlap and converge on the primary attributes, knowledge domains, and skills that nurse leaders need to lead people and manage organizations in health care.

Leadership is an activity of human engagement and a relationship experience founded in trust, communication, inspiration, action, and "servant-hood." The leadership role is so important because it embodies commitment and forward-reaching action. Arising from a drive to make things better, leaders use their power to bring teams together, spark innovation, create positive communication, and drive forward toward group goals. Leadership has been described by others in many ways:

> *Great necessities call forth great leaders.*
>
> -Abigail Adams

> *Leadership: the art of getting someone else to do something you want done because he wants to do it.*
>
> -Dwight D. Eisenhower

> *Leadership is the special quality which enables people to stand up and pull the rest of us over the horizon.*
>
> -James L. Fisher

> *Leadership and learning are indispensable to each other.*
>
> -John F. Kennedy

> *Leadership is lifting a person's vision to higher sights, the raising of a person's performance to a higher standard, the building of a personality beyond its normal limitations.*
>
> -Peter F. Drucker

> *The first step to leadership is servanthood.*
>
> -John Maxwell

> *The first responsibility of a leader is to define reality.*
>
> -Max DePree

> *Leadership has a harder job to do than just choose sides. It must bring sides together.*
>
> -Jesse Jackson

> *The only test of leadership is that somebody follows.*
>
> -Robert K. Greenleaf

> *Leadership is getting people to work for you when they are not obligated.*
>
> -Fred Smith

> *The main characteristics of effective leadership are intelligence, integrity or loyalty, mystique, humor, discipline, courage, self sufficiency and confidence.*
>
> -James L. Fisher

Leadership is important to study, learn, and practice in today's complex, rapidly changing, turbulent, and chaotic health care work environment. Such an environment generates challenges to the nurse's identity, coping skills, and ability to work with others in harmony. It also presents the opportunity to lead, challenge assumptions, consolidate a purpose, and move a vision forward. Leadership is important for nurses because they need to possess knowledge and skill in the art and science of solving problems in work groups, systems of care, and the environment of care delivery. The effectiveness of an individual nurse depends partly on that individual's competence and partly on the creation of a facilitating environment that contains sufficient resources to accomplish goals. The nurse leader combines clinical, administrative, financial, and operational skills to solve problems in the care environment so that nurses can provide cost-effective care in a way that is satisfying and health promoting for patients and clients. Such an environment does not simply happen; it requires special skills and the courage and motivation to move a vision into action. Thus the study of nursing leadership and care management focuses critical thinking on what it takes to be a nursing "environment architect," transition leader, and manager of care delivery services.

THE TWO ROLES OF A NURSE

Nursing is a service profession whose core mission is the care and nurturing of human beings in their experiences of health and illness. Nurses have two basic roles: care providers and care coordinators. The first role is more often the role that is recognized. In the United States, the acute care medical model in hospitals over time came to be the primary focus of attention and jobs for nurses. In this illness-focused model, the nurse's care provider or "doing" role was the most important and valued aspect of nursing. Little reward came from the "thinking" and integrating skills nurses were capable of. With a shift to managed care, the nurse's care management role has become more prominent, needed, and valued. The delivery of nursing services involves the organization and coordination of complex activities. Nurses use managerial and leadership skills to facilitate delivery of quality nursing care.

THE LEADERSHIP ROLE

Leadership is a unique role and function. It can be part of a formal organizational managerial position, or it can arise spontaneously in any group. Certain characteristics, such as being motivated by challenge, commitment, and autonomy, are thought to be associated with leadership. Effectiveness is a key outcome of leadership efforts in health care. It has been suggested that there is a scarcity of leaders and a crisis in leadership in nursing. The IOM has raised awareness about patient safety and quality of care issues, and the Magnet Recognition Program® is one evidence-based nurse response. In times of chaos, complexity, and change, leadership is essential to provide the guidance, direction, and sense of stability needed to ensure followers' effectiveness and satisfaction.

The focus on leadership as a crucial need arises from the impact of significant changes that have occurred in the organization, delivery, and financing of health care during this period of time that has been characterized as "turbulent" and "tumultuous" because of "waves of chaos." Under such circumstances, nurses are challenged to respond with leadership. Nurses can best respond by adapting to changes, seeking new tools for dealing with the new health care environment, and leading the way with client-centered strategies.

Both nurses and the health care delivery systems in which they practice need leaders. The current health care environment is in a period of profound transition characterized by competition, conflict, consumer orientation, rapid communication, and chaos (Hagenow, 2001). Potential health care leaders likely will possess "a passion to make things better, a commitment to values, a focus on creativity and innovation, and the knowledge and skills necessary to identify health care needs and then to mobilize and array the human and other resources necessary to achieve goals and effect outcomes" (Huber & Watson, 2001, p. 29). Exhibiting quiet but respected competence, a leader may be the "wise" or "go-to" person within the group, a superior problem solver, a strategic communicator, or someone who is emotionally intelligent and strong in interpersonal relationship skills. Leaders may grow gradually out of a smoldering issue or erupt through a crisis event. Clearly, "something changes as leadership blossoms" (Huber & Watson, 2001, p. 29).

LEADERSHIP OVERVIEW

Leadership is a natural element of nursing practice because the majority of nurses practice in work groups or units. Possessing the license of an RN implies certain leadership skills and requires the ability to delegate and supervise the work of others. Leadership can be understood as the ability to inspire confidence and support among followers, especially in organizations in which competence and commitment produce performance.

Leadership Skills

Leadership is an important issue related to how nurses integrate the various elements of nursing practice to ensure the highest quality of care for clients. Every nurse needs two critical skills to enhance professional practice. One is a skill at interpersonal relationships. This is fundamental to leadership and the work of nursing. The second is skill in applying the problem-solving process. This involves the ability to think critically, to identify problems, and to develop objectivity and a degree of maturity or judgment. Leadership skills build on professional and clinical skills. Hersey and colleagues (2008) identified the following three skills needed for leading or influencing:

1. *Diagnosing:* Diagnosing involves being able to understand the situation and the problem to be solved or resolved. This is a cognitive competency.
2. *Adapting:* Adapting involves being able to adapt behaviors and other resources to match the situation. This is a behavioral competency.
3. *Communicating:* Communicating is used to advance the process in a way that individuals can understand and accept. This is a process competency.

Among the important personal leadership skills is emotional intelligence. Based on the work of Goleman (1997, 2000), relational and emotional

PART I

integrity are hallmarks of good leaders. This is because the leader operates in a crucial cultural and contextual influencing mode. The leader's behavior, patterns of actions, attitude, and performance have a special impact on the team's attitude and behaviors and on the context and character of work life. Followers need to be able to depend on role consistency, balance, and behavioral integrity from the leader. The four skill sets needed by good leaders are as follows:

1. *Self-awareness:* Ability to read one's own emotional state and be aware of one's own mood and how this affects staff relationships
2. *Self-management:* Ability to take corrective action so as not to transfer negative moods to staff relationships
3. *Social awareness:* An intuitive skill of empathy and expressiveness in being sensitive and aware of the emotions and moods of others
4. *Relationship management:* Use of effective communication with others to disarm conflict, and the ability to develop the emotional maturity of team members

These interpersonal relationship skills are crucial to the work of leadership. The chaos and complexity of the seismic shifts in health care structure, delivery, form, technology, and content have made visible the urgent need for leaders to emerge, mobilize, and encourage followers. Leaders are pivotal to bridging the efforts of followers with the goals of organizations. This is both tricky and risky and may be overwhelming (Porter-O'Grady, 2003). However, good leaders are anchors to the vision and the larger goal, guides to coping and being productive, and champions of energy and enthusiasm for the work.

Leadership and Care Management Differentiated

In nursing, leadership is studied as a way of increasing the skills and abilities needed to facilitate working with people across a variety of situations and to increase understanding and control of the professional work setting. A long history and rich literature surround leadership theories, much of it from outside of nursing. Nursing has drawn from both classic and contemporary thinkers. Bennis (1994) made a strong argument for leadership, stating that quality of life depends on the quality of the leaders. He noted three reasons why leaders are important: the character of change in society, the de-emphasis on integrity in institutions, and the responsibility for the effectiveness of organizations. Fiedler and Garcia (1987) argued that leadership is one of the most important factors that determine the survival and success of groups and organizations. *Effective* leadership is important in nursing for those same reasons, specifically because of its impact on the quality of nurses' work lives, being a stabilizing influence during constant change, and for nurses' productivity and quality of care.

Leadership theory often is discussed separately from management theory. Their area of overlap may not be clear or explained. Some have seen management as a subset of leadership. The premise of this textbook is that leadership and management are not identical ideas. This can be seen in their distinct definitions. They are distinct, and yet they overlap. Both leadership and management will be explored separately in this chapter and in Chapter 2, and their intersection will be developed within each of the chapters to better integrate the two concepts with nursing practice.

If the delivery of nursing services involves the organization and coordination of complex activities in the human services realm, then both leadership and management are important elements. The leader's focus is on people; the manager focuses on systems and structure (Bennis, 1994). Thus although both are processes used to accomplish goals, each focus is different. For example, a nurse may use leadership strategies or management strategies to motivate others but the desired outcome of the motivation is likely to be different. There are, however, similarities between leadership and management in an area of overlap. In this area of overlap, the processes and strategies look similar and may be employed for a similar outcome or blended together to accomplish goals.

DEFINITIONS

There are a variety of definitions of leadership. **Leadership** is defined here as the process of influencing people to accomplish goals. Key concepts related to leadership are influence, communication, group process, goal attainment, and motivation. Hersey and colleagues (2008) defined leadership as a process of influencing the behavior of either an individual or a group, regardless of the reason, in an effort to achieve goals in a given situation. Burns (1978) noted that leadership occurs when human beings with motives and purposes mobilize in competition or conflict with others to arouse, engage, and satisfy motives.

Most leadership definitions incorporate the two components of an interaction among people and the process of influencing. Thus leadership is a social exchange phenomenon. At its core, leadership is influencing people. In contrast, management involves influencing employees to meet an organization's goals and is focused primarily on organizational goals and objectives. Bennis (1994) listed a number of distinctions between leadership and management. He noted that the leader focuses on people, whereas the manager focuses on systems and structures. The leader innovates and conquers the context. Another distinction is that a leader innovates whereas a manager administers. Kotter (2001) noted that managers cope with complexity whereas leaders cope with change.

Management is defined as the coordination and integration of resources through planning, organizing, coordinating, directing, and controlling to accomplish specific institutional goals and objectives. Hersey and colleagues (2008) defined management as the "process of working with and through individuals and groups and other resources (such as equipment, capital, and technology) to accomplish organizational goals" (p. 5). They identified management as a special kind of leadership that concentrates on the achievement of organizational goals. If this idea were visualized, it would be in concentric circles—not depicted as overlapping separate circles.

Leadership is a broad concept and a process that can be applied to any group. Grant (1994) noted that leadership, management, and professionalism have different but related meanings, as follows:

- *Leadership:* Guiding, directing, teaching, and motivating to set and achieve goals
- *Management:* Resource coordination and integration to accomplish specific goals
- *Professionalism:* An approach to an occupation that distinguishes it from being merely a job, focuses on service as the highest ideal, follows a code of ethics, and is seen as a lifetime commitment

ROLES

A distinction can be made between leadership and management roles. Management activities are concerned with managing the resources of an organization. The idea of management

LEADING & MANAGING **DEFINED**

Leadership

The process of influencing people to accomplish goals.

Management

The coordination and integration of resources through planning, organizing, coordinating, directing, and controlling to accomplish specific institutional goals and objectives.

Leadership Styles

Different combinations of task and relationship behaviors used to influence others to accomplish goals.

Followership

An interpersonal process of participation.

Empowerment

The act of giving people the authority, responsibility, and freedom to act on what they know.

can generate a negative reaction when it is equated with the "command and control" concept of authoritarian and bureaucratic organizations. These management models do not fit well with an environment experiencing constant change. Some pressures influencing the role of the manager and demanding new skill sets to facilitate clinical work include the pace of technology out-running clinicians' ability to learn and the phenomenon of managing temporary workers employed by others (e.g., outsourced functions and agency nurses). The demands of management work are increasing in amount, scope, complexity, and intensity and thus causing increased role stress and leaving less time to plan and focus on unit management (Porter-O'Grady, 2003).

BACKGROUND

Terms related to leadership are *leadership styles, followership*, and *empowerment*. **Leadership styles** are defined as different combinations of task and relationship behaviors used to influence others to accomplish goals. **Followership** is defined as an interpersonal process of participation. **Empowerment** means giving people the authority, responsibility, and freedom to act on their expert knowledge and skills.

Leadership can be best understood as a process. Much attention has been focused on leadership as a group and organizational process because organizational change is heavily influenced by the context or environment. Nurses need to have a solid foundation of knowledge in leadership and care management. This applies at all levels: nurse care provider, nurse manager, and nurse executive. However, the depth and focus of care management roles and skills may vary by level. For example, the nurse care provider concentrates on the coordination of nursing care to individuals or groups. This may include such activities as arranging access to services, direct care provision, referrals, and family support. At the next level, the nurse manager concentrates on the day-to-day administration and coordination of services provided by a group of nurses. The nurse executive's role and function concentrate on long-term administration of an institution or program that delivers nursing services, focusing on integrating the system and building a culture (Mintzberg, 1998).

LEADERSHIP: FIVE INTERWOVEN ASPECTS

Hersey and colleagues (2008) noted that the leadership process is a function of the leader, the followers, and other situational variables. The leadership process includes five interwoven aspects: (1) the leader, (2) the follower, (3) the situation, (4) the communication process, and (5) the goals (Kison, 1989). Figure 1.1 shows how these components relate to one another. All five elements interact within any given leadership moment.

Process Part 1: The Leader

The values, skills, and style of leaders are important. Their internalized pattern of basic behaviors influences actions and the ability to lead. Leaders' perceptions of themselves, their roles, and their expectations also have an impact on their followers. Self-awareness is crucial to leadership effectiveness and is the focus for many leadership exercises. Internal forces in leaders that impinge

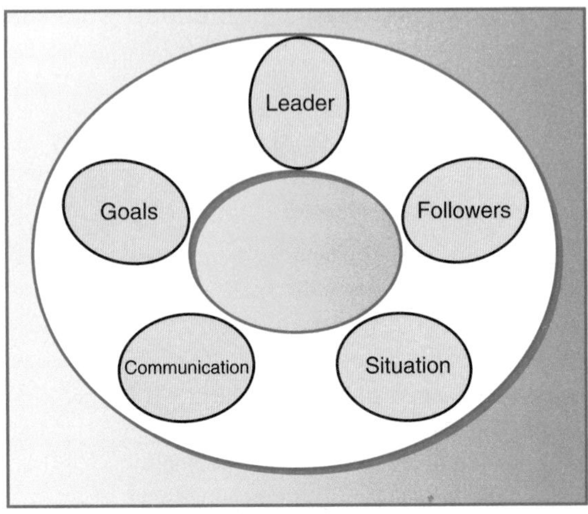

Figure 1.1
Components of a leadership moment.

on leadership style are values, confidence in employees, leadership inclinations, and sense of security in uncertainty (Tannenbaum & Schmidt, 1973). Interpersonal, emotional, and social intelligence skills also contribute to the effective leadership of knowledge workers (Goleman, 1997, 2000, 2007; Porter-O'Grady, 2003).

Process Part 2: The Follower

Followership is the flip side of leadership. It is likely that without followers there is no leadership. Followers are vital because they accept or reject the leader and determine the leader's personal power (Hersey et al., 2008). Followers also need self-awareness to know themselves and their expectations. Situations in which members of a group are not accustomed to working together or do not hold shared expectations frequently lead to conflict. Groups have personalities that include a discernible level of trust. The wise leader assesses the trust and readiness to change levels of the group.

Process Part 3: The Situation

The specific circumstances surrounding any given leadership situation will vary. Elements such as work demands, control systems, amount of task structure, degree of interaction, amount of time available for decision making, and external environment shape the differences among situations (Hersey et al., 2008). Organizational culture and ethos also are important factors in the situation. For example, in one setting the culture may resemble one big happy family, with an emphasis on teamwork and morale boosting. The cultural aspects of that leadership situation are different from those of an organization in which there is a fast-paced tempo and people seem very busy. Environmental or cultural differences also cause the leadership situation to vary. The leadership situation in a group that is knowledgeable and experienced in solving problems is very different from the leadership situation in a group that is not experienced at the task or at working together. The personality styles of both superiors and subordinates have an influence on the situation, the work demands, and the amount of time and resources available.

Process Part 4: Communication

Communication processes vary among groups regarding the patterns and channels used and how open or closed the communication flow is. Communicating is basic to the process of influencing and thus to leadership. Through communication, the leader's vision and message are received by the followers. After choosing a channel, the sender transmits a message. However, the message is filtered through the receiver's perception. Communication is transmitted through both verbal and nonverbal modes. Organizations include a variety of communication structures and flows. These may be downward, upward, horizontal, grapevines, or networks. Communication may be formal or informal (Hersey et al., 2008). Certain acts performed by leaders have positive effects and make people feel more respected; listening and informal chatting are prime examples (Alvesson & Sveningsson, 2003).

Process Part 5: Goals

Organizations have goals, and individuals working in organizations also have goals. These goals may or may not be congruent. For example, the goal of the organization may be to decrease costs or increase revenue. In contrast, the goal of the individual nurse may be to spend time counseling and teaching clients because that is what is seen by the nurse as the most important activity. Goals may thus be in conflict, in which case there is tension and a need for leadership.

Summary

Clearly, leadership is a complex and multidimensional process. Nurses need to be aware of the interacting elements in any leadership situation. Critical thinking can be applied to:

1. Diagnosing and analyzing the five elements,
2. Adapting to the situation, and
3. Communicating for effectiveness.

For example, if a nurse works in a situation in which there is a high level of frustration, it may be time to step back and analyze the basic five elements. Doing so sets the stage for better decision making about change strategies and strategic management.

LEADERSHIP THEORIES

Hersey and colleagues (2008) have done a thorough overview of leadership and organizational theory since the early 1900s. From an early awareness of the leader's need to be concerned about both tasks and human relationships (output and people) sprang a long history of leadership theories that can be grouped as *trait, attitudinal*, and *situational* (Hersey et al., 2008). The trait approach focuses on identifying specific characteristics of leaders. The attitudinal approach measures attitudes toward leader behavior. The situational approach focuses on observed behaviors of leaders and how leadership styles can be matched to situations. Leadership theories have evolved away from an early focus on the traits or characteristics of the leader as a person because it was found that it is not possible to predict leadership from clusters of traits. However, several authors have developed lists of traits common to good leaders (Bass, 1982; Bennis & Nanus, 1985; Yukl, 1981), and interest remains in the characteristics to look for in good leaders. Further background on the history of leadership research can be found online (e.g., *www.sedl.org/change/leadership/history.html*).

Trait Theories

Characteristics of Leadership

In the trait approach, theorists have sought to understand leadership by examining the characteristics of leaders. Presumably, leaders could be differentiated from non-leaders. The trait approach has generated multiple lists of traits proposed to be essential to leadership. Bennis (1994) identified a recipe for leadership that contained six ingredients: a guiding vision, passion, integrity (including self-knowledge, candor, and maturity), trust, curiosity, and daring. Leaders arise in a context, and they are said to be "made," not "born." They appear to learn leadership skills in stages (Bennis, 2004). Thus leadership skills can be both taught and learned. It is important for nurses to recognize that they can learn, practice, and improve their personal leadership competencies.

Drucker (1996) noted that effective leaders know the following four things:

1. The only definition of a leader is someone who has followers.
2. Popularity is not leadership; results are.
3. Leaders are visible and set examples.
4. Leadership is not rank but responsibility.

Leaders ask questions such as these: What needs to be done? What can I do to make a difference? What are the goals? What constitutes performance and results? Thus leaders do not need to know all the answers, but they do need to ask the right questions (Heifetz & Laurie, 1997).

Leaders are active, not passive. The risk-taking element of leadership involves taking action. Leaders engage their environment with behaviors of doing, influencing, and moving. These are action terms. Pagonis (1992) noted that to lead successfully a leader must demonstrate two active, essential, and interrelated traits: expertise and empathy. Leaders are those who talk about adventures into new territory and take the risks inherent in innovation (Kouzes & Posner, 1987). Leadership means giving guidance and using a focused vision.

A leader may see the need to chart a course that is new or unknown, unpopular, or risky because it challenges those with vested interests who have much to lose. In a way, nursing's struggle for greater economic parity in health care is courageous and risky. Clancy (2003) noted that leaders need to "consistently find the courage to hold true to their beliefs and convictions" (p. 128). Both ethical fitness and moral courage form the backbone of making necessary and hard—but right and unpopular—decisions. Cost containment, patient's rights, safe staffing, stress and anger, and ethical dilemmas all challenge the leader to identify right from wrong and act from his or her sense of conviction. The leadership courage continuum runs from "good coward" (cannot muster courage to make tough choices) to "reckless courage" (shoot from the hip). Leaders need to be willing to make tough choices plus overcome the fear associated with them.

Research by Bennis and Thomas (2002) indicated that extraordinary leaders possess skills required to overcome adversity and emerge stronger and more committed. They suggest that "one of the most reliable indicators and predictors of true leadership is an individual's ability to find meaning in negative events and to learn from even the most trying circumstances" (Bennis & Thomas, 2002, p. 39). "Crucible" experiences shape leaders. These are trials, tests, and transformative experiences that force leaders to question themselves and what matters and to hone their judgment. Consequently, leaders come to a new or altered sense of identity. "Crucible" experiences can occur from positive or negative triggers, but leaders see them as opportunities for reinvention. Great leaders possess the following four essential skills:

1. The ability to engage others in shared meaning
2. A distinctive and compelling vocal tone
3. A sense of integrity
4. A combination of hardiness and ability to grasp context, called "adaptive capacity"

Characteristics such as knowledge, motivating people to work harder, trust, communication, enthusiasm, vision, courage, ability to see the big picture, and ability to take risks are associated with important leadership qualities in research findings. For example, Bennis and Nanus (1985) studied 90 chief executives from 1978 to 1983 and found

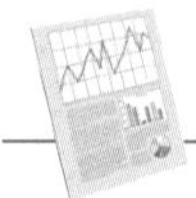

Research Note

Source: Upenieks, V. (2003). Nurse leaders' perceptions of what compromises successful leadership in today's acute inpatient environment. *Nursing Administration Quarterly, 27*(2), 140-152.

Purpose

The purpose of this research was to explore nurse leaders' perceptions of the value of their roles and their beliefs about how power and gender interface with leadership success. Data were gathered via interviews with 16 nurse leaders: 7 from Magnet™ institutions and 9 from non–Magnet™-designated hospitals. Qualitative content analysis techniques were used. The theoretical framework guiding the study was Kanter's Structural Theory of Organizational Behavior.

Discussion

The results showed that 83% of the nurse leaders validated that access to power, opportunity, information, and resources created an empowered environment and fostered leadership success and aided job satisfaction of nurses. In addition, four other factors contributed to leadership success and role worth: supportive organizational culture committed to the professional expertise of nurses, leadership qualities of the nurse leader, teamwork among physicians and other providers, and compensation reflecting the value of nursing. Leadership traits deemed essential were being visible, accessible, influential, visionary, credible, honest, articulate, knowledgeable, and supportive of advancement and educational opportunities.

Application to Practice

Leadership, particularly when coupled with organizational position, is an opportunity for nurses to accomplish group goals. Certain organizational structural characteristics predispose nurse leadership success. Nurse leaders need to seek to develop, acquire, or elicit access to power, opportunity, information, and resources. Once this foundation is laid, nurse leaders need to mobilize their personal leadership skills and abilities, such as visibility, responsiveness, passion, and business astuteness to create and nurture a supportive organizational culture, collaborative interdisciplinary teamwork, and a meaningful compensation structure for nurses. To do so should affect nurse satisfaction and retention. Magnet™ research studies support the transformational leadership style as the most often reported type used in Magnet™ hospitals and a work environment that fosters professional nursing practice as an essential element for increasing nurse job satisfaction. Strategic leadership applications make a difference.

that there were two key leadership traits. One is a guiding set of concepts, and the other is the ability to communicate a vision. Kouzes and Posner (1987) defined the following five behaviors that correlated with leadership excellence:

1. *Challenging the process:* Leaders go beyond the status quo to search for opportunities, experiment, and take risks to achieve lofty goals.
2. *Inspiring shared vision:* Leaders envision the future and enlist others in sharing the dream.
3. *Enabling others to act:* Leaders foster collaboration and develop and strengthen others so that the whole team performs well.
4. *Modeling the way:* Leaders set an example and structure events so that incremental progress is celebrated as small wins.
5. *Encouraging the heart:* Leaders appreciate and recognize individual contributions and formally celebrate accomplishments.

These five practices can be seen as the way leaders get extraordinary things done through people in an organization. The practices and qualities of leadership help nurses enrich their own style and contribute to a more productive workplace. The following list identifies qualities that people say they want to see in their leaders (Curtin, 1989) and is as valuable today as in 1989:

- *Visibility:* People want to see their leaders and have frequent, casual contacts with them.
- *Flexibility:* People learn from leaders who can "roll with the punches," tolerate ambiguity, and have a sense of personal empowerment.
- *Authority:* This is the right to make decisions, give direction, and accept/administer criticism. Authority is recognition granted from below.
- *Assistance:* This occurs by serving those who serve, create, or produce and by creating the environment and resources necessary to do the job.
- *Feedback:* People want their leaders to listen to them and give them quality feedback as they go about their particular work.

The following eight competencies of leaders are synthesized from the literature by Murphy and DeBack (1991):

1. Managing the dream
2. Mastery of change
3. Organizational design
4. Anticipatory learning
5. Taking the initiative
6. Mastery of interdependence
7. Holding high standards of integrity
8. Exercising broad-perspective decision making

One research-based nursing model (Mathena, 2002) identified the following six core behaviors critical for nursing leadership success:

1. Visioning
2. Interdisciplinary team building
3. Workload complexity analysis
4. Work process analysis
5. Stakeholder analysis
6. Interactive planning

Vision and Trust

Although the lists of leadership characteristics and competencies vary somewhat, the functions of visioning, setting the direction, inspiration, motivation, and enabling systems and followers are at the core of leadership activity. Bennis (1994) discussed what has come to be called "the vision thing." The one specific defining quality of leaders is vision—the ability to create a vision and put it into operation.

Leadership is founded on trust: "Trust is the emotional glue that binds leaders and employees together and is a measure of the legitimacy of leadership" (Malloch, 2002, p. 14). Organizations that focus on sustaining a healing culture rebuild organizational trust by focusing on trust in relationships with employees. Behaviors that build trust include sharing relevant information, reducing controls, and meeting expectations. Trust-destroying behaviors include being insensitive to beliefs and values, avoiding discussion of sensitive issues, and encouraging competition via winners and losers. Nurses can be aware of the crucial nature of trust in the leadership and management relationship. Trust goes both ways and needs to be nurtured. Nurses can start by examining their own behaviors and then taking deliberative actions to strengthen trust in the environment.

Followers expect that leaders will provide a sense of vision and a sense of direction with standards for achieving the group's goals. Leaders can create an environment that is positively charged for productivity or allow followers to languish without direction or mission. It is possible that leaders can create a negative climate that becomes destructive to the group. If the leader plays a major role in creating a group's culture and ethos, then closing down communication, breeding distrust and competition, and neglecting positive motivation can sow the seeds of group disintegration. Thus the characteristics possessed and used by the leader can make a crucial difference in the functioning and effectiveness of any group.

Leadership "Dos and Don'ts"

The long history of leadership theory has highlighted the importance of focusing on both of the two basic leadership elements of tasks and relationships. These are core to all leadership in all situations. The Trait Approach has led to long lists of skills and characteristics associated with successful leaders. These can be distilled into leadership "dos and don'ts."

A profile of leaderships "dos" includes honesty, energy, drive, tenacity, creativity, flexibility, visibility, emotional stability, knowledge, conceptual skills, and leadership motivation. Among these characteristics, honesty (defined as trustworthiness) and energy are at the top of the list. Leadership is founded on trust and does not survive without it. Leadership is hard, sustained work that requires a great deal of energy and sputters without it.

A profile of leadership "don'ts" includes untrustworthiness, insensitivity to others, aloofness, overmanaging, abrasiveness, inability to think strategically or staff effectively, inability to build a team, and focusing on internal organizational politics (overly ambitious). Among these characteristics, untrustworthiness is a fatal flaw and insensitivity to others is a likely cause for ineffective leadership (Hersey et al., 2008).

In summary, leadership is a dynamic process. To be effective, leadership styles need to match the situation. Styles of leadership range from authoritarian to permissive to democratic and from transactional to transformational. The individual nurse's task is to determine in which environments he or she functions best and is most comfortable or where he or she most likely will succeed. This facilitates placement for success and a better match between leader and follower.

Attitudinal Theories

As leadership theories evolved, leadership came to be viewed as a dynamic process and an interaction among the leader, the followers, and the situation. Leadership theory began to move beyond a focus on traits to explore the concept of leadership styles. Leadership styles are discussed next, followed by a discussion of attitudinal leadership theories.

Leadership Styles

Leadership styles are defined as different combinations of task and relationship behaviors used to influence others to accomplish goals. They are sets or clusters of behaviors used in the process of effecting leadership. Leaders need to be concerned about both tasks to be accomplished and human relationships in groups and organizations. Hersey and colleagues (2008) said that leadership styles are the consistent behavior patterns exhibited in influencing the activities of others by working with and through them, as perceived by those others. Different styles evoke variable responses in different situations. The way people influence others through actions taken and the perspectives of other people is related to leadership efforts and constitutes leadership style. The two major leadership terms are *task behavior* and *relationship behavior*, and a leader's leadership style is some combination of task and relationship behavior. Hersey and colleagues (2008) defined these terms as follows:

- *Task behavior:* The extent to which leaders organize and define roles, explain activities, determine when, where, and how tasks are to be accomplished, and endeavor to get work accomplished

- *Relationship behavior:* The extent to which leaders maintain personal relationships by opening communication and providing psychoemotional support and facilitating behaviors

Tannenbaum and Schmidt (1973) suggested that a leader might select one of many behavior styles arrayed along a continuum. The continuum ranges from democratic to authoritarian (or subordinate-centered to leader-centered). Their work suggested that there are a variety of leadership styles (Figure 1.2) or points along the continuum. They discussed three distinct styles: authoritarian, democratic, and laissez-faire. Some individuals are able to integrate styles and flexibly match to the situation at hand, but this is rare.

Authoritarian

The authoritarian leadership style uses primarily directive behaviors. Decisions of policy are made solely by the leader who tends to dictate tasks and techniques to followers. Leaders tell the followers what to do and how to do it. This style emphasizes a concern for task. Authoritarian leaders are characterized by giving orders. Their style can create hostility and dependency among followers; it may also stifle creativity and innovation. On the other hand, this style can be very efficient, especially in a crisis.

Democratic

This approach implies a relationship and person orientation. Policies are a matter of group discussion and decision. The leader encourages and assists discussion and group decision making. Human relations and teamwork are the focus. The leader shares responsibility with the followers by involving them in decision making. In nursing, interdisciplinary teamwork is a major element in effectiveness. The democratic style makes output appear to move more slowly and is thought to take longer than using an authoritarian style. Group consensus needs time and facilitation to be fostered. Furthermore, the needs of disenfranchised minority groups must be balanced. Intergroup cohesion is a focus with this style. The challenge of the democratic style is to get people with different professional backgrounds, personal biases, and psychological needs together to focus on the problem and next action steps.

Laissez-Faire

This style promotes complete freedom for group or individual decisions. There is a minimum of leader participation. A leader using this style may seem to be apathetic. Because the style is based on noninterference, a clear decision may never be formulated. The laissez-faire style results in a decision, conscious or otherwise, to avoid interference

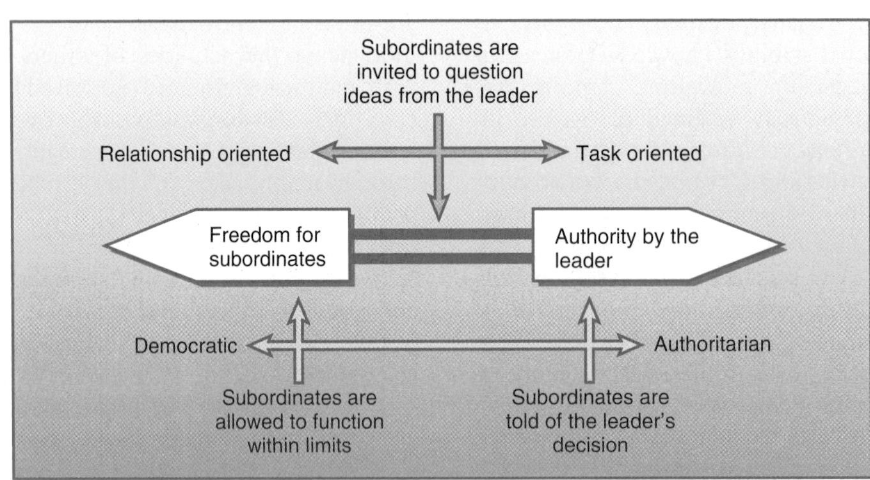

Figure 1.2
Continuum of leader behavior.

and let events take their own course. The leader is either permissive and fosters freedom or is inept at guiding a group. Followers may need greater structure than the leader gives them. Despite its potential drawbacks, this style has advantages when used with groups of fully independent care providers or professionals working together.

One style is not necessarily better than another. Each has advantages and disadvantages. There are situational and contextual factors to consider when choosing a style. Styles should vary according to the appropriateness of the situation with reference to an evaluation of effectiveness. Flexibility is important. For example, if a nurse prefers to operate in a democratic style yet suddenly a code situation occurs, then the nurse must rapidly switch from a democratic to an authoritarian style. Some democratic leaders cannot vary their style sufficiently to handle crises. On the other hand, in a staff meeting, an authoritarian leader may be ineffective with a group of professionals and would need to be flexible enough to switch to a democratic or laissez-faire style, depending on the circumstances. The basic needs are for leader self-awareness and knowledge of the group's ability and willingness levels before examining the situational elements and choosing a leadership style. Self-awareness is key to strategically using leadership styles.

Attitudinal Leadership Theories

Hersey and colleagues (2008) identified a second approach to leadership research that focused on the measurement of attitudes or predispositions toward leader behavior. Occurring mainly between 1945 and the mid-1960s, the attitudinal approaches began with the Ohio State Leadership Studies and included the Michigan Leadership Studies, Group Dynamics Studies, Likert's Management Systems, and Blake and McCanse's Leadership Grid.

Leader behavior was described as having two separate dimensions, as follows:

1. Initiating structure and consideration in the Ohio State Leadership Studies
2. Employee-orientation and production-orientation in the Michigan Leadership Studies

These dimensions are similar to the authoritarian (or task) and democratic (or relationship) ideas of the leader behavior continuum. The Group Dynamics Studies highlighted goal achievement (similar to task) and group maintenance (similar to relationship) elements of leadership behavior (Cartwright & Zander, 1960). Likert (1961) studied high-performance managers to develop an understanding of a general pattern of management. He found that close supervision was less associated with high productivity. High productivity was associated with clear objectives and transmitting to the subordinates an idea about what is to be accomplished and then giving them the freedom to do the job. He described a continuum of management styles, called *System 1 through System 4*, from no trust in subordinates through condescending confidence, substantial but not complete confidence, to complete trust and confidence in subordinates. This parallels the task-to-relationship continuum. Notice here the focus shifts to management, yet the theory applies to leadership as well.

Blake and Mouton (1964) used task and relationship concepts in their grid, which was later modified by Blake and McCanse (1991). The following five types of leadership or management styles, based on concern for production (task) and concern for people (relationship), emerged:

1. *Impoverished:* This style uses minimal effort to get the work done.
2. *Country club:* This approach emphasizes attention to the needs of people to effect satisfying relationships.
3. *Authority-obedience:* This style strives for efficiency in operations.
4. *Organizational man:* This approach works on balancing the necessity to accomplish the task with maintaining morale.
5. *Team:* This style promotes work accomplishment from committed people and interdependence through a common cause, leading to trust and respect.

Hersey and colleagues (2008) noted that Blake and Mouton's (1964) conceptualization tended to be an attitudinal model that measured the values and feelings of managers whereas the Ohio State model

PART I

included both attitudes and behaviors and focused on leadership. Both the leadership style (task versus relationship) and the attitude of the leader about leadership behaviors are important. However, attitudinal theories still did not fully capture the leadership experience because the environment and its complexity were not factored in.

Situational Theories

A third phase of leadership theories grew out of a group of contingency theories whose central idea was that organizational behavior is contingent on the situation or environment. This means that which one is the best all depends on the situation at hand. What is needed by the leader is diagnostic ability. The leader observes and analyses which abilities and motives are present in the followers. With sensitivity, cues in the environment can be identified and used to make choices regarding leadership style. One choice a leader has is to alter his or her own behavior and the leadership style used. Personal flexibility and leadership skills are needed to vary one's style when the followers' needs and motives change or vary. The ability to diagnose, choose, and alter behavior to implement a leadership style best matched to the situation is a critical skill needed for leadership for effectiveness. Thus no one leadership style is optimal in all situations. The nature of the situation needs to be considered. Styles can be chosen to match the situation (Hersey et al., 2008).

Fiedler's Contingency Theory

As situations become more complex, leadership becomes more difficult. Fiedler (1967) developed a Leadership Contingency Model to explain how to apply this idea. He classified group situational variables of leader-member relations, task structure, and position power into eight possible combinations, ranging from high to low on these three major variables. *Leader-member relations* refers to the type and quality of the leader's personal relationships with followers. *Task structure* means how structured the group's assigned task is. *Position power* refers to power that is conferred on the leader by the organization as a result of the assigned job. Fiedler examined the favorableness of the situation from the perspective of the leader's influence over the group. The most

Practical Tips

Tip # 1: Learn About Yourself

Doing an honest personal appraisal of your own leadership styles, skills, and preferences gives you power through self-knowledge. Many leadership style instruments are available. Be honest with yourself. Rather than focusing on what is a right or a wrong profile, use the information to manage yourself with the aim of being more effective in your work situation.

Tip # 2: Flex Your Style

Armed with the information from Tip #1, try flexing your style when the situation suggests it. If you are a democratic-type leader by nature, practice, using role playing or other methods, what you would do or say when an authoritarian style was needed (e.g., code blue). In this way, you can become more comfortable with a style that is not your natural one well ahead of an actual situation occurring.

Tip # 3: Prepare for Performance Appraisals

Begin a portfolio of documented positive performance elements that you will keep up for 1 year at a time. Follow your job description's outline or major categories. Include leadership exemplars, such as those suggested in Tips #1 and #2. Submit these at the time of formal performance evaluations.

favorable situation occurs with good leader-member relations, high task structure, and high position power. The least favorable situation occurs when the leader is disliked, has an unstructured task, and has little position power. With Fiedler's model, group situations can be analyzed to determine the most effective leadership style.

Fiedler (1967) examined which style (task-oriented versus relationship-oriented) would be most effective for each of eight situations. A key general principle is that the need for task-oriented leaders occurs when the situation is either highly favorable or very unfavorable. A task-oriented style is needed for situations on the extremes, whereas a relationship-oriented style is needed when the situation is moderately favorable.

For example, a staff nurse goes into a nursing unit meeting not wanting any extra assignments but hoping that some of the ongoing problems will be solved. If the nurse has a reasonably good relationship with the leader, the leader should use a high-relationship style with the nurse. The leader should use selling, convincing, encouraging, and motivating strategies. The leader should make the nurse feel good about his or her ability to accomplish a task, provide something of quality, and work with other people. If, however, the staff nurse's mind is closed about any changes or if passive-aggressive or subversive actions occur, then the leader needs be more directive. A possible reaction might be to give the nurse an assigned task. On the extremes of highly favorable or highly unfavorable situations, leaders need to use task-oriented behavior to get the work moving. In the middle of the continuum, a high-relationship style is needed, again to foster productivity.

In Situational Leadership®* theory, leadership in groups is never a static circumstance. The situation is dynamic and subject to change. In a very difficult situation, relationships may be the leader's preferred emphasis. However, if interpersonal relationships are not an immediate problem or if the group is on the verge of collapse, then strong authoritative direction is needed to get the group moving and accomplishing. For this situation, the task-oriented leader is a more effective match between leader and job. However, groups do not remain static; they move back and forth through stages. When the problem no longer is just the need to get the group moving but also includes solving numerous interpersonal conflicts, a relationship-oriented leader is better matched to the situation. Eventually, as the situation progresses, a relationship-oriented leader can become less effective. This occurs because once the group has less conflict, individuals may begin to coast along and positive motivation may be lost as individuals become apathetic. Once again, a task-oriented style is called for—challenging individuals by using the motivation they need to continue to produce. Because of the factor of constant change, maintaining good leadership is complicated for any group. One way to foster effective leadership is to evaluate leaders according to Fiedler's contingency model (1967) and then use this information to increase leaders' awareness of their natural style tendency: relationship-oriented or task-oriented. Fiedler's measure for leadership style is the Least Preferred Coworker (LPC) scale (Fiedler & Chemers, 1984). The LPC is an 18-item semantic differential scale that is the personality measure of Fiedler's contingency model (Fiedler & Garcia, 1987).

Favorable or unfavorable situations are determined in part by the receptivity of the followers, but they are also determined by whether the larger environment is positive or negative. An example of an unfavorable situation in nursing is the following:

> A nurse's job is to lead and manage a hospital's critical care area, which has serious morale problems. The nurse is new and has a master's degree but soon discovers that a majority of the followers have long tenure on the unit and both educational and experiential backgrounds that are very different. There may be values clashes between the leader and the followers. The task is to change the environment, but the nurse discovers that this work group has maintained its traditions over a long period.

This is an unfavorable situation and a leadership challenge. Fiedler's theory (1967) suggests that the

*Situational Leadership® is the registered trademark of the Center for Leadership Studies in Escondido, CA 92025.

PART I

best leadership style under unfavorable circumstances is task-oriented.

Hersey and Blanchard's Tri-Dimensional Leader Effectiveness Model

Hersey and colleagues (2008) described the Tri-Dimensional Leader Effectiveness Model first developed by Hersey and Blanchard. First, a two-dimensional model was constructed, in which task behavior and relationship behavior were displayed on a grid from high to low and were divided into four quadrants: (1) high task, low relationship; (2) high task, high relationship; (3) high relationship, low task; and (4) low task, low relationship (Figure 1.3). These quadrants represent four basic leadership styles: telling, selling, participating, and delegating. As applied to the continuum of authoritarian versus democratic styles, telling would be authoritarian and participating would be democratic. The two most common leadership styles are selling and participating. Selling requires the most from a leader, who must provide high amounts of guidance and support. Movement into a participative leadership style requires much less structure and task-directive behavior from the leader because the individual or group is performing but is not quite confident enough in its own ability for the leader to completely let go. The individual or group wants to talk about things.

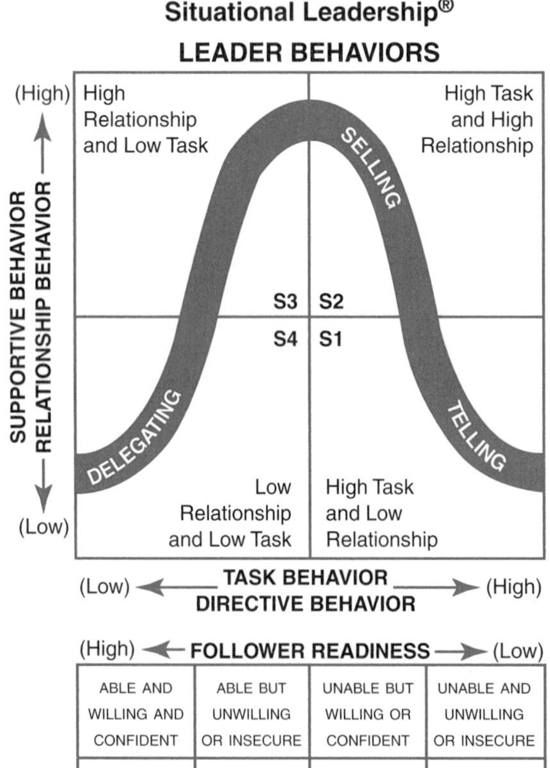

Figure 1.3
Expanded Situational Leadership® model. (© Copyright 2006. Reprinted with permission of the Center for Leadership Studies, Inc., Escondido, CA 92025. All rights reserved.)

To choose an appropriate style, the leader needs to be knowledgeable about the readiness of the followers. This leads to the third dimension of effectiveness. *Effectiveness* is defined as how appropriately a given leader's style interrelates with a given situation. The third dimension is the environment in which a leader operates and that interacts with the leader's style.

Overlaid on the basic grid is a continuum of readiness ranging from low to high. Readiness has two aspects: ability and willingness. Job *ability* is based on the amount of past job experience, job knowledge, problem-solving ability, ability to take responsibility, and ability to meet deadlines. This forms a composite of the ability to do the job. The other part of readiness is psychological *willingness*, which means being willing to take responsibility and have a positive attitude toward accepting the obligation to complete a task. Psychological readiness is manifested by willingness to take some risk and by accepting the job requirements. It includes achievement motivation, wanting to do well, persistence, a work attitude, and a sense of independence. These factors create a willingness to take on and complete a job. Hersey and colleagues (2008) combined ability and willingness into four levels of readiness. Level 1 is unable and unwilling or insecure. Level 2 is unable but willing or confident. Level 3 is able but unwilling or insecure. Level 4 is able and willing or confident. These readiness levels can be matched with the corresponding leadership styles of level 1 with telling, level 2 with selling, level 3 with participating, and level 4 with delegating. Thus readiness assessment can help predict appropriate leadership style selection.

Hersey and colleagues (2008) emphasized the importance of the readiness of followers. Readiness can be applied to a work group. Have the members worked together for a long time in the job, or are they new employees? The culture is more solidified in a work group that has worked together for many years on a particular unit. The leader's leadership style would have to take into account where the followers are in terms of their readiness as a critical factor for determining the style to choose. Using leadership theory, leaders assess themselves, look at the followers' readiness, and assess the situation to determine whether it is favorable or unfavorable. Then a telling, selling, participating, or delegating style is selected.

For example, telling is an appropriate leadership style to use with followers who are at the novice level and with followers who are not able or willing. For example, a nurse is appointed as chair of a committee. First, the nurse might undertake a leadership analysis to determine whether this group needs high-relationship behaviors. If they do not know each other and the situation is politically charged, the nurse leader needs to help people become comfortable with each other. If the nurse leader is a task-oriented person, a high-relationship person may need to be called on to assist the group process so that it is facilitated and becomes effective.

One currently accepted view of organizational behavior describes leadership as situational or contingent and concerned with what produces effectiveness. Hersey and colleagues (2008) noted that the common themes include the following: the leader needs to be flexible in behavior, able to diagnose the leadership style appropriate to the situation, and able to apply the appropriate style. Thus there is no one best way to influence others or one best style. Their Situational Leadership® is a synthesis of the interplay among task behavior, relationship behavior, and the readiness of the followers.

TRANSACTIONAL AND TRANSFORMATIONAL LEADERSHIP

After the eras of trait, attitudinal, and Situational Leadership® theories, an interest arose in how leaders produced quantum results. Burns (1978) and Dunham and Klafehn (1990) broadened the concept of leadership styles to include two types of leaders: the transactional leader and the transformational leader.

A *transactional leader* is defined as a leader or manager who functions in a caretaker role and is focused on day-to-day operations. Such leaders survey their followers' needs and set goals for them based on what can be expected from the followers. A transactional leader is focused on the maintenance and management of ongoing and routine work.

A *transformational leader* is defined as a leader who motivates followers to perform to their full potential over time by influencing a change in perceptions and by providing a sense of direction. Transformational leaders use charisma, individualized consideration, and intellectual stimulation to produce greater effort, effectiveness, and satisfaction in followers (Bass & Avolio, 1990). Figure 1.4 distinguishes between transactional and transformational leadership.

The transactional leader is more common. This type of leader approaches followers in an exchange posture, with the purpose of exchanging one thing for another, such as a politician who promises jobs for votes. Burns (1978) said that transactional leadership occurs when the leader takes the initiative in contacting others for the exchange of valued things. Therefore transactional leadership is comparable to a bargain or contract for mutual benefits that aids the individual differences of both the leader and the follower. Key characteristics are contingent rewards and management-by-exception. Expected effort and expected performance are the outcomes. The transactional leader works within the existing organizational culture and is an essential component of effective leadership (Bass & Avolio, 1990). In nursing, an example would be the exchange of a salary for the services of a nurse to provide care (Barker, 1991). Another example occurs when a leader offers release time or paid

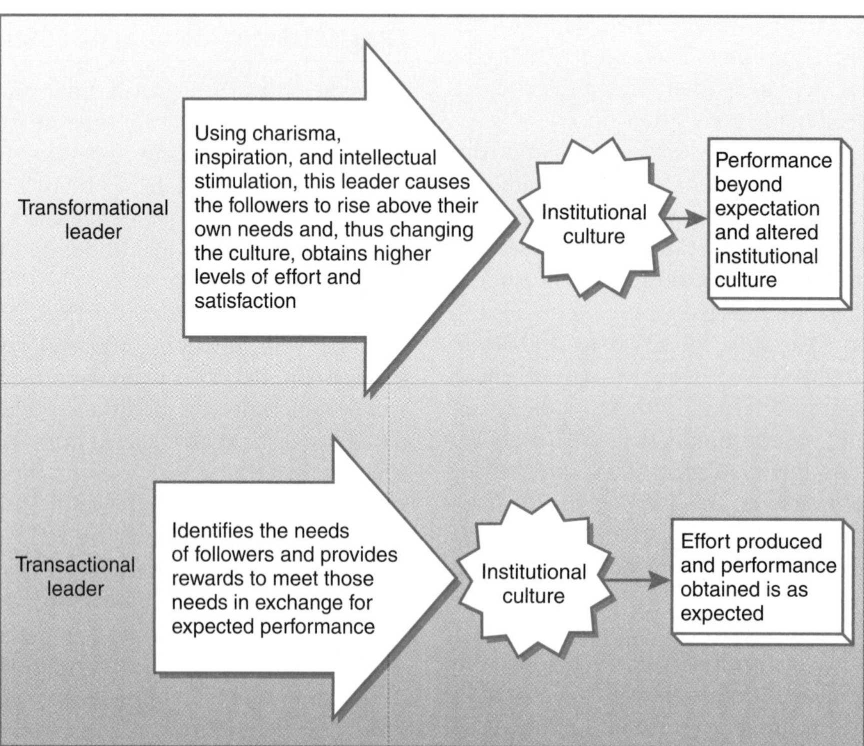

Figure 1.4
Transactional and transformational leadership.

time to entice staff members to do project or committee work. Continuous or incremental change, the first order of change, can be handled well at the transactional level.

Transformational leadership occurs when persons engage with others so that leaders and followers raise each other to higher levels of motivation and ethical decision making (Burns, 1978). Instead of emphasizing differences between the leader and the followers, transformational leadership focuses on collective purpose and mutual growth and development. Transformational leadership augments transactional leadership by being committed, having a vision, and empowering others to heighten motivation in a way that attains extra effort beyond performance expectations. Transformational leadership is used for higher-order change and to change the organization's culture. Circumstances of growth, change, and crisis call forth transformational leaders (Bass & Avolio, 1990).

The American Nurses Credentialing Center's (ANCC) Magnet Recognition Program® has emphasized transformational leadership. The revised 2008 Magnet™ model has clustered the 14 Forces of Magnetism into five key components: transformational leadership; structural empowerment; exemplary professional practice; new knowledge, innovations, and improvements; and empirical outcomes (ANCC, 2008). This evidence-based 2008 Magnet™ model clearly identifies the core parts of successful nursing leadership and management. For the nursing department of a hospital to be Magnet™ recognized, its nursing leadership needs to exhibit more than leadership—specifically, transformational leadership. A transformational leadership style has been shown to generate greater follower commitment, follower satisfaction, and overall effectiveness (Kleinman, 2004). As health care is transforming, so too must nurse leaders transform organizational values, beliefs, and behaviors to lead people to where they need to be for the future. The ANCC (2008, p. 22) noted: "Such leadership requires vision, influence, clinical knowledge, and expertise as well as an understanding that transformation may require atypical solutions and create turbulence." Based on the original work by McClure and colleagues (1983), the ANCC Magnet Recognition Program® has a website with a helpful checklist for self-assessment before beginning an application *(www.nursecredentialing.org/Magnet.aspx).*

Transformational leadership is a concept that is useful and applicable to nursing. The finding that leadership quality is a key element in developing a culture of excellence among Magnet™ hospitals is important for nursing management (Kramer, 1990). Organizations with a transformational leader would exhibit characteristics such as pride and satisfaction in the work, enthusiasm, team spirit, a sense of accomplishment, and nurse satisfaction (Barker, 1990). Bennis and Nanus (1985) identified the following four activities for transformational leadership:

1. Creating a vision
2. Building a social architecture that provides meaning for employees
3. Sustaining organizational trust
4. Recognizing the importance of building self-esteem

Three factors underlie effectiveness as a transformational leader: individual consideration, charisma, and intellectual stimulation (Bass et al., 1987; McDaniel & Wolf, 1992). In one comparative study, nurse executives' transformational scores were found to be higher than those of general managers (Bass, 1985; Dunham & Klafehn, 1990). Other research has been done to test transformational leadership theory in nursing (McDaniel & Wolf, 1992). Transformational leadership was the type of leadership most often reported in Magnet™ research studies (Upenieks, 2003a, 2003b). Transformational leadership qualities appear to be better suited to the work of professionals and important for leadership in nursing.

CONTEMPORARY LEADERSHIP

Society has moved into the information age, and there has been a metamorphosis in health care organizations as they transform into knowledge or learning organizations. Nurses are knowledge workers who use expertise and specialized knowledge in the care of patients. They need matching organizations that will value, nurture, and foster the acquisition of the data, information, and knowledge needed for effectiveness. Today's health care environments demand that front-line workers such as nurses have and maintain the expertise and the information necessary to take action to solve problems (Drucker, 1994). In this milieu, leadership is interactional, relational, transformational, and needed at all levels.

Arising in conjunction with the application of complexity theory and chaos theory, the new view of leadership was described by Wheatley (1992) as being simpler, less stressful, and more appropriate to complex organizations in the midst of chaos. Her view of leadership emphasized the importance of connectedness and relationships within self-organizing systems. Nursing has a natural niche within interactional and relationship leadership theories. Optimal health care delivery is truly interdisciplinary and holistic. When connections and relationships are strong, patients benefit.

Quantum Leadership

Contemporary definitions of leadership describe leadership as the result of a relationship between leaders and followers in which a distinct set of competencies is used to allow the relationship to achieve shared goals (Wilson & Porter-O'Grady, 1999). This is complex and requires nurses to be creative and flexible. Old ways of leading and managing are insufficient to present circumstances. Thus it is proposed that quantum leadership is needed to produce results in today's health care environment. Quantum leadership is about discovering—it is an ongoing process of exploration, curiosity, and asking questions (McCauley, 2004). The elements of quantum leadership are discovering, authenticity, passion, creating, relationship, inquiry, and fiscal astuteness. Driven by organizational stress and the feeling that something more and different in work life is needed, quantum leadership is one type of leadership strategy that helps nurses focus on the future, stretch and break boundaries, and encourage breakthrough thinking to solve problems in a complex and fluid care environment.

Servant Leadership

Another popular contemporary leadership concept is called *servant leadership*. Greenleaf (2002) used the term to describe leaders who choose first to serve others and then to be a leader, as opposed to those who are leaders first (often because of a power drive or need to acquire material possessions) and later choose to serve. Servant-leaders put others first. They choose to make sure that other people's highest-priority needs are being served in a way that promotes personal growth and helps others become freer and more autonomous. When applied to health care, servant leadership is an attractive alternative to the traditional bureaucratic environment experienced by nurses. The servant leadership model draws attention to the necessity for leaders to be attentive to the needs of others and is a model that enhances the personal growth of nurses, improves the quality of care, values teamwork, and promotes personal involvement and caring behavior.

FEMINIST LEADERSHIP PERSPECTIVE

Leadership styles appear to have a gender component. The feminist perspective on leadership was presented by Helgeson (1995a, 1995b). She identified female leadership as a weblike structure—dynamic and continuously expanding and contracting. It is characterized by a concern for family, community, and culture. The inclination is for a democratic power style, and the emphasis is on the importance of establishing relationships, maintaining connections with others, and deriving strength from empowering others. By contrast, leadership approaches described by men tend to be influenced by the military and participating in team sports. Men tend to spend their time on meetings and tasks requiring immediate attention, focusing on completion of tasks and achievement of goals. Women tend to focus on process; men tend to focus on achievement and closure. Women tend to be more flexible and value cooperation, connectedness, and relationships. Exploring the feminist perspective on leadership is valuable in that it provides food for thought as health care organizations and the nurses working in them struggle with not wanting to let go of the familiar hierarchy management style yet needing to reconfigure to the circular or web structure to be effective.

GOOD TO GREAT BUSINESS MODEL

In the business world, leadership is important for building and maintaining companies that return investment to stockholders. Interesting research was done by Collins (2001) to study the leaders of 11 companies who followed a "good-to-great" growth pattern of cumulative stock returns. He found that the behaviors and competencies of leaders settled into one of five hierarchical levels. Individuals can move among levels, but results in the business world appeared to differ according to the level of leadership exhibited by the leader. The five levels of leadership are as follows:

1. Highly capable individual
2. Contributing team member
3. Competent manager
4. Effective leader
5. Executive

The level-5 leader builds enduring greatness and is characterized as having a paradoxical blend of personal humility and professional will. The level-5 leader first addresses "who" by getting the right people in the right jobs and then addresses the "what" by figuring out the best path to greatness. By contrast, the level-4 leader first addresses the "what" by setting a vision and developing a plan and then addresses the "who." Level-5 leaders also confronted brutal facts without losing faith, transcended the curse of competence, created a culture of discipline, and pioneered the application of carefully selected technology. It is not known whether or how Collins' (2001) work applies to nursing and health care, but the emphasis on people as assets is also important for nursing care management.

Leadership research in nursing has revealed the following factors central to successful nursing leadership (Upenieks, 2003a, 2003b):

- Formal and informal power
- Access to information and resources
- Opportunity to grow from new challenges
- Supportive organizational cultures in which nurses are valued for their expertise
- Visibility, responsiveness, a passion for nursing, and business astuteness shown by nurse leaders
- Respectful and collaborative teamwork
- Adequate compensation representing value

Many of the factors crucial to successful nursing leadership are similar to those identified in the business world. These have been synthesized into a competency framework. In 2005, the American Organization of Nurse Executives (AONE, 2005) identified five core nurse executive competency domains: (1) leadership, (2) communication and relationship management, (3) professionalism, (4) knowledge of the health care environment, and (5) business skills and principles. Each domain was further elaborated with specific skill categories. This conceptualization provides a roadmap for curriculum and continuing education and a blueprint for nurse executive self-assessment and evaluation. Leadership effectiveness theories and skills can be explored by nurses who seek to learn and improve their personal leadership competency.

EFFECTIVE LEADERSHIP

Effective leadership is an integrated blend of leadership principles and characteristics with management principles and techniques. Longest (1998) identified six core management competencies needed to manage an integrated health system: conceptual, technical managerial/clinical, interpersonal/collaborative, political, commercial, and governance. Using this model, Tornabeni (2001) outlined practical leadership techniques for the nurse leader. Table 1.1 displays practical actions for nurses to take to improve leadership skills. Nurses can grow such skills by knowledge and awareness (e.g., through assessment tools) and then putting knowledge and skills to work through guided exercises and mentored experiences.

Table 1.1

Tornabeni's Practical Advice

Longest's Category	Tornabeni's Advice
Conceptual	Have a vision. Gather information. Broaden your scope. Take risks.
Technical managerial/ clinical	Devise a step-by-step approach and plan. Generate buy-in. Delegate tasks. Motivate continuously by recruiting competent people; developing them; giving them appropriate tools, authority, and resources; holding them accountable; and rewarding "right" behavior.
Interpersonal/ collaborative	Build your team. Look for talent within. Pick the cream of the crop. Establish a sense of collegiality. Help your people cope with change.
Political	Understand the politics. Build an internal network.
Commercial	Build an external network. Exchange ideas and challenges with outside colleagues.
Governance	Trust your intuition. Have a sense of purpose. Do the hard work (perspiration). Have passion.

Data from Tornabeni, J. (2001). The competency game: My take on what it really takes to lead. *Nursing Administration Quarterly, 25*(4), 1-13.

PART I

Leadership effectiveness is based on the ability to adapt in a complex and chaotic environment. Adaptive problems arise from change and chaos and often are systems problems that affect people, planning, institutional operations, or work processes. Adaptive solutions engage followers in confronting the issue and the situation. Effective leadership for adaptive problems includes the following types of behaviors (Heifetz & Laurie, 1997):

- Giving direction to identify the issue, key questions, and appropriate discussion
- Protecting the group by regulating distress
- Maintaining disciplined attention
- Managing conflict
- Shaping norms and group adaptation through learning

Effective leaders have a grasp of themselves, their team, their goals, nursing and health care, and important evaluative data for "dashboards." They use their personal style, vision, and energy to focus on goal attainment and group satisfaction. Starting with whatever natural talent a nurse possesses, essential leadership skills can be practiced over time for greater effectiveness. Effective leadership uses empowerment. For nurses, empowering means that the power over clinical practice decisions is invested in staff nurses, enabling them to do what they do best. This process is similar to nurses empowering clients. Leadership involves elements of vigor and vision and can be understood as a dynamic combination of competence, willingness to take responsibility, and strength of character to do what is right because it is the right thing to do.

FOLLOWERSHIP

Pagonis (1992) noted that, by definition, leaders do not operate in isolation. Instead, leadership involves cooperation and collaboration. The basic nature of leadership is interactive; it revolves around the interpersonal relationships among leaders and followers. Therefore cooperation and collaboration between leader and followers and between followers and the leader enhance the group's effectiveness.

Followership is an interpersonal process of participation. It implies an engagement of the follower with the leader, and possibly a group, by which the follower takes guidance and direction from the leader to accomplish group goals. The importance of followership is emphasized because leadership requires the presence of followers. The relationship between the leader and the followers defines leadership. The corollary to leadership is followership, or helping to get the job done. A good leader clearly needs good followers (Brakey, 1991). Bennis (1994) noted that followers need three things from leaders: direction, trust, and hope. With these three elements in place, followers are empowered in their participation efforts.

It may be that as nurse leadership becomes recognized as a vital element in meeting future challenges, nurse followership will assume a greater importance in practice. At one level, the nurse functions as a leader within the nurse-patient relationship and within the framework of care management. However, within nursing the staff nurse often is viewed as being at the level of a follower in the nursing organizational hierarchy.

There are different degrees of followership engagement. Murphy (1990) reviewed Kelley's (1988) model of five categories of followers and applied them to nursing. "Sheep" are followers who lack initiative, sense of responsibility, and critical thinking. "Yes-people" lack enterprise and yield to the opinions, will, or decisions of others. "Alienated" followers are capable of independence and critical thinking but appear passive because they resist open opposition; the result is frustration and disillusionment. "Survivors" never make waves or take risks; they check which way the wind is blowing. "Effective" followers have initiative and think for themselves. They manage themselves well and are responsible and well balanced. They are competent and committed. Effective followers are an asset to be nurtured, developed, and valued. Effective followers contribute to success in organizations. Nurses can and should examine their own behavior and ask themselves the following: "In this situation, what kind of follower am I?"

Guidera and Gilmore (1988) stated that the enlightened follower incorporates the cohesiveness of collective group thought without being afraid to be candid or to criticize objectively. Self-awareness is an important aspect of both leadership and followership. This means that nurses can assess themselves to better understand their own style and leadership characteristics. Self-assessment tools are available to assist nurses in awareness of both leadership and followership behaviors. One example is the LEAD instruments developed by Hersey and colleagues (2008). Leadership self-assessment instruments can be found online (e.g., *www.nwlink.com/~donclark/leader/survlead.html*). Other instruments include the Leader Behavior Description Questionnaire, or LBDQ-12 (Stodgill, 1963), the Least Preferred Coworker Scale (Fiedler & Chemers, 1984; Fiedler & Garcia, 1987), the Leadership Practices Inventory (Kouzes & Posner, 1988), the Multifactor Leadership Questionnaire (MLQ) (Bass & Avolio, 1990), the Self-Assessment Leadership Instrument (Smola, 1988), and multiple training instruments. Leadership-related research instruments were identified, compared, and evaluated by Huber and colleagues (2000). Some instruments are useful for research and others for leadership training or self-diagnosis. A wide variety of tools are available. Individuals can increase their effectiveness through greater awareness and subsequent honing of both their leadership and followership skills.

LEADERSHIP AND MANAGEMENT IMPLICATIONS

Leadership is a key element in operating successful groups and organizations. It is a key resource for the improvement of nursing services. The following five practices are common to most exceptional leadership achievements (Kouzes & Posner, 1990):

1. Challenging the process by searching for opportunities, experimenting, and taking risks
2. Inspiring a shared vision by envisioning the future and enlisting the support of others
3. Enabling others to act by fostering collaboration and strengthening others
4. Modeling the way by setting an example and planning small successes
5. Encouraging the heart by recognizing contributions and celebrating accomplishments

LEADERSHIP & MANAGEMENT **BEHAVIORS**

Leadership Behaviors

- Shows followers how to think about old problems in new ways
- Treats followers as unique individuals
- Stimulates critical thinking
- Inspires followers
- Demonstrates expertise and empathy
- Is visible to followers
- Is flexible
- Provides assistance and feedback (coaching)
- Communicates a vision
- Establishes trust
- Motivates the group to achieve goals
- Promotes innovation and risk taking
- Empowers followers
- Masters change
- Mentors followers
- Is creative and innovative

Management Behaviors

- Makes decisions
- Communicates
- Plans and organizes
- Manages changes
- Motivates followers

Overlap Areas

- Exercises broad-perspective decision making
- Communicates with followers
- Motivates followers

PART I

Nurse leaders can read, learn, and practice leadership skills. For example, the five practices identified through research as being associated with exceptional leadership can serve as an assessment guide for leadership situations. Furthermore, they can form the basis for strategic plans and activities to improve a given nursing work environment. Individuals can use this information for self-assessment.

As nurses work in a rapidly changing practice environment, leadership is important because it affects the climate and work environment of the organization. It affects how nurses feel about themselves at work and about their jobs. By extension, leadership is thought to affect organizational and individual productivity. For example, if nurses feel goal-directed and think that their contributions are important, they are more motivated to do the work. Important for the professional practice of nurses is how they feel about themselves and how satisfied they are with their jobs. Both aspects have implications for how well nurses are retained and recruited. Leadership cannot be overlooked because leaders function as problem finders and problem solvers. They are people who help everyone else overcome obstacles. The leadership role is one of bridging, integrating, motivating, and creating organizational "glue."

Leadership in nursing is crucial. *First*, it is important to nurses because of the size of the profession. Nurses make up the largest single health care occupation and one that is experiencing critical shortages. Pressures, including costs, in the health care environment are rapidly thrusting nurses into leadership roles in highly complex and stressful work situations.

Nurses are the largest group of health care professionals in most settings of service delivery and represent the largest human resource expenditure in most care settings (O'Neil et al., 2008). Besides volume, nurses also are distributed both horizontally and vertically and in leadership roles throughout care delivery systems. Nurses are found at the first level of caregiving process management and on up to executive level of leadership and strategic decision making. Given the challenges of cost containment, an aging population needing more health care services, and issues of access and quality of care, nurse leaders are experiencing greater pressure to perform and produce more effective alignment of key processes, functions, and resources. Organizations have under-invested in nursing leadership skill development, leaving them at risk of under-performing, especially in the three strategic challenges of finance, workforce, and patient safety (O'Neil et al., 2008).

Second, nursing's work is complex, often conducted in complex settings. Tremendous changes in nursing have occurred in the past 25 years. These are changes in philosophy, knowledge base, technological complexity, ethical dilemmas, and impacts from constant change and societal pressures. Thus leadership is needed to guide and motivate the nurses and health care delivery systems toward positive achievements for better patient care. Leadership in nursing is needed to influence the organizational context of care for greater effectiveness and productivity. Contextual aspects include culture, leadership, and organizational infrastructure (Marchionni & Ritchie, 2008). Leaders establish norms and values, define expectations, reward behaviors, and reinforce culture (Shirey, 2007). Authenticity and caring are valued in nurse leaders and are exhibited by people who are genuine, trustworthy, reliable, and believable and who create a positive environment (Pipe, 2008; Shirey, 2006).

Third, nurses enter the practice of nursing by licensure but they come from a variety of educational backgrounds. A baccalaureate degree or certification as a clinical nurse leader (CNL) does not automatically confer advanced leadership skills. However, without a baccalaureate degree at minimum, nursing as a profession is disadvantaged when compared with other professions whose minimum preparation is uniformly baccalaureate or above. Thus nurses will need strong leadership to resolve the interprofessional dilemmas derived from educational diversity and issues related to professionalization and employment. For example, each nurse will need to develop leadership skills in relating to peers who have different educational backgrounds and value systems. Nursing needs strong leadership for public policy advocacy on behalf of nursing as a profession and for its own growth and advancement in the provision of cost-effective patient care.

Nursing's leadership challenge includes developing strategies that help followers cope with change and develop the ability to adapt in positive and productive ways. Indeed, "one of the future leader's most important functions is to cultivate the human capital of their organization" (Anderson, 1997, p. 334). Leaders help create an environment for followers to be able to use innovation, creativity, and collective problem solving. An important role for the leader is to instill confidence in followers. The leader needs to be able to encourage, coach, and question to increase the learning and growth of followers (Anderson, 1997).

Recent research has brought to light the gaps, barriers, and needs related to developing nursing leaders as a human capital asset (O'Neil et al., 2008). The top five competencies identified by nurse leaders were the following (O'Neil et al., 2008):

- Building effective teams
- Translating vision into strategy
- Communicating vision and strategy internally
- Managing conflict
- Managing focus on patient and customer

Barriers to expanding leadership training for nurses were the inability to get released time away to attend and the budget to fund attendance. Thus "budget and release time were rate-limiting realities" (O'Neil et al., 2008, p. 182).

Nurses are knowledge workers in an information age. Knowledge workers respond to inspiration, not supervision. Although professionals require little direction and supervision, what they do need is protection and support (Mintzberg, 1998). This is best manifested in the covert leadership of the unobtrusive actions that permeate all the things the leader does. Inspiration also can come from a focus on results. Leaders need to model what they want. Positive leadership outcomes are balanced, strategic, lasting, and selfless (Ulrich et al., 1999).

CURRENT ISSUES AND TRENDS

Four current issues and trends have significance for leadership in nursing. The first is the dramatic U.S. demographic data related to the aging of the "Baby Boom" generation. Next is the demographic profile of nursing in the United States. Also important are issues of collective action and ethical leadership in nursing.

Comprehension of a major societal and public policy issue related to the aging of a large demographic bulge (commonly known as the "Baby Boom" generation) is beginning to reach into the awareness of the U.S. general public. Called the "2030 problem" (Knickman & Snell, 2002), this socioeconomic and demographic phenomenon is real, looming, urgent, and fraught with health care challenges. Current statistics show that there are approximately 37 million Americans ages 65 years and older, representing 12.4% of the population, or 1 in 8 Americans (U.S. Census Bureau, 2008). The percentage of Americans 65 years of age and older has tripled since 1900. Issues related to health burdens and chronic illness are characteristic of older adults. In fact, persons 85 years of age and older may spend up to half of their remaining lives inactive or dependent.

U.S. population and health trends are assessed and monitored by governmental agencies such as the U.S. Census Bureau, Centers for Disease Control and Prevention, Bureau of Labor Statistics, and Health Resources and Services Administration. The statistics related to the Baby Boom generation are impressive. As of the 2000 U.S. census, Baby Boomers represented 28% of the U.S. population (U.S. Census Bureau, 2001). Born between 1946 and 1964, Baby Boomers in 2030 will be between the ages of 66 and 84 years and are projected to number 61 million people. In addition to Baby Boomers, the U.S. population in 2030 is projected also to include 9 million people born before 1946. This predictable tidal wave will make chronic illness and long-term care a huge economic burden. Knickman and Snell (2002) suggested that there are four key "aging shocks": (1) uncovered costs of prescription medications, (2) uncovered medical care costs, (3) private insurance costs for the "Medi-gap," and (4) costs of long-term care. They projected that there will be an overwhelming economic burden if tax rates need to be raised dramatically, economic growth is retarded because of high service costs, or future generations of workers have worse general well-being because of service costs or income transfers. Nurses will be challenged to find evidence-based care delivery and service systems models and strategies that address the projected growth industry in chronic illness.

Examining the demographic profile of nursing in the United States offers a clue about nursing followership. The average age of a licensed, registered professional nurse in the United States was 43 years in 1992 (Rosenfeld, 1994). This figure rose to 44.3 years in 1996 as the federal government's RN sample surveys documented the aging of the RN population (U.S. Department of Health and Human Services [USDHHS], 1997). The Seventh National Sample Survey of Registered Nurses was conducted in 2000 and published in 2002 (USDHHS, 2002). An estimated 2,714,671 licensed RNs were in the United States, and 81.7% were employed in nursing. The RN population continues to age. The average age of the total RN population was 45.2 years in 2000. Only 9.1% were younger than 30 years, with 18.3% younger than 35 years and 31.7% younger than 40 years.

By 2004, the most recent available statistics from the Health Resources and Services Administration (HRSA) National Sample Survey of Registered Nurses indicated that 2,915,309 licensed RNs were in the United States; 83.2% were employed in nursing; the average age of the total RN population was 46.8 years; 8% were younger than 30 years; and 41.1% were 50 years old or older. The increase in the 50+ age category is striking: 25.1% in 1980, 33% in 2000, and 41.1% in 2004 (USDHHS [HRSA], 2008). The profile of RNs revealed that fewer young nurses were entering the workforce, large cohorts of the RN population were moving into their 50s and 60s, few minorities were in the profession (10.7%), and even fewer men were in the profession (5.8%).

The highest educational preparation for RNs is 17.5% diploma, 33.7% associate degree, 34.2% baccalaureate, and 13% master's or doctoral degree. However, a look at just the recent (past 5 years) graduates shows a dramatically different profile: 56.7% associate degree and 39.9% baccalaureate degree or higher. Hospitals remain the major employer of nurses (56.2%), down from a peak of 68% in 1984. Public and community health (10.7%), ambulatory care (11.5%), and other noninstitutional settings had the largest percentage gain in RN employment from 1980 to 2004. The average actual annual earnings of full-time RNs was $57,785 (USDHHS, 2008). This implies that nurses are going to need to look at how nursing is structured and organized, because nursing is no longer a young person's profession, on average. The bulk of nursing's population is advancing each year in average age. Therefore roles, deployment, and workforce utilization in nursing may need to shift to accommodate nursing demographics.

The direction of current trends indicates that major changes in nursing practice demographics will occur in the twenty-first century. The number of diploma nurses is dramatically decreasing, enrollments in nursing schools are fluctuating, and there are only small increases in the number of men (4.3% to 5.8% from 1992 to 2004) and minorities (about 10% in 1996 to 10.7% in 2004) in nursing. More advanced practice nurses are being prepared as nurse practitioner programs increase and as primary care becomes emphasized. Practice is increasingly complex, and practice settings are evolving.

The strength of a profession lies in its internal unity and ability to mobilize collective action. Yet less than 5% of all RNs belong to the American Nurses Association (ANA), which is the organization that represents nursing at the national level. This is a problem for leadership and followership in nursing. The fact that there are more than 2.9 million RNs yet few belong to the major organization that speaks for nursing reflects a potential dilution of the power of the profession. Individual nurses who are not members are effectively cut off from participation in the collective and from information that can help them in their practice. However, there are many specialty groups in the nursing profession. These groups have organized into national organizations of specialty groups in nursing, such as the Nursing Organizations Liaison Forum (NOLF), and are linked with the ANA through the Tri-Council for Nursing. At the national level, the many nursing groups have banded together so that when there are issues that are relevant to all nurses, nursing can speak with a united voice.

Under conditions of health care reform, turbulence, pressures for cost containment and better management of care, and constant change, ethical leadership becomes crucial. For instance, there are consequences to the changes being undertaken to achieve the goal of containing costs. The downsizing of nursing personnel in the 1990s led to an awareness of medical errors and patient safety issues. Yet solutions were costly and sometimes prohibitive. Nurses will find themselves in positions of both formal and informal leadership when ethical issues arise. There may be questions of advocacy for both patients and nurses. For example, must nursing services be targeted for downsizing? When downsizing occurs, how are justice, fairness, respect for persons, and prevention of harm handled? How are scarce nursing resources allocated and advocated? What institutional mechanisms help or hinder ethical decision making (Aroskar, 1994)? How can hospitals and other institutions remain financially viable during intense reimbursement reductions? Remarkably parallel issues arise over the management of scarce resources in long-term care, ambulatory care, home health care, case management, and other nursing care settings. How nurses incorporate ethics into their leadership styles and decision making affects nurses, nursing, and the delivery of patient care.

Leadership is considered key to the success of health care organizations. Nurses are pressed to demonstrate the outcomes of their care and provide evidence of the effectiveness of their service delivery. The link between leadership style and staff satisfaction highlights the importance of leadership in times of chaos. A nurse leader needs to be dynamic, show interpersonal skills, and be a visionary for the organization and the profession. The ability to inspire and motivate followers to carry out the vision is crucial.

Summary

- Effective leadership is important in nursing.
- Leadership principles can be learned through education and practice.
- Leaders must know themselves and their followers, the situation, the communication process, and goals, and they must be flexible enough to make necessary adaptations.
- Leaders are those who innovate and take the risks inherent in new approaches.
- Effectiveness means matching leadership behaviors to the environment and then adapting within that environment.
- Leaders who never vary their style are probably ineffective some of the time.
- Leadership involves a concern for task and a concern for people.
- Good leaders need good followers.

CASE STUDY

Nurse Kathryn Gardner has worked for 5 years as a staff nurse providing care to patients with developmental disabilities. She now has the opportunity to apply for her "ideal" job as the director of an innovative program funded by a local charity. Nurse Gardner has obtained the job description and related application forms. The request to write a description of her philosophy of leadership and management has her stuck. She believes in patient empowerment for self-care management. Unsure of how to translate this into a leadership statement, Nurse Gardner consults the literature. As she reads, she comes across a leadership style assessment instrument. Using this tool, she identifies herself as higher on task than relationship style. With further reading and some coaching, she begins to formulate the germ of an idea: her leadership style uses activities of bridging, integrating, motivating, and creating organizational "glue" to empower nurses to help patients achieve self-management skills. She writes several drafts. When she believes that the document is polished, she completes the rest of the paperwork to apply for the job. She now feels more confident about presenting herself well in a job interview.

CRITICAL THINKING EXERCISE

Nurse Victoria Munoz has been reading leadership theory. She had hoped to be inspired by this new knowledge and discover better ways to solve some problems in the nursing work environment. Instead, Nurse Munoz is puzzled. The real work environment is dramatically different from what the theory says it should be. Many articles call for strong, motivating leadership in nursing with shared leadership and empowerment of staff nurses. However, in the health care environment in which Nurse Munoz works, nursing units have been consolidated and reorganized. The inpatient nurse managers are now responsible for multiple nursing units. The nurse managers of the ambulatory clinics have been realigned to report to a physician Director of Clinics. Everyone has a new role, position, boss, and followers.

Furthermore, the nurses of the inpatient clinical departments have been exhausted from work overload and now feel angry and devalued because of the effects on the Department of Nursing. The final straw comes when they realize that the new directors of the nonclinical departments have been promoted within 3 months of the organizational changes, whereas the nurse managers remain at their previous level.

1. What is the problem?
2. What are the key issues?
3. How should Nurse Munoz handle the situation?
4. What should Nurse Munoz do first to demonstrate leadership?
5. What leadership style would be most appropriate in this situation?
6. What leadership and management strategies might be helpful?

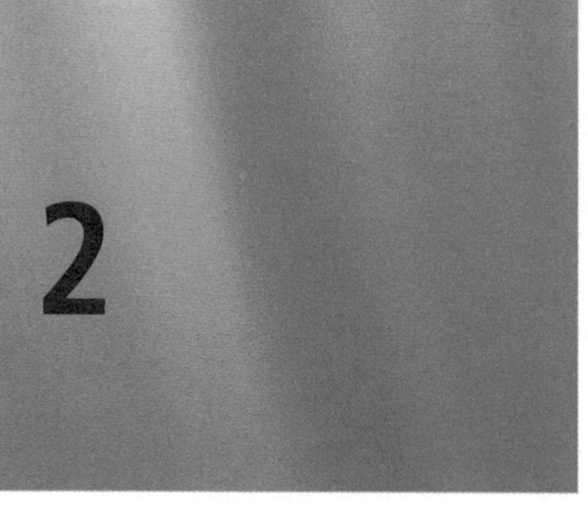

2 Management Principles

Diane L. Huber

PART I

CHAPTER OBJECTIVES

- Define and describe management and nursing management
- Formulate the management process
- Critique the nature of managerial work
- Analyze the roles a manager plays
- Distinguish classic management thought from contemporary theories
- Relate management concepts to nursing leadership and management
- Review legal aspects of management
- Exercise critical thinking to conceptualize and analyze possible solutions to a practice exercise

The global information age has engulfed our society, yet challenges to health care management linger. Along with an array of opportunities, such as instantaneous communication across vast distances, health care organizations and the people in them struggle with an ever-accelerating rate of change, knowledge explosion, and information flow. The context for health care management includes a nurse shortage and fierce competition, doing more with less, waves of technology revisions, information proliferation, consumerism, generational values differences, and cultural diversity. The recruitment, development, deployment, motivation, and leveraging of human capital (nurses) as scarce resources and prime assets are critical management issues for service industries in general and nursing and health care specifically.

At the core, managers manage people and organizations. People's time and effort, as well as organizations' money, facilities, and supplies, need to be directed in a coordinated effort to achieve best results and meet objectives. Following are some thoughts about management:

> *The conventional definition of management is getting work done through people, but real management is developing people through work.*
>
> -Agha Hasan Abedi

> *My main job was developing talent. I was a gardener providing water and other nourishment to our top 750 people. Of course, I had to pull out some weeds, too.*
>
> -Jack Welch

> *I mean, there's no arguing. There is no anything. There is no beating around the bush. "You're fired" is a very strong term.*
>
> -Donald Trump

> *Executives owe it to the organization and their fellow workers not to tolerate nonperforming people in important jobs.*
>
> -Peter Drucker

Never tell people how to do things. Tell them what to do and they will surprise you with their ingenuity.
-George S. Patton

The best executive is the one who has sense enough to pick good men to do what he wants done, and self-restraint enough to keep from meddling with them while they do it.
-Teddy Roosevelt

Things may come to those who wait, but only the things left by those who hustle.
-Abraham Lincoln

LEADERSHIP AND MANAGEMENT DIFFERENTIATED

Leadership and management are equally important processes. Because their focus is different, their importance varies according to what is needed in a specific situation. They are overlapping but distinct ideas. However, some have viewed them as almost identical or very similar. For example, Hersey and colleagues (2008) thought that leadership was a broader concept than management. They described management as a special kind of leadership. This view would position management as a subpart of leadership, not as a distinct concept. However, according to the definitions, characteristics, and processes, the concepts of leadership and management are different, but at the area of overlap they look similar. For example, directing occurs in both leadership and management activities (the area of overlap), whereas inspiring a vision is clearly a leadership function. Both leadership and management are necessary, although some have proposed the death of management altogether (Porter-O'Grady, 1997) and a shift to process leadership. This may be similar to Mintzberg's (1994) idea of nursing management occurring in an interactive model rather than following a step-by-step list approach.

An evidence-based approach to differentiating nursing leadership from management is to identify discrete competencies through an integrative content analysis of the literature base (Jennings et al., 2007). In 140 articles reviewed, they found 894 competencies, of which 862 (96%) were common to both leadership and management. Thus the overlap area appeared to be larger than previously thought. However, leadership and management do serve distinct purposes. Perhaps it is time to apply leadership and management concepts and competencies by setting, level of role responsibility, career stage, and social context to more fully apply the evidence base to practice.

In a similar fashion, Bass and Avolio (1990) distinguished transactional leadership from transformational leadership, in which transactional leadership resembles what has been called *management*. They noted that there is a similarity between what they called *transactional leaders* and traditional descriptions of managers. Transformational leaders, however, reflected the "strong forces" of leadership. Transactional leaders, or in this case, managers, focused on maintenance of the quality and quantity of performance, reduction in resistance to change, and the implementation of decisions in a specific situation. By contrast, increasing effort, making leaps in performance, changing group values and needs, creating innovative ideas, and improving quality were described as the activities of transformational leaders. In this model, the transactional process occurs first and appears to be essential to effective leadership in that it provides the traditional management functions that are so important for day-to-day operations. It would appear that *transactional leadership* is another name for *management functions* and that this theory sees management as a process leading to expected outcomes. The area of overlap with leadership is not addressed, but there is presumed to be some overlap along this continuum. Distinctions between leadership and management are important for choosing an effective style that is matched to the situation.

Under conditions of maintenance and stability, transactional management appears to be needed. For growth, crisis, or change, transformational leadership is a major component of effectiveness. Thus management and leadership do not appear to be identical. The focus of each is different. It is possible that management is focused on task accomplishment and leadership is focused on human relationship aspects. They may be sequential, and they are interrelated. Clearly, a balance of the two is necessary. There is a "gray area" in which the foci of their outcomes overlap. This overlap occurs where the two processes are integrated or synthesized to accomplish goals and where the same strategies are employed even though the goals may differ.

In 2008, the American Nurses Credentialing Center (ANCC) presented a new model for its Magnet Recognition Program® based on a statistical analysis of hospital reviews (American Nurses Credentialing Center [ANCC], 2008). The five evidence-based components are transformational leadership; structural empowerment; exemplary professional practice; new knowledge, innovation, and improvements; and empirical quality results. The key managerial component is structural empowerment. Based on extensive nursing research, solid structures and processes that are developed by influential leaders and where professional practice flourishes are important for the organization. This is accomplished through the strategic plan, structure, systems, policies, and programs.

DEFINITIONS

Management is defined here as the process of coordination and integration of resources through activities of planning, organizing, coordinating, directing, and controlling to accomplish specific institutional goals and objectives. Management has been viewed as an art and a science related to planning and directing human effort and scarce resources to attain established objectives. Management has been viewed in a variety of ways. Another definition of management is a process by which organizational goals are met through the application of skills and the use of resources. Hersey and colleagues (2008) defined management as "the process of working with and through individuals and groups and other resources (such as equipment, capital, and technology) to accomplish organizational goals" (p. 5).

Management, then, applies to organizations. The definition of leadership emphasizes actions that influence toward group goals; the definition of management focuses on organizational goals. The achievement of organizational goals through leadership and manipulation of the environment is management. In a systems approach to management, the inputs would be represented by human resources and physical and technical resources. The outputs would be the realization of goals (Figure 2.1). Koontz (1961) concluded that management is the art of the following:

- Getting things done through and with people in formally organized groups
- Creating an environment in an organized group in which people can perform as individuals yet cooperate to attain group goals

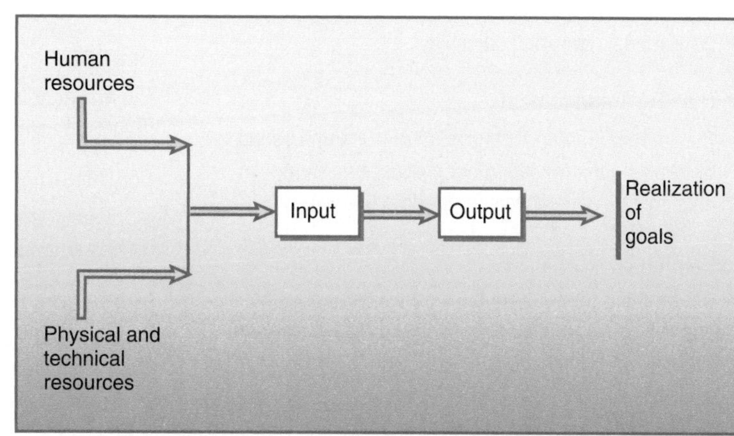

Figure 2.1
Systems view of management.

- Removing barriers and roadblocks to performance
- Optimizing efficiency in effectively reaching goals

Thus management is a separate function with a specific purpose and related roles but one that is focused on organizations. To achieve organizational goals, managers are involved in activities such as analyzing issues, establishing goals and objectives, mapping out work plans, organizing assets and supplies, developing and motivating people, communicating, managing technology, handling change and conflict, measurement, analysis, and evaluation. Without talent and attention to these functions, effectiveness and morale drop.

Effective managers are thought to be those who can weave strategy, execution, discipline, inspiration, and leadership together as they unite an organization toward achieving its goals. Sull (2003) found that successful managers may vary in personal attributes but all excel at managing commitments. Managerial commitments may be capital investments, hiring or firing decisions, public statements, or other strategy decisions. A commitment is defined as "any action taken in the present that binds an organization to a future course of action" (Sull, 2003, p. 84). Commitments give employees a clear sense of focus for prioritization and motivation; however, they limit flexibility. The most enduring commitments tend to be strategic frames, resources, processes, relationships, and values.

Drucker (2004) suggested that effective executives do not need to be leaders. "Great managers may be charismatic or dull, generous or tightfisted, visionary or numbers oriented. But every effective executive follows eight simple practices" (Drucker, 2004, p. 59). These eight practices are divided into the following three categories:

Practices That Give Executives the Knowledge They Need

1. They asked: "What needs to be done?"
2. They asked: "What is right for the enterprise?"

Practices That Help Executives Convert Knowledge to Action

1. They developed action plans.
2. They took responsibility for decisions.
3. They took responsibility for communicating.
4. They were focused on opportunities, not problems.

LEADING & MANAGING DEFINED

Management
The coordination and integration of resources through activities of planning, organizing, coordinating or directing, and controlling to accomplish specific institutional goals and objectives.

Nursing Management
The coordination and integration of nursing resources by applying the management process to accomplish nursing care and service goals and objectives.

Planning
Determining the long-term and short-term objectives and the corresponding actions that must be taken to achieve these objectives.

Organizing
Mobilizing the human and material resources of the institution to achieve organizational objectives.

Directing
The managerial function of establishing direction and then influencing people to follow that direction.

Coordinating
Motivating and leading personnel to carry out the desired actions.

Controlling
Comparing the results of work with predetermined standards of performance and taking corrective action when needed.

Practices That Ensure That the Whole Organization Feels Responsible and Accountable

1. They ran productive meetings.
2. They thought and said "we," not "I."

Effective management also appears to be a result of artful balancing. Managers need to function at the point at which reflective thinking combines with practical doing (Gosling & Mintzberg, 2003). Described as managerial mind-sets within the bounds of management, managers interpret and deal with their world from the following five perspectives (Gosling & Mintzberg, 2003):

1. *Reflective mind-set*: Managing self
2. *Analytic mind-set*: Managing organizations
3. *Worldly mind-set*: Managing context
4. *Collaborative mind-set*: Managing relationships
5. *Action mind-set*: Managing change

These five mind-sets were described as being like threads for the manager to weave. The process is as follows: analyze, act, reflect, act, collaborate, reanalyze, articulate new insights, and act again.

Management is central to the work of nursing. **Nursing management** is defined as the coordination and integration of nursing resources by applying the management process to accomplish nursing care and service goals and objectives.

BACKGROUND: THE MANAGEMENT PROCESS

An organization can be any institution, agency, or facility. Working to achieve an organization's goals involves the process of management. The principles that guide the process of management need to be identified to be useful for greater effectiveness. A Frenchman named Fayol (1949) reasoned that management could be taught if there were basic principles. To explain the management process, Fayol formulated the principles that created a basis for management practice. He said that managers perform unique and discrete functions: they plan, organize, coordinate, and control. Fayol's ideas were revolutionary in that, for the first time, management was seen as a unique and separate activity from the work of producing a product. Workers labor to produce the product; managers labor to manage organizations toward goal achievement. Someone needs to monitor financial indicators; hire, train and evaluate personnel; improve quality; coordinate work and effort; fix systems problems; and ensure that goals are met. In nursing, this means that nurses do the work of providing nursing care while nurse managers coordinate and integrate the work of individual nurses with the larger system.

The four steps of the management process are as follows (Fayol, 1949; Figure 2.2):

1. Planning
2. Organizing
3. Coordinating or directing
4. Controlling

These functions make up the scope of a manager's major effort. Planning involves determining the long-term and short-term objectives and the corresponding actions that must be taken. Organizing means mobilizing human and material resources to accomplish what is needed. Directing relates to methods of motivating, guiding, and leading people through work processes. Controlling has a specific meaning closer to the monitoring and evaluating actions that are familiar to nurses. The management process can be compared to an orchestra performing a concert or a team playing a football game. There is a plan and an organized group of players. A director manages the performance and controls the outcome by making corrections and adjustments along the way. The management process

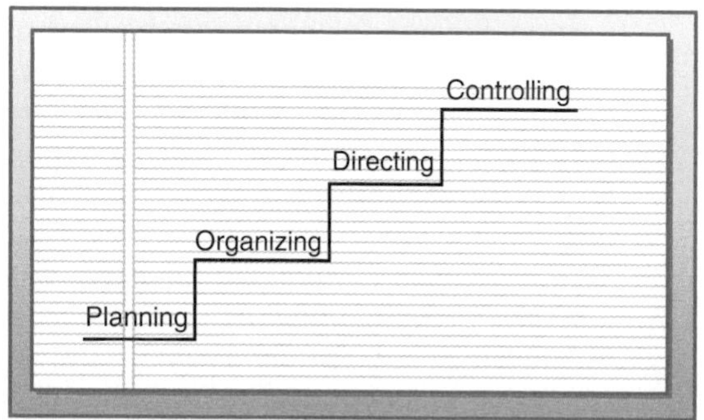

Figure 2.2
Four steps of the management process.

PART I

is a rational, logical process based on problem-solving principles. Fayol's classic management process idea remains the core framework around discussions about what management is and does.

Planning

Planning is the managerial function of selecting priorities, results, and methods to achieve results (McNamara, 1999a). It is setting the direction for a system and then guiding the system to follow the direction (McNamara, 1999b). **Planning** is defined as determining the long-term and short-term objectives and the corresponding actions that must be taken to achieve these objectives. Steiner (1962, p. 28) described planning as "the conscious determination of courses of action to achieve preconceived objectives." Planning can be detailed, specific, and rigid, or it can be broad, general, and flexible. Planning is deciding in advance what is to be done and when, by whom, and how it is to be done. Hersey and colleagues (2008) described planning as involving the setting of goals and objectives and developing "work maps" to show how they are to be accomplished. Planning activities include identifying goals, objectives, methods, resources, responsible parties, and due dates.

The two types of planning are as follows (Levenstein, 1985):

- *Strategic planning:* More broad-ranged, this approach means determining the overall purposes and directions of the organization (see Chapter 37). This is often focused on mission, vision, and major goal identification. Scenario planning may be used in the strategic planning process to help participants see the "big picture" and analyze multiple chaotic influences (see Chapter 5 for more information on scenario planning).
- *Tactical planning:* More short-ranged, this type means determining the specific details of implementing broader goals. Examples are project planning, staffing planning, and marketing plans.

Three errors can create planning flaws: (1) errors of fact: the plan is based on misinformation; (2) errors in assumption: the plan is based on incorrect assumptions; and (3) errors of logic: the plan is based on faulty reasoning. Planning flaws carry over into organizing, directing, and controlling activities.

An alternative conceptualization to the model of planning that views it as an orderly, top-down sequence is the model proposed by Hayes-Roth and Hayes-Roth (1979). Their idea was that opportunistic planning approaches are used to face complex planning tasks. Planners, under conditions of complexity, pursue whatever seems opportune or promising at the time. A plan becomes multidirectional and develops by increments. This approach may appear chaotic compared with systematic planning, but it leads to better plans in complex task situations. Similar to the interactive planning that nurses do with patients, interactive planning between nurses and nurse managers also is the best strategy for effective planning. This may be due in part to the phenomenon of an environment of chaos.

Planning is a process that heavily depends on the decision-making process. Part of planning is choosing among a number of alternatives. Thus in nursing, the manager often must balance the needs of clients, staff, administrators, and physicians. Because resources are limited, planning involves an analysis of how to best proceed under the given constraints (Kepler, 1980).

Planning involves considering systems inputs, processes, outputs, and outcomes. The process of planning in its larger context means that planners work backwards through the system. Starting with the results, outcomes, or outputs desired, they then identify the processes needed to produce the results and then identify the inputs or resources needed to carry out the processes (McNamara, 1999b). Typical planning phases include the following:

- Identify the mission.
- Conduct an environmental scan.

- Analyze the situation (e.g., SWOT analysis of strengths, weaknesses, opportunities, and threats).
- Establish goals.
- Identify strategies to reach goals.
- Set objectives to achieve goals.
- Assign responsibilities and timelines.
- Write a planning document.
- Celebrate success and completion.

Many plans fail because of incompletion; thus it is important to focus on ensuring that the plan is carried out or that deviations are recognized and managed. Recommended guidelines are as follows (McNamara, 1999b):

- Involve the right people in planning.
- Do a written plan, and communicate it widely.
- Establish goals and objectives that are specific, measurable, acceptable, placed in a time frame, stretching, and rewarding.
- Build in accountability (regular review).
- Note deviations, and replan.
- Evaluate the planning process and the plan.
- Conduct ongoing communications.
- Make the planning process compatible with the preferences of the planners.
- Acknowledge and celebrate results.

The planning process is intimately involved with establishing objectives. Fayol (1949) identified planning as examining the future and drawing up a plan of action. Activities involved include the laying out of the work to be done, determining the use of resources, and establishing the standards for evaluation. Levenstein (1985) argued that the role of the nurse manager as planner is critical to the successful functioning of the institution and the care of clients. This is because the overall plan of any client's care is shaped and reshaped with nursing input and then implemented by the nursing staff. Thomas (1983) noted that the institution is held or glued together by the nurses, enabling it to function. The nurse is engaged in a constant mental planning operation when deciding what specific things are to be accomplished for the client. The same is true for the nurse manager who is deciding how to devise, implement, and maintain a positive and productive work environment for nurses.

Planning is a function that assumes stability and the ability to predict and project into the future. Yet the current environment is turbulent, making planning difficult. Learning and adapting are important abilities in a changeable environment. Interactive planning has been suggested as an approach to planning in complex situations and changing environments (Ackoff, 1981; Foust, 1994). Interactive planning takes a developmental approach. Problems are viewed as interrelated. Interactive planning principles emphasize the importance of participation among participants, a nonlinear view of relationships called *systems thinking*, and a focus on creating a desired future outcome. Interactive planning can contribute to effective care planning and to effective care management by nurses (Foust, 1994).

Organizing

Organizing is a management function related to allocating and configuring resources to accomplish preferred goals and objectives. It is the activities done to collect and configure resources to effectively and efficiently implement plans (McNamara 1999a, 1999c). **Organizing** can be defined as mobilizing the human and material resources of the institution to achieve organizational objectives. Fayol (1949) noted that the organizing function was concerned with building up the material and human structures into a working infrastructure. Authority, power, and structure are used for influence. The goal is to get the human, equipment, and material resources mobilized, organized, and working. Organizing so that the goals and objectives can be accomplished includes forging and strengthening relationships between workers and the environment. The first step is to organize the work; then the people are organized; finally the environment is organized.

Organizing closely follows the planning process. In fact, these terms are often referred to together: *planning* and *organizing*. Organizing encompasses activities designed to bring together an array of various resources including personnel, money, and equipment in a manner that is the most effective for accomplishing organizational goals. There are a variety of ways to do this, but the essence of organizing is the integration and coordination of resources (Hersey et al., 2008).

There are a wide variety of topics related to organizing, which is considered to be one of the major functions of management. Lack of organization can be a major source of stress. McNamara (1999a, 1999c) identified the following categories under managerial organizing:

- Organizing yourself, your office, your files
- Organizing a task, job, or role through task and job analysis, job descriptions, and time management
- Organizing various groups of people such as staff, committees, meetings, and teams
- Organizing human resources through benefits, compensation, staffing and deployment, and training and development
- Organizing facilities and technology

Organizing can be thought of also as a process of identifying roles in relationship to one another. Thus organizing involves activities related to establishing a structure and hierarchy of jobs and positions within a unit or department. Responsibilities are assigned to each job. The complexity of this aspect of organizing is related to the size of the organization and the number of employees and jobs. For nurse managers, the activities of budget management, staffing, and scheduling are all organizing activities that are interrelated and tied to role relationships (Kepler, 1980). Organizing in nursing also relates to other human resources and personnel functions such as developing committees and bylaws, orientation, and staff in-service. Organizations organize by establishing a structure, such as a hierarchy with divisions or departments, and by developing some method for division of labor and subsequent coordination among subunits.

Directing

Directing is the managerial function of establishing direction and then influencing people to follow that direction. Directing can also be called *leading* (McNamara, 1999a) or *coordinating*. **Coordinating** is defined as motivating and leading personnel to carry out the desired actions. Fayol (1949) identified coordination as including activities of binding together, unifying, and harmonizing the activity and effort of various personnel.

Along with communicating and leading, motivation often is included with the description of the activities of directing others. Motivating is a major strategy related to determining the followers' level of performance and thereby to influencing how effectively the goals of the organization will be met. The amount of employee effort that can be influenced by motivation is thought to be from 20% to 30% at the low end and as high as 80% to 90% for highly motivated people (Hersey et al., 2008). A wide range of effort can be influenced through motivation. Motivation is a complex activity, but it is a critical managerial function. (See Chapter 9 for more information on management theories related to motivation.)

On a day-to-day basis, coaching is used as a technique to direct and motivate followers. The manager delegates activities and responsibilities when making assignments. The function of directing involves actions of supervising and guiding others within their assigned duties. The use of interpersonal skills is required to delicately balance the need to direct and supervise with the need to create and maintain a motivational climate (Kepler, 1980). Nurses with disabilities have become a special case of managerial directing. Federal laws now apply (i.e., Americans with Disabilities Act), and managers have to manage accommodations for some when balancing overall assignments.

Within nursing there is a legal aspect to the managerial directing function. In some state licensing laws, supervision is a defined and regulated legal element of nursing practice. Delegation and supervision are viewed legally as a part of the practice of nursing. Thus nurses have a specific need to know and understand this area of nursing responsibility within their scope of practice.

Practical Tips

Tip # 1: Get the Tasks Accomplished

Stop and check out your management style. If you work in a high-stress or crisis-oriented environment, are you constantly chasing chaos? What aspects of management theories can you use to stimulate greater participation by all staff in the management of the unit's work? Develop one strategy for converting authoritarian delegation to empowerment for getting the tasks accomplished.

Tip # 2: Motivate Staff

Do a survey of all staff about motivation and management style by asking each one the following: (1) What motivates you? (2) What management style do you prefer? Analyze the data, and integrate this knowledge into your management strategies. Evaluate the effectiveness of any changes you make.

Nurses carry responsibility and accountability for the quality and quantity of their supervision, as well as for the quality and quantity of their own actions in regard to care provision. Nurses also are being tapped for their important role as care coordinators. Nurse managers carry the added responsibility and accountability for the coordination of groups of nurse providers and assistive or ancillary personnel. Nurse managers also have an overall responsibility to monitor and provide surveillance or vigilance regarding situations that can lead to failure to rescue, patient safety errors, or negligence. Too many hours worked, nurse fatigue from stress, too heavy a patient workload, and other systems problems are situations to monitor with regard to legal accountability.

Controlling

Controlling is the management function of monitoring and adjusting the plan, processes, and resources to effectively and efficiently achieve goals. It is a way of coordinating activities within organizations by systematically figuring out whether what is occurring is what is wanted (McNamara, 1999a, 1999d). The controlling aspect of the managerial process may seem at first to carry a negative connotation. However, when used in reference to management, the word *control* does not mean being negatively manipulative or punitive toward others. Managerial controlling means ensuring that the proper processes are followed. Fayol (1949) called this the activity of seeing that everything occurs in conformity with established rules. In nursing, the term *evaluation* is used to refer to similar actions and activities. Control or evaluation means ensuring that the flow and processes of work, as well as goal accomplishment, proceed as planned. **Controlling** is defined as comparing the results of work with predetermined standards of performance and taking corrective action when needed. This means ensuring that the results are as desired and, if they are not up to standards, then taking some action to modify, remediate, or reverse variances.

The coordination of activities of a system is one aspect of managerial control, along with financial management, compliance, quality and risk management, feedback mechanisms, performance management, policies and procedures, and research and trend analysis. These control activities are used by managers to communicate to reach a goal, track activities toward the goal, guide behaviors, and coordinate efforts and decide what to do. Managerial coordination and control are important to the success of any organization (McNamara, 1999a, 1999d). Ongoing, careful review using standardized documents, informatics systems, and standardized measures avoids drift and the waste of time and resources that occur when direction is vague. Well-exercised, managerial control is flexible enough to allow innovation yet present enough to effectively structure groups and organizations toward goal attainment.

The management function of controlling involves the feeding back of information about the results and outcomes of work activities, combined with activities to follow up and compare outcomes with plans. Appropriate adjustments need to be made wherever outcomes vary or deviate from expectations (Hersey et al., 2008). In nursing, when a critical path is used to track client care, the variances are analyzed and corrected as a function of managerial control. The controlling function of management has been described as a constant process of reevaluation to see whether what is currently happening meets needs, plans, and standards, as well as to identify where improvements might be possible (Kepler, 1980).

In summary, by using the four steps of the management process, goals can be accomplished by and through other people. These managerial functions are aimed primarily at the productivity element of an organization. For nursing, within a human services industry, managerial skills are employed to enhance the utilization of human resources (Kepler, 1980).

MANAGEMENT IN NURSING PRACTICE

Nurses have two major components to their role: care provider and care integrator. McClure (1991) called these the *caregiver* and *integrator* roles. The image of the "bedside nurse" emphasizes the care provider aspect of nursing. The integrator role is a complementary function that arises from nursing's central positioning in the day-to-day coordination of service delivery and central location at the hub of information flow regarding care and service delivery. This linkage relationship is depicted visually in Figure 2.3. Although the coordination of care has always been a key nursing function, it is becoming more visible and valued in health care and as nurses assume case management roles that focus on integrating clinical care. However, the relative proportion of the nurse's role that is devoted to management and coordination functions varies within nursing according to the job category. One useful way to analyze nursing jobs is to assess the relative balance of the two role components in any job.

At the lowest levels of an organization, employees are hired for some technical or professional skill. In highly technical, constantly changing fields such as nursing, it takes nearly all of a nurse's time to be clinically and technically competent. Yet for a middle manager, only a part of the work time can be spent being clinically and technically competent. The other part is spent carrying out the work of management: planning, organizing, coordinating or directing, and controlling the work of nursing and other personnel. With advancement to the highest nurse executive level, the job change inevitably results in the nurse executive becoming the least competent technician because the job demands an increasing focus on specialized management and leadership activities, which have

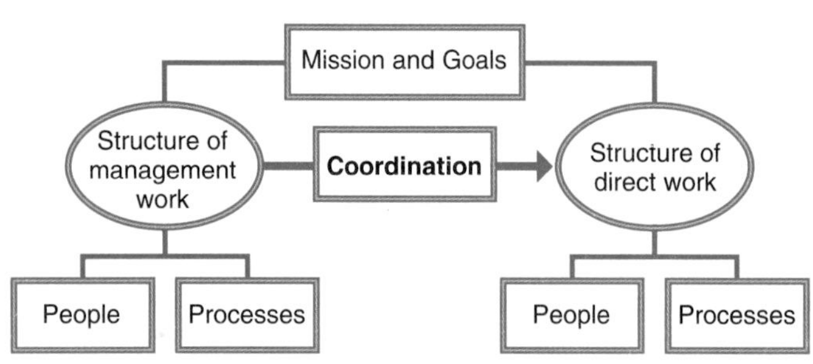

Figure 2.3
Linkage of clinical and management domains.

their own set of skills and expertise. These are normal organizational dynamics. They occur because management is a discrete function. Part of the task is to link the top of the organization to the bottom and vice versa in a two-way street. The bottom also has to know what the top is doing and recognize the fact that managers manage while technicians complete their assigned tasks, and together the group accomplishes individual and organizational goals (Organizational Dynamics, 1975). This view highlights the value of investing in infrastructure that organizes and supports the work that nurses do. Managers in nursing perform discrete and important functions that provide an environment and climate to facilitate delivery of client services. Mintzberg (1994) described this managing as *blended care.*

For nursing, Mintzberg (1994) compared management as cure, which is intermittent and interventionist, with management as care, which is continuous and involved. Management as care is thought to be more effective. In this modality, nurses are postulated to be able to move more easily and naturally into management because of nursing's roots in caring. Mintzberg noted that in this sense the focus of nursing is management, as contrasted to medicine with its focus on cure. Mintzberg's ideas (1994) coincide with a contemporary view of organizations and their management. Organizations are living entities composed of people in relationships. Management becomes a view of work as being accomplished through relationships and people who are self-organizing. Skill at facilitation becomes a major management role (Crowell, 1998). Porter-O'Grady (1997) called this process *leadership.*

One part of managing people and relationships in organization is to manage the expression of emotion. The management of emotions, called *emotional intelligence (EI)*, has come to be recognized as foundational for organizational health and its four components of strategy, capability, viability, and spirit (Metts, 2008). Emotional intelligence is the intersection of thinking and emotion. Skill building and training in positive thinking and a focus on positive emotions assist nurses to better listen, encourage, motivate, and create connections. The goal is to achieve optimal outcomes.

In nursing, the management process is directed primarily toward the human element, or the management of human resources. It is through this dynamic and interactive process that the work of nursing is accomplished. Nurse managers balance two competing needs: the needs of the staff related to growth, efficiency, motivation, morale, and accomplishment; and the needs of the employer for productivity, quality, and cost-effectiveness. Desired outcomes include staff satisfaction and productivity (Kepler, 1980).

MANAGEMENT IN ORGANIZATIONS

The Nature of Managerial Work

Lewin (1947) said that the behavior of human beings is a function of individual psychology, the needs patterns of people, and the environment in which they work. Behavioral theory and its applications to the management of people focuses on organizing and processing work and accomplishing organizational objectives at a targeted minimum cost and minimum waste. The responsibility for doing that lies with management. Managers manage people and the environment. One view of management suggests that the manager's behavior, the role, and the situation created for people to work in actually trigger or cause followers' behavior. Thus the manager's role is distinct and important for individual and organizational outcomes because of its direct impact on how and what gets done.

Mintzberg (1973, 1975) reformulated Fayol's ideas about the nature of managerial work. Mintzberg's synthesis of research findings about managers in general revealed the following:

- Managers work at an unrelenting pace at activities characterized by brevity, variety, and discontinuity. Managers are strongly action-oriented.
- Managers handle exceptions and perform regular work, such as ritual and ceremonial duties, negotiation, and processing of soft

information linking the organization to its environment.
- Managers prefer oral communication.
- "Judgment" and "intuition" describe the procedures managers use to schedule time, process information, and make decisions.

Zaleznik (1992) noted that managerial culture emphasizes rationality and control—a manager is a problem solver. He noted that it takes neither genius nor heroism to be a manager. What is needed is persistence, tough-mindedness, hard work, intelligence, analytical ability, tolerance, and goodwill. Some would suggest that positive interpersonal relationship skills also are necessary for success. Drucker (1954) suggested that the three jobs of management are to manage a business enterprise, manage managers, and manage workers and work. The skills needed by nurse managers include conceptual or thinking skills, clinical technical skills in nursing methods and techniques, and group and human relations skills (Katz, 1955).

Mintzberg (1975) described the manager's job in terms of ten roles or sets of behaviors. Derived from the formal authority and status of the position are three interpersonal roles: figurehead, leader, and liaison. As the nerve center of the organizational unit, information processing is a key part of the role. Informational roles are monitor, disseminator, and spokesperson. Information is the basic input to decision making. The decisional roles are entrepreneur, disturbance handler, resource allocator, and negotiator (Figure 2.4). Mintzberg suggested a number of important managerial skills, as follows:

- Developing peer relationships
- Carrying out negotiations
- Motivating subordinates
- Resolving conflicts
- Establishing information networks and disseminating information
- Making decisions in conditions of extreme ambiguity
- Allocating resources

If management is important to achieving organizational goals, then the skills, abilities, functions, actions, and strategies used by managers to manage are important to know and understand. Kepler (1980) suggested that the managerial skills to be

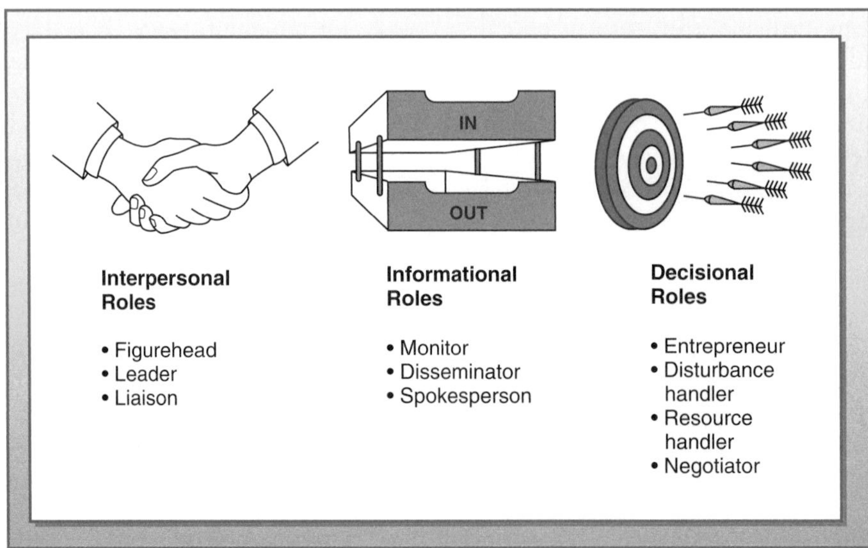

Figure 2.4
Mintzberg's 10 managerial roles. (Data from Mintzberg, H. [1975]. The manager's job: Folklore and fact. In M. Matteson, & J. Ivancevich [Eds.], *Management classics* [3rd ed., pp. 63-85]. Plano, TX: Business Publications.)

mastered are processes of understanding, communication, and effective use and manipulation (through selective use of rewards and punishment) of personnel.

Mintzberg (1994) elaborated his earlier work on the nature of managerial work by expanding it to an interactive model (Figure 2.5). The model uses concentric circles. At the core is a person who is in a job. The person has some unique set of values, experiences, knowledge, and competencies. The combination of the person and the job creates a frame composed of the job's purpose, the person's perspective about what needs to be done, and selected strategies for doing the job. The frame can range across two continua: from vague to very specific and from person-selected to externally imposed. The frame results in an agenda of work issues and time scheduling. Placed at the center of the figure, these elements form the core of the job of a manager. Managerial roles and behaviors at this level include conceiving the frame and scheduling the agenda.

Growing out of the core are three concentric circles—from abstract to concrete. These are called the *information, people*, and *action levels* of managerial work. At the most abstract level, the manager processes information and uses it to drive the action. At the next level, the manager works with people to encourage work activities. At the most concrete level, the manager manages the action.

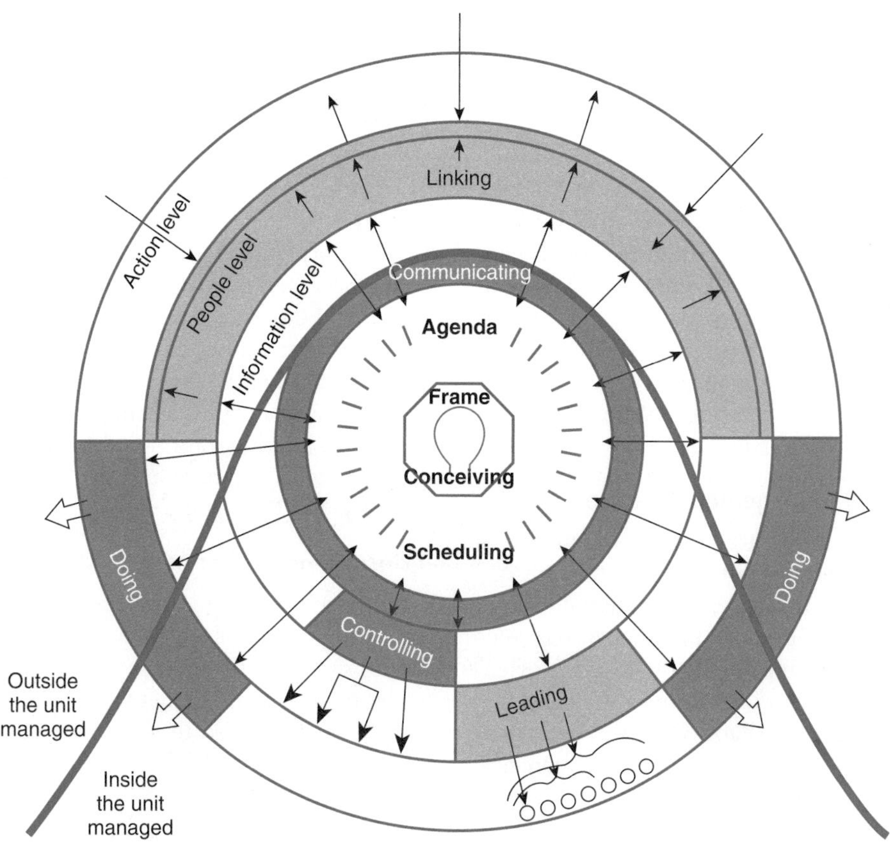

Figure 2.5
Mintzberg's Model of Managerial Work. (Redrawn from Mintzberg, H. [1994]. Managing as blended care. *Journal of Nursing Administration, 24*[9], 30.)

At the information level, the associated managerial roles are communicating information and controlling by using information to control the work of others. At the people level, the managerial roles are leading and linking. Leading involves encouraging and enabling individuals (by mentoring and rewarding), groups (by team building and conflict resolution), and the whole organization (by building a culture). The linking roles have the manager relating to the external environment by building networks of contacts and acquiring information from the environment to transmit back to the unit. At the action level, the associated managerial role is called *doing* or *supervising*. Behaviors include doing, handling disturbances, and negotiating (Mintzberg, 1994).

Mintzberg's (1994) interactive model provides a visual display of a way of thinking about managerial work and associated roles and activities. The model could be used as a basis for self-assessment and can be applied to specific managerial jobs. Nurses who strive to apply the concepts to their managerial work could use the model to examine and analyze managerial styles, behaviors, and roles. As managers, nurses manage both people (clients, themselves, and other staff or providers) and the environment of client care delivery. An understanding of the management process and the roles related to the work of a manager can assist nurses to improve their personal effectiveness and their organization's productivity.

Contemporary Management Theories

Human organizations are complex in nature. It is tricky to provide overall direction for an organization in times of rapid environmental change. The recent focus of leadership theory has been on interactional, relational, and transformational leadership to guide organizations through successful change and chaos. However, less attention has been focused on how to advise managers who are working toward the organization's goals and trying to use resources effectively and efficiently under conditions of change, scarcity, and complexity. It is thought that the nature of how the four managerial functions of planning, organizing, coordinating or directing, and controlling are carried out needs to change to accommodate a new management paradigm. Because of forces such as technology, the Internet, increasing diversity, and a global marketplace, organizations have experienced pressure to be more sensitive, flexible, and adaptable to stakeholders' expectations and demands (McNamara, 1999e, 1999f).

The result has been a reconfiguration or restructuring of many organizations from the classic hierarchical, top-down, rigid form to a more fluid, organic, team-based, collaborative structure. This has had an impact on how managers manage. Managers cannot control continued rapid change. Old familiar plans and behaviors no longer provide clear direction for the future. Managers now need to focus on two major aspects of management: managing change through constant assessment, guidance, and adaptation; and managing employees through worker-centered teams and other self-organizing and self-designing group structures (McNamara, 1999f). Bureaucratic management is out; organic and virtual management is in.

A variety of contemporary theories of management have arisen to help organize management thought. Four major management theories now predominate: contingency theory, systems theory, complexity theory, and chaos theory. Each one contributes principles useful for nursing management and administration and for nurse managers working to coordinate and integrate health care delivery. The following is a brief overview.

Contingency Theory

Contingency theory is considered to be a leadership theory, but it also applies to management. The basic principle is that managers need to consider the situation and all its elements when making a decision. Managers need to act on the key situational aspects with which they are confronted. Sometimes described as "it all depends" decision making, contingency theory is most often used for choosing a leadership or management style. The "best" style depends on the situation (McNamara, 1999g).

Systems Theory

Systems theory has helped managers to recognize their work as being embedded within a system and to better understand what a system is. Managers have learned that changing one part of a system inevitably affects the whole system. General systems theory was derived from the work of Ludwig von Bertalanffy (1968) as a way of thinking about studying organizational wholes. General systems theory uses the following concepts:

- Organization
- Wholeness
- Control
- Self-regulation
- Purposiveness
- Environment
- Boundaries
- Equilibrium
- Steady state
- Feedback

A system is a set of interrelated and interdependent parts that are designed to achieve common goals. Systems contain a collection of elements that interact with each other in some environment. The elements of an open system and related examples in health care are shown in Table 2.1.

A key principle of systems theory is that changes in one part of the system affect other parts, creating a ripple effect within the whole. Using systems theory implies a rational approach to common goals, a global view of the whole, and an emphasis on order rather than chaos. The input-throughput-output model exemplifies this linear thinking aspect of general systems theory.

Systems theory is easy to understand but difficult to apply in bureaucratic systems or organizations with strong departmental "silos." This is because coordinators and integrators with sufficient organizational power to cross the system are needed but often not deployed. Without integrators, systems parts tend to make changes without consideration of the whole system. Shifting to systems theory thinking helps managers view, analyze, and interpret patterns and events through the lens of interrelationships of the parts and coordination of the whole (McNamara, 1999g).

Table 2.1

Open System Elements and Health Care Examples

Open System Elements	Health Care Examples
Inputs to the system (resources)	Money, people, technology
Transforming processes and interactions (throughputs)	Nursing services, management
Outputs of the system	Clinical outcomes, better quality of life
Feedback	Customer and nurse satisfaction, government regulation, accreditation, lawsuits

In health care, concepts such as interrelatedness and interdependence fit well with multidisciplinary teamwork and shared governance professional models. However, concepts of attaining a steady state and equilibrium are difficult to reconcile with the reality of uncertainty, risk, change, and ambiguity that characterize the turbulence of the change occurring in the health care delivery environment. Previously, managers were advised to draw up 5-year and even 10-year plans; managers today have seriously shortened their strategic planning and other related time lines in response to the rapidity of change. An example of the use of systems theory is basing an analysis of a planned change, such as implementing a new program, on systems concepts by identifying inputs, throughputs, outputs, and feedback loops to more effectively plan how the new program fits into the existing system. Sometimes this process is used for short time frame rapid response team projects.

Complexity Theory

Arising in scientific fields such as astronomy, chemistry, biology, geology, and meteorology and involving disciplines such as engineering, mathematics, physics, psychology, and economics, literature is growing since the late 1980s on the behavior of complex adaptive systems (Rosenhead, 1998). Complexity theory is a more general umbrella theory that encompasses chaos theory. The focus of complexity theory is the behavior over time of certain complex and dynamically changing systems. The concern is about the predictability of the behavior of systems that under certain conditions perform in regular and predictable ways but in other conditions change in irregular and unpredictable ways, are unstable, and move further away from starting conditions unless stopped by an overriding constraint. What is most intriguing is that almost undetectable differences in initial conditions will lead to diverging reactions in these systems until the evolution of their behavior is highly dissimilar. Thus stable and unstable behavior is the focus of interest (Rosenhead, 1998).

Stable and unstable behavior can be thought of as two zones. In the stable zone, a disturbed system returns to its initial state. In the unstable zone, any small disturbance leads to movement away from the starting point and further divergence. Which subsequent type of behavior will occur depends on environmental conditions. The area between starting and divergence is called *chaotic behavior*. This refers to systems that have behavior with certain regularity yet defy prediction based on that regularity. The classic example of this is weather prediction (Rosenhead, 1998).

Before the formulation of complexity theory, the unpredictability of systems was attributed to randomness that was measured by statistical probability. It is now understood that a small difference in starting conditions can result in apparently random, quite different trajectories that are highly irregular but not without some form. Plotted over time, the apparently random meanderings of these systems can show a pattern to the movements; but the variation stays within a pattern that repeats itself (Rosenhead, 1998).

Complexity theory has informed classical management theories. Previous management theories heavily emphasized rationality, predictability, stability, setting a mission, determining strategy, and eliminating deviation. Discoveries from complexity and chaos theories include the fact that the natural world does not operate like clockwork machinery. Key findings of complexity theory are the "effective unknowability" of the future and an understanding of the role of creative disorder. Managers need to alter their reflexive behaviors, put an emphasis on "double-loop learning" that also examines the appropriateness of operating assumptions, foster diversity, be open to strategy based on serendipity, welcome disorder as a partner, use instability positively, provoke a controlled ferment of ideas, release creativity, and seek the edge of chaos in the complex interactions that occur among people. Change management takes on a very different form when complexity theory is used (Rosenhead, 1998).

The selection of a management theory and related managerial activities may be seen as more appropriately based on ordinary versus extraordinary management needs (Stacey, 1993). Ordinary management would be selected for day-to-day operations and problem solving. It would use classic, rational linear management theory and Fayol's (1949) framework for planning and management, with control at the center. To deliver cost-effective outcomes, competent basic management is necessary (Rosenhead, 1998). Extraordinary management would be used to transform organizations under conditions of open-ended change. This form of management seeks to unlock and activate the hidden knowledge and the creativity that is potentially available within the people who make up organizations. Informal groups and self-organizing teams are used. The focus is on learning and adapting. Both ordinary and extraordinary management are needed and have to be enabled to coexist for maximum effectiveness (Rosenhead, 1998; Stacey, 1993).

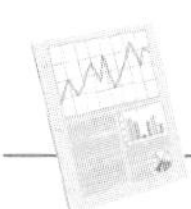

Research Note

Source: Ebright, P.R., Patterson, E.S., Chalko, B.A., & Render, M.L (2003). Understanding the complexity of registered nurse work in acute care settings. *Journal of Nursing Administration, 33*(12), 630-638.

Purpose

Complexity in nursing comes from multiple goals, obstacles, hazards, missing data, and behaviors surrounding care situations. To keep things from going wrong, nurses make decisions to adapt and manage complexity in the midst of a changing environment. The purpose of this research was to investigate RN work complexity in an acute care setting using a human performance framework. Field observations followed by semistructured interviews were the methods used with a purposive sample of eight expert RNs. The research question was this: "What human and environmental factors affect decision making by expert RNs on medical-surgical acute care units?"

Discussion

Content analysis resulted in the emergence of 22 patterns across participants that were grouped into the following three main categories:

1. Patterns of work complexity (n = 8) that are human and environmental factors affecting work, such as disjointed supply sources, repetitive travel, and interruptions
2. Patterns of cognitive factors driving performance and decisions (n = 8), such as maintaining patient safety and knowing unit routines and work flow
3. Patterns of care management strategies (n = 6), such as stacking and stabilizing and moving on. The results revealed multiple patterns that characterize RN work on medical/surgical acute care units and how RNs cope and adapt to manage workload demands.

Application to Practice

This study examined the actual work of RNs in the context of patient assignments within conditions of unpredictability, missing information, and unreliable access to resources and processes. The rich data suggested ways to redesign systems to decrease or better manage work complexity. The human performance framework helped uncover routine aspects of the daily management of work that came to be seen as a series of gaps and discontinuities that serve to distract RNs from focusing on critical role functions such as clinical reasoning about patient care. Managerial actions to fix these systems gaps support the work of nursing and avoid wasting large amounts of valuable time.

Chaos Theory

Chaos is seen as a particular mode of behavior within the more general field of complexity theory (Rosenhead, 1998). Sometimes the two are used together: chaos and complexity. Chaos, as used in complexity theory, is not utter confusion and disorder but, rather, a system that defies prediction despite certain regularities. Chaos is the boundary zone between stability and instability, and systems in chaos exhibit bounded instability and unpredictability of specific behavior within a predictable general structure of behavior. They may pass through randomness to evolve to a higher order of self-organized complex adaptive structures (Rosenhead, 1998). At first, this seems to make no sense. However, chaos theory principles can be applied in health care.

As many health care organizations move away from bureaucratic models and recognize organizations as whole systems, more organic and fluid structures are replacing the older ones. Sometimes referred to as "learning organizations," these structures are tapping into the inherent capacity for individuals to exhibit self-organization. In the transition, experiences of change, information overload, entrenched behaviors, and chaos reflect human reactions to organizations as living systems that are adapting and growing (Wheatley, 1999). Complexity and a sense of things being beyond one's control create a search for a simpler way of understanding and leading organizations.

Randomness and complexity are two principal characteristics of chaos. There is a paradox in the fact that even in the simplest of systems, it is extraordinarily difficult to accurately predict the course of events; yet some order arises spontaneously even in these simple systems. Patterns form in nature—some are orderly, and some are not orderly. Concepts of nonlinearity and feedback help explain situations of complexity without randomness (with order). Chaos theory suggests that simple systems may give rise to complex behavior, and complex systems may exhibit simple behavior. At the essence of chaos is a fine balance between forces of stability and those of instability. Two examples are snowflake formation and the behavior of the weather.

It is difficult for minds trained in linear thinking to grasp chaos theory. In the past, the effects of nonlinearity were discounted. Much of scientific thought was based on assumptions of linearity and beliefs that small differences averaged out, slight variances converged toward a point, and approximations could give a relatively accurate picture of what could happen. It was assumed that predictability would come from learning how to account for all variables and a greater level of detail. However, the wholeness of systems resists being studied in parts. Both chaos and order are important elements in the powerful and unpredictable effects created by iteration in nonlinear systems (Wheatley, 1999). An example of chaos theory in action is when a seemingly small change, such as using assistive personnel instead of professionals, in effect creates ripples and larger impacts on the system than preplanning would seem to indicate.

There are many implications of chaos theory for health care delivery systems. The slightest variation can have enormous results in a dynamic and changing system. What is important is the quality of the system, its complexity, its distinguishing shapes, how it develops and changes, and how it differs from or compares with another system. In many ways, this highlights what nurses have known: the whole of nursing is complex and crucial to health care delivery systems in which nurses are major care coordinators.

A search for ever-finer measures for discrete parts of the system probably is futile. Looking for themes or patterns rather than isolated causes is encouraged. Clearly, predictability still exists. However, for nonlinear variables and systems, randomness plays a key role in the creation of patterns of complexity and harmony of form (Wheatley 1999).

Chaos theory can be applied to management in health care organizations. Viewing the organization as similar to a living organism, taking a holistic approach, and trusting in a natural organizing phenomenon, the manager combines expressed expectations of acceptable behavior and the grant of the freedom to individuals to assert themselves in nondeterministic ways. Guiding principles or values create powerful motivation. The manager's job is to reveal and handle the mostly hidden dynamics of the system and forge a direction for the organization as a complex adaptive system. The goal is for a self-managed system with people capable of engaging in cooperative behavior, using feedback to learn and adapt, self-organizing, and operating with flexibility.

LEADERSHIP AND MANAGEMENT IMPLICATIONS

It can be argued that all nurses are managers. Staff nurses are the employees at the most critical point in fulfilling the purpose of health care organizations: they are in close and frequent contact with the client, and they coordinate the delivery of health care services.

The administration of nursing services is divided into two basic levels: the nurse manager and the nurse executive. Both have the responsibility to create a work environment that facilitates and encourages nursing staff and nursing practice. The nurse manager manages one or more defined areas of nursing services and is responsible to a nurse executive. Nurse managers allocate available resources, coordinate activities, facilitate interactive management, and have major responsibility for implementing the vision, mission, philosophy, goals, plans, and standards of the organization and nursing services (American Nurses Association [ANA], 2004; ANCC, 2004).

The nurse executive is responsible for managing organized nursing services from the perspective of the organization as a whole and for transforming values into daily operations to produce an efficient, effective, and caring organization. The nurse executive is accountable for the environment in which clinical nursing practice occurs. The nurse executive provides leadership and direction for all aspects of nursing care (ANA, 2004; ANCC, 2004).

The work of nursing is complex, and the role of the nurse manager is influenced by human and environmental factors in complex organizations. Being on the front lines of health care, nurse managers collaborate with others and carry out activities such as the following:

- Managing clinical nursing practice and care delivery
- Coordinating care with other disciplines to integrate services
- Managing the budget
- Managing human resources
- Being responsible for staffing and scheduling
- Evaluating the quality and appropriateness of care
- Orienting and developing employees
- Ensuring compliance with regulatory and professional standards
- Maintaining patient safety

Because of chaos, complexity, and change, client care management has needed new structures and managerial behaviors. Predicated on trust

LEADERSHIP & MANAGEMENT BEHAVIORS

Leadership Behaviors

- Is visible
- Communicates a vision
- Motivates followers
- Seeks out new resources
- Evaluates outcomes

Management Behaviors

- Coordinates client care
- Plans daily operations
- Makes assignments
- Sets goals for subordinates
- Hires staff
- Responds to needs/desires of subordinates as long as the work is accomplished
- Exchanges rewards for work effort
- Manages resource allocation
- Monitors work and quality processes
- Takes corrective actions
- Counsels subordinates
- Manages change
- Handles conflict situations
- Communicates among levels

Overlap Areas

- Exercises broad-perspective decision making
- Communicates
- Motivates subordinates
- Evaluates process and outcomes

and cooperation in human relations, managers are challenged to promote consistency and stability and be anchors in an unstable world. Curtin (2000) suggested the following 10 ethical principles that might help managers reconcile perspectives and interests while centering on mission and core values:

1. Frugality and sophisticated therapeutic skill (doing the most with the least resource expenditure)
2. Clinical credibility through organizational competence
3. Presence (visibility)
4. Responsible representation at highest levels
5. Loyal service
6. Deliberate delegation
7. Responsible innovation
8. Fiduciary accountability
9. Self-discipline
10. Continuous learning

Clearly, both nurse managers and executives need a background and ability in the day-to-day fundamentals of management to achieve goals. Beyond this, skill and ability in "extraordinary management" will serve to enhance individual and collective competence. Balancing day-to-day operations with transformative management and leadership is a creative synthesis of the best of the "old" with the best of the "new" management theories.

Management has been described as a discipline that uses a set of tools to achieve desired outcomes. It becomes nursing management when the desired outcomes are nursing goals. If management occurs at all levels of nursing, the nursing profession needs methods for assisting nurses to develop competence in management (Genovich-Richards & Carissimi, 1986). One beginning step is to measure and evaluate managerial behavior. For example, a measurement instrument was developed by Morse and Wagner (1978) to identify specific behaviors and activities characteristic of managerial work. Built around Mintzberg's nine managerial roles (1973), the final instrument contained 51 items tapping six role factors. Although managerial roles are somewhat distinct, testing this instrument revealed that the factors are interrelated to a moderate degree. The final six role factors are (1) managing the organization's environment and resources, (2) organizing and coordinating, (3) information handling, (4) providing for growth and development, (5) motivating and conflict handling, and (6) strategic problem solving. This instrument can be used to measure and evaluate similarities and differences in managerial work, such as before and after restructuring occurs.

Using a conceptual framework of three domains of nursing management behaviors—client care management, operational management, and human resources management—Genovich-Richards and Carissimi (1986) described the use of a management assessment center technique for nursing. The following seven key areas were the focus of an intensive 1-day session using exercises, simulations, and management activities for practice:

1. Leadership ability
2. Decision-making skill
3. Analytical ability
4. Organizational ability
5. Group performance skill
6. Personal characteristics such as sensitivity, flexibility, and competitiveness
7. Self-awareness

A management assessment center technique is one tool that nurses can use to develop individuals and enhance their managerial skills and abilities. It could become a staff development or in-service program. This tool could be used for growth and self-assessment for staff who desire or contemplate advancement along a nursing administration career track. Management skills also need to be taught to nursing students and novice nurses. A combination of simulated and practice-based experiences that apply management content can be created by using a flexible assignment plan and clinical resources.

Legal Aspects of Management

The managers of any health care organization are responsible to the policy-making body of the organization. Managers also have an obligation to comply with the laws of society at local, state, and national levels. Managers are responsible for ensuring that laws are adhered to—both in the actions of management itself and in the actions of those employees who assist the managers in carrying out the mission of the organization. Concern for the law involves three general areas: personal negligence in clinical practice, liability for delegation and supervision, and organizational liability related to employment issues.

Activities of clinical client care involve corresponding legal accountability and risk. Errors do happen. Some lead to injury to a client. At minimum, nurses have an ethical obligation to nonmaleficence (to do no harm to clients). This duty is discharged in part by remaining competent in knowledge and skills, the standards of practice, and use of evidence-based practice. Nursing negligence occurs when nurses' actions are unreasonable given the circumstances or fail to meet the standard of care or when the nurse fails to act and causes harm. Harm can arise from acts that are unintentional, such as omissions or negligence, or it can result from acts that are intentional, such as defamation, invasion of privacy, assault and battery, false imprisonment, or intentional infliction of emotional distress (Aiken, 1994).

Four elements of negligence are required for malpractice: a duty owed to the client (e.g., to render nursing care), breach of duty, proximate cause or causal connection to the nurse, and damages. Common clinical practice areas of negligence or liability include the general areas of treatment, communication, medication, and monitoring/observing/supervising/surveillance. Examples of common negligence allegations in nursing malpractice suits include client falls, use of restraints, medication errors, burns, equipment injuries, retained foreign objects, failure to monitor, failure to ensure safety, failure to take appropriate nursing action, failure to confirm accuracy of physician's orders, improper technique or performance of treatments, failure to respond to a client, failure to follow hospital procedure, and failure to supervise treatment (Aiken, 1994).

Beyond personal liability for clinical practice, nurses and nurse managers have accountability and liability for their acts of delegation and supervision. Both nurses and nurse managers carry an obligation to report incompetent practice that occurs at any point in the care delivery process. Nurse managers have a duty to train, orient, and evaluate the ability of nursing staff to perform specific functions and tasks. Health care organizations have a duty to monitor the competence and ability of nursing and medical professionals and to inquire about their credentials (Aiken, 1994). Both nurses and nurse managers have a duty to follow policies and procedures when reasonable. Nurse managers are advised to review policies and procedures carefully, including the language used, to adhere to legal and ethical parameters more closely. Clearly, management in nursing practice means that nurses must fulfill obligations and duties both to clients and to the organization. This means using knowledge, skill, and decision-making abilities to reduce the incidence of negligence and malpractice by employees as a way to reduce harm to clients and legal risk to the organization. As the primary care coordinators, nurses need to manage the environment of care delivery. Ensuring staff competence and reporting incompetent practice are key activities. For example, in nursing, legal and ethical issues arise when a nurse is impaired by substance abuse. The overall consideration is protecting the client from harm. Confronting a staff member suspected of substance abuse must be done carefully. However, when an incident occurs, the nurse manager has a responsibility to intervene.

Organizations are constrained by specific laws related to employment issues. Although the various health care providers and their employing organizations have specific legal and ethical obligations to clients, such as informed consent and preserving patients' rights as outlined in the Patient Self-Determination Act of 1990, organizations carry specific legal and ethical obligations to employees. The employer has an obligation to provide a safe and secure care delivery environment (Aiken, 1994). For example, the Occupational Safety and Health Administration's (OSHA's) rules and regulations must be followed. As a branch of the U.S. Department of Labor, OSHA has become involved with issues related to protecting health care workers from exposure to blood and body fluid–borne pathogens such as hepatitis B (HBV) and human immunodeficiency virus (HIV), the virus that causes acquired immunodeficiency syndrome (AIDS). By enforcement of universal precautions among health care workers, the principal idea is to prevent the transmission of pathogens from worker to client or client to worker, thus providing a safer work environment. Guidelines from the Centers for Disease Control and Prevention (CDC) were adopted by OSHA. The mandates include use of universal precautions, employer provision of protective equipment, inspection procedures, and risk management of potentially exposed employees. The employer incurs the costs of HBV vaccine, protective equipment and supplies, and exposure prevention and management. OSHA uses the mechanisms of surprise inspections and steep fines to enforce compliance.

Employment decisions are subject to liability for wrongful failure to hire, wrongful failure to advance, and wrongful discharge. Title VII of the U.S. Civil Rights Act of 1964, the Age Discrimination and Employment Act (ADEA) of 1967, and the Americans with Disabilities Act (ADA) of 1990 are some specific pieces of federal legislation that affect hiring and employment. In addition, other federal statutes, governmental mandates, and state and municipal laws prescribe and proscribe various actions that are part of or relate to the employment process.

The Equal Employment Opportunity Commission (EEOC) is a federal agency that enforces many of the federal mandates concerning discrimination. Other federal agencies, including funding agencies, also have enforcement responsibilities in this area. Most states and many municipalities also have antidiscrimination enforcement agencies, and some laws provide the individual employee with the opportunity to bring private litigation through the courts.

The antidiscrimination statutes, in general, were designed to protect employees from discrimination in the workplace when it is based on race, color, sexual orientation, religion, gender, pregnancy, national origin, age, or physical or mental disability. In some cases, discrimination based on some of these characteristics is legally acceptable if it is based on what the law describes as a bona fide occupational qualification (BFOQ). The use of BFOQs to justify discrimination is usually defined in very narrow fashion. Two examples of gender discrimination in employment that can be justified as BFOQs are "wet nurse" and "sperm donor."

Management policies and procedures must be in compliance in the areas of hiring, performance appraisal, management of employees with problems, and termination (Aiken, 1994). Lawsuits also have formed the basis for the standards to be met for the termination of employees. Discharges may occur for lack of adherence to employer-established policies or standards, "good cause" per institutional policy, illegal activity, assault, insubordination, or excessive absenteeism. Written notice and the reasons for termination avoid misunderstandings and show justice through due-process procedures. Careful documentation is important. If the employee is a member of a protected group, the employer may be required to submit formal justification for the termination (Aiken, 1994).

The various legal and ethical considerations of nursing management span client, provider, and employer rights and obligations. Both nurses and their employing organizations are responsible for knowing and following the various applicable laws and regulations. In-service education can increase knowledge and awareness. Nurse managers need to manage the environment of nursing care to ensure client safety, provider justice and safety, and organizational compliance with the law.

CURRENT ISSUES AND TRENDS

The classic notions of management and managerial work were developed in a sociopolitical era of industrialization and bureaucratization. Currently in business and industry, competitive pressures and economic forces are compelling organizations to adopt new flexible strategies and structures. Organizations are being urged to become leaner, more entrepreneurial, and less bureaucratic. This trend has created levels of complexity and interdependency.

The result has altered conventional ideas and realities of managerial work, including shifts in roles and tasks. Traditional sources of power are eroding, and some motivational tools are less effective than they used to be. The erosion of power from hierarchical positions is perceived as a loss of authority and may create confusion about how to mobilize and motivate staff (Kanter, 1989). Kanter noted that in a leaner and flatter corporation there are many more channels for action, and managers need to work synergistically with other departments. Managers' strategic and collaborative roles become more important as they serve as integrators and facilitators, not as watchdogs and interventionists.

Current and emerging issues in health care are complex and ethically challenging for managers. The "big three" issues of access, cost, and quality continue to be organizing themes that affect any organization's internal operations. Insurance coverage is an issue of access, as is the geographic location of facilities, providers, and services. Increased complexity and technology prompt provider specialization and affect cost. Consumer preferences and increased health care awareness affect both cost and quality. Critical medical errors and patient safety issues create pressure related to the need for quality. Complexity, randomness, and chaos created by change all call for new management and leadership strategies.

Within health care delivery systems, issues and trends facing today's managers include the following:

- Management of populations with chronic illnesses
- Resources to acquire technology on an ongoing basis
- The need for primary and preventive services and programs, including complementary and alternative programs
- Integration and seamlessness of clinical and financial services and information
- Protection of consumers' privacy
- Shortages of key personnel, especially registered nurses
- Financing structures such as capitation and managed care
- Care delivery and process management
- Management of knowledge workers and personal accountability
- Pressures for quality and sustainable outcomes
- Leadership skills related to change management

Herzliner (1998) predicted a managerial revolution in the U.S. health care sector. He critiqued vertically integrated systems and managed care organizations and noted that they cannot provide the convenient, supportive, moderate-cost health care that is desired by the U.S. public. It is likely that "focused factories" will arise in response to the "everything-for-everybody" current situation. In health care, these focused organizations would consist of a multidisciplinary team of health care providers who have frequent interaction to achieve focused goals such as delivering services for complex medical problems. Other foci might include care for a chronic disease, handling a high volume of diagnoses, or providing information and support. This phenomenon has been manifested in the rise of case management and disease management processes and programs. These structures will proliferate if there is sufficient market pressure for them.

Drucker (1988) used the hospital, the university, and a symphony orchestra as models for organizations evolving in today's society. As health care reconfigures, health care delivery settings will likely be knowledge-based organizations composed

PART I

primarily of specialists whose performance is directed by organized feedback from colleagues, clients, and headquarters. Nurses are positioned at the care coordination intersection and have needed skills for facilitating flow and integrating care delivery. Nurses' roles may change, but their need for managerial competence will remain. Nurses are well prepared to serve as integrators and facilitators of client care. Thus nurses appear to move easily into management and blend care into management for effectiveness (Mintzberg, 1994).

Summary

- A manager's job is to coordinate and integrate resources.
- Classical management theory defined the management process as planning, organizing, coordinating or directing, and controlling.
- Mintzberg described 10 roles that managers play.
- Mintzberg developed a model of managerial work that elaborated on managerial roles.
- New managerial theories emphasize contingency, complexity, and chaos.
- All nurses are managers; they coordinate and deliver health services to clients.
- As institutions adopt new flexible strategies and structures, managerial roles and tasks are being reconfigured.
- Nurses have valuable related skills of coordination and integration.

Case Study

Nurse Anthony Kaufman is the director of Ambulatory Clinic A. Last year he participated in strategic planning for all the ambulatory clinics. A plan for Clinic A also was developed and approved. This year Nurse Kaufman concentrated on fine-tuning the management of the clinic. He developed a data tracking system, and trend data are now in. One disturbing trend is the rise in visit cancellations. Although the rate of cancellations is not a threat to clinic management, the increase needs to be evaluated. He does further analysis and discovers that the increase has been occurring mostly among adult females of the Muslim religion. Nurse Kaufman needs to determine the root cause: Is this an issue of individual staff cultural sensitivity, a systems problem, or some other cause?

The data are shared with the staff, and a brainstorming session occurs. One of the staff has a terrific idea: to use community contacts and internal group leaders to help inform the clinic staff as to the problem(s). The marketing and social services departments are enlisted to help. They set up roundtable gatherings, championed by the local leaders among Muslim women. One major concern emerges from these meetings: the traditional hospital gown is too revealing, unacceptable, and embarrassing. Many Muslim women had cancelled appointments for this very reason. The information is eye-opening for Nurse Kaufman. First, he is glad that it was not a staff performance issue. Second, it had never occurred to him. Hospital gowns have been the same for a very long time, and no one questions them. He calls another meeting, explores the results with staff, and asks for creative solutions. This seems like a simple managerial move. However, as the mostly female staff members begin to analyze the issue, they become excited about the possibility of a needed change. Nurse Kaufman is afraid that things might spin out of control as nurses discuss hospital gown redesign options, such as contacting New York name-brand designers. Eventually the process is worked through, using multidisciplinary collaboration, and a new gown design with extra coverage is approved and ordered.

CRITICAL THINKING EXERCISE

Nurse Su-lin Zhang sits down to the computer and opens up a new document file. It is time to put some thoughts down in writing. The long-term care facility where she works recently merged with a private, for-profit integrated delivery system dominated by administrators from the acute care hospital. In the aftermath of the merger, a form of program or product-line management was instituted that uses interdisciplinary teams. In addition, her long-term care facility will be competing against the other ones in the network based on "best practices" benchmarks that have not yet been specified. Nurse Zhang wants to be sure that her facility comes out in first place.

1. What problem(s) do you see in this scenario?
2. Why is this a problem?
3. What are the issues involved?
4. How might Nurse Zhang handle the situation?
5. What should Nurse Zhang do with her text when it is completed?
6. What management role would be best suited to this situation?
7. What management strategy might be most effective?

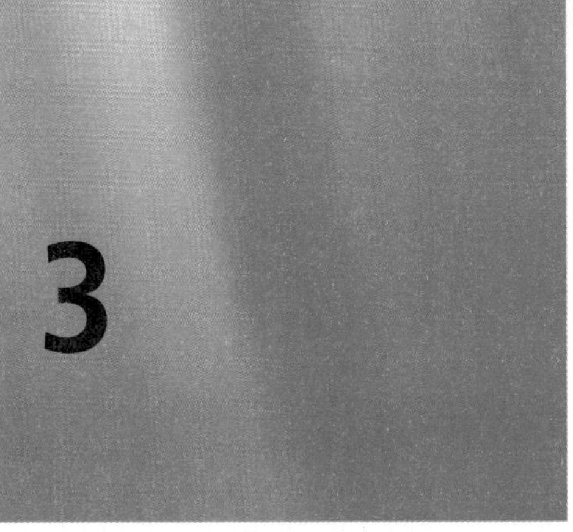

Change and Innovation

Maryanne Garon

PART I

CHAPTER OBJECTIVES

- Stimulate thinking about change and resistance
- Define and describe differing perspectives on change, including planned change and emergent views on change
- Synthesize the concepts of change and innovation
- Describe leaders' and managers' roles in change
- Explain the advantages of participatory approaches to change
- Distinguish among Lewin's steps in the process of planned change
- Explain a force field analysis
- Associate Rogers' five phases to the adoption of change
- Compare Lippitt's and Havelock's elements of the process of change
- Define and discuss resistance to change
- Analyze emotional responses to change
- Analyze effective approaches to change
- Analyze major areas of rapid change in health care and nursing
- Exercise critical thinking to conceptualize and analyze possible solutions to a practice exercise

Change is a pervasive element of society, of today's health care environment, and of life. Many words are used to describe change, including *constant, inevitable, pervasive, universal,* and *powerful.*

> *Nothing endures but change.*
>
> -Heraclitus

> *Change alone is eternal, perpetual, immortal.*
>
> -Arthur Schopenhauer

> *It is change, continuing change, inevitable change, that is the dominant factor in society today.*
>
> -Isaac Asimov

> *Change is the law of life. And those who look only to the past or the present are certain to miss the future.*
>
> -John F. Kennedy

> *We participate in a world where change is all there is. We sit in the midst of continuous creation, in a universe whose creativity and adaptability are beyond comprehension. Nothing is ever the same twice, really.*
>
> -Margaret Wheatley (2007, p. 84)

Some of the following common sayings reflect the pervasiveness of change:

- "Nothing is sure but death and taxes."
- "The more things change, the more they stay the same."
- "Let's go back to the good old days."

Change is inevitable in health care, just as it is in life. Nurses today are accustomed to change in their environments. Many have seen changes in the acuity of patients, changes in both practice models and skill mixes, a change to evidence-based practice, changes in educational requirements, and changes within their own roles. Some nurses report that changes in practice are so frequent that they are taken for granted (Copnell & Bruni, 2006).

Yet they also indicate that the very basis of nursing, providing care and support for patients, has not changed (Copnell & Bruni, 2006).

Organizational change can be initiated in response to external pressures, or it may come from within. In health care, change has often been externally imposed because of changes in reimbursement, regulatory changes, requirements of accrediting bodies, and marketplace demands. Changes in health care organization can also originate internally. Examples of internally initiated changes might include a unit that wants to change its practice model or a nursing service that wants to incorporate evidence-based practice.

Change is seldom easy. It can be complex and irrational. Even when it is the individual's own decision to make a change, it can be difficult. When someone makes a change, such as deciding to stop smoking, to lose weight, or to go back to school, initiating, following through, and sustaining that change is challenging. Initiating and sustaining organizational change is even more difficult. When change is seen as unnecessary, imposed from above, or threatening workers' sense of security, the process is even more difficult. To guide the change process, nurse managers and leaders need a thorough understanding of change grounded in theory, applicable research, and reports of successful change processes.

Two approaches or models of change are commonly found in the literature: planned change theories or models and emergent models (Shanley, 2007). Critiques of the planned approach highlight the prominence of the top-down approach and overemphasize the role of managers in the process. In addition, the emphasis on cookbook-like approaches portrays change itself as linear, rather than complex and multidimensional.

In emergent approaches, the complex and multidimensional view of change is central. The emphasis is on principles or processes of change because there is little support for one particular strategy or number of steps being more effective than another (Shanley, 2007). Emerging views of change also emphasize the importance of the participatory process in change. Therefore, in this model, it is essential for nurse leaders to understand the role of the recipients in creating and sustaining change. Viewing change and resistance as two opposing forces can result in *stereotyping* one group as irrational resistors, rather than as partners in and co-creators of change.

DEFINITIONS

Change is defined as an alteration to make something different. This activity of alteration can be haphazard or planned, obvious or subtle, radical or incremental, left to chance or occurring by drift. *Planned change* is defined as a process of intentional intervention to create something new. In general, it is a process by which new ideas or programs are created and developed, diffused through communication and intervention, and result in consequences of adoption or rejection.

When discussing change, several other terms are often used to describe change itself or the process of change. These terms are *innovation, transition,* and *transformation.* In recent years, innovation has often been used to describe organizational change. **Innovation**, while implying introduction of something new, is also about change. The word **transition**, defined as a process of change, is also used in descriptions of change in organization. Finally, **transformation** is also used to describe change but often is used in terms of more radical changes such as "to change completely the appearance or character of something or someone, especially so that they are improved" (Cambridge Advanced Learner's Dictionary, 2008).

From an organizational perspective, planned change is a decision to make a deliberate effort to improve the system. Many authors (Balogun, 2006; Lippitt et al., 1958; Rogers, 2003) added another factor—utilizing an assigned person to help make a deliberate effort to improve the system—to the definition of change. The most commonly used term has been *change agent.* According to Lippitt and colleagues (1958), the **change agent** is the outside helper used to plan and implement the change process. The term has come to mean a person who functions as a change facilitator. Other terms used similarly to describe the role of a change facilitator are *change ambassador* and *opinion leader.*

LEADING & MANAGING DEFINED

Change

An alteration to make something different; a complex process that occurs over time and is influenced by any number of unpredictable variables.

Innovation

The use of a new idea or method.

Transition

A change from one form or type to another.

Transformation

The use of new ideas, innovation, and creativity to change fundamental properties or the state of a system.

Resistance

To refuse to accept or be changed by something.

Change Agent

A person or thing that produces a particular effect or change.

Leadership

An influence relationship in which leaders and collaborators with mutual purposes intend real change.

Data from Cambridge Advanced Learner's Dictionary. (2008). Retrieved July 28, 2008, from http://dictionary.cambridge.org/define.asp?key=84436&dict=CALD; Pettigrew, A.M. (1990). Longitudinal field research on change: Theory and practice. *Organizational Science, 3*(1), 267-292; and Rost, J. (1991). *Leadership for the 21st century*. New York: Praeger Publishers.

Rogers (2003) defined a change agent as someone who influences innovation decisions in a direction deemed desirable. Some definitions of **leadership** incorporate the idea of someone who works with followers to create change (Rost, 1991).

BACKGROUND

According to Wheatley (2007):

> In the 1990s, surveys began reporting disappointing failures with organization change. CEOs reported that up to 75 percent of their organizational change efforts did not yield the promised results. These change efforts fail to produce what had been hoped for yet always produce a stream of unintended and unhelpful consequences. Leaders end up managing the impact of unwanted effects rather than the planned results that do not materialize. (p. 83)

Change has long been a topic of interest to individuals and organizations. Much of the writings on organizational change have emphasized a top-down planned change strategy. In most of these, the focus was on the role of administrators and top managers in the change process. Change was seen as initiated by administrators who formulate a plan for the change and communicate it to middle managers and others. Strategies for disseminating the change, informing staff, and dealing with resistors (often viewed as stubborn and irrational) are developed and implemented (see Table 3.1 for contrasting views of change).

Alternative views emerged that promoted the idea that top-down change is not just undesirable, it does not work (Balogun, 2006). Staff and other "recipients" of change must be viewed as integral to the process rather than as potential obstructions to be influenced and acted upon (Porter O'Grady & Malloch, 2007). All levels need to be involved in planning for and sustaining change, and ideas for change can come from all levels. In addition, when considering the processes of change, issues of power and how individuals make sense of the change are essential.

Evidence supports this emergent view of change (Shanley, 2007). Although there is minimal literature showing that various approaches to planned change actually work, there is evidence on what *does* work (Balogun, 2006). The literature points to the decreased importance of executives and increased importance of those affected by any change. It is said that the planned approach is too simplistic, takes too much for granted, and does not allow the analysis of the complex aspects of change over time (Pettigrew, 1990).

Table 3.1

Contrasting Views of Change

	Planned Change (traditional view)	Emergent View
Direction	Top-down, linear	Multidirectional, multidimensional
Initiator	Leader initiated	Diffuse
Process	Planned, step-by-step process	Principles to guide process
Organizational culture	May be considered	Essential to consider
Power issues	Not considered, or not spoken	Essential to consider
Role of staff/ recipients of change	Resistors	Participants in change process
View of the change recipients	May be assessed so they can be changed or manipulated	Essential to process

Theories of change that focus on the human side of change are important to consider. The leader-collaborator relationship needs to be central to the process. In addition, leaders must assess and understand the participants' response to change, political and power issues that affect initiation of change, and how to develop organizational or unit cultures that facilitate and sustain change.

PERSPECTIVES ON CHANGE

Types of Change

Two major types of change are applied both to individuals and to organizations. They are first-order and second-order change. The terms were first popularized by Watzlawick and colleagues (1974) in a book based on their work in family therapy. In their definitions, a first-order change is one within a given system in which the system itself is unchanged. The terms *first-order change* and *second-order change* can be applied to individuals, small systems, and organizations.

First-order change occurs in a stable system and is characterized by rational step-wise processes. It is seen as a method for maintaining stability in a system while making small incremental adjustments. First-order change is not seen as a vehicle for innovation, nor would it achieve organizational transformation (Alas, 2007). For an organization, it is adaptation based on monitoring the environment and making purposeful adjustments. At the industry level, this is evolution as a response to external forces such as markets. An example in nursing is when a new evidence-based protocol is developed and put into use in clinical practice. This is adaptation and adjustment.

Second-order change is discontinuous and radical and occurs when fundamental properties or states of systems are changed. Second-order change calls for transformation, using innovation, new ideas, and creativity. In a second-order change, however, the occurrence changes the system itself. Watzlawick and colleagues (1974) found that second-order change often appears strange, unexpected, and even nonsensical.

At the organization level, second-order change is described as *metamorphosis*. The entire organization is transformed, reconfigured, or moved along its life cycle. At the industry level, second-order change occurs when an entire industry is revolutionized or experiences quantum change such as emergence, transformation, or decline. An example in health care is the widespread implementation of computerized physician order entry (CPOE) technology in response to the Institute of Medicine's recommendations for patient safety reforms.

Organizational Change

Literature on organizational change is extensive. Lewin's (1947, 1951) unfreezing, moving, and refreezing three stages of change theory is the classic model. Related research and theory development have been done on topics such as strategic planning, adaptive learning, decision theory, management, diffusion of innovations, social-psychological response and adaptation, process improvements, how members manage and achieve change, and weighted factor importance of project selection models (Gustafson et al., 2003).

An additional concept in organization change is that of learning organizations. Learning organizations are ones that learn to adapt to change (Alas, 2007). How organizations adapt is related to their ability to be open, dynamic, and responsive to changes in the environment. The success of the learning organization is directly related to the people within the organization and their own learning. Workers need to be empowered themselves to be open and responsive to changes and to become "lifelong learners" (Senge et al., 1994).

Within the learning organizations, Senge and colleagues (1994) described the following five learning disciplines:

- **Personal mastery:** Refers both to individual capacity to create desired results and to the creation of an environment or culture in which others can do the same
- **Mental models:** How individuals develop, create, and project the personal vision they have of the world and understanding how these personal views affect their decisions and actions
- **Shared vision:** Sharing preferred future visions within a group for developing plans to get to that preferred future
- **Team learning:** A sharing of learning skills and conversations so that the group can develop skills and learning greater than the individual parts
- **Systems thinking:** Envisioning the organization as an inter-related system, rather than unrelated parts

Learning organizations are about change and helping people embrace change. Although Senge and colleagues (1994) noted that change and learning are certainly not synonymous, they believe they are clearly linked.

Systems theory, complexity theory, and chaos theory are all models or worldviews that influence organizational change. These models suggest that the behaviors of complex systems are nonlinear, spontaneous, and self-organizing. Small changes can often produce larger dynamic (and sometimes unintended) effects. These models help us promote different understandings of changes in complex systems and how systems adapt to change (Porter O'Grady & Malloch, 2007). However, these are not prescriptive models; instead, the focus is on interrelationships, processes, and systemic behavior.

CHANGE THEORIES

Lewin's Change Process

The basic concepts of the change process were outlined by Lewin (1947, 1951). Most nurses have heard of Lewin and his three elements for a successful change: (1) unfreezing, (2) moving, and (3) refreezing (Figure 3.1). It might also be tempting to relegate

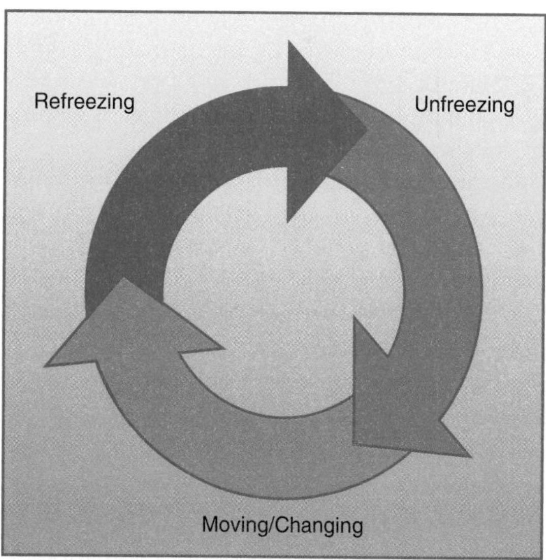

Figure 3.1

Elements of a successful change. (Data from Lewin, K. [1947]. Frontiers in group dynamics: Concept, method, and reality in social science; social equilibrium and social change. *Human Relations, 1*[1], 5-41; Lewin, K. [1951]. *Field theory in social science: Selected theoretical papers*. New York: Harper & Row.)

Lewin's ideas to the older, more traditional views of planned change (Burnes, 2004). However, Lewin was not only a remarkable thinker but also a humanitarian who believed that it was essential for democratic values to permeate all aspects of society. His model is also meant to help increase understanding about how groups and organizations change, not as a rigid strategy to impose change. Lewin's basic change process is still useful and applicable today.

Lewin coined the term *planned change* to distinguish the process from accidental or imposed change (Burnes, 2004). Lewin's (1947, 1951) theory of change used ideas of equilibrium within systems. *Unfreezing*, the first stage of change, can be characterized as a process of "thawing out" the system and creating the motivation or readiness for change. An awareness of the need for change occurs. This first stage is cognitive exposure to the change idea, diagnosis of the problem, and work to generate alternative solutions. A change agent needs trust, respect, and rapport to unfreeze individuals and groups effectively. Education, motivation, enthusiasm, and team building are leadership strategies. Awareness of the need for change is generated from the following:

- Unmet expectations (lack of confirmation)
- Discomfort about action or inaction (guilt or anxiety)
- Removal of an obstacle to change (psychological safety)

The unfreezing stage is considered to be finalized when those involved in the change process understand and generally accept the necessity of change.

The second change stage is *moving*. This means proceeding to a new level of behavior, which implies that the actual visible change occurs in this stage. When the individuals involved collect enough information to clarify and identify the problem, the change itself can be planned and initiated. Lewin (1951) observed that a process of "cognitive redefinition," or looking at the problem from a new perspective, occurs. As a first step to launch a change, a pilot test may be done so that the change can be pretested and a transition period launched.

The final change stage is *refreezing*. In this stage, new changes are integrated and stabilized. Reinforcement of behavior is crucial as individuals integrate the change into their own value systems. It is important to reward change behavior. Leadership strategies of positive feedback, encouragement, and constructive criticism reinforce new behavior. Leaders point the way throughout the process of change.

Lewin's (1947, 1951) planned change process stages can be compared to the nursing process and the generic problem-solving process (Table 3.2). Unfreezing is like assessing in the nursing process and like problem identification and definition in the problem-solving process. Moving is similar to planning and implementing in the nursing process and similar to problem analysis and seeking alternative solutions in the problem-solving process. Refreezing is like evaluation in the nursing process and like implementation and evaluation in the problem-solving process.

Table 3.2

Similarities of Change, Nursing Process, and Problem Solving

Change	Nursing Process	Problem Solving
Unfreezing	Assessing	Problem identification and definition
Moving	Planning and implementing	Problem analysis and seeking alternatives
Refreezing	Evaluation	Implementation and evaluation

Data from Workman, R., & Kenney, M. (1988). The change experience. In S. Pinkerton, & P. Schroeder (Eds.), *Commitment to excellence: Developing a professional nursing staff* (pp. 17-25). Rockville, MD: Aspen.

Individuals and systems naturally strive for equilibrium. Lewin (1951) saw this as a balance between driving forces that promote change and restraining forces that inhibit change. Both driving and restraining forces impinge on any situation. The relative strengths of these forces can be analyzed. To create change, the equilibrium is broken by altering the relative strengths of driving and restraining forces. A force field analysis facilitates the identification and analysis of driving and restraining forces in any situation. Unfreezing occurs when disequilibrium is introduced into the system to disrupt the status quo. Moving is the change to a new status quo. Refreezing occurs when the change becomes the new status quo and new behaviors are frozen.

The process of change may flow back and forth among stages. It is not a simple linear process in which one step follows the preceding one. The process may move rapidly, or it may stall in any one phase. The goal of planned change is to plan, control, and evaluate the change.

Lewin's (1947, 1951) work forms the classic foundation for change theory. Other change theorists have elaborated further understandings and applications of change theory. Bennis and colleagues (1961) assembled a book of readings on planned change that emphasized planner-adopter cooperation and high levels of adopter participation.

Because actually implementing planned change is more dynamic and complex than Lewin's model, Lippitt (1973) refined and expanded Lewin's (1947, 1951) work on unfreezing, moving, and refreezing to identify the following seven phases of the change process that more fully describe planned change:

1. Diagnosis of the problem
2. Assessment of motivation and capacity to change
3. Assessment of the change agent's motivation and resources
4. Selecting progressive change objectives
5. Choosing an appropriate role for the change agent
6. Maintaining the change once it is started
7. Termination of the helping relationship with the change agent

The first three steps can be compared to Lewin's unfreezing (1947, 1951). Steps 4 and 5 match moving, and steps 6 and 7 are comparable to refreezing. Similar to Lippitt (1973), Havelock (1973) listed the following six elements in the process of planned change:

1. Building a relationship
2. Diagnosing the problem
3. Acquiring relevant resources
4. Choosing the solution
5. Gaining acceptance
6. Stabilization and self-renewal

The first three steps correspond to the unfreezing stage of change, the fourth and fifth are similar to the moving stage, and the last relates to refreezing. The various conceptualizations of the stages of the process of change bear similarity to one another but vary in emphasis (Table 3.3).

Innovation Theory

Change and *innovation* are companion terms, but innovation has been differentiated from change. Change is a disruption; innovation is the use of change to provide some new product or service (Romano, 1990). An innovation is defined as

Table 3.3

Comparisons of the Process of Change Theories

Lewin	Rogers	Lippitt	Havelock
Unfreezing	Awareness, interest, evaluation	Steps 1, 2, 3	Steps 1, 2, 3
Moving	Trial	Steps 4, 5	Steps 4, 5
Refreezing	Adoption	Steps 6, 7	Step 6

something new—the introduction of a new process or new way of doing something. Innovation also has been viewed as the use of a new idea to solve a problem (Kanter, 1983).

Kanter (1983) said that innovation refers to the process of bringing any new or problem-solving idea into use. Innovation is often linked with creativity. Organizations need to promote environments that encourage creativity and opportunities for innovation (Hughes, 2006).

Leaders are essential to innovation because they must help create the environment and opportunities for innovation.

Purposeful innovation must start with a review and analysis of the environment and the opportunities for innovation. A purposeful and organized search for change is the basis for systematic innovation. A careful analysis of the opportunities for change is the best hope for successful economic or social innovation. This occurs because successful innovations exploit change. Thus Drucker (1992) came to describe innovation as the systematic use of opportunity from changes in the economy, technology, and demographics. He noted that the challenge today is to make institutions capable of innovation. This can be approached from the viewpoint of innovation as systematic and hard work having little to do with genius and inspiration. Innovation, Drucker (1992) noted, depends on "organized abandonment" (p. 340). This is a process of eliminating the obsolete and the no longer productive efforts of the past. Clearly, a willingness to view change as an opportunity is needed.

Drucker (1985, 1992) identified seven sources for innovation opportunities: the unexpected, incongruity, process needs, changes in industry or market structure, demographics, new knowledge, and changes in perceptions or moods. He likened the seven sources to windows on a building in that just as windows let in light and air, innovation can be infused into an organization by these various sources. In an information-based organization in which innovation needs to be systematized, the leader or manager will find four skills important: (1) get outside the organization for facts and perspective, (2) take responsibility for one's own information needs, (3) focus for effectiveness, and (4) build learning into the system.

In nursing, theories of planned change and nursing research are used for conceptualization and research on innovations. In one analysis of the nursing literature, Lewin's (1947, 1951) change theory and Rogers' (2003) diffusion theory were the most frequently cited theories (Tiffany et al., 1994). However, popular change theories may be incomplete or inadequate to meet the needs of nurse change agents in practice. This is because popular theories overlook social systems problems or focus on analyzing and watching change rather than being theories of change planning (Tiffany et al., 1994).

Rogers (2003) described a cognitive innovation-decision process through which individuals and groups pass. The five stages of innovation-decision are as follows (Rogers, 2003):

1. First knowledge of an innovation's existence and functions
2. Persuasion to form an attitude toward the innovation
3. Decision to adopt or reject
4. Implementation of the new idea
5. Confirmation to reinforce or reverse the innovation decision

The innovation-decision process is a series of actions, behaviors, and choices over time as a new idea is evaluated and a decision is made whether to incorporate this into practice. The perceived newness and associated uncertainty are distinctive aspects of the innovation.

According to Rogers (2003), most change agents concentrate on creating awareness-knowledge. However, a more important role could be played by concentrating on how-to knowledge, which adopters need to test out an innovation. Using Hersey and colleagues' (2008) four levels of change concept, the change agent would first work on awareness-knowledge, then address attitudes and emotions, and then work on how-to skills to create a change in individual behavior.

Individual members of a group or social system will adopt an innovation at different rates. This time element of the adoption of an innovation usually follows a normal, bell-shaped curve when plotted over time on a frequency basis. However, if the cumulative number of adopters is plotted, an S-shaped curve appears (Rogers, 2003). The normal adopter frequency distribution was segmented into the following five categories (Rogers, 2003):

1. Innovators
2. Early adopters
3. Early majority
4. Late majority
5. Laggards

Change agents can anticipate these five categories as an expected phenomenon, identify followers as to likely adopter category, and target interventions accordingly. This means that for effective change, nurse leaders can recognize that there will be individual variance in "warming up" to an innovation, plan for this with targeted strategies to decrease resistance, and capitalize on the power of innovations and early adopters.

Individuals need to be interested in the innovation and committed to making change occur. The outcomes of change are either that the change is accepted or adopted or that the change is rejected. If the change is accepted, it can be either continued or eventually dropped. If the change is rejected, it can remain rejected or be adopted later in some other form. Rogers' theory (2003) described change as more complex than Lewin's (1947, 1951) three stages. The following five factors determine successful planned change (Rogers, 2003):

1. *Relative advantage:* The degree to which the change is thought to be better than the status quo
2. *Compatibility:* The degree to which the change is compatible with existing values of the individuals or group
3. *Complexity:* The degree to which a change is perceived as difficult to use and understand
4. "*Trialability*": The degree to which a change can be tested out on a limited basis
5. *"Observability"*: The degree to which the results of a change are visible to others

The *diffusion of innovations* is a term derived from Rogers' work (2003) that is used to discuss the adoption of a new idea or process. Innovations create consequences. To move a new idea to the level of dissemination and adoption requires information, enthusiasm, and authority (Romano, 1990). Four elements to consider in an innovation diffusion are the innovation itself, communication channels, time, and the members of the social system (Romano, 1990).

McCloskey and colleagues (1994) analyzed organizational and management changes in nursing and defined management innovations as "new strategies, structures, or processes for the organization, delivery, and financing of quality care" (p. 36). They identified five categories of nursing managerial innovations: (1) the introduction of new technology, (2) personnel development, (3) changes in the organization of work, (4) changes in rewards/incentives, and (5) implementation of quality improvement mechanisms.

Hughes (2006) presented a review of innovations developed by nurses worldwide. The examples given were grouped in categories of historical examples, research, clinical practice, business, education, technology, public health, and policy. The following are some examples:

- The establishment of Mobile Surgical Services, a mobile cataract service in New Zealand
- The development of a prone positioner, the Vollman Prone Positioner, to assist critically ill patients to lie prone, which improves oxygenation
- An Interdisciplinary Neighborhood Team project, which developed teams of public health nurses and community outreach workers to mobilize community-driven, population-based projects

Hughes (2006) found that nurse innovators share some common characteristics. They are as follows:

- Self-confident
- Conscientious
- Ambitious

Furthermore, these nurses demonstrated the following:

- A strong desire to acquire recognized qualifications
- Motivation to learn

PART I

- Perseverance
- Initiative
- Tenacity
- Determination
- A willingness to take risks

Hughes also found that innovation is both achievable and cost-effective. She believed that reporting the number of innovations that nurses have created worldwide will show increased understanding of the role that nurses take in creating innovation.

In times of constant change and with pressures for cost containment and quality enhancement, nurses need to be able to evaluate innovations for effectiveness and efficiency. No systematic evaluation method exists. Therefore innovations lack the systematic analysis element advocated by Drucker (1985, 1992) and may be adopted primarily according to managerial trends. Because of the energy and resources needed to make a change, careful evaluation is crucial to positive outcomes.

LEADERSHIP AND CHANGE

> *Never doubt that a small group of thoughtful, committed citizens can change the world. Indeed, it is the only thing that ever has.*
>
> -Margaret Mead

> *Change will not come if we wait for some other person or some other time. We are the ones we've been waiting for. We are the change that we seek.*
>
> -Barack Obama

Leaders are an essential part of the change process. The approach, skills, and values that individual leaders bring to change efforts are integral to the success of process. Some authors have even used change as part of the definition for leadership. Burns (1978), credited with introducing the idea of transformational leadership, emphasized that leadership is about transformation. Transformational leadership is a model of leadership that embodies change. Rost (1991) conceived leadership not as positional but as a process that moves people to work together to make real change in their lives. The value of Rost's definition is that leaders do not depend on an organizational position and the leader role may rotate depending on the change desired and the approach taken. These views of leadership are more consistent with the emergent view of change.

Within health care, with the continuous and rapid rate of change, nurse leaders need skill in working with the change process. In the nurse executive's competencies from the American Organization of Nurse Executives (AONE) (2005), understanding change and innovation and how to manage it is an essential leadership competency for nurses. Shirey (2007) presented 10 tips for expert, effective leadership, based on the AONE's competencies. Number four was *"Be a change agent and advocate for innovation"* (p. 169).

Despite the fact that change is ever-present and necessary, leaders/managers still find it one of the most difficult aspects of their role. In fact, managers

Practical Tips

Tip # 1: Work on Reframing Your View of "Resistors"

Include them early in the change process as participants. Consider the positive aspects of resistance: Think of those who speak up as the "canaries in the coal mine." They can be an early warning system, letting you know if more resistance is brewing. This is because if the resistors are vocal, they communicate what the staff is thinking. If one person is open in complaining, there may be ten others who remain silent.

Tip # 2: Make the Change Process Participative and Democratic, As Much As You Are Able

It does take more time initially, but you will save time by not having to deal with the unintended consequences of imposed change.

often report that their reactions to change and the need to initiate change are emotions similar to and as strong as those associated with disasters, catastrophes, and even abuse (Shanley, 2007). Also, change can have multiple negative outcomes, including low morale, stress, and low self-esteem.

Leadership Roles in Change

Nurse leaders may take a number of roles in the process of change. Nurse executives and administrators are essential for providing the vision of a preferred future, initiating change, and helping guide the direction of change. Middle-level and first-level managers and staff, as the recipients of change, may also take roles in initiating and sustaining change. In addition, nurses in a variety of roles, from educators to clinical nurse specialists to staff nurses, may take on roles of change agents, opinion leaders, and early adopters of innovations. This often resembles a brokering or buffering role.

Leaders As Change Agents

Change agents can follow a number of steps in the process of change, as follows:

- Articulate a clear need for the change.
- Have the group participate by leaving details to those people who have to implement the change.
- Provide reliable information and the details to those who are to implement the change.
- Motivate through rewards and benefits to help the change along.
- Do not promise anything that cannot be delivered.

For example, when implementing a planned change to a new care delivery system, the change agent would need to be clear about the need for and the benefits of the change. This might include greater autonomy for nurses. The details of implementation should be left to the group, but only after reliable and detailed information is communicated to them. Rewards and benefits, not threats about performance appraisal, should be the basis of the motivation to change.

Participation itself may be motivating. Promised benefits from the change should be limited to what the change agent can reasonably deliver.

POWER AND POLITICS

Power issues and politics are central in considering change and have often been overlooked. Leaders need to consider power issues when planning for change. Shanley (2007) suggested that change initiators ask, "Whose needs are being met by the change, and whose interests are being served by the change?" In addition, many of the usual approaches to planned change reinforce hierarchical managerial practices and top-down control, thus making change more difficult to implement.

Some past changes in health care, such as the restructuring efforts of the 1990s, created change that was negative for nurses and, eventually, organizations and patients. These changes were externally imposed, reportedly for cost-containment because of reimbursement changes. The top-down destructive influences of those changes were demoralizing to nurses and had long-term, unintended consequences, including changed staffing ratios and increased usage of unlicensed personnel, and possibly even contributed to the current nursing shortage. Claire Fagin (2001) prepared a report for the Milbank Memorial Fund, documenting the decline in quality and availability of nursing services in hospitals. This decline was related to the restructuring of hospitals in response to financial pressures from managed care companies. One particularly poignant story told of an outside consultant who was brought in to help an organization change its structure in the 1990s for cost-containment. As Fagin (2001) described:

> I once had a chance conversation with a man who, I learned, had in the past worked for one of the major consulting companies and had been deeply involved in the restructuring of a number of hospitals. Learning that I was a nurse, he said, somewhat sheepishly, "I'm one of the bad guys." He told me about what he described as his "naive and dangerous period" and was filled with guilt over the restructuring recommendations he had made in his former job. His awakening, he said, had come when his wife had had a baby who required intensive, long-term neonatal care. During the hours and days the couple spent at the hospital visiting their critically vulnerable infant, they had a chance to see nurses at work expertly

> caring for—and ultimately saving—their child. In the process, he came to understand what nurses do and how important their job is. (p. 5)

In implementing change, considerations of power may be one of the most difficult areas for nurse leaders. Powerful economic or political interests may pressure nurse leaders to make organizational changes or enact restructuring to alleviate immediate problems. Unfortunately, the long-term effects of these changes may be difficult to foresee or to quantify. Nurses, at all levels, must learn to speak up, articulate, and support the value of their role and evaluate change for the long term.

THE PROCESS OF CHANGE

Change in health care has been shown to be continuous and rapid. It may appear to be like a continuum from haphazard drift at one end to a structured, planned change at the other. Change can occur by drift as things and people unilaterally change in an uncontrolled way. At the other end of the continuum, change can be deliberate and planned, as occurs when an organization identifies a plan to adopt and implement any new program. This is a conscious decision that is implemented through a planned change process. In the middle are ad hoc or active approaches to change based on strategies of education, emotional arousal, or coercion.

Planned Change

The amount of change and the rapidity of change disrupt and disorganize people. Because of the rapidity of change in areas such as computer software, it is easy to slip into the perception that history is what occurred 2 years ago and ancient history refers to 5 years ago. Obsolescence occurs before people have had a chance to adapt to the last round of changes. The inevitable result is stress on individuals as they try to cope. These dynamics affect nurses in their roles as care providers and care managers and profoundly influence the profession of nursing through employment and compensation fluctuations. One method to enhance nurses' productivity and decrease stress from turbulence in the environment is to strategically use planned change.

The use of planned change is a nursing management intervention strategy. The nurse uses diagnosis and intervention in clinical practice: the nurse assesses, diagnoses, develops a plan for the client's care needs, and selects an intervention that is matched to that assessment and diagnosis. Managers also assess, diagnose, and plan interventions to meet organizational needs and goals. They look at resource allocation and deployment of people in using planned change as a management intervention. Planned change theories are engineering theories in that they use social science principles to plan change (Tiffany & Lutjens, 1998). Planning and managing the change process may focus on any or all of the following situational elements: organizational structure, people, or resources.

"Two basic kinds of change theories exist: theories that help people watch change and theories that help people cause change" (Tiffany & Lutjens, 1998, p. 15). *Planned change* refers to deliberately engineered change in groups. A planned change theory is a set of logically interrelated concepts that explain how change occurs, predict forces and effects, and help planners control variables in a change process (Tiffany & Lutjens, 1998). In their review and analysis of the change theory literature, Tiffany and Lutjens (1998) identified three theories popular in nursing and one in a non-nursing model. The three main theories used in nursing are Lewin's (1947, 1951) planned change theory, writings by Bennis and colleagues (1961, 1976), and Rogers' (2003) theory of diffusion of innovations. One model not used in nursing is Bhola's (1994) configurations, linkages, environment, and resources (CLER) systems model. Lewin's (1947, 1951) theory ranks as the most popular change theory among nurses (Tiffany & Lutjens, 1998).

Change Management

To ensure that the process of change is effective, it is important to understand how unintended consequences can result from top-down planning or ineffective communication. Balongun (2006) shared of the following implications for leaders on the process of change based on her extensive research on organizational change:

- Executives and administrators do not direct change, but they do initiate and influence the direction of change.
- The recipients of change (middle managers and staff) translate and edit plans for change.
- The main method by which recipients interpret what the change is all about is through informal communication with peers (not top-down or official information channels).
- Senior managers need to monitor these communications and learn to engage in the lateral, informal communications. Some of this can be accomplished using "management by walking about."
- More explicit attention must be given to open discussions and storytelling in communication about change.
- The recipients of change will mediate the outcomes, so senior managers need to acknowledge this and actively engage with them.
- In large organizations, using change ambassadors to help with the engagement/discussion process may be helpful.
- Finally, senior managers need to "live the changes" they want others to adopt. The recipients of change are quick to notice inconsistencies between the action, words and deeds of the leaders.

Balogun (2006) asserted that the meaning of "managing" change needs to be reconsidered. The idea needs to change from one of top-down control to one of participation and communication.

Another useful strategy for preplanning the management of change is to assess readiness for organizational change. One inventory to use is the Organizational Change-Readiness Scale (OCRS) (Jones & Bearley, 1996). The 76-item inventory was designed to analyze the ability of an organization to manage change effectively. The five dimensions of structure, technology, climate, system, and people are assessed for barriers and supportive conditions. The five dimensions tend to influence each other. A Lewin-type force field analysis is applied to the results.

Research by Gustafson and colleagues (2003) resulted in a short survey instrument and a companion statistical model to predict the potential for successful implementation of a health system change. It was shown to be effective in predicting the outcome of actual improvement projects. Called the *Organizational Change Manager* (OCM), it used 18 factors to predict organizational change success in health care (Box 3.1). The factors were displayed on a survey instrument. Each factor is rated for high, medium, or low performance based on definitions of success as rated by the opinions of experts who completed the survey. A Bayesian statistical model was used to predict the probability of success before implementation. This model could help in decision making about whether a change is worth it, strengthening critical aspects before implementation, and in evaluating and tracking a change process.

Box **3.1**

Factors That Predict Organizational Change Success

1. Mandate/project launch
2. Leader goals, involvement, and support
3. Supporters and opponents
4. Middle manager goals, involvement, and support
5. Tension for change
6. Staff needs assessment, involvement, and support
7. Exploration of problem and understanding customer needs
8. Change agent prestige and commitment
9. Source of ideas
10. Funding
11. Relative advantages
12. Radicalness of design
13. Flexibility of design
14. Evidence of effectiveness
15. Complexity of implementation plan
16. Work environment
17. Staff change required
18. Monitoring feedback

Data from Gustafson, D.H., Sainfort, F., Eichler, M., Adams, L., Bisognano, M., & Steudel, H. (2003). Developing and testing a model to predict outcomes of organizational change. *Health Services Research, 38*(2), 751-776.

PART I

The Human Factor: Resistance

If you want to make enemies, try to change something.
-Woodrow Wilson

Do not conquer the world with force, for force only causes resistance. Thorns spring up when an army passes. Years of misery follow a great victory. Do only what needs to be done without using violence.
-Tao Te Ching

The path of least resistance makes all rivers, and some men, crooked.
-Napoleon Hill

It's not so much that we're afraid of change or so in love with the old ways, but it's that place in between that we fear. . . . It's like being between trapezes. It's Linus when his blanket is in the dryer. There's nothing to hold on to.
-Marilyn Ferguson

Resistance to change should be expected as integral to the whole process of change. Like the Peanuts© cartoon character, Linus, human beings need something to hang on to. The old ways may indeed need to be changed, but the natural fear of what will replace them may cause people to cling to the old. People may fear being disorganized or having their routines interrupted. Some may have a vested interest in the status quo. Others may believe that a change may diminish their own status or disrupt their network of interpersonal relationships.

Almost all changes encounter some resistance as a natural phenomenon. Resistance may be rooted in anxiety or fear. For example, some individuals fear expenditure of the energy needed to cope with change. Some fear a loss of status, power, control, money, or employment. Misconceptions and inaccurate information about what the change might mean and individuals' emotional reactions create resistance to change. Although resistance is characterized as a challenge, a negative behavior, or something to be overcome, not all resistance is bad. It may be a warning to the change agent to re-evaluate the change, clarify the purpose, or increase communication. The leader or change agent may need to re-conceptualize his or her approach to the change, anticipate resistance, determine why it is occurring, and better understand the perspective of the resistors.

To fully understand the concept of resistance, it is helpful to re-conceptualize staff nurses as the solution in initiating change rather than as the problem. Too often, nurses have been characterized as the targets of change, irrational resistors, and problems to overcome rather than as co-creators of change. Nurses are central to change within health care. They are the largest group of health care providers. They play a key role in the initiation, planning, and sustenance of change (Leeman et al., 2007). In fact, because of their numbers and their key role in the process, nurses were found to be the only viable agents of sustaining change (Balfour & Clarke, 2001).

Resistance Reframed

One way to reframe perceptions of resistance is to consider the positive effect that resistors and resistance have played in history and in the development of the United States. From the actions of the rebels in the Boston Tea Party to the anti-slavery abolitionists in the nineteenth century to the Civil Rights activists of the 1960s, resistance has shaped our history. Furthermore, some individuals have contributed to our views on resistance. They include Thoreau, who in 1849 wrote his classic essay "Civil Disobedience" and contributed the underlying idea that acting from principle, on the belief of what is right, is above the law. John Woolman, a Quaker, spent his life convincing other Quakers to give up slavery by personally visiting them one by one and discussing their views of morality. Sojourner Truth, an African-American woman born as a slave, worked tirelessly for the rights of African Americans. Martin Luther King, Jr., led the Civil Rights movement in the 1960s and inspired with his words on passive resistance. All of these "resistors" were leaders who inspired others to work for change. So, as leaders, how do we inspire others to work for change rather than impose organizational change from above? This is the challenge.

Re-conceptualizing staff and others as the co-creators of change instead of resistors not only provides an alternative view of change and resistance but also can point to new strategies for moving organizations toward change. In viewing resistance from the emergent view, it is important not to dichotomize initiators and recipients of change. It is essential to the change process to involve all. The success and sustainability of the change depends on the commitment to the change by those at the level of the change.

Nurses live with change daily. The common belief that nurses resist change has not upheld. Instead, nurses have reported that changes occur so frequently that they could not remember all of them (Copnell & Bruni, 2006). Falk-Rafael (2000) found that the nurses in her qualitative study had six different orientations to change. Three of these were ways they ended up accepting change: critical approval, insidious assimilation, wounded acquiescence. She found that nurses used judicious circumvention and constructive opposition when they believed that changes could jeopardize their clients' health (Falk-Rafael, 2000). The final orientation was nurses initiating change themselves through what she labeled "visionary transformation" (Falk-Rafael, 2000, p. 336). Her findings countered some commonly held beliefs about nurses' resistance to change.

Box 3.2

Emotional Stages of Change

1. *Equilibrium:* There is a sense of balance and inner peace before change occurs.
2. *Denial:* Energy is drained by denial of the reality of a change.
3. *Anger:* Energy is used to ward off the change.
4. *Bargaining:* Energy is used in an attempt to eliminate the change.
5. *Chaos:* Energy is diffused, with a loss of identity and direction.
6. *Depression:* No energy is left to produce results.
7. *Resignation:* Energy is expended to accept change passively.
8. *Openness:* Renewed energy is available.
9. *Readiness:* There is willingness to use energy to explore new events.
10. *Reemergence:* Energy is rechanneled, producing empowerment.

Data from Perlman, D., & Takacs, G. (1990). The 10 stages of change. *Nursing Management, 21*(4), 33-38.

EMOTIONAL RESPONSES TO CHANGE

Within nursing, Perlman and Takacs (1990) focused on how individuals cope with change and work through the changes that affect them. Although individuals must devote personal resources and energy to accomplish change, organizations tend to overlook the human emotions associated with an organizational change. Using the death-and-dying literature as a foundation, Perlman and Takacs (1990) described 10 stages in the emotional realm of the process of change (Box 3.2).

Another view of the emotional stages of change was suggested by Manion (1995), who identified the following seven stages people go though during personal transitions:

1. *Lose focus:* Confusion and disorientation abound.
2. *Minimize the impact:* Deny or pretend the change is not significant.
3. *The pit:* Feelings of anger, discouragement, resentment, and resistance arise.
4. *Let go of the past:* Energy returns as the end of the change process is seen.
5. *Test the limits:* More optimism is gained, and the individual tries out new skills or seeks new experiences.
6. *Search for meaning:* The individual reflects on the change process and recognizes what was learned.
7. *Integration:* The transition is completed, and the change is integrated into daily life.

Both Perlman and Takacs' (1990) and Manion's (1995) stages resemble the general grief model. However, Manion's model is more customized to change. Stages 5 through 7 mirror the process of coping that occurs as attitudes reconfigure and individuals work to produce positive outcomes.

Individuals proceed through the emotional stages at various rates (Perlman & Takacs, 1990). Somewhere between stage 7 (resignation) and stage 8 (openness) the individual begins to heal and cope with the change. Any organizational change process involves continual letting go of the status quo and emotional grief reactions. Change is more successful as the intellectual and emotional issues involved in change phases are recognized and addressed.

Although most people inherently distrust change, change can be viewed either positively or negatively. Viewing change as an ending entails an understanding of the concept of loss. To help individuals adapt, support needs to be provided along with encouragement that they can control their own response to change. Those who view change as a beginning are more optimistic. The four positive responses to change are uninformed optimism, informed pessimism, hopeful realism, and informed optimism. Communication, open discussion, sharing information, and respect for values and input are helpful strategies (Bonalumi & Fisher, 1999).

The emotional response to change is a psychological process related to an individual's attitude toward change and is one factor over which the individual has control. In times of chaos and stress from change, the ability to manage one's own attitude is a key skill for success.

> *If you don't like something, change it. If you can't change it, change your attitude. Don't complain.*
>
> *-Maya Angelou*

> *Some people change when they see the light, others when they feel the heat.*
>
> *-Caroline Schoeder*

> *Everyone thinks of changing the world, but no one thinks of changing himself.*
>
> *-Leo Tolstoy*

> *The release of atom power has changed everything except our way of thinking ...*
>
> *-Albert Einstein*

Spencer Johnson's (1998) book *Who Moved My Cheese?* used the parable of four mice (Snif, Scurry, Hem, and Haw) who look for cheese to eat. Cheese is a metaphor for anything people desire or think will make them happy. When change occurs, individuals suffer trauma if what they want is taken away. There are both simple and complex ways to respond to change. The book helps readers think about ways of looking at and responding to change and understanding that attitudes and behaviors are choices that can be altered when necessary. So doing reduces stress.

EFFECTIVE CHANGE

Ineffective responses to change do not allow the change process to go forward. They include being defensive, giving advice, and prematurely persuading. The way to deal with emotionality is to allow people to express themselves while avoiding action based on the emotionality. Trying to immediately persuade people cuts off their ability to vent emotions. Without venting, they may not be able to work through the stages. Censuring, controlling, or punishing probably drives resistance underground. The more that a planned change is driven by authoritarian actions, the more that the seeds of future discontent are sown. The most effective managers possess self-confidence, knowledge of the change process, and the interpersonal skill to help participants accept, allow, and see the process of change as natural, thereby enhancing coping while facilitating planned change.

Change cycles can be either participative or directive. In a participative change, new knowledge is made available to participants to trigger change. Personal power is used to trigger knowledge, attitude, individual behavior, and group behavior change. Directive change occurs when a change is imposed by some external force. Position power is used to trigger group behavior, individual behavior, attitudes, and knowledge change (Hersey et al., 2008).

The probability of effectiveness of the change process can be increased through several techniques, as follows:

- Explain the rationale for a change so that individuals understand it.
- Allow emotions to be worked out.
- Give participants all the information they need.
- Help individuals cope with change.

The following actions should be avoided when implementing a change within an organization:

- Simply announce a change without bothering to lay a foundation.
- Ignore or offend powerful people in the organization.
- Violate the authority and communication lines in the existing organization.
- Rely only on formal authority in implementing a change.
- Overestimate your formal authority.
- Make a poor decision about what change is needed, and do not be open to people critiquing the decision.
- Communicate ineffectively.
- Put people on the defensive.
- Underestimate the perceived magnitude of the change.
- Do not deal with the people's fears about insecurity or change of status.

Concerns, insecurities, and resistance are predictable as a part of change. Effectiveness and success are increased as these reactions are anticipated and strategies to cope are developed. The leader's role is to recognize, accept, and help followers process, adapt, and cope with these emotional stages to deal effectively with change. The leader's behaviors are crucial to helping followers with the disruption and reintegration that occur during any change. Thus leaders need to focus on people, considering factors such as the following:

- The time and effort it takes to adjust
- The possibility of less desirable outcomes
- Fear of the unknown
- Tolerance for change capacity
- Trust levels
- Needs for security
- Leadership skills
- Vested interests
- Opposing group values
- How coalitions form
- Strongly held views
- Existing relationship-dynamics disruptions

Davidhizar (1996) suggested that people make nine common mistakes in coping with organizational change. Knowing these areas helps nurses to proactively plan to avoid them and thereby work to ensure effective change processes. These nine mistakes are as follows:

1. Assuming management should keep them comfortable
2. Expecting someone else to reduce the stress
3. Shooting for a low-stress work setting
4. Trying to control the uncontrollable
5. Failing to abandon the expendable
6. Fearing the future
7. Picking the wrong battles
8. Psychologically unplugging from the job
9. Avoiding new assignments

As the leader focuses on followers to help them transition a change, the followers need to take responsibility for their own behavior. The stress of change is felt by both leaders and followers, and both are part of successful outcomes.

How is change effective? A positive and constructive group process needs to be established. Interpersonal relationships are very important. Given the number of changes going on in the environment, empowerment involves using change successfully. Successful change empowers participants. Nurses are empowered when change increases their responsibility, authority, and accountability and gives them the mechanisms to make decisions to be able to affect client care.

LEADERSHIP AND MANAGEMENT IMPLICATIONS

Because of the complexity and extent of change, knowledge and skill in applying systems principles are needed by nurses who are leading and managing change. An organization that is committed to changing itself as required needs continuous learning and adaptation as a systems value. As described earlier, this is a *learning organization*. These innovative and creative organizations need to foster their commitment to change and innovation. In their 2007 text, Porter-O'Grady and Malloch (2007) move away from discussion of structural components of change and, instead, emphasize four practices for current workplaces, as follows:

LEADERSHIP & MANAGEMENT BEHAVIORS

Leadership Behaviors

- Models the change they want to see
- Envisions a changed future
- Enables change to progress constructively
- Models healthy adaptation to change
- Develops mutual goals with followers
- Uses influence strategies with followers
- Communicates the need for change
- Initiates changes
- Evaluates the impact of change and innovation

Management Behaviors

- Models the change they want to see
- Plans change with others; sustains change
- Organizes the group and the environment to implement change
- Influences directions of change
- Adapts to change
- Uses influence strategy with followers
- Evaluates changes
- Communicates the need for change

Overlap Areas

- Models the change they want to see
- Initiates and influences the direction of changes
- Uses influence strategy with followers
- Evaluates changes
- Communicates the need for change

1. Empowerment
2. Shared decision making
3. Self-direction
4. Shared governance

Change is implied in the definition of leadership. If leadership is defined as influencing others, then the activity of influencing is directed toward some change. The ability to envision and communicate a changed future is part of the definition of leadership. Numerous authors have noted that change is an inevitable fact of life, but leaders and managers can cope by developing processes that allow them to initiate and influence change. The essentials of leadership that are needed are an ability to envision the change needed, reflection on the issues inherent in the change, positive communication skills, an ability to promote cultures that encourage creativity and change, and showing that they actually "walk-the-talk."

Transformational change is a part of organizational transformation. To produce strategic change, transformational leaders work with others to ignite a vision, change structure and culture, change mindsets and power structures, and empower others (Robbins & Davidhizar, 2007). Both leaders and managers can be effective in initiating and influencing organizational change. Anyone in the organization can be the focal point for making appropriate and effective change, but the employees in staff positions need to enlist the cooperation and support of the administrative hierarchy.

Because of constant change, nurses and health care systems have had to learn and adapt. To view the scope of change surrounding nursing in perspective, four areas of major change can be identified—organizational structures, nursing labor force, reimbursement, and information systems (Figure 3.2). First, organizational structures have been changing and reconfiguring in response to the environment and financial pressures. For example, population-based care, case management, patient-centered care, and patient safety initiatives are elements reflecting change in regard to client care systems redesign. In health care, bureaucratic systems endured for a long time but were not well suited to the work of professionals. The empowerment of staff to result in outcomes of quality is the goal. Clearly, national health care reform is an issue creating uncertainty and change throughout the health care delivery system and its organizations. Changes also are occurring in health care as integrated networks form and care increasingly is moved into community settings. Changing organizational structures are occurring in the midst of a

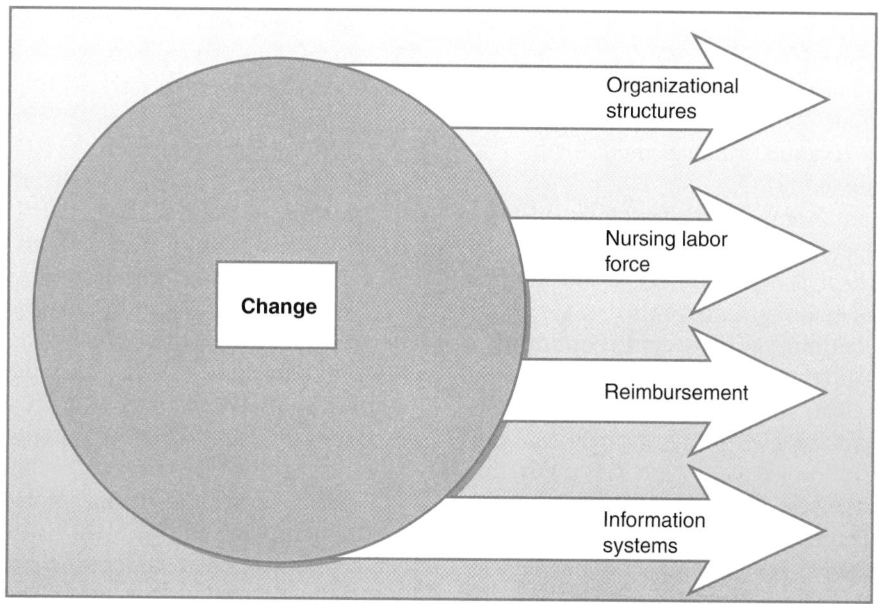

Figure 3.2
Areas of major change in health care and nursing.

nurse shortage. The complexion of the nurse workforce is changing, and recruitment and retention, education, and staff deployment alternatives are being explored.

Another area of important change in health care is reimbursement. For example, reimbursement (payment) for physicians has been changing, driven by the federal government's relative value units determinations and now pay-for-performance. Reimbursement for nurse practitioners currently is allowed under Medicare/Medicaid. However, managed care, with its capitated reimbursement structure, has changed payment to all forms of health care providers. Payment reforms are likely to continue and change. The cost areas are physician payment, already being ratcheted down; pharmaceutical costs; and equipment and technology costs. The government will continue to review and explore the amount of dollars spent and the way those dollars are spent in an effort to reduce a huge national budget deficit fueled partly by health care costs. An increase in governmental intervention and regulatory control can be predicted in health care.

Present and future changes will bring an increasing use of information systems. A massive increase in computerization is urgent in a managed care environment. For example, a national practitioner's data bank was created from quality concerns. Any physician or nurse who has been party to a lawsuit must have this information reported. Large national databases of all licensed nurses also are being compiled. Powerful computers and sophisticated software programs have a pattern of undergoing updates and generational changes within a few years or sooner, creating challenges of compatibility, archival retrieval, maintaining currency, and staff training.

CURRENT ISSUES AND TRENDS

The character of the changes occurring in health care approach a paradigm shift rather than an adaptation. In 1996, Issel and Anderson, identified the following six interconnected transformations that are major areas of change still influencing health care today:

1. From person-as-customer to the population-as-customer
2. From illness care to wellness care and prevention
3. From revenue management to cost management
4. From autonomy of professionals to their interdependence
5. From client as nonconsumer to consumer of cost and quality information
6. From continuity of provider to continuity of information

Nurses can create new environments or establish new organizational forms that will lead and shape the direction of health care. It is a question of which are the best courses of action and how to best direct the transformations.

Change drivers for nursing and health care include cultural diversity, the aging U.S. population, new services and technologies, health care costs, and the public policy of posting information about quality of care (Wakefield, 2003). These changes have and will continue to alter the health care delivery system. They present both opportunities and challenges, and nurses need to be able to anticipate and monitor trends for their immediate and long-term effects on practice.

It is a new era for leadership with new rules (Porter-O'Grady & Malloch, 2007). This means that leaders need to be able to guide others through this new reality as they experience transition and change. Porter-O'Grady and Malloch (2007) said that the leader acts as a good signpost reader in a transition time (e.g., as we are now living); they anticipate the path of change and guide others in the direction that the change is moving to continue to work and survive in these turbulent times when the environment is ever-changing. Wheatley (2007) suggested that principles are needed, not techniques or models. The four core principles of change she proposes are the following (Wheatley, 2007):

- *Participation is not a choice:* Engaging people in the change from the beginning can prevent unintended consequences in the end.
- *Life always reacts to directives; it does not obey them:* This principle suggests offering invitations for others to work with us, rather than issuing directives or orders or even giving "visionary" messages.
- *We do not see "reality"; we create our own interpretation of what is real:* This principle stresses the importance about not arguing who is right or who is wrong, but understanding that each one of us filters reality through our own lenses.
- *To create living health in a living system; connect it to more of itself:* This principle is based on a strong respect for systems, and it supports the leader's task of strengthening communication and connections within the system.

The health care environment has been described as turbulent because of the rapid rate of change and the perceived constancy of change. However, change can be growth-producing, renewing, and invigorating for individuals and organizations. This occurs as individuals and organizations enlist creativity to derive an innovation that improves the environment or client care delivery. "Leadership *is* the leading of creativity which leads to creative change" (Kerfoot, 1998, p. 99).

An investment in creativity and innovation, with resulting change, provides strategic advantage. Creativity withers in hostile environments in which all of the time is spent thinking about survival. Strategies to develop a culture that fosters creativity and change include the following (Kerfoot, 1998):

- Promoting conversations and dialogue
- Providing access to information
- Building relationships
- Teaching rethinking, questioning, and innovation
- Creating a culture of innovation
- Orchestrating and executing

In an organizational context, creativity means producing novel and useful ideas by an individual or a group. It is the basis of invention and innovation. Creativity in organizations is influenced by

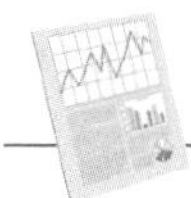

Research Note

Source: Hayman, B., Cioffi, J., & Wilkes, L. (2006). Redesign of the model of nursing practice in an acute care ward: Nurses' experiences. *Collegian, 13*(1), 31-36.

Purpose

This study reported on the experiences of nurses in a unit implementing a new practice model in a 30-bed surgical unit in Australia. Because restructuring or redesign of hospital units has been found to cause psychological stress and job dissatisfaction, these researchers believed it was important to address the nurses' experiences in this change. The new model of care redesigned by the nurse managers was a team model with increased numbers of assistive personnel and decreased numbers of registered nurses. It included a clinical coordinator—an RN who coordinated staff and provided clinical support.

Discussion

The change studied in this case was initiated by the managers and implemented without apparent input from the staff involved. The qualitative findings showed that the nurses tried to remain open to "trialing" the new model but that they were not satisfied, in the end, with the change. They perceived the change forced on them by management without consideration of their input. The registered nurses believed that quality of patient care had been compromised and thus their own job satisfaction had decreased.

Application to Practice

The health care environment has been described as turbulent because of the rapid rate of change and the perceived constancy of change. However, change can be growth producing, renewing, and invigorating for individuals and organizations. This occurs as individuals and organizations enlist creativity to derive an innovation that improves the environment or client care delivery. "Leadership *is* the leading of creativity which leads to creative change" (Kerfoot, 1998, p. 99).

management practices and creativity-relevant work group skills. Creativity is one important aspect of organizational innovation (Gilmartin, 1999).

Summary

- Change is a pervasive element of society, of today's health care environment, and of life.
- Change is defined as an alteration to make something different.
- Planned change is defined as a process of intentional intervention.
- A change agent is a facilitator used to plan and implement the change process.
- The amount of change and the rapidity of the pace of change disrupt and disorganize humans.
- The use of planned change is a nursing management intervention strategy.
- Lewin's theory of change uses ideas of equilibrium within systems.
- A successful change involves Lewin's three elements: unfreezing, moving, and refreezing.
    - Unfreezing is the first stage of change and can be characterized as a process of thawing out the system.
    - The second stage of change is moving to a new level of behavior.
    - The final stage of change is refreezing new changes so that they are integrated and stabilized.
- Both driving and restraining forces impinge on any situation.

- To create change, the equilibrium is broken by altering the relative strengths of driving and restraining forces.
- Rogers identified five phases to the adoption of change and five factors that determine successful planned change.
- Lippitt identified seven phases of the change process.
- Havelock's six elements to the process of planned change are building a relationship, diagnosing the problem, acquiring relevant resources, choosing a solution, gaining acceptance, and stabilization and self-renewal.
- Perlman and Takacs describe 10 stages in the emotional voyage of the process of change.
- Resistance is a natural response to change.
- Participatory approaches to change can decrease resistance
- Ineffective responses to change do not allow the change process to proceed.
- Innovation is the use of change to provide some new product or service.
- Rogers' theory of innovation diffusion helps to understand how to create changes in clinical practice and organizational management.
- The ability to envision and communicate a changed future is part of the definition of leadership.

Case Study

Nurse Rebecca Romero was director of a large ambulatory care service in a not-for-profit medical center. Over the years, increasing numbers of services were moved to ambulatory care, and her span of control and workload had increased. She knew that a profound change in the organization of her department, the structure of the work, and the role of various staff members was needed to keep the department moving forward. She had given some thought and had some ideas but was committed to a participatory leadership style.

Fortunately, this department of nursing had embraced a decentralized style. Nurse Romero shared her concerns and some of her ideas with the registered nurse (RN) group at their staff meeting. The RNs had noticed some of the same issues that Rebecca had, and they began to brainstorm their own ideas for change. However, Nurse Romero reminded the RNs that all levels of staff would be impacted by these changes and they needed to be involved in planning.

Having gained the support of the RN group, Nurse Romero called a full-staff meeting. In this meeting, she began with a review of some the current economic and environmental issues impacting the department. She stated that she thought that the department needed to consider how to make changes that would improve some of the current problems yet be acceptable to all the staff. Then, rather than suggest specific changes, she asked for a representative committee from the staff to work with her on the change. Several of the RNs, licensed vocational nurses (LVNs), and one nursing assistant (NA) and clerk volunteered to work on the change committee with Nurse Romero.

Over the next several months, the committee met weekly. They outlined the needs for changes and proposed solutions. They worked out the pros and cons of each solution. In the end, they had two alternatives to present to the rest of the staff. With Nurse Romero's support, the committee presented their work, including the two proposed alternatives. Each member spoke up about how others in their type of position would be affected. The staff came to consensus that the first model presented had the most positive outcomes and agreed to carry out the implementation plan. The ambulatory care staff was able to implement a transformational change in their department with virtually no resistance.

CRITICAL THINKING EXERCISE

Nurse Nancy Chang works in an intermediate care unit in a large, integrated delivery system. The nurses on the unit have been dealing with ever-increasing patient acuity. In addition, a new state law will mandate a change in RN-to-patient ratio by 2010. Nurse Chang is called into a meeting with the unit director, who tells her that the decision has now been made to implement a new staffing pattern: an all-RN staff. Nurse Chang will need to introduce this change and encourage the staff to participate in the change. Nurse Chang knows the potential benefits in the long run but worries about the impact on all levels of staff. This will mean hiring more new graduates, so there will be more nurses to orient. The nursing assistants will have to leave their unit and area of comfort, and the way in which care is delivered will greatly change. She is trying to decide what to do first.

1. What is (are) the problem(s)?
2. Whose problem is it?
3. What should Nurse Chang do?
4. What theory or model might be useful?
5. How might she best plan this change process?
6. How might she prevent or decrease resistance of other staff?

The process for change utilized by Nurse Romero and the committee included the following:

1. A thorough internal assessment, including future departmental growth, space, patient needs, and staff roles, including a review of the health care system's strategic plan to ensure that it was congruent
2. A change process that incorporates the governance structure and consensus decision-making style of the department
3. New role descriptions for RNs, consistent with their current positions, because they would take on more of a coordinator role for their clinics
4. Continuing to build trust and relationships within the staff and to reassure administration, patients, and families that the changes will result in improved patient care
5. Changes consistent with space considerations
6. Efficient and effective infrastructure and operating processes
7. Recognition that the need for staff acceptance and participation outweighs the need to move quickly
8. No increases in budget or resources

Using these 8 points as a guideline, Nurse Romero and the staff together began to implement their plan for organizational change and transformation.

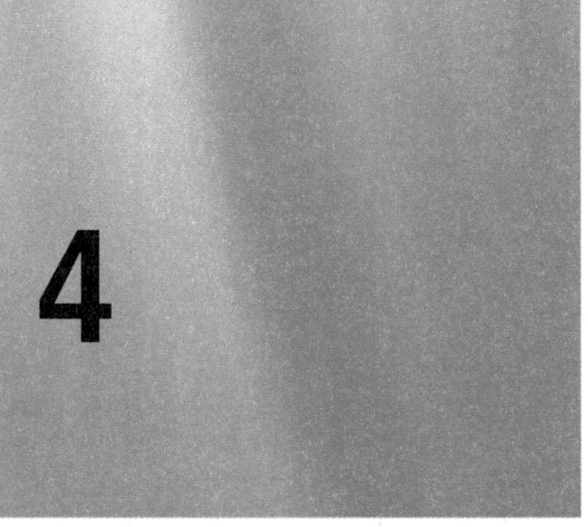

4 Organizational Climate and Culture

Mary K. Anthony

PART I

CHAPTER OBJECTIVES

- Describe the forces behind a changing health care culture
- Delineate the significance of organizational culture
- Define and differentiate organizational culture and climate
- Describe characteristics of emerging climates
- Evaluate influence of unit-based nursing teams on culture and climate in nursing practice
- Synthesize leadership factors important to creating positive climates
- Analyze the importance of culture across contemporary factors in nursing practice
- Exercise critical thinking to conceptualize and analyze possible solutions to a practice exercise

In the past several decades, health care organizations have needed to respond to economic, social, and financial changes that have caused a redirection in how health care providers think and deliver care. Each change progressively led health care organizations to move beyond the era of restructuring to compete in a marketplace based on their ability to demonstrate lean performance, increased efficiency, and safe quality outcomes. Consider the impact of the following changes. The payment structure for health care has shifted from fee-for-service to a prospective payment system to pay-for-performance. In 2001, the Institute of Medicine's (IOM) *Crossing the Quality Chasm* (IOM, 2001) described the challenge for redirection in the twenty-first century that includes moving from provider-centered care to patient-centered care. Inclusion of patient and family values, norms, customs, and need for participation is becoming a dominant force in making treatment decisions. The recent focus on issues related to patient safety emphasized not only outcomes but also scrutiny of the processes and behaviors that achieve safe care. The potential that the information technology explosion holds will change the speed and transparency of knowledge and information. The recognition that professionals who work together in teams rather than within their own disciplinary silos achieve better outcomes has changed the nature of interdisciplinary relationships. The impact of a supply-based nurse shortage, the demand for nursing care, and mandate for evidence-based practice are changing the face of nursing care. Taken together, these forces have redefined and redirected health care and combined to create a "perfect storm" in which nurses are challenged to navigate in these turbulent waters. In the perfect storm, nurses may wonder how these factors link with culture and their role as nurses and leaders.

Culture represents an important phenomenon that has to be understood to practice nursing effectively, no matter where the practice environment exists. Nurses' insight into culture enables them to better understand staff behaviors and relationships, norms, change processes, expectations, and communications. This holds true for all levels of nurses from novice to expert practitioner and manager.

Nurses have a pivotal role in care delivery. Diers (2001) stated, "Nursing is two things: the care of the sick (or the potentially sick) and the tending of the entire environment within which care happens" (p. 1).

Tending to the environment implies that nurses need to understand the culture of the setting in which they practice. The reason for the existence of the modern hospital is to provide nursing care, although this is not overtly recognized in our culture. This means that the explicit and implicit vision, mission, values, priorities, and strategic direction of the organization have to be recognized, understood, and aligned with realities of daily practice and care priorities. This chapter provides an overview of culture and focuses on the factors that affect the culture within an organization and how nurses working together can effectively respond. The chapter discusses organizational culture and climate and their relationship to the nursing work environment, workforce, and practice.

DEFINITIONS

Culture

Organizational culture is rooted in anthropology, psychology, sociology, and management theory and first appeared in the academic literature in 1952 (Scott et al., 2003). **Culture** is the set of values, beliefs, and assumptions that are shared by members of an organization. An organization's culture provides a common belief system among its members. The purpose of culture is to provide a common bond so that members know how to relate to one another and to show others who are outside of the organization what is valued. Scott and colleagues (2003) described organizational culture as an amalgamation of symbols, language, dress, symbols of authority, myths, ceremonies, rituals, practices, assumptions, and behaviors. The variables make up an intricate cluster of interactive components that overtly manifest themselves in a setting. Culture is sometimes likened to an iceberg in that only the top of the iceberg is visible and the invisible part of the iceberg runs deep into the ocean (Daft, 2001). The top of the iceberg can be thought of as being the mission statement, policies, procedures, organizational charts, the way people dress, and the language they use. The invisible part of the iceberg can be what is implicit in the organization such as the unwritten rules and customs that pervade the work environment (most easily missed yet critical to know). Collectively, these variables define the character and norms of the organization.

Some easy ways to understand culture are illustrated with the following examples. A symbol representing excellence in nursing care is recognition as a Magnet™ hospital. The care delivery model that guides nursing practice is another observable that helps interpret the culture. For instance, when a relationship-based nursing care model is used, it represents an underlying belief in patient-centered care. Open visiting hours in ICUs conveys the importance of family as partners. How new nurses are oriented expresses values about the socialization of new nurses. Are organizational commitment to learning, professional career development, a designated preceptor, and a clear individualized orientation plan discussed? Is a mentor assigned? The visible aspects of culture shape the underlying values of the organization.

Culture is a multifaceted phenomenon, difficult to comprehend and unravel. The acute care hospital constitutes one of the most complex organizations in our current social environment. Health care relationships in hospitals depend on communication and collaboration between and among caregivers to facilitate intricate processes linked to the delivery of patient care. One way to better understand such relationships is to appreciate how the hospital culture affects nursing units, nursing practice, and patient outcomes. For a nurse to function effectively in an organization, whether as a staff nurse or manager, a solid grasp of organizational culture, characteristics, and operations is essential.

Climate

Organizational climate is a concept that is closely linked to the organization's culture and is sometimes confused with it. Although many people use *culture* and *climate* interchangeably, the terms are in fact not the same. **Climate** is an individual perception of what it feels like to work in an environment (Snow, 2002). It is how nurses perceive and feel about practices, procedures, and rewards (Sleutel, 2000). People form perceptions of the work environment because they focus on what is important and meaningful to them. This explains why some aspects of culture may be interpreted differently. Climate is easier to quantify than culture, and so climate refers to the aspects of the work environment that can be measured. Researchers who study climate describe various components of the work environment that influence outcome behaviors (Sleutel, 2000). Some characteristics that are often used to study climate are decision making, leadership, supervisor support, peer cohesion, autonomy, conflict, work pressure, rewards, feeling of warmth, and risk (Litwin & Stringer, 1968; Stone et al., 2005). Within organizations, it is common to identify other types of subclimates that focus on very specific aspects of the organizations (e.g., climates related to patient safety, ethics, and learning).

Culture-Climate Link

Regardless of the practice setting, a link exists between culture and climate and that link is what is important in understanding attitudes, motivations, and behavior among nurses (Stone et al., 2005). The common links between culture and climate can be described as the interaction of shared values about what things are important, beliefs about how things work, and behaviors about how things get done (Uttal, 1983). Research has shown that among nurses, culture or climate affects job satisfaction (Hart & Moore, 1989), intent to turnover (Hemingway & Smith, 1999), and needlestick and near misses (Clarke, Rockett, Sloane, & Aiken, 2002; Clarke, Sloane, & Aiken, 2002). One interesting aspect of climate that has receivedattention over the past several years is workforce diversity. Four generations of nurses are in the current workforce: "Veterans" (the oldest nurses), "Baby Boomers," "Generation X," and "Millenials" (the youngest working nurses). There is consensus that nurses from different generations have values that were shaped by the social, economic, political, and historical forces during the era in which they grew up. It is not well established whether nurses from different generations also perceive the work climate differently.

Nursing Work Group

Although organizations usually have a single culture, many climates can exist within that culture. Groups and organizations exist within society and develop a culture that has a significant effect on how members think, feel, and act. Culture becomes a learned product of the group experience. In general, nurses work together in a group such as on a nursing unit, in home care, in long-term care, or in communities. The nursing unit, or **nursing work group,** is a small geographical area within the larger hospital system where nurses work interdependently to care for a group of patients. On units, groups of nurses work together, spend time together, and set up their own norms and values and ways to communicate with each other (Brennan & Anthony, 2000). These factors contribute to that unit having its own climate or perception of what it feels like to work on that unit. Climate is evident in staff perceptions of policies, practices, and goal

LEADING & MANAGING DEFINED

Culture

Shared beliefs, values, and ways of thinking that guide how people relate to one another.

Climate

Perceptions held by individuals about what it feels like to work in a certain environment; climate influences behavior.

Nursing Work Group

Nurses working in a common geographical area within a larger organization work interdependently to care for a group of patients and develop their own norms and values.

achievement. Some authors describe this as a work group subculture (Coeling & Simms, 1993). Understanding culture from the unit perspective offers an unprecedented view of nurses' work. The importance of creating a unit environment with a culture or climate that empowers nurses to practice in ways that effect and sustain a positive practice environment, such as collaborative relationships, relates to how climate and culture can be managed so they will improve quality care and nurse and patient outcomes.

BACKGROUND

Organizational culture has been studied as both something an organization *has* and something an organization *is* (Mark, 1996). Peters and Waterman's *In Search of Excellence* fueled a renewed business focus on culture as the means to achieve organizational success and competitive advantage (Peters & Waterman, 1982). Industry leaders in the corporate world quickly realized that the philosophy and values of an organization could determine success and secure market advantage (Wooten & Crane, 2003). The health care industry has been slower than the corporate world to embrace culture as a means to optimize organizational performance.

Schein (1996) is a renowned sociologist who has defined organizational culture as a shared value system developed over time that guides members on how to problem solve, adapt to the external environment, and manage relationships. The mission statement for an organization offers a snapshot of strategic priorities and is an important way to get a sense of organizational values. How does the mission get communicated? Is it evident in organizational decisions? Schein suggested that a deeper understanding of cultural issues in organizations is necessary not only to understand what goes on but also, more important, to affect outcomes.

Organizational culture affects both quality and quantity of nursing care and patient outcomes. Shared meanings, the taken-for-granted practice and assumptions of a work unit group, can exert a significant effect on performance and outcomes. Basic underlying assumptions are those that are never questioned and make up an integral part of the fabric of an organization that extends to the unit work level, such as a commitment to excellence and to the surrounding community. Each organizational unit has cultural norms and values that blend the social realities and features that shape interactions among staff, patients, and families. The manner in which the staff perceives organizational culture, manages boundaries, and translates implied values to a unit level has a direct effect on the production of patient care (Alderfer, 1980).

Measurement of organizational culture and climate is fraught with difficulties, and there is no single best instrument. Qualitative methods are often used for culture, and quantitative measures are used for climate. A range of measurement tools is available; however, all have limitations in scope, ease of use, or scientific properties. The choice of a measurement instrument should be directed by definition, purpose, and context for cultural assessment (Scott et al., 2003).

RESEARCH

A growing body of research confirms that the relationship between nurse staffing and patient outcomes is influenced by culture or climate and the organizational characteristics of the structure in which nurses practice (Aiken, Sloane, & Lake, 1997; Mitchell & Shortell, 1997; Needleman et al., 2001; Seago, 2001; Sovie & Jawad, 2001). In the past several years, studying the impact of culture has shifted from the hospital level to the unit level where caregiver relationships, communication, and autonomy intersect to inform care decisions that affect outcomes. Boyle (2004) found that nurse autonomy/collaboration, practice control, manager support, or continuity/specialization was significantly related to adverse events. To understand how the culture of the organization and climate of a unit are related to professional practice, three contemporary trends in achieving a culture/climate of quality are discussed here: Magnet Recognition Program®, patient safety climate, and learning climate.

Magnet™ Recognition

The American Nurses Association's (ANA) American Nurses Credentialing Center (ANCC) is the home for the esteemed Magnet Recognition Program® (ANCC, 2008). The focus of this program is to recognize nursing services in health care organizations that provide excellent nursing care and attract and retain professional nurses. The process of Magnet™ recognition uses appraisal of the 14 Forces of Magnetism, which are qualitative factors first identified in 1983 via research and derived from evidence-based knowledge and the ANA's (2004) standards of nursing practice for nurse administrators.

In 1983, the ANA's American Academy of Nursing's Task Force on Nursing Practice in Hospitals studied nursing service "best practices" by surveying 163 hospitals. The goal was to identify and describe those factors that, when present, created an environment that attracted and retained qualified RNs who delivered quality care. The 41 best hospitals were called "Magnet™ hospitals" because of their clear ability to attract professional nurses. The characteristics they displayed were identified and called "Forces of Magnetism." Since 1983, the Magnet Recognition Program® has blossomed and become the "gold standard" in nursing. In 2008, a new model for this program was unveiled, again based on research and practice evidence. In Magnet™-designated hospitals, a strong visionary nurse leader nurtures a nursing professional environment and advocates for and is supportive of excellence in nursing practice. The facility's reputation is enhanced, and the profession of nursing is elevated to greater esteem.

Magnet™-designated hospitals have been recognized over the years for excellent patient care, support of strong nursing practice environments, and the ability to attract and retain nurses (ANA, 1997; Kramer & Hafner, 1989). The term *Magnet™ hospital* was derived from a policy study commissioned in 1982 by the American Academy of Nursing. The study examined the organizational characteristics of U.S. hospitals successful in the recruitment and retention of nurses during a national nursing shortage—hence the name (McClure et al., 1982).

Aiken and colleagues (1994) transformed the initial Magnet™ hospital work into a program of research congruent with quality of care and organizational effectiveness through study of the links between hospital organizational culture and care outcomes. Magnet™ hospitals were conceptualized as those institutions that have a specific organizational culture with characteristics of autonomy, practice control, and collaboration. Aiken and colleagues (1994) examined mortality rates in 39 Magnet™ hospitals and 195 control hospitals using multivariate matched control sampling. Magnet™ hospitals had a significantly lower mortality rate (4.6% lower) for Medicare patients than that of control hospitals. The Magnet™ hospital culture provided higher levels of autonomy and control of practice and fostered stronger professional relationships among nurses and physicians than did non-Magnet™ hospitals.

Magnet™ hospital research and the organizational framework developed by Aiken, Sochalski, and Lake (1997) provide the means to better understand the link between the unit culture characteristics and adverse events. A nursing unit culture that supports and values nurse autonomy and the provision of adequate resources and effective communication among providers most likely constitutes an environment in which practice excellence is the norm. Effects of nursing interventions are mediated by such organizational characteristics at the unit level (Aiken & Fagin, 1997). Magnet™ hospitals are an example of a positive culture that affects nurses and patient outcomes. Magnet™ recognition is considered the gold standard for excellence in nursing (Wolf, 2006) and is sought by nurses, physicians, hospitals, and the public.

Today, the interrelationships among culture, climate, and outcomes are under scrutiny. Hospitals wanting to achieve Magnet™ status must meet the 14 Forces of Magnetism identified by the American Nurses Credentialing Center (ANCC, 2004, 2008). Research that measures the Hospital Magnet™ Standards focuses on eight characteristics of an excellent work environment: clinically competent peers, collaborative nurse-MD relationships, clinical autonomy, support for education, perception of adequate staffing, nurse

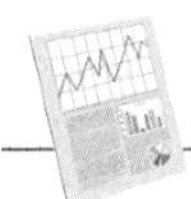

Research Note

Source: Stone, P.W., et al. (2006). Organizational climate and intensive care nurses' intention to leave. *Critical Care Medicine, 34,* 1907-1912.

Background

The shortage of nurses is particularly evident in a critical care unit where nurses with specialized knowledge and skills are needed to meet the care requirements of complex patients. A work environment that is satisfying to the needs of nurses promotes retention of nurses in these units with traditionally high turnover rates.

Study Methods and Design

Purpose: The purpose of the study was to evaluate the incidence of nurses working in an ICU who intended to leave their unit because of working conditions and then to identify factors that could be used to predict intention to leave.
Design: This descriptive study was part of a larger study to evaluate ICU nosocomial infections. *Sample:* The sample was composed of 2323 registered nurses working in 110 ICUs across 66 hospitals. On average, nurses were 39.5 years old, had a total of 15.6 years of experience, and worked in their current position for 8.0 years.
Instruments: The Perceived Nurse Working Environment Scale, developed from the Nursing Work Index Revised (NWI-R), had seven subscales measuring unit climate and included the following: professional practice, staffing/resource adequacy, nurse management, nursing process, nurse-physician collaboration, clinical competence, and positive scheduling climate. Nurses were asked to respond to the item "Do you plan to leave your current position in the coming year?" If they responded positively, they were asked to describe their reasons. For nurses who indicated their intention to leave, their responses were analyzed and divided into two groups: those leaving because of retirement or promotion and those intending to leave because of working conditions.
Results: Seventeen percent of nurses (n = 391) indicated they were intending to leave within the next year. Of those 391, 202 (52%) gave their reason for leaving as being related to working conditions. The other 48% of nurses indicated their reason for leaving was associated with a career opportunity, personal or family, retirement, or no reason given. In general, nurses who were intending to leave because of the work environment rated all of the organizational climate dimensions lower than all other responding nurses. Three of the climate factors were statistically significant in predicting nurses' intention to leave. Professional practice (measured as nurses' involvement in hospital decision governance and opportunities to advance), nurses' perception of the competence of other nurses, and experience were found to decrease the likelihood of intention to leave by 48%, 39%, and 3% respectively.

Application to Practice

In a time when hospitals struggle to fill RN vacancies, the findings strengthened the premise that the climate of the work environment is an important predictor of nurses' intention to leave the unit. Although response rates were low, in ICUs, which are noted for their difficulty in recruiting and retaining nurses, these findings validate the importance of creating a unit climate in which nurses have opportunities to participate in practice decisions, can professionally develop, and value the contributions of their peers.

manager support, control of nursing practice, and patient-centered values (Schmalenberg & Kramer, 2008). From a broader perspective, Stone and colleagues (2005) developed an integrated structure-process-outcome model of relationships among factors describing organizational climate and its effect on outcomes. They identified leadership values, strategy and style, and organizational structure aspects such as communication, governance, and technology as the structural components of climate. Likewise, the process elements of climate include supervision, work design, group behavior, and emphasis on quality that is driven by patient centeredness, safety, innovation, and evidence-based practice. Taken together, these components are likely to have an effect on nurse and patient outcomes.

Patient Safety Culture and Climate

Since the publication of the Institute of Medicine report *To Err is Human: Building a Safer Health System* (Kohn et al., 2000) suggesting that 98,000 persons die in hospitals because of errors, an emphasis on an organization's patient safety culture and climate has driven both research and change in hospital practices. A safety culture is an outgrowth of the larger organizational culture and emphasizes the deeper assumptions and values of the organization toward safety, whereas the safety climate is the shared perception of employees about the importance of safety within the organization (DeJoy et al., 2004). Like organizational climate, the safety climate has a number of different components including leadership, involvement, blameless culture, communication, teamwork, commitment to safety, beliefs about errors and their cause, and others (Blegen et al., 2005).

Safety climate refers to keeping both patients and nurses safe. Keeping an "eye out" for patients is at the heart of safety. Nurses, who are on the front line of patient care, are in the best position to monitor patients to prevent adverse events or near misses of adverse events. The ability of nurses to know the patients and recognize early critical warning signs is a skill derived from knowledge, not a simple task application. Astute recognition of deviations from normal and timely intervention signify that nurses know their patients and are capable of rescuing them from an adverse event. Knowledge of the patient is derived through subjective, objective, and intuitive observations that are honed as nurses develop a level of expertise in working with specific patient populations. Factors that influence nurses' ability to watch over patients to avoid errors and adverse events include being short staffed or fatigued from working overtime or lacking education and experience (Hinshaw, 2008).

Included in the concept of a safety climate is a focus on nurses' health. Nurses working in hospitals have one of the highest rates of work-related injuries, especially back injuries and needlesticks (Mark et al., 2007). As with patient safety, when fewer nurses are working, less help is available to provide care to patients. This results in more work needing to be done in a shorter time. Both of these factors can lead to taking shortcuts that can result in injury.

Regardless of whether the focus of safety is on the patient or the nurse, the likelihood of injury can be lessened where there is a cohesive team. When there is a shared perception among a group of nurses about the value and importance of safety, they are more likely to work together effectively toward common goals. In believing that the safety climate values learning in preventing, detecting, and mitigating the effect of errors and injuries, the likelihood of improving outcomes increases. As nurses work together as a team, they share information, can anticipate events, and are more likely to respond positively to unanticipated events.

One major shift in an organization's safety climate is the move from a punitive environment to one that is characterized as a fair and just culture. David Marx (2001) suggested that in a just culture, organizational, individual, and interpersonal learning are balanced with personal accountability and discipline. In a fair and just culture, expectations for system and individual learning and accountability are transparent. Underlying these beliefs, an organizational strategy needs to be identified that can effectively implement just such a fair and just culture. When an organization, such as a hospital, can freely discuss mistakes with the intention of learning from them and when it takes the time and resources needed to understand the mistakes (e.g., root cause analysis), the organizational culture changes from a "who dunnit?" to an environment that is respectful and open to learning (Connor et al., 2007). Within a systems-oriented approach, learning from adverse events and unproductive successes can lead to new wisdoms and new ways of doing things. When a systems approach underlies learning and is the concern of everyone, knowledge that is gained from it becomes widespread for common use by everyone (Institute of Management Administration, 2000).

Learning Culture and Climate

Access to new information is occurring at a record pace, and organizations need to keep up with new information and ways of practicing. In a learning culture, the norms and assumptions for learning lead to behaviors that support continuous learning (Daft, 2001). A learning climate is characterized by a shared and positive perception of the value of learning to enhance practice, quality, and outcomes. The emphasis on developing a culture of learning stems from at least three major trends affecting health care. The first is the focus on patient safety in which learning and accountability are guideposts for error control. Second is the emphasis on evidence-based research and translating findings into practice, and third is the explosion of information technology in health care delivery that increases access and transparency of care.

One area that is motivating and sustaining a learning environment for nurses is linked to a hospital's aspiration to achieve Magnet™ status. In the journey toward Magnet™ designation, research, and evidence-based practice become important in meeting the core criteria. Cultures in which continuous learning is valued are less likely to become outdated and stale. In the past, it was not unusual to hear nurses say in relation to their practice, "We have always done it that way." Today, a learning environment fosters nurses to propose new ideas. Moving new research findings into practice has historically taken many years. In a continuous learning culture, nurses are challenged to ask, "How can this be done better?" Nurses interact with many patients on a daily basis. Patients are experts about themselves, and nurses are expert about nursing practice. Blending these areas of expertise best positions nurses to ask the question "How can practice and the environment in which practice occurs be improved?" Nursing practice becomes a daily venue for generating questions that are important to practice.

Culture and group norms can have a profound impact on the shared values that are expressed by nursing staff on individual work units in the hospital setting (Koerner, 1996). The formation of the team at the unit level holds a collective vision for continuous learning. In turn, the norm for learning intersects with the desire for good practice and forms a cohesive unit that shares a value for learning that generates excitement for moving beyond traditional practice. Cultures and climates in which knowledge is freely shared can have a groundswell effect. Examples of outward and visible signs that support nurses-shared values for inquiry include journal clubs, unit presentations, poster displays, and participation in evidence-based research teams.

LEADERSHIP AND MANAGEMENT IMPLICATIONS

Culture is characterized by complexity, tangibles, and intangibles and is relatively enduring, making it hard to change. Climate, on the other hand, is easier to change. Regardless, the basic elements that constitute culture and climate must be understood before any change. Change that begins at the unit level may be most influenced by nursing leadership. Nurses have the ability to create or change a work culture or climate to accomplish a change that may affect productivity, satisfaction, and safe quality patient-centered care.

The role of a nursing leader extends well beyond a formal title into the realm of informal influence to affect culture and the climate. A primary task of the leader is to create a vision so convincing that the entire team is inspired to engage and move forward. Values drive behaviors. The leader communicates this vision by influencing norms and values and creating a shared perception through role modeling and ensuring role clarity, accountability, and a work environment that promotes safe patient-centered care.

Nursing unit leadership, particularly that of the nurse manager, is key to creating a positive unit climate that promotes effective unit functioning and quality care (Sorrentino et al., 1992). Unit-based nurse managers serve as bridges between the senior nursing leadership and their staff who are frontline providers. By virtue of their position, they are instrumental in shaping and managing the core values of their staff (Anthony et al., 2005). "Nurse managers have multiple and competing demands that they must balance in defining, prioritizing, and implementing their role responsibilities to meet the goals of the organization as well as those of the profession" (Anthony et al., 2005, p. 146). Increasingly, studies are showing that the nurse manager is important in retention (Anthony et al, 2005; Boyle et al., 1999; Taunton et al., 1997), professional practice (Manojlovich, 2005), and work environments (Upenieks, 2003). However, this influence is diluted when nurse managers are managing too many units or across too many areas and need to create and support a climate unique to each unit (Kimball & O'Neill, 2002).

Key areas within the leader's scope of control are recruiting and retaining staff, welcoming new staff, providing orientation, celebrating and recognizing staff accomplishments, facilitating change, and promoting a learning environment. Unit climate is evident in how policies are enacted, unit norms, dress code and appearance, environment, communication, and teamwork. The nurse manager can articulate the vision, mission, and goals of the organization and work with staff to translate them into unit-level values for performance, thus linking the context of the organization to clinical practice.

Values drive the way resources are distributed. They contribute to a general attitude and sense about the quality of working life and reflect the organization's core goals. Clues can be gleaned from organizational documents such as philosophy statements and meeting minutes. Caring values of the organization are reflected in the way the organization treats its staff. Organizational values may not mirror professional values. The leader's role is to bridge such values with the values of individual team members to construct unit climate. Values support the mission and the related vision, which support strategies and action plans. The key platform is shared values. Given the complexity and diversity of the nursing workforce, developing and sustaining a set of shared values is no easy task and requires leadership skill.

Leaders are expected to chart a clear course for change and mobilize staff to accomplish

LEADERSHIP & MANAGEMENT BEHAVIORS

Leadership Behaviors

- Envisions a dynamic culture
- Inspires a creative climate
- Models constructive interpersonal relationships
- Enables followers to be productive
- Influences others to work together
- Creates shared values
- Develops stories, rituals, and metaphors
- Bridges organizational, unit, and professional goals
- Promotes values that emphasize safety and learning

Management Behaviors

- Manages the structure to affect culture positively
- Models constructive interpersonal relationships
- Acts with equity and justice
- Maintains rituals and ceremonies
- Influences employees to work together
- Promotes values that emphasize safety and learning
- Builds teams that are proactive and can handle unexpected situations

Overlap Areas

- Models constructive interpersonal relations
- Influences the group to work together
- Promotes values that emphasize safety and learning

organizational goals. This means implementing change effectively. Effective cultural change requires communication, passion, and sense of the whole. The nurse manager can create such opportunities through using focus groups, holding team meetings, coaching and mentoring, posting minutes from staff meetings, consulting communication books, and empowering staff by soliciting their input. The value of communication cannot be overstated. Much of the work is common sense, but the importance of doing this work lies in carefully attending to the basic change process as a way to avoid the need for damage control later.

Peters and Waterman (1982) stressed that the greatest need people have is to find meaning in their work life. The job of managers is to help better create meaning through the use of stories, slogans, symbols, rituals, legends, and myths that convey the values, beliefs, and meanings shared among the staff. These managers have to function as passionate leaders to motivate staff.

The challenges of leadership belong to every nurse, not just those in formal management roles. Leadership at the staff level may simply take a different form—for example, a staff nurse adapting to a challenging patient assignment, taking initiative to change practice through performance improvement, or challenging the status quo is participating in unit culture construction. Further, staff nurses are critical to founding and maintaining a Magnet™-designated organization.

Implications

Nurse leaders armed with a valid and reliable assessment of current work cultures can identify strategic target areas for change. A thorough understanding of organizational culture and unit climate is a powerful diagnostic tool that may be used to identify both troubled units and high-performance areas. An effective organizational culture empowers nurses to practice fully within the scope of their knowledge and education. This may be seen in failure-to-rescue rates. Variance in failure-to-rescue rates for adverse events may signal key differences in work cultures within a hospital structure (Aiken et al., 1994).

The culture of a nursing unit practice environment may exert a significant and independent effect beyond that of staffing and skill mix by enhancing or impeding interventions once problems are detected. Nurses serve as the surveillance system for early detection of adverse events. The *right* number of nurses may have less influence on patient outcomes than the organization and structure of the work environment itself for nurses, including the perceived level of autonomy, the amount of control over their practice, and effective collaboration with physicians (Aiken et al., 2001; Sochalski et al., 1999; Sovie & Jawad, 2001).

CURRENT ISSUES AND TRENDS

At the beginning of the chapter, a number of forces were identified that have had significant influence in changing the culture of health care delivery. Several of these forces have particular impact on nursing care, and a brief discussion of them follows.

Patient-Centered and Family-Centered Care

The Institute of Medicine's *Crossing the Quality Chasm* (2001) has identified that the culture of patient care must transition from care that is driven by providers to care that is patient-centered and family-centered in which patient and family norms, values, and preferences are respected. The National Healthcare Quality Report from the Agency for Healthcare Research and Quality (2002) defined two aspects of patient-centered care: the patient experience and patient partnerships. The patient's experience of care includes communication, care, and understanding of the meaning of his or her illness. This approach changes the perspective from a patient with a disease to that of an individual with an experience.

Patient partnerships, the second dimension of patient-centered care, are formed when nurses are responsive to patient needs, values, and preferences and then customize the care to the patient. For example, when doing discharge teaching, information that is of high importance and value to the patient is addressed first in a patient-centered model of care. As patient advocates, nurses can be leaders in transitioning an organizational culture from provider-driven care to care that is truly patient-centered.

Generational Diversity and the Nursing Shortage

The importance of a positive work climate on organizational, patient, and nurse outcomes is firmly established and evidence-based. However, creating a work environment for nurses that meets their personal and professional values is a challenge for most nursing leaders. Nurses from the Baby Boomer generation and Generation X make up more than 80% of the nursing workforce (U.S. Department of Health and Human Services, 2004). Because nurses from each of these generations were raised with a different set of priorities and values, a work environment supportive to each generation is an important retention strategy. For example, Baby Boomer nurses value rewards. Recognition and pay may be motivators for them. In contrast, Generation X nurses are concerned with a better balance of work and life (Duchscher & Cowin, 2004). In its 2002 report "Health Care's Human Crisis: The American Nursing Shortage," the Robert Wood Johnson Foundation provided a comprehensive overview of the nurse shortage. A core recommendation was the need to reinvent work environments to address and appeal to needs and values of both new and experienced generations of nurses (Kimball & O'Neill, 2002).

Tailoring the work environment to meet generational and life-stage needs is a recurrent theme in being able to successfully address the shortage and deliver the desired care system. The current and future workforce shortages are compelling realities that have relevance for organizations and leaders who must create cultures that promote a positive work environment for all employees.

Models of Care

A movement is underway to shift from restructuring to developing unit-level models of care that will transform health care systems. Multiple internal and external forces require financial accountability, competitive posture, and change in the structure of care processes. Ensuring the delivery of safe and effective quality care demands flexibility and engagement of leaders and staff nurses in changing work processes. The term *model of care* surfaces frequently; however, the specifics of how to construct such a model seem elusive. A direct link exists between this concept and *culture.*

Practical Tips

Tip #1: Examine the Socialization of New Nurses

Examine the practices of how new nurses are socialized to your unit. Do the practices reflect the values of your unit? Of your organization?

Tip #2: Understand Unit Climate and Diverse Workforce

At the next staff meeting, ask your staff to identify three areas that would improve the climate of the unit. Note whether nurses from different generations focus on different aspects of the work environment.

Tip #3: Generate Enthusiasm for Learning

For the next month, listen to what staff members mention during report, in rounds, or in general conversation about ways to improve practice. Write down this information, and keep a running list. At a subsequent staff meeting, let staff know how often they had ideas to improve practice and the content of their suggestions. Form a task force of interested staff to choose one of those suggested improvements and begin a search for the evidence.

PART I

Development of a new model must be preceded by assessment of the unit culture, an understanding of the patient population, what members of the staff need to care for them, and what roles are required to form the unit team. There is no one right model, nor does one size fit all settings. The work entails a deliberative process to facilitate change that will improve outcomes. Culture development must be an essential component of any new model development.

Summary

- Understanding organizational culture is important for successful functioning.
- Culture gives meaning to behavior and influences decision making.
- Culture is shared values and beliefs.
- Culture is determined by organizational factors that are both visible and invisible.
- Climate is the perception of what it feels like to work on a specific unit.
- Climate has elements that can be identified and measured.
- Cultures and climate can and should be built and sustained by nurse leaders with staff.
- Culture and climate elements can influence patient outcomes and retention.
- A positive patient safety climate is one in which there is a balance of learning and accountability.
- Learning climates value curiosity that leads to new ideas, thinking, and practices.

CASE STUDY

In response to an anticipated workforce shortage, the patient service leadership team of one organization elected to collaborate with human resources to develop a strategy for future success. It quickly became clear that planning for the shortage translated to crafting a plan for the future and was far greater than recruitment and retention. The work evolved into a broad initiative with a vision, guiding principles, core strategies, expected outcomes, and development of a leadership infrastructure. This work, called *Striving for Excellence*, was intended to change the culture. The work plan included extensive communication of the vision, identification of key stakeholders, assessment of the current and desired future state, gap analysis, and implementation plan. The vision was translated into actionable concrete steps that engaged nurse managers and staff at the unit level in the change process.

A nurse manager identified patient safety as a high-risk issue for the population of children on an inpatient psychiatric unit. A review of the literature substantiated that traumatic sequelae resulted from the use of restraints. Furthermore, regulatory agencies mandated a reduction in the use of restraints.

Challenges facing this manager were cultural resistance, knowledge deficits, and a changing patient population. The *Striving for Excellence* vision served as a unifying concept, and change theory provided the framework for mobilizing staff commitment. Psychodynamic concepts helped ensure that the change was integrated into clinical practice. Use of restraints was viewed as a treatment failure, and staff experienced a shift in thinking; that is, interventions moved from stopping aberrant behavior through use of restraints to reflection about what the behavior meant. Outcomes demonstrated a 60% reduction in the use of restraints; this resulted in a sustained change in practice for that nursing unit and has been recognized as a best-practice model. The nurse manager astutely summarized the real work as culture change.

CRITICAL THINKING EXERCISE

Hospital Y made a strategic decision to transform a 12-bed rehabilitation unit that had operated for 30 years and was a recognized leader in excellent multidisciplinary care for patients and families. The experienced nursing staff had low turnover and enjoyed strong partnerships with physicians, social workers, physical therapists, and occupational therapists.

The new unit was designed to meet the acute care needs of older patients with medical diagnoses. The change introduced an entirely new patient population and called for development of a new model of care for acutely ill older patients who would experience a significantly shorter length of stay than would a rehabilitation patient population. Subsequently, a new team of caregivers had to be identified to create new processes of care to ensure effective outcomes.

1. What is the problem?
2. Identify challenges faced by the manager and staff.
3. What steps would you take to define the new model of care?
4. How will the culture of this unit change?
5. What can the staff do?

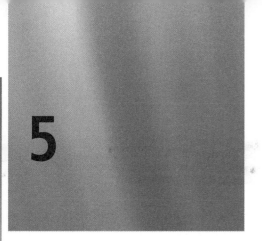

5

Critical Thinking and Decision-Making Skills

Betsy Frank

CHAPTER OBJECTIVES

- Define and describe critical thinking, problem solving, and decision making
- Explore the relationship between critical thinking, problem solving and decision making in nursing practice, leadership, and management
- Understand why critical thinking, problem solving, and decision making are foundational skills for nurse managers and leaders
- Describe various models for problem solving and decision making
- Exercise critical thinking and decision-making skills to conceptualize and analyze possible solutions to a practice exercise

PART II

Critical thinking, problem solving, and decision making are important skills for nurses caring for patients and for nurse leaders and managers (Thomas & Herrin, 2008a). In a fast-paced health care delivery environment, staff nurses, leaders, and managers must be able to analyze and synthesize a large array of information to solve complex problems that occur in complex health care delivery systems. To deliver effective patient care, they also must be able to use critical thinking and decision making to solve organizational system and bedside patient care problems (see Figure 5.1) (Grossman, 2007).

Nurses are a cadre of knowledge workers within the health care system. As such, they need information, resources, and support from their environment. The environment surrounding this system has moved from a process-oriented system characterized by a reliance on procedures and controlled by the providers to a system that is outcome-driven, evidence-based, best practice–oriented, and controlled by the user (Porter-O'Grady, 2003). The emergence of managed care as a dominant form of health care financing and delivery has created upheaval in clinical practice. However, the savings from managed care have disappeared as health insurance premiums have experienced double-digit inflation (Emmanuel, 2002). In acute care hospitals and other health care delivery settings, complexity, change, and unpredictability in the environment have left nurses with increased uncertainty and a perception that critical information for decision making has been lacking (Peters, 2002). With the Magnet™ hospital and other quality initiatives, nurses are coming to expect that they will participate in shared decision making among themselves and other health care providers (Thomas & Herrin, 2008b). Therefore participation in concert with others in decision making within health care organizations requires that nurses have expertise in critical thinking and problem solving, an expertise that use skills and knowledge, as well as creativity and intuition. Just as intuition is part of expert clinical practice (Benner, 1984), intuition plays an important role in developing managerial and leadership expertise (Shirey, 2007). In fact, all problem solving and decision making may have an intuitive component (Gladwell, 2005).

DEFINITIONS

Critical thinking can be defined as a set of cognitive skills including "interpretation, analysis, evaluation, inference, explanation, and self-regulation" (Facione, 2007, p. 1). Using these skills, nurses in direct patient care and leaders and managers can reflect analytically, reconceptualize events, and avoid the tendency to make decisions and problem solve hastily or on the basis of inadequate information. Facione also pointed out that critical thinking is not only a skill but also a disposition that is grounded in a strong ethical component.

Critical thinking in nursing can be defined as the following (Scheffer & Rubenfeld, 2000):

> ...an essential component of professional accountability and quality nursing care. Critical thinkers in nursing exhibit these habits of the mind: confidence, contextual perspective, creativity, flexibility, inquisitiveness, intellectual integrity, intuition, open-mindedness, perseverance, and reflection. Critical thinkers in nursing practice the cognitive skills of analyzing, applying standards, discriminating, information seeking, logical reasoning, predicting and transforming knowledge. (p. 357)

Furthermore, critical thinking in nursing, unlike Facione's more general definition, involves creativity, intuition, and transforming knowledge (Rubenfeld & Scheffer, 2006). Critical thinking is a higher-order mode of thinking (Lemire, 2002) and is much more than the just the five steps of the nursing process (Tanner, 2000).

A **problem** is defined as a deficit or surplus of something that is necessary to achieve one's goals. It can be thought of as a difference or gap between what exists and a goal. Thus a problem is a deficiency or undesirable current state (Le Storti et al., 1999). Solving problems involves moving from an undesirable to a desirable state (Chambers, 2009). Given this broad definition, no wonder Le Storti and colleagues stated that all nursing practice is problem solving. Chambers reinforced this notion by stating that problem solving occurs in a variety of nursing contexts including case management, direct client care, and team leadership. Problems exist where outcomes need to be achieved (Pesut & Herman, 1999). Problems present opportunities for decision making and change and require critical thinking to arrive at the best solution (Finkelman, 2001). The logical extension of this would be that **problem solving** is the process of fixing something that needs to be fixed. Nurses are challenged to supplement traditional problem-solving techniques with creative thinking (Chambers, 2009; Rubenfeld & Scheffer, 2006).

A **decision** is a choice among alternatives. Drummond (2001) states that **decision making** is making choices that will provide maximum benefit.

LEADING & MANAGING DEFINED

Critical Thinking
Interpretation, analysis, evaluation, inference, explanation, and self-regulation.

Problem
A deficit or surplus of something that is necessary to achieve one's goals.

Problem Solving
The process of fixing something that needs to be fixed.

Decision
A choice among alternatives.

Decision Making
The process of making choices that will provide maximum benefit.

He goes on to say, however, that those making decisions can never be sure of the outcome of their actions.

Decision making can also be defined as a behavior exhibited in selecting and implementing a course of action from alternative courses of action for dealing with a situation or problem. It may or may not be the result of an immediate problem. The problem-solving process is initiated as the result of an immediate problem. Decision making, however, may occur some time later. Both problem solving and decision making use information and draw conclusions about that information. Both require critical thinking. Values, life experiences, and individual thinking preferences create variability in these processes. Problem solving includes a decision-making step. Because problems change over time, decisions made at one point in time may need to be changed (Choo, 2006).

The process of selecting one course of action from alternatives forms the basic core of the definition of decision making. Choo (2006) noted that all decisions are bounded by cognitive and mental limits, how much information is processed, and values and assumptions. In other words, no matter the decision-making process, all decisions are limited by a variety of known and unknown factors. As a result, all decisions will have unanticipated consequences.

BACKGROUND

Critical Thinking

Critical thinking is both an attitude toward handling issues and a reasoning process. Critical thinking is not synonymous with problem solving and decision making (Figure 5.1), but certainly effective problem solving and concurrent decision making cannot occur without critical thinking (Lemire, 2002). Figure 5.2 illustrates the way obstacles such as poor judgment or biased thinking create detours to good judgment and effective decision making. Critical thinking helps overcome these obstacles. Critical thinking skills may not come naturally. The nurse who is a critical thinker has to be open-minded and have the ability to reflect on present and past actions and to analyze complex information.

Critical thinking is a skill that is developed for clarity of thought and improvement in problem-solving effectiveness. The roots of the concept of critical thinking can be traced to Socrates, who developed a method of probing questioning as a way of thinking more clearly and with greater logical consistency. He demonstrated that people often cannot rationally justify confident claims to knowledge. Confused meanings, inadequate evidence, or self-contradictory beliefs may lie below the surface of rhetoric. Therefore it is important to ask deep questions and probe into thinking sequences, seek evidence, closely examine reasoning and assumptions, analyze basic concepts, and trace out implications. Other thinkers, such as Plato, Aristotle, Thomas Aquinas, Francis Bacon, and Descartes, emphasized the importance of systematic critical thinking and the need for a systematic disciplining of the mind to guide it in clarity and precision of thinking. In the early 1900s, Dewey equated critical thinking with reflective thought (The Critical Thinking Community, 2008). Critical thinking, then, is characterized by thinking that has a purpose, is systematic, considers alternative viewpoints, occurs within a frame of reference, and is grounded in information (The Critical Thinking Community, 2008).

Questioning is implicit in the critical thinking process. The following are some of the questions to be asked when thinking critically about a problem or issue (Elder & Paul, n.d.):

- What is the question being asked?
- Is this the right question?
- Is there another question that must be answered first?

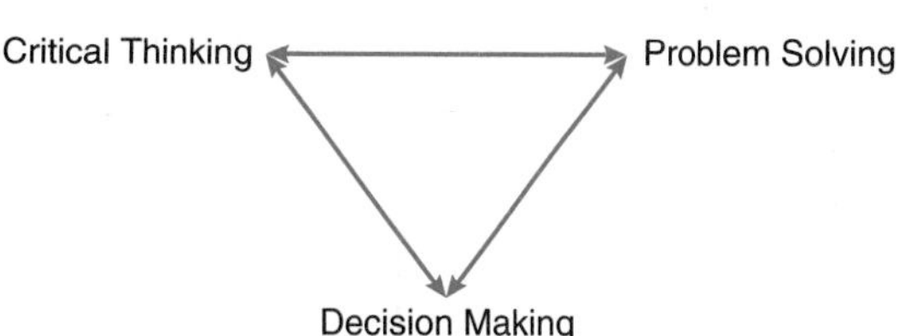

Figure 5.1
Differences and interactions among critical thinking, problem solving, and decision making.

PART II

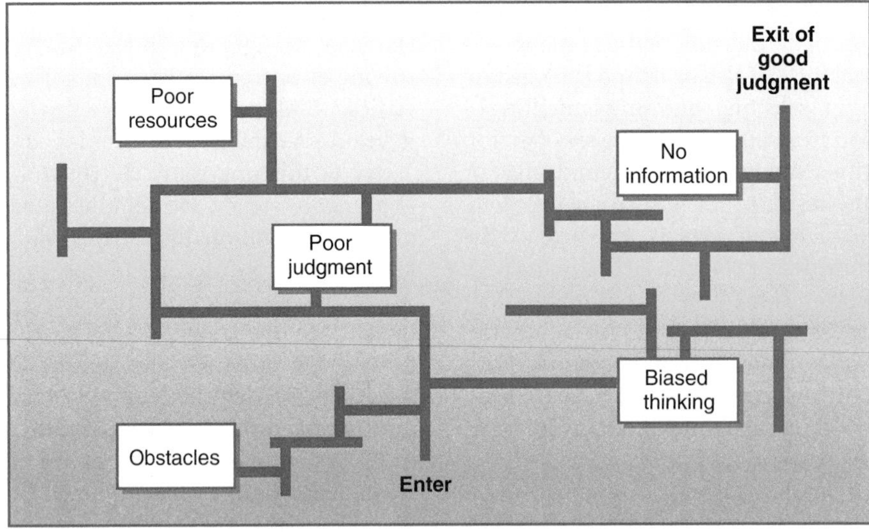

Figure 5.2
The problem-solving maze.

- What information is needed?
- Given the information, what conclusions are justified?
- Are there alternative viewpoints?

No matter what questions are asked, critical thinkers need to know the "why" of the thinking, the mode of reasoning (inductive or deductive), what the source and accuracy of the information is, what the underlying assumptions and concepts are, and what might be the outcome of the thinking (The Critical Thinking Community, 2008).

Critical Thinking in Nursing

Nurses in clinical practice continually make judgments and decisions based on the assessment and diagnosis of client needs and practice problems or situations. Clinical judgment is a complex skill grounded in critical thinking. Clinical judgment results in nursing actions directed toward achieving health outcomes (Pesut & Herman, 1999). Scheffer and Rubenfeld (2000) have stated that habits of the mind that are characteristic of critical thinking by nurses include confidence, contextual perspective, creativity, flexibility, inquisitiveness, intellectual integrity, open-mindedness, perseverance, and reflection. Emphasizing the value of expert experience and holistic judgment ability, Benner (2003) cautioned that clinical judgments must not rely too heavily on technology and that the economic incentives to use technology must not come at the expense of human critical thinking and reasoning in individual cases.

Critical thinkers have been distinguished from traditional thinkers in nursing. A traditional thinker, thought to be the norm in nursing, preserves status quo. A critical thinker challenges and questions the norm. Unlike traditional thinkers, critical thinkers are creative in their thinking and anticipate the consequences of their thinking (Rubenfeld & Scheffer, 2006). As McNichol (2002) noted, creative thinking leads to a more responsive and effective health care system because more solutions to problems are generated.

Nurse leaders and managers have an obligation to create care delivery climates that promote critical thinking, which leads to innovative solutions to problems within the system of care (McNichol, 2002; Porter-O'Grady et al., 2005). Such a climate encourages deep reflection, especially so that nurses feel safe to learn from mistakes, and encourages nurses to ask questions and consider a variety of viewpoints and alternative solutions to problems.

What specific strategies can be used to promote a climate in which critical thinking is fostered? First and foremost, the nurse manager/leader, in the role of mentor, coach, or preceptor, should encourage questions such as "Is what you are doing or proposing based on sound evidence?" (Ignatavicius, 2008). As managers, allowing staff and self "think time" is essential for reflection and is a key component of critical thinking (Albarran, 2004; Hader, 2005). Albarran suggested other strategies such as facilitating creative problem solving and having an "idea of the month," which promotes innovation. He went on to say that the use of evidence-based practice protocols is important but should not negate creative implementation of the protocols in order to accommodate individual patient responses to interventions.

Coaching new and experienced nurses to develop expertise in clinical judgment is critically important. Many new nurses, in particular, need to further develop their critical thinking skills (del Bueno, 2005; Etheridge, 2007). In addition to having preceptors and others ask questions of new nurses, nurse managers and leaders can use other strategies to enhance critical thinking in nursing staff. Use of critical pathways and the development of other cognitive shortcuts can foster a proactive approach to management of clinical problems, and critical thinking helps the nurse evaluate the appropriateness of care delivered within the critical pathway framework (Ferrario, 2004).

Developing concept maps is another useful strategy to promote critical thinking. Although typically used in pre-licensure programs (Ellermann et al., 2006), nurse managers can encourage their preceptors to use concept maps with orientees (Toofany, 2008). Developing concept maps in concert with others further develops a nurse's critical thinking through the process of dialogue. Simulations also promote critical thinking or "thinking like a nurse" (Tanner, 2006). According to Tanner, simulations can promote clinical reasoning, which leads to making conclusions in the form of clinical judgments and, thus, effective problem solving. The use of human patient simulators is well known in educational settings. Simulators may also be useful in orienting new graduates to the acute care setting (Ackermann et al., 2007). Ackermann and colleagues have reported that the use of simulators as part of the orientation process may promote role socialization and subsequent job retention.

Problem Solving

Creativity and problem solving are inextricably linked. Creative problem solving is defined as "thinking directed toward the achievement of a goal by means of a novel and appropriate idea or product" (Le Storti et al., 1999). This statement implies that if leaders and managers act without thinking, results may be less than desirable (Menkes, 2006). Although, traditionally, problem solving has emphasized rational, logical thought, creativity is essential if the best clinical outcomes are to be achieved.

Creative problem solving rests on two principles: *deferred judgment* and *divergent-convergent thinking sequences.* Deferred judgment means the temporary suspension of criticism or evaluation. This is important for the generation of unique and useful ideas. Deferring judgment helps eliminate bias and jumping to quick conclusions (Le Storti et al., 1999). Divergent-convergent thinking sequences are an opening up to possibilities, followed by the subsequent selection of the most promising ones. This means that several alternative problem statements are generated in such a way as to offer different perspectives and different senses of direction for solving a problem. The divergent questions are then evaluated, and selection converges on one path to take (Le Storti et al., 1999). The goal is to develop innovative problem-solving strategies that are productive and useful. Brainstorming is one strategy for generating multiple solutions to problems at hand (Buhler, 2004).

Another aspect of effective problem solving is incorporating cultural sensitivity into defining and solving problems (Smith-Trudeau, 2006). When nurse leaders and managers fail to consider differing cultural interpretations of issues, respect may be perceived as lacking, conflict may arise, and consequently the problem solving can be sabotaged. Not taking ownership for problems can also derail effective problem solving (Cox, 2005). Effective teams need to ask why, what, and how. However, asking who and acknowledging that the "who" may be a team member facilitate the problem-solving process.

Problem-solving activity has been conceptualized from two points of view: (1) individual or clinical problem solving and (2) managerial problem solving. At the level of an individual, problem solving is viewed as intimately related to how the individual processes information. In health care, a concern about accuracy and effectiveness has placed an emphasis on diagnostic reasoning and clinical decision making. Problem solving becomes more complex for managers in organizations because of multiple stakeholders and the dynamic state in which it occurs; thus managerial problem solving rests on an understanding of general systems theory (Lemire, 2002). General systems theory postulates that a change in one part of a system affects all other parts of the system. Because of these dynamic effects, problem-solving effectiveness requires the incorporation of what systems effects will result from a decision. Frequently, groups, often interdisciplinary (Forman, 2006), are involved in problem solving, so the need is greater for interaction, a slower process, and a consensus. Problems may have to be solved at the best possible level rather than at an ideal level.

Problem solving as a process can be linked to the delivery of nursing care and the organizational change process. A classic problem-solving model has been proposed by deChesnay (1983). Some situations produce problems (a difficulty), others create problems in which conflicts arise (a dilemma), and yet others become problems in which the solution appears to not have a logical path (a paradox). The complexity of decision making and its psychological impact increase as the situation moves along a hierarchy from difficulty to paradox. Thus problems can be categorized by their level of complexity. Once categorized, the nursing process and the change process can then be applied to strategically enhance problem solving. The problem can be framed as either an individual's problem or a system's problem. The evaluation of the outcome of problem solving involves an assessment of effectiveness. If the problem is resolved, the problem-solving process would be judged as effective. It would be judged ineffective if the problem stayed the same or worsened (deChesnay, 1983).

Because each situation is different in complexity, managing a difficulty, dilemma, or paradox may require different strategies depending on the situation. A difficulty may be only a minor problem and may need only a straightforward solution. A dilemma results from the combination of a difficulty plus conflict. One example occurs with values differences, such as when professional values clash with the values of the client. For example, a nurse may decide that being with a spouse undergoing medical tests is more important than being on the job, whereas the nurse manager may view the situation otherwise (Smith-Trudeau, 2006). In this case, both the nurse and the nurse manager need to use critical thinking to resolve the inevitable conflict. A paradox is a situation in which no logical solution to the problem exists (deChesnay, 1983). In practice, paradoxes are found commonly within ethical issues. Ethical principles often are applied in critical thinking and decision making, especially when there is no clear right answer.

Newell and Simon (1972) defined human problem solving as *information processing*. Information-processing behavior depends on the characteristics of the problem solver and the task. In nursing, the concepts of the nursing process, clinical decision making, and nursing informatics are discussed in relation to problem solving as information processing.

The nursing process is a generic problem-solving strategy widely applicable in practice, but the delivery of nursing care that is approached solely on a rigidly standardized step-by-step nursing process has been called into question (Tanner, 2000, 2006). According to Tanner, who has built on earlier work by Benner (1984), step-by-step approaches must incorporate pattern recognition or an "intuitive clinical grasp" (p. 205). Moreover, Taylor (1997) showed that novice nurses differed from more expert nurses in their diagnostic rea-

Practical Tips

Tip #1: Make Time to Reflect

Reflection is a key component of critical thinking. Make time in your day to think about your practice and reflect upon what could be improved.

Tip #2: Perform a Critical Review of Practice Protocols

Creativity and the use of evidence-base practice protocols are important tools for managerial and clinical decision making. The use of critical thinking skills will help you know when established protocols or policies should be altered in their implementation.

Tip #3: Create Collaboration

A key characteristic of complex adaptive organizations/Magnet™ hospitals is collaboration. Each person can foster shared decision making and promote a climate in which creative problem solving can take place.

soning abilities used in clinical problem solving. In some instances, novice nurses did not independently problem solve but, rather, copied a more expert nurse's performance. Kennedy (2002) found that nurses use cue interpretation from data presented before a patient encounter to begin to define the problem at hand. This highlights the complexity of problem solving and decision making in nursing practice.

Problem-Solving Styles

Many organizational interactions occur around the need to identify, define, and solve problems. Individuals appear to have a relatively stable personality-related problem-solving style. It appears that problem-solving styles have an influence on how well people can work together. Furthermore, personality style relates to how an individual acquires, stores, retrieves, and transforms information (Kirton, 1994). Thus a relationship may exist between problem-solving style and effectiveness in any given situation. As with leadership style, no one style is optimal. The effectiveness of a style is situational, determined by what is appropriate to the circumstances.

The Kirton Adaption-Innovation Theory identified two types of problem solvers: adaptors and innovators. Adaptors seek solutions to problems in tried and accepted ways. They are focused on resolving problems rather than finding them. They rarely challenge rules and are methodical, reliable, and efficient. Innovators are the opposite. They seek solutions to problems in original, creative, and challenging ways. They discover problems and avenues for resolution. Innovators question current practices and promote changes. Kirton's theory supports the characteristics of critical thinkers as having various problem-solving styles. Although different ways of thinking about problem-solving styles exist, by using the critical thinking skills of reflection and analysis, a nurse can increase self-awareness and knowledge about alternative ways of acting on problems.

Steps in the Problem-Solving Process

The steps of the problem-solving process are listed somewhat differently in various literature sources. Box 5.1 provides a seven-step general framework for problem solving drawn from various sources (Davidhizar & Bowen, 1999; Facione, 2007; Finkelman, 2001). In no way, however, is it implied that the process is linear or assumed to occur in a straight-line fashion from step 1 to step 7. In fact, the process is iterative. This means that

Box 5.1

Seven Steps of Problem Solving

1. Define the problem.
2. Gather information.
3. Determine desired outcome.
4. Develop solutions.
5. Consider consequences.
6. Make decisions.
7. Implement and evaluate solutions.

information and activities of one step feed back into the dynamic process, and the cycle of steps may start over again before completing all steps. For example, as information is gathered, a problem might have to be redefined; as solutions are generated, new information may come to light that, in turn, may yet again redefine the problem. The seven steps can be interpreted as follows:

1. *Define the problem.* Does a problem really exist that requires an investment in time and resources to solve? Perhaps an already existing protocol can be used to deal with the issue at hand. On the other hand, perhaps the problem in question really consists of more than one problem, or perhaps what appears to be a problem may not require action at all (Davidhizar & Bowen, 1999). Clearly, formulating the problem may be helped by refining a written statement of the problem (e.g., "The problem is …").
2. *Gather information.* The problem solver cannot overestimate the critical importance of this step. Too often, people start the problem-solving process without having spent enough time gathering information about the problem. It is important to start by gathering as much input and information as possible from a variety of sources. Shortening the information-gathering process to save time may cause difficulty later. The information must be analyzed by separating important from peripheral information, and timetables of prior events may need to be determined to gain a full understanding of the problem (Finkelman, 2001). Part of gathering information includes defining the context of the problem (Facione, 2007).
3. *Determine the overall goal or desired outcome.* This step guides decision making and actions toward the desired outcome. An outcomes focus contributes to the effectiveness of chosen activities. In fact, determining the overall goal can illuminate the need for more information, as well as facilitate the generation of possible solutions (Pesut & Herman, 1999).
4. *Develop solutions*. Notice that the word *solutions* is plural. A problem suggests more than one alternative solution (Davidhizar & Bowen, 1999; Finkelman, 2001). People have choices, and problems have solutions. It may be that in the whole array of multiple solutions to any problem, none of them are particularly enticing. However, solutions or multiple options to any given problem situation always exist. Expanding the ability to look at problems as always having a potential for multiple solutions is a key conceptual element in dealing with problems. It helps avoid knee-jerk reactions that occur when the problem is identified without careful deliberation or critical thinking. It may be seductive to shortcut the time and energy involved with careful problem analysis and take an easily available solution, but this jeopardizes effectiveness.
5. *Consider the consequences.* This step should be done carefully for each alternative solution. The first action is to list the potential consequences. This is a critical thinking strategy. It requires a broad perspective that includes all potential consequences. The problem solver's values will play a role in the analysis and evaluation of the consequences. For example, a consequence seen as very negative by one person may be perceived as less so by another. A careful analysis of the available options is essential (Facione, 2007).

6. *Make a decision*. This is the decisive action stage. At some point, analysis needs to be brought to closure and a decision made. Various techniques are useful for driving decision making to one selected choice. One useful strategy is to explicitly list why certain choices were chosen over another (Facione, 2007).
7. *Implement and evaluate the solution*. This is the action and feedback stage. The results of the problem-analysis and decision-making cognitive processes now culminate in the direct action determined as necessary to be taken. This step may require risk and courage. Periodic checks on effectiveness need to be made and then fed back into the problem-solving process. Some people can never seem to get to this stage. They cannot seem to generate solutions. Observe your colleagues. Are they problem identifiers? Some people have great difficulty clearly identifying the problem. Others can easily figure out what the problem is but then cannot get beyond problem identification. Are individuals solution generators? Or are they locked into preformed ideas, a type of "hardening of the concepts"? If they are able to generate solutions, can they then move into the risk-taking steps of making a decision and implementing a solution? The evaluation aspect involves doing a check and asking whether anything was missed. This self-correcting measure will help ensure that the best decision has been made (Facione, 2007).

Some questions to ask during problem solving that promote critical thinking include the following:

- What specifically is the problem?
- Why, how, and to whom is it a problem?
- Why should anything be done about it?
- What are the facts, and what do they mean?
- What are the possible solutions?
- Which solutions are acceptable?
- What is the ideal or preferred solution?
- What is the best solution?
- Will it work? Is it worth doing?
- Is it the right thing to do?

Problem solving starts with an awareness of a problem. Perhaps a nurse announces that there is a problem, such as not having enough linen on the night shift in a hospital. The questions just listed might be asked of the nurse as a clarification process. An example of the problem-solving process in action is the following:

- What are the facts? Linens usually run out before 4 AM.
- What do the facts mean? Was not enough linen ordered? Is linen being horded in patient rooms?
- What kind of solution should be sought? Should the linen cart always have sufficient linen? Should nurses remove linen only as needed? There are inventory costs to consider.
- Is the optimal or ideal solution desired, or is it best to look for a solution that is just adequate? Is any solution that comes along acceptable? Is having more than enough or just enough linen the goal?
- What are the possible solutions? Should linen be ordered twice a day? Should nurses be more careful in removing linen from the cart?
- Which one is the best solution? Will it work, and is it worth doing? Does a new process need to be formulated when current procedures may really be adequate? Does more linen really need to be ordered? If so, what are the budgetary consequences?

This process of critical thinking aids careful deliberations and forms the foundation for effective decision making.

Decision Making

Decision making is the essence of leadership and management. It is what leaders and managers are expected to do (Keynes, 2008). Thus decisions are visible outcomes of the leadership and management process. The effectiveness of decision making is one criterion for evaluating a leader or manager. Yet, staff nurses and nurse managers and leaders must make decisions in uncertain (Drummond, 2001) and complex (Clancy & Delaney, 2005) environments.

Within a climate of uncertainty and complexity, nurse managers and leaders must also understand that all decision making involves high-stakes risk taking (Clancy & Delaney, 2005; Keynes, 2008). If poor decisions are made, progress can be impeded, resources wasted, harm or damage caused, and a career adversely affected. The results of poor decisions may be subtle and not appear until years later. Take, for instance, a decision to reduce expenses by decreasing the ratio of registered nurses to nurses' aides. There may be a short-term cost savings, but if not implemented appropriately, this tactic may result in the gradual erosion of patient care over time. Unintended effects may include higher turnover of experienced nurses, increased adverse events such as medication errors, decreased staff morale, and lower patient satisfaction scores. The long-term outcome of this decision may actually result in the opposite of the original objective—that of reducing expenses. Thus it is vital for nurses to understand decision making and explore styles and strategies to enhance decision-making skills. "Effective decision-making, however, is contingent on many factors, not the least of which is the unique information processing of individual staff" (Clancy & Delaney, 2005, pp. 194-195).

Decision making, like overall problem solving, can be thought of as a process with identifiable steps yet influenced by the context and by whether there is an intuitive grasp of the situation. Nurses make decisions in personal, clinical, and organizational situations and under conditions of certainty, uncertainty, and risk. Various decision-making models and strategies exist. Nurses' control over decision making may vary as to amount of control and where in the process they can influence decisions. Awareness of the components, process, and strategies of decision making contributes to effectiveness in nursing leadership and management decision making. The basic elements of problem solving and decision making can be summarized into the following two parts: (1) identifying the problem and (2) making the decision. According to Finkelman (2001), the steps of the decision-making process are as follows (p. 55):

- Recognize and define the process.
- Gather relevant data or information.
- Identify possible solutions or options to solve a problem or deal with an issue.
- Reach a decision.
- Evaluate the results.
- Test or assess the solutions.

Notice, then, how these steps are analogous to the problem-solving process. In other words, step 6 of the 7-step problem solving process, called "Make a Decision," involves the problem-solving process. Thus decision making is used to solve problems.

But decision making is *more* than just problem solving. Decision making may also be the result of opportunities, challenges, or more long-term leadership initiatives as opposed to being triggered by an immediate problem. In any case, the processes are virtually the same but their purposes may be slightly different. Nurse managers use decision making in managing resources and the environment of care delivery. Management of decision making involves an evaluation of the effectiveness of the outcomes that result from the decision-making process.

Whether nurse managers are the sole decision makers or facilitate group decision making, all the factors that influence the problem-solving process also impact how decisions are made: who owns the problem that will result in a decision, what is the context of the decision to be made, and what lenses or perspectives influence the decision to be made? For example, the chief executive officer may frame issues as a competitive struggle not unlike a sports event. The marketing staff may interpret problems as military battles that need to be won. Nurse executives may view concerns from a care or family frame that emphasizes collaboration and working together. Learning and understanding which analogies and perspectives offer the best view of a problem or issue are vital to effective decision making. It may be necessary for nurse managers to expand their frame boundaries and be willing to consider even the most outlandish ideas. Obviously, it is important to begin the problem definition phase with staff members who are closest to the problem. However, it is wise to then consider adding individuals who have no connection with the issue whatsoever. Often it is these "unconnected" staff members who bring new decision frames to the meeting and have the most unbiased view of the problem. Often, decisions can originate within the confines of the shared governance system that may be in place within an organization (Dunbar et al., 2007). One of the core competencies for health professions education as outlined from the Institute of Medicine (IOM) (2003) is working in interdisciplinary teams. Therefore using interdisciplinary teams for problem solving and decision making can be assumed more effective in many instances. No matter who is involved in the decision-making process, the basic steps to arrive at a decision or resolve problems remain the same.

DECISION OUTCOMES

One critical aspect of both problem solving and decision making is to determine the desired outcome. The desired outcome may vary—from an ideal or short-term resolution to covering up the situation. What is desired may be (1) for the problem to go away forever, (2) to make sure that all involved in this problem are satisfied with the solution and gain some benefit from it, or (3) to obtain an ideal solution. Sometimes a quick decision is desired, and researching different aspects of the problem or allowing for participation in decision making is not appropriate. For example, in disaster management, the nurse leader will use predetermined procedures for determining roles of the various personnel involved (Coyle et al., 2007).

Desired decisions can be categorized into two end points: minimal and optimal. A minimal decision results in an outcome that is sufficient, satisfies basic requirements, and minimally meets desired objectives. This is sometimes called a *"satisficing" decision.* An *optimizing decision* includes comparing all possible solutions with desired objectives and then selecting the optimal solution that best meets objectives (Choo, 2006). In addition to these two strategies, Janis and Mann (1977) described two other strategies: mixed scanning and incrementalism. *Incrementalism* is slow progress toward an optimal course of action. *Mixed scanning* combines the stringent rationalism of optimizing with the "muddling through" approach of incrementalism to form substrategies. *Optimizing* has the goal of selecting the course of action with the highest payoff (maximization). Limitations of time, money, or people may prevent the decision maker from selecting the more deliberative and slower process of optimizing. Still, the decision maker needs to focus on techniques that will enhance effectiveness in decision-making situations.

Just as critical thinking and problem solving are not truly step-by-step processes, neither is decision making. Barriers exist and, once identified, can lead to going back through the decision-making process. Flaws in thinking can create hidden traps in decision making. These are common psychological tendencies that create barriers or biases in cognitive reflection and appraisal. Six common distortions are as follows (Hammond et al., 1998):

1. *Anchoring trap:* When a decision is being considered, the mind gives a disproportionate weight to the first information it receives. Trends and old numbers may become anchors, giving too much weight to past events. It is human nature to focus on an event that leaves a memorable or strong impression. All individuals have preconceived notions and biases that influence decisions in a variety of ways. For instance the Institute of Medicine (IOM, 2001) endorsed the use of computerized physician order entry (CPOE) as one solution to reduce medication errors. Following close on the heels of the IOM's report, the Leapfrog Group, a consortium of Fortune 500 companies, announced that use of a CPOE would be included as one of three criteria used to evaluate a health system's quality practices. Since both the IOM's and Leapfrog Group's announcements, the number of health systems purchasing CPOE systems has significantly increased. Aside from

the financial costs involved, human-factor errors and work-flow issues can hamper successful implementation (Campbell et al., 2006). Nurse executives should consider possible consequences carefully when evaluating new technology (Benner, 2003).

2. *Status-quo trap:* Decision makers display a strong bias toward alternatives that perpetuate the status quo. Often this is the result of accelerating change in the work environment. Past practices that exhibit any sense of permanence provide managers with a feeling of security. Maintaining the status quo thus holds a magnetic attraction.
3. *Sunk-cost trap:* Past decisions become sunk costs, and new choices are often made in a way that justifies past choices. This may result in becoming trapped by an escalation of commitment. Because of rapid, ongoing advances in medical technology, managers are frequently pressured to replace existing equipment before it is fully depreciated. If the new equipment provides a higher level of quality at a lower cost, the sunk cost of the existing equipment is irrelevant to the decision-making process. However, managers may delay purchasing new equipment and forgo subsequent savings because the equipment has yet to reach the end of its useful life.
4. *Confirming-evidence trap:* This bias leads people to seek out information that supports an existing instinct or point of view while avoiding contradictory evidence. A typical example is favoring new technology over less glamorous alternatives. A decision maker may become so enamored by technological solutions (and slick vendor demonstrations) that he or she may unconsciously decide in favor of these systems even though strong evidence supports implementing less costly solutions first.
5. *Framing trap:* The way a problem is initially framed profoundly influences the choices made. Different framing of the same problem can lead to different decision responses. A decision frame can be viewed as a window into the many and varied reasons a problem exists. As implied by the word *frame,* individuals may perceive problems only within the boundaries of their own frame. The human resources director may perceive a staffing shortage as a compensation problem, the chief financial officer as an insurance reimbursement issue, the director of education as a training issue, and the chief nursing officer as a work environment problem. It is obvious that all issues may contribute, in part, to the problem; however, each person, in looking through his or her individual frame, sees only that portion with which he or she is most familiar.
6. *Estimating and forecasting traps:* People make estimates or forecasts about uncertain events, but their minds are not calibrated for making estimates in the face of uncertainty. The notion that experience is the parent of wisdom suggests that mature managers, over the course of their careers, learn from their mistakes. It is reasonable to assume that the knowledge gained from a manager's failed projects would be applied to future decisions. As logical as this sounds, there is a tendency in human behavior to disregard negative outcomes and remember the positive ones (Belsky & Gilovich, 1999). Whether right or wrong, humans tend to take credit for successful projects and find ways to blame external factors on failed ones. Unfortunately, this form of overconfidence often results in overly optimistic projections in project planning. This optimism is usually buried in the analysis done before ranking alternatives and recommendations. Conversely, excessive cautiousness or prudence may also result in faulty decisions. Dramatic events may overly influence decisions because of recall and memory exaggerating the probability of rare but catastrophic occurrences. It is important that managers objectively examine project planning assumptions in the decision-making process to ensure accurate projections. Because misperceptions, biases,

and flaws in thinking can influence choices, actions related to awareness, testing, and mental discipline can be employed to ferret out errors in thinking before the stage of decision making (Hammond et al., 1998).

DECISION-MAKING SITUATIONS

The situations in which decisions are made may be personal, clinical, or organizational (Figure 5.3). Personal decision making is a familiar part of everyday life. Personal decisions range from multiple small daily choices to time management and career or life choices.

Clinical decision making in nursing relates to quality of care and competency issues. According to Tanner (2006), decision making in the clinical arena is called *clinical judgment.* In nursing, as with all health professions, clinical judgments should be patient-centered, use available evidence from research and other sources, and use available informatics tools (IOM, 2003). These crucial judgments should take place within the context of interdisciplinary collaboration. Within a hospital or other health care agency, a social network forms that is multidisciplinary (Tan et al., 2005). This social network has to collaborate for positive change within the organization and to make clinical decisions of the highest quality.

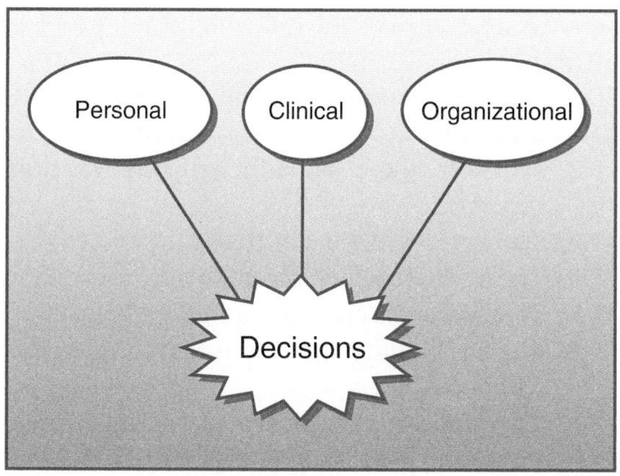

Figure 5.3
Decision-making situations.

Nurses manage care and make decisions under conditions of certainty, uncertainty, and risk. For example, if research has shown that, under prescribed conditions, the selection of a specific nursing intervention is highly likely to produce a certain outcome, then the nurse in that situation faces a condition of relative certainty. An example would be the prevention of decubitus ulcers by frequent repositioning. If little knowledge is available or if the specific situation is more complex or variant from the usual, then the nurse faces uncertainty. Risk situations occur when a threat of harm to clients exists. Conditions of risk occur commonly relative to the administration of medications, crisis events, infection control, invasive procedures, and the use of technology in nursing practice. Furthermore, these conditions also apply to the administration of nursing care delivery, in which decision making is a critical function.

Conditions of uncertainty and complexity are common in nursing care management. Over time, the complexity of health care processes has increased as a natural outgrowth of innovation and new technology. With computerized integration of billing, physician ordering, results of diagnostic tests, information about medications and their actions and side effects, and critical pathways and computerized charting, complexity may actually increase. Trying to integrate so many data points in care delivery can overwhelm the care provider who is making clinical judgments. As a result, subtle failures in any part of the information system can go unnoticed and have catastrophic outcomes (Perrow, 1984). For example, if a laboratory technician inputs the wrong diagnostic test results, treatment decisions based on those results could bring about an adverse patient outcome. In addition to the information available in the organization's information system, ready access to the Internet and online library sources can further create complexity in the decision-making process.

Wading through vast amounts of data can be literally overwhelming to managers. In fact, terms such as "data smog" and "information overload" are creeping into the literature in response to the onslaught of mounting information (Shenk, 1997). It is imperative that technology be harnessed for nurses to augment data analysis and information delivery.

Nurse leaders are coming to understand that innovation and new technology are the driving forces behind the discovery of new knowledge and improvements in patient care. However, because earlier technology acts as the foundation for newer technology, future processes within the health care system will continue to show increasing complexity. Overlapping, unclear, and changing roles for nurses as a result of new technology and services create complex decision-making situations and impact the quality of care delivered (IOM, 2003).

ADMINISTRATIVE AND ORGANIZATIONAL DECISION MAKING

According to Choo (2006), organizations use information to "make decisions that commit resources and capabilities to purposeful action" (p. 1). Nurse managers, for example, make staffing decisions and thus commit financial resources for the purpose of delivering patient care.

Etzioni (1989) noted that the traditional model for business decisions was rationalism. However, he further asserted that as information flow became more complex and faster-paced, a new decision-making model based on the use of partial information that has not been fully analyzed had begun to evolve. He called this model "humble decision making."

This approach arises in response to the need to make a decision when the amount of data exceeds the time available to analyze it. For instance, predicting the outcome of clinical and administrative decisions in health care is problematic because such processes are collectively defined as complex adaptive systems (CAS). A CAS is characterized by groups of individuals who act in unpredictable, nonlinear (not cause and effect) ways, such that one person's actions affect all the others (Holden, 2005).

In CASs, humans do behave in unpredictable ways (Tan et al., 2005). Therefore the use of traditional planning tools that assume a linear cause-and-effect outcome often results in inaccurate predictions (Perrow, 1984). The consequences of such forecasts can be serious adverse outcomes. For example, if an organization commits to implementing a CPOE system without adequate resources devoted to physician buy-in, errors in treatments may actually increase rather than decrease (Sengstack & Gurerty, 2004). Another, perhaps unanticipated, consequence of a decision has been the adverse effect on patient care when the registered nurse staff has been decreased to save personnel dollars (Kane et al., 2007).

Decision making is also influenced by the manager's leadership style. A democratic/collaborative style of leadership and decision making works best in a complex adaptive system, such as a hospital, which is characterized by a large array of social relationships. However, the full array of leadership styles may at some time be used in the decision-making process. Vroom and Yetton (1973) proposed a managerial decision-making model that identified five managerial decision styles on a continuum from minimal subordinate involvement to delegation. Their model uses a contingency approach, which assumes that situational variables and personal attributes of the leader influence leader behavior and thus can affect organizational effectiveness. To diagnose the situation, the decision maker examines the following seven problem attributes:

1. The importance of the quality of the decision
2. Whether there is sufficient information/expertise
3. The amount of structure to the problem
4. The extent to which acceptance/commitment of followers is critical to implementation
5. The probability that an autocratic decision will be accepted
6. The motivation of followers to achieve organizational goals
7. The extent to which conflict over preferred solutions is likely

The nurse manager has a full range of decision-making styles available. The choice of style depends on the context for the decision to be made. The decision style should be matched to situational needs so the probability of effective decision making increases.

PROBLEM-SOLVING AND DECISION-MAKING TOOLS AND STRATEGIES

Various strategies are used for problem solving and decision making. These strategies are based on time and mental structure variations (e.g., fast, slow, impulsive, intuitive, or logical). Some formal decision-making strategies are discussed.

Trial and Error

In using trial and error, a shoot-from-the-hip or dart-throw type of solution is put into effect. A solution that seems attractive is chosen and simply tried out. Those managers who use trial and error as the usual strategy for decision making often are seen as ineffective. They are perceived as poor problem solvers. Evidence-based practice protocols have largely replaced trial-and-error decision making at the bedside (Cannon et al., 2007).

Pilot Projects

Pilot projects involve experimentation with limited trials. Pilot projects or carefully defined trials are used to experiment by trying out a solution alternative on a small or restricted basis to see whether major problems will occur and to reduce risk. Pilot project strategies may resemble research projects. These projects may also be linked to quality improvement initiatives.

Creativity Techniques

Creativity techniques include brainstorming sessions, the Delphi process, and nominal group techniques, in which a group gathers for free-thinking exercises (Van de Ven & Delbecq, 1974). They are especially suited to a complex problem that appears to have no good solution. Creativity techniques are used as a way to generate solutions, ideas, and thoughts by approaching the problem with freedom from preformed bias. Such techniques often are team-based strategies.

Decision Tree

A decision tree is a graphic model that visually displays the options, outcomes, and risks to be anticipated (see the Case Study at the end of this chapter). A decision tree starts to the left and flows to the right or starts at the top and flows to the bottom. A question or problem is posed, and the possible options become branching nodes. Thus decision paths can be traced through option points and beyond. For example, a very simple decision tree might start with the question "Are you committed to becoming a nurse?" The answer to that question is *yes* or *no*. Depending on the answer, the corresponding path is followed as mapped out on the decision tree. The tree enables visualization of the alternatives and their consequences. It helps with decision making through analysis and clarity (Pidgeon & Gregory, 2004).

Critical paths are similar to decision trees. Critical pathways are descriptions of the specific protocol steps needed for critical or key incidents that must occur in a predictable or timely order to keep the expected outcomes, length of stay, and overall costs appropriate. They are designed to be used with a defined patient population and are grounded within evidence-based practice (De Bleser et al., 2006). Critical pathways are designed to incorporate multidisciplinary perspectives and to display and track the client's entire expected course of treatment and expected outcomes. Variances are identified immediately and managed by the health care provider. Perhaps because critical paths are implemented within complex adaptive systems, their true effect on patient care outcomes has not been definitively demonstrated (Vanhaecht et al., 2006).

As nursing evolves in sophistication and knowledge base, with better identification of nursing diagnoses and the array of matching nursing interventions, standardized languages could be incorporated into decision trees that are readily accessible to nursing staff (Clancy et al., 2006).

Group Problem Solving and Decision Making

In the group problem-solving and decision-making technique, the leader calls the group together to discuss and participate in solving a problem. The leader invites participation, either in the problem-identification or the problem-resolution part of the decision-making process. Personality and leadership style appear to influence the effectiveness of group or team problem solving and decision making (Saulo, 1996). There are a number of models of group decision making. The four general models are as follows:

1. The rational model, based on an economic perspective of decision making and maximum utility
2. The political model, based on power, influence, negotiation, bargaining, and interest group influence
3. The process model, which uses standard operating procedures and guidelines
4. The "garbage can" model, characterized by difficult problem identification and difficult problem resolution under circumstances of ambiguity, complexity, and non-rationality

All these models can be used at one time or another, either singly or in combination, depending on the nature of the issue at hand. For example, when a problem involves budgetary allocations, the political model might be used. After an evidence-based practice guideline has been agreed upon, the process model might be used to implement the guideline.

Scenario Planning

Scenario planning is a problem-solving and decision-making strategy given an uncertain and changing future. It is a group process strategy that encourages group participants to create "possible future" stories. Thus it is forward-looking and appropriate for fluid and changing environments in which there are many possible futures. This technique asks the question "What if . . . ?"; then different stories of the future are described (scenarios). In this way, a wide array of perspectives is gathered and the entrenched mindset is overcome. Stories of the future are constructed in a way that highlights pathways, driving forces, turning points, and deep behavioral forces. Scenario planning helps illuminate early warning signs, trigger new opportunity ideas, and may protect from some risks.

Worst-Case Scenario

Worst-case scenario is especially helpful in making decisions that involve risk. Risky decisions frequently, but not always, relate to the use of money or prestige. In this technique, the "worst case" (i.e., everything that could go wrong does go wrong) is determined. The worst case is outlined for each known alternative. Then the alternative with the best result—when, or if, everything possible does go wrong—is selected. So if money or reputation is on the line, the "least of all the evils" is chosen. For instance, CPOE systems, if used correctly, have been shown to significantly reduce medication errors. However, because of the enormous cost and social change required to implement such systems, establishing an adequate return on the investment has been difficult. Unfortunately, documented savings from avoidable and unavoidable adverse drug events may be thought of as "soft" numbers and open to speculation. By determining the absolute worst that could happen and working backward from that scenario, the decision maker chooses the best alternative for the situation to minimize potential anticipated risk or damage.

In their book *Smart Choices,* Hammond and colleagues (1999) recommended creating a "consequences table" for addressing multiple alternatives. To develop such a table, list the problem consequences objectives along the left side of a page and the various alternatives along the top. To rate the ability of each alternative to meet the desired objective, create a standardized key that ranks each alternative. For example, consider the following problem statement regarding medication errors:

> *The rate of adverse drug events has exceeded the benchmark rate for three consecutive quarters. This has coincided with two sentinel events that required extended patient hospitalization and potential litigation.*

After a period of analysis, a cross-functional team lists the following alternatives as potential solutions to the medication error problem:

- Develop an automated medication administration system that includes bar coding, automated storage and control units on the floors, and robot technology.
- Implement CPOE with decision support.
- Standardize all medication abbreviations on order sheets.
- Remove high-risk drugs such as potassium chloride from ward stock, and place pharmacists on the floor to assist with medication orders.

Table 5.1 displays the desired objectives and a standardized key to analyze and rank them.

By ranking the various alternatives through a standardized key, a fair comparison among alternatives can assist managers eliminate undesirable choices. When developing a consequences table, it is important to view the long-term or downstream effects of implementing specific alternatives. Make sure to "play out" different scenarios and the tactics needed to overcome them. For instance, in evaluating whether to implement CPOE, several scenarios may result and need to be evaluated in planning and management. As shown in Table 5.2, identifying how one action can lead to another makes it possible to preempt significant barriers to implementation.

Computerized Decision Making

In the arena of decision-making strategies and analytical tools, there are also sophisticated and computerized forecasting techniques, such as linear programming models and mathematical techniques such as predictive modeling that assign a probability to each possible outcome and then run multiple analyses on multiple combinations. However, traditional analytic methods fail to capture the dynamic and nonlinear aspects of complex systems such as hospitals. Too often, as the number of variables and stochastic (i.e., containing random variables) cross-level interactions increases (as in human organizations), the computer time to solve the problem rises exponentially. As a result,

PART II

Table 5.1

Desired Objectives Analysis

Objective	Alternative A	Alternative B	Alternative C	Alternative D
1. Reduces the number of medication transactions	5	4	2	3
2. Enables medication administration through automation	5	4	2	2
3. Meet or exceeds net present value target	3	2	5	3
4. Meets regulatory standards	3	3	3	3
5. Improves accuracy	4	4	5	4
Total Score	**20**	**17**	**17**	**15**

1, Does not meet objective; *2,* meets some aspects of objective; *3,* meets objective; *4,* exceeds objective; *5,* significantly exceeds objective.

Table 5.2

Scenario Analysis: Implement CPOE on All Inpatient Units by a Given Date

Result Period #1	Result Period #2	Result Period #3
Physician response to training is poor, resulting in ...	Difficulty in operating the system, resulting in ...	The nursing staff having to use both a paper and an online record, leading to ...
There are many computer interface problems, resulting in ...	A slow, unreliable, and cumbersome system, leading to ...	Refusal of the staff to use the system, leading to ...
Physicians have to change their medication ordering practice, leading to ...	Longer patient rounding time, resulting in ...	A perception of less physician productivity, leading to ...

CPOE, Computerized physician order entry.

complex system problems quickly become intractable using standard statistical analysis tools. One tactic suggested in the IOM report to overcome this problem was to increase the use of simulation (computational modeling) as a decision tool in designing safer processes within complex hospital systems (IOM, 2001).

Computational Modeling

A computational modeling approach views organizations (hospitals and other community agencies) as a collection of computer-simulated agents that are both intelligent and adaptive. By conducting "virtual experiments," computational models can provide a "what-if" analysis of various tactics aimed at decision making. Although a variety of methods may be used, the general process for computational modeling begins with encoding a series of statements in propositional calculus, or "if . . ., then . . ." format, into a computer program. Using a series of computer algorithms, these statements can represent various theories and be analyzed to produce output that simulates corresponding social behavior. A computer modeling simulation has been used to demonstrate how a smallpox epidemic could be contained under various projected scenarios (Burke et al., 2006).

Six Sigma

Another group problem-solving and decision-making approach is *Six Sigma* (Morgan & Cooper, 2004). This statistical approach to problem solving reduces actions that can lead to errors and that have an adverse impact on patient outcomes and organizational financial outcomes. Precise data are gathered and analyzed statistically. Based on the data, process improvements are made. With this approach, the goal is a virtually error-free health care delivery environment.

LEADERSHIP AND MANAGEMENT IMPLICATIONS

Critical thinking skills enhance the quality of clinical judgment, problem solving, and decision making. Critical thinking skills are one of the top-rated competencies required for staff nurses (del Bueno, 2005) and nurse leaders and managers (Lemire, 2002) within this chaotic health care delivery system. Nursing problems may be complex and high-risk, necessitating thorough deliberation and some creativity. Problems can be solved and decisions made using a variety of tools and strategies. The nurse manager does not have to personally solve all the patient care problems that occur on a day-to-day basis. The focus of leadership and management decision

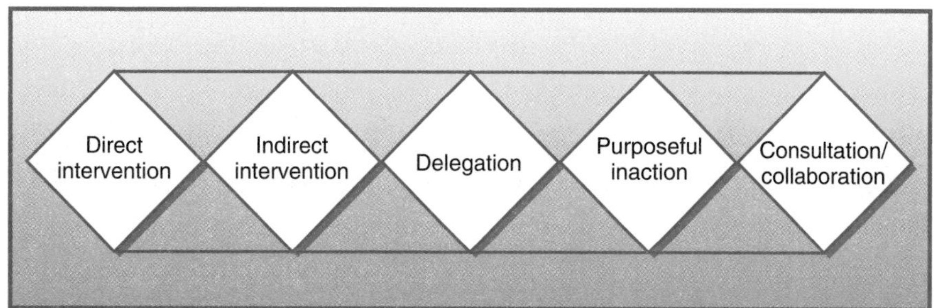

Figure 5.4
Strategies for problem solving.

making is more closely related to the nurse's role as care coordinator and systems problem solver.

Some problems, such as those requiring disciplinary action, do require the manager's *direct intervention.* In conflicts between staff members or between family and staff members, the manager might use negotiation and other forms of conflict management that could be viewed as *indirect intervention* because the manager does not actually solve the problem but, rather, persuades others to solve the problem themselves. The nurse manager might *delegate* the problem solving to others. For example, a unit manager might ask a team of staff nurses and the unit secretary to figure out when is the best time to order supplies for the unit.

Sometimes, the nurse manager might choose *watchful waiting.* A particular staff member might be causing some interpersonal difficulties. If the staff member has submitted his or her resignation, dealing with the behavior might not be worth the energy.

Most problem solving and decision making should take place within the confines of *collaboration and consultation.* Shared governance initiatives have shown that collaboration and consultation result in high-quality patient care delivery systems. Therefore a critical role for nurse managers and leaders is *facilitation* by fostering a climate that encourages creativity and interdependence.

Modeling desired critical thinking behaviors is also important. For example, in hospitals, nurse leaders and managers can use change-of-shift reports to promote critical thinking and subsequent problem solving by using the Socratic method and asking who, what, when, and where questions such as "What nursing interventions have been effective?" or "What will happen if this course of action is chosen?" Another strategy for promoting critical thinking is to create a climate in which mistakes can be made and then analyzed without fear of punishment (Cohen, 2002). Figure 5.4 summarizes these strategies.

Nurse managers and leaders have many competing demands on their time. Deciding which problems need immediate attention and which can wait involves the ability to prioritize one's actions. Clinical decision-making skills can be focused and enhanced by the use of critical thinking. Nurses can and do use decision making in all aspects of care management, but the nurse manager deals more with system-level issues rather than the day-to-day direct patient care decisions (Sherman et al., 2007).

Clearly, all nurses are on information overload. Ways to capture the available data and use it for effective problem solving and decision making are critical. Hospital information systems can be used to capture data such as length of stay, skill mix, case mix, patient and employee job satisfaction, and other variables that can be important when decisions need to be made (Junttila et al., 2007).

Complexity and Chaos

Nurse managers and leaders solve problems in complex systems in which all decisions carry some amount of risk. Complexity and chaos theory has application to leadership and management decision making. The behavior of nurses is governed, to some extent, by the rules (formal and informal), information flow, diversity, and interconnectedness of the organization (Chu et al., 2003). This complex web of interdependence and mutual causality among nurses, physicians, and support staff results in a complex adaptive system characterized by open boundaries, multiple levels of organization, and rule sets that serve as the organization's operating procedures. The system changes over time as it adapts to changes in external and internal environments. Multiple feedback loops exist, and new ways of organizational behavior emerge (Minas, 2005). One example of this type of complex adaptive system is how hospitals have adapted to a changing reimbursement environment such that the majority of surgeries, in many places, are done on an outpatient basis. For hospitals and other health care organizations to survive, nurse managers and leaders must use critical thinking skills when considering the vast array of choices that can be made when determining an organization's future.

The "good old days," when life was more predictable and less chaotic and patients routinely stayed 3 to 5 days as inpatients, have disappeared. History has shown that past technological innovations combine to form new technological innovations; and with each iteration, complexity increases (Waldrop, 1992). For example, discharge teaching must now begin *before* admission, not after the patient is admitted for surgery. Patients may be at the hospital or surgery center for only 1 to 2 hours after the surgery has ended; thus they are still under the influence of anesthetics or analgesics and cannot comprehend or remember the instructions that were given. Because change is occurring so rapidly, past practices that exhibit any sense of permanence may provide managers with a feeling of security. Leading in a world of complexity does not necessarily require a new set of management tools. Rather, nurse leaders must first learn to recognize complex, nonlinear systems and then assess which management strategies are most effective in dealing with them.

Just like complex patient care scenarios, complex social organizations, like hospitals, produce patterns that can be difficult to recognize (Wheatley, 1999) unless one is an expert critical thinker (Benner, 1984; Shirey, 2007). Expert nurse leaders can quickly and intuitively grasp organizational patterns without going through a step-by-step analysis of a situation.

Inevitably, some mistakes will be made; but nurse managers and leaders who look upon mistakes as learning opportunities help promote adaptive systems.

CURRENT ISSUES AND TRENDS

More than 10 years ago the Pew Health Professions Commissions (1998) identified that critical thinking was an essential skill for health care providers in the twenty-first century. The American Association of Colleges of Nursing (1998) has endorsed critical thinking as a key skill for baccalaureate-prepared nurses. Yet many nurses still exhibit a lack of critical thinking skills (del Bueno, 2005). Nurse leaders and managers are essential to promoting a climate that encourages critical thinking and innovative problem solving and decision making (Currie et al., 2007). New staff nurses, in particular, need support to develop confidence in learning to think like nurses (Etheridge, 2007). Promoting critical thinking is critical to thinking like a nurse.

Whether critical thinking is even promoted in nursing education programs is controversial, as is its measurement (Adams, 1999; Walsh & Seldomridge, 2006). Some standardized measurement instruments are available, such as the Watson-Glaser Critical Thinking Appraisal (Watson & Glaser, 1994) and the California Critical Thinking Skills Test, the California Reasoning Appraisal (Insight Assessment, 2008a). But these instruments are not specific to the discipline of nursing. A new instrument, the Health Sciences Reasoning Test (Insight Assessment, 2008b) has potential for more accurately appraising critical thinking skills in nurses.

Clearly, more research needs to be done. Nevertheless, nurturing, developing, and demonstrating evidence of critical thinking skills remain important issues in nursing education and practice. Nurse managers and staff nurses must form

LEADERSHIP & MANAGEMENT BEHAVIORS

Leadership Behaviors

- Provides a climate that fosters critical thinking skills
- Influences group and individual decision-making and problem-solving activities
- Inspires others to collaborate to make decisions and solve problems
- Envisions creative alternatives to problems
- Motivates the group to innovate in response to identified problems
- Models good problem-solving and decision-making behavior
- Encourages proactive thinking in decision making not related to immediate problems
- Networks with nurse colleagues

Management Behaviors

- Acts to resolve problems
- Plans for projected organizational deficits and surpluses
- Organizes the environment to decrease problems
- Directs individuals in problem resolution
- Delegates tasks and responsibilities
- Controls levels of conflict
- Makes decisions about resource allocation
- Motivates subordinates to come to consensus
- Plans day-to-day operations
- Resolves selected problems
- Organizes the work through priority setting
- Evaluates productivity

Overlap Areas

- Uses critical thinking, problem-solving processes and decision-making strategies to accomplish goals
- Motivates individuals and groups to solve problems and make decisions
- Solves problems and makes decisions

partnerships (Kerfoot, 2006) and create a climate in which critical thinking can occur. Such a climate encourages creativity and innovation (Albarran, 2004).

Despite the need for creativity, a certain amount of standardization must occur if safe patient care is to be delivered (Clancy et al., 2006; Kerfoot, 2006). Decision-making activities in nursing include standardization of care and improving quality and safety through evidence-based protocols. The standardization of care, through adoption of standardized languages, is one strategy nurse administrators can use to reduce the complexity of care and enable nurses to make better decisions (Clancy et al., 2006). Linking standardized care procedures to patient safety initiatives is vital if health care providers and patients are to safely navigate complex care environments.

Nurse leaders need to advocate for a preferred future for nursing and evaluate the effectiveness of decision making in practice. Both are aimed at making careful projections about what decisions to make, given uncertainty, to improve organizational and system performance. In times of change, nursing has an opportunity to make decisions that proactively direct the future. Nursing has demonstrated its value to the health care system. When staffing levels are unsafe, patient care suffers (American Nurses Association, 2008). Therefore nurse leaders must be a party to all decisions regarding how care is delivered in health care organizations via shared governance arrangements.

Many hospitals are applying for Magnet™ recognition from the American Nurses Credentialing Center. One of the 14 Forces of Magnetism involves management style and another promotes interdisciplinary collaboration. These two elements of a management style that is collaborative and the promotion of interdisciplinary staff input in decision making are evidence-based "best practices" (Thomas & Herrin, 2008b).

The efficiency, efficacy, and effectiveness of health care decisions will continue to enjoy a strong focus in nursing, with shifts toward outcomes

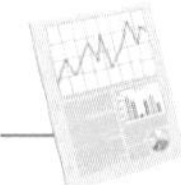

Research Note

Source: Terzioglu, F. (2006). The perceived problem-solving ability of nurse managers. *Journal of Nursing Management, 14*(5), 340-347.

Purpose

The aim of this descriptive study was to determine the perceived problem-solving ability of nurses working in the hospital as managers.

The majority of the nurse managers in this study were very experienced, having more than 11 years experience. However, 69.5% had no management education. Most did not read management journals. Nurses who attended meetings, had formal management education, and read management journals perceived themselves as more competent in problem solving.

Application to Practice

A high level of critical thinking and problem-solving abilities is necessary if nurse managers are to be effective decision makers in complex organizations. Without focused education, much of the decision making that takes place may be trial and error and not based on principles of effective problem solving and decision making. Therefore those appointed to managerial positions should have either formal or continuing education relevant to their roles. In addition, nurse managers should attend yearly conferences to keep their skills updated.

specification. As performance improvement specialists, nurses will be challenged to make decisions that directly affect quality, access, cost, productivity, and the "bottom line." Effective approaches to decision making are needed when care is delivered in a complex system in which multiple stakeholders need to be served, time is constrained, and the amount of information is overwhelming.

Summary

- Critical thinking is the basis for good problem solving.
- All nurses, including nurse leaders/managers, need skills in critical thinking and problem solving to make effective decisions.
- A problem is a situation in need of resolution.
- Problem solving is a process of coming to a solution for the problem.
- The steps of the problem-solving process involve decision making.
- There are multiple strategies for solving problems.
- Decision making is a key aspect of leadership and management.
- Decision making involves the act of choosing and implementing a course of action from among alternatives.
- Decision making may or may not be the result of an immediate problem.
- Decision making is a process with identifiable steps.
- Decision-making situations are personal, clinical, or organizational.
- There are various administrative decision-making models.
- There are different decision styles and strategies.
- Creativity and innovation promote effective decision making in complex systems.
- Standardization of care is one aspect of a safe patient care environment.

CASE STUDY

Effective decision making relies, in part, on analyzing alternative levels of uncertainty or risk. In addition to making "apples to apples" comparisons through such tools as present value calculations, estimating the probability that each alternative will actually occur can be helpful. For instance, a hospital interested in improving nurse vacancy rates analyzed nursing salaries under the following four scenarios: (1) no change over current rates, (2) adjusting rates to the local market, (3) adjusting rates slightly above the local market, or (4) adjusting rates well above the market. For each alternative, the net present value of the savings from decreased recruitment costs offset by the increased salary expense over 5 years was calculated. Using studies from similar markets, the probability that each alternative would achieve the desired vacancy rate was estimated. The hypothetical results of the four alternatives are summarized in Figure 5.5.

As noted on Figure 5.5, alternative 2 (matching the nurse's salaries to the current market rate) has the highest estimated savings (adjusted by its probability) of the four alternatives. It is important to note that relying on just the net present value without considering its probability can be misleading. Alternative 1 (doing nothing) actually has the highest present value, but the probability of achieving the desired outcome is only 25%. Thus alternative 1's estimated total savings are actually the lowest of the four alternatives.

Figure 5.5 is an example of a "decision tree." Diagrams such as decision trees can be invaluable in understanding complicated alternative solutions. New research into knowledge representation has shown that human cognition is more effective through visualization rather than text. Decision trees, fishbone diagrams, problem continuums, and flow charts are frequently used as visualization tools in problem analysis. To assist in visualization techniques, managers should consider placing a large "grease board," dry-erase board, or flip chart in their office to quickly map out various alternatives.

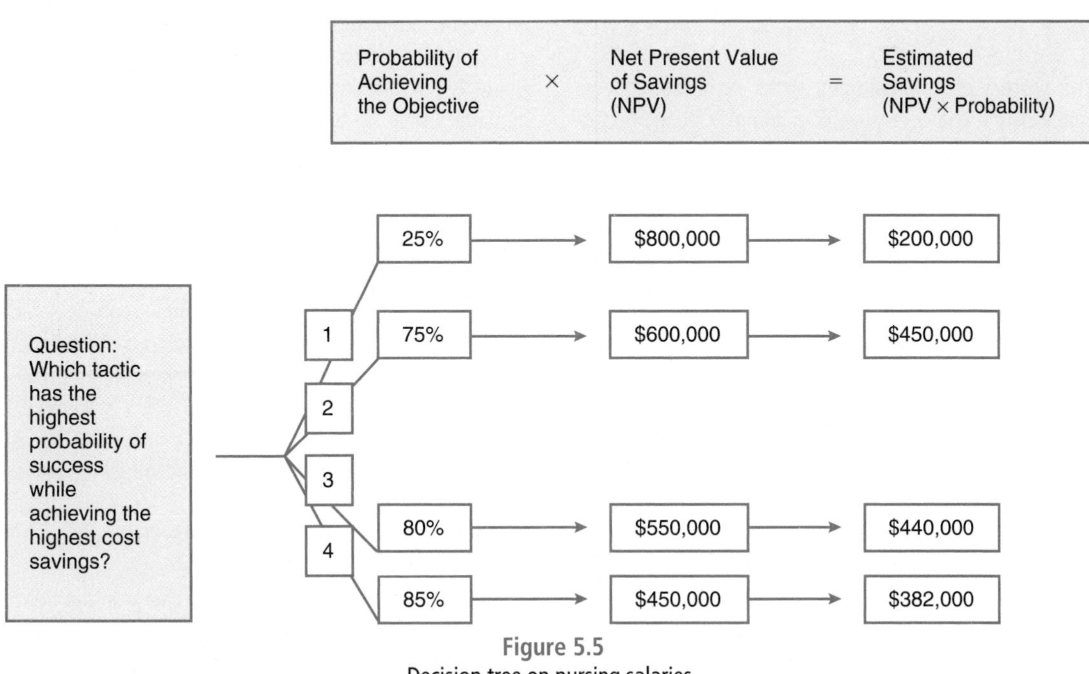

Figure 5.5
Decision tree on nursing salaries.

CRITICAL THINKING EXERCISE

Scenario 1

Nurse Brad Flint works the 12-hour evening shift on a busy surgical unit in a 200-bed community hospital. He has been employed on this same unit for 5 years. During this past year, he has been late six times and he often receives several calls per shift from his children. Unit Manager Susan Smith has verbally counseled Nurse Flint and placed a disciplinary warning in his personnel file. If Nurse Flint does not consistently arrive on time for his shift over the next 3 months, he will be suspended without pay and perhaps lose his job.

1. What is the problem?
2. Why is it a problem?
3. Who owns the problem?
4. What are the key issues?
5. What cultural issues may be involved?
6. What should the unit manager do first when dealing with Nurse Flint?
7. How should critical thinking be used?
8. What problem-solving strategies should Unit Manager Smith use with Nurse Flint?

Scenario 2

The process of nurse staffing within a hospital meets many of the characteristics of a complex adaptive system. Numerous agents (nurses) interact in a diverse social network (patients, physicians, therapists) that overlaps multiple hospital systems (admission, care, treatment, evaluation, discharge) to safely provide the appropriate number of trained staff throughout the hospital. The staffing system, constrained by rules (policies and procedures), is managed through the hierarchal management structure of the hospital.

Floating, a subprocess of the staffing system, is often used to redistribute nursing staff from overstaffed to understaffed units. In a stable environment, floating process behavior may settle into a reoccurring pattern of (1) the daily assignment of float staff to units, (2) communication to individual nurses about their assignments, and (3) a productive feedback loop between nurses and management regarding patient assignments. However, in an unstable environment, floating process behavior may take on an entirely different form. For instance, if float nurses are routinely expected to manage unfamiliar patients on unfriendly, foreign units without appropriate orientation and training, a reoccurring pattern of negative behavior may develop (a reinforcing positive feedback loop). In this case the pattern may be characterized by (1) the daily assignment of float staff to units, (2) communication to individual nurses of their assignments, (3) resistance by staff to float, and (4) a daily feedback loop of escalating conflict between management and float staff.

In complex systems such as staffing, any small disturbance in a positively reinforcing feedback loop may amplify in a "nonlinear" fashion throughout the system. Examples of a small disturbance may include changes in floating policies, miscommunication between management and staff, or even one nurse having a particularly negative floating experience. The cascading effect of disturbances within the complex social network of staff may result in unanticipated outcomes. For example, the pattern may manifest itself as staff refusing to float or demands for premium pay when floating. Regardless of its pattern, the emergence of new staff behavior is the result of multiple agents (staff) spontaneously self-organizing in an effort to adapt to the current environment.

Complex systems are nonlinear and unpredictable. However, by altering or "tuning" system parameters, managers may be able to "steer" system behavior in such a way that staff self-organize in a desired direction (Minas, 2005). For instance, if done correctly, the implementation of simple rules can create positively reinforcing feedback loops that allow self-organization and emergence to occur.

In the floating example, nurse administrators could allow staff to develop "a code of floating conduct" that requires all nurses to adhere to the following five simple rules:

1. Treat float staff cordially when on a unit.
2. All float staff are assigned a resource nurse from the floor.
3. The resource person must orient the float nurse using a standardized form.
4. The resource nurse must regularly check on the float nurse.
5. Both the float and resource nurses must fill out an evaluation form at the end of the shift.

To reinforce behavior, nurse administrators would review all evaluation forms daily. If a negative floating experience is noted, the nurse administrator would follow up with the float nurse, resource nurse, and manager of the unit within 24 hours. In addition, all evaluation forms would be trended for problems and presented to a committee of staff nurses on a monthly basis. If a particular unit showed a problem trend, the data would be shared with the manager and unit staff and follow-up action to alleviate the problem would be required. Data also would be shared with units that consistently scored high on float evaluations as a reward.

By tuning the rules, information flow, and communication parameters, nurse administrators can steer the system toward a positively reinforcing feedback loop and a new attractor that incorporates the five rules. The result, demonstrated in Figure 5.6, is a self-policing float system. Units that consistently score poorly on float evaluations self-organize to improve their image and prevent being labeled an unfriendly area. Eventually a new culture will "emerge" throughout the organization as units naturally compete among themselves to improve.

Although seemingly simple, the float example illustrates an alternative strategy for managing in a CAS environment. Rather than using management strategies that concentrate on enforcing top-down complicated policies and procedures, the CAS uses simple rules to enable naturally occurring, bottom-up self-organization and emergence. Instead of attempts to force system elements directionally, emphasis is on creating a climate for positive change but with an understanding that the final outcome remains uncertain.

1. For what undesirable patterns should managers be on the alert when implementing change in a complex process such as floating?
2. What key parameters within the floating process can managers "tune" to move the system in a desirable direction?
3. Describe examples of tactics that could be employed to control parameters surrounding the floating process.
4. How might managers create positively reinforcing feedback loops that enable staff to "self-organize" around attractive solutions?
5. What computerized data might be available to evaluate the outcome of the floating process?

PART II

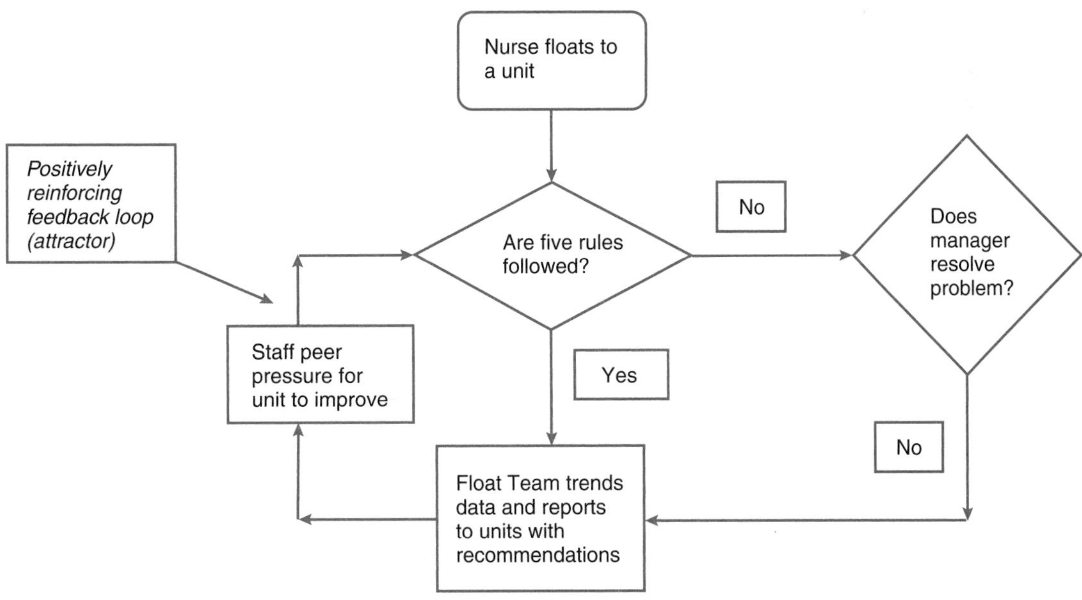

Figure 5.6
Tuning system parameters to steer the float system toward a new attractor.

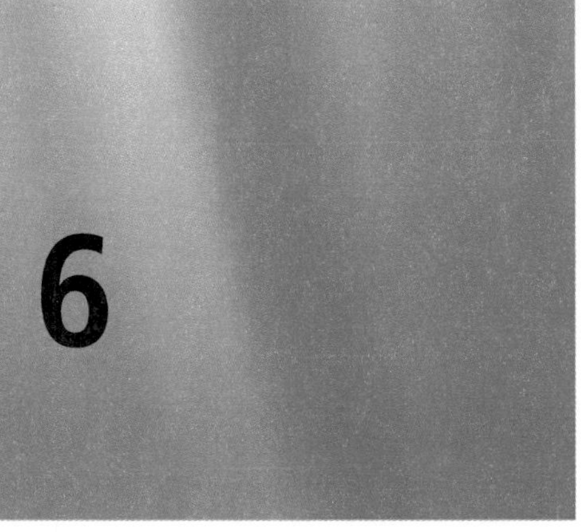

6

Managing Time and Stress

Karen S. Cox   Susan R. Lacey

CHAPTER OBJECTIVES

- Create a recognition of time management issues and possibilities
- Define time management
- Examine time management processes
- Construct an array of time management strategies and techniques
- Define and describe stress, job stress, and burnout
- Illustrate a general model of stress
- Compare stress mediators
- Analyze sources of stress in nursing
- Analyze coping and adaptation in nursing
- Discuss the link between stress, nursing workforce, and quality
- Exercise critical thinking to conceptualize and analyze possible solutions to a practice exercise

 TIME MANAGEMENT

"Time controls and limits how we use our other resources. Thus, it is often referred to as our most valuable resource" (Ferner, 1995, p. 8). Time may be the most precious resource to manage. There is an old saying that time is money. In health care, time affects both money and quality (Severance & Cervantes, 1996). For each nurse there is a finite and identifiable limit to the hours and minutes available to do the work. With the same 60 seconds in every minute, nurses need to find ways to stretch the time available to meet the needs that arise. Time pressures are a key source of stress and an area in which nurses have the most to gain by learning management techniques.

Many nurses complain about needing more time. They are stressed and frustrated. At any point in time, nurses juggle work and other roles such as student, partner, parent, child, or friend. As workplaces are restructured for efficiency and employ fewer people, personal work-role stress rises. Effective time management is needed.

The temptation is strong to apply superficial slogans and gimmicky solutions to the issue of time management. It is easy to suggest that nurses learn to work smarter, not harder. However, quick fixes result in temporary solutions, because the problem of time management is pervasive and the solutions often appear elusive (Ferner, 1995). Nurses can relate to Covey and colleagues' (1994) description of feeling caught between what they have to do (the clock) and what they believe is right to do (the compass). For example, paperwork and scheduled tasks are clock aspects of work. Developing a relationship with patients and meeting their spontaneously arising needs are compass aspects of nursing (Severance & Cervantes, 1996). Somehow the balance needs to be found and the increasing scarcity of time brought under control.

DEFINITION

We all have only 24 hours in a day and 168 hours in a week. In that time, certain activities are conducted by necessity and to fulfill commitments and goals. Typical activities include personal time (to eat, sleep, get dressed, and do personal maintenance), job or work time, free time, and time for personal growth, leisure, and family (Ferner, 1995). When competing demands create a time conflict, time management becomes important.

Time management is defined as the accomplishment of specified activities during the time available. It is the process of managing the things an individual does with his or her available time. In reality, time management is self-management (Ferner, 1995).

BACKGROUND

The goal of time management is the efficient use of time resources to be effective in achieving goals. Principles of analysis and planning need to be used. This may be difficult because time management is personal, cultural, and a matter of individual style and circumstances. However, success in time management is tied to analysis, planning, and commitment to a course of action. It must be internalized and become a habit. Difficult as it may be, successful time managers control interruptions, say no, and delegate (Ferner, 1995).

Time management has been linked to success and the achievement of goals. The perception of being successful is linked to the perception of how time is spent (Noreiko, 1996). Awareness and analysis of goals and objectives is a beginning step. Goals and objectives may be short-term (1 week to 3 months), medium-term (3 months to 1 year), or long-term (1 to 5 years). They should be specific, measurable, achievable, realistic, and defined in terms of time (Noreiko, 1996). Overall, serious attempts to improve time management require commitment to new habits, analysis based on data, planning effort, and follow-up re-analysis (Ferner, 1995).

THE TIME MANAGEMENT PROCESS

Time management is a deliberative process of identifying and focusing on the activities needed to accomplish tasks and goals. This is important to nurses and nurse managers, who need to organize and be productive in personal time and also need to manage and coordinate the work of others. Individuals cannot control time itself; therefore they need to learn to manage the available time more efficiently and effectively. This can be learned; however, it may be difficult, especially when comfortable habits need to be changed. The first step is to mobilize willingness and determination to examine personal characteristics and habits. Then attention must be given to making changes that will result in each person being in charge of what actually occurs with the time available. Improved ability to manage time can come from the following (Arnold & Pulich, 2004):

- Examining attitudes toward time
- Analyzing time-wasting behaviors
- Developing better time management skills

Managing Your Time

In Julie Morgenstern's book *Never Check E-mail in the Morning: And Other Unexpected Strategies for Making Your Work Life Work* (2004), the author outlined ways to be more productive given the constant bombardment of competing demands for limited time. This is particularly important in the Internet age. It is not unusual to open up work and/or personal e-mail accounts and have hundreds of e-mails that await attention. However, do they all need responses and do they need to be checked the first thing in the morning? Much of this depends on the culture of the organization. There may be an expectation that you process e-mail as soon as you arrive. However, this may be negotiable to some extent.

For e-mail specifically, Morgenstern (2004) discussed leaving the first hour of the day e-mail–free. It is amazing how much time can be lost when trying to respond to the overwhelming number of items. She stated that e-mail is the biggest "time-suck" of the day. She also offered detailed information for how best to sort and organize e-mail by sender so that time is focused on the most important e-mails needing attention. According to Morgenstern (2004):

> E-mail plays a leading role in the development of our supremely impatient culture, where everything has to be "now, now, now!" People expect immediate responses, because an immediate response seems possible. Or you may feel driven to return your boss's or colleagues' e-mails first

> thing in the morning so that they will know you are in the office. But, just because messages arrive instantaneously in your box doesn't mean that you have to respond immediately. (p. 97)

Other ways exist to be reached for more emergent issues, such as a mobile pager. If your staff need you quickly, they always have the option to page you. Set aside time in your day to respond to your e-mail, but some items may need thought and processing for an effective response. If you want to avoid knee-jerk responses about a topic that should be considered carefully, you can send a quick reply that lets the sender know when he or she will have a more thorough response.

One place to start is in self-awareness. Time management habits are embedded in personal preferences, childhood experiences, and cultural influences that may be unconscious or rarely consciously examined. For example, individuals have personal work and management styles that may be based in gender, culture, or personal preferences. One example is the monochronic/polychronic continuum (Hahn, 2008).

Monochronic or Polychronic Continuum

Individuals vary according to what they prefer and how they choose to approach work task organization. This preference appears to be mediated by cultural and gender influences. As a result of natural human diversity, discord or conflict may arise if opposites are assigned together and not assisted to understand these differences and how to harmonize style preferences. These preferences array across a continuum.

At one end is the monochronic style. This style is characterized by working through each part of a project in an orderly fashion and completing one task before starting on the next. Orderly, sequential, linear, and logical, persons using this style approach work with specific and detailed plans and schedules to which they are highly committed (highly monochronic) or with an organized approach that addresses tasks in an analytical and prioritized way (moderately monochronic). They tend to be individualistic and prefer an isolated and uninterrupted work place (Hahn, 2008). Because this is a linear model, it may have disadvantages in work environments of chaos and complexity, such as in nursing.

At the opposite end is the polychronic work style, in which people tend to do multiple tasks simultaneously. They approach work projects multidimensionally, with flexible and adjustable plans and shared responsibilities. They work on many different parts of a project at the same time and are flexible, spontaneous, and adaptable (highly polychronic). If moderately polychronic, individuals prefer performing many activities at the same time, working in teams and within a general competition timeframe, flexibly approaching project implementation (Hahn, 2008). If not skillfully managed, however, the polychronic style can deteriorate into chaos.

Awareness of individual work and task styles enhances personal effectiveness, planning, and decision making about personal choices and team harmony. Self-tests are available, such as the Monochronic/Polychronic Self Test. Illustrated in Figure 6.1, this test is a set of 16 items, each rated on an anchored descriptor scale from A through E.

ANALYZING AND MANAGING TIME

Time management is like any general management endeavor. It involves the skills of planning, organizing, implementing, and controlling. The time management process is continuous and ongoing and involves a cycle of analyzing, planning, reanalyzing, and replanning with the following eight steps (Ferner, 1995):

1. Analysis of current time use with time logs
2. Analysis of time logs to identify time problems, causes, and solutions
3. Self-assessment
4. Setting goals and establishing priorities
5. Developing action plans that define tasks, resource needs, and time frames
6. Implementing action plans via planning guides, schedules, and to-do lists
7. Developing techniques and solutions to improve time management problems
8. Follow-up and reanalysis

Text continued on p.129

A Monochronic/Polychronic Self-Test

This instrument is designed to assist you in understanding your personal cultural preferences, with respect to both work style and management style. It may serve as an indicator of how you might adapt in certain organizations and global regions.

Pick the letter that best describes your preferred opinion or behavior in an organizational situation. The letters A through E are a scale with C representing the midpoint between the two extremes. As best you can, determine where your opinion or behavior would occur most consistently on the scale for each of the situations below.

1. When working on a project, you find it most effective to:

A	B	C	D	E
Work through each part of the project in an orderly fashion.				Work on many different parts of the project at the same time.

2. You work most effectively in an organization when:

A	B	C	D	E
You are seldom interrupted by and rarely interact with other employees.				You are constantly interacting with and interrupted for discussions by other employees.

3. When you are assigned a project that is due at a specific time, you:

A	B	C	D	E
Establish a specific plan for achieving the project by the deadline, if not before.				Create a flexible plan which may or may not accomplish the project by the exact deadline.

Figure 6.1
A monochronic/polychronic self test. (From Innovations International. [2008]. *A monochronic/polychronic self test.* Salt Lake City, UT: Author. Retrieved October 24, 2008, from www.innovint.com/downloads/mono_poly_test.php/.)

4. Organizational information is most efficiently shared and disseminated through:

A	B	C	D	E
Detailed or written memos or internal communication systems.				Informal interoffice verbal communication among employees.

5. To be successful, an organization must focus most on:

A	B	C	D	E
Reaching projected goals and accomplishing task objectives.				Developing each worker and establishing quality relationships among employees.

6. The best project results are produced when everyone agrees:

A	B	C	D	E
To a detailed plan which is executed and completed according to the original design.				To an informal plan that is adjusted as the project proceeds.

7. When you want to discuss something with a co-worker whose office door is closed, you would probably:

A	B	C	D	E
Walk away, assuming he or she does not want to be disturbed.				Knock, open the door, and ask for a few minutes to discuss your concern.

Figure 6.1 cont'd

Continued

8. With respect to your valued possessions, you:

A	B	C	D	E
Almost never lend them to anyone.				Lend them often and easily.

9. When you are late for a scheduled appointment, you feel that:

A	B	C	D	E
You should apologize for being late.				You should not apologize, assuming that he/she will understand that something important came up.

10. In general, after you no longer serve a valued client, you tend to:

A	B	C	D	E
Lose contact with him/her because of your busy schedule and/or you no longer work with him/her directly.				Stay in communication to know how his/her life is progressing.

11. A sign of a good manager is her or his ability to:

A	B	C	D	E
Solicit employee input, but use executive decision making where vital business and policy issues are concerned.				Extensively involve employees in deciding vitally important business and policy-making issues.

Figure 6.1 cont'd

12. Your business presentation style tends to be:

A	B	C	D	E
Orderly, sequential, and logical.				Flexible, spontaneous, and adaptable.

13. Businesses run best when job responsibilities are:

A	B	C	D	E
Fixed and uniquely adapted to each employee.				Constantly changing and overlapping between employees.

14. In a fast-paced, decentralized, information-oriented society, important business matters:

A	B	C	D	E
Require immediate and decisive decision making.				Demand sufficient time for discussion, consensus, and deliberation.

15. The most successful business ventures are dependent upon:

A	B	C	D	E
An in-depth analysis and thorough discussion of all information relevant to the transaction.				The people involved and their ability to work together effectively.

Figure 6.1 cont'd

Continued

16. The most effective way to contribute to an organization is to:

A	B	C	D	E
Specialize in one area and become an expert on a subject.				Accumulate cross-disciplinary knowledge in as many areas as possible.

Scoring Instructions

For each letter chosen, A, B, C, D, or E, write the number of times it was circled next to the appropriate letter in the spaces below, and multiply this number by the figure shown. For example, if B was circled five (5) times, write "5" in the blank space beside B and complete the multiplication, "5" × 2 = "10". Finally, add the products in this column to obtain a total numerical score.

A _____ × 0 = _____

B _____ × 2 = _____

C _____ × 5 = _____

D _____ × 8 = _____

E _____ × 10 = _____

TOTAL _______

Interpretation of Scores

0-40 Highly Monochronic = A to B range on the scale.

These individuals approach work with specific and detailed plans and schedules, to which they are highly committed. The realization of business objectives is their highest priority, and personal relationships are one dimension among many toward this end. These individuals prefer specialized and unique work responsibilities, private working conditions, and short-term, formal work relationships. They are inclined to communicate impersonally and in low context. Their decision making tends to be individualistic, timely, and based on their position of influence within the organization. The essence of leadership is the individualistic vision of the future.

41-80 Moderately Monochronic = B to C range on the scale.

These individuals demonstrate an organized approach to projects and are committed to their completion on time. They ultimately prioritize the successful completion of projects, and tend to address tasks in an analytical and information-oriented manner. These individuals tend to prefer an isolated and uninterrupted work environment; social interaction has its appropriate time and place. Their significant communications are usually to the point, logical and written. Though group input is an important element in these individuals' decision-making process, they ultimately rely on personal judgment to make important final decisions.

Figure 6.1 cont'd

81-120 Moderately Polychronic = C to D range on the scale.

These individuals tend to assign work projects into a general time frame for completion, flexibly approaching project implementation and readily adjusting its execution when something more important comes along. They prefer performing many activities at the same time and working in teams. These individuals develop many informal, long-term working relationships as their means to realizing goals. Their communication of information tends to be personal and informal, rather than through official channels. They solicit and rely heavily on employee input for most decision making.

121-160 Highly Polychronic = D to E range on the scale.

These individuals multidimensionally approach work projects with flexible, adjustable plans and shared responsibilities. They tend to believe success of business transactions is ultimately determined by the individuals involved and their cohesiveness as a team. Work is founded upon quality interpersonal interaction and long-term investment in community, which takes precedence over all forms of activity. Communication tends to be spontaneous and high context. Decision making is based on extensive group involvement, discussion, and consensus. The essence of leadership is the subtle balance of group consensus and personal vision.

Figure 6.1 cont'd

Time	Activity	Notes
7:00 AM	Arrived on unit, changed into scrubs	
7:15 AM	Joined report	
7:35 AM	Conference with nurse manager	
7:45 AM	Phone call from patient's family	
7:55 AM	Began initial assessments	
8:10 AM	Responded to request from physician	
8:15 AM	Medication rounds	

Figure 6.2
Activity log for the beginning of an RN shift.

The first step is to analyze how time is currently being spent by keeping a time log. This is a running account of what was actually done and how much time it took. Include activities as you do them, such as open mail, chat with co-workers, or make coffee. This log can be analyzed by day, week, month, or year, depending on the circumstances. For example, if the focus is on a work shift, it might be most useful to analyze by the hour for a week. If the focus is on implementing a new project, an overview may be by the month for a year. Figure 6.2 shows a sample activity log for the start of a hospital-based RN's work shift. Recording time use makes the abstract idea of time become a concrete reality and identifies time wasters (Pagana, 1994), specifically where time is lost. Time wasters keep an individual from doing other things that have more value or importance. The two general categories of time wasters are (1) external ones, such as phone calls and drop-in visitors, and (2) internal, or self-generated, ones.

Lack of self-discipline, failure to delegate, procrastination, indecision, and personal disorganization are examples of self-generated time wasters that are within an individual's power to solve. The goal is to control the cause of wasting time by strategies such as deferring a task when there is something more important to do, diminishing the time spent on the task, or eliminating selected parts of the task (Ferner, 1995). Diaries, calendars, organizers, personal digital assistants (PDAs), and integrated software scheduling tools are all devices to help manage time.

Keeping track of all completed tasks and starting a daily planner to log all tasks that need to be completed initially focus an individual on personal time management reality. Next comes self-assessment regarding why time is lost or not used effectively. Effective time management is blocked by procrastination, perfectionism, and an inability to prioritize (Rocchiccioli & Tilbury, 1998). Procrastination may occur because of any of the following (Business Town.com, 2004):

- You are not really committed to doing the job.
- You are afraid of the job.
- You do not place enough priority on the activity.
- You do not know enough to do the task.
- You simply do not want to do the job.

The following strategies can help overcome the reasons just listed:

- Examine motivation and personal benefit; then either do what needs to be done to get out of it or do it anyway for your own reasons.
- Identify and confront the fear, and act despite the fear.
- Recast it in positive motivation, and either act or resign yourself to living with the consequences of inaction.
- Gather the information you need, and plunge into the task.
- Tough it out, or farm it out.

In summary, overcoming procrastination is a combination of identifying the reasons, confronting attitudes and fears, and weighing the consequences. Then mobilization to action is required.

Perfectionism is the need to do everything exactly right—to be perfect. It can lead to procrastination over the fear of making a mistake. The antidote to perfectionism is to set acceptable and realistic standards for goal achievement.

Prioritization is a key aspect of time management. After analysis of personal characteristics, attitudes, and behaviors that may block time management effectiveness comes setting goals and establishing priorities. One way to approach this is to analyze what needs to be done immediately and what can wait. Goals and activities can fall into one of the following four categories (Rocchiccioli & Tilbury, 1998):

1. Important and urgent
2. Important but not urgent
3. Not important but urgent
4. Not important and not urgent

Analyzing and managing time takes concentrated effort and an openness to rethinking habits and routines. Often a small amount of effort yields large returns, so changes are important. Reframing situations also helps. For example, establishing an approximate hourly cost for your time (e.g., hourly salary figure plus benefits) and then multiplying this by the number of hours spent in meetings helps clarify why actions need to be taken to make meetings more efficient and effective. Assessing personal strengths and weaknesses might help focus personal choices for projects or job duties, such as joining a team. Fundamental motivation, such as doing what you enjoy, also helps time management decisions. Balance is a final consideration. Setting realistic goals, preserving contingency-for-the-unexpected time, and carefully identifying essential tasks in the right order are strategies that help achieve balanced time management.

TIME MANAGEMENT STRATEGIES

Closing the gap between how an individual would like to be spending time versus how the time is actually spent depends on the deployment of an array of time management strategies. Two fundamental strategies universally recommended are analyzing the workday and prioritizing the workload.

In nursing, care needs and work assignments can fluctuate daily, making organizing the workday a challenge (Sherry, 1996). Some general strategies can be identified. Their use depends on the individual situation, available resources, and safety considerations, as follows:

- Take control of your calendar by analysis and prioritization.
- Minimize time spent in the office in nonproductive behavior or away from client care.
- "Tame the telephone" through effective clerical support.
- Simplify documentation using technology.
- Plan ahead.
- Save time for others.

Pagana (1994) created a list of time management techniques useful for nursing students, including the following:

- Omission by decision: deciding what not to do
- Learning to say no: refusal because of time constraints and prioritization
- Blocking interruptions, especially by visitors and phone calls
- Guarding an individual's best or prime time
- Programming blocks of time, especially for large projects
- Organizing work space
- Managing committee meetings
- Delegating
- Planning the use of time

Inpatient nursing is challenging. The shortened lengths of stay have resulted in higher overall activity for nurses. The first and last days of a hospital stay are traditionally the most labor-intensive. However, given shortened lengths of stay, every day of a patient's stay is now likely to be labor-intensive. An example of nurses' time compression is the need to start discharge planning at admission.

When confronted with a workload that is overwhelming, a nurse can try several tactics. First, it is crucial to take 15 to 20 minutes to plan the day. Skipping this will cost time throughout the shift because of the downtime to do extra steps that could have been economized or the rework time of redoing tasks. The tasks that must be accomplished need to be prioritized at the outset. As the day progresses and priorities change, the high-priority items will be the guide for making the best decisions under time limits. Often when a person is overwhelmed, he or she is tempted to focus on a less important task such as making a bed when those 10 minutes could best be used reviewing home care planning with a family.

Asking for help is an important time management strategy. Often nurses see this as a sign of inadequate performance and thus may wait too long to engage others. Before asking for help, the nurse should consider what specific task would be most helpful for another to do.

Nurse managers face multiple and competing priorities on a daily basis. It is not unusual to feel overwhelmed and unsure about what to do first. Not unlike what occurs in a direct care role, planning is key for managerial time management. What are the tasks that are critical to accomplish today? Keeping these goals in the forefront will help throughout the day when the unexpected occurs and new tasks are added to the to-do list.

Keeping a close handle on how the unit staff members are doing can pay off in time management. By building in opportunities for daily communication, many issues can be addressed before they become major problems. There is no substitute for the nurse manager being available, especially for staff members who work off-shifts and frequently feel neglected by administration.

Many time management strategies surround the analysis, setting of priorities, motivation, planning, and follow-up structure of effective time management. Analysis is a detailed and honest look at what actually occurs during an allotted period as opposed to extracting only what is productive from among what occurs. Deciding priorities based on the importance and urgency of goals and then developing action plans and schedules can help better align time use with desired outcomes. Motivation is an internal strategy to overcome potential barriers and delays. Planning and follow-up are needed to ensure that goals are met within the set time frames.

Often when individuals feel that they have more tasks than they can complete, they have difficulty realizing that reorganizing their workload may result in successfully fulfilling their responsibilities. For instance, many students find the requirements of a class overwhelming until they break them down into manageable segments. Registered nurses (RNs) often have a sense of being overwhelmed by the rapid-fire needs and wants of patients, families, co-workers, and bosses until they apply analysis, prioritization, organization, and delegation to the chaos. Some time management tips and strategies are as follows:

- Continually analyze and examine how time is spent. What can be dropped or delegated?
- Keep a time log, calendar, or other scheduling device.
- Develop a specific statement of major goals: short-term, intermediate, and long-term. Focus on goal attainment.
- Focus on getting yourself started and keeping yourself motivated.
- Keep daily to-do lists, and continually reprioritize them.
- Aim to keep a balanced lifestyle. Take breaks. Find your productive time and maximize this.
- Learn when and how to decline to participate in time-wasting activities. Instead, ask others to cooperate with you in productive activities.
- Anticipate unexpected events and be realistic but stay organized.
- Capitalize on technology to assist time management.
- Work to conduct and keep meetings effective.
- End the workday as close to on-time as possible.

Many projects can be more successfully time-managed by the use of checklists, division into smaller tasks or steps, tracking progress, using Gantt charts, and managing group meetings. Figure 6.3 displays a Gantt chart, which is a common project planning time-line visual display. Control over time empowers individuals and frees up energy to handle multiple competing demands (Pagana, 1994). The practice and improvement of time management habits can increase goal achievement and reduce stress.

STRESS MANAGEMENT

Nurses are healers. They focus on activities related to caring in the diagnosis and treatment of human responses to health and illness. However, inherent in this caring occupation are numerous sources of built-in stress that become occupational hazards for nurses. For example, dealing with human illness and suffering, life-and-death situations, and clients who are demanding or in pain, making critical judgments about interventions and treatments, and balancing work and family commitments become forces that realistically generate stress in nurses (Aurelio, 1993). Furthermore, the organizations that employ nurses may become stressful work environments. For example, organizational cultures may devalue nurses, policies and deployment practices may prevent nurses from using their knowledge and skills, and job and professional autonomy may be restricted (Aurelio, 1993). Empowerment of staff nurses has been significantly related to lower burnout and higher work satisfaction (Laschinger, Finegan, & Shamian, 2001; Laschinger, Finegan, Shamian, & Almost, 2001). Clearly, for nurses, it is important to have work-related empowerment strategies in place.

Under conditions of restructuring, reengineering, and a nurse shortage, nurses feel threatened and concerned about their workload. Real or perceived short-staffing and increasing workloads raise concerns about client safety and the nurse's ability to cope and deliver adequate service to clients (Sovie & Jawad, 2001). As with the level of conflict, the level of stress needs to be neither too high nor too low. Moderate levels should be the target. At stress levels that are too low, nurses may become apathetic or nonproductive. If the stress level is too high, energy is absorbed in trying to deal with stress and is therefore diverted from productivity. Performance drops as stress reaches high levels. Clearly, both nurses and their employers have a stake in managing stress and stressful environments.

Activities	Days of the Month															
	1-2	3-4	5-6	7-8	9-10	11-12	13-14	15-16	17-18	19-20	21-22	23-24	25-26	27-28	29-30	31
Activity #1	X	X														
Activity #2		X	X													
Activity #3						X	X									

Figure 6.3
Monthly activities.

DEFINITIONS

Stress is one concept that links the effects of behaviors (e.g., poor eating habits, lack of exercise) to health consequences. **Stress** is defined as "a physical, mental, psychological, or spiritual response to a stressor" (Narasi, 1994, p. 73). A **stressor** is defined as an experience in a person-environment relationship that is evaluated by a person as taxing or exceeding resources and threatening the sense of well-being (Dietz, 1991; Lazarus & Folkman, 1984). Stress has been seen as a stimulus, a response, or a transaction (Lyon & Werner, 1987) that is either internal or external.

Selye's (1965) general stress theory forms the theoretical background for understanding stress. According to Selye (1965, 1976), stress is a nonspecific state composed of a variety of induced changes in the human biological system. Thus stress is a syndrome with a characteristic set of symptoms. It can lead to acute and chronic health problems. Stress also is described as a personal response and a phenomenon that occurs inside a body as a reaction to the stimulus of a stressor. The body's emotional and physical responses are a result of a "fight-or-flight" syndrome (Woodhouse, 1993).

The concept of stress has been applied from Selye's (1965, 1976) biophysiology framework to psychosocial states in individuals. For example, stress has been viewed as something that occurs when individuals interact with their environment in such a way that they are presented with a demand, a constraint, or an opportunity for behavior (McGrath, 1976).

Occupational or **job stress** is defined as a tension arising in a person that is related to the demands

LEADING & MANAGING DEFINED

Stress

Physical, mental, psychological, and spiritual responses to any stressor.

Stressor

An experience in a person-environment relationship that is evaluated by a person as taxing or exceeding resources and threatening the sense of well-being.

Occupational or Job Stress

A tension arising in a person that is related to the demands of the role or job.

Burnout

Responses to chronic emotional stress that have three components: (1) emotional or physical exhaustion, (2) lowered job productivity, and (3) overdepersonalization.

of the person's role or job (McVicar, 2003). Job stress, or "disquieting influences," can accumulate into levels that are too high and reach the point of burnout (Hinshaw & Atwood, 1983). **Burnout** is defined as "a response to chronic emotional stress with three components: (a) emotional and/or physical exhaustion, (b) lowered job productivity, and (c) overdepersonalization" (Perlman & Hartman, 1982, p. 293). Burnout in nursing is described as being the terminal phase of the individual's failure to resolve work stress or the accumulated inability to cope with day-to-day job stresses (Smythe, 1984). Levels of job stress that are too low or too high decrease individual productivity (Benson & Allen, 1980; Hinshaw & Atwood, 1983).

BACKGROUND

Stress is a pervasive part of everyday life and a common theme in nursing. Many of the effects of stress are personal and individual. It is necessary for nurses to understand stress both on a personal level and in relation to their work (Schwab, 1996).

From the work of Selye (1965, 1976), stress is known to have biophysiological effects on humans. However, in nursing practice, stress is most often applied to a discussion of the psychosocial state of persons as they interact with their environment. Demands, constraints, and opportunities occur that trigger stress (McGrath, 1976).

One general model of stress portrays stress along a continuum from potential stressor to consequences or outcomes (Elliott & Eisdorfer, 1982). At one end is a potential stressor, such as a demanding client. Then come mediators, such as social support, coping behaviors, or defense mechanisms; the individual's psychological reactions, such as emotional states of anxiety or fear; and biological reactions, such as an increase in catecholamines. Finally, there are consequences or outcomes, such as physical illness, burnout, or coping. In this model, stress is pictured as a dynamic process across a continuum and the result of an interaction between an individual and the environment (Lowery, 1987) (Figure 6.4).

In general, two important processes appear to mediate the person-environment relationship: coping and cognitive appraisal. Coping is the individual's actions and activities for adapting to the situation as presented. Coping relates to the means or methods used to deal with or manage a perceived stressful event (Dietz, 1991). The other major mediator is cognitive appraisal. This is the individual's assessment or interpretation of the stressor or potential stressor. Cognitive appraisal relates to the individual's evaluation or perception of whether and to what degree any event or transaction is stressful (Dietz, 1991; Lowery, 1987). Coping strategies can be either active or inactive. Active strategies work toward resolving or reducing the stress. Inactive strategies are focused on avoiding the stress (Simoni & Paterson, 1997).

Stress responses vary widely from one person to another. Lazarus (1966) suggested that perception

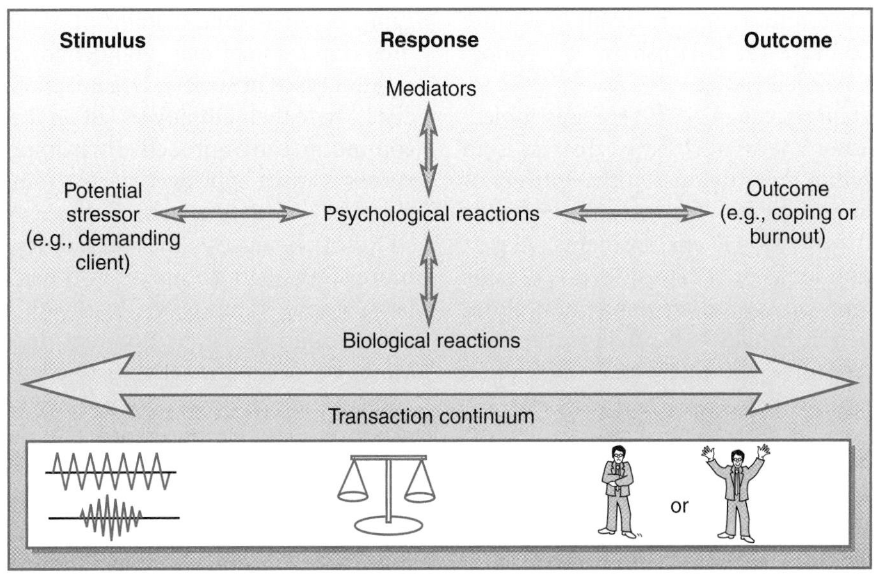

Figure 6.4

General model of stress. (Data from Elliott, G., & Eisdorfer, C. [1982]. *Stress and human health.* New York: Springer; Lowery, B. [1987]. Stress research: Some theoretical and methodological issues. *Image, 19*[1], 42-46; and Lyon, B.L., & Werner, J.S. [1987]. Stress. *Annual Review of Nursing Research, 5,* 3-22.)

and cognitive appraisal of the stress factor are key to understanding the psychological stress response. Thus psychological stress is based on a relationship between the person and the environment that is appraised by the person as taxing or exceeding coping resources (Lazarus & Folkman, 1984). The stress phenomenon includes the objective stressor, the person's perception, the context of the situation, intervening processes, residual stimuli, and the manifestations of the stress response (Pollock, 1984). This means that a stress event is a complex interaction and that the psychological response is under the individual's control via his or her cognitive framing or interpretation. Theoretically, changing the cognitive interpretation could change the stress response and increase coping and adaptation ability.

Nurses have studied a variety of stress reactions that occur as emotional and psychological manifestations of failed defense and coping. Chief among these are anxiety and depression. Often overlooked in research are the consequences or outcomes of exposure to stress. The outcomes can be either positive or negative. It is not known whether exposure to stress helps immunize the individual against severe reactions to future stressors or whether the individual becomes worn down and more susceptible to being overwhelmed by the next stressor. Mastery of stress is advocated but is not easily translated into simple techniques (Lowery, 1987). In nursing, hardiness and burnout have been investigated as stress outcomes.

SOURCES OF STRESS IN NURSING

Stress is associated with the work of nursing. Individual nurses may experience internal tension, conflict, or stress. Occupational or job stress derives from the jobs and organizations that employ nurses. Stress in nursing is an occupational and managerial concern (Huber, 1994). Individual nurses' health, job satisfaction, absenteeism, and turnover, along with client welfare, are thought to be affected by high levels of work-related stress (Norbeck, 1985). For an in-depth background on stress in nursing, at least three articles extensively analyze the theoretical and research literature (Hardy & Conway, 1988; Hinshaw & Atwood, 1983; Lyon & Werner, 1987).

It is important to recognize that stress is subjective, and a person's level of stress or distress is an interaction within an individual in the entirety of his or her environment. This includes both the personal and professional environments. A person's perception of his or her stress level is in large part a reflection on his or her perception about being equipped to handle it. Because perceptions change, a stressful event today may be viewed differently a month from now (McVicar, 2003).

Contemporary Sources of Stress

One of the biggest challenges we all face, regardless of our profession, is finding ways to balance our time well—not just at work, but *between* work and home. By the year 2010, approximately 40% of nurses will be older than 50 years (Health Resources and Services Administration, 2002). Although each generation has issues of competing personal and work demands, perhaps no generation has experienced this phenomenon to the extent that older nurses are at this moment in history. Rosabeth Kanter (1977), a noted sociologist, described this concept in 1977 as "spill-over"; however, it is just as relevant today. Spill-over occurs when a person tries to compartmentalize his or her work and home demands. Invariably, these spheres are merged not only cognitively but also while managing one's finite resources of time, energy, and money. Nursing leaders would do well to consider this framework when designing and implementing management policies in health care settings today.

Each generation has unique developmental issues associated with engagement in the workplace; however, given the shear number of nurses born between 1946 and 1964 (e.g., "Baby Boomers"), the largest group of actively working nurses, solutions are needed to retain these valuable employees and reduce their stress. Baby Boomers are often called the "Sandwich Generation" (CBS Broadcasting Inc., 2006). The Sandwich Generation is individuals who are *sandwiched* between pressures to assist aging parents while helping transition their children (and sometimes grandchildren) into their rightful place in society. Organizations that appreciate where their employees fall on the generational continuum can be proactive in helping reduce these stressors when spill-over starts to impact individual or organizational performance.

Research suggests that these nurses experience more stress than do nurses in other cohorts. Two large studies (Santos & Cox, 2000; Santos et al., 2003) found that Baby Boomer nurses had worse scores on occupational adjustment (stress, strain, and coping), compared with other nurse cohorts, using quantitative measures. The first study had staff nurse participants ($n = 413$) from one institution, and the second study included participants from four diverse institutions ($n = 694$). In addition, focus group findings indicated that the Boomer cohort had a sense of hostility toward younger nurses aligned with their perception that younger nurses, those born between 1965 and 1979 (i.e., "Generation Xers"), were not as committed to the organization as they were. Indeed, this coincides with the generational conflict that has been characterized in the popular press as the "live to work" (Boomers)–"work to live" (Generation Xers) paradox (Lancaster & Stillman, 2002).

As much as it would be desirable to create strict boundaries between work and home lives, this continues to be a struggle, especially as parents are living longer and with more chronic conditions. We would do well as leaders within our organizations to create environments that not only help our staff find ways to keep the balance they need to be productive in their jobs but also assist them when they are facing issues with family members. The Family and Medical Leave Act enacted in 1993 (Department of Labor, 2007) provided this tangible support for employees to manage emergent issues within their immediate families; however, research suggests that organizations must do more than fully comply with this act if they are to keep valuable employees (Rocco et al., 2006). For years it has been known that having programs or assistance in place for staff in times of need reduces their stress and makes them more

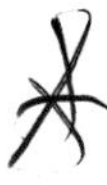
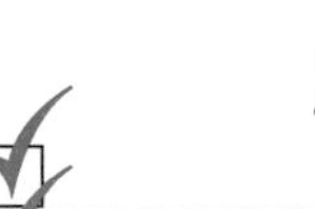

Practical Tips

This chapter is heavily sprinkled with hidden practical tips. The theory has been well known for a long time, but nurses still need guidance about how to customize strategies that will work for them. Here are some basic tips.

Tip # 1: Assess Use of Time

Start with an honest assessment of what you do with your time for 1 workday and 1 non-workday. You don't have to reveal this to anyone but yourself, but do it.

Tip # 2: Analyze Stressors

Choose 1 day this week to sit down with a piece of paper (can be with your computer or laptop) and make two columns. In the first column, list all the things that cause your stress. It is okay to start with "Not enough time for …". Do this column first. In the second column, list actions you might take to alleviate the stressors.

Tip # 3: Make a Change

Analyze your reflections after looking at the results from Tips #1 and #2. Choose one thing and make a change that will reduce the time spent and ease some of the stress.

loyal employees (Iaffaldano & Muchinsky,1985). This is particularly true in a time when the majority of seasoned employees struggle to keep up with many competing demands on their time and energy.

The Robert Wood Johnson Foundation (RWJF), the largest philanthropic organization that funds research and programs to address the health care industry's key issues, commissioned a report about older, more seasoned nurses (2006). Specifically this report outlined ways to retain these valuable staff members in a time when the physical and mental demands of the nurse are exponentially increasing. The following are ways in which innovative organizations can retain their most knowledgeable nurses (p. 57):

- Social interaction with peers and patients
- More control over work setting
- Participation in decision making
- Work recognition, encouragement, and positive feedback from supervisors
- Favorable work schedules
- Economic incentives
- Less strenuous jobs that use their experience
- Ergonomically friendly, safe, and effective workplaces
- Retirement programs that make working longer attractive
- Innovative new nursing roles

Individual Sources of Stress

Sources of stress that arise from the individual nurse can be either internal or external in origin. For example, the individual nurse may bring to work internal personal emotional conflicts or the need to balance work and family roles. Similar to intrapersonal conflict and tensions in women's careers, the pressure to balance multiple roles in life may create an internal tension that is manifested by personal stress (Huber, 1994). Stress on the individual nurse from an external source may be derived from the characteristics of an individual's personality. For example, the individual's personality may not fit in or match a given work situation (Getzels, 1958). This is an external stress source in that the external work situation impinges on the individual.

Potential outcomes or consequences of the sources of stress that arise from the individual nurse include hardiness (McCranie et al., 1987; Rich & Rich, 1987; Wagnild & Young, 1991), burnout

(Bailey, 1980; Stehle, 1981), and reality shock (Kramer, 1974; Kramer & Schmalenberg, 1977; Schmalenberg & Kramer, 1979). Hardiness is a personality characteristic composed of commitment, control, and challenge. This outcome of withstanding high job stress is a variable that may reduce or buffer burnout. Buffering occurs because the higher the personal hardiness, the lower the burnout (Simoni & Paterson, 1997).

Burnout has been described as a syndrome of emotional exhaustion, negative attitudes, and cynicism toward clients that afflicts individuals in the helping professions (Maslach & Jackson, 1981). Apathy, alienation, job dissatisfaction, and depersonalization of clients are associated with burnout (Tarolli-Jager, 1994). In the new graduate, the movement from school to active practice can create an incongruence or conflict in the values and behaviors of the two subcultures in nursing, termed "reality shock." Reality shock can create feelings of helplessness, powerlessness, frustration, and dissatisfaction. This crisis of role transformation may be resolved by adopting organizational values, returning to school, limiting personal involvement or commitment, becoming burned out, hopping from job to job, abandoning nursing, or becoming bicultural and working with the best of both worlds (Schmalenberg & Kramer, 1979). Burnout is a condition that develops from continuous job-related stress, but not all nurses under stress develop burnout (Schwab, 1996). Mediation or stress-resistance resources include hardiness and the use of social resources (Sawatzky, 1998). A person's self-esteem may be the most important personal factor predicting burnout potential (Schwab, 1996).

Organizational Sources of Stress

In contrast to the sources of stress generated within or from an individual, nurses experience stress that comes from the nature of nursing and the organizations that typically employ nurses. Sources of stress that arise from the job or occupational environment relate either to the intrinsic nature of the work or to a specific work environment. The intrinsic nature of nursing's work is recognized as stressful. This includes bedside nursing care delivery to ill or hospitalized clients (Laschinger, Finegan, & Shamian, 2001).

Work environments and organizations that employ nurses also generate stress for nurses. For example, the role of the nurse can be a source of stress and strain (Dewe, 1987). Organizations can and do generate multiple and conflicting demands on nurses, resulting in a job experience that generates numerous stressful situations. Energy and coping resources are devoted to the task of adapting and mastering the stress of role pressures and competing role expectations.

Role stress and role strain have been important leadership and management topics for many years. Hardy (1978) developed a typology of seven sources of role stress: role ambiguity, role conflict, role incongruity, role overload, role underload, role overqualification, and role underqualification. *Role Theory* (Thomas & Biddle, 1966) is a collection of concepts and hypotheses that predict how an individual will perform in a given role. It indicates the circumstances under which certain types of behavior can be expected (Conway, 1988).

Role stress and role strain have been linked to stress in social systems (Hardy, 1978; Miller, 1971). Role expectations, location of the role in the social structure, inadequate resources, and the social context create role difficulties and stressors. Role stress arises from sources external to the role occupant. It is a social structural condition generated from role obligations that are vague, irritating, difficult, conflicting, or impossible to meet. Role strain is a subjective state of emotional arousal that occurs in response to external conditions of social stress (Charnley, 1999; Hardy & Hardy, 1988; Huber, 1994). The organizations that employ nurses can create role ambiguity when role expectations are unclear, role conflict when role expectations are incompatible, role incongruity when the nurse's professional values conflict with role expectations, role overload when too much is expected in the time available, or role underload when highly expert nurses are underutilized. Thus role stress and strain are common to nursing practice.

Specific characteristics present in health care work environments and organizations also generate stress in nursing. For example, the physical and technical environment, patterns of interpersonal relationships, professional-bureaucratic role conflict, multiple expectations, management, leadership style, communication patterns, staffing and workload, negative client outcomes, relationships with physicians, lack of participation in policy decisions, and inadequate knowledge and skills for role functions each can be a source of stress (Hinshaw & Atwood, 1983; McGrath, 1976). Clearly, the dynamics between nurses and physicians contribute to nurses' satisfaction with their jobs (Mills & Blaesing, 2000). Leatt and Schneck (1980) categorized the organizational sources of stress as derived from either role-based or task-based situations. Huckabay and Jagla (1979) categorized intensive care unit (ICU) nursing stressors into the four categories of interpersonal communication problems, knowledge-base stressors, environmental stressors, and patient care situations.

Hospitals and health care organizations have environmental contexts with elements that may help or hinder the work of nurses (McClure et al., 1983). Structural, procedural, and contextual factors cause stress and conflict (Landstrom et al., 1989). Stress interrelates with other organizational variables, such as organizational climate, group cohesion, job satisfaction, turnover, productivity, conflict, change, and organizational restructuring (Hinshaw & Atwood, 1983; Hinshaw et al., 1987; Huber, 1994). Job strain has increased in many nursing environments because of increased workload and higher acuity (Laschinger, Finegan, Shamian, & Almost, 2001).

Job satisfaction and turnover have been the major outcome variables of organizational stress that have been studied (Hinshaw et al., 1987; Irvine & Evans, 1995; Landstrom et al., 1989; McCloskey & McCain, 1987; Price & Mueller, 1981; Weisman et al., 1981). Job satisfaction is a major predictor of anticipated turnover or intent to stay or leave. Anticipated turnover is a major predictor of actual turnover (Hinshaw, 1989). Job stress is an individual factor that influences job satisfaction, thereby having an indirect effect on anticipated turnover (Hinshaw et al., 1987). In critical care environments, perceived stress is related to job satisfaction and psychological symptoms (Bratt et al., 2000).

Turbulence and organizational change create stress. Regionalization and integration transform simple organizations into complex networks of community health care systems. As health care organizations change in response to social, consumer-related, governance, technology, and economic pressures, chaos and opportunities arise (Schumacher & Larson, 1993). With dramatic changes in the structures and functions of health care organizations, stress has become an ongoing reality for staff (Santos & Cox, 2000).

A new concept described in the nursing literature is operational failures (Tucker, 2004). Operational failures are defined as disruptions or errors in the supply of needed information or materials. These failures are frustrating; however, nurses tend to figure out how to compensate for them rather than bring them to the attention of managers.

A sense of perceived control over related work pressures is critical to perceived stress and stress outcomes. External forces beyond a nurse's control that interfere with the ability to deliver quality care increase occupational stress. For example, some nursing stressors are lack of control over staffing patterns and staff mix, lack of resource availability such as supplies and equipment, and lack of autonomy (McVicar, 2003). Furthermore, as organizations create and deploy work teams to deliver quality care, interpersonal stressors from the group dynamics of teams may create stress for both staff and managers (American Hospital Association [AHA], 2002). Implementing strategies and structures for empowerment is a major technique for organizational innovations designed to increase participation and decrease burnout, as evidenced by the research in Magnet™-designated environments (Laschinger et al., 2003).

COPING AND ADAPTATION

Stressors are demands or threatening experiences from either the internal or external environment of an individual that create disequilibrium. Restoration and balance are sought as a result of stressors (Keenan et al., 1993). Excessive occupational stress can lead to the undesirable outcome of burnout. Burnout in nurses undermines the nurse's helping relationship. Therefore it is counterproductive for organizations to allow occupational stress to flourish without checks and balances. A preferable outcome goal is for nurses to function as self-dependent innovators who operate within realistic expectations and exercise control within a stressful work environment (Grant, 1993).

The array of coping strategies is vast, but not all coping strategies elicit an adaptive response. Generalized resistance resources include personality characteristics, predispositions, social supports, and health practices. Each can function as a buffer. Consequently, some individuals who experience high stress levels do not become ill and may actually thrive on stress (Sawatzky, 1998). Social support and the personality characteristic of hardiness were key mechanisms of Pollock's 1984 "Adaptation Nursing Model."

The concept of hardiness grew out of the observation that high stress does not create illness in all people and that a modest relationship exists between stressful life events and illness symptoms (Kobasa et al., 1982). Hardiness is a personality style that contains elements of commitment, control, and challenge and that affects coping by buffering the stress-illness relationship. It also appears to affect adaptation by influencing the individual's perception of the stressful event and strategies and resources chosen (Sawatzky, 1998).

An individual's coping ability is the major variable modulating stress and its outcome. Coping strategies are key elements of nurses' stress reactions. The coping process is composed of the perception of stress, conditions and situational factors affecting cognitive appraisal, assessment of coping mechanisms, and the selection of a coping strategy (Harris, 1989). Nurses need to learn to manage or cope effectively with daily work stressors by evaluating and moderating response patterns. For example, attitudes and skills, habits or typical approaches to problems, and specific actions for stress management all can be used to intervene between stress and the outcome. Effective coping actions reduce emotional distress, resolve or diminish problems, and maintain or enhance the sense of self (Woodhouse, 1993).

There have been various recommendations for nurses for coping with and managing stress. For example, the development of an internal warning system to alert the individual to stress and provide a choice of responses has been recommended (Hartl, 1989). Nurses need to test the subjective and objective boundaries of stress and be willing to look after their own best interests. This may be a competing value to the concept of altruistic, unselfish service to others. However, guilt may be used by organizations to induce nurses to respond in ways that serve primarily the interests of the institution (Woodhouse, 1993). The most recent version of the Code of Ethics for Nurses, developed by the American Nurses Association (2001), makes it clear that nurses must consider their own needs as well as those of the patients they serve. The fifth principle of the Code of Ethics states that the nurse owes the same duty to self as to others and this includes the responsibility to preserve integrity and patient safety.

Stress management techniques range from those focused on the individual to those focused on the organization. Some coping strategies used by nurse executives include spending time on non–work-related interests, using a personal support network, being active in the larger professional arena, identifying resources for problem solving, manifesting somatic symptoms, walking away from situations to gain perspective, considering resigning, adhering rigidly to rules, complying, and participating in dysfunctional competition (Scalzi, 1988). Humor in communication can also be used as a mechanism for coping with stress and thereby enhancing morale and productivity (Woodhouse, 1993).

A comprehensive stress management plan may be needed for organizations. It begins with a baseline stress assessment to determine the levels and types of occupational stress. Interactions of departments and availability of support systems can be analyzed in relationship to nursing stress levels. Educational programs can be developed around universal stress and coping themes, such as work overload, time management, decision making, prioritization skills, and change management. Assessments of nurses' perception of their workload may help target changes where the most impact will be felt (Cox, 2002).

Other methods of personal or organizational strategies for coping with stress include physical activity; nutritional control; environmental control; psychological strategies to improve attitudes, self-esteem, and self-mastery; and interpersonal strategies related to social support. Exercise, sports, hobbies, meditation, relaxation, and spiritual exercises are advocated. Stress audits can be personal assessments or organization-wide reports. Balancing an increase in personal control with coping with what is beyond control is a key strategy. Monitoring the effects of caffeine, nicotine, and sleep/rest is advocated to increase coping. Intervention techniques can be focused on filtering, buffering, and adapting to stress.

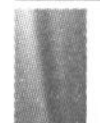

LEADERSHIP AND MANAGEMENT IMPLICATIONS

Time management is a central strategy for reducing stress and improving coping ability. Stress is an important concern for leaders and managers in nursing. It is a pervasive fact of organizational operations. Both personal and occupational stresses create consequences for leaders and managers that also may affect meeting goals and levels of productivity. The list of work-related and non–work-related stressors is long. Leaders and managers will need to assess the levels and types of stress in individuals and in the environment to begin to moderate stress toward useful levels.

Stress at a level that is too high reduces nurses' coping and adaptive abilities and is counterproductive. Nurse leaders and managers may have a role to play in caring for the psychological needs of the staff. Identifying and addressing prevalent operational failures at the department level can decrease many daily frustrations. Personal hardiness may be augmented by increased awareness. Leaders and managers can provide counseling, support groups, team-building activities, and stress management programs. Generational differences should be considered in developing targeted interventions (Santos & Cox, 2000).

Nurse leaders and managers have a stake in assessing and diagnosing the sources of nursing occupational stress. As much as possible, nurse leaders should use psychometrically sound instruments to evaluate both developing and assessing the impact of interventions (Huber et al., 2000). This becomes the foundation for planning, implementing, and evaluating strategies to manage job stress. Within organizations, nurse productivity, job satisfaction, and retention improve when occupational stress is managed. Some stressors can be modified, improved, or reduced by making structural or organizational changes. Adequate staffing, correcting problems in the physical environment, and facilitating positive communication are suggested strategies for nurse leaders and managers. Internal organizational systems may be malfunctioning and need correction. For example, organizational structures, client care variables, availability of support services, and nursing care delivery modalities may create stress and be amenable to modification for stress reduction. Organizational remedies should be founded on staff input and be directly related to improving the system (Huber, 1994; Norbeck, 1985).

Nurse leaders and managers may need to find strategies for nurses coping with an environment that creates stress because of the threat of personal danger. For example, nurses who work in abortion clinics may be personally threatened with harm. Instances arise in which infants are kidnapped from hospital nurseries. Clients may physically assault caregivers. Caregivers may be involved in fistfights or throwing objects. Policies and procedures need to be in place to protect nurses and clients from physical injury or harm.

Leaders can inspire hope and a vision for the future. They must role-model the ability to balance personally and professionally. They can communi-

LEADERSHIP & MANAGEMENT BEHAVIORS

Leadership Behaviors

- Role-models workload prioritization
- Enables followers to cope with stress
- Models personal stress management
- Uses humor
- Encourages adaptation and growth
- Mentors and provides social support
- Communicates ways of coping
- Envisions the future
- Inspires hope
- Influences greater personal and group control

Management Behaviors

- Uses humor
- Manages personal stress
- Plans for stress assessment
- Organizes the environment to decrease stress
- Evaluates individual and occupational stress
- Influences followers to manage time and cope with stress
- Plans goals and activities within time targets
- Organizes work space for efficiency

Overlap Areas

- Uses humor
- Manages personal stress
- Creates ways to constructively manage time

cate with humor and inspire others to adapt to stress. Managers can plan and organize the environment to modulate organizational stress. This includes restructuring to increase nurses' access to formal and informal power and to information, resources, and support (Kanter, 1993; Laschinger et al., 2003). Leaders and managers can manage personal stress and influence others toward enhanced coping and support of one another. Thus both individual and occupational stress can be managed.

CURRENT ISSUES AND TRENDS

Important parallel research is being conducted that can add to our understanding of time management and stress, specifically how improving nursing resources can increase patient and organizational outcomes; this goal can be directly linked to better time management and reduction of stress throughout the organization. Empirical findings strongly suggest that a link exists between a higher concentration of nursing resources and better patient outcomes (Kane et al., 2007). In March of 2007, the Agency for Healthcare Research and Quality (AHRQ) released findings from a meta-analysis of 94 observational studies conducted between 1990 and 2006 that suggested that increased nursing resources in hospitals are associated with decreased patient mortality, shorter lengths of stay, and lower risk of adverse events. This verifies once again that quality patient outcomes are linked to the numbers of available RNs.

The national quality agenda is in full swing. It is difficult to imagine quality outcomes without good nursing care. Therefore it is imperative that leaders within organizations seek ways to reduce stress among staff nurses. This will ultimately translate into better patient outcomes and will become cyclical and reinforcing. A by-product of better outcomes for patients will be reductions in stress levels among the leaders themselves. This occurs because leaders respond to internal and external stakeholders in the age of "transparency" and "mandated" outcomes reporting about the work that nurses perform. Reporting positive results produces lower levels of external pressure, and therefore stress drops.

This is a unique time in nursing. The vast amount of literature that links nursing care with outcomes has impacted policies of the largest payer of health care in the United States, the Centers for Medicare and Medicaid Services (CMS), as evidenced by their latest recommendation regarding hospital reimbursement. In August 2007, CMS proposed specific changes in reimbursement that are linked to patient outcomes and nursing care (CMS, 2008). This proposal outlines plans to reduce reimbursement for organizations in which patients experience adverse events that are nurse-sensitive. If that is the case, a next logical step should flow from such a position. Hospitals, specifically those with nursing departments that have consistently better nurse-sensitive outcomes, should receive higher reimbursement rates than those that do not. This new reimbursement schema should put leadership on high alert that decisions made that influence staffing and support structures for nurses impact the organization's bottom line and lead to transcending the historical framework of nursing services being part of the daily bed charge (Welton et al., 2006).

Few nurses have risen to positions of national prominence in the national quality agenda; however, in every day of a professional staff nurse's life, he or she affects the quality agenda *one patient at a time*. Translating knowledge about the link between the work that nurses do and quality care with the science of time and stress management should be a core competency for nursing leaders in today's complex health care environment.

Health care reform and economics are creating stress and pressure for nurses both directly and indirectly. The turbulence and change that occur as health delivery systems merge, integrate, regionalize, and restructure in turn cause uncertainty, anxiety, role ambiguity, and stress. Pervasive stress is inevitable with such large-scale reforming processes of systems. Nurses must cope with new ways of thinking and delivering care. Individual stress responses, turf battles, and conflicts occur as the friction surfaces among individuals. For example, teamwork and collaboration may ultimately provide a fertile ground for systems improvement, but teamwork may be a new mode of operating and therefore a source of stress. Individuals are likely to feel helpless, anxious, and out of control when faced with massive systems changes (Huber, 1994).

Leaders and managers may themselves be under sufficient stress and thereby have less energy to devote to helping their staff through difficult psychological transitions. Cost-containment pressures may result in decisions to eliminate staff education for stress management. Institutional remedies may be substantially diminished.

It is difficult to prescribe methods for work-related stress management during periods of high environmental turbulence. Educating and supporting staff nurses, reducing paperwork, changing organizational climates, enhancing nurses' participation in decision making, and reducing workloads, all positive strategies for reducing nurses' stress, may not be implemented by organizations during unstable environmental conditions. Furthermore, under health care reform initiatives, there have been major redesigns of roles and tasks in nursing and health care. Role ambiguity has become a major source of stress, directly related to both advanced practice nurses and unlicensed assistive personnel. With so many focal points for stress, nursing as a profession is challenged to create a vision for the future and strategies for today.

Stress and conflict also may create opportunities for nursing. Clarity of direction for the profession in carving out key nursing roles and responsibilities in a community-based, managed care environment is a key stress and coping strategy. For example, case management has become a growth area for nursing as payers begin to value and pay for cost-effective care coordination and management. Changes prompt the need to adapt. Building and nurturing teams, managing change, and providing strong leadership can create a climate for innovation and creativity as one productive response to uncertainty and stress. Conflicts and changes generate stress. Positive and proactive responses help nurses cope and adapt to stress in a way that produces growth and productivity.

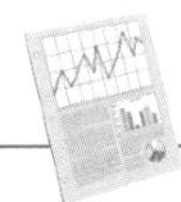

Research Note

Source: Shader, K., Broome, M.E., Broome, C.D., West, M.E., & Nash, M. (2001). Factors influencing satisfaction and anticipated turnover for nurses in an academic medical center. *Journal of Nursing Administration, 31*(4), 210-216.

Purpose

This quantitative study examined the relationship between work satisfaction, stress, age, cohesion, work schedule, and anticipated turnover. Determining the impact of these relationships on intent to leave could provide nurse leaders with the knowledge to design interventions to improve work environment and retention.

Discussion

In one academic medical center, a variety of factors believed to influence satisfaction and anticipated turnover were studied using a cross-sectional survey of nurses using three self-report instruments. Job stress, work satisfaction, group cohesion, and weekend overtime were all individually predictive of anticipated turnover. However, there were differences in these predictors based on age of the nurse. Also, the more job stress, lower group cohesion, and work satisfaction, the higher the anticipated turnover. Many of the findings are supportive of previous work environment research.

Application to Practice

This study considered a number of important aspects in the nursing work environment. However, some key issues embedded in the surveys as discrete concepts such as manager support, workload, and nurse-physician relationships were not analyzed. Regardless of this, important relationships were confirmed. It is important to assess nurses' perceptions of the work environment to make significant changes. Without pre-intervention and post-intervention assessments, nurse leaders won't know the actual impact of changes.

Summary

- Time is a scarce and valuable resource.
- Time management is self-management of activities.
- Time management strategies are aimed at organizing and mobilizing effective activities.
- Planning, analysis, and prioritization are key elements of time management.
- The current health care environment is turbulent and stressful.
- Stress is inherent in healing occupations.
- Stress needs to be neither too high nor too low.
- Stress is an individual response to a stressor.
- A stressor is an experience that is taxing or threatening.
- Occupational stress is a tension related to the job or role.
- Burnout is a response to chronic stress.
- Stress moves from potential stressor to outcomes and consequences.
- Coping and cognitive appraisal mediate stress.
- Stress consequences are either positive or negative.
- Sources of stress are individual or organizational.
- Multiple factors cause stress in nursing.
- Stress outcomes take different forms—from positive to negative.
- Coping modulates stress and its outcome.
- There are both individual and organizational stress-management techniques.
- Leaders and managers can influence stress and stress management.

CASE STUDY

Nurse Maria Vasquez is thrilled with the results of the time management training she recently received. A year ago, when she became the new nurse manager for both the operating rooms and the trauma center, she felt that everything was crashing in on her. She would arrive for work to find 15 to 20 phone messages to return, a 5-inch stack of mail to open, and 50 e-mail messages waiting on the computer. Nurse Vasquez found that on most days her attention was diverted by numerous "brush fires" that kept cropping up. In addition to the daily complaints from her staff about the normal employee concerns, there had been rumors that some nurses were talking about forming a collective bargaining unit as protection against short staffing and layoffs.

Nurse Vasquez went to her nursing director and asked for help. The director suggested that she take a couple of days and attend a time management class to see if it would give her any ideas to help in organizing her work and improving her efficiency.

Once she completed the class, Nurse Vasquez was excited about the idea of using an activity log to record her daily activities as a first step toward increasing her efficiency. She discussed the idea with the nursing supervisors who report to her, and they were interested in using the activity log idea themselves. Since then, Nurse Vasquez and her supervisors have found that by using the activity logs and identifying what is consuming their time, they have been better able to organize and have increased their efficiency as a result.

CRITICAL THINKING EXERCISE

Nurse Whitney Gould was initially very excited about her recent promotion to nurse manager of a 50-bed regional intensive care nursery. Before this promotion, she had been a charge nurse for 5 years on the unit. She felt this had prepared her for the position, but things have not fallen smoothly into place for her. Every time she enters her office, she is greeted with 50 e-mails, a stack of mail, and several voice messages. Each day she thinks this will be the day she finally has time to regroup and get organized.

Today was a good example of how that just never works out. Nurse Gould arrived at 6:30 AM to find the night charge nurse and nursing supervisor disagreeing about day staffing. The charge nurse also told her that several night nurses were taking a patient care concern to the ethics committee if she did not intervene. A surgeon called and voiced issues about a specific nurse that required immediate investigation. A recently hired graduate nurse called in tears because she failed boards. Staffing was short for the upcoming night shift. The chief nursing officer called and requested that Nurse Gould not only give a tour for some potential donors in the unit but also complete her staffing variance report before the end of the day. It is now 6 PM and she is heading out the door, physically and emotionally exhausted and wondering whether tomorrow will be just more of the same.

1. What problem(s) do you see in this scenario?
2. Why is this a problem?
3. What should Nurse Gould do first?
4. What factors should Nurse Gould assess and analyze?
5. What sources of stress are present?
6. How does Nurse Gould's stress affect the stress of nurses in the unit?
7. What strategies could be employed to control stress and enhance coping?

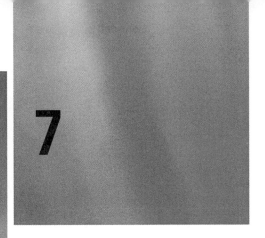

7

Legal and Ethical Issues

Robert W. Cooper

CHAPTER OBJECTIVES

- Explain how the law and professional codes of ethics confer autonomy—both authority and accountability—on nurses and nurse managers
- Identify and describe the grounds on which nurses, nurse managers, and health care organizations can be found legally liable for harm caused to others by civil wrongs
- Compare the sources of legal liability to which nurses and nurse managers are exposed in clinical practice with those encountered in carrying out their responsibilities related to delegation and supervision
- Describe the various steps nurse managers can take to protect themselves, the staff nurses reporting to them, and their facilities from legal liability and its related costs
- Define judicial risk, and explain its potential effects on the litigation process
- Identify the key sources of ethical conflict encountered in clinical health care, and describe the resources available for use in deciding how to resolve the resulting dilemmas
- Describe the conflict faced by nurse managers due to the clash between clinical and organizational ethics
- Explain the various steps nurse managers can take to prepare themselves and the staff nurses reporting to them for dealing effectively with the dilemmas arising from the clash between clinical and organizational ethics
- Exercise critical thinking to conceptualize and analyze possible solutions to a practice experience

A major advantage of being viewed as a profession is the societal grant of autonomy in practice. In professional terms, *autonomy* means that the occupational group has control over its own practice. The American Nurses Association's (ANA) original *Nursing: A Social Policy Statement* (1980) identified two mechanisms that frame autonomy: the legal regulation of nursing practice via state licensure laws, and the professional regulation of nursing practice via standards and ethical codes of practice.

Although some laws can be unethical, laws generally provide minimum standards of acceptable conduct that are binding on individuals, groups, and businesses in dealing with other members of society. Many situations, however, are either not covered by specific laws or involve issues so complicated that, although the law can provide general guidelines for conduct, the issues cannot be fully resolved by the legal system alone. In these cases, ethical codes for a profession provide standards of conduct that serve as guidelines for decision making by the members of the profession.

By the very nature of their work, nurses and nurse managers are decision makers constantly faced with making choices in personal, clinical, and organizational situations. These decision-making situations are commonly fraught with legal and ethical issues that often become entwined. As members of a profession, nurses and nurse managers are guided by both legal and ethical considerations in making decisions.

LEGAL ASPECTS

There are extensive legal aspects to both nursing practice and nursing management. For example, nurse practice acts exist for each state and govern the legal practice of nursing, including delegation and supervision. The legal regulation of nursing via nurse practice acts and related administrative rules arises because society needs to have safeguards that protect the health and safety of citizens. In regard to health care, the public demands assurance that health care providers, including nurses, are properly prepared and competent to deliver needed services. Thus to practice nursing, the person must hold a valid license issued by the state. Therefore it is illegal to practice nursing without a license. State licensure confers autonomy on nurses to the limit of legal standards of practice.

Autonomy involves accountability, as well as authority, for one's decisions and actions. As professional autonomy and responsibility increase, so does the level of accountability and liability. To the extent that nurses are subject to malpractice lawsuits and carry malpractice insurance, nurses are held accountable (Aiken, 2004).

The legal aspects of nursing management center around decision making and supervision. Because all nurses retain personal accountability for their own acts and the use of knowledge and skills in the provision of care, personal accountability cannot be assumed by another. Nurse managers keep their own personal accountability for their own specific acts, but they are accountable also for their acts of delegation and supervision. Nurse managers carry the major responsibility for developing and upholding the standards of care for the staff.

Nurses and nurse managers carry the accountability for the supervision of others, who are often unlicensed assistive personnel. Supervision includes monitoring the tasks performed, ensuring that functions are performed in an appropriate fashion, and ensuring that assigned tasks and functions do not exceed competency or require a license to perform.

Nurse managers use their autonomy to make decisions about practice situations. They are accountable for carrying out supervisory responsibilities; proper notification; assessing the competency of staff; training, orientation, and evaluation of staff; reasonable staffing decisions; and monitoring and maintenance of professional treatment relationships with clients, called *nonabandonment* (Aiken, 2004; Guido, 2006).

DEFINITIONS

In addition to law included in the federal and state constitutions, United States law is composed of **statutory law** (law enacted by the U.S. Congress, state legislatures, and local government bodies), **administrative law** (regulations promulgated and adopted by federal or state agencies to implement statutory law adopted by Congress or state legislatures), and **common law** (decisions of courts setting precedents to be followed, at least in that court's jurisdiction, until overturned by a higher court). The law recognizes two classes of wrongful acts that may cause harm. These are **criminal acts** (conduct that is offensive or harmful to society as a whole) and **civil acts** (wrongs that violate the rights of individuals by tort or by breach of contract). Persons found guilty of crimes are generally fined and/or jailed, whereas persons who commit civil wrongs are usually required to pay monetary damages to those who are wronged.

Nurses, nurse managers, and health care facilities are all subject to being found **legally liable** (i.e., legally responsible) for harm caused to others by civil wrongs. More specifically, liability is created when the law imposes a civil obligation on a wrongdoer to compensate an injured party for the consequences of a wrongful act. As shown in Figure 7.1, there are two sources of legal liability—torts and contracts.

The most common source of legal liability for nurses and nurse managers is a *tort*—that is, a wrongful act (other than breach of contract) committed against another person or organization or their property that causes harm and can be

LEGAL LIABILITY
A civil obligation imposed by law on a wrongdoer requiring compensation of an inured party through money damages or some other legal remedy for the consequences of a wrongful act

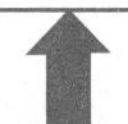

"JUDICIAL RISK" FILTER
Various aspects of the litigation process that can introduce further uncertainty and additional cost into the determination of legal liability
- Witnesses' perceptions of the facts can change over time
- Courtroom conditions can influence the jury

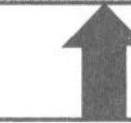

TORTS
Tort—a wrongful act (other than a breach of contract) committed by one person that causes harm to another by invading a legally protected right
- **Personal (Direct) Liability**—liability imposed on the person who committed the wrongful act
- **Vicarious Liability**—a person or organization that has not behaved wrongfully can be held legally liable for torts committed by others

CONTRACTS
- **Breach of Contract**—if a party to a contract does not perform as promised, the other party can sue for money damages or seek the remedy of specific performance
- **Hold Harmless or Indemnity Agreements**—one party assumes the liability of another party for damage in situations in which the first party would not otherwise be liable

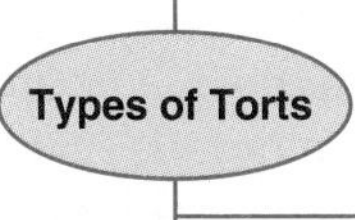

Negligence
- An unintentional tort
- Negligence—failure of a person to exercise the degree of care that an ordinary prudent person would have exercised under similar circumstances
- Malpractice—failure of a professional person to act as other prudent professionals with the same knowledge and education would have acted under similar circumstances

Intentional Torts
- A wrongful act that was intended to cause harm
- Examples
  - Assault and battery
  - False imprisonment
  - Defamation—libel and slander
  - Invasion of right of privacy
  - Fraud
  - Intentional torts against property (trespass, conversion)

Strict Liability Torts
- Tort liability imposed when the defendant acted neither negligently nor with intent to cause harm
- May be applied in cases involving dangerously defective products—medical devices, use of unlicensed medicines

Figure 7.1
Sources of legal liability.

PART II

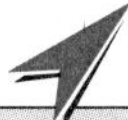

LEADING & MANAGING DEFINED

Statutory Law

Law enacted by the U.S. Congress, state legislatures, or local government bodies and signed (approved) as required by the President, governor, or local equivalent such as a mayor.

Administrative Law

Rules and regulations adopted by federal or state agencies to implement statutory law adopted by Congress or state legislatures.

Common Law

A system of laws or principles based on court decisions and on customs and usages rather than on statutory written laws.

Criminal Acts

Conduct that is offensive or harmful to society as a whole and violates statutes prohibiting such conduct; persons found to have committed criminal acts are typically fined or jailed.

Civil Acts

Conduct that violates the rights of individuals by tort or by breach of contract; there may or may not be in existence statutes prohibiting such conduct; persons who have committed civil wrongs are usually required to pay money damages to those who were wronged.

Legally Liable

When the law imposes a civil obligation on a wrongdoer to compensate an injured party for the consequences of a wrongful act.

Negligence

Failure to exercise the proper degree of care required by the circumstances.

Malpractice

Failure of a professional person to act as other prudent professionals with the same knowledge and education would act under similar circumstances.

remedied by a civil (rather than criminal) lawsuit. Although torts most commonly give rise to *personal* (or *direct*) liability for the person committing the wrongful act, in some cases another person or organization may also be held *vicariously* liable for the same wrongful act they did not commit. For example, when a nurse commits a tort, the nurse may be found to be directly liable and the nurse's employer also may be found to be vicariously liable for the nurse's wrongful action.

As indicated in Figure 7.1, determination of legal liability as a result of a tort depends on more than just the various technical elements of the tort that must be proved by the injured party (plaintiff), the presentation of various available defenses by the defendant, and the formal rules of the judicial system regarding the litigation process. In the case of torts, the legal outcomes are often influenced also by what may be termed *judicial risk*—various aspects of the litigation process that can introduce further uncertainty and additional cost into the determination of legal liability. Judicial risk can result in findings with respect to legal liability that are not based solely on the merits of the case nor on the rules of law applicable to the case.

There are three categories of torts: negligence, intentional torts, and strict liability torts. **Negligence** is the failure to exercise the proper degree of care required by the circumstances. In general, the standard of care is defined as that which a reasonably prudent person would exercise under the circumstances to avoid harming others. Malpractice is a special type of negligence that applies only to professionals and employs a higher standard of care than ordinary negligence. **Malpractice** is the failure of a professional person to act as other prudent professionals with the same knowledge and education would act under similar circumstances. Depending on the nature of the situation involved, nurses and nurse leaders may be subject to either ordinary negligence or malpractice. An example of ordinary negligence would be a situation in which a nurse saw that food had been spilled on a client's floor but failed to have it cleaned up, and as a result, the client slipped and broke her hip. Because this is an act not requiring the exercise of professional judgment, the standard of care in determining negligence would be the degree of care that an ordinary prudent person would exercise under the circumstances. However, if the client had fallen and broken her hip because a nurse had failed to raise the side rails on the client's bed, the standard of care in determining malpractice would be the degree of care other prudent professionals with the same knowledge and education could be expected to exercise under similar circumstances.

Although negligence involves unintentional wrongful acts that harm another person or his or her property, *intentional torts* are voluntary and willful acts intended to cause harm by interfering with another person's rights. Common intentional torts occurring in the health care field include, among others, assault and battery, medical battery (surgical procedures performed without patient consent), false imprisonment, trespass to land, conversion of property, and intentional infliction of emotional distress.

In some cases, tort liability can be imposed without the defendant acting either negligently or with intent to cause harm. *Strict liability* requires that the responsibility for some accidents automatically rests with the defendant. With strict liability, anyone who engages in an activity known to endanger others assumes responsibility for any resulting damages. In general society, situations requiring strict liability include such activities as blasting, keeping dangerous animals, and selling dangerously defective products. In the health care field, the concept of strict liability has been applied in some cases involving harm caused by, among other things, the use of unlicensed medicines, defectively designed medical devices, tainted or contaminated drugs, and the prescription of dangerous combinations of drugs without obtaining a sufficient medical history to ensure that problems do not occur.

As shown in Figure 7.1, contracts are also a source of legal liability. In most states, employment of nurses generally follows the employment-at-will doctrine in which there is no written contract specifying the term of employment. However, in some cases, nurse managers, especially those at higher levels in an organization, negotiate written employment contracts. In addition, a few courts have ruled that contracts existed on the basis of language used in advertisements and statements made during the interviewing process. Courts also have held that contracts may arise after employment based on statements made in employee manuals and handbooks. With an increasing number of nurses negotiating various types of consulting arrangements with facilities, working as independent contractors and operating their own privately owned businesses, contracts are playing an even greater role in nursing.

Legal liability based on contracts can arise in two ways: breach of contract, or an agreement to assume another party's liability. The most common is *breach of contract*, in which one party to the contract fails to perform as promised in the contract. In this case, the injured party can either sue for monetary damages or seek the remedy of specific performance in which the court orders the party that caused the breach to do what was promised by the contract. For example, if a nurse has an employment contract stating that he or she can be discharged only for incompetence but then is discharged for another reason, the nurse can bring a suit for wrongful discharge under contract law due to breach of contract. Less likely to be encountered by nurses is legal liability arising from *an agreement to assume another party's liability*. An example of such an agreement is a "hold harmless" agreement commonly found in leases. For example, in signing a lease for property needed to carry on his or her privately owned business, the nurse likely would be agreeing to assume responsibility for all injuries occurring on the premises, including any caused by the owner of the property.

LAW AND THE NURSE MANAGER

The managers of any health care organization are responsible to the policy-making body of the organization. The managers also hold an obligation to comply with the laws of society at local, state, and national levels. Managers are responsible for ensuring that laws are adhered to in the actions of management itself and also in the actions of those employees who assist the managers in carrying out the mission of the organization. Concern for the law involves three general areas: personal negligence in clinical practice, liability for delegation and supervision, and liability of health care organizations.

Personal Negligence in Clinical Practice

Activities of clinical client care involve corresponding legal accountability and risk. Errors do happen. Some lead to injury to a client. At minimum, nurses have an ethical obligation to nonmaleficence, or to do no harm to clients. This duty is discharged in part by remaining competent in knowledge and skills and the standards of practice. Nursing negligence/malpractice occurs when the nurse's actions are unreasonable given the circumstances or fail to meet the standard of care or when the nurse fails to act and causes harm. In nursing, harm related to clinical practice commonly arises from negligent acts or omissions (unintentional torts) and a variety of intentional acts (intentional torts) such as invasion of privacy or assault and battery (Aiken, 2004).

To establish legal liability on the grounds of malpractice (professional negligence), the injured client (plaintiff) must prove the following four elements:

1. A duty of care was owed to the injured party.
2. There was a breach of that duty.
3. The breach of the duty caused the injury (causation).
4. Actual harm or damages were suffered by the plaintiff.

Critical in determining liability for malpractice (professional negligence) is the definition of the duty (standard) of care owed by the nursing professional to the client. The standard of care, the minimum requirements that define an acceptable level of care, is "the average degree of skill, care, and diligence exercised by members of the same profession under the same or similar circumstances" (Aiken, 2004, p. 39). Standards of care can be found in the state nurse practice act, standards published by the American Nurses Association, other professional organizations and specialty practice groups, federal agency guidelines and regulations, and the facility's policy and procedure manuals. In malpractice cases, the standard of care owed to the injured client is commonly introduced into evidence by expert witnesses and the impact of that evidence is ultimately determined by the jury after receiving instructions from the judge on the law applicable to its use.

Common clinical practice areas that give rise to allegations of malpractice include the general areas of treatment, communication, medication, and the broad category of monitoring/observing/supervising/surveillance. Examples of common negligence allegations in nursing malpractice suits include patient falls, use of restraints, medication errors, burns, equipment injuries, retained foreign objects, failure to monitor, failure to ensure safety, failure to take appropriate nursing action, failure to confirm accuracy of physicians' orders, improper technique or performance of treatments, failure to respond to a patient, failure to follow hospital procedure, and failure to supervise treatment (Aiken, 2004).

Because intentional torts differ in nature from negligence (unintentional torts), establishing legal liability for these intentionally harmful acts is based on elements different from those used in proving malpractice. To establish liability on the grounds of an intentional tort, the injured client (plaintiff) must prove that a voluntary and willful act by the nursing professional (defendant) was intended to interfere with the plaintiff's rights and was a substantial factor in doing so. Unlike negligence, intent is necessary in proving intentional torts. However, proof of actual injury or damage is not required, because intentional torts interfere with another person's rights. Also, there is no need to determine duty or standards of care in proving intentional torts.

Liability for Delegation and Supervision

Over and above personal liability for clinical practice, nurses and nurse managers have accountability and liability for their acts of delegation and supervision. Both nurses and nurse managers are obligated to report incompetent practice that occurs at any point in the care delivery process. Nurse managers have a duty to train, orient, and evaluate the ability of nursing staff to perform specific functions and tasks. Health care organizations have a duty to monitor the competence and ability of nursing and medical professionals and to inquire about their credentials (Aiken, 2004).

Both nurses and nurse managers have a duty to follow policies and procedures when reasonable. Nurse managers are advised to review policies and procedures carefully, including the language used, in order to adhere to legal and ethical parameters more closely. Clearly, management in nursing practice means that nurses must fulfill obligations and duties both to clients and to the organization. This means using knowledge, skill, and decision-making abilities to reduce the incidence of negligence and malpractice by employees as a way to reduce harm to clients and legal risk to the organization. As primary care coordinators, nurses need to manage the environment of care delivery. Ensuring staff competence and reporting incompetent practice are key activities. For example, in nursing, legal and ethical issues arise when a nurse is impaired by substance abuse. The overall consideration is protecting the client from harm. Confronting suspected abuse must be done carefully. However, when an incident occurs, the nurse manager has a responsibility to intervene.

Liability of Health Care Organizations

In addition to the liability faced by nurses and nurse managers arising out of malpractice in clinical practice and negligence in the process of delegating and supervising, health care facilities face extensive exposure to legal liability from several sources. These sources include negligence of their employees, negligence of independent contractors, corporate negligence arising out of the facility's responsibilities to hire qualified employees and monitor and supervise their activities, and failure to comply with numerous laws and regulations, especially those related to employment issues. Nurse managers have important roles to play in helping their organizations control facility liability arising from each of these sources.

Under the doctrine of *respondeat superior* (meaning "let the master answer"), an employer may be held vicariously liable for the negligent act or omission of an employee. For the employer to be found vicariously liable, the employee's act or omission must occur both during the course of employment and while the employee was acting within the scope of employment. For example, if a nurse negligently injured a client during the course of and within the scope of employment, not only would the nurse be directly liable for damages but also the health care organization would be vicariously liable. Because of their "deep pockets" (their ability to pay larger settlements or judgments) and the concept of vicarious liability, health care facilities are almost always named as defendants in malpractice suits. Nurse managers can play a key role in assisting facilities to avoid payments for vicarious liability by ensuring that the nurses they supervise deliver competent care to clients while following facility policies and procedures (Guido, 2006).

Under the doctrine of ostensible authority (or apparent agency), facilities may also become liable for the negligence of an independent contractor if it would appear to a reasonable client that the independent contractor is a facility employee. For example, a hospital might be held liable for the negligence of an agency nurse who appeared to a client to be a nurse employed by the hospital. Guido (2006) recommended that when dealing with agency or temporary personnel, nurse managers should, among other things, do the following:

- Consider their skills, competencies, and knowledge when delegating tasks and supervising their actions.
- Ensure that they are made aware of facility policies and procedures, resource materials, and documentation procedures.
- Assign a resource person to each temporary staff member to serve in the role of mentor and help prevent potential problems from occurring because of a lack of familiarity with institution routine or where to turn for assistance.

A relatively new area of law being created by the courts, the doctrine of corporate liability, holds health care organizations themselves legally responsible for "ensuring that competent and qualified practitioners will deliver quality heath care to consumers" (Guido, 2006, p. 281). Under this doctrine, facilities can be held liable for a variety of activities that are beyond the control of any single employee, including the following (Aiken, 2004):

- Failure to check references, educational credentials, license status, disciplinary actions, and criminal record for applicants
- Failure to protect the clients from health care providers who can cause harm
- Failure to monitor the quality of care provided by all medical and nursing personnel within the facility
- Failure to periodically review staff competency
- Failure to terminate an employee who has harmed a client and then injures another client.

Nurse managers can help the facility avoid corporate liability by, among other things, ensuring that those who report to them remain competent and qualified and have current licensure. Nurse managers should also report to appropriate managers dangerously low staffing levels or incorrect mixes of staff for effectively meeting the health care needs of clients, as well as report incompetent, illegal, or unethical practices to appropriate authorities (Guido, 2006).

In addition to facility liability arising from vicarious liability, the doctrine of ostensible authority, and the doctrine of corporate liability, health care organizations are constrained by specific laws related to employment issues. Although the various health care providers and their employing organizations have specific legal and ethical obligations to clients, such as executing informed consent and following the Patient Self-Determination Act of 1990, organizations carry specific legal and ethical obligations toward employees. The employer has an obligation to provide a safe and secure care delivery environment (Aiken, 2004).

Management policies and procedures must be in compliance in the areas of hiring, performance appraisal, management of employees with problems, and termination (Aiken, 2004). Lawsuits also have formed the basis for the standards to be met for the termination of employees. Discharges may occur for lack of adherence to employer-established policies or standards, "good cause" per institutional policy, illegal activity, assault, insubordination, or excessive absenteeism. Written notice and the reasons for termination avoid misunderstandings and show justice through due-process procedures. Careful documentation is important. If the employee is a member of a protected group, the employer may be required to submit formal justification for the termination (Aiken, 2004).

The various legal and ethical considerations of nursing management span client, provider, and employer rights and obligations. Nurses and their employing organizations are responsible for knowing and following the various applicable laws and regulations. In-service education can increase knowledge and awareness. Nurse managers will need to manage the environment of nursing care to ensure client safety, provider justice and safety, and organizational compliance with the law.

LEADERSHIP AND MANAGEMENT IMPLICATIONS

As indicated previously, nurses, nurse managers, and the facilities that employ them face legal liability from a wide array of sources. Although it is not possible to avoid legal liability in all cases, nurse managers can take a number of steps to protect themselves, staff nurses reporting to them, and their facilities where possible. The first step is summed up in a statement often attributed to football coach Vince Lombardi: *The best defense is a good offense.* Nurse managers can do a number of things in applying this strategy of using a good offense to defend against problems leading to legal liability. First, because problems generally can be dealt with more effectively if anticipated, nurse managers should see that both they and the staff nurses who report to them are knowledgeable concerning the most common problem areas related to malpractice and the other sources of legal liability, especially new ones that have not yet been experienced within the unit. Providing this information to staff nurses and using examples will probably improve both recognition and retention. In addition to the previous brief discussion of the sources of legal liability faced by nurses and nurse managers, extensive information, including examples, is available from numerous sources. These include books (e.g., Aiken, 2004; Brothers, 2005; Guido, 2006), nursing journals (e.g., Eskreis, 1998; Frank-Stromborg & Christensen, 2001a; Miller & Glusko, 2003; Trott, 1998), and a variety of websites (e.g., Croke, 2003; Nurses Service Organization [NSO], 2007; Wetter, 2007).

Next, nurse managers should ensure that both they and their staff nurses are aware of the many prevention activities that can aid them in avoiding these legal liability problems. In addition to facility guidelines, numerous ideas for reducing potential liability are available to the nurse manager and staff nurses in a variety of resource, such as the following:

- Books that focus on legal and ethical issues in nursing (e.g., Aiken, 2004; Guido, 2006)
- Articles in nursing journals (e.g., Frank-Stromborg & Christensen, 2001b; Miller & Glusko, 2003)
- Websites that present articles and continuing education materials providing recommendations for avoiding malpractice (e.g., Croke, 2003; NSO, 2007; Wetter, 2007)

Many, if not most, of the lawsuits seeking to determine legal liability involve the alleged failure of nurses to meet appropriate standards of care, especially those reflected in the policies and procedures of their facility. Therefore nurse managers must not only ensure that they and their staff nurses know the standards of care that apply to them and are competent to satisfy them but also actively participate in facility committees as well as those at the state, national, and even international level that make decisions as to the standards of care to which nurses will be held.

Although the first step in defending against problems of legal liability involves taking positive action in an effort to prevent them from arising, it is not possible for nurses, nurse managers, and health care facilities to avoid legal liability in all cases. This is so, if for no other reason than the existence of what might be termed *judicial risk.*

PART II

LEADERSHIP & MANAGEMENT BEHAVIORS

Leadership Behaviors

- Serves as spokesperson to the media on legal and ethical issues
- Guides others toward safe, legal, and ethical decision making
- Role-models ethical behavior
- Empowers followers to apply ethical decision-making models
- Facilitates autonomy
- Inspires multidisciplinary teams to discuss and resolve legal or ethical issues

Management Behaviors

- Assesses degree of implementation of laws governing practice
- Interprets the meaning of laws
- Revises policies and procedures following legal and ethical principles
- Establishes an ethics committee
- Manages violations of the law per procedure

Overlap Areas

- Scans the environment for trends and new laws
- Disseminates information to others about legal and ethical nursing practice
- Establishes mechanisms to handle legal and ethical issues

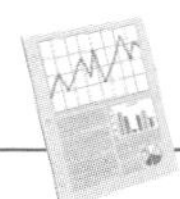

Research Note

Source: Eskreis, T.R. (1998). Seven common legal pitfalls in nursing. *American Journal of Nursing, 98*(4), 34-41.

Purpose

Malpractice is a type of negligence for which nurses have been sued. The purpose of this article is to present and analyze legal case studies in seven areas of malpractice allegations commonly brought against nurses.

Discussion

The seven common legal pitfalls in nursing are patient falls, failure to follow physician's orders or established protocols, medication errors, improper use of equipment, failure to remove foreign objects, failure to provide sufficient monitoring, and failure to communicate. The author presents and discusses actual cases arising under each category. Analysis of the actions that lead to a breach of practice includes tips for avoiding problems. In addition, a box of legal definitions of terms is provided. Most useful is a display box titled "Tips for Avoiding Common Legal Pitfalls" in which nursing actions for prevention and risk reduction are presented.

Application to Practice

A negligent professional act that causes injury is known as *malpractice*. For a successful lawsuit, the injured party must prove that the nurse's conduct lacked due care. Knowledge of the most common problem areas, the use of examples, and the display of prevention tips aid the nurse in avoiding problems. A caring nurse-client relationship is an important preventive measure.

Judicial risk can result in findings with respect to legal liability that are not based solely on the merits of the case or on the rules of law applicable to the case. In the case of torts, aside from all the lists of elements that must be proved by injured plaintiffs, all the legal defenses available for attempting to block their arguments for damages, and the formal rules of the judicial system regarding the litigation process, legal outcomes also are often influenced by judicial risk—that is, various aspects of the litigation process that can introduce further uncertainty and additional cost into the determination of legal liability. The following are some examples:

- Any client can sue a staff nurse, nurse manager, and/or health care facility for a tort, and if no response is filed within the legal time frame, the court will enter a default judgment against the defendant. Thus, at a minimum, regardless of the apparent validity of the grounds for the lawsuit, the defendant must incur defense costs or lose.
- Given the typical lengthy period between the defendant's act or omission and the introduction of evidence into the trial, many things can happen that will alter the perception of the facts. Witnesses, for example, may be questioned repeatedly, coached, or simply forget exactly what they witnessed. (See Case Study 1.)
- Conditions in the courtroom can also influence the jury. Some jury members may be influenced by the dress or behavior of the defendant's attorney and form subsequent opinions despite the facts (e.g., a high-priced lawyer with an arrogant attitude may elicit feelings such as "We'll show him"). Or the appearance of the plaintiff may influence

jurors (e.g., "How could a little old man like that be partly responsible for his own injuries, and besides, who cares anyway since the defendant has liability insurance?").

- Often more than one principle of law applies to a case, and the outcome may be influenced by which one the judge uses in giving his or her instructions to the jury.
- In suits such as those alleging malpractice in providing or failing to provide proper end-of-life care, juries and even judges can be sufficiently influenced by their emotions so as to rationalize a finding of legal liability against the defendant, especially when, as is generally the case, liability insurance is available to pay the judgment. In fact, in some cases, a jury can actually change the law of a jurisdiction in making its decision. (See Case Study 2.)

In some cases, the elements of judicial risk make impossible even one's best efforts to prevent legal liability from being imposed on them and/or their facility. Thus all nurses, whether staff or managers, should carry adequate professional liability insurance to protect themselves against defense costs and liability judgments (or settlements). Although nurses are often covered as employees under a facility's professional liability policy, a number of reasons exist why they should also carry their own individual professional liability insurance. An employer can sue a nurse found guilty of malpractice for reimbursement (indemnification) of any damages the facility was required to pay as a result of vicarious liability. In addition, because a facility's professional liability insurance protects a nurse only while acting within the scope of employment or the nurse practice act, individual liability coverage would be required by private-duty nurses and off-duty nurses providing volunteer services. Although a facility's policy may provide only a single attorney to represent the different interests of the facility and the nurse, an individual policy will provide an attorney to specifically represent the nurse's interests. An individual policy will also provide funds to cover a nurse's defense costs and a portion of the judgment (or settlement) in the event that the total judgment exceeds the limits of liability of the facility's coverage. Individual policies generally provide coverage for personal injuries such as libel, slander, assault, battery, and violation of privacy, which may not be covered for employees in facility policies. Despite the large size of potential judgments and thus the high limits of liability required to adequately protect against them, many nurses can obtain individual coverage with limits of $1 million per claim and $6 million aggregate for an annual tax-deductible premium of less than $100 (less than $50 if within 12 months of graduation).

ETHICAL ISSUES

In addition to potential legal concerns, nurses and nurse managers are often faced with ethical dilemmas in connection with decision making. Ethical dilemmas require that decisions be made about what is right and wrong in situations in which an individual has to make a choice between equally unfavorable alternatives. Traditionally, nurses, like other health care professionals, have faced ethical dilemmas arising primarily out of clinical practice. These dilemmas have involved conflicts among principles and/or rules attributable to common morality (socially approved norms of human conduct), standards articulated in professional codes of ethics, public policies promulgated by government agencies, and in some cases, the personal values of the health care professionals themselves (Beauchamp & Childress, 2001). More recently, ethical dilemmas faced by nurses and nurse managers have increasingly involved clashes between the principles, rules, values, and standards of clinical/professional ethics and those of organizational/business ethics (Austin, 2007; Johnson, 2005).

Although the domain of clinical ethics is the care of clients, the domain of organizational ethics is a facility's business-related activities, including, among others, marketing, admissions, transfer, discharge, billing, and the relationship of the facility and its staff members to other health care providers, educational institutions, and payers. These are activities that all directly affect the care of patients

(Spencer, 1997). Organizational ethics reflect a health care facility's basic values that serve as guides for proper and acceptable behavior in decision making and thus help ensure that the facility "conducts its business-patient care practices in an honest, decent, and proper manner" (Joint Commission on Accreditation of Healthcare Organizations [JCAHO], 1996, p. 95). Together, clinical and organizational ethics reflect a health care facility's concern that, whether related to the continuum of care or the continuum of services related to that care, ethical dilemmas should be resolved based on principles of right action (Blake, 1999).

ETHICAL DECISION MAKING IN CLINICAL HEALTH CARE

Many of the decisions nurses and nurse managers make on a daily basis have an ethical component and may involve conflicts among ethical responsibilities. These conflicts may involve clashes between the following:

- Two ethical duties to the client (e.g., duty to respect autonomy and duty to benefit the client)
- The client rights and benefits (e.g., withholding or withdrawing treatment in respect for a client's right to die by forgoing treatment at any time and treating or continuing treatment that is expected to produce more good for the client)
- Duties to self and duties to the client (e.g., a nurse's desire to remain on the same shift because of parental responsibilities and the need to advocate for better treatment of the clients by some health care practitioners on that shift)
- Professional ethical provisions and religious ones (e.g., a professional code requiring the recognition of the client's right to self-determination and a nurse's religious beliefs prohibiting abortion)

When ethical dilemmas are encountered in dealing with clinical matters, health care professionals commonly refer to various principles, rules, and standards for guidance in making moral decisions. Principles and rules are normative generalizations that provide guidance in ethical decision making. Although rules are more specific in content and restricted in scope than principles, neither can fully guide action but, rather, must be complemented by judgment for a decision to be made (Beauchamp & Childress, 2001; O'Neill, 2001).

Definitions

Like other health care practitioners, nurses apply four fundamental morality principles and a number of related rules in dealing with ethical dilemmas encountered in clinical practice on a daily basis. The four principles that form the cornerstone of biomedical ethical decision making are (1) autonomy, (2) beneficence, (3) nonmaleficence, and (4) justice. **Autonomy** refers to the client's right of self-determination and freedom of decision making. **Beneficence** means doing good for clients and providing benefit balanced against risk. **Nonmaleficence** means doing no harm to clients. **Justice** is the norm of being fair to all and giving equal treatment, including distributing benefits, risks, and costs equally (Aiken, 2004; Beauchamp & Childress, 2001; Guido, 2006).

Biomedical ethics also recognizes a number of rules that are related to the four fundamental principles and, likewise, provide guidance in dealing with ethical dilemmas (Beauchamp & Childress, 2001). Examples of commonly applied rules are fidelity, veracity, confidentiality, and privacy. **Fidelity** means being loyal and faithful to commitments and accountable for responsibilities. **Veracity** is the norm of telling the truth and not intentionally deceiving or misleading clients. **Confidentiality** prohibits some disclosures of some information gained in certain relationships to some third parties without the consent of the original source of the information. **Privacy** is a right of limited physical or informational inaccessibility (Aiken, 2004; Beauchamp & Childress, 2001; Guido, 2006).

Code of Ethics

In addition to these basic moral principles and rules of biomedical ethics, nurses are also provided

LEADING & MANAGING DEFINED

Autonomy

An individual's right of self-determination and freedom of decision making.

Beneficence

Doing good for clients and providing benefit balanced against risk.

Nonmaleficence

Doing no harm to clients.

Justice

Being fair to all and giving equal treatment, including distributing benefits, risks, and costs equally.

Fidelity

Being loyal and faithful to commitments and accountable for responsibilities.

Veracity

Telling the truth and not intentionally deceiving or misleading clients.

Confidentiality

The prohibition of some disclosures of information gained in certain relationships without the consent of the original source of the information.

Privacy

A right of limited physical or informational inaccessibility.

standards of conduct by professional codes of ethics. For example, the ANA's *Code of Ethics for Nurses: With Interpretive Statements* (2001) provides nonnegotiable standards as to the ethical obligations and duties of those who enter the nursing profession. The ANA (2001) indicated that the Code "provides a framework for nurses to use in ethical analysis and decision-making" (p. 3).

As with the principles and rules just discussed, the Code's provisions and accompanying interpretive statements, for the most part, do not focus on giving precise answers to specific ethical problems but, rather, provide general guidance as to how to act when faced with ethical dilemmas. The Code does, however, identify and provide somewhat more specific advice related to several currently unresolved ethical problems such as those involving the following:

- Practitioner decisions surrounding a client's right to die
- The introduction of incentive systems to decrease spending
- Responding to questionable and impaired practice
- Handling situations in which a client's needs are beyond a nurse's qualifications and competencies
- The existence of organizational barriers to ethical practice

Decision-Making Model

Although a number of decision-making models and processes have been proposed for use in resolving ethical dilemmas encountered in clinical practice (Aiken, 2004; Guido, 2006), they are all essentially modified versions of the six-step problem-solving model traditionally used in business, as follows:

1. Define the problem.
2. Develop alternative courses of action.
3. Evaluate each alternative course of action.
4. Select the best course of action.
5. Implement the selected course of action.
6. Monitor the results.

Because an ethical dilemma is merely a type of problem, specifically one that involves conflict, the six-step problem-solving model provides a process for making a decision when a moral dilemma arises in clinical practice. The ethical principles, rules, and standards just discussed are moral resources that can be used along with practitioner judgment to evaluate the alternative courses of action in step 3 of the problem-solving process to provide a basis for selecting the most appropriate course of action for resolving the dilemma.

THE CLASH BETWEEN CLINICAL AND ORGANIZATIONAL ETHICS

In today's rapidly changing health care environment, the traditional clinical ethical principles of autonomy, beneficence, nonmaleficence, and justice are being severely tested as they compete with demands for financial performance (Mohr & Mahon, 1996). External financial pressures arise out of the reliance by health care facilities on market competition as a vehicle for cost control as derived from social policy (American Medical Association [AMA], 2000). By the very nature of their work, nurse managers play two different and often conflicting, roles: a professional caregiving role and an organizational role involving responsibilities associated with the management of nursing care or other aspects of a health care facility. Harvey Fineberg, former dean and professor at the Harvard School of Public Health, observed the following (Buerhaus et al., 1997):

> These two roles, joined together in a single person, require a constant balancing and juggling act that requires coming to grips with the tensions and pulls between putting the patient first in the tradition of nursing and caretaking, versus the responsibilities and obligations of institutional leadership, which bring into play other human, financial, and institutional forces and needs. (p. 13)

Dilemmas arising from the clash between clinical/professional ethics and organizational/business ethics are experienced daily by nurses and nurse managers (Austin, 2007; Johnson, 2005). Unfortunately, despite the passage of time, they continue to present major challenges to the delivery of professional nursing care in many, if not most, health care facilities (Cooper et al., 2002; Cooper et al., 2004; Miller, 2006). Specific examples of nurses' ethical dilemmas include the practice of pulling or floating nurses to areas in which they are not cross-trained, an action that also increases the client-to-nurse ratio to greater limits. Nurse managers may be asked to reduce expenditures by leaving specialty areas, such as labor and delivery, uncovered when no clients are present. Organizations may refuse to purchase equipment or provide support services on off-shifts. Home visits may be refused if reimbursement cannot be captured. Time for teaching and counseling clients may be denied via staffing practices. Nurses may experience responses of "there is no money" for nursing care needs while the hospital takes over the office space occupied by nursing services to renovate for a new physicians' lounge and private dining room. A physician may request that a nurse manager deploy a hospital nurse to the physician's private practice office to help with clients. Along with their ethical concerns, most, if not all, of these dilemmas also have the potential to give rise to unfavorable legal consequences if resolved improperly.

Perceptions of Staff Nurses and Nurse Managers

Studies conducted by Cooper and colleagues provide some evidence as to the perceptions of staff nurses (Cooper, 2004) and nurse managers (Cooper, 2002) regarding the importance of the clash between clinical ethics and organizational ethics and its key effects on the delivery of quality health care. In each study, randomly selected participants were presented with a list of ethics-related statements that were referred to as *ethical issues* for simplicity (33 issues for staff nurses and 40 for nurse managers). Participants were asked to rate each issue on a 5-point scale, with "5" meaning that the issue was a major ethical problem for heath care organizations and "1" meaning that it is not a problem. The high positive correlation coefficient for the group means of staff nurses and nurse managers for the 32 ethical issues common to both studies was 0.9023, which suggests that the order of the 32 issues in terms of the extent to which they present problems for health care facilities is quite similar for the two studies.

Another area of similarity is reflected in 4 of the 8 ethical issues rated in the top 10 by both staff nurses and nurse managers. Both the 325 responding staff nurses and 295 responding nurse managers identified failure to provide service of the highest quality (defined by both groups of respondents as service that is inconsistent with both the standards of the nursing profession and the ANA Code of Ethics) as a major problem facing health care facilities. Moreover, the respondents to both studies indicated that this disappointment with the quality of service was felt not only by those in the nursing profession and the clients for whom they care but also by other health care providers employed by the organization.

Three other ethical issues rated in the top 10 by both the staff nurses and the nurse managers suggest a potential cause of this purported widespread disappointment with the quality of service provided by health care facilities in general. In both studies, the ethics-related statement rated first in terms of the extent to which it causes problems for health care organizations was the failure to provide service of the highest quality because of economic constraints determined by the organization. This issue is a direct reflection of the conflict between clinical ethics, with its primary focus on the delivery of high-quality client care, and organizational ethics, which has been heavily influenced in recent years by cost constraints imposed by the market (Johnson, 2005; Miller, 2006). Both the staff nurses and nurse managers also rated quite high an ethics-related statement pointing even more directly at the ongoing ethics clash, that of conflict between organizational and professional philosophy and standards (Cooper et al., 2002; Cooper et al., 2004). Finally, in rating department closings and layoffs among the top-10 issues in both studies, staff nurses and nurse managers identified an important problem stemming directly from the conflict between clinical ethics, with its focus almost exclusively on health care needs of individual clients, and organizational ethics, with its focus on the responsibility of facilities to provide health care to patient populations by responding to market pressures to remain competitive through cost control (AMA, 2000). These findings appear to suggest that the yet unbridled conflict between clinical and organizational ethics may be a major if not the key cause contributing to the perceived failure of many health care facilities to provide service of the highest quality as anticipated by the standards and codes of ethics of professional nursing.

LEADERSHIP AND MANAGEMENT IMPLICATIONS

Nurse managers have a responsibility to prepare themselves and those reporting to them to deal effectively not only with the yet unresolved issues of clinical ethics, such as full disclosure and end-of-life care, but also with the many unresolved dilemmas arising from the ongoing conflict between clinical and organizational ethics (Andrews, 2004). A study of nurse managers (Cooper et al., 2003) provided suggestions of where the emphasis should be placed to be most productive. The study found that, after their own personal moral values and standards, nurse managers tended to find several aspects of their organizational environment to be more helpful in dealing with ethical dilemmas than resources related to the professional environment. Resources related to the professional environment include the current ANA Code of Ethics (which was rated least helpful among 17 personal, organizational, and professional resources), professional publications/resources on ethics, literature on ethics/professionalism, and professional meetings in which ethical issues can be discussed.

Within the organizational resources, informal factors related to organizational climate were viewed as being more helpful in dealing with ethical dilemmas than formal organizational resources such as a facility's statement on ethics, the organization's policy for identifying and resolving ethical issues, a contact person within the organization to

Practical Tips

Tip #1: Prepare Yourself First

Before you can prepare those reporting to you to respond effectively to the ethical challenges encountered daily, it is essential that you have or develop the skill for doing so. Carefully assess and, where indicated, strengthen your own abilities to, among other things, identify the ethical dilemmas and conflicts encountered in nursing practice, apply ethical problem solving/decision making skills in responding to them, engage in conflict resolution where needed, advocate effectively for needed change, identify relevant sources of information related to these activities, and create an environment that encourages others to discuss their ethical concerns with you as well as their colleagues.

Tip #2: Be a Role Model

As a nurse leader/manager, you can also contribute significantly to the ethical development of those reporting to you by serving as a positive role model by exhibiting an unwavering commitment to ethical behavior. Among the ways you can exhibit this commitment is to always act with integrity, exhibit ethical decision-making skills, participate actively in advocating for nurse empowerment and other needed change, be willing to act with moral courage despite personal risk, participate in organizational services available to resolve ethical issues, and work continually to establish and maintain an ethical climate in your area of responsibility that provides the support and protection necessary to encourage collegial discussion and resolution of nurses' specific ethical concerns.

which unethical activity can be reported, and ethics training provided by the organization (which was rated next to last out of 17 possible resources). Involving merely the *absence* of pressure to compromise one's own ethical standards, the two top-rated factors—the fact that your boss does not pressure you into compromising your ethical standards and an organizational environment/culture that does not encourage you to compromise your ethical values to achieve organizational goals—suggest that an important way health care facilities and their managers can assist nursing professionals in resolving ethical dilemmas effectively is by neither explicitly nor implicitly pressuring them to go against their own ethical values (Cooper et al., 2003). Other informal organizational factors rated as being more helpful in dealing with ethical dilemmas than the formal resources provided by one's facility included the organization's culture and management philosophy, management's clear communication of appropriate ethical behavior, and the ability to go beyond one's boss, if necessary, for information and advice on ethical issues. These are all factors that, despite any personal risk involved, nurse managers at all organizational levels can and must continually work to improve and maintain if a culture that encourages and supports ethical behavior is to exist within their facility. In even a broader sense, Miller (2006) pointed out, "Creating a positive culture in which nurses can flourish is the responsibility of leaders in the profession who model the behaviors that support good work in nursing" (p. 482). Shirey (2005) presented a list of strategies for consideration by nurse leaders working to create a positive ethical climate for nursing practice within health care organizations.

In addition to the need for nurse managers to prepare staff nurses and others working for them to identify and otherwise deal effectively with ethical issues encountered in their health care facilities (Porter-O'Grady, 2003; Zuzelo, 2007), in recent years, the nursing ethics literature has called on nurse managers to encourage participation by staff nurses, as well as increase participation themselves, on facility ethics committees, especially those dealing with issues of organizational ethics and conflicts between clinical and organizational ethics (ANA, 2001; Guido, 2006; Zuzelo, 2007).

Even more directly, the ANA's *Code of Ethics for Nurses: With Interpretive Statements* stated, "Nurse administrators must ensure that nurses have access to and inclusion on institutional ethics committees" (2001, p. 7). The ANA Code continues, "Nurses must bring forward difficult issues related to patient care and/or institutional constraints upon ethical practice for discussion and review" (2001, p. 7). In their role of responsible representation, nurse managers should also ensure that "the clinical and ethical concerns of nurses are heard at the highest levels of organizational decision making" (Curtin, 2000, p. 12).

To "markedly expand the boundaries of nurses' ethical roles in hospitals" (Dodd et al., 2004, p. 16), nurses have been called on to engage in *ethical activism* in an effort to make facilities more willing to encourage their participation in ethical deliberations, and *ethical assertiveness* to expand their participation in deliberations that shape ethical decisions even when not invited to do so. Finding that "nurses are more likely to employ ethical assertiveness and ethical activism in settings that are already receptive to nursing involvement" and where written protocols mandating nursing involvement in ethics deliberations already exist, Dodd and colleagues (2004) called on nurse managers to "focus on generating administrative support for nursing involvement" and "to make efforts to ensure that nurses experience their setting as receptive to their participation in ethical deliberations" (pp. 25-26).

Although increased and improved training would undoubtedly contribute to better preparing staff nurses and nurse managers to carry out these activities (Zuzelo, 2007), the key factor for success is an organizational culture that encourages, supports, and rewards ethical behavior (Goodstein & Carney, 1999; Lachman, 2002; Pentz, 1999; Upenieks, 2003). In this context, organizational culture can be defined as a set of shared core values that members of an organization have reflected on, articulated, and accepted as normative (Silverman, 2000). As principles of right action, these shared core values serve as guides for proper and acceptable behavior in making decisions within the organization. Creating an organizational culture that will serve as a resilient base for a successful organizational ethics initiative requires that the core values not only be identified and effectively communicated to the organization's members but also be championed and demonstrated by the organization's top managers (Douglas, 2007; Goodstein & Carney, 1999; Pentz, 1999; Shirey, 2005).

In reality, the organizational cultures of health care facilities are arrayed along a continuum ranging from those based on letter-of-the-law compliance with regulatory and accrediting requirements to those that encourage, support, and reward ethical behavior. Therefore nurses and nurse managers will face varying types and degrees of challenge in their efforts to carry out the activities related to knowledge, participation, disclosure (Douglas, 2007), activism, and assertiveness mentioned previously. In many cases, it will take pressure from nurse managers to encourage senior management to recognize the need and provide their support for these activities of staff nurses and nurse managers. In facing this challenge, nurse managers should remember that, among other things, leaders are expected to have courage and to take risks in constantly challenging the status quo. Nurse managers should also encourage risk taking among the nurses reporting to them by defending and supporting them when they do (Porter-O'Grady, 2003).

In view of the significant degrees of change and uncertainty associated with the legal and ethical aspects impacting decision making in nursing care management, there is certainly no shortage of current issues and trends in this area. A major current issue, of course, is the nursing shortage and the disturbing expectation of its continuation and growth in the future (Auerbach et al., 2007; PricewaterhouseCoopers [PWC], 2007). This issue gives rise to a number of legal and ethical challenges for nurse managers and staff nurses. Resulting largely from increases in cost-cutting measures and other financial constraints, as well from deterioration of working conditions (American Hospital Association [AHA], 2002; Gordon, 2005; O'Neil & Seago, 2002), the nursing shortage has resulted in a major problem called *short staffing*. This refers to the use of an insufficient nursing staff on a unit or in a facility for the number of patients requiring care at various acuity levels (Aiken, 2004; Guido, 2006). Consequences commonly associated with short staffing (Cooper et al., 2004) include the following:

- Deterioration of patient outcomes in terms of increased mortality and failure-to-rescue rates (Agency for Healthcare Research and Quality [AHRQ], 2004, 2007; Aiken et al., 2002)
- A general decline in the quality of patient care (Buerhaus et al., 2005, 2006, 2007; Hassmiller & Cozine, 2006)
- Deterioration of nurse outcomes resulting from increased burnout and greater job dissatisfaction (AHRQ, 2004; Aiken et al., 2002)
- Increases in organizational costs resulting from increased turnover (AHA, 2002; Hassmiller & Cozine, 2006; PWC, 2007)
- Legal liability

In an effort to deal with short staffing, nurse managers are often required to do the following: float nurses to areas in which they are not cross-trained, an action that also increases the client-to-nurse ratio closer to staffing requirements; use agency (temporary) personnel; and use unlicensed personnel. Staff nurses, nurse managers, and health care facilities all face numerous possibilities of legal liability, as well as dilemmas involving conflicts between clinical and organizational ethics, as a result of short staffing and actions taken in an effort to temporarily solve this problem.

Potential legal and ethical problems are encountered also in connection with unresolved issues of clinical practice such as decisions about withholding or withdrawing life-support systems. Just as the AMA's Code of Medical Ethics (AMA, 1994) provides physicians with guidance in dealing with issues related to the withholding or withdrawing of life-sustaining medical treatment, the ANA's Code of Ethics provides guidance for nurses regarding the responsibilities they may face in dealing with key issues associated with end-of-life care. For example, the ANA Code addresses (1) respecting the client's right of self-determination, which is consistent with the ethical principle of autonomy, (2) ensuring that the client is fully informed and understands his or her options, (3) enlisting the use of a surrogate if the client's comprehension is questionable, and (4) handling conflicts between the moral standards of the profession and the nurse's own moral values.

Despite this guidance and the best efforts to apply it to end-of-life care, claims of legal liability against a nurse, nurse manager, and/or the facility that employs him or her (not to mention the physician) can arise from a variety of alleged torts related to the withholding or withdrawal of life support. For example, economic, non-economic (emotional distress), and/or punitive damages might be claimed for negligence (including malpractice) arising out of the following:

- Failure to adequately inform the client in a manner that facilitates an informed judgment
- Failure to obtain proper consent for an organ donation
- Provision of life-prolonging treatment against the client's wishes
- Failure to provide life-sustaining treatment when it is requested by the client
- Failure to recognize that the client's standardized advance directive document did not deal with CPR even though the client was a candidate for a DNR order
- Failure to properly interpret the client's advance directive document because of its unreadable legal language
- Denial of proper medical care
- Failure of a nurse to make timely arrangements for another nursing practitioner to take over a particular client's care when the nurse's own moral values conflict with those of the profession

Damages might also be sought on the grounds of intentional torts such as medical battery for tissue burns, broken bones or other harm arising out of resuscitation, or intentional infliction of emotional distress. A nurse may also be named in a lawsuit filed primarily as a result of a physician's alleged malpractice or intentional tort. Being named in this lawsuit would at least give rise to costs associated with the nurse's defense. Finally, even when the basic rules to avoid negligence or intentional tort have been closely followed, a nurse, nurse manger, and/or facility may still be found legally liable for payment of damages as a result of judicial risk. As mentioned earlier, in some cases, juries and even judges can be sufficiently influenced by their emotions so as to rationalize a finding of legal liability against the defendant, especially when, as is generally the case, liability insurance is available to pay the judgment.

Nurses need to focus on their use of expert judgment in practicing the highest legal and ethical standards in the quest for high-quality care and services. In some instances, they may also be called upon to demonstrate moral courage—the courage to honor ethical core values in the face of personal risk (Lachman, 2007a, 2007 b).

Summary

- As members of a profession, nurses and nurse managers are guided by both legal and ethical considerations in making decisions.
- Most commonly, nurses and nurse managers are subject to legal liability arising from malpractice and intentional torts they personally commit in clinical practice, from negligence in their acts of delegation and supervision, from failure to follow policies and procedures when reasonable, and from breach of contract.
- Critical to the determination of legal liability for malpractice (professional negligence), standards of care can be found in the state nurse practice act, standards published by the American Nurses Association, other professional organizations and specialty practice groups, federal agency guidelines and regulations, and the facility's policy and procedure manuals.
- Health care facilities can be held legally liable for malpractice or intentional torts committed by nurses and nurse managers they employ under the doctrine of respondeat superior, for malpractice and intentional torts committed by independent contractors (e.g., agency personnel) under the doctrine of ostensible authority, and for failing to ensure that competent and qualified practitioners are hired and that they deliver quality health care to clients under the doctrine of corporate liability.
- Judicial risk can result in findings with respect to legal liability that are not based solely on the merits of the case or on the rules of law applicable to the case.
- The four principles of autonomy, beneficence, nonmaleficence, and justice; several closely related rules of biomedical ethics; and standards of conduct provided by professional codes of ethics provide guidance to nurses and nurse managers when faced with ethical dilemmas arising in the course of clinical practice.
- Many ethical dilemmas encountered in today's health care environment involve a conflict between clinical ethics with its primary focus on the delivery of high-quality client care and organizational ethics reflecting a number of other human and financial considerations, including the reliance of health care facilities on market competition as a vehicle for cost control.
- In preparing themselves and those reporting to them to deal effectively with yet unresolved dilemmas of either clinical ethics or the conflict between clinical and organizational ethics, nurse managers should work toward the establishment of an organizational culture that encourages, supports, and rewards ethical behavior in both their own area of responsibility and the entire health care facility.

Case Study

Case 1

This strange case was personally experienced by the author in Las Vegas, a city with high population turnover. It provides an even more extreme example of what complications can occur because of the long delay that is typical between an accusation of negligence and the actual trial. In this case, the individual who showed up in court claiming to be the plaintiff was not of the same race as the injured individual who had actually filed the lawsuit 2 years earlier. The obvious error regarding who was the injured person was not even recognized by the defense attorney, who was assigned the case shortly before the trial. Had the defendant not pointed out the situation to the judge, who appeared annoyed at having to recognize the defendant at the beginning of the trial, the trial would have continued.

Case 2

In another example, the author served as foreman on a jury in a contributory negligence state. The jury was instructed by the judge that if the plaintiff (a very elderly man who would be spending the rest of his life in some type of health care facility as a result of injuries caused by an auto accident) was even partially at fault for his own injuries, the jury had to find in favor of the defendant and the plaintiff would be awarded no damages. During 6 hours of deliberation, feeling sympathy for the plaintiff, all jury members except the foreman repeatedly ignored the fact that the testimony of witnesses had indicated that the elderly man was completely at fault and voted continually to find that the plaintiff's injuries were completely the fault of the defendant (a trucking company and its driver) who had insurance and thus could afford to pay. Because the foreman was concerned that the viewpoint of the other jurors was not consistent with the judge's instructions regarding the state's law and thus not faithful to legal instructions, he held out until the issue essentially became one of whether the jury should return and continue deliberations the next day. In the next round of voting, the entire jury properly applied the state's contributory negligence law and found for the defendant. This case illustrates two aspects of judicial risk. First, the radical change in the jury members' votes was clearly not based solely on the merits of the case but, rather, on their desire to not have to return the next day for further deliberations. Second, if, instead, the jury foreman had changed his vote to provide a unanimous verdict for the plaintiff, the jury would have essentially changed the state's law in reaching its verdict by not applying the contributory negligence doctrine to the facts of the case.

CRITICAL THINKING EXERCISE

Ms. Anna vanDahm, one of the wealthiest and most influential people in town, was placed in the hospital's intensive care unit (ICU) after undergoing kidney replacement surgery. Because of the inability to deliver high-quality care as a result of financial constraints and a high turnover rate because of nurse discontentment with the dictatorial leadership styles of ICU nurse managers, the ICU was regularly short of qualified staff nurses. As a solution to this problem of short staffing, nurses from other units with lower levels of client acuity were routinely floated to the ICU, often without regard to whether or not they were cross-trained to take on ICU responsibilities.

Abigail Friendly, an RN without prior training or experience in caring for ICU clients, was floated to the ICU, where she was assigned to provide care for Ms. vanDahm, who had responded very poorly to her surgery and was put on a life-support system by a physician just before Nurse Friendly's arrival. While Nurse Friendly was caring for her, Ms. vanDahm communicated, in the presence of her oldest son, that she did not want to be resuscitated in the event of cardiopulmonary arrest.

When her shift ended a few minutes later, Nurse Friendly, exhausted and overwhelmed by what she had just experienced, left for home. Shortly thereafter, Ms. vanDahm sustained a cardiopulmonary arrest; however, in the absence of proper documentation and notification, she was resuscitated. Subsequently, the son, angry that his mother's request had not been followed, consulted an attorney, who promptly contacted the hospital's CEO. The next day, Nurse Friendly, who had

CRITICAL THINKING EXERCISE—cont'd

always received highly positive performance evaluations over the 5 years she was employed by the facility and also was subject to protection under the provisions of an antidiscrimination statute, was told by the manager of her unit that she was being fired effective immediately.

1. Nurse Friendly
   a. On what grounds could Nurse Friendly be found legally liable for malpractice?
   b. What actions should have been taken by Nurse Friendly to prevent malpractice in this type of situation?
   c. What ethical dilemma(s) did Nurse Friendly face in this situation?
   d. What factors should have been considered by Nurse Friendly in dealing with the ethical dilemma(s) encountered in this situation?
2. Manager of Nurse Friendly's unit
   a. On what grounds could the nurse manager be found legally liable?
   b. What actions should have been taken by the nurse manager to prevent legal liability in this type of situation?
   c. What ethical dilemma(s) did the nurse manager face in this situation?
   d. What factors should have been considered by the nurse manager in dealing with the ethical dilemma(s) encountered in this situation?
3. Nurse manager of the ICU
   a. On what grounds could the nurse manager be found legally liable?
   b. What actions should have been taken by the nurse manager to prevent legal liability in this type of situation?
   c. What ethical dilemma(s) did the nurse manager face in this situation?
   d. What factors should have been considered by the nurse manager in dealing with the ethical dilemma(s) encountered in this situation?
4. Hospital
   a. On what grounds could the hospital be found legally liable?
   b. What actions should have been taken by the hospital to prevent legal liability in this type of situation?

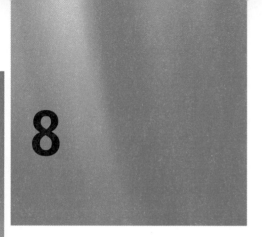

8 Communication, Persuasion, and Negotiation

Bonnie Weaver Battey

CHAPTER OBJECTIVES

- Describe the varying degrees of the implementation of holistic health care in nursing practice
- Develop a plan for implementing new criteria for spiritual care of patients
- Appreciate the role of communication, persuasion, and negotiation in inter- and intra-professional relationships
- Apply Chaos Theory and Complexity Theory as appropriate to management in nursing
- Apply Situational Leadership®* Theory in the practice of nursing leadership
- Apply Humanizing Nursing Communication Theory (HNCT) in providing spiritual care to patients and facilitating attitudes of enthusiasm, mutual respect, and collegiality among nursing staff
- Facilitate appropriate communication networks in a task group process
- Exercise critical thinking to conceptualize and analyze possible solutions to a practice exercise

The purpose of this chapter is to introduce a preferred role of nursing leadership in goal setting, communicating, persuading, and negotiating in the implementation of change in a complex context.

DEFINITIONS

- **Human Being:** An existential being who is a complex whole (holistic; body-mind-spirit). Living beings capable of symbolizing, perceiving the negative, transcending the environment by inventions, ordering the environment, striving for perfection, making choices, and engaging in self-reflection. Human beings are composed of an interacting set of characteristics: living, communicating, negativing, inventing, ordering, renaming, choosing, and self-reflecting. These characteristics are not necessarily unique to the species but are of particular concern to nursing (Duldt et al., 1984; Duldt & Giffin, 1985).
- **Humanizing Nursing Communication Theory:** A nursing theory describing the manner of communicating that acknowledges the unique characteristics of the holistic human being. The communication patterns of interaction (communing, asserting, confronting, conflicting, and separating) are conveyed with an attitude that can be identified on the humanizing-dehumanizing continuum (Battey, 2006, 2007, in press; Duldt, 1989; Duldt & Giffin, 1985). Humanizing Nursing Communication Theory (HNCT) is based on "normal" as opposed to "therapeutic" and includes not only professional-client but also inter- and intra-professional communication.
- **Interpersonal Communication:** A two-way level of communication concerned with the face-to-face interactions between people who are consistently aware of each other. Each person assumes the roles of both

*Situational Leadership® is the registered trademark of the Center for Leadership Studies in Escondido, CA 92025. All rights reserved.

PART III

sender and receiver of messages, involving constant adaptation and spontaneous adjustment to the other person (Patton & Giffin, 1981).

- **Leadership:** A process of influencing the behavior of either an individual or a group, regardless of the reason, in an effort to achieve goals in a given situation (Hersey et al., 2008).
- **Nonverbal Communication:** Unspoken, this communication is composed of affective or expressive behavior.
- **Persuasion, Negotiation, and Bargaining:** Persuasion is the conscious intent by one individual to modify the thoughts or behaviors of others (Bettinghaus, 1968). Negotiation is a dialogical discussion between two or more parties to arrive at an agreement about some issue. To bargain is to make a series of offers and counteroffers about what each party will do, give, receive, etc., until an agreement is reached to the satisfaction of all. All three of these involve communication. Persuasion uses argumentation and appeals to logic, whereas negotiation and bargaining may involve some sense of compensation and perhaps coercion, such as bullying or condescending behaviors.
- **Spiritual Assessment:** Information needed by nurses resides within each patient, and the professional nurse seeks to use the patient's own definition in developing individualized plans of care. This information may be obtained through informal conversation or a formal assessment interview.
- **Spiritual Care:** Interpersonal communication. It exists in the relationship between the caregiver and the care recipient. Whether the spiritual care exists at all is determined by the perceptions of the one receiving the care. The implication of this definition is that nurses need specific communing skills to establish and maintain the relationship.
- **Spirituality:** A dimension of all human beings that is relational in nature, with a higher being and/or with other human beings; may include spiritual and religious practices, perhaps within an organized faith community.
- **Verbal Communication:** Includes both written and spoken communication.

BACKGROUND

Communication is a process in which information, perception, and understanding are transmitted from person to person. As an integral part of any relationship, communication is important to nurses. Nurse leaders and managers can view communication as a tool to accomplish work and meet goals. The significance of communication revolves around its effectiveness and the climate in which communication occurs. Effective communication is enhanced by clear, direct, straightforward, and frequent message transmission. Trust, respect, and empathy are the three ingredients needed to create and foster effective communication.

For leaders, communication is a key element of the role. Leaders are in charge of vision, and the vision needs to be communicated as a compelling image. Such a compelling image is thought to induce enthusiasm and commitment in others. Thus a major part of the leader's role is to communicate a vision. Leaders shape values and norms in a way that binds and bonds individuals and groups. Communication is key to this effort. Visions are communicated by means of managing meaning and creating understanding, commitment, and ownership of a vision. Leaders use communication as a tool for building trust. Trust is the glue that holds leaders and followers together.

Communication is a basic and essential skill for leaders and managers. Communicating, along with diagnosing and adapting, is one of the three basic competencies of influencing and leadership (Hersey et al., 2008). It is a critical and important tool for effectiveness in engaging and motivating people and in getting work done through others. Structuring messages so that people understand them clearly and avoiding emotion-laden triggers enhance the communication effectiveness of a manager. For example, the communication of accurate (correct, truthful, precise), adequate (sufficient, consistent, repetitious), and applied (useful and appropriate to the nurse's individual needs) information was necessary for directing managed care changes (Apker & Fox, 2002). These communication techniques can foster stronger organizational affiliation while maintaining nurses' strong identification with nursing.

Health care organizations are complex and exist in uncertain environments. Nurse leaders and managers play a crucial role in the management of information and communication for the purpose of effective care coordination and the avoidance of unsafe and error-prone care situations. Medical errors and patient safety in hospitals have been a focus of the Institute of Medicine. Clearly, providers need high-quality information and effective communication. Nurse administrators are responsible for developing care delivery systems with adequate structure and an effective communication system that enhances care coordination. These systems of communications need to enable patient rescue and safety by coordinating care, preventing information loss, and improving methods of surveillance (Anthony & Preuss, 2002). Interventions have been initiated to augment nurse and physician collaboration in intensive care units (Boyle & Kochinda, 2004) and to capture communication patterns in OR nurses to facilitate automation to reduce adverse events (Moss & Xiao, 2004).

A related concern for the management of information and communication is how to prevent breaches of patient confidentiality. The Health Insurance Portability and Accountability Act (HIPAA) provisions have heightened awareness about and strategies to protect patients' privacy and data security in health care transactions. For example, fax transmissions need to be secure and security measures need to be taken to protect computerized databases and electronic transmissions. In a series of interviews with 51 patients, Brann and Mattson (2004) identified both internal and external confidentiality breaches, which were categorized into a typology table. Health care providers' actions that disseminate confidential information can harm patients. Systems, processes, and structures can be altered to prevent many of these situations.

Acquiring interpersonal relationship skills, including the ability to communicate, is as essential to a leader's personal set of leadership skills as psychomotor skills are for a clinical nurse. Leadership and management ability is predicated on a facility for communication. In nursing leadership and management, skillful communication is essential for effective implementation of the change process. It is an intervention that leaders and managers in nursing use to accomplish their goals. Communication is a key component of case management practice.

Language is used by leaders to give meaning to work. Farley (1989) identified six areas of organizational communication that can be assessed for communication problems (Box 8.1). Communication problems may be a source of dissatisfaction. Research has indicated that a positive communication atmosphere, positive communication between staff nurses and immediate superiors, and personal feedback on job performance are related to nurse job satisfaction (Pincus, 1986).

Communication effectiveness becomes crucial in times of disaster. In fact, often one of the key outcomes of disaster drills is to identify breaks in the communication system so they can be fixed before a real-time event occurs. Argenti (2002) found that in times of extreme crisis, the internal communication to employees took precedence. It was most important for the leader to effectively rebuild the morale of employees so that they could then serve customers. The five strategies he recommended are as follows:

Box 8.1

Communication Assessment

- Accessibility of information
- Communication channels
- Clarity of messages
- Span of control
- Flow control/communication load
- The individual communicators

Data from Farley, M. (1989). Assessing communication in organizations. *Journal of Nursing Administration, 19* (12), 27-31.

1. Get on the scene to lead, decide, and show compassion.
2. Choose your channels carefully because normal flows often are disrupted due to destroyed phone and power lines.
3. Stay focused on the business.
4. Have a contingency and disaster plan in place.
5. Improvise, but from a strong foundation of values, preparation, and training.

A couple of examples from nursing leadership and management are worth considering. In hospital nursing, situations occur in which nurses are sent (*pulling, floating,* and *farming* are the terms used) from the unit in which they normally work to another unit. The person who has to deliver the often unpleasant news determines whether to call the unit and leave a brief note on the assignment sheet or go to the nurse to talk directly about the change. Some might offer to take the nurse to the other unit, introduce the person to the charge nurse, and smooth out the transition. There are different ways to structure and deliver the message to be effective in difficult situations.

One leadership situation occurs when a nurse presents a proposal to a committee who must be convinced to release the money for a project that is vital to the care of clients. Strategic planning and a written business plan are used to determine how to maximize the message delivery. This may include knowing how to structure the communication, nonverbally as well as verbally, so that a positive impression is created to set the stage for a full and impartial hearing.

Leaders and managers always communicate in basic ways, whether they want to or not—they always communicate their attitude and their goals and expectations. Trust or distrust is communicated. Leaders communicate a vision, subtly or directly, and a sense of where they are going and what they expect from their followers.

One technique used for interpersonal effectiveness in groups, collaborative teams, and interdisciplinary work situations is persuasion. The tactics of persuasion are useful when an authoritarian leadership style is not appropriate and the nurse has to convince colleagues to work together.

Harvey (1990) suggested that skillful, positive questioning can persuade people to accept change. People are more willing to commit themselves when they see personal benefits. Positive questioning capitalizes on this fact to establish hopeful, affirmative attitudes. Inviting agreement, commitment, and realization of benefits facilitates necessary changes. Setting a positive and cooperative tone within a work group is each member's responsibility. Nurses frequently may be in situations in which they need to persuade others to cooperate. Therefore they will need to use strategies of persuasion and negotiation.

The work of successful nurses and managers depends on the ability to negotiate. Nurses need to be able to articulate needs, positions, and justification for resources. The different techniques of conflict resolution and influencing in nursing include bargaining and negotiation as one method of gaining power and persuading others to grant autonomy by using individual and collective action. The use of collective action at both the work group and the larger profession levels can make a difference in terms of autonomy in professional practice, job satisfaction, and a general positive feeling about the profession of nursing.

Human interaction issues are the general arena in which leaders and managers spend most of their time. Power and conflict become important focal points of human interaction in organizations that may need management or resolution through persuasion or negotiations. Both conflict resolution and negotiation techniques can and should be used to manage change. As nurses are confronted with the impact of mergers, downsizing, restructuring and reengineering, and alterations in skill mix, negotiation skills are needed. These skills can help improve relationships and aid managers to function in their designated roles.

Negotiation is used to educate clients and other professionals about nurses' roles and contributions, to get a fairer exchange in decision-making autonomy, to interact with vendors, to deal with client complaints, to interact with integrated health systems and group health care purchasers, to deal with unionized employees, to respond to the media, and to negotiate with medical staff and managed care groups to consolidate contracts (Sherer, 1994).

COMMUNICATION LEADERSHIP

Implementing spiritual care in clinical practice within an agency is an example of communication leadership. Spirituality is in itself complex, unique, and difficult. As a leader, nurses are responsible for their area of knowledge, power, and influence. Nurses cannot expect to change other professions and disciplines but can set realistic goals about major issues within the scope of nursing leadership influence and make a difference in patient care. A plan to address the spiritual dimension of holistic care is offered based on theories, supporting research, and the study of spirituality in healing (Battey, 2006, 2007, in press). This is *not* to be considered *the* final answer but merely an initial way to provide one perspective in developing a plan most appropriate to situational leadership needs. The following discussion looks more specifically at the problem, an approach to solving it, and potential outcomes.

The Issues

New Criteria to Be Met

One issue for leaders in nursing is to implement holistic care—the spiritual dimension of this paradigm in particular. Some may just add the word *holistic* to the mission statement and continue business as usual. This is not enough. The holistic paradigm is becoming the desired mode of health care delivery.

In the 2005 manual for hospitals, The Joint Commission (TJC) (formerly The Joint Commission on Accreditation of Healthcare Organizations [JCAHO]) included requirements about spirituality care (TJC, 2008). Nurses are now charged to define and record social, *spiritual*, and cultural variables influencing the patient's health in their initial assessment. The American Nurses Association (ANA) (2005) has published similar guidelines. The North American Nursing Diagnosis Association (NANDA) (2008) manuals for nursing diagnoses cite Spiritual Distress as an accepted nursing diagnosis. Many facilities have pastoral care departments to provide spiritual care.

Pastoral Care

Departments of pastoral care are commonly found in hospitals, and clinical chaplaincy is now recognized as a certified, ecumenical, and multicultural role in bringing pastoral care to any patient's bedside. This care is to be provided for all patients. It is a daunting task to become familiar with all the different beliefs systems and comparative religions. Data from www.adherents.com shows the breakdown of the major world religions and lists the following statistics of adherents by religion:

- Christianity: 33%
- Islam: 21%
- "Nonreligious": 16%
- Hinduism: 14%
- Primal-indigenous: 6%
- Chinese traditional: 6%
- Buddhism: 6%
- Sikhism: 0.36%
- Judaism: 0.22%

Duldt (2002) described the roles of chaplains and others in a hospital pastoral care department. Unfortunately, there are not enough chaplains to meet patients' needs, so the use of laymen as volunteers has increased. In the past 5 years, some hospitals have eliminated chaplaincy programs because positive "outcomes" attributable to chaplains are difficult to identify and quantify. The economic "bottom line" considerations prevail. Consequently, many hospitals have lists of clergy and laymen in the community who are to be called upon to minister to the spiritual needs of patients who are members of their own faith community. However, plans for pastoral care tend to be nonexistent for those patients without such an affiliation (Kraus & Holmes, in press). In addition, many theological seminaries are following this trend and are removing studies in pastoral theology and pastoral care from their curricula (Paul Kraus, personal communication, June 4, 2007).

Spiritual Care of Nurses

If spirituality is defined as relational and if spiritual care is interpersonal communication, then the spiritual care of the nurses also is important. Extensive documentation in the literature exists regarding the disruptive and distracting communication interactions not only between nurses and between nurses and professional colleagues (e.g., physicians, pharmacists, administrators) but also between nurses and patients. The research, the literature, and common knowledge from reading the daily papers indicate that nursing personnel experience high turnover rates, job dissatisfaction, and burnout; many RNs are leaving the profession. The shortage of nursing personnel in most areas of the United States is having a negative effective on retention of nurses and recruitment of students to nursing (Buerhaus et al., 2005; Buerhaus, 2007). The work environment is described as hostile to nurses, and patient outcomes of increased severity of illness and mortality have been directly related to poor communication skills of the staff (Kramer & Schmalenberg, 2003). The clinical ambiance and interpersonal communication received by nurses need to change. Leaders can set realistic goals within the scope of their leadership influence and make a difference where nurses live and work.

Are Leaders Prepared to Deliver Outcomes?

The challenge of this issue of leadership and communication, persuasion, and negotiation revolves around *who* is to change *what, when, how, with whom,* and *with what outcome?* How can the leaders (the "who") who are to implement holistic care—especially spiritual care (the "what")—throughout the nursing organization somehow (the "how") involve all nursing professionals (the "with whom") so that nurses will be able to provide spiritual care to patients (the "with what outcome")?

Leaders, to a significant degree, are alumni of an educational system that historically did not teach these concepts. If they did, nursing education about spirituality was likely to be an hour's lecture by a chaplain or minister. In fact, the current literature reveals a wide range of perspectives, including the position that spiritual care is not to be provided by nurses. Fortunately, most nurses are creative, "renaissance" people who are talented in examining, learning, reviving, and adapting to meet new challenges.

Management Approaches

There is a great need in the health care professions to provide holistic care (body, mind, and spirit) to all clients, regardless of religious, ethnic, or cultural characteristics, in a humane (nonjudgmental and compassionate) manner. Yet today's American health care system emphasizes certain business and management concepts such as efficiency, accuracy, and economy. This is expected in the use of sophisticated medical terminology and highly skilled specialists who operate modern equipment, but the technical and disease-oriented language that is used is often ineffective in aiding some patients to understand their health conditions.

The Hostile Workplace

Registered nurses are often overlooked in the power and decision making arenas. Nurses represent the largest licensed professional health care provider group in America. The professional nurse traditionally has had the closest and longest interpersonal contact with patients compared with most other health care providers. In this same health care system, technology rules in a labor-intense service industry, as seen in all the buildings, equipment, and sophisticated monitoring machines that need to be operated by human beings. Yet nursing colleagues, as well as other health care professionals, overlook the need to communicate with one another in a holistic and humanizing way. Ulrich (2004) urged nursing leaders to limit the "fear factor" in nursing practice for the welfare of the patients as well as the staff. The Institute for Safe Medication Practices (ISMP) (*www.ismp.org*; and *www.ismp.org/msaarticles/intimidationprint.htm)* reported a survey indicating the role that intimidation plays in the safe administration of medications.

Childers (2004) described the hostile work environments in which professional colleagues behave as "bullies." Lindeke and Sieckert (2004) focused on the nurse-physician collaborative communication and noted that the intentional sharing of knowledge of patients leads to improved patient outcomes as well as increased workplace satisfaction among staff. Namie and Namie (2008), social psychologists and founders of the Workplace Bullying and Trauma Institute *(www.bullyinginstitute.org/)*, say that although many good nurses have been driven out by toxic environments, many other nurses have just accepted those environments. The Namies' studies indicated that 70% of the people targeted by a bully have to quit either because of health (33%) or because they are victims of manipulated negative performance reviews (37%). Keefe (2007) noted that the age-old problem of nurses "eating their young" is bullying and new graduates do not need to go through a trial by fire when beginning a new job. In a second report, plans for changing the culture are outlined by the Institute for Safe Medication Practices (2008). The plans involve long, expensive administrative processes to establish a zero-tolerance policy, a reporting system, conflict resolution, and educational programs *(www.ismp.org/msaarticles/intimidation2print.htm)*. However, polices are limited in changing the way people feel about one another and how they interact. Toxic workplaces are expensive and need to be addressed for nurses and other health care providers.

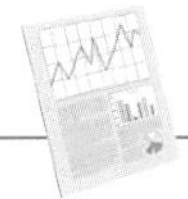

Research Note

Source: Boyle, D.K., & Kochinda, C. (2004). Enhancing collaborative communication of nurse and physician leadership in two intensive care units. *Journal of Nursing Administration, 34*(2), 60-70.

Purpose

Poor nurse-physician collaborative communication is one of the factors in increased risk-adjusted mortality and length of stay in ICUs. The purpose of this study was to test an intervention designed to enhance collaborative communication among nurse and physician leaders in two different ICUs. The Analytic Model for Studying ICU Performance was the framework for the study. In this model, nurse-physician collaborative communication is one of four predictor variables of ICU outcomes. The study used a pretest-posttest, repeated measures design with follow-ups at baseline, intervention, and 6 months after. ICUs in two hospitals participated. The Collaborative Communication Intervention was targeted to the five dimensions of nurse-physician collaborative communication: leadership, communication, coordination, problem solving/conflict management, and team-oriented culture. The intervention consisted of 23.5 hours of training using six standardized curriculum models: leadership, core skills for communication, guiding conflict resolution, helping others adapt to change, teams, and trust. Evaluation data were gathered pretest and posttest, using a vignette test and a self-perception and staff-perceptions questionnaire.

Discussion

The intervention proved feasible and useful. After the intervention, nurse and physician leaders' communication skills significantly increased. Six months after intervention, scores on unit outcome measures showed improvement, including a decrease in personal stress. This was a pilot study and small in scope, but it was intervention-focused and attempted an experimental design.

Application to Practice

ICU nurse and physician leaders have the responsibility to create an environment of collaborative communication as a way to effect a positive work environment and affect outcomes. In this study, collaborative communication improved after a training intervention. Individual skills increased. Other ICUs and potentially other units could benefit from similar skills training interventions.

Communication

Health care providers in general, and nursing as a discipline and practice profession in particular, are basically humanitarian—that is, concerned with and focused on the well-being of people. Yet an unfortunate trend, reported by both health care consumers and providers, appears to be a growing lack of concern for one another. People frequently describe unpleasant encounters that leave them confused, insulted, irritated, and indignant when they seek care. Why this happens and is tolerated is not clear.

An old and basic interpersonal communication model is operative in human communication:

Speaker → Message → Receiver

In this model, the person who initiates the communication is referred to as the "Speaker" and the person to whom the message is directed is the "Receiver." Effective communication occurs when the receiver interprets the speaker's message in the same way the speaker intended it (Patton & Giffin, 1977). Box 8.2 displays the ten characteristics of interpersonal communication. In the nursing context, the model looks like this:

Nurse and other health care providers	→	Message (Bad News)	→	Patient/ Client

By the very nature of being a nurse or other health care provider, messages to patients or clients may be characterized as "bad news." The messages may be about delayed meals, unpleasant and even painful procedures, and distressing revelations about illness. The age-old pattern of "blaming the messenger" may be in effect and disrupt relationships. Clients confronted with their own unhealthy lifestyle and poor health practices may be unable to understand or may just reject the messages they receive. This creates a greater potential for consumers' dissatisfaction. Too often consumers question the accuracy of the therapy and, being so unsure, may not comply with directions. When medications, an MRI, and other tests cost more than they can afford, particularly those without health insurance, the consumers do not know where to turn.

Box 8.2

Ten Characteristics of Interpersonal Communication

The following characteristics are presented to stimulate discussion and help identify the dimension of interpersonal communication as opposed to other dimensions such as small group, organizational, and mass communication (Patton & Giffin, 1981, pp. 12-20):

1. Communication is unavoidable and inevitable when people are aware of one another.
2. In interpersonal communication, both the sender and the receiver of "meaning"* must be present.
3. Each person assumes roles as both sender and receiver of messages in interpersonal communication.
4. The choices that a person makes reflect the degree of that person's interpersonal communication competencies.
5. In interpersonal communication, the sender and the receiver are interdependent.
6. Successful interpersonal communications involve mutual needs to communicate.
7. Interpersonal communication establishes and defines the nature of the relationship between the people involved.
8. Interpersonal communication is the means by which we confirm and validate self.
9. Because interpersonal communication relies on behaviors, we must be satisfied with degrees of mutual understanding.
10. Interpersonal communication is irreversible and unrepeatable and almost always functions in a context of change.

***Note:** "Meaning" is what a word, sign, or symbol means or what the sender or senders want to convey. It refers to the implications of the content of the message. The receiver needs to understand what the sender intends to convey by the message or what he means in order to avoid misunderstandings.

Regretfully, there appears to be a trend for people to interact in a dehumanizing manner in the health care system, and this trend can be expected to continue. Too often it is unpleasant for the consumer as well as the professional care provider. In the twenty-first century, U.S. society is moving toward a nationwide shift in the financing and lack of availability of health care resources, the increased numbers of clients, the increasing complexity of care, and the lack of personnel in nursing and other heath care professions (Johnson, 2000). Health care providers, especially nurses, are experiencing reality shock, anger dismay, job dissatisfaction, and burnout. They frequently choose to resign, resulting in high annual turnover and high inactivity rates among practitioners.

Dehumanizing processes can be counteracted by effective interpersonal communication, the key to humanizing relationships between people. *To humanize* means to recognize the individual's human characteristics and to address the presented health care issues with dignity and respect. To implement the spiritual aspect of holistic health care, concerted effort is needed by health care leaders in both education and practice to guide people in a careful exploration of interpersonal communication processes that are known to promote humanizing relationships not only between the nurse and client but also between and among health care colleagues.

IMPLEMENTING SPIRITUAL CARE

It is the position of this author that each profession needs to define spiritual care within its own discipline's knowledge base. Nurses are not chaplains. Professional limitations are needed for the role of the professional in administering spiritual care. The proposed definition of spirituality useful for nurses is that spirituality lies within each patient, and the professional nurse seeks to use the patient's own definition in developing individualized plans of care. Ethically, as nurses strive to deliver just holistic care, they need to keep their own spiritual/religious beliefs to themselves and avoid proselytizing. Although definitions of spirituality are endless, *nurses need be responsible for only five dimensions: beliefs, values, meanings, goals, and relationships (BVMGR).* The BVMGR rubric is proposed as the most appropriate guide or assessment tool for nurses. Nurses can be alert to the BVMGR topics during routine care of patients.

The core of spiritual care is supporting the following position: **the definition of spirituality that is relevant to a particular patient/client can be found only within that person.** Therefore it should not matter whether the nurse is a Buddhist or whether the hospital is owned by Jews or Catholics or Adventists or whether this happens to be a public hospital in the middle of the Christian "Bible Belt" of the southern United States. What is relevant to the health care decisions to be made for a particular patient is what he or she Believes, Values, finds Meaningful in life, maintains as life Goals, or has as special interpersonal Relationships. For nursing assessment, it is the rubric of BVMGR—the dimensions of a patient's spirituality—that forms the basis for spirituality care.

Spirituality in Education

In medical education, two consensus conferences were held by the American College of Physicians, and a strong stance was taken in the late 1990s. They concluded that physicians should address not only the physical dimension of suffering but also the psychological, spiritual, and existential dimensions (Puchalski, 2004). The Medical School Objectives Project, lead by M. Brownell Anderson of the Association of American Medical Colleges, proposed curriculum changes to include spirituality issues. Puchalski, a physician and a Carmelite nun who served as co-chairperson with Anderson, initiated one of the first courses on spirituality and health in the United States at George Washington University School of Medicine. Puchalski's course has become a requirement in that curriculum, and it has served as a model for over 60% of the U.S. medical schools that now offer courses on spirituality and health. The medical students are taught the FICA rubric for spiritual assessment as developed by Puchalski:

F — Faith, Belief, and Meaning
I — Importance and Influence
C— Community
A— Address/Action in Care

Medical students are required to complete the spiritual assessment interview in 10 minutes or less in the "social history" section of the patient's history.

In comparison, the approach in nursing education is diffused and fragmented. Historically, spiritual care has long been associated with nursing. Florence Nightingale (1959) identified addressing spiritual needs of patients as a part of the nursing role. However, because the concept of spirituality is not well defined and is ambiguous in meaning, a debate is developing in the nursing literature about whether to teach it in nursing programs (McSherry & Cash, 2004). For example, only two theorists are specifically addressing spirituality as a major concept: Betty Neuman's systems model (1982) and Madeleine Leininger's "Transcultural Nursing" (1978). In a review of textbooks by McEwen (2004), many definitions of *spirituality* were found, but definitions of *spiritual care* are sparse. Number of pages devoted to spiritual issues ranged from 0% for most to a high of 13%. Only two texts were exceptions. Carson (2000) integrated spiritual care throughout her psychiatric nursing text. Hitchcock and colleagues (2003) had a chapter in their community nursing text. A third noteworthy exception is "Kozier & Erb's Fundamentals of Nursing" text (Berman et al., 2007). Berman wrote a chapter devoted to an in-depth presentation of spirituality, providing a strong support to defining the spirituality and spiritual care as a dimension of nursing's body of knowledge.

Lemmer (2002) conducted a survey of U.S. baccalaureate nursing programs. Faculty reported that content about spirituality is included but few had definitions of spirituality or spiritual care. Teachers reported being uncertain about understanding the spiritual dimension of nursing and feeling uncomfortable teaching this content. Although one third of programs used role modeling as a method of teaching, faculty can best teach students using tools such as spiritual care mapping (Mitchell et al., 2006).

The following definition is drawn from religious rather than health care scholars and offered as a benchmark for nursing. According to Kraus and Holmes, spiritual care is not technique, technology, maps, guidelines, drugs, or directives that make the impact; rather, *spiritual care is defined as interpersonal communication.* Spiritual care occurs within the relationship between the caregiver and the care recipient. Whether the spiritual care exists at all is determined by the perceptions of the one receiving the care (Kraus & Holmes, in press). The implication of this definition is that nurses need to develop specific communing skills. Two theories, *Humanizing Nursing Communication Theory* and *Communication Ethics Theory,* offer solid direction to nurses for interacting in a compassionate manner with spiritually distressed clients (Battey, 2006, 2007, in press; Duldt, 1991).

Spirituality in Practice

The literature reveals there are many questions about the ways in which spirituality assessments are conducted and whether one assessment tool can prove adequate in measuring the significance of spirituality in the lives of individuals, all of whom may interpret its meaning differently. Power (2006) indicated it is unlikely that tools can be developed that are widely applicable for identifying and assessing spirituality. A research report by Baldacchino (2006) identified main competencies of nurses for spiritual care: (1) delivery of spiritual care by the nursing process, (2) nurses' communication with patients, (3) interdisciplinary team and clinical/educational organizations, and (4) safeguarding ethical issues in care. New standards reflect the importance of chaplaincy service, yet inadequate spiritual assessment, unsupportive organizational structure and climate, and lack of understanding of chaplains' role can prevent these services from being fully utilized. Nurses need to recognize when to make referrals to chaplains and how to help develop the organizational infrastructure to support processes of spiritual care (McClung et al., 2006).

Spirituality and Health

It is well known that spiritual care is needed when individuals face emotional stress, physical illness, or death. People may experience disharmony of mind, body, and spirit and may need to enhance their personal spiritual coping strategies (McEwen, 2004). Facilitating spiritual health promotes healing

(Taylor, 2002). Research on allostasis (a new term for stress) and allostasis loading has demonstrated the direct influence of spiritual health on development and/or progress of physical and mental illnesses. When spiritual self-care interventions are used upon perceiving and/or experiencing stress, changes in the chemistry of brain/body can diminish allostasis loading and increase resiliency (McEwen, 2000; McEwen & Seeman, 1999). It enables individuals to transcend the current situation for higher meaning and purpose, provides hope, and promotes experiencing connectedness with others (McEwen, 2004). When the goal of nursing leadership is to implement a program of spiritual care in nursing practice, it needs to be grounded in theory and research.

LEADERSHIP AND MANAGEMENT IMPLICATIONS

Choosing Theories for Leadership

There are numerous theories about leadership and management of business and organizations that nursing leaders can use. Chapter 1 overviews leadership principles and contains further background. It is useful to recall that communication is a central competency of leadership. A critique of selected leadership models that emphasize communication follows.

Certain criteria are necessary for evaluating theories. For example, the theoretical statements of relationship between concepts need to be logical and agree with known data. The concepts need to be well defined and capable of being operationalized, and the statements that describe how the concepts relate to one another need to be testable and provide direction for research. It is helpful if the statements intuitively agree with one's own experiences and are clear, simple, and useful. The theoretical relationship statements are required to do at least one of the following: describe, explain, predict, and/or control phenomena (Duldt, 2002). Three theories are highlighted and evaluated. The first—Chaos Theory and Complexity Theory—are currently in vogue and are the front-runners of theoretical discussions in many disciplines. The second and third theories, Situational Leadership® Theory and Humanizing Nursing Communication Theory, have been

LEADERSHIP & MANAGEMENT BEHAVIORS

Leadership Behaviors

- Communicates a vision
- Structures messages to inspire
- Motivates by communication strategies
- Projects a professional image
- Models positive communication
- Influences frequent communication
- Coaches followers
- Structures symbols and shared meanings
- Persuades followers to accomplish goals
- Convinces followers to work together
- Invites agreement and commitment
- Negotiates common understandings

Management Behaviors

- Communicates with superiors and subordinates
- Structures messages for clarity
- Directs the performance of others by communication strategies
- Manages organizational goal accomplishment by communicating
- Persuades subordinates to accomplish organizational goals
- Bargains for scarce resources
- Exchanges ideas and plans
- Negotiates agreements and contracts

Overlap Areas

- Communicates with others
- Promotes effective communication
- Persuades others
- Negotiates with others

Table 8.1

Criteria for Evaluating Theories

Criteria	Chaos Theory/ Complexity Theory	Situational Leadership® Theory	Humanizing Nursing Communication Theory
1. Logical relationship statements	Maybe	Yes	Yes
2. Agrees with known data	No	Yes	Yes
3. Concepts well defined; can be operationalized	No	Yes	Yes
4. Provides direction for research; testable	Not yet	Yes	Yes (needs more research)
5. Intuitively easy to use and understand	Not yet	Yes	Yes

Data from Duldt, B.W. (2001). *Anatomy of a theory: Theoretical perspectives for nursing and health care professionals.* A computer assisted instructional program; student workbook (pp. 11-13). St. Louis: A.S.K. Data Systems, Inc. (www.askdatasystems.com).

overlooked in nursing contexts but have much to offer given the current conditions in nursing practice (Table 8.1).

Chaos Theory and Complexity Theory

Most would agree that one characteristic of nursing is its unpredictability, its chaos and complexity. To use a theory about chaos and complexity is intuitively attractive. Sometimes, no matter how hard nursing leaders try to maintain consistency and control, things do become chaotic. Projects seem to take off "on their own" and defy direction. Chaos is commonly known as disorganization and disorderliness, but the meaning for this concept in Chaos Theory is quite different. It refers to behavior that is unpredictable in spite of certain regularities. As described by Lorenz (1993), the Chaos Phenomenon differs from the predictable swinging of a pendulum of a clock. Instead, it is more like the unpredictable random patterns of weather. A meteorologist, Lorenz was preparing for presenting the weather report when he decided to run the numbers through the computer once more to update the information. He initiated the program a short time later than his original run, and the outcome was quite different. This illustrates a fundamental observation of Chaos Theory: changing the starting point of a computer analysis of the weather can result in a change in the outcome. Lorenz (1993) presented a paper entitled "Does the Flap of a Butterfly's Wing in Brazil set off a Tornado in Texas?" in which he described this phenomenon of chaos. This "butterfly wing flap" label is often referred to in the literature when discussing Chaos Theory.

Chaos has become a concept of Complexity Theory. Over the past three or four decades, Complexity Theory has been the focus of scientific disciplines such as astronomy, chemistry, physics, evolutionary biology, geology, and meteorology. Systems studied in these disciplines have phenomena in common, which seem to pass from an organized state, through a chaotic phase, and "emerge" or to evolve into a higher level of organization. Examples of this emergence is not unlike Darwin's evolutionary theory of "natural selection." The theory originated at the Santa Fe Institute, a "think tank" involving the "top 10 percent" of scientists from numerous countries and of diverse disciplines. The Institute, incorporated in 1984, has been funded by a large number of individuals as well as private foundations to study the "emerging synthesis of science" (Waldrop, 1992, p. 79).

Complexity Theory is seen by some as replacing the reductionist, Newtonian logic of the seventeenth to twentieth centuries with a new, all-encompassing theory of science for the twenty-first century (Waldrop, 1992). Some authors are pondering how this theory can be applied to nursing (Dombeck, 2002; Haigh, 2002; Lowenstein, 2003; Velde et al., 2002). A new journal publication, *Complexity and Chaos in Nursing*, has begun, and there is a website for a large listing about using Chaos Theory in the nursing literature *(www.southernct.edu/chaos-nursing/chaos_bib.htm)*.

Nursing as a profession is very interested in research-based nursing practice. When considering the evidence supporting Complexity Theory, mathematical computer models seem to provide the only validation in the biological and physical sciences, and essentially *no research studies* support the theory to date. Analogies (identifying similarities and differences between two different systems) and metaphors (a descriptive term transferred from one idea to another that is not really applicable) are being used primarily to enlighten and stimulate new understandings in applying Complexity Theory to disciplines other than the biological and physical sciences, such as economics and education. The primary application to management seems to be that organizations are supposed to operate at the edge of chaos. Rosenhead (1998) noted that this is little more than crisis management or functioning between order and disintegration. However, Pediani (1996) pointed to examples from the sciences, such as pharmacology, in which Chaos Theory and Complexity Theory seem relevant to some patients' responses to drugs. This newer theory may have broad application in relation to clinical cases.

In management, the traditional focus for leaders is to identify organizational goals and to make decisions facilitating goal achievement. Control is central to logical management processes. However, in Complexity Theory, the idea of control is considered a delusion because of uncertainty and deviations are denied and disregarded. The natural world, according to this theory, does not operate this way and is continually evolving to a higher level of complexity. In Complexity Theory, the future is so unpredictable that long-term planning is not helpful. Rather, it is suggested that managers need to look for instability and complex interactions between people so that learning occurs and the best result "emerges." Management needs to be alert to creative approaches and allow some ambiguity among ideas (Waldrop, 1992). The idea of interconsecutiveness of the parts (people) of the whole suggests that communication among the parts (people) is a key feature of Complexity Theory.

However, for nursing leaders to consider this approach when initiating a new program, spiritual care, for example, may be risky. The way to incorporate this new theory is not yet supported by solid research and "emerged" intelligent practices. As many nurses may remember, the nursing process was introduced about 30 years ago with little testing, evaluation, and orientation. The staff viewed this new approach to charting and thinking about care as difficult and time consuming. The outcome of this project was poor; this was not anticipated by the advocates of the nursing process. Yet, the idea of interconnectedness of things does fit the concept of holistic care, and it can also "make important contributions toward restructuring and reorganizing nursing" (Walsh, 2000, p. 39).

In summary, a plan for spiritual assessment and care by nurses needs to have pilot studies and evaluation. There are management theories from which to choose that are well supported by research and practice. Situational Leadership® is one such theory that has a long history of research and development.

Situational Leadership® Theory

One result of World War II was a serious, national interest in studying leadership and group behaviors. Flight crews (pilot, co-pilot, flight engineer, navigator, bombardier, and up to five gunners) in the B17, B24, and B29 bombers had to get along. Each had a specific job, and if the crew did not work together, they would not reach their target and/or all could die. Experts were called to Washington, D.C., to provide guidance. The research started in earnest, and by the mid-1950s, the science of small

PART III

task groups and organizational management courses were being offered in Ohio State, Michigan, and other university business research centers. The names of early researchers included Drucker, Tannenbaum, Argyris, Bennis, Blake and Mouton, Stogdill, and Cartwright and Zander. In the past 40 years, the theories, research, practice, and consulting about leadership and task group behaviors have developed a strong scientific base that is readily available to nursing leaders. For example, the text by Hersey and colleagues (2008) provides an excellent introduction to leadership studies, synthesizing the theories and research into their own theory of Situational Leadership®.

Bureaucratic organizational cultures lead to poor, shallow, and mistrustful relationships according to Argyris (1962). "Without interpersonal competence or a 'psychologically safe' environment, the organization is a breeding ground for mistrust, intergroup conflict, rigidity, and so on, which in turn leads to a decrease in organizational success in problem solving" (Argyris, 1962, p. 43). In contrast, early in the study of organizational management it was recognized that if humanistic or democratic values are upheld in an organization, then trusting, authentic relationships become the favored mode of communication. Typically, this focus on humanistic values results in an increase in interpersonal competence, intergroup cooperation, flexibility, and ultimately, organizational effectiveness. People are treated as human beings, and they are enabled to develop to their full potential in working and in living these values (Argyris, 1962; Hersey et al., 2008). Communication, persuasion, and negotiation are central to organizational effectiveness.

Situational Leadership® is based on the assumption that there is no singularly successful leadership style but, rather, that leaders need to use a variety of styles that can be adapted to the unique combination of variables present in each situation.

The communication of the leader to individual followers is divided into four styles. The first two are leader-focused, and the second two are focused on the follower. The leader selects the style appropriate to the diagnosis of the maturity of the follower. Although many leaders are found to have one dominate style, the more effective leader is one who can flex among styles, depending of the situation. The Leadership Styles are as follows (Hersey et al., 2008):

- *Style 1: Telling.* Here the leader tells the follower "what to do, when to do it, where to do it, and how." The directions are clear and the follower is supervised closely. The follower is at Readiness Level 1, has little ability to do the task, and is seldom willing.
- *Style 2: Selling.* The leader explains the rationale for the task and answers the follower's questions for clarification. The follower at Readiness Level 2 has some ability but is only occasionally willing to do the task.
- *Style 3: Participating.* The leader engages in dialogue with the follower to share ideas and help make decisions. At Readiness Level 3, the follower now has quite a bit of ability and confidence in performing the task and often is willing to do so.
- *Style 4: Delegating.* The leader now trusts the follower and turns over the responsibility for decisions and performance regarding completing the task. At Readiness Level 4, the follower now has much experience completing the task and is typically very willing to complete it.

Communication, persuasion, and negotiation are core skills in leadership. Research shows that the most important variable in leadership is the communication that occurs between the leader and the follower(s) (Sanford, 1950). This is the focus of Situational Leadership®.

Situational Leadership® focuses on three competencies deemed necessary for a leader's success. These are summarized as follows (Hersey et al., 2008):

- *Diagnosing is a cognitive—or cerebral—competency.* It is the understanding of what the situation is now and knowing what it can reasonably be expected to be in the future. The discrepancy between the two is the problem to be solved. This discrepancy is what the other competencies are aimed at resolving.

- *Adapting is a behavioral competency.* It involves adapting behavior and other resources in a way that helps close the gap between the current situation and what the leader wishes to achieve.
- *Communicating is a process competency.* Leaders need to communicate effectively. If leaders cannot communicate in a way that people can understand and accept, they will be unlikely to meet their goals.

Situational Leadership® for Groups

Research in small task group process has also revealed movement from an initial organization through a period of disorganization or chaos to reorganization at a level that achieves a goal. A group is defined as two or more people, and it exists to meet the needs of each individual in the group so that each will be satisfied. The leader's four major styles of communication used with task groups are similar to those for individual followers (telling, selling, participating, and delegating). The process includes moving from defining, clarifying, and involving to empowering according to the leader's diagnosis of the maturity level of the group (Hersey et al., 2008).

Group readiness levels include four stages: forming, storming, norming, and performing. At the forming readiness level, the group needs direction in defining task goals and objectives as opposed to personal goals. The members are uncertain and insecure about their role in the group. This initial period is chaotic. During the storming period, there is more willingness to accept the group goals and objectives but there are still differences of opinion, competition for recognition, and attempts to influence the group. During the norming period, there is greater agreement on the task goals as the group develops cohesiveness and adjusts to the group and task. Finally, during the performing period, the members are thinking as one and willingly performing the task. There is camaraderie and team spirit as the group becomes self-managing (Hersey et al., 2008).

When combining the leadership style and the group readiness levels, the descriptions may be summarized as follows (Hersey et al., 2008):

- *Level 1: Group Readiness:* The group is described as uncertain and in chaos, without a common goal. The leader's Style 1, monological communication of "defining," concentrates on setting goals and providing descriptions of roles and responsibilities.
- *Level 2: Group Readiness:* The group members compete for recognition and influence during this storming phase as they begin to bring their personal goals into agreement with the group goal. The leader's Style 2, "clarifying," fine-tuning details of the group's responsibility. The leader's position is central within the circle of the group members.
- *Level 3: Group Readiness:* Group members begin to come together, "norming," as the individuals accept the group goal; they emerge toward cohesiveness. The leader's Style 3, "involving," is dialogical and located within the circle of members of the group. The leader becomes more involved with goal setting and serves as an active member.
- *Level 4: Group Readiness:* The group members begin to function together, "performing" in synergy with one another toward goal attainment. The leader's Style 4, "empowering," lets the team become self-managing. The leader steps outside the group circle to serve as the conduit of communication between the group and the organization and/or its other groups.

Overview of Groups

Hersey and colleagues' (2008, p. 261) definition of a group is "two or more individuals interacting, in which the existence of all (the existence of the group as a group) is necessary for the individual group members' needs to be satisfied." It is important to note that individual group members have differing needs to be satisfied by being a part of the group. As a principle, the degree to which individual need satisfaction is achieved differentiates effective from ineffective groups; the greater the individual's satisfaction, the higher the probability of group effectiveness (Hersey et al., 2008). According to workplace specialists, job satisfaction has been found to include much more than salary increases, decreased overtime, and tangible rewards. Appreciation, trust, and respect do not have direct costs. These, as well as support for individual growth and a sense of purpose, have been identified as important factors in job satisfaction. Job satisfaction means having a leader who is fair and honest, listens to concerns, and helps the followers in developing knowledge, attitudes, and skills to advance their careers. Some have suggested that nurses probably do not leave agencies; they leave dehumanizing nursing leaders (Gardner, 2008). Nurse leaders need to be in touch with the degree to which nursing staff are satisfied. Job satisfaction has again become an important issue in the workplace environment, given the current nurse shortage (Aiken et al., 2001; Buerhaus et al., 2007).

Members assume a variety of roles within the process of a group. Most are constructive in nature, contributing to the discussion, solving the problem, and achieving the group goal. These roles may be questioning, suggesting possibilities, taking notes, and summarizing the group's progress. However, some roles are not helpful. The most disruptive periods in group process are probably in Readiness 1, "forming" with uncertainty and chaos; and Readiness 2, "storming" with intergroup dissonance and competition. It is at these levels that members may behave in roles that hinder group effectiveness, such as criticizing, attacking, or name calling. The leader needs to intervene as appropriate with discussions of goals, standards, and feedback on behavior and progress for individuals or the group, depending on the situation. The degree to which roles are not helpful probably influences member satisfaction, and certainly interferes with communication and collaboration (Hersey et al., 2008).

The workplace does not have to be hostile. There is support on a national level to promote effective communication and collaboration. It is important that positive interdisciplinary relationships are active in the organizational culture.

According to the U.S. Department of Health and Human Services (2008, p. 6), "the U.S. Congress has provided for support to programs that enhance collaboration and communication among nurses and other health care professionals and promote nurse involvement in health facilities' organizational and clinical decision-making."

Further, "As a means of assisting with nurse retention and with enhancing patient care, Section 831 was also amended to call for grants related to collaboration and communication among nurses and other health professionals, and to promote nurse involvement in decision-making in health care facilities. Considerable documentation exists that demonstrates the increased job satisfaction that comes from these practices" (U.S. Department of Health and Human Services, 2008, p. 13).

Humanizing Nursing Communication Theory (HNCT)

For most of the past century, concern for the manner by which human beings are treated has increased, not only on an international and national level but also in business and industry. The need for humane behavior toward people, especially in communication behavior, is particularly important as health care evolves into a larger and more complex industry. In a conference report (Troupin, 2001) from the Durban South Africa meeting of the World Organization of Family Doctors, David Satcher, the former U.S. Surgeon General, reviewed the history of health care for the past 100 years. His message to family physicians was to take an active role in improving the overall quality of health through focused efforts. He noted that health resources can be more equitably distributed if leadership is directed to improving and humanizing problems in the health care system.

It is proposed that if health care personnel, especially nurses, are regarded in a manner that acknowledges all characteristics of human beings, then these personnel will tend to regard the patients, clients, peers, and professional colleagues in a similar manner. Because registered nurses constitute the largest health care occupation in the United States, with 2.5 million jobs of the 4,585,000 people employed in hospitals in the United States (U.S. Department of Labor, Bureau of Labor Statistics, 2008), humanizing efforts become important to the fabric of health care.

Numerous theories of communication have been developed for nursing practice, usually in clinical psychiatric and mental health contexts. Attitudes are an important factor. Nurse leaders can become intellectually aware of and sensitive to the wide range of humanizing and dehumanizing attitudes (Box 8.3) that can be used with different patterns of communication interaction (Figures 8.1, 8.2, and 8.3). The list of attitudes was developed by searching the literature for concepts commonly used in promoting relationships and in counseling; then the antonyms were identified using a thesaurus. The patterns of interactions were identified from the discipline of communication studies and are known to be commonly used in everyday communication.

At the core of the patterns of interaction model is the most humanizing communication, **"communing,"** that involves four necessary elements: **trust, self-disclosure, feedback,** and **listening** (see Figure 8.2). For example, the patient (or follower) needs to trust the nurse (or leader) enough to self-disclose personal concerns often not revealed to anyone else. The nurse (or leader) needs to respond by providing feedback that is

Box 8.3

Humanizing-Dehumanizing Continuum of Attitudes

Humanizing	Dehumanizing
Dialogue	Monologue
Individual	Categories
Holistic	Parts
Choice	Directives
Equality	Degradation
Positive Regard	Disregard
Acceptance	Judgment
Empathy	Tolerance
Authenticity	Role-playing
Caring	Careless
Irreplaceable	Expendable
Intimacy	Isolation
Coping	Helpless
Power	Powerless

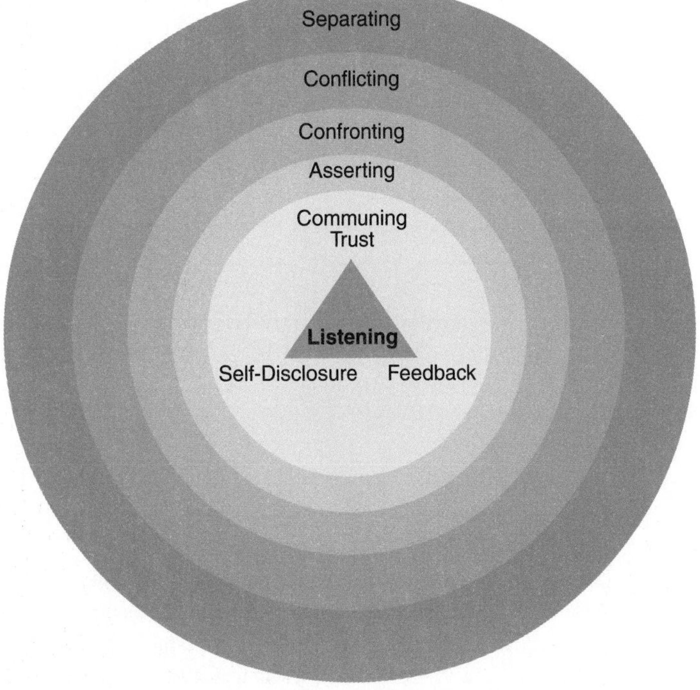

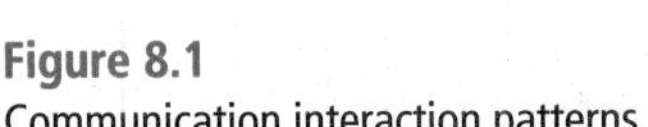
Figure 8.1
Communication interaction patterns.

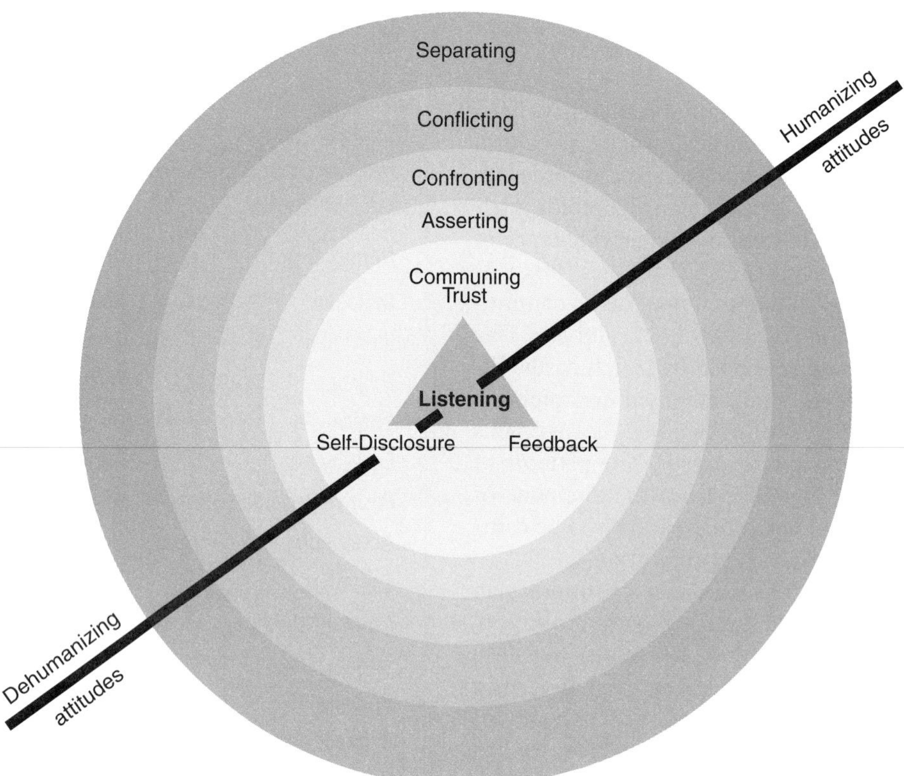

Figure 8.2
Interaction of communication interaction patterns and continuum of attitudes.

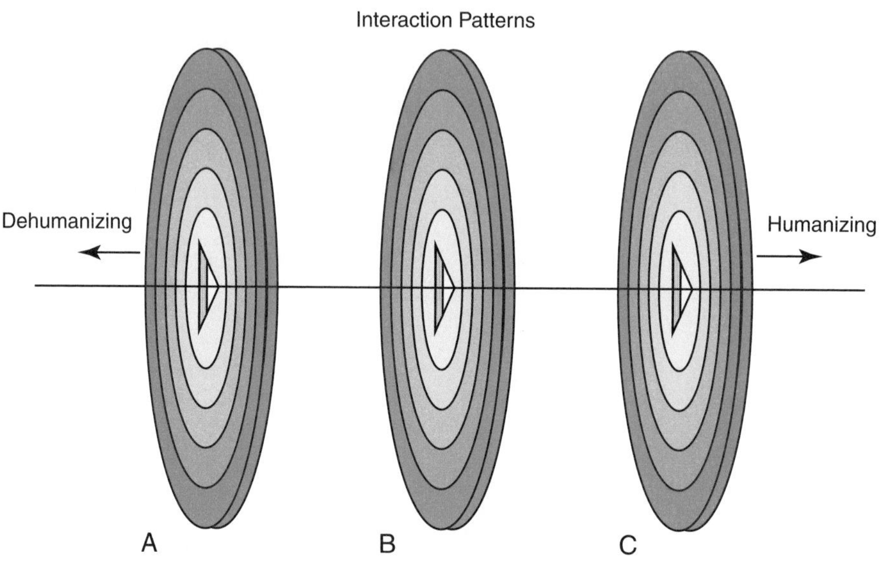

Figure 8.3
Communication continuum of choices.

informative yet supportive to the patient (or follower). Both need to listen with intentionality to what is being said (Figure 8.4). This is communing, and by the definitions offered earlier, this is dialogue and this also is spiritual care.

As one moves outward on the model of patterns of interaction (see Figure 8.2) to assertiveness, confrontation, and conflict, perceptions increasingly differ, ultimately ending the relationship in separation, if dehumanizing attitudes are consistently used. However, to the degree that humanizing attitudes are used at any level, the relationship can return to the communing level (Box 8.4). Agendas, such as **s**ituation, **b**ackground, **a**ssessment, and **r**ecommendation (SBAR), de Shazer's (1985) solution-focused brief therapy (SFBT), and many "crucial conversation tools" as suggested by Patterson and colleagues (2002) may be used within the patterns of interaction and attitudes continuum. The *Nursing Communication Observation Tool Instruction Manual* (Duldt, 1989) may be helpful in research and in teaching HNCT.

In group process as described in Situational Leadership®, the communing or dialogue of HNCT can be chosen by design for a high probability of positive outcomes in a group as it moves through the forming, storming, norming, and performing sequence of group process.

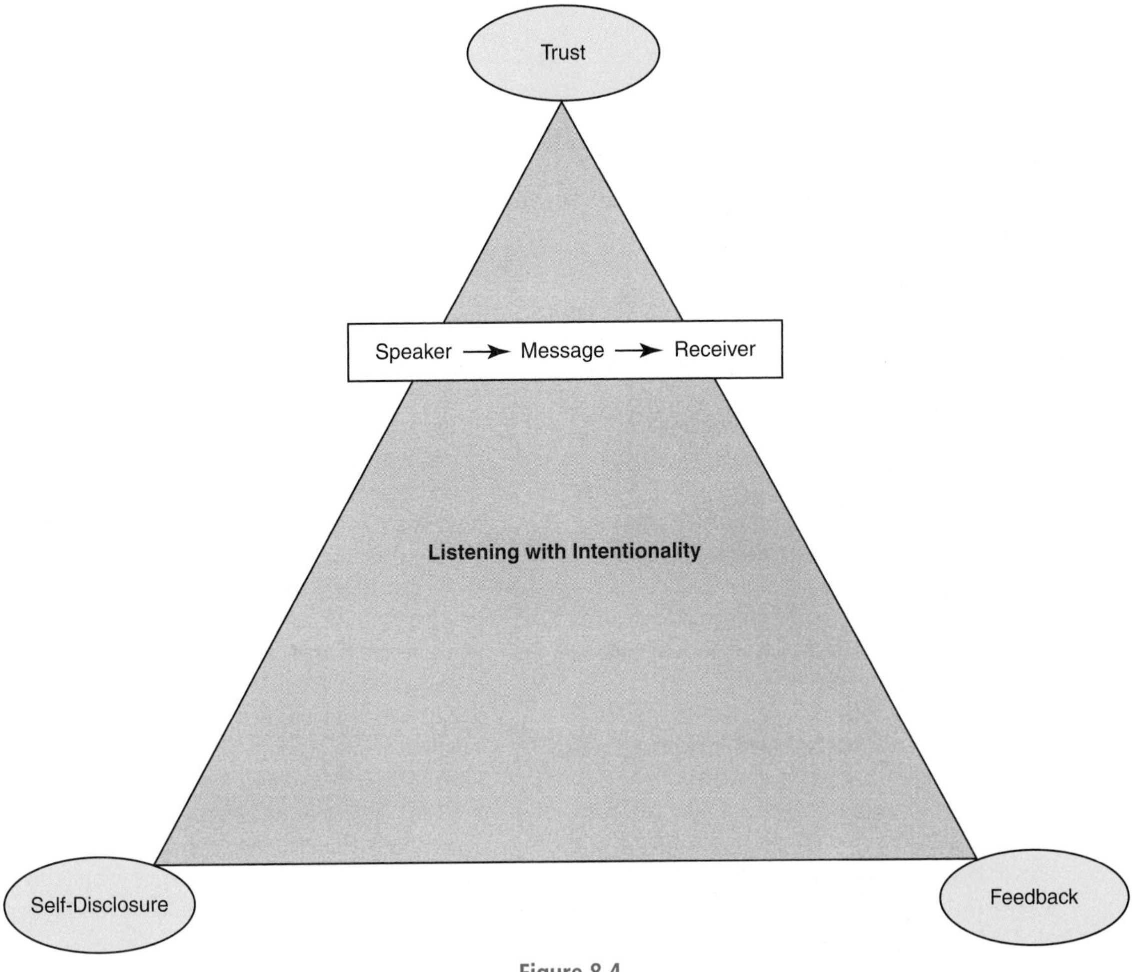

Figure 8.4
Communing tripod.

PART III

LEADING & MANAGING DEFINED

Communing

Dialogical, intimate communication occurring between two or more people; the heart of humanistic communication. The central tripod of communing is trust, self-disclosure, and feedback.

Listening

The core of communing; involves making a conscious effort to attend to what another person is saying, particularly to expressions of feelings, meanings, and perceived implications. When listening with "intentionality" or wanting to help, this becomes *compassionate listening.*

Trust

One person relying on another, risking potential loss in attempting to achieve a goal, when the outcome is uncertain; and the potential for loss is greater than for gain if the trust is violated.

Self-Disclosure

Risking rejection in telling how one feels, thinks, and so on, regarding "here and now" or existential events.

Feedback

Describing how another's behavior, beliefs, and so on are perceived; giving one's evaluation or feelings.

Box **8.4**

Theoretical Relationship Statements of Humanizing Nursing Communication Theory

1. To the degree to which one receives humanizing communication from others, to that degree one will tend to feel recognized and accepted as a human being.
   a. While applying the nursing process, to the degree to which a nurse is able to use humanizing communication, to that degree will the client, peer, or colleague tend to feel recognized and accepted as a human being.
   b. In a given environment, if a critical life situation develops for a client, to the degree the nurse uses humanizing communication attitudes and patterns while applying the nursing process, to a similar degree will the health of the client tend to move in a positive direction.
2. To the degree that listening, trust, self-disclosure, and feedback occur, to that degree humanizing communication or communing also occurs.
3. In the event one tends to experience dehumanizing communication (e.g., monological rather than dialogical communication, categorical rather than individualistic), then one tends to move outward (on the model) to the next pattern of interaction.
4. In an interpersonal relationship of trust, self-disclosure, and feedback, to the degree that dehumanizing communication attitudes are expressed by another, to that degree one tends to use assertiveness as a pattern of interaction.
5. To the degree that assertiveness tends not to re-establish trust, self-disclosure, and feedback and to the degree that dehumanizing attitudes are expressed by another, to that degree one tends to use assertiveness as a pattern of interaction.
6. To the degree that confrontation tends not to re-establish trust, self-disclosure, or feedback and to the degree that dehumanizing communication attitudes continue to be expressed by another, to that degree one tends to use conflict resolution as a pattern of interaction.
7. To the degree that conflict tends to not re-establish trust, self-disclosure, and feedback and to the degree that dehumanizing communication attitudes continue to be expressed by another, to that degree one tends to terminate the relationship by separation.

Box 8.4

Theoretical Relationship Statements of Humanizing Nursing Communication Theory—cont'd

8. To the degree that humanizing communication attitudes occur in a relationship, in the event of separation, the relationship can be resumed to the same degree of closeness regardless of the separation.
9. To the degree to which a nurse uses humanizing communication, to that degree will the nurse tend to receive humanizing communication from others—clients, peers, colleagues, and leaders.
10. To the degree that one is aware of one's own choice (and motives) about interaction patterns, to that degree one can develop communication skills and habits that tend to have predictable results in establishing, maintaining, and terminating interpersonal relationships.

Implementing Spiritual Care in Nursing

The Goal

The nursing leader needs to communicate the need to formally design a way to fulfill the holistic health criteria for spiritual care not only to the nurses but also to other disciplines and groups within an agency (see the Practical Tips box). It is vital to have the support of the nurse leader's leaders (i.e., heads of departments within the agency, top administrators, perhaps the board of directors). The more people outside the nursing group who are supportive, the easier it will be to implement change. One can expect some criticism, such as "Nurses are not chaplains!" or "The clergy in the community take care of that!" or "We have a Chaplain!" or "The doctors and admitting office personnel get that information." With supporting comments from the leader's leaders, the nurse leader garners support.

Broad goals need to be identified. For example, the approach to spiritual care needs to be ecumenical or all-inclusive. The wide variety of religious and spiritual belief systems need to be acknowledged and respected. This needs to include those who may not have support from a faith community, such as atheists or agnostics. The ethics of spiritual care need to be established early. The patient's perspective of spirituality is to be the guide for providing individualized care, not the nurse's. This may occur in a Jewish hospital by a Christian or Buddhist nurse when caring for an atheist, Mormon, Islamic, or Hindu patient. The nurses cannot be expected to know about each one of these belief systems, but they need to learn what to ask and to listen for the individual's beliefs that have an impact on the patient's health care (Boxes 8.5 and 8.6).

The Task

One strategy for implementing spiritual care is for the nurse leader to ask for five nurse volunteers to serve on a special spiritual care task team. By having an odd number (e.g., 5 or 7 or 9 members), the group composition may enable achieving a majority vote and tends to facilitate the progress of the team. It also tends to give the team a timeline for completing the project. Having those nurses who are initially interested in the task involved as early adopters will tend to increase their involvement as well as satisfaction with the outcome. Because this is to be a nursing function, the nurses need to have ownership of their group. Other professionals, such as chaplains or oncology physicians, may be invited to serve as consultants or provide educational resources to the group.

As noted in Situational Leadership® Theory, the leader needs to be aware of the degree of job satisfaction each group member is experiencing. The leader may use the Job/Communication/Satisfaction/Importance (JCSI) survey and research

PART III

Practical Tips

Recommendations for Implementing a Program of Spiritual Care

1. Secure the support of the leader's leader and other agency leaders as appropriate.
2. Persuade followers to accept goal of program; ask for five volunteers from the total group to serve on a small group task group to design the program.
3. Establish communication with other agency leaders, especially the chaplain and others who may serve as resource people for the task group.
4. Use Situational Leadership® Styles 1-4 and Follower/Group Maturity Levels 1-4 to diagnose appropriate way to communication with the group.
5. Establish the goal of the group: to develop an ecumenical, multicultural program, guidelines, and policies for spiritual care of all patients.
6. Analyze the group patterns of communication within the agency culture and the task group (i.e., star or circle). Encourage the circle pattern rather than the star pattern within the group if deemed appropriate.
7. Require pilot studies and evaluation of the proposed program before implementing throughout the agency.
8. Upon implementation, request that items be added to the patient evaluation form to receive feedback on how the spiritual care program is perceived by the consumers of health care.
9. Make announcements to the community at large as appropriate.

Box **8.5**

The Five "Rs" Rubric for the Role of the Nurse

The role of the nurse can be seen as limited to the five "Rs": Recognizing, Responding, Recording, Reporting, and Referring.

Nurses need to *recognize* symptoms of spiritual distress, and they need to know the ways of *responding* to these distressed patients in a manner that has a high probability of success in comforting these persons. Then nurses need to figure out what to *record* and to *report* while considering the legal, ethical, and "need to know" confidentiality issues. Finally, nurses need to know to whom *referrals* are to be made to meet the needs of each situation.

The chaplain's role consists of continued assessment to identify specific spiritual issues and to develop a treatment plan addressing each issue. The chaplain would then implement the plan and evaluate the patient's response, adjusting the plan as indicated. This process may continue over considerable time. Upon dismissal from the hospital, the patient may be referred to a community resource, particularly if the patient is a member of a faith community.

From Battey, B.W. (in press). *Spiritual assessment for nurses and other health care professional: A computer assisted instructional program with instructor's manual and student handbook.* Antioch, CA: Author. Computer assisted instructional tools are available from A.S.K. Data Systems, Inc. (www.askdatasystems.com).

tool (Battey, in press; Duldt, 1980). This tool may be helpful in monitoring followers' satisfaction with their job and organizational communication, as well as the perceived importance of each aspect involved.

Role of the Nurse Leader

The nurse leader will probably find a careful study of Situational Leadership® helpful. The relationship styles, defining, clarifying, involving, and empowering describe the highest probability of

Box 8.6

Role of the Nurse in Spiritual Care

Nurses are not chaplains. It is proposed that the *definition of spirituality for use by nurses lies within each patient and that the professional nurse seeks to use the patient's own definition in developing individualized plans of care.* Ethically, nurses must keep their own spiritual/religious beliefs to themselves, avoiding proselytizing. The focus is on what the patient believes, not the nurse.

Although definitions of spirituality seem to be endless in the literature, *the nurse needs to be responsible for five major dimensions: beliefs, values, meanings, goals, and relationships.* These dimensions include the following kinds of information:

- Beliefs—Whether an "other" exists; that there is a universal force or power or energy that is creative and renewing. Who or what is my God or god(s)?
- Values—What is of ultimate importance in my life? How have I prioritized my resources?
- Meanings—What would I give up my life for? What are the significances or implications of my life's events, and what is happening to my body and mind?
- Goals—What is my "mission" in life? What am I called to do? What goals are appropriate? Where am I needed? What have I accomplished? What can I accomplish now?
- Relationships—What is the ultimate relationship or power in my life? What relationships do I need? What changes will occur as relationships are initiated, maintained, or ended, given what is happening to my body and mind?

The BVMGR rubric is proposed as the most appropriate guide or assessment tool for nurses. Specific lists of questions are to be asked or just noted if a formal assessment interview is deemed inappropriate. It is suggested that a formal interview may not be necessary because nurses are "there" 24/7; nurses just need to be alert to the BVMGR topics that might be mentioned during routine care of patients. The number of minutes may vary, since the conversation may be very brief (e.g., in the ER or ICU), or continue for a long time (e.g., perhaps hospice or rehabilitation contexts). Finally, not all patients' spiritual issues become salient while under nursing care, so it may not be appropriate to hold formal interviews with everyone.

Modified from Battey, B.W. (in press). *Spiritual assessment for nurses and other health care professionals: A computer assisted instructional program with instructor's manual and student handbook* (lesson 1, Definitions). Antioch, CA: Author. Computer assisted instructional tools are available from A.S.K. Data Systems, Inc. (www.askdatasystems.com).

success for the manner in which the leader relates to the group.

Communication Within the Group

Classic research by Bavelas (1953) revealed the best way to communicate within a group for effectiveness in task performance, as well as for group morale. The communication patterns he tested were (1) the autocratic, hub, or star pattern and (2) the democratic, circle pattern.

Five members were in each experimental group. In the star pattern, members wrote messages only to the leader at the center or hub of the group—a one-way communication pattern. This pattern proved to be fastest but could have negative effects on morale. All the messages went from one member to the leader; the members could not send messages to one another. With each experimental trial, the members developed a low opinion of themselves (except for the leader), and they became dissatisfied. Some sabotaged the task by writing messages in foreign languages or just tearing up messages. The leader at the hub of the group was happy getting all of the messages and participated effectively. However, when confronted with an emergency, the members tended to avoid responsibility and to look to the leader to solve the problem; the group did not perform well. Still, overall, this group proved to solve the problem faster and accomplished more than the circle group.

In contrast, in the democratic circle group, members could send messages to one another—the two-way communication or dialogical pattern. The progress was described as slow and inaccurate, but the members were happy. No one wrote messages in foreign languages and the like, but they seemed to like the task even though they were critical of their own work. No one leader emerged. Because more messages were sent, the circle group had the advantage of check-backs and opportunities to find and correct errors. In the event of an emergency, the members became cohesive and were able to solve the problem, coping with the situation much better than those in the star pattern.

These experiments show how communication can affect how people feel about their own and the group's job performance, participation, satisfaction, and responsibility. Although experienced nursing leaders may feel comfortable using the circle pattern, leaders with less experience may feel more comfortable with the star pattern. It may be appropriate to use both patterns, depending on the situational variables within the organization as a whole. It is suggested that the circle pattern would be most appropriate in introducing a change in order to develop commitment and involvement of the members. Using the star communication pattern may tend to result in resentment and opposition, and it is to be avoided if a democratic circle pattern of communication is currently in place. Before implementing change, the nurse leader is well advised to first analyze the communication pattern currently in place (Hersey et al., 2008).

CURRENT ISSUES AND TRENDS

Teaching Communication

There are many approaches to teaching communication skills to nursing students. Most approaches are based on procedures, techniques, and/or rubrics that provide an agenda of topics for specific case situations. Communication seems to be such a broad topic that it is unclear what to include. In addition, teaching communication skills is particularly challenging under conditions of cultural diversity.

What is needed is a general communication theory specifically for nursing that will provide a framework from which to teach communication skills to nursing students. The HNCT perspective of communication is believed to be useful in all situations in nursing practice, and thus it can serve as a "benchmark" theory. This theory aids the nurse in coping with the wide range of messages containing *facts* and *feelings* as well as *patterns of interaction* and *attitudes* experienced in the practice of nursing. This nursing theory can be utilized in conjunction with other nursing theories to provide a unique perspective of the communication dimension of interpersonal interactions. The HNCT is realistic in that it recognizes the humanizing as well as dehumanizing attitudes of communication with nurses, clients, and others. This theory is an "is" rather than a "should be" theory. It provides the nurse with options to choose along a continuum of humanizing to dehumanizing attitudes, and nurses can intervene by design so that there can be an escape from negative patterns of communication. It provides direction to change relationships into humanizing interaction patterns and attitudes. Although this theory is easily understandable for clinical nurses, it is not widely used and warrants further research.

There is a need to determine a theoretically based and research evidence–supported approach to teaching communication. It is important that this approach be most effective in developing interpersonal communication skills in nursing students to ensure that they have the highest probability of responding in a humanizing manner with patients in critical life situations. The criterion for determining the degree of humanizing or dehumanizing that has occurred is what is experienced by the receiver of the speaker's message, which is the response of the receiver. This is analogous to the recipient of the sexual harasser's message determining the meaning of the message regardless of the speaker's intent. The dehumanizing message is perceived as unattractive; the receiver's body language indicates defensiveness and distancing from the speaker, and posture and facial expression changes.

Documentation in the literature is extensive regarding disruptive and distracting communication interactions not only between nurses and between nurses and professional colleagues (e.g., physicians, pharmacists, administrators) but also between nurses and patients. The research indicates that nursing personnel experience high turnover rates, job dissatisfaction, and burnout; many RNs are leaving the profession. The work environment is described as hostile to nurses, and patient outcomes of increased severity of illness and mortality have been directly related to poor communication skills of the staff. There is some evidence that this is an issue in many parts of the world, not just in the United States. The clinical ambiance needs to change. Research by DeMarco and colleagues (2007) on the concept "self-silencing" reveals that women are socialized to value relationships to the degree that they choose not to reveal their needs or feelings to avoid disagreements and potential loss of the relationship. Findings indicate this is a gender issue and may limit the degree to which RNs can be independent and in control of their professional practice. It is suggested that research is needed about the use of assertiveness, confrontation, and conflict as HNCT patterns of interaction.

There is a need for research to determine the distribution of nursing students and staff communication on the humanizing and dehumanizing continuum. One way to do this is to use the Nursing Communication Observation Tool (NCOT), which is designed for use in data collection within the framework of HNCT. Data can be obtained by having groups or subjects view a video, such as "Wit" or "The Doctor," and then identify patterns of interaction and attitudes on the NCOT. Analysis may show a range of sensitivity that would provide direction for educational interventions. How can nurses (and others) be "inoculated" to increase their resilience to a hostile workplace? How can nurses be instructed in the "every day" communication skills necessary in clinical practice and not just in specialized communication as is taught in psychiatric nursing? HNCT is designed to suggest directions for educational interventions, but more research is needed.

Summary

- Communicating, along with diagnosing and adapting, is one of the three basic competencies of influencing and leadership.
- Communication is the art of being able to structure and transmit a message in a way that another can easily understand and/or accept.
- Communication is defined as the degree to which information is transmitted among the members and parts of an organization.
- Verbal communication is both written and spoken (oral).
- Nonverbal communication is unspoken and is composed of affective or expressive behaviors.
- Interpersonal relationships include an element of communication.
- Communication occurs in a variety of interactive patterns.
- Group dynamics and the interaction of multiple people provide complexity and challenges to the communicative process and the influence of perception in organizations.
- Persuasion and negotiation are influence techniques.
- Persuasion is human communication designed to influence another to modify attitudes or alter behaviors by using argument, reasoning, or entreaty.
- Communication is the core of leadership; influencing is achieved through persuasion.
- Negotiation is a give-and-take exchange to resolve conflicts.
- The work of a leader or manager depends on the ability to negotiate.
- Humanizing Nursing Communication Theory is applicable to providing spiritual care.
- Organizational and work communication needs to be collegial, respectful, and positive.

CASE STUDY

As director of the nursing education department in a large hospital, Evelyn Sullivan is responsible for providing the educational component for nursing staff. The current educational program for the entire nursing staff is spiritual assessment and care. The staff is composed of nurses of a wide variety of Christian religious affiliations. One concern about the content of the workshops Evelyn is planning is conveying convincingly the ethical standards to be maintained (i.e., autonomy, beneficence, confidentiality). Of particular concern is the issue of respecting the patients' beliefs and avoiding proselytizing or trying to convert patients to the nurses' own religion. Nurses are to listen for what patients believe as it is relevant to their health care and try to work within these beliefs. Evelyn devised the following plan.

A group of 30 nurses would be attending the first workshop on spirituality and spiritual care. In an introductory lecture, the purpose of the spiritual assessment is to learn the following:

1. How spirituality/religion influence health care
2. How beliefs help patients cope with illness and stress
3. What spiritual needs can be identified and addressed
4. What referrals are needed to the chaplain, priest, or religious official
5. What the scope of the patients' support systems is

Evelyn's plan was to ask nurses to write on the provided index card how they defined spirituality and spiritual care. After about 5 minutes, Evelyn would then ask the nurses to meet in small groups to share their ideas and briefly discuss their definitions.

Rather than following the usual method, Evelyn decided to not have the small groups report about their discussions or definitions. Rather, she would ask them to keep this information to themselves by putting the index card in their pocket. That card contains what they personally believe, and they could use this as a reminder about spiritual care principles. In considering spirituality, the nurses were to listen carefully for the **b**eliefs, **v**alues, **m**eanings, **g**oals, and **r**elationships, the BVMGR, to what the patient says comprises spirituality. Although the patient may profess being a member of a certain religious organization, the patient may not believe exactly what is commonly known about that religion or accept all the tenets of that religion.

On the basis of this information, a "designer" spiritual care plan can be developed to provide spiritual comfort to the patient. The focus is to be on the patient's definitions of spirituality, not the nurse's. The rationale for this is based on the ethical principles of autonomy, beneficence, and confidentiality.

Evelyn followed this plan in the presentation of the first workshop. The nurses had no difficulty writing their beliefs and briefly discussing them with one another. Everyone followed her instructions and put the index cards in their pockets. In the remainder of the workshop, the five "Rs" role of the nurse and the role of chaplains and community church leaders were discussed at length as spiritual care plans were developed for case situations. Evelyn was relieved to note that the nurses did not discuss their own beliefs but did, in fact, think about how patients they had known thought about and practiced spirituality.

CRITICAL THINKING EXERCISE

Nurse Aminta Parra is in charge of an interdisciplinary team at Sunrise Hospital. The nurses at Sunrise have identified a need to develop a critical pathway for ventilator-dependent patients who are about to be discharged to home with home health care. Nurse Parra knows that these patients have multiple complex care needs. It is urgent that information flow be specific and detailed to make "seamless" the care transfer between the hospital and home care, wherever this may be. First, Nurse Parra had to manage a few physicians who flatly stated that they would not follow a "cookbook" concocted by nurses. Then the dietary representative presented the team with dietary's protocols and suggested that nurses integrate these since nurses were in charge of the pathway maintenance. Next, Nurse Parra discovered why the local home health care representative was not returning phone calls and could not come to team meetings for quite a while: the group was planning a move in 1 month and was just notified of that The Joint Commission (TJC) would be visiting in 3 months.

1. What is the problem?
2. Whose problem is it?
3. What should Nurse Parra do?
4. What mode of communication should Nurse Parra use?
5. How can Nurse Parra structure a clear message?
6. To whom should Nurse Parra communicate first? Who else needs to be involved in the communication flow?
7. What leadership and management strategies should Nurse Parra use?

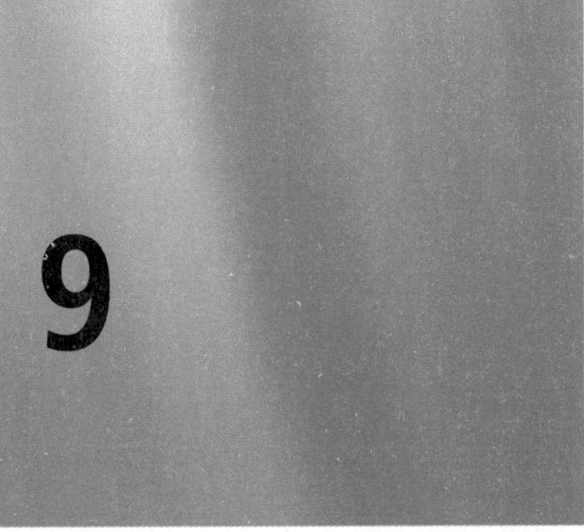

9 Motivation

Richard W. Redman

CHAPTER OBJECTIVES

- Define and describe motivation
- Examine the content and process motivation theories
- Differentiate between internal and external motivation
- Critique classic theories of motivation
- Analyze motivation in organizations
- Evaluate motivation in nursing
- Analyze the link between motivation and leadership and management
- Exercise critical thinking to conceptualize and analyze possible solutions to a practice exercise

The concept of motivation seems to pervade daily life. It may manifest in a negative way, as when someone is *not motivated* to do something, or more positively, as when someone is particularly "pumped" (i.e., excited and motivated) to get something done. A central characteristic of motivation is some type of energy, drive, or will to behave in a certain way or to accomplish something.

Motivation is a multidimensional phenomenon. It can be viewed from biological, physiological, and psychological perspectives. The biological and physiological explanations are helpful but inadequate when the importance of the psychological perspective is considered. Psychological insights range from cognitive mechanisms to the attitudinal perspective. Motivation theory even has a philosophical perspective when one considers concepts such as the fully functioning individual and self-actualization (Petri, 1996).

Motivation has been described as the ability to get individuals to do what one wants them to do—when and how one wants it done. Motivated people have a sense of forward drive as an identifying characteristic; they also exhibit energy, enthusiasm, and goal-directedness.

Motivation is central to a number of issues important to nurses and nursing practice. It is a factor in how nurses feel about professional issues and affects the workplace or practice setting. It has implications for leadership as nurses struggle with the challenge of how to get members of a team or work group to do something they may not want to do. Also, motivation theory can provide insights into the process of trying to understand how patients' behaviors are related to health and illness activities and the challenge this relationship presents to nurses as they help patients take on more responsibility for their health.

First, this chapter examines the large body of motivation theory and reviews some of the different approaches to explaining motivation and behavior. Next, some applications of these theories are considered from the perspective of nursing and health services research. Finally, key principles from motivation theories are presented and applied to professional nursing practice.

DEFINITIONS

The term **motivation** comes from the Latin word *movere*, meaning "to move." Although it has multiple definitions, three common components are embodied in the term *motivation*. Motivation describes factors that are believed to energize human behavior in some way. It also refers to the mechanisms of how and where that behavior will be directed. Finally, it encompasses insights on how that behavior is sustained over time. Essentially, motivation means the degree to which an individual is moved or aroused to expend effort to achieve some goal or purpose (Rainey, 2001).

Motivation also is used to describe the process of activating human behavior. It implies a sense of movement, excitement, and expectancy. Motivation is a catalyst to move individuals toward goals.

The basic unit of human behavior is an **activity** or a discrete action. People vary in both their ability and their willingness to do any activity. Motivation is the willingness aspect. **Motives or needs** are the wants, drives, or impulses within an individual. They are the drives to action and the reasons for behavior. Motives are directed toward goals and are the energizing forces that become an incentive to strive for the desired rewards outside the individual. Activity is generally focused on the need(s) with the greatest strength at any given point in time.

Motivation to work is the degree to which members of an organization are willing to fulfill their role or to do their job. Energizing forces within individuals drive them to behave, and environmental forces trigger these drives. The idea of goal orientation means that human behavior is directed *toward* something. To analyze motivation from a systems orientation means to look at the forces within individuals, as well as those in the environment that feed back to either reinforce the intensity of a drive or to discourage a course of action and redirect efforts. For example, motivation can be sparked as a result of persuasive communication that occurs between a leader and a follower.

The most powerful source of motivation is thought to be internal, intrinsic drives. To effectively motivate, leaders need to discover in their followers some internal or external need or trigger that arouses a desire, energizes the will, and serves as a basis for action or thought.

MOTIVATION THEORY

A large body of literature that includes several theories of motivation has developed over the years. Although these theories initially focused on behavior in general, the primary focus eventually shifted to motivation as it relates to work; thus most motivation theories are focused on motivation and behavior in the workplace and are found in the business and organizational sciences literature. Motivation theory permeates nearly all aspects of management sciences today, including elements of leadership, teams, job performance, change management, and decision making. It is seen by managers as an essential component in the job performance equation on all levels. Researchers see theories of motivation as fundamental to developing evidence-based policies and

LEADING & MANAGING DEFINED

Motivation

The degree to which an individual is moved or aroused to achieve a goal or purpose.

Activity

A basic unit of human behavior.

Motives or Needs

Wants, drives, or impulses.

Motivation to Work

The degree to which members of an organization are willing to work.

guidelines for effective management practices that can be applied in all types of work environments (Steers et al., 2004).

Rainey (2001) described motivation theories as the foundation for thousands of research studies on the topic. However, the volume of theories and research projects has not resulted in one single theory that everyone agrees on. Rainey (2001) noted that motivation is best viewed as an umbrella construct that embraces a set of concepts and issues rather than a single variable or theory with a precise operational definition.

Motivation theories often reflect an interaction between processes or factors internal to the individual and stimuli or forces in the external environment. Each of these components is emphasized and valued to varying degrees in a given theory. As the social, behavioral, and biological sciences have matured over time, motivation theories have reflected these developments. Some theories focus primarily on personality and genetic characteristics, explaining motivation as primarily originating in innate characteristics of the individual. Eventually, theories became more social in their orientation, recognizing the importance of work groups or cultural factors as influencing variables in shaping motivation within an individual (D'Aunno et al., 2000). Today, theories generally contain elements that are found within individuals, as well as in the social or professional environment in which individuals work.

Given the large number of motivation theories that are available, schemas for grouping them have been developed. Box 9.1 presents two ways to categorize the large number of motivation theories that exist. The more common method is to group them as either content or process theories. Content theories describe behavior based on factors that exist primarily within the individual. Most of these factors focus on needs, drives, or forces within an individual that result in the person directing behavior in some particular way. Process theories examine behavior as a function of human decision-making processes and often include components in the environment that motivate people to behave in various ways (Porter et al., 2003).

Box 9.1

Approaches to Categorizing Motivation Theories

I. Schema developed by Porter and colleagues (2003)
   A. Content theories (factors primarily within the individual)
      1. Maslow's hierarchy of needs
      2. McClelland's needs for achievement, power, and affiliation
      3. Herzberg's two-factor theory
   B. Process theories (focus on the psychological or behavioral processes)
      1. Operant conditioning
      2. Vroom's expectancy theory
      3. Goal-setting theory
II. Schema developed by Mitchell & Daniels (2003)
   A. Internal motivation theories
      1. Thoughtful (based on cognitive approaches)
         a. Expectancy theory
         b. Goal-setting theory
      2. Not rational (non-cognitive; based on individual differences)
         a. Personality theory
         b. Genetic theory
   B. External motivation theories
      1. Job design or characteristics model
      2. Social theories: groups and culture

Development in this area of theory progressed gradually over the past century. Initially, theories focused on instincts as a driving force and included concepts such as fear, curiosity, or sociability. The theories were referred to as *content theories* and eventually evolved into a variety of need theories. Eventually, the theories became more oriented toward drives and reinforcement through interaction with the environment, thus becoming more behaviorally oriented. These theories view individuals in a learning relationship between their actions and consequences for those actions. This behavioralist view of individuals is still a central theme in many motivation theories today. As theories developed more of a focus on process, they became more cognitive in their underpinnings, attempting to explain and understand the thought processes involved in determining how people will behave, especially in the workplace. This work culminated in a focus on goal-setting theory, which is the dominant perspective today (Steers et al., 2004).

Regardless of the particular theoretical perspective on work motivation, most researchers would agree that the best way to view work performance is as an interaction effect between abilities and motivation (O'Reilly & Chatman, 1999). It might be seen in terms of the following simple formula:

$$\text{Performance} = \text{Ability} \times \text{Motivation}$$

An individual can have strong abilities to perform a task or fulfill a set of responsibilities, but if the individual is not motivated to perform or to do them well, he or she will not do so. The reverse can also be envisioned, in which someone is highly motivated to do his or her best but the person simply does not have the abilities or skill to successfully perform a task or carry out a set of responsibilities. In this sense, motivation might best be viewed as a moderator of ability.

There are too many motivation theories available to examine all of them here. Instead, a few examples from the content and process categories have been selected with the intent to depict how they are used to explain and predict behavior.

Content Theories

The content theories are based on factors that exist primarily within the individual. These often describe instincts, needs, drives, or attitudes within the individual that result in an individual behaving in some particular manner. The classic theory in this category was called the *need satisfaction model.*

Need Satisfaction Model

To motivate is not an easy task. Knowledge about how individuals pursue the satisfaction of needs helps nurses understand motivation. A special process is involved with motivation. First, a need is felt. For example, a felt need is something like needing to get a job or earn money. Next, there is some sort of activity or behavioral response to the felt need. Then the goal is either attained or blocked. If the goal desired to reduce the feeling of need is blocked, frustration results. At this point, another round of the process is initiated in an attempt to reduce the frustration. This process forms the core of the need satisfaction model (Schweiger, 1980) (Figure 9.1). For example, a nurse assesses that a client is in pain and determines that comfort measures are not sufficient to alleviate the pain or the client-felt need. The nurse, in a behavioral response, contacts the physician for an analgesic prescription. This results either in attaining the goal if successful or in frustration if unsuccessful. If unsuccessful, new behaviors are called for because frustration has become the new felt need.

In general, motivational theories are based on the relationship of attitudes, needs, and behaviors. Motivation can be either internal or external, called *intrinsic* or *extrinsic. Internal motivation* is that which arises from within an individual and is aimed at a sense of personal accomplishment. *External motivation* is motivation that arises from outside an individual, in which something or somebody

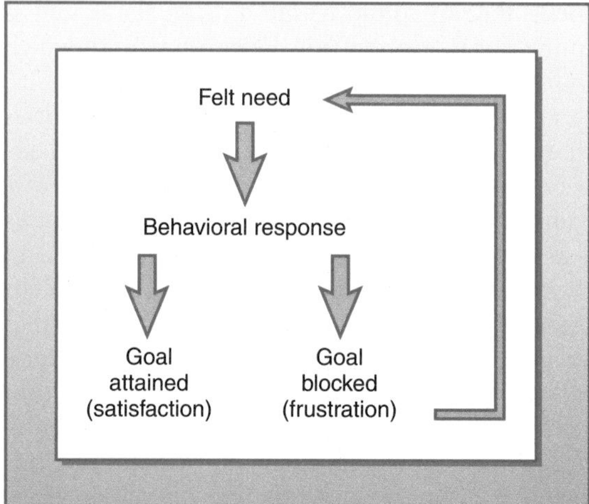

Figure 9.1
Need satisfaction model. (Data from Schweiger, J. [1980]. *The nurse as manager*. New York: John Wiley & Sons.)

becomes an incentive. External motivation is related to the application of rewards or punishments. For example, a grade given for performance on an examination is an external motivator. Weight loss, smoking cessation, and chemical dependency rehabilitation programs all deal with internal rather than external motivation and the challenge of finding the right combination to overcome strong urges and behavioral or lifestyle choices.

A person's attitudes and values create the internal versus external orientation. Some circumstances involve a combination of both internal and external motivators. For example, nurses may work at a rapid pace because they enjoy feeling a sense of achievement, an internal motivator, but also because they are given an external motivator in the form of a heavy assignment. Personal philosophy, values, beliefs, and assumptions are the foundations for motivation. To understand an individual's internal motivation, one must understand the person's beliefs, values, and assumptions (Figure 9.2).

The need satisfaction model provides insight into understanding human behavior. This model has been the basis for many theories of motivation, including Maslow's (1954) hierarchy of needs theory, Alderfer's (1969) ERG theory, Herzberg's (Herzberg et al., 1959) motivation-hygiene theory, and McClelland's (1961, 1976) need for achievement theory. Some theorists have focused on specific human drives deemed to be important. Some examples are the achievement motive, the affiliation motive, the need for equity, the need for activity and exploration, the need for competence, and the self-actualization motive (Lawler, 1973).

Going beyond a description of needs, one group of motivation theories uses a cognitive premise as its base. The cognitive theories assume that individuals reason, think, and consider the consequences of their behavior. Thus the focus is on the thought and evaluative processes individuals use in participating and performing in the workplace. These theories examine the attractiveness of outcomes to individuals and are categorized as *expectancy theories*. Expectancy, equity, and goal-setting theories are included, although goal setting has been viewed primarily as a technique rather than a theory. Vroom's (1964) expectancy theory is a major example of the cognitive theories (Lawler, 1973; Steers & Porter, 1987). As applied to working in organizations, theories of motivation are discussed in connection with job satisfaction. Herzberg's theory is an example. Job satisfaction is an internal subjective state related to an affective reaction to motivated job behavior. It is related to organizational outcomes

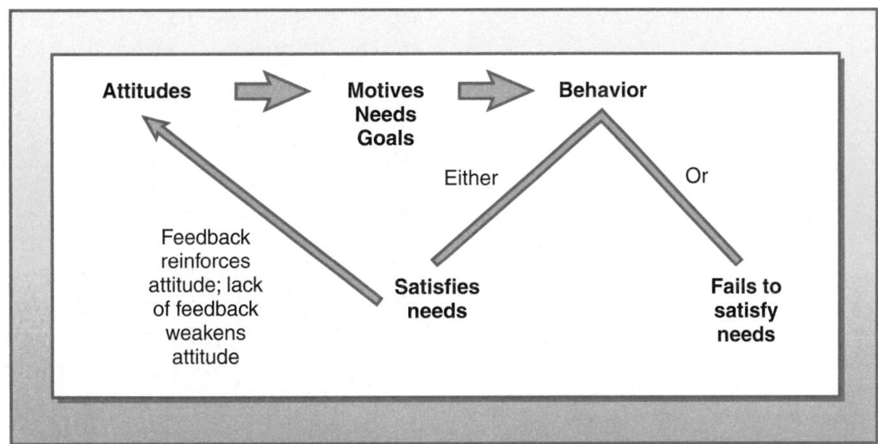

Figure 9.2

Relationship of attitudes, motives, and behavior. (Data from Schweiger, J. [1980]. *The nurse as manager*. New York: John Wiley & Sons; and Steers, R., & Porter, L. [1987]. *Motivation and work behavior* [4th ed.]. New York: McGraw-Hill.)

such as absenteeism and turnover, which are costly to organizations and influence their effectiveness (Lawler, 1973; Price & Mueller, 1986). Motivation as applied to the work environment also is the focus of Hackman and Oldham's (1979) job characteristics theory. Finally, McGregor's (1960) Theory X and Theory Y are related to motivation. Not truly a theory of human motivation, McGregor's Theory X and Theory Y describes managerial attitudes toward employees and is more specific to assumptions about what motivates people to work. Three examples of content theories that will be described in more detail here are Maslow's, Herzberg's, and McClelland's theories.

Maslow's Hierarchy of Needs Theory

Maslow (1954) arrayed human needs along a hierarchy from most basic to most sophisticated. This progression can be thought of as stair steps or as a pyramid (Figure 9.3). At the bottom, or base, are the most basic needs, the *physiological* drives for food, sleep, clothing, and shelter. These needs are usually associated with the survival needs for which humans seek to acquire money. The majority of an individual's activity will be at this level until the needs are fulfilled sufficiently to sustain the body. When physiological needs are fulfilled, other levels of needs emerge and dominate.

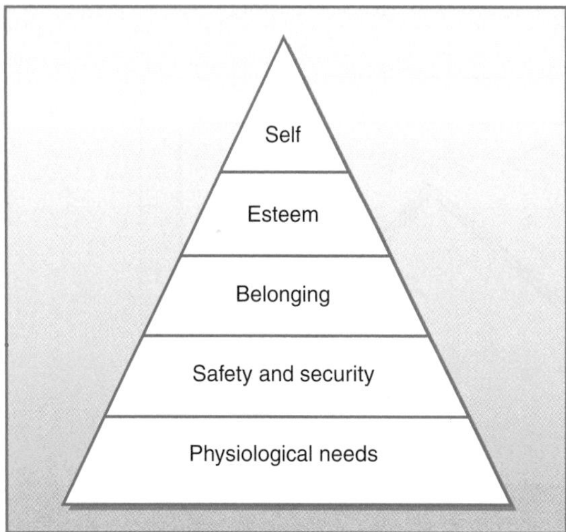

Figure 9.3
Maslow's hierarchy of human needs. (Data from Maslow, A. [1954]. *Motivation and personality*. New York: Harper & Row.)

The second level in the Maslow's hierarchy is *safety and security* needs. These are needs to be free of the fear of physical harm and deprivation of basic physiological needs. Employee benefit plans are aimed at security needs. The third level is *belonging* needs that relate to the drive for affiliation and love. These are social needs. In nursing, work group social support and cohesion meet some belonging needs. The next level is *esteem and ego* needs. These are needs to achieve independence, respect, and recognition from others. Satisfaction of esteem needs results in prestige, self-confidence, power, and a feeling of usefulness. Recognition is an important esteem motivator in nursing. The highest level of the hierarchy of needs, at the apex, is *self-actualization* needs. These relate to the need to maximize one's potential and achieve a sense of personal fulfillment, competence, and accomplishment. This need is individual and internal. In Maslow's theoretical framework, needs at the lower levels must be fulfilled before those at a higher level can emerge and have energy devoted to them (Maslow, 1954). Maslow's theory applies to people in general and is not specific to work or organizational behavior.

Alderfer (1969) modified Maslow's (1954) work by collapsing the five hierarchical levels into three sets of needs: existence needs, relatedness needs, and growth needs. According to Alderfer's model, existence needs are those human needs specific to sustaining life. Maslow's physiological and safety/security needs would be included in existence needs. Relatedness needs are needs for meaningful interpersonal relationships, similar to Maslow's belonging needs. Growth needs are the needs for self-esteem and self-actualization, similar to Maslow's self-actualization needs. Alderfer's (1969) model has been called the *ERG theory*, the acronym standing for existence, relatedness, and growth needs. The ERG theory added the dimension of a frustration-regression process that occurs when higher-level needs are continually frustrated.

Maslow's theory is familiar to nurses because it is often used to explain patient or client behavior.

However, it is one of the early theories that, over time, has diminished in value. Although Maslow's theory is quoted extensively, it has not held up well when research has been conducted to test it. The five-step hierarchy has never been confirmed through research, although studies have provided some support for a two-step hierarchy with lower-level needs that deal with material and security needs and higher-level needs that deal with an emphasis on achievement and challenge. The theory remains attractive, in spite of its lack of empirical verification. The idea that individuals have growth needs and motives and that some needs are more important than others continues to hold intuitive appeal. Although Maslow's theory is not used in management sciences today, as one of the early motivation theories, it has had a significant influence on the development of many other content theories (Rainey, 2001).

Herzberg's Motivation-Hygiene Theory

Herzberg (Herzberg et al., 1959) applied Maslow's general theory of motivation specifically to work motivation. Herzberg's motivation-hygiene, or two-factor, theory proposed that there are two different categories of needs, which are independent and affect behavior in different ways: hygienes and motivators (Figure 9.4). The hygiene or maintenance factors are security, status, money, working conditions, interpersonal relations, supervision, and policies and administration. The hygienes are related to the environment and conditions of the job. They are not growth-producing motivators for employees; they only prevent lost productivity due to job dissatisfaction. On the other hand, the motivators seem to be effective in motivating toward superior performance and positively affecting job satisfaction. They are related to the job itself. The motivators are growth and development, advancement, increased responsibility for work, challenging work, recognition, and achievement.

In Herzberg's theory, work motivation is seen as composed of job satisfaction and dissatisfaction. Satisfaction is not a continuum, with satisfaction on one end and dissatisfaction on the other. Rather, satisfaction and dissatisfaction were seen as two independent continuums: (1) no satisfaction to high satisfaction and (2) no dissatisfaction to high dissatisfaction. The hygiene factors are essentially equivalent to Maslow's lower-level factors, whereas the motivators are higher-level factors (Figure 9.5). In other words, there must be enough of the hygiene factors so that the employee is not dissatisfied. Enough of the motivators need to be present to be personally rewarding.

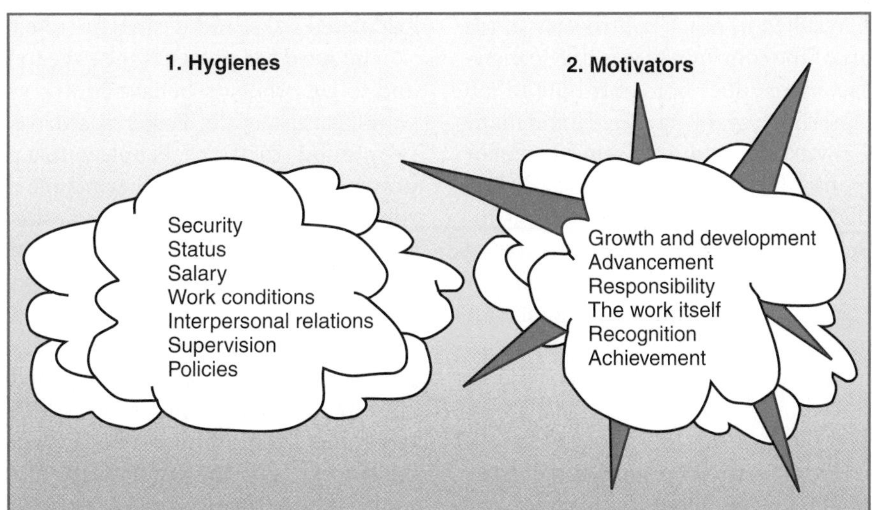

Figure 9.4
Herzberg's factors. (Data from Herzberg, F., Mausner, B., & Snyderman, B. [1959]. *The motivation to work*. New York: John Wiley & Sons.)

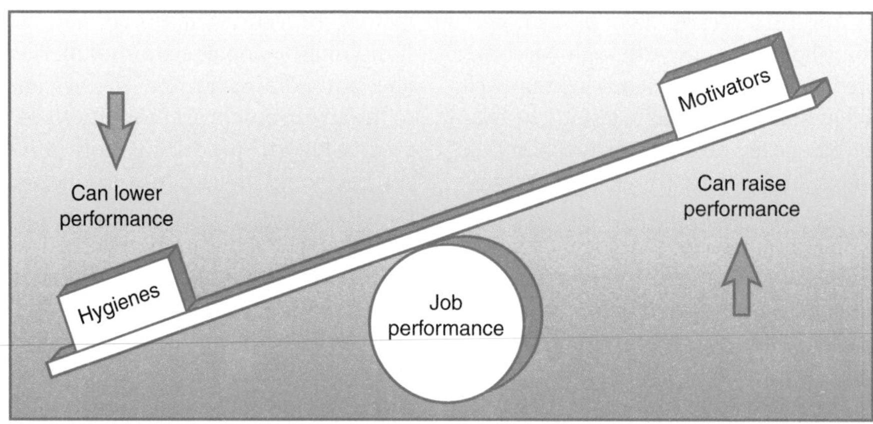

Figure 9.5
Herzberg's two-factor theory. (Data from Herzberg, F., Mausner, B., & Snyderman, B. [1959]. *The motivation to work*. New York: John Wiley & Sons.)

Herzberg's two-factor theory was one of the first motivation theories to be developed that focused specifically on work motivation and the identification of ways that jobs might be enriched to address motivational needs that employees bring to the workplace. Herzberg's earliest work appeared in 1959 and was refined extensively through the 1970s. The theory has been referred to as a "job enrichment" theory because it sparked a number of strategies to enrich jobs as a means to address the motivator factors and, it is hoped, job satisfaction (Herzberg, 2003; Miner, 2002).

This theory resulted in much controversy in the workplace. Part of the controversy was due to viewing pay as a factor that does not contribute to job satisfaction. Most surveys rank pay highly, and many employees see pay as an indicator of achievement or increased responsibility. Thus some critics do not see conceptual clarity between intrinsic and extrinsic rewards. Regardless, the theory has contributed to an increased understanding of the importance of restructuring work so that it is interesting and stimulating and provides opportunities to satisfy motivation for growth and fulfillment (Rainey, 2001).

McClelland's Theory

McClelland (1961, 1976) identified three basic needs that people possess in varying degrees: the need for achievement, the need for power, and the need for affiliation. Each person tends to have one predominant need. The **need for achievement** is the strong desire to overcome challenges, to excel, to advance or succeed, and to grow. The need for achievement can be identified and assessed. Individuals with a high need for achievement set moderately difficult but achievable goals and like to take personal responsibility for finding solutions to problems. Included is a need for competence, or a strong desire to make a contribution or to produce some visible outcome and to do quality work. Those who exhibit high need for achievement are eager for responsibility, take calculated risks, and desire concrete feedback.

The **need for power** is the urge to be in control and to get others to behave contrary to what they would naturally do. Power is a drive to influence people and situations. People with a pure need for power need to control other people and the environment around them. They desire to make an impact, be influential, be in charge, and gain personal influence and prestige more than they desire productivity.

The **need for affiliation** is the desire to work in a pleasant environment and the need for friendly, close relationships. Affiliation is a drive to relate to people. People who have a high need for affiliation seek out meaningful friendships, want to be respected and liked, avoid decisions that oppose the group, and are more interested in high morale than productivity.

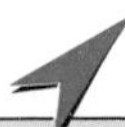

LEADING & MANAGING DEFINED

Need for Achievement

The strong desire to overcome challenges, to excel, to advance or succeed, and to grow

Need for Power

The need to be in control and to get others to behave contrary to what they would naturally do

Need for Affiliation

The desire to work in a pleasant environment and the desire for friendly, close relationships

McClelland and Boyatzis (1982) studied individuals with long tenure in management positions and found a "leadership motive pattern" that enabled effectiveness at higher levels of an organization. The features of a leadership motive pattern are moderately high levels of the need for power and low needs for affiliation, with high levels of self-control. Absent is the need for achievement motive, which was associated with managerial success at lower management levels in nontechnical areas (Henderson, 1993). Thus theories of needs motivation have been related to leadership and management by investigating which characteristics or combinations of characteristics can be used to predict job "fit" or success.

Henderson (1993) found that nurse managers' and nurse executives' profiles did not fit the profile of successful managers described by McClelland and Boyatzis (1982). Specifically, about one third of respondents showed no power motive preference. There may be a variety of explanations for this, such as differences in industry versus service sector, female role socialization, the position of nurse executives in the hierarchy, individual characteristics of age or education, or the type, complexity, or culture of the setting. It is possible that profiles change over time. Measurement tools may not be precise or setting-specific enough to detect relationships. Thus theories and measures need to be evaluated as data are gathered for decision making and prediction.

McClelland's (1961, 1976) framework can be used for self-assessment and to assess and influence others. Self-assessment is an analysis of which of these types most represents an individual. Once self-assessment has been completed, others in the environment can be evaluated for their highest need motivation. Communication is enhanced and conflicts are diminished as effective strategies are employed to meet individuals' needs. People are motivated by different needs, and understanding the basic types helps nurses learn to work with diverse personalities in actual work situations. The idea is to match the individual's need structure to the assignment in the organization. To plant individuals in a place where they will grow is a key to productivity and success.

Process Theories

Process theories of motivation concentrate on behavioral and psychological processes in motivation as opposed to needs and drives that may influence motivation. Three classic process theories are highlighted in this chapter: (1) operant conditioning, (2) expectancy theory, and (3) goal-setting theory.

Operant Conditioning

A classic approach to motivation that focuses primarily on processes in the external environment is operant conditioning. Nurses are familiar with behavior modification, which also derives directly from operant conditioning theory. In this theory, behavior and motivation are shaped primarily as the result of responses to stimuli in the environment. People respond to stimuli that they view as rewarding, and they avoid stimuli that they view as undesirable or punishing. Generally, this theoretical perspective does not focus to any degree on the internal processes operating within the individual and emphasizes the process of shaping behavior through environmental stimuli such as rewards. In the business literature, a series of books on the "one minute manager," based on operant conditioning, have been published (e.g., Blanchard et al., 1999).

Expectancy Theory

Expectancy theory is built on the basic premise that individuals seek to do what they think will produce desirable results and minimize undesired results. This theory poses that individuals in the work setting will engage in behaviors that they expect will lead to valued outcomes. Different work-related activities are viewed as having positive or negative valences (similar to the electron valences in chemistry). Outcomes of behavior are viewed as having positive or negative assessments, and an employee will be motivated to perform those behaviors with the highest valences, or the highest probability of leading to very good results (Pinder, 1998).

Lewin (1935) described behavior as a function of characteristics in both the person and the environment. Thus motivation can be influenced by the nature of the individual and by the policies and practices of the organization. Lewin (1935) introduced the concept of valence, defined as the attractiveness of an outcome. Later theories introduced the concept of expectancy, defined as the likelihood that an action will lead to a certain outcome. The general expectancy theory framework views behavior as determined by the multiplication of valence with expectancy.

Vroom's (1964) VIE theory is the most well-known expectancy theory and is the one applied to work settings (VIE stands for valence-instrumentality-expectancy). Instrumentality is a belief about the probability that behavior will lead to other second-level outcomes. All three VIE variables are beliefs held by individuals related to what they expect will happen. Vroom (1964) postulated that behavior results from conscious choices among alternatives. The choice behaviors are related to perception and the formation of attitudes and beliefs. Humans naturally choose to maximize pleasure and minimize pain. The combinations of VIE, which Vroom represented symbolically by mathematical equations, interact to create a motivational force for action. In the context of work, individuals will pursue the level of performance that they believe will maximize their overall best interest (Steers & Porter, 1987).

Vroom's (1964) VIE theory was refined by Porter and Lawler (1968), who found that employee effort was determined jointly by two factors: (1) the individual's assessment of the value of certain outcomes and (2) the degree to which there is a belief that the person's effort will lead to the attainment of valued rewards. Both beliefs must be in place for further effort to be elicited. However, there is a distinction between actions and outcomes effort may not result in job performance. Furthermore, performance and satisfaction may or may not be related, depending on a variety of factors (Lawler, 1973; Steers & Porter, 1987).

Nurses attempting to use VIE theory try to structure rewards on an individualized basis. However, it is difficult to assess the actual needs of employees, so their values and attitudes are assessed as a proxy for actual needs. Managers work to assign personnel to jobs that they are capable of performing. For example, nurses would operationalize this theory when delegating to unlicensed assistive personnel by structuring assignments to meet needs and preferences. However, nurses' control over the work environment may be constrained in organizations by policies and procedures or union contracts.

Expectancy theory is a prominent and well-regarded theory of work motivation, even though it has not held up well in research. This is probably because of the complexities of trying to identify and measure, in terms of valences, what is important to the individual. The theory also proposes that individuals compute complex equations in their mind before they act, which is also difficult to measure (Rainey, 2001). Nonetheless, expectancy theory is viewed as an important conceptual framework that has made valuable contributions and insights regarding motivation in the workplace. The fact that perceptions about reward expectancies exist is an important contribution.

Goal-Setting Theory

Goal-setting theory is currently the most prominent motivation theory. Its basic premise is simple: goals serve as targets for human behavior. In turn, difficult, specific goals lead to higher performance than vague or nonexistent goals. Difficult goals direct attention and effort toward the task, serve to mobilize action, and motivate the individual to search for strategies that will lead to effective performance. A component of this theory is self-efficacy, a concept that is quite familiar to nurses and used to describe health behaviors in patients. Self-efficacy relates to a person's confidence and sense of capability in accomplishing goals. Self-efficacy is enhanced by the goals that are set before an individual. This approach to motivation relies heavily on cognitive processes. Because behavior is intentional, it arises from the deliberate actions and conscious choices to accomplish specific goals. In essence, people act in ways that are consistent with their intentions and goals (Pinder, 1998).

This theory fits nicely into many work settings in which goals are used to help individuals define their performance and grow over time. Many management principles are based on collaborative goal-setting between employee and manager as a way to guide work behavior and to set a framework for evaluation of performance (Rainey, 2001). The use of periodic feedback is an important tool to help individuals attain their desired goals and to encourage or motivate them to continue to strive to accomplish targeted goals.

JOB CHARACTERISTICS MODEL

The job characteristics model describes how the characteristics of a job and individual differences among workers interact to affect motivation, job satisfaction, and productivity at work (Hackman & Oldham, 1979). The model is often used as a framework to analyze the design of jobs and how this affects motivation and job satisfaction in workers. Frequently, the redesign of work in health care organizations is based in the diagnostic methods that are part of the job characteristics model (Redman & Ketefian, 1995).

The job characteristics model depicts core dimensions of any job (skill variety, task identity, task significance, autonomy, and feedback), psychological state of the worker (the meaningfulness of work to the employee, the degree of responsibility an employee has for the outcomes of his or her work), and personal or work outcomes (level of performance, job satisfaction). These factors interact in ways that influence both how employees feel about their work and their motivation to perform at certain levels of productivity (Hackman & Oldham, 1979). When using this approach to redesign work, attempts are made to increase the motivation potential of a job. This might be done, for example, by increasing the employee's autonomy or the esteem of his or her work. The job characteristics model is viewed as an important framework for enriching jobs in a way that could affect employee motivation, satisfaction, and productivity.

RELATED THEORIES OF WORK MOTIVATION

Organizations that employ nurses seek to manage scarce human resources in a way that best coordinates and motivates nurses as employees. However, the best way to do this is not immediately obvious. Traditional bureaucratic organizations use close supervision and tight control of employees. Human relations or human resources models use limited participation or decentralization to enhance employee morale and cooperation. Because motivation is a complex yet critical element, it has been extensively investigated. Two related theories of work motivation are McGregor's Theory X and Theory Y and the famous Hawthorne studies.

McGregor's Theory X and Theory Y

A manager's philosophy about people, attitudes, and assumptions plays a role in his or her choice of motivational strategies. The assumptions about the nature of people that Theory X managers bring to the workplace are based on a belief that people who work for an employer are lazy. These managers assume that employees dislike responsibility, prefer to be directed, resist change, and want safety. At the same time, however, Theory X managers assume that employees are rational in that they can be motivated. The accompanying belief is that people are motivated by money and the threat of punishment. Thus if the workers are lazy, management must be active. Managers need to impose structure and control and closely supervise employees, since external control is necessary to deal with unreliable, irresponsible, and immature workers. This view of human nature and motivation is called *Theory X* (McGregor, 1960).

Challenging the conventional Theory X view of the day, McGregor (1960) proposed Theory Y (Box 9.2). In a democratic society, the Theory X view of human nature and the managerial practices based on it may not be correct and appropriate. Thus management approaches based on Theory X may fail to motivate individuals toward organizational goals. Theory Y assumes that people are not lazy and unreliable by nature but, rather, that people can be self-directed and creative if they are properly motivated.

Box 9.2

Managerial Assumptions in McGregor's (1960) Theory X and Theory Y

Theory X

People:

- Dislike work
- Need control and force to make them work
- Like to be directed
- Lack ambition

Theory Y

People:

- Like to work
- Can be self-disciplined for objectives to which they are committed
- Will accept responsibility

Theory Y acknowledges that the behavior of people is complex. Under certain conditions people will accept responsibility; they are not necessarily passive; and creativity exists in all levels of the organization. Theory Y managers truly believe that motivation can be unlocked by creating and fostering an environment that is motivating. They view this as their job as managers. These managers think people do like to work, can be self-directed, and will accept responsibility given an environment in which to grow, accomplish, and feel a sense of self-esteem and autonomy. It is the manager's job to create a motivating environment within the system of work. McGregor's (1960) Theory X and Theory Y is not so much a motivation theory as it is a theory about managers' beliefs, which then translates into the ways they choose to motivate their employees.

Hawthorne Studies

Industrial efficiency experts have been interested in determining what mix of physical conditions, work hours, and work methods is ideal to stimulate maximum productive output by workers. Unlocking the secrets of the motivation to work and the relationship between motivation and productivity has been a universal management concern.

In 1924, a famous experiment that came to be known as the *Hawthorne studies* was conducted at the Hawthorne plant of Western Electric, outside Chicago. A team of researchers went into the plant to find out what motivated people. The purpose of the study was to test the effect of working conditions, including such diverse variables as lighting and pay, on productivity.

The researchers had reliable data on the production line, and they knew exactly how long it took a worker to wire a telephone. The regular production line was used as a control. For the experiments, the researchers pulled five workers off the assembly line and put them in a room, creating a mock production line so that the researchers could control and manipulate variables. The first variable was lighting. When more lights were added, production went up. Other variables included scheduled rest periods, company lunches, and shorter work weeks. After introduction of each variable, production went up. To test the strength of association of working conditions and productivity, all the innovations were suddenly withdrawn. Surprisingly, production went up to a new all-time high. All the researchers were able to conclude was that changes in physical working conditions alone had nothing to do with productivity. It must have been something else: specifically, productivity must be tied to the human aspects, such as the attention lavished on the workers. At this point, the research was refocused and employee interviews were conducted to explore the human relations aspects.

The Hawthorne studies resulted in a new awareness about the need to study and understand human interpersonal relationships at work. The most significant factor affecting organizational productivity was job-related interpersonal relationships, not just pay or working conditions. When informal groups identified with management and the workers felt competent, productivity increased. Furthermore, the findings pointed to involving workers in the planning, organizing, and controlling of their own work as a way to secure workers' positive cooperation. Out of the Hawthorne studies came the phrases "the Hawthorne effect," to refer to attention paid to employees, and "the informal organization," to denote the web of interpersonal relationships beyond management control. Insights gained from the Hawthorne experiments began the human relations era of management theory with its emphasis on human motivation at work.

Clearly, the behavior of people is complex. Therefore motivation is not a simplistic matter.

Practical Tips

Tip #1: Know Yourself

Whether you are thinking of yourself as a student, a professional nurse, an employee, or a potential leader, knowing what motivates you in terms of goals, rewards, values, or trigger factors in the environment is essential. These are related to how you approach your responsibilities and your work and also how colleagues will approach you. Reflecting about yourself periodically is important in terms of how your motives and behaviors are interacting in your life in general and at work in particular.

Tip # 2: Know Where You Are Going

Having a clear sense of where you are going relates very closely to your motives and goals. Rather than drifting along, you can realign your behavior and motives in a way that will chart the course for important next steps in your career. It is actually your personal motives and goals that are a major determinant of what you can accomplish. Although rewards and environment are important, they are just part of the equation. Be your own "life coach," and develop a motivating plan for action.

Tip #3: Be Flexible and Open to Change

It is clear that rapidly changing environments are here to stay, whether we are looking at work environments or broader society. Recognize what you can control and influence and how that affects your motivations and goals. By being unwilling to consider how things might be done differently, you run the risk of seeing everything from a pessimist's perspective, which in turn will affect your motivation, attitude, and behavior. If you find yourself in an overwhelmingly negative environment that always seems to be on a downward spiral, find a new environment that is more aligned with your personal values and motives. You control these decisions. You alone have the power to change yourself and choose how you respond in any given situation.

The motivation of human beings is not reducible to a formula as simple as "people are motivated by money." The differences in motivation stem from the differences in people. However, in creating circumstances in which people are more likely to become self-motivated, managers can consider the following list of needs that employees expect of their employers (McConnell, 1998):

- Capable, respected leadership
- Decent and safe surroundings
- Acceptance as a member of a group
- Recognition and other feedback
- Fair treatment
- A reasonable sense of job security
- Knowledge of the results of individual effort
- Knowledge of the organization's policies, rules, and regulations
- Recognition for special effort
- Respect for individual beliefs
- Assurance that others are doing their fair share of the work
- Fair monetary compensation

Although nurses can identify and prioritize motivating aspects, no simple protocol automatically motivates nurses. This is because motivation is internal to the individual and driven by unique combinations of complex factors.

RESEARCH FINDINGS ON MOTIVATION IN NURSING

A number of examples of research addressing work motivation in nursing practice can be found in the literature. Typically, the focus of work motivation research looks at how motivation of employees is associated with various dependent variables such as job satisfaction, desire to continue in one's job, or commitment to the organization. Often the focus is on conditions of the work environment that may have a positive or negative impact on nurses in terms of how they feel about their work, their positions, and the organization in which they are employed. A few studies are highlighted here to illustrate the diversity of studies and the different motivation theories that frame the investigations.

Rantz and colleagues (1996) conducted a series of interviews with nurses in different types of roles to find out what types of factors in their jobs were most closely related to their motivation. Interpersonal relations with colleagues at work ranked as the most important factor. Recognition at work, the amount of responsibility, and the nature of the work itself were also identified as critical motivating factors. These factors were deemed as areas that could be addressed in the work setting to enhance the motivation and job satisfaction of nurses (Rantz et al., 1996). This study used Herzberg's two-factor theory as its framework.

Home health care nurses were studied to examine the impact of increasing workloads on the motivation of the nurses. These increased workloads had created a variety of additional demands and stress for the public health nurses. These changes had a direct effect on the motivation of the nurses: motivation decreased when the nurses felt that responsibilities and the workload were overwhelming. In this study, information about work goals was a strong predictor of positive work motivation (Laamanen et al., 1999). These findings fit nicely with goal-setting theory.

Tzeng (2002) studied staff nurses in acute care hospitals to identify what factors would predict the nurses' intent to stay in their positions at the hospital. The most significant predictor was the work motivation of the nurses and how they thought their jobs provided opportunities for them to meet their motivational needs. The quality of the work environment moderated their levels of work motivation. Those nurses who felt rewarded had positions in which they were involved in decision making and felt valued by the hospital; they also had increased levels of motivation and were less likely to leave their position. This study contains elements of Herzberg's two-factor theory, expectancy theory, and goal-setting theory.

A similar study found that various aspects of the work environment have a greater impact than personality variables on how individuals feel about their work (Laschinger et al., 2001). In general, work experiences are a strong predictor of affective feelings about work and, based on various theories of motivation, can have an impact on employee motivation and job performance.

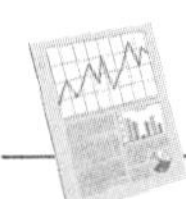

Research Note

Source: Laschinger, H.K., Finegan, J., & Shamian, J. (2001). The impact of workplace empowerment, organizational trust on staff nurses' work satisfaction and organizational commitment. *Health Care Management Review, 26*(3), 7-23.

Purpose

The purpose of this study was to assess the impact of current hospital restructuring and job reengineering on nurses who are directly affected by these initiatives. Specifically, the investigation tested a model that links staff nurses' workplace empowerment, organizational trust, job satisfaction, and commitment to the organization. All of these factors are related directly or indirectly to work motivation in nurses. Five research instruments were distributed to 600 staff nurses in urban tertiary care hospitals in Ontario, Canada. A response rate of 69% (412 nurses) was obtained.

Discussion

The analyses indicated that nurses perceived their work settings to be only moderately empowering and they did not perceive their jobs to offer a high degree of formal power over decision making and clinical judgment. They reported higher confidence and trust in their peers than in their managers. In addition, they were not very satisfied with their jobs. The testing of the proposed model revealed that the degree of workplace empowerment, or ability to make decisions that affect their work, perceived by the nurses was strongly related to their trust of management, job satisfaction, and a willingness to exert effort in the workplace as well as continue to work at the same organization. The results suggest that fostering work environments that increase nurses' perceptions of empowerment will have positive effects on the organizational members, as well as increase organizational effectiveness.

Application to Practice

The factors addressed in this study continue to demonstrate the important relationship between creating motivating work environments and how nurses feel about their jobs. The creation of work environments that encourage professional nursing practice by giving nurses control over their decision making will improve job satisfaction and the motivational attitudes that affect job performance, ultimately leading to improved quality of patient care. The implication for managers is to focus less on control and more on facilitation of nurses' work. Both nurses and managers must be willing to work together to create work environments that foster motivation, work satisfaction, and commitment to organizational goals to provide high-quality nursing care.

The issue of quality of the work environment and its relationship to how nurses feel about their jobs and the organizations they work for is a consistent finding in the research literature. This is a major theme in the Magnet™ hospital program, which is based on the idea that hospitals that create positive working environments supporting professional nursing practice will have more committed employees, have a better employee retention rate, and provide better patient care (McClure & Hinshaw, 2002). These research findings relate to the various motivation theories on how work and the work environment interact with motivational needs and desires of the employee. The focus for results is on improved work performance and better quality work.

LEADERSHIP AND MANAGEMENT IMPLICATIONS

Motivation is a key concept of leadership and management in nursing. The art of leading and managing groups of professionals requires creative, interesting, and continuous ways to make people feel good

PART III

about what they are doing. In a service industry with professional employees, human relations variables are important for productivity, since the work depends on the knowledge, skill, and work effort of human beings. Motivation is important for understanding why people work and why some people are highly productive and others are not, as well as for comprehending complex relationships related to teamwork and productivity in organizations. Organizations have a vital interest in productivity. The trend in work life is to emphasize working harder and being more effective. This requires some internal or external force to move human beings to continuous high levels of productivity. Motivation, along with the structures set up in organizations to motivate human beings, has an effect on outcomes such as performance, turnover, and absenteeism.

Recent work has been done on personal characteristics and how they relate to motivation (Apter, 2007). For example, optimism, or the expectation that good things will happen, is seen as one characteristic related to motivation. A growing literature supports the view that expectations for the future have an important impact on individual motivation and how one responds to adversity or challenging situations (Carver & Scheier, 2002). Another example can be found in work on empathy and altruism, both important aspects of the work in nursing. Evidence indicates that individuals who feel empathy toward people in need also feel an altruistic motivation to help (Batson et al., 2002). This is likely closely linked to leadership behavior in which the good of the group or team is advanced beyond the personal goals of the leader (Collins, 2001).

Nursing leaders are in a critical position in terms of creating environments that recognize and use the unique talents of all individuals in the work team. The work environment is a very important component in empowering and motivating employees, and work environments in which each employee can achieve personal satisfaction and professional fulfillment can be designed (Moore & Hutchison, 2007). Leadership behavior and individual motivation are linked in essential ways.

Clearly, no single theory or model fits all situations or predicts with accuracy what motivates individuals or how they will behave in a given situation. A variety of theories exist, each one providing some insight. Over time, the earlier theories have influenced and helped refine the theories developed at later points in time. Human motives are multiply determined, and the complexity of factors that motivate human beings remains to be

LEADERSHIP & MANAGEMENT **BEHAVIORS**

Leadership Behaviors

- Enables others through high expectations
- Recognizes contributions
- Celebrates accomplishments
- Creates social support networks
- Fosters collaboration
- Communicates an inspiring vision
- Motivates followers
- Sets an example of high motivation
- Provides opportunities for growth and development

Management Behaviors

- Plans motivating rewards
- Links rewards to performance
- Directs others to achieve organizational goals
- Evaluates effectiveness of motivation strategies
- Motivates subordinates
- Provides opportunities for subordinates to achieve
- Provides valued rewards

Overlap Areas

- Motivates others
- Provides opportunities for need satisfaction

worked out (Petri, 1996). Given the complexities of human behavior and the rapid pace of change in contemporary work environments, it is unlikely that a definitive theory on motivation will be developed in the near future. That notwithstanding, it is possible to derive some general principles from the various motivation theories that exist to serve as guides for both work behavior and nursing practice. Generalizations from motivation theory follow:

- *The complexities of human behavior will likely never be explained by one simple theory.* However, motivation theories help nurses identify that individuals, in general, will seek outcomes that are positive for them and try to avoid outcomes that are negative. Knowing this, motivation theory suggests how important it is for nurses to understand what it is that they value as positive and negative outcomes for themselves (Amabile, 1997). The same applies to work with patients. Motivation theory is likely to provide important insights in terms of how and why nurses behave as they do. Although it may not explain the *why*, it likely will predict the *what*. Nurse leaders and managers can use this theory to create positively motivating work environments.
- *Nurses are aware of individual differences as they work with patients.* This same variation in behavior is evident in motivation and work behavior as well. Although it seems simplistic, more often than not, nurses expect all employees to work in the same way or perform at the same level. However, individuals vary on almost every dimension because of fundamental factors such as values, needs, personality, and culture. Individuals have unique genetic and personal backgrounds that shape who they are—including wants, reactions, and motives (Mitchell & Daniels, 2003). Given this variation, it is very important that time be spent getting to know oneself, colleagues, and patients and reflecting on how the unique components of every individual can come together to influence his or her motives and behavior. Recognizing the variation and uniqueness in those with whom they work will help nurses and leaders and managers understand their motivations and why they behave as they do.
- *Goals are important, regardless of the task at hand.* Whether focusing on team members or patients, it is always important to have established goals that are understood by all in order to see successful behavior (Nicholson, 2003). There is no guarantee that people will perform accordingly because of the phenomenon of individual variation. However, it is quite likely that if shared goals do not exist, not everyone will behave in a predictable manner. Goals are a major motivating factor, and specific goals are generally preferred to ambiguity. Setting goals and contracts with individual employees is a powerful way to motivate individuals (Rousseau, 2004). Once goals have been set, preferably in collaboration with those who will be affected by them, there is a higher probability that individuals will be motivated to perform accordingly.
- *Incentives and rewards are always important.* Regardless of the motivation theory that seems to work best for a given situation, nurse leaders and managers need to remember the importance of giving feedback to individuals so that they receive cues on how they are doing and what else they might need to do. Nurses value recognition for doing a task well, and rewards work well in recognition programs (Kane & Montgomery, 1998). Rewards do not have to be monetary; being recognized and praised is often as important as money (Morse, 2003). This is especially important in the current health care environment, which is continually challenged by diminishing resources.
- *Equity is important.* Nurses are social beings, and all people tend to compare themselves with those around them. This is equally true in the workplace. If variations in performance are noted yet rewards and recognition are given to all, even individuals who

may be performing at a substandard level, nurses will likely have a negative reaction. Nurses want to be treated fairly and want to see consistency from leaders and managers when they compare themselves with others. Motives can vary, but nurses anticipate that, as individuals, they will be treated fairly and equitably.

CURRENT ISSUES AND TRENDS

Although the work on theory development about motivation seemed to slow down by the 1990s, the need for further work in this area is growing (Ambrose & Kulik, 1999; Locke & Latham, 2004). In an assessment of the state of motivation theory development, Steers and colleagues (2004) pointed out that not all of the insights to be made about motivation have been accomplished. One reason is the dramatic changes that have occurred in the workplace over the past decade. Companies, including the health care industry, have downsized and restructured with regularity. The workforce is increasingly diverse, information technology has dramatically changed how much of a nurse's work is transacted, and the distribution of power and the role of teams keep evolving. All of these forces have an impact on the motivation of employees, regardless of the theory that seems to fit best in a given situation.

Another major challenge for motivation theory is the rapid diversification in society. Cultural differences can have a profound impact on motivation and job attitudes, although is it not always clear why or how culture influences motivational processes. Often differences are seen in behavior across national boundaries, but the underlying dynamics are not obvious. Nearly all motivational theories have been developed in the United States and, as a result, have integrated American cultural values extensively (Lachman, 1997). When these theories are applied in other countries or with workers of different cultures, they often do not work well to explain or predict motivation or behavior in the way we would expect. Cultural differences are important variables that influence both individual behavior and environmental characteristics. A growing body of evidence suggests that cultural differences influence work values, motivation, and job attitudes. The degree to which values, attitudes and behaviors are emphasized in various cultures, and how they are prioritized, varies considerably across cultures (Heine, 2007). This evidence suggests that existing motivation theories need to be reexamined and that new theories of motivation no doubt need to be developed (Hofstede, 1993; Sanchez-Runde & Steers, 2001). As society becomes increasingly diverse, this need will become more critical within health care delivery systems.

Summary

- Motivation is important in a service industry such as nursing.
- Motivation and human relations variables are important for productivity.
- Motivation is a state of mind in which a person views goals.
- Motivation is a process of activating human behavior.
- Motivation to work is the willingness to work.
- Motivation is a process of felt need, behavior, goal attainment/blockage, frustration, and cycle repetition.
- Motivation can be either internal or external.
- There are many theories of motivation.
- Maslow described a hierarchy of five levels of needs.
- Alderfer collapsed Maslow's theory into three levels.
- Herzberg applied Maslow's theory to work motivation.
- Herzberg identified hygiene and motivator factors related to satisfaction and dissatisfaction.
- McClelland identified three basic needs.
- Vroom's work represents cognitive motivational theories.
- McGregor differentiated managers' attitudes into Theory X and Theory Y.

- The Hawthorne studies highlighted the importance of human interaction factors in work motivation.
- Personal and economic rewards are powerful motivators in nursing.
- The core of what motivates nurses is the work itself.
- Motivation is complex.
- The manager's job is to create an environment that fosters motivated behavior.

CASE STUDY

John Smith is in his third year as a staff nurse in the surgical ICU at a large teaching hospital. The acuity level of the patients continues to increase as the number of staff nurses available in the ICU continues to decrease. The nursing shortage has affected the staffing ratios in the hospital and in Nurse Smith's unit. Increasingly, he is working mandatory overtime, has fewer days off, and is exhausted. Nurse Smith notices that the ICU is relying increasingly on external agency nurses. The agency nurses make more money, have better control over their schedules, and do not have to work mandatory overtime. He feels as though the hospital and nursing administration do not recognize the depth of the staffing problem and are doing little to address the working conditions. Morale on the unit continues to decline, staff nurses are quitting, and no new hires are found to take their place. Nurse Smith, too, is ready to quit and go to work for an agency where he will make more money and have better control over his schedule.

1. What are the key factors in the ICU work environment, and how are they affecting the staff nurses?
2. How might motivation theories be used to analyze the situation?
3. What next steps would you take if you were the nurse manager in this ICU?

PART III

CRITICAL THINKING EXERCISE

Staff nurses in a coronary step-down unit feel as though they are spending most of their time "performing tasks" and moving patients quickly to discharge. They have little opportunity to be involved in patient education activities. The nurses want to be involved in designing programs that will educate patients about risk factors and lifestyle changes that will promote better health in the future. However, the nurse manager and the physicians do not see this as important. The job satisfaction of the nurses continues to decline on the unit.

1. How would you characterize the work environment on this unit?
2. What insights might be obtained from motivation theories?
3. What kinds of change might be implemented that would improve job satisfaction and increase the motivation of the staff?

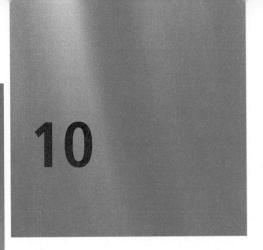

10 Team Building and Working with Effective Groups

Jo Manion Diane L. Huber

PART III

CHAPTER OBJECTIVES

- Highlight the emergence of teamwork as a knowledge work strategy
- Define a group, committee, team, and team building
- Outline the elements of group interactions
- Evaluate the reasons why people join groups
- Compare the advantages and disadvantages of using groups in organizations
- Identify the points on the continuum of group decision-making power
- Explain committee structure and function
- Differentiate among work groups, pseudoteams, and true teams
- Examine the dynamics of work groups and interdisciplinary teams
- Relate the leader's function in committee work and effective meetings
- Discuss constructive group member roles
- Identify the types of disruptive group members
- Exercise critical thinking to conceptualize and analyze possible solutions to a practice exercise

Nurse leaders in today's health care organizations must be skilled group facilitators with an exquisite ability to manage and lead the collective work of people. A significant percentage of work completed in organizations today is done through collective efforts, either in work groups, committees, or teams. Understanding the characteristics of each of these entities and basic principles for attaining successful outcomes increases the leader's effectiveness.

In the 1990s, many health care organizations attempted to convert their traditional hierarchical, bureaucratic structures to a team-based structure, with varying degrees of success. Many of these efforts were less than successful at the broad organizational level; yet the factors driving these changes still exist. "The appreciation of 'teamwork' intensified during these years and has developed as a major management concept" (Spitzer, 1998, p. 169). Teamwork is the new imperative for various reasons. Changing reimbursement, managed care organizations, increasing complexity, technology advances, rapid information dissemination at the worker level, and the shift to a knowledge worker–based service society are some of the social and economic forces operative in health care. These forces converged to create great change in health care delivery.

A major trend in the late 1990s, creating successful teams was thought to provide the strength and structure to deal with work complexities and changes (Brown, 1998). When the redesign, integration, merger, and partnering strategies settle, a decentralized and organic structure called the *knowledge organization* emerges with a growing emphasis on the role of teams. Although interdisciplinary teams have always played an important role in home care, hospice, and other community settings, hospitals and large health care organizations are placing more emphasis on teams as a part of their core structure.

"Knowledge has become so complex and specialized that virtually no single individual can be effective alone" (Sorrells-Jones & Weaver, 1999, p. 15). Because knowledge workers are specialists, the only way for them to be adequately productive is to work in groups or teams. Thus as the focus shifts to building knowledge work teams, a tandem concern is raised about how to help these teams be more effective and productive (Drucker, 1993; Sorrells-Jones & Weaver, 1999).

Developing effective teams of professionals from different disciplines has proven to be difficult. However, effective knowledge work teams can create a form of synergism in which the outcome is greater than the sum of individual efforts. Such synergism confers a competitive edge and boosts productivity under conditions of constrained resources. Developing a team-based structure is one way to enlist employee participation. Such teams capitalize on possibilities for improved productivity, better decisions, and process innovation. Thus the development of flexibility and responsiveness in well-designed teams holds the potential for positive solutions to health care delivery problems (Manion et al., 1996). Team building is a strategy for designing, implementing, developing, and nurturing work teams in organizations. These work teams are a specialized subset of the many types of groups that form or are formed in organizations. Group work is a major managerial strategy for accomplishing work through others.

Nurses do not work in isolation. In many nursing care delivery settings, nurses function in a work group environment or as a part of a team. Although often these teams are composed of all nursing personnel, nurses are increasingly becoming involved in interdisciplinary and cross-functional work teams. In some occupations, people work in relative isolation from others, but that is not the reality of the work of nursing. As health care restructures and becomes more complex, a greater value is being placed on high-performing and cohesive work groups. This is because complexity and cost-control factors in the health care environment have dictated the use of interdisciplinary and cross-functional work teams. Therefore nurses need to learn how to function constructively in group situations and continually build their skill set in team collaboration.

In nursing, group process theory relates to both how to be therapeutic with clients and how to work as an employee within an organization that is often large and complex. Nursing has at its core both a caring and a coordinative function. The nurse's coordinative role is at the hub of all client care information. For example, nurses collect, process, and integrate the initial assessment and laboratory data; handle the tracking of all therapeutic interventions for the client; are at the bedside in hospitals for surveillance of minute-by-minute changes; and are the major point of contact for clinical care delivery in many settings and sites. For example, if analgesics are given in a hospital, nurses track whether that intervention has worked, whether alternative pain strategies might be needed, and what psychological reaction the client might have. Clients and families note that a physician may visit a hospital unit once a day and may not recognize the fine distinctions of change in a client's condition. Nurses predominate in actual client care in home health, long-term care, hospice, and many other settings. The nurse is involved more intimately and more proximately than any of the other health care providers in managing the total health care of the client. Therefore understanding and developing skill in group process and group dynamics is essential within the context of leadership and management in nursing because of the group functioning and coordinative aspects of nursing practice.

Nurses have to work collaboratively, not only with other nurses and their nurse manager but also with people who do not share the same professional background, such as those in the administrative structure of the organization, other providers, the supply department, or the legal staff. These interpersonal and collaborative activities shape the essence of nursing practice. In addition, generational differences and issues of cultural diversity (see Chapter 13) contribute to how people frame issues differently and thus affect how people work in groups. Therefore as the environment of health care becomes more collaborative, nurses need strong group process and interaction skills to communicate clearly and collaborate effectively with a variety of health care workers.

DEFINITIONS

A **group** is defined as any collection of interconnected individuals working together for some purpose. Groups are important in organizations not only because of informal network dynamics but also because of the formation and functioning of formal committees and teams.

A **committee** is a relatively stable and formally composed group. Committees are a specific type of group in that they are stable, meet periodically, and have an identified purpose that is part of the organizational structure. There is a mechanism for maintaining and selecting members. Typically, committees have official status and sanction within an organization. For example, there is a policy and procedure committee or a quality assurance/improvement committee.

Team building is defined as the process of deliberately creating and unifying a group into a functioning work unit so that specific goals are accomplished (Farley & Stoner, 1989). A **team** was defined by Katzenbach and Smith (1993) as "a small number of people with complementary skills who are committed to a common purpose, performance goals, and approach for which they hold themselves mutually accountable" (p. 45). Manion and colleagues (1996) modified this definition slightly for health care by noting that the members need to be consistent. This was in reaction to confusion in terminology for many people in health care with a history of team nursing, in which whoever was present on a given shift was on the team. In this type of team nursing model, members could vary from shift to shift and from day to day, reducing the overall performance outcomes of the team. Team nursing was an assignment pattern and work allocation methodology rather than a true team model as seen in business and industry.

The distinction between a work group and a true team is crucial. The mistake made by many health care leaders is assuming that simply calling a group a *team* actually makes it a team. As Katzenbach and Smith (1993) noted repeatedly, the group becomes a true team only by doing its collective work. The team goes through a developmental process that takes time and the investment of energy to materialize. Many collective entities in today's organizations are called a *team* yet clearly function more as a work group than a true team.

LEADING & MANAGING DEFINED

Group

Any collection of interconnected individuals working together for some purpose.

Committee

A relatively stable and formally composed group; a subset of a group.

Team Building

The process of deliberately creating and unifying a group into a functioning work unit so that specific goals are accomplished.

Team

A small number of consistent people with complementary skills, a shared purpose that entails collective work, specific performance goals, common approaches to the work, and who hold themselves mutually accountable for outcomes.

Work Group

Collection of individuals who are led by a strong and focused leader.

Pseudoteam

A group of people who think they are a team but are not; characterized by confusion over purpose or a highly politicized purpose, dysfunctional and unhealthy interpersonal relationships and communication patterns, lack of clarity about goals, and no evaluation criteria.

A **work group** is a collection of individuals who are led by a strong, clearly focused leader. They come together to share information and ideas, and they may even mutually make some decisions. However, the members of the work group have individual work products for which they are responsible and these consume their major focus and effort. For example, in a patient care unit, the unit secretary has certain responsibilities as does the charge nurse, the patient care nurse, and the manager. The boundaries remain fairly clearly separated when the collective entity is a work group. Each person may feel individual accountability, but there is little to no collective accountability.

This is in contrast with a true team, which is a collective entity in which the leadership rotates and is shared by various members of the team, depending on appropriateness and fit of skills and abilities. In a true team, there are collective work products—for example, the provision of quality patient care to all of the patients housed in the department. There is group as well as individual accountability. If one member of the team is having a problem, it is not just that person's problem but, rather, is the problem of and for the whole team to resolve. An example of team thinking is "No one sits down until we can all sit down" or "No one goes home until we all go home." If quality outcomes are difficult for one team member, all team members are affected by this and become engaged in helping the affected team member meet expectations. In the management book *The Goal* (Goldratt & Cox, 2004), the author tells a parable about taking a Boy Scout troop on a hike. When it was discovered that Herbie was slowing the whole group down, the weight in his backpack was redistributed and the troop sped up. This is how a high-performing team works.

Another collective entity apparent in many organizations is a **pseudoteam**. This is a group of people who believe they are already a team, although clearly they fall short of the definition of a true team. Characteristics of a pseudoteam include confusion over their purpose, unhealthy or toxic interpersonal issues and communication patterns, members who put individual needs and ambition above the needs of the team, the presence of hierarchical rituals that preclude full participation of all members, unclear goals, and a lack of evaluation criteria. The true danger of pseudoteams is that members think they are already a team and thus see no need for improvement. As a result, they do not grow and develop but, rather, just become more and more dysfunctional with the passage of time.

BACKGROUND

Group interactions are a pervasive element of the health care environment in which nurses work. A basic understanding of groups helps nurses function more effectively. These principles apply to any group, whether an actual team, a committee, or an informal group effort. Group interactions are composed of the following elements (Book & Galvin, 1975) (Figure 10.1):

- The *process* that the group undergoes to reach outcomes: This relates to the unique way the group interrelates and begins to work together. The leader can assess group process through observation. What is the process that occurs while accomplishing its task?
- The *standards* that regulate the group's behavior: This relates to the specific values and norms that are chosen for group processing. Which ones are chosen; which are discarded?
- The process of *problem solving* or *decision making* that the group adopts: Does the group solve problems? How are decisions made? Are they group decisions made by consensus, or are they individual decisions made with group input (as occurs when the group participates but the decision is made by a leader or manager)?
- The *communication* that occurs among group members: What are the internal patterns and styles of communication used by group members? To whom does the group communicate? Do they report as a subcommittee to a full committee? If a team, does the team have frequent communication with external team leaders? What are the internal and external modes of communication for group input and output?

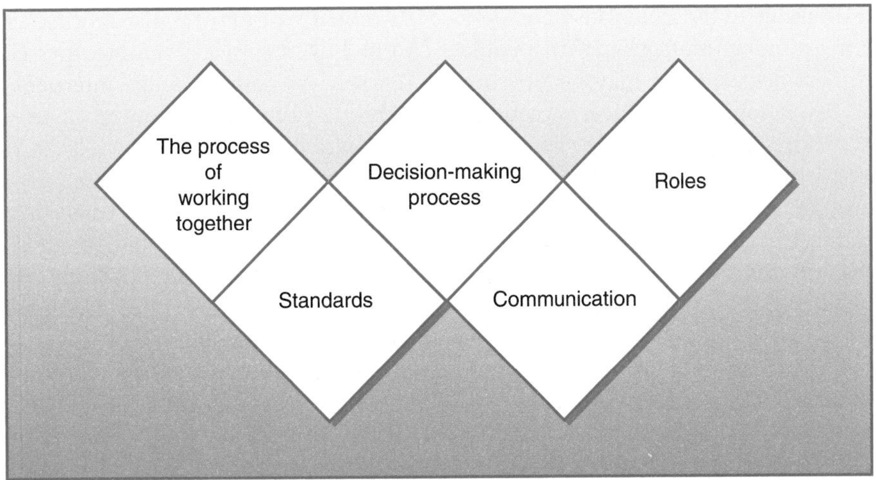

Figure 10.1
Group process elements. (Data from Book, C., & Galvin, K. [1975]. *Instruction in and about small group discussion*. Falls Church, VA: Speech Communication Association.)

- The *roles* played by each member: Members will adopt a variety of group roles within the group, but roles are fluid. Members may take on different roles in different situations. For self-awareness, knowing what part one played in his or her family helps an individual recognize roles that he or she might gravitate toward in groups. It is important to remember when assessing group interactions that roles in the group are not always clearly established by the leader or the group. In this situation, each group member moves in and out of group roles that best suit him or her. Clarity in the more formal roles such as team leader, facilitator, recorder, and time-keeper is important to avoid confusion and unnecessary conflict.

Groups tend to go through a series of stages in their work and development. Farley and Stoner (1989) identified these as (1) orientation, (2) adaptation, (3) emergence, and (4) working. The *first stage*, orientation, occurs when the group first forms and the members begin to relate to one another and the task. The group needs to develop trust and define boundaries in order to establish involvement and identification. The *second stage*, adaptation, occurs as the group begins to develop a collective identity and differentiate roles. The group needs a facilitative structure and climate to maximize its processing and to work through the establishment of roles, rules, norms, and a common language. The *third stage*, emergence, occurs as control issues arise. Disputes, disagreements, confrontations, alliances, and power struggles mark this stage of determining control over the group in order to emerge with a more consolidated identity. The *final stage*, working, occurs when conflict and dissension dissipate and the group achieves greater cohesion through negotiation. The group is now focused primarily on decision making and productivity. The stages may overlap and are not necessarily sequential. The group leader pays attention to the stage of the group as a way of monitoring the group's development and progress. For example, in the orientation stage, the leader may need to be more alert to the need to intervene personally than would be the case in the working stage when the group has achieved a higher level of maturity.

WHY PEOPLE JOIN GROUPS

The reasons why people join groups are many and may include, for example, a desire to satisfy psychological drives and primary needs; or it may be an assignment of job expectation. Group participation can be desirable to individuals for a variety of reasons. For example, interaction with people and a sense of self-achievement may result from participating. Psychological satisfaction can be derived from making a contribution, being with people, accomplishing goals, and demonstrating outcomes through group participation. Groups provide an outlet for affiliation needs—to make friends or meet and mix with people. Groups at all levels fulfill socialization and friendship needs in a number of ways.

In nursing, the formation of groups occurs primarily for one of two reasons: (1) to provide a personal or professional socialization and exchange forum, or (2) to provide a mechanism for interdependent work accomplishment. Groups can be social, professional, or organizational in purpose. The following are some reasons why groups would be established in organizations:

- Group activities can create a sense of status and esteem.
- Groups allow an individual to test and establish reality.
- Groups function as a mechanism for getting a job done.
- The work to be accomplished requires the complexity of knowledge and skill possible only in a group configuration.

"The ebb and flow of work done by groups is a major part of the working environment of hospital nurses" (Leppa, 1996, p. 23). The work group provides an institutional and professional identity for an individual nurse, and work groups become a focus for interpersonal relationships, support, and social integration. Interpersonal relationship elements such as work group cohesion, communication, and social integration remain consistent moderate-level predictors of nursing job satisfaction (Blegen, 1993; DiMeglio et al., 2005). In addition, being part of a healthy group or team is also related to the level of organizational commitment by the employee. Individuals with an emotional connection to their work group have lower levels of turnover (DiMeglio et al., 2005; Manion, 2004).

Work groups can be disrupted by factors such as downsizing, reorganization, absenteeism, and turnover. Work group disruption has been shown to be linked to negative outcomes (Leppa, 1996). In a study of four hospitals, interpersonal relations were found to be an important part of nurses' job satisfaction. There was a relationship between work group disruption and interpersonal relations (Leppa, 1996). Things get done because of relationships among people; nurses need to build successful collaborative relationships among multiple levels of colleagues, key people, organizations, and clients (Laramee, 1999).

A breakdown in working relationships can lead to a strike vote in a collective bargaining environment (Ponte et al., 1998). Furthermore, informal work group norms exert a strong influence on nurses' behavior and can contribute to forms of nursing deviance. Work group relationships can reinforce behaviors and reinforce rationalization, thus leading to deviant behaviors becoming passively or actively accepted. Such strong work group norms can be seen in the extreme. For example, in one study of nurses in practice, nurses used work group norms to neutralize opposition to and reinforce behaviors of drug theft and use (Dabney, 1995). Clearly, there is a strong relationship between work groups, interpersonal relationships, and outcomes such as nurses' behaviors and perceptions. Work group relationships are a powerful mechanism influencing both good and bad outcomes in nursing practice.

ADVANTAGES OF GROUPS

There are advantages to group work. For example, groups are one vehicle for solving problems. Veninga (1982) identified the following five major advantages of group problem solving over individual problem solving:

1. *Greater knowledge and information*: Obtaining a broader and wider range of knowledge and experiences creates a higher-quality input into group problem solving. The insights of one member can stimulate the thinking of others (Beachy & Biester, 1986). With the increased specialization of health care workers today, this is especially true.

2. *Increased acceptance of solutions*: If there is a decision to be made in an organization, people can get together in a group to talk about it so that the people themselves are more committed to the decision. When individuals who are going to be affected by a decision are part of the decision-making process, they do not have to be convinced of the rightness of the decision and are more likely to be committed to implementing it.
3. *More approaches to a problem*: Complex problems typically are more manageable when a number of perspectives are mixed together to address the problem. The advantages include blending and complementing individual learning and problem-solving styles to capitalize on strength through diversity.
4. *Individual expression*: Groups allow for individual expression, and in organizations specifically, there may be few mechanisms for expression of individual perspectives. Sharing information and getting input are done best in groups (Veninga, 1982). Sometimes groups allow people to express themselves—for example, if they are anxious about a change or if morale is low.
5. *Lower costs*: If the group is functioning in a positive and constructive manner, the use of a group can be less expensive than the use of individual effort to accomplish a task. Group decision making is cost-effective if it saves time. For example, when a group meets for one session as opposed to the leader meeting multiple times with multiple individuals, the leader and possibly the group members save time. Furthermore, cost-effectiveness may result through the division of labor (Beachy & Biester, 1986).

It is imperative that the purpose of the group be established and assessed, especially when the group is part of a larger organization. This means that all members need to have a clear definition of the work of the group. Either the leader needs to disseminate this information or the followers need to ask for clarification. Then the stated purpose should be evaluated periodically. Is it a functioning group? Is it accomplishing the task to which it was assigned? If not, should the group be disbanded? Sometimes when the work output of a group of nurses is analyzed, meetings appear to be very costly endeavors. For example, when the number of hours spent by all committee members is multiplied by their individual hourly salary and fringe benefit cost and added together to compute a committee total, the sum of costs for the group may be astounding (Table 10.1). This is another reason for paying attention to how well the group is functioning.

Table 10.1
Committee Cost Analysis

Members	Salary/ Hour($)	Benefits/ Hour($)	Cost/ Hour($)
Nurse 1	25	7	32
Nurse 2	25	7	32
Pharmacist	37	9	46
Nurse manager	30	8	38
Physician	120	N/A	120
			TOTAL: **268**

A well-tuned and functioning group is positive for an organization. Often such a group is less expensive and time-consuming in terms of solving complex problems. Participation and involvement in a group decision typically results in individuals being more committed to a decision, even if there is disagreement.

DISADVANTAGES OF GROUPS

Group decision making can be derailed at a number of points in the process. The three disadvantages commonly noted about group decision making are the potential for premature decisions, individual domination, and disruptive conflicts (Veninga, 1982).

Premature Decisions

The disadvantages of group work include the fact that decisions can result from pressure. Once a majority vote is taken, the minority experience an element of pressure because of psychological dynamics related to subtle pressure for group acceptance and conformity. This is often referred to as "groupthink." It may be difficult to be a "devil's advocate" or to adopt the role of bringing alternative critique points to the group for consideration because of a concern about not being personally socially accepted. For example, derision and humiliation can occur if members react with strong negative opinions. This response stifles further input.

Individual Domination

Some of the disadvantages of groups relate to the possible emergence of dominating or argumentative members who obstruct the group process. These members make it an unpleasant experience for all involved. In a sense, they sabotage the work of the group. An example occurs when the group is not functioning well or the members are not adhering to the task of the group because of a chronically negative individual or other distractions (e.g., socializing, avoiding the task, not preparing themselves). It becomes costly and time-consuming for the group to divert its energy and productivity to working out interpersonal dynamics rather than moving forward on the group's task.

Disruptive Conflicts

If people perceive an adverse effect on a group member or members or if they feel threatened, conflicts usually emerge. Conflicts can accelerate in a competitive environment when members vest in their own position. Conflicts may also occur over personality differences, differences of opinion, or clashes of values. Although it may seem contradictory, conflicts can serve as a control mechanism in a group and may actually result in far superior outcomes. When group members are comfortable respectfully disagreeing with each other, a premature acceptance of decisions can be avoided because opposing viewpoints are considered. However, group members and leaders need to become skilled and comfortable in handling interpersonal dynamics.

GROUP DECISION MAKING

Group work can be, and typically is, a slow process. It takes more time for a group to arrive at a decision than for one person to make the decision.

In addition, a continuum of decision-making power may be vested in a group (Figure 10.2). A group or committee has certain powers, tasks, and functions, as well as certain parameters or latitude in terms of how far to go in making a decision. Decision power is a matter of degree, with four distinct points on the continuum of authority for decision making: autocratic, consultative, joint, and delegated.

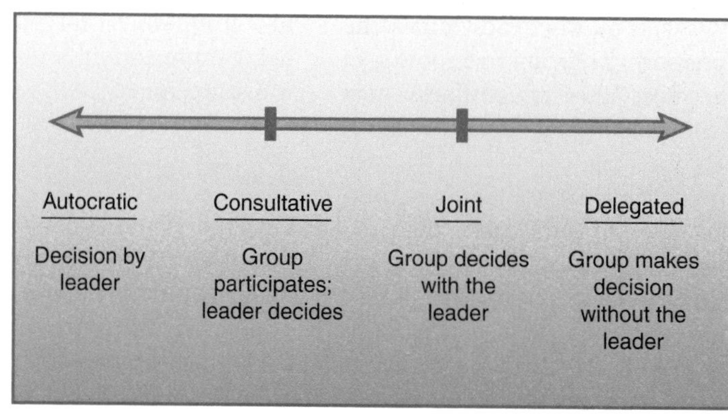

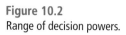

Figure 10.2
Range of decision powers.

On one end of the continuum is an *autocratic decision procedure* in which the leader makes all of the decisions. In this process there is input, perhaps, but not necessarily a vote. For example, in certain legislative committees the chairperson may or may not be able to put forth legislation or block a bill. It may be the case that an autocratic leader controls the power and the committee exists mainly for the sake of appearance. This type of committee is set up for reasons other than making participative decisions. It is hoped that very few of these structures are found in human service organizations because they can generate increased cynicism.

A *consultative decision procedure* occurs when decisions involve employee participation but the leader still makes the final decision alone. Group members may make certain recommendations, but these must then go to the leader, chairperson, or head of the group, who makes the final decision. There is more participation with this type of procedure, but the ultimate decision is not under the control of the group members.

Some decision procedures result in *joint decision making*. In this approach, the entire group decides, whether by a two-thirds vote, simple majority, consensus, or some other process. In a joint decision procedure, the employees have as much influence as the leader. The leader has one voice, one vote. The leader can use persuasion, but when it comes to the final vote, the leader's vote is equivalent to that of any other member of the group. This is fundamentally different from the leader making the decision with group input.

Finally, at the other end of the decision continuum is the *delegated decision procedure*. This occurs when the committee chair or leader allows participants to make the final decision. For example, in true self-scheduling, the leader may set up the basic parameters but the staff members (usually through the work of a smaller, designated team) actually decide what schedule they work. The true test of a delegation decision procedure is whether the leader overrides the followers' decision. Technically, the leader would not have the authority to veto or override. If it is truly a delegation situation, the leader would go forward with the approach that the decision is the choice of the group. An indication of this type of delegation is when the leader responds: "I am authorized by the group to, do ...." The leader becomes the advocate and the spokesperson but not the decision maker. Hersey and colleagues (2008) labeled these same four procedures as *authoritative, consultative, facilitative*, and *delegative* decision-making styles.

It is advisable for the followers in any group to determine who has the authority to make decisions. Knowledge about what type of group it is and what delegation or decision procedures can be anticipated is critical to participation. A leadership or conflict moment may occur when a group assumes that the decision procedure rule in effect is delegation and the decision is *its* to make but the leader has a different idea. Clarity before beginning work on an issue avoids unnecessary conflict and augments productivity.

WORK TEAMS

In health care, interdisciplinary care teams are a matter of survival. High-performance teams are essential to an organization's efficiency and effectiveness because collaboration and teamwork are essential to achieving high-quality work outcomes and cost control.

Three types of teams found in health care are (1) primary work teams, (2) leadership teams, and (3) ad hoc teams. Primary work teams include all forms of client care teams such as an emergency department trauma team. In the operating room, teams are often based on the specialty (e.g., a cardiovascular or an orthopedic team). The senior executive team is an example of an executive or management leadership team. At the hospital department level there may be a leadership team that is composed of the nurse manager, the charge nurses, and perhaps an educator. Continuous quality improvement teams, project teams, and problem-solving teams are examples of ad hoc teams found across settings and sites. Specific problem-solving teams in departments are other examples of ad hoc teams. The chief characteristic of these teams is that they are created to perform a very specific piece of work. When that work is completed, the team dissolves. Among all types of teams, any team may become a self-directed work team. This is a group that accepts increasingly higher levels of authority for its area of responsibility. A self-directed work team is fully responsible for delivering a well-defined segment of a finished product or service (Manion et al., 1996). It has the requisite capacity and authority for the work undertaken.

Designing, building, and implementing effective work teams requires a specific methodology and process. A primary work team fails if it behaves like a collection of individuals operating from narrowly defined jobs; if it is composed of the wrong mix of members, size, structure, responsibility, or expertise; or if it cannot fluidly shift activities and adapt to changes. The following four steps are key to designing a highly effective health care team (Manion et al., 1996):

1. Define the total pool of work for the team.
2. Differentiate responsibilities within the pool.
3. Narrow the design options to attractive alternatives.
4. Identify the single best design to implement.

These principles apply regardless of the type of team being formed. After the team has been carefully designed for the work it is to accomplish, the next step is to build the team by incorporating the essential elements needed to function. These elements are meaningful purpose, consistent membership, specific performance goals, commitment to a common approach, complementary and overlapping skills, and mutual accountability for outcomes.

Managing this development process is a key leadership function. This means that the leader guides the team in the development of its purpose. The team members are more likely to coalesce into a strong team if they have been given the time and opportunity to carefully reflect on their purpose and agree on what they do and for whom they do it. The team becomes a true team by doing its work. Specific performance goals give it direction and also provide evaluative criteria by which the team's success can be measured. Although it is simplistic to say that the team has common working approaches, unnecessary conflict occurs in this area if the leader and team members have not established these key processes. Agreement is needed about how things are going to be done and by whom. This ranges from the establishment of team behavioral norms to agreement on procedural issues. This step usually requires a significant amount of time and will continue to be addressed throughout the lifetime of the team. By laying a foundation carefully, effective teams can emerge (Manion et al., 1996).

The dynamics of interdisciplinary teams create some unique issues. Regrouping people into multidisciplinary groups can create anxiety and fear. A lack of common vocabulary and understanding about other disciplines' practices may become apparent. It has been said that professionals simply do not know how to work together in teams (Sorrells-Jones, 1997). Other perils and pitfalls occur when teams are assigned, not designed. Additional errors may include the following (Manion et al., 1996):

- Confusion occurs about the team's work.
- The team lacks real authority.
- Structural team building is not done.
- Dysfunctional behavior occurs.
- Team-based outcome measures and coaching are lacking.

Trust and communication are critical elements of building effective work teams. It is not enough to simply structure the team. Team members need to work collaboratively and interdependently first before striving to work synergistically. Key to moving away from independent action and toward synergistic work teams is to change the use of power among team members toward finding synergistic solutions that address divergent needs (Gage, 1998). An infrastructure of open communication with an emphasis on information sharing enables team members to understand and believe in the team's strategies. Teams benefit from a communication critical path and the valuing of individual accountability for communication (Page, 1998).

Team performance and effectiveness are important managerial concerns. Dysfunctional team behaviors can occur. Lencioni (2002) identified five key dysfunctions of a team as absence of trust, fear of conflict, lack of commitment, avoidance of accountability, and inattention to results.

Teams form, grow through stages, and mature. Team dynamics change throughout this process. Teams benefit from team building and developmental training. Articulating and negotiating expectations for healthy interpersonal behavior benefits team development. For example, active listening and demonstrating mutual respect promote an open environment. Direct communication and honest feedback, addressing conflict, and negotiating for win-win solutions facilitate healthy interpersonal dynamics in teams and enhance their productivity and performance (Manion et al., 1996; Page, 1998). A key characteristic of an emotionally intelligent team is one that has established norms that guide team member behaviors (Cherniss & Goleman, 2001).

Team norms are best established when the team initially forms. They are continually revisited, modified, and expanded throughout the life span of the team. The process for developing norms is usually leader-initiated and begins with a conversation within the team about how members expect each other to behave and contribute. The norms are usually developed during a group meeting in which ideas are shared, refined, and finally negotiated with all team members. Appropriate topics for behavioral norms include, but are not limited to, expectations around the following:

- Communication, both at the individual and group levels
- How team members treat each other
- How support is to be demonstrated
- Decision-making process
- How conflict is to be handled

For example, one team developed the following expectations of each other:

I expect you to:

- Communicate in an open, honest, and direct manner with me.
- Give me feedback when my behavior creates a difficult or uncomfortable situation for you.
- Persist and work with me on difficult issues until we reach a mutually agreeable resolution.
- Pitch in gladly, provide help when asked, and look for ways to help each other out.
- Respect confidences and not share sensitive information we discuss with others without my knowledge or permission.
- Be trustworthy as evidenced by honoring and meeting commitments made, by being loyal to absent team members, and by presenting me in the best light to others.

Often these norms are referred to as the *team operating agreement*, the *code of conduct*, or *articulated expectations*. In many teams, once they are identified, team members sign on to them, indicating agreement, and they often are posted in sight in the workplace. These norms are more than just a paper exercise. They signify that the team member agrees to live by the expectations and address other team members who do not.

Katzenbach and Smith (1993) looked at the spectrum of teams and plotted the following five discrete points along a team performance curve:

1. A working group in which there is no incentive to form a team
2. A pseudoteam that has no common purpose or set of goals
3. A potential team in which significant incremental performance is needed
4. A real team that fits their definition
5. A high-performance team that outperforms other teams and has members deeply committed to one another's growth and success

The greater the performance, the greater is the advantage to the group and the organization.

Performance in teams is linked to productivity, but the direct applicability to the delivery of nursing care remains a complex challenge (Sheafor, 1991). For example, Schmeiding's (1990) research indicated that staff nurses may prefer dependence on those in higher hierarchical positions. Some nurses were not motivated, prepared, or inclined to assume a high level of personal responsibility for decision making in client care coordination and

Practical Tips

Tip #1: Use Self-Reflection

Think about the groups on which you serve, and make a list. What is the purpose of each of these groups? How would you categorize each group (i.e., whether it is a committee, a team, or a work group)? What are the attributes that caused you to put the group in one category or the other? How well does the type of group fit its primary purpose? Would any of these groups be more effective if they were developed into another type of group (e.g., a work group that would be more effective as a team, a group that needs to become a formal committee)?

Tip #2: Evaluate Committees

Create a list of committees on which you serve or have served in the past. Evaluate each for its effectiveness in accomplishing its primary mission and goals. Identify interventions that could have helped the committee be more effective.

Tip #3: Deal With Difficult Group or Team Behavior

At your next committee, group, or team meeting, sit back and observe the behavior of the members. What are effective and ineffective behaviors you see? If you are the facilitator, develop a plan or actions for dealing with the ineffective behaviors or for reinforcing the positive and constructive behaviors. If the group has not established their group norms, initiate a conversation about these and lead their development.

work group administration. This has implications for leadership and management of professional nurses and for decentralization and shared governance. Furthermore, it is not known whether these attitudes are still valid or have shifted with time.

Nurse leaders need to learn how to manage in a team-centered environment; staff nurses must learn how to be effective team players (Sovie, 1992). Interactive leadership is needed to create a group identity. Participatory management; sharing power and information; and generating trust, mutual respect, and enhanced self-worth are seen as key elements in successful performance teams. Teamwork begins with members who are well prepared and personally competent. Teamwork then includes shared ownership and decision making (Sovie, 1992). Nurses often begin with experiences on client care teams and ad hoc problem-solving teams or continuous quality improvement teams, moving later to senior leadership and interdisciplinary or cross-functional teams (Farley & Stoner, 1989).

Group process is a framework by which to understand team development (Farley & Stoner, 1989). Sovie (1992) identified four essential components of high-performing teams: roles, activities, relationships, and the environment. This means that highly effective teams establish positive roles among the members, who are able to focus their activities toward productivity. To become highly effective, the relationships of the team members need to become cohesive. The team requires a facilitative and supportive environment in which to work through the task and relationship elements. Management of team building and team performance includes skill in the process of conflict management. Diverse backgrounds and varying views result in the potential for differences, conflicts, turf battles, and office politics. The leader's repertoire must include strategies of conflict resolution, empowerment, collaboration, and coordination. Sovie (1992) called the manager "a gatekeeper at the critical boundary of team and organization" (p. 97) who has to keep com-

Box 10.1

Team Performance Checklist

✓ Small in number
✓ Adequate levels of skills
✓ Meaningful purpose
✓ Specific goal(s)
✓ Clear working approach
✓ Sense of mutual accountability

Data from Katzenbach, J., & Smith, D. (1993). *The wisdom of teams: Creating the high-performance organization.* New York: Harper Collins.

munication, objectives, and needs flowing both ways. Diplomacy, negotiation, and power-based strategies or alliances may be employed in team building (Farley & Stoner, 1989). Lencioni (2006) promoted the idea that to overcome the common turf battles and the tendency team members have to function in their own narrow scope (silo thinking), the team needs to have a pressing, time-constricted goal upon which to focus.

The complementary skills that are needed, in the right mix, to do the team's task fall into at least three categories: technical or functional expertise, problem-solving and decision-making skills, and interpersonal skills. To assess and strengthen team performance, Katzenbach and Smith (1993) recommended an analysis of each of their six basic elements of teams: small in number, adequate levels of complementary skills, a truly meaningful purpose, specific goal(s), clear working approach, and sense of mutual accountability (Box 10.1). The characteristics of highly effective teams include a common purpose or clear, elevating goal; agreed-on performance goals or results-driven structure; competent members; a common approach for the work; a unified commitment; complementary skills; a collaborative climate; mutual accountability; standards of excellence; external support and recognition; and principled leadership (Katzenbach & Smith, 1993; Manion et al., 1996).

COMMITTEES

An essential part of any nurse's role is to be involved in committee and group work. Work is accomplished through people, and the coordination of care is furthered through committee actions. It also is important to nurses' job satisfaction and autonomy to have an avenue of involvement and participation in which to actively solve problems and retain autonomy over nursing care. Shared governance models incorporate staff nurse participation in groups and committees as a core element of how work gets accomplished.

Some people react negatively to committees because they dislike the time involved and because they are frustrated with the psychodynamics of group process and decision making. However, committees are a mainstay of organizations and can be an important way to make changes in clinical practice. Lencioni (2004) believed there is no substitute for a good meeting—one in which there is passionate, dynamic, and focused engagement—to gather the collective wisdom of the group. Understanding committee workings facilitates the process of being a more effective nurse.

Committee structures are preferable in the following two kinds of situations:

1. *Situations in which each member's input is needed to attain a certain goal.* For example, a committee may be set up to implement self-scheduling or to start a new program to benefit clients. If the work cannot be done alone or if there is a need to have everyone's agreement, then a committee is probably appropriate.
2. *Situations in which diverse representation facilitates implementation of proposed activities.* To have a diverse group of people provide input in order to get the job done, a committee should be created. For example, a multidisciplinary products committee could be established to develop a process in which products would be reviewed before a large amount was purchased. This approach avoids the nurses at the care delivery site using products that are potentially unsafe or unusable, and thus costly.

Several types of committees are found in organizations. One kind is the standing committee, which, as the name implies, is a constant, ongoing part of the organizational mission, performing critical and essential functions. For example, policy committees are standing committees because there always are policies to write and review. The same is true for quality assurance/improvement committees because quality improvement activities are ongoing and continuous.

Contrasted to a standing committee is the task force, also called a *project team* or *ad hoc committee*. This is a committee that is developed in response to some emergent or immediate need. A need arises, and a group is formed. A task force is not part of the organizational core mission. It is formed in response to a specific circumstance that arises or to study a specific problem. The committee is expected to disband when the issue is resolved. Examples are a search committee to replace an advanced practice nurse or a problem-solving group dealing with, for example, patient flow issues or bed space availability in the emergency department, which subsequently affects the entire hospital.

Some groups or committees are structured to gather together members based on organizational position or job position. For example, all the nurse managers may belong to a group of nurse managers or staff nurses may belong to a staff nurse council. By holding the position of nurse manager, the person belongs to that committee. This provides an opportunity for peer interaction, support, and problem solving.

There are multidisciplinary interdivisional committees. A multidisciplinary committee includes participants from several divisions or specialties. The participants may all be from within the institution or from both inside and outside the organization. These committees often are used to coordinate and eliminate boundary conflicts. Some examples are a products committee, a risk-management committee, or a medical liaison committee in which nurses and physicians work together to improve patient care and reduce interprofessional conflicts. In some cases, multidisciplinary teams are formed using a committee structure (e.g., to develop a critical pathway). Other committees may be cross-functional (e.g., nurses meeting with members from the information technology or facilities management department to discuss and resolve issues).

Within organizations, committees perform a central role in the implementation of the strategic plan. A committee is a group that can assume accountability for planning, implementing, and evaluating the outcomes of a strategic goal translated to the operational level. Committees accomplish some departmental activities and provide a mechanism for increasing staff participation in decision making. In an environment characterized by complex work, committees become a major vehicle for resolving issues related to the organization's mission. Two elements promote efficient and effective committee decision making: appropriate representation (by including people affected by changes) and delegation of an appropriate level of authority to the committee (Wilson et al., 1999).

Committees evolve over time. To remain vital, committees need to be evaluated regularly for congruence with organizational mission and contribution to outcomes. Occasionally, environmental changes or internal restructuring creates a situation forcing reexamination of the coordination and focus of committees. Both restructuring and revitalization of committees can be accomplished through strategic planning, multidisciplinary forums, enhanced communication, a phased process, and evaluation of the changes (Deveau & McCabe, 1996; Wilson et al., 1999).

If asked to be on a committee as a unit representative, it is advisable for the nurse to explore the nature and characteristics of the committee. The nurse needs to determine the authority level delegated to this particular committee, remembering that this delegation may be formal or informal. Another factor involves assessing who is on the committee and whether the nurse has a positive or negative relationship with the other members. Other factors include whether the people on the committee are highly motivated, whether they are task- or relationship-oriented people, and what committee politics exist. The feedback mechanisms and the committee's productivity are key characteristics. The track record of the committee is reflected in its output. These characteristics are important for the nurse to understand before deciding to participate. Preparation for followership enhances both personal and committee productivity. It is also helpful to clarify any expectations for the committee role being considered. For example, is the nurse there to share individual opinions or to represent others in the department? This role requires more active solicitation of colleagues' opinions and ideas.

EFFECTIVE MEETINGS

Meetings are common occurrences in health care organizations. Whether a meeting involves a group, a committee, or a team, the leader's role is to maximize the benefits of the meeting. Structuring a meeting for effectiveness requires preparation and effort. To manage effective meetings, the leader should consider the purpose for which they are organized. There are several purposes for meetings (Jacobs & Rosenthal, 1984). The first type of meeting is held for *information dissemination*. For example, the designated leadership person calls the group together to let the members know that direction has come down to cut the budget by 10% because of fiscal retrenchment. A meeting is called to disseminate information about what is happening and to provide time for questions and answers. Perhaps there has been an organizational change, such as the decision that one unit is going to be consolidating with another unit or that a new building, department relocation, or merger is being planned.

Second, there are meetings held for the purpose of *opinion seeking*. The goal of these meetings is open dialogue to solicit group opinions and ideas on specific topics or issues. This purpose does not imply that decision making is the prerogative of the group. Seeking opinions is an input strategy and may be used only for gathering data or testing group reactions. For example, an opinion-seeking meeting may be called to invite input on equipment purchases for budget requests.

The third type of meeting is held for the purpose of *problem solving*. The meeting is structured to solicit help in clarifying, analyzing, and solving a specific problem. This type of meeting is more action-oriented. Group participation in decision making is encouraged. For example, group problem solving or unit meetings may be called to discuss ways to solve problems related to disruptive or manipulative clients or family members. Meetings for the purpose of problem solving must follow a methodical structure; otherwise, they are likely either to deteriorate into a complaint session or to result in ineffective or unacceptable recommendations. Effectively leading these groups requires strong facilitation skills and knowledge in problem-solving techniques.

Several team-related functions of group meetings can contribute to effectiveness. For example, a meeting provides a structure to facilitate a sense of identity and to help the team more fully achieve its purposes. A meeting is a forum for updating shared knowledge among a team. A meeting reinforces the collective goals and objectives of the team. Furthermore, a meeting can create a sense of commitment to group decisions. It can be an opportunity for a manager to be perceived as a leader. A true team uses the meeting time to accomplish a collective work product as compared with a committee or work group who uses meeting time to discuss issues and then delegate the work outside of the actual meeting time. However, a meeting is a waste of time for all concerned unless they clearly understand what the meeting is intended to achieve (Jay, 1982).

Beachy and Biester (1986) discussed restructuring meetings toward effective group management. As nursing department meetings became unmanageable, one organization developed a questionnaire to survey the group and evaluate the meetings. Aspects such as the cost/benefit ratio of attending meetings, group process, decision making, and relevancy of agenda items were examined for individual members' feelings about effectiveness. The group then discussed ideas for restructuring the meetings. Active participation was seen as being the essence of effective meetings. Certain elements of time management, group process, and decision making are related to effectiveness in meetings (Beachy & Biester, 1986).

Jay (1982) outlined guidelines for conducting meetings. For example, in a meeting held to achieve specific objectives, each agenda item can be identified as being for information (e.g., progress reports), for development (e.g., new policy or strategy plan), for implementation (e.g., formulating a detailed action plan), or for change within the organization (e.g., changing documentation forms used by multiple user groups). Identifying on the agenda the category of each item helps clarify and focus the group discussion. Using a timed agenda can also facilitate the process. This involves identifying on the agenda, next to each item, the anticipated amount of time allotted for discussion. This should serve as a guideline rather than a rigid parameter and must not be substituted for good judgment when a particular discussion is productive but takes longer than anticipated.

The leader of the group can facilitate meeting effectiveness by preparing and dealing with both the task and the people involved. The leader needs to listen carefully, process the interactions, control the flow, and keep the meeting directed toward accomplishing the objectives. The ideal size of a group is 4 to 7 people, with 12 being the upper limit (Jay, 1982). Members should be carefully selected for best input and potential contribution to the work. The leader needs to start on time and be alert to seating positions. The leader can facilitate effectiveness by controlling the compulsive talkers, drawing out the silent members, protecting the junior members, encouraging the clash of ideas, discouraging the clash of personalities, avoiding the squashing of creative ideas, and closing on a note of achievement (Jay, 1982). The leader also needs to attend to careful meeting wrap-up. Summarizing after the meeting the group's accomplishments and verifying task assignments going forward are important leader responsibilities. Box 10.2 presents a checklist for leading effective meetings.

Box **10.2**

Effective Meetings Checklist for Leaders

- ✓ Identify the purpose of the meeting:
  - Information dissemination
  - Opinion seeking
  - Problem solving
- ✓ Prepare an agenda and related materials
- ✓ Identify the category of each agenda item:
  - For information
  - For development
  - For implementation
  - For change in the system
- ✓ Set the size at four to seven people
- ✓ Carefully select members (based on skill and expertise)
- ✓ Distribute agenda well in advance of meeting
- ✓ Start on time
- ✓ Listen carefully
- ✓ Process the interactions
- ✓ Control the flow of interactions
- ✓ Keep the meeting directed toward accomplishing objectives

Data from Jay, A. (1982). How to run a meeting. *Journal of Nursing Administration, 12*(1), 22-28.

Without thought and preparation, people go into a meeting focused on their own issues, biases, and perspectives; they may not be tuned in to how to be productive within the meeting. However, even in a negative situation, individuals may choose to participate in a way that assists or enhances the process by making constructive suggestions about how things could be done better. This is an ideal situation—one to be encouraged, structured, and facilitated by the leader.

The duties of the chairperson include preparation of the physical environment. Comfort and convenience engineering is part of the leader's responsibility in terms of preparing an environment that is conducive to people being satisfied, productive, positive, and working together. The worst-case situation occurs when members have to sit in an uncomfortable chair in a room that is too cold, too hot, or too noisy because of construction; when members cannot hear or talk to other people; or when the technology does not work. Consider how to facilitate group work through hosting functions related to breaks, food, and beverages. It is human nature for members to be more relaxed and productive in comfortable surroundings.

As all nurses are pressured to do more with less under severe time and travel constraints, conducting meetings assisted by technology has become a major strategy. Speaker phones, videoconferencing, Internet hook-ups, real-time (synchronous) discussion boards, and related audio or video technology strategies are commonly employed. They become useful ways to save time by eliminating travel to an in-person site. However, specific problems may occur such as technology incompatibility, speed of transmission, hook-up failures, or other delays in transmission that result in people talking over one another or hesitancy in speaking, a lack of interpersonal modulation due to absence of body language, or a tendency to forget about people who are not actually in the room. Despite these known issues, nurses in the future will increasingly experience meetings assisted by technology.

A leader has a responsibility to prepare and motivate participants. The participants' responsibility is to read and be prepared, show up on time, and attend to the task at hand. The leader needs to prepare an agenda with handouts and background materials and distribute them to the members, giving the members time to read them. The better-prepared the members are, the more they can participate, increase the quality of decisions, and be more effective.

The leader's preparation activities include reviewing the status of agenda topics as part of preparing the agenda. Questions to ask include the following:

- Where are we?
- What else needs to be done?
- What supporting materials might help the committee?
- Who should be invited?

A leader who comes to the meeting and distributes a handout for a quick look before discussion, input, or a vote violates the participants' ability to think through what is being presented. This may be done as a tactic to avoid thorough deliberation by pressuring for the immediacy of a decision, but more often this behavior results from disorganization or lack of attention to leader responsibilities.

CONSTRUCTIVE GROUP MEMBERS

People in groups assume a variety of roles. Lancaster (1981) identified both group building roles and group maintenance roles as being a part of group interactions. Group building roles include initiator, encourager, opinion giver, clarifier, listener, and summarizer. Group maintenance roles include tension reliever, compromiser, gatekeeper, and harmonizer. The group building roles concentrate more on relationship functions than on task functions; the group maintenance roles focus more on task functions than on relationship functions.

One positive way to handle meetings is to identify a facilitator. Often this is the formal group leader or individual in a position of authority, but it does not have to be. If this is a true team, the role of facilitator may rotate among team members. In a committee, the facilitator is probably the committee chairperson. A facilitator conducts the meeting, ensuring that everyone has the opportunity to speak, maintains the focus of the meeting, and ensures that group dynamics remain positive.

Also needed is a group recorder. The task of taking minutes or summarizing discussion and decisions may need to be delegated to a clerical support person (if possible) if group members are averse to taking on the task of recording outcomes. However, a recorder who is a group member technically can do far more than just take minutes. This person should be in tune with the group processing and with the inputs and roles of group members and help keep the group on time. The recorder can provide feedback to the facilitator in terms of how to improve the process. One key tip is to construct a standardized meeting record (or minutes) form to facilitate the process and flow documentation. It is helpful to decide in advance the level of detail required in the minutes to avoid lengthy minutes and potentially unnecessary effort. One useful way to expedite group work is to use a laptop computer to directly enter draft minutes.

Finally, group members are needed. In this instance, *group members* means active participants, each with equal status in the meeting. The three components of facilitator, recorder, and group members contribute to the design of a positive working group.

DISRUPTIVE GROUP MEMBERS

Another role that the group leader assumes is that of process facilitator. The leader must observe group member actions and be prepared to control or redirect disruptive behaviors. Following are common types of disruptive group members that are encountered (Jacobs & Rosenthal, 1984), with strategies for the leader to use in managing dysfunctional members.

Compulsive Talkers

The leader needs to identify individuals who are compulsive talkers and consider how their behavior can be modified. One suggestion is to thank them for their input and then ask to hear from others on that same topic before they are given permission to speak again, as a way of guiding and opening up the meeting to be more effective. If this behavior continues to impact the group negatively and the individual is not receptive to this subtle feedback, meeting with the person after the group work and giving direct, constructive feedback about the negative impact of his or her behavior may be necessary.

Nontalkers

The nontalkers are the quiet ones. The leader can ask them to write down and submit their ideas or ask to hear their thoughts on the matter at hand. The leader can specifically ask them questions to draw them out and thereby open up a broader range of group input. Preparing members in advance by posting the agenda or letting them know where their input will be crucial is also a way to include the nontalkers. Sometimes these people need time to think through their thoughts before they engage in a conversation, unlike their more spontaneous and verbal peers.

Interrupters

The leader has to control the interrupter because this person is demonstrating a lack of self-control. The interrupter can be a problem in groups because the person who is interrupted feels violated and wonders why he or she is not given the courtesy of finishing a thought and having his or her full input considered. The leader needs to halt the interruption and control and redirect the interrupter. This can easily be accomplished by saying "Let's let Joan finish what she was saying."

Squashers

Squashers try to squash an idea before it is even developed. Suggestions about processes or procedures that have not been proven or even tried are much easier to criticize than are facts or opinions. Persons who are averse to change may have a litany of reasons why a potential solution would never work or why this proposed project simply cannot or should not happen. Often these are people who do not want to take a personal risk or undergo the personal effort of making a change, so it is easier to squash everything and maintain the status quo. Especially during brainstorming sessions, the leader must be alert to and have a method for containing the squasher. An easy way to influence this is to set the expectation at the beginning of the session by saying, for example, "For this exercise, please do not engage in analyzing or saying anything negative about the ideas thrown out until we have them all identified." In some selected instances, the leader may choose to allow the negative input for a certain amount of time and then move the group beyond it. One method to move the group is to direct an equal amount of time to exploring the positive benefits and potentials of the proposal. The leader may need to express a vision or ideal future and challenge the group to take up the opportunity.

Busybodies

Busybodies really are not committed to the group's work. They frequently arrive late, leave early, take personal messages or cell phone calls during the meeting, never read the agenda, are passive-aggressive, and simply want to show up for a few minutes for the purpose of appearances but do not contribute any effort. They are meeting their needs by showing up, but they are not contributing to the ongoing group work or the task at hand; nor are they invested in the group's goals. The leader needs to find creative mechanisms to engage the busybodies, perhaps by giving them a concrete assignment with accountability. If this does not work, they may need to be released from the group or placed in an advisory role.

MANAGING DISRUPTIVE BEHAVIOR IN GROUPS

The most useful way to affect these negative behaviors is to lead the group through the clarification of their working expectations. When group members have clearly identified what they need from each other to work together productively in a group setting, they have established the norms for acceptable and non-acceptable behavior.

Another key way the group leader can control disruptive group behavior is to take advantage of several creativity techniques to heighten both the content and the process of group work. Because perceptions and biases may cloud individuals' ability to generate creative ideas or solutions, the techniques of brainstorming, Delphi survey, or nominal group technique (NGT) can be employed (Van de Ven & Delbecq, 1974). Brainstorming is the encouragement of the generation of large numbers of diverse ideas, free from critique or labeling in regard to practicality or feasibility. A Delphi survey technique employs sequential rounds of questionnaires to collect the judgment and consensus of opinion of experts on a topic. It often is used for prioritization purposes.

The NGT (Van de Ven & Delbecq, 1974) avoids social exchange contamination by following a process of silently gathering ideas in writing, using round-robin feedback from group members to identify ideas, clarifying and evaluating each identified idea, and individually voting on priority ideas. The group decision is derived mathematically. An example of NGT would be when a nurse leader of a hospital nursing unit calls a staff meeting to develop the department's goals and strategies for the following year based on the organizational strategic plan. The first step is to have group members write down key goals or initiatives silently and independently. Then, going around the group, the ideas about potential goals that were identified by group members are written on a flip chart, one at a time. Next, each recorded idea is discussed by the group to clarify and evaluate. Then group members vote privately in the form of ranked priorities of which initiative is the most important and fundamental. Individual priority rankings are displayed. A group decision is made about the department's key priorities based on these ratings, and an action plan is then developed. The structure provided by using these creativity techniques often serves to influence and increase commitment by the group.

Thus the nurse leader can take an active role in structuring group work for positive processing and effective outcomes. It is important to control the flow to modulate disruptive group members without humiliating them. Another way is to structure positive and constructive group roles among members. The leader also may choose to involve the group in managing dysfunctional members. This can be done by agreement on behavioral norms (e.g., respect for all persons' input) and on how the group collectively will enforce them. Peer pressure also is a powerful group behavior modification tactic. The leader's vision, enthusiasm, interpersonal relationship skills, and empowerment of followers all facilitate group effectiveness.

LEADERSHIP AND MANAGEMENT IMPLICATIONS

The leadership and management role in groups, teams, and committees includes strategically considering the work to be accomplished, determining the structure most suited to doing the work,

LEADERSHIP & MANAGEMENT BEHAVIORS

Leadership Behaviors

- Encourages group members to participate
- Communicates enthusiasm and vision of group goals
- Motivates followers to accomplish group goals
- Models constructive group participation
- Inspires team collaboration
- Facilitates constructive group roles
- Monitors group process

Management Behaviors

- Plans committee agenda and task accomplishment
- Enables group members to participate
- Organizes a team
- Delegates group work and assigns tasks
- Arranges support services
- Communicates through reporting structure
- Handles conflict situations

Overlap Areas

- Communicates to further the group's productivity
- Monitors the group's movement toward goal accomplishment

putting the structure in place, and facilitating the work process. This requires a leader who understands the basic differences among work groups and teams, committees, and informal groups. The leader also must be able to think carefully about the work to be accomplished and determine whether it is primarily collective or individual work.

The leader's role includes inspiring members to participate, preparing critical questions, developing agendas and background materials, continually coaching the group for effective functioning, and guiding the long-range strategy. This is a planning, coordinative, and tracking function. Leaders and managers address questions such as the following: What is the task? What is the best way for this task to be accomplished? Is collective work involved? Do we need a team, or will a good work group or committee suffice? How many meetings will it take? How much effort is required? How can the tasks be divided? How can they be delegated?

In planning for meetings, a good leader puts in the time and effort to prepare all the members so that when they come to the meeting, they know what the issues are and they are familiar with the background of the task to be accomplished. The leader facilitates the group coming to some agreement about norms for decision making, length of discussion, when to vote or use consensus, and the process through which the task is completed efficiently and effectively. This is done as a deliberate agenda item that the leader initiates, opens for discussion, and brings to closure. Nurses may find that the group leader role challenges them to plan, organize, coordinate, and evaluate the work of the group.

An effective leader understands that a process is involved in creating effective work teams, highly functioning groups, and committees. The process requires facilitation and a significant amount of coaching from the leader. The leader's style must fit the development stage of the group, with the leader providing more extensive structure and direction in early stages and minimal structure and direction in later stages. Coaching involves the transfer of responsibility to the team or the group. Skill, capability, and readiness of the group must be assessed.

CURRENT ISSUES AND TRENDS

Workforce Shortages

Workforce shortage issues are a primary workforce deployment and health policy concern that is likely to only worsen in the future as retiring Baby Boomers decimate the current workforce. Organizations are struggling with approaches to

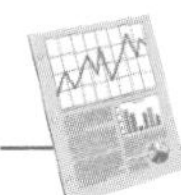

Research Note

Source: Kuhar, P., Miller, D., Spear, B., Ulreich, S., & Mion, L. (2004). The meaningful retention strategy inventory: A targeted approach to implementing retention strategies. *Journal of Nursing Administration*, 34(1), 10-18.

Purpose

Nurses' values often determine whether they remain working with an organization. The purpose of this study was to explore retention strategies that are meaningful for staff nurses.

Discussion

The authors developed, tested, and implemented a tool, the Meaningful Retention Strategy Inventory, in a multihospital system to determine which retention strategies would be of most interest to staff nurses. Both staff nurses and nurse leaders were surveyed. The instrument consisted of 59 items related to job satisfaction that were elicited from an extensive literature review. Among all staff nurses (n = 971), the top three strategies were as follows:

1. Teamwork—staff members' ability to work together to get the job done, 79.6%
2. Periodic increases in salary, 78.5%
3. Support from co-workers, 77.0%

Nurse leaders ranked the following top three strategies:

1. Teamwork, 84.6%
2. Support from co-workers, 80.2%
3. Periodic salary increases, 76.9%

When these factors were compared across various age-groups of staff nurses, teamwork and co-worker support were the most highly rated strategies by all nurses older than 36 years. Younger nurses rated these two strategies in their top four picks.

Application to Practice

The findings of this study support the basic premise of this entire chapter. Not only do nurses work interdependently in the workplace, in groups and teams, but also they highly value teamwork. They identified it as one of the most meaningful retention strategies that could be implemented. Closely related and valued is co-worker support. Although co-worker support can come in a variety of ways, one very effective mechanism is through working together collectively in groups or teams. Thus any managerial or leadership intervention that focuses on developing good and healthy working relationships, strengthening effective group processes, and obtaining meaningful outcomes of group work has a direct impact on reducing turnover rates and increasing the retention of staff nurses.

attract qualified individuals into nursing, but just as important are the strategies needed for retaining them. Unless the workplace environment is positive and affirming, many new practitioners leave all too quickly (Manion, 2005). A key aspect of a positive work environment is the relationships one has with colleagues and co-workers. Groups and teams with healthy interpersonal relationships help foster a strong sense of connection and community among people (Manion, 2004; Manion & Bartholomew, 2003). Another aspect of a positive workplace related to groups is people's need to see problems solved and difficult aspects of work resolved so that conditions improve over time. Effective problem-solving groups are a crucial aspect of making this happen (Manion, 2005).

Collective Leadership and Interdisciplinary Teams

Collective leadership teams are receiving renewed attention as the need for increased leadership capacity in our organizations reaches a crisis. The scope of the nurse manager's role is expanding to include responsibilities for multiple departments and increased strategic leadership demands. Collective leadership is an alternative that increases the capacity of an individual nurse manager struggling to effectively juggle multiple responsibilities. Sharing leadership responsibility is also a way to increase leadership capacity organizationally because it facilitates leadership ability developing at every level in the organization.

Interdisciplinary teams are considered to be essential for the effectiveness of health care organizations and for patient safety. Most patient safety initiatives focus directly on effective communication within the team as a way to reduce errors.

New Methods of Compensation

As health care organizations restructure, reorganize, and implement team-based collaborative practice, new methods of employee compensation are needed. Compensation programs that reward employees only for individual effort become counterproductive to the rewards and incentives needed for effective work teams. Innovative approaches to pay and rewards are needed. The way a compensation program is structured sends a clear message to employees. The old system of compensation needs to morph into a menu of compensation offerings that address both individual and team efforts and productivity.

Using Groups for Innovation

Groups and committees are used as vehicles to promote innovation and change in organizations. One example in nursing is the institution of research-based nursing practice by using a planned change process and a research utilization committee to facilitate the process of incorporating evidence-based practice in nursing. Groups that are skilled in creativity techniques and understand the process of innovation can be very effective in disseminating and implementing evidence-based practice changes.

Other examples of innovation groups and committees are total quality management (TQM) initiatives, continuous quality improvement (CQI) methods such as TQM, and business techniques such as "Lean," "Six Sigma," and rapid-response teams. These techniques are used as ways of addressing problems related to cost and quality. Total quality management is a concept that comes from the work of Deming (Aguayo, 1990; Darr, 1989), who emphasized moving decision making to the worker level. The worker who is closest to actually producing the work is the one with the greatest knowledge and the greatest potential for solving production problems. Deming further recommended work group problem-solving teams. Problems, in Deming's methodology, were defined as systems problems. By contrast, a common way of thinking about problems is to look for an individual to blame. The result of systems thinking is to capture the energy of teams to tackle systems problems.

Following the Institute of Medicine's report *To Err Is Human: Building a Safer Health System* (Kohn et al., 2000), the entire health care delivery system has been challenged to focus on systems problems and review and improve processes and procedures. This work is often done in groups and committees. The overall focus on quality has led to adoption of business management concepts such as "Lean" and "Six Sigma." These are customer-focused and data-driven approaches to deriving best practices. The focus is on reducing process variation and then on improving process capability. Lean focuses on process speed; Six Sigma focuses on process quality.

Whether CQI, TQM, Lean, Six Sigma, or some related program, staff nurses are expected to participate more actively in multidisciplinary teams. In an organization that looks at problems as systems problems, the next step is to acknowledge that anyone involved in that part of the system needs to be engaged in solving the problem. Therefore coordinating client care and solving problems through interdisciplinary committees and groups with people of equal status is the strategy best suited to solving systems problems.

The basic strategy behind each of these systems-based approaches is to bring together interdisciplinary collaborative groups. This means that if there is a problem in client care, the physicians, nurses, ancillary staff, and any other direct caregivers are involved. They get together and collaborate about problems with the client care delivery system and discuss how these problems can be fixed. The facilitator does not have to be a content expert or the person with the most expertise in that problem area. In fact, having the most expertise in a problem area can actually be problematic when functioning as a facilitator because it becomes too tempting to take over the process. The individual's facilitation skills are crucially important.

Establishing equality among peers regardless of status and using expertise and responsibility result in a different way of looking at work, which has implications in terms of how nursing practice may change. It also means nurses are going to continue to be involved more substantially in groups, committees, and teams. To increase effectiveness, a current trend is to address the serious issue of professionals not knowing how to work together in teams (Sorrells-Jones, 1997). For example, one study demonstrated the positive outcomes, including improved physician/nurse communication, by the use of a collaborative approach to standardized protocol development and implementation (Lassen et al., 1997).

Nursing Organizations

An example of a nationwide group approach to problem solving in nursing is the Tri-Council. For years, one of the problems of organized nursing has been that nurses have not spoken with one unified voice. Despite that more than 2 million people are licensed as RNs in this country, nursing previously had not unified to speak on issues of health care policy, acquiring resources for nursing, or responding to the larger profession's needs and directions. The Tri-Council comprises four core groups: the American Nurses Association (ANA), the National League for Nursing (NLN), the American Organization of Nurse Executives (AONE), and the American Association of Colleges of Nursing (AACN). Several states have actually employed this same model to increase the collaboration among these key groups at the local level. The Tri-Council is a network of groups in which representatives of large nursing organizations link together to tackle national professional nursing issues and problems. It is a good example of how the group process can be used positively and constructively and how much clout can be generated by working together and speaking in unity.

There is also an organization of specialty groups in nursing called the *Alliance*, which brings together the interests of all nurses in the various specialties. Formed in 2001 by the Nursing Organizations Liaison Forum (NOLF) and the National Federation of Specialty Nursing Organizations (NFSNO), the Alliance includes a broad range of membership. It allows for joint efforts among associations and nursing groups who have aligned interests. Clearly, the profession of nursing is working to capitalize on the positive synergy and power of collective action that groups and teams provide.

Summary

- Nurses are involved in and accomplish their work through participation in a variety of groups.
- There are many types of groups in health care organizations, including informal groups, work groups, teams, and committees.
- Group interactions are composed of process, standards, problem solving, communication, and roles.
- Groups tend to go through a series of developmental stages that are predictable.
- People join groups to fulfill primary needs and psychological drives.
- There are both advantages and disadvantages to the use of groups in organizations.
- Meetings can be structured for effective group participation.
- The purpose of a group meeting may be for information dissemination, opinion seeking, or problem solving.

- Decision-making power in groups is delegated along a continuum from none to all.
- A group may be formally structured into a committee, a relatively stable group, to accomplish an organizational goal.
- The committee leader has certain tasks and responsibilities to perform in managing the group toward productivity.
- One leadership role is to control disruptive group members.
- Group participation has become an increasingly large part of the nurse's role in practice because of increased complexity of nurses' work, the issues experienced in the workplace, and the increased use of multidisciplinary work groups in complex organizational structures.
- True teams require a great deal of developmental time and effort but are capable of moving the collective performance of a group to a higher level than a work group.

CASE STUDY

Instituting a Nurse-Managed Clinic

Changes in health care require proficient use of resources. Nurses today must actively seek opportunities to make changes in ways that favorably affect their work and patient care. Although we do not always have a say in whether to change the way we work, we have a choice in the way we respond to change. The use of groups to solve efficiency problems is one technique used to bring about effective and efficient change.

One treatment option for advanced prostate cancer patients is monthly hormone therapy. This treatment blocks the body's utilization of testosterone, thereby "starving" the prostate of testosterone and stopping cancer growth. These patients require monthly treatment for the rest of their lives. The population of these patients in our clinic had grown such that the volume was unmanageable. It was evident that a change was required.

Each nurse had his or her own caseload of patients who were seen each month. The norm was that, no matter what the nurse was doing, when his or her patient arrived for an appointment, the nurse would quit what he or she was doing and see the patient. This method of patient care management was adequate until more physicians were added to the department and there was an extraordinary increase in all areas of clinic activity, including procedures, treatments, and clinic visits. The fact that the patient's primary nurse would "drop" whatever he or she was doing when the patient arrived became incredibly disruptive to patient flow in all areas of the clinic. It was obvious that a new method of patient care management was needed.

There was a long history of "each nurse has his or her own patients" to overcome; it was the norm for years. Resistance was expected in changing this norm and instituting a new one. Although most nurses realized the difficulties with the current system, some had fears. For the change to be effective, these fears had to be addressed and all had to participate in the process of defining and implementing the change.

A series of staff meetings were held to address the problem. It was important that the entire staff was present so that each person could participate, voice opinions, and identify fears and uncertainties. With everyone joining in with suggestions, more ideas with which to work were produced. A clinical nurse specialist (a nurse with a master's degree in nursing) in urological oncology was invited to attend the meeting. She had a long history of working with the group when there were difficult patient situations. She also was a former nurse manager, and her management experience was invaluable. She supported the need for a change.

The manager presented the idea of the need for a change and asked the group for suggestions. Ideas were voiced and were augmented by other members until the concept of an innovative nurse-managed clinic, where the bulk of the 90 patients would be seen on a single day, came about. Monday, the day of least patient activity in the clinic, was chosen. The entire concept was a direct result of seeking member involvement; the finalized idea was better than any one person's individual idea. Now that the basic concept of a nurse-managed clinic had been identified, it was time to address the nurses' concerns about this clinic. These fit into three main categories: the adequacy of patient follow-up, decreased patient satisfaction, and the loss of the nurse-patient relationship. All these concerns involved giving up "control" of the patient care and trusting other staff to maintain the quality of care each nurse gave. In the past, each nurse maintained his or her own caseload and had direct control over the patient's care. Each nurse also enjoyed close interpersonal relationships with patients in her caseload.

The group discussed the fact that adequate follow-up was crucial, because if the patient missed a dose of his or her medication, the cancer could spread. Each nurse had previously used his or her own method of scheduling follow-up, and it became obvious that standardization was now essential. This was addressed by standardizing what was documented each visit, including follow-up appointments, by use of a rubber stamp.

Decreased patient satisfaction was another concern. It was evident that patients enjoyed having one nurse to call with questions and that a rapport had developed. This concern also affected nurse satisfaction in that nurses might lose the close relationships with patients and their families that had developed. It was feared that patients would be deeply dissatisfied if they had a different nurse at each monthly visit. As one group member said, "After all, these are cancer patients and they have special needs." The group discussed these fears and agreed that, if possible, patients should see only two or three nurses in hopes of maintaining rapport and trust. This concern was addressed by assigning each nurse a day of the week to see patients. Because the hormone injection was given every 28 days, patients had the opportunity to schedule their visit on the same weekday each month. This compromise also allowed nurses to maintain some of their relationships with patients and their families.

Implementation took about 6 months. Nurses had to change their concept of patient care, but so did the patients. It was each nurse's responsibility to discuss the new care management system with his or her patients and move their appointments to Monday, the chosen day of the new clinic. Surprisingly, few patients resisted.

A standardized documentation and assessment system removed the concern of poor follow-up and standardized the tracking of worrisome patient systems.

Patients are more educated about their disease because the same assessment questions are asked each visit. Patients call with early changes in status, preventing permanent sequelae. Patients usually see one of three nurses when they come for the monthly visit. Some physicians have changed their follow-up of these patients from twice a year to once a year, evidencing their trust in the nursing staff's ability to assess patients and identify problems. A file card system has been implemented to give the nurse immediate access to patient symptoms and information when patients telephone and the patient record is not available. Patient satisfaction has been monitored in a quality assurance study with the result of 100% of patients being "satisfied" or "very satisfied" with their nursing care. This study is repeated biannually.

PART III

CRITICAL THINKING EXERCISE

Organize into a small group; then select a leader. Take a few minutes to do this, and then select or appoint a process recorder. The leader's role is that of a nurse manager at Our Lady of Sorrow Community Hospital. The leader has just been informed that she must cut two nurse jobs immediately. This is part of an immediate reduction in force (RIF) at the hospital to meet some very serious financial reversals. To accomplish the task, the leader has called together your group (the nurses of the unit). The leader has the task of deciding how to cut the nursing personnel budget and must now lead your group to develop a plan while preserving a sense of teamwork. The process recorder is to prepare a summary of the group's work and report as requested.*

Continued

CRITICAL THINKING EXERCISE—cont'd

1. Observe the process the group uses to select its own leader. Did anyone try to avoid selection? Was someone an enthusiastic volunteer? How long did the process take? Were the selection criteria discussed? What were the selection criteria?
2. What method was used to select/appoint a process recorder? What power strategy was used to make this decision?
3. What is the problem identified in the task?
4. What did the group leader do to handle the situation?
5. What should the group leader do to handle the situation?
6. How did group members respond to the task?
7. What leadership and management strategies might be effective?
8. What could the leader and followers consider changing in the situation?
9. How did group members feel about what happened?

Follow up this exercise with one that tackles a similar problem: this time the leader has just been informed of a serious staffing crisis. Nurse turnover during this time of nursing shortage has created a serious coverage problem. Some nurses who have been working 80 hours per week in double shifts are now threatening to quit. A plan for safe coverage needs to be developed.

Involving members in change helps both members and management. Members benefit because they are involved in what affects their work. Management benefits because involvement tends to reduce resistance and increase ownership of the change. The health care delivery system benefits as high-performing teams tackle and solve systems problems and improve patient safety.

*Case study provided by Lynne A. NezBeda, BSN, RN, CURN, Nurse Manager, Urology, Cleveland Clinic Foundation, Cleveland, Ohio.

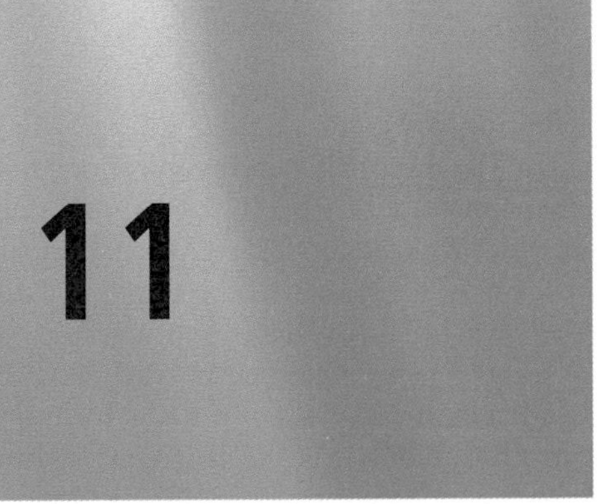

11 Delegation

Maureen T. Marthaler   Diane L. Huber

CHAPTER OBJECTIVES

- Define and describe delegation, delegator, delegate, and supervision
- Analyze the relationships among delegation, responsibility, and accountability
- Outline the seven elements of delegation
- Examine the five steps in the process of delegating
- Evaluate delegation pitfalls
- Identify solutions to delegation pitfalls
- Analyze the legal and regulatory aspects of delegation, assignment, and supervision
- Analyze the use of and delegation to licensed practical nurses/licensed vocational nurses and unlicensed assistive personnel
- Exercise critical thinking to conceptualize and analyze possible solutions to a practice exercise

Delegation is a fundamental aspect of every nurse's job when working with unlicensed assistive personnel (UAP). The effective delegation of work to others is essential in every type of health care setting and organization. Effective delegation skills also are important for managers whose function is to get work done through the labor of others (Poteet, 1989). For most nursing jobs, the zone of responsibility exceeds one person's ability to complete all the tasks (Figure 11.1). This is especially true for the care coordination aspects of nursing care management. Thus nurses need to delegate parts of nursing care delivery to others because, at some point, it becomes impossible to do it alone.

In the 1800s, delegation was defined by Florence Nightingale (1859) as a critical skill: "But then again to look at all these things yourself does not mean to do them yourself.... But can you not insure that it is done when not done by yourself?" (p. 17). Nurses have delegated to paraprofessionals in the health care environment, whether to students, licensed practical nurses/licensed vocational nurses (LPNs/LVNs), orderlies or technicians, corpsmen, medication assistants-certified, nursing assistants, or some other form of nurse extender.

Due to the current and projected registered nurse shortage, a pressing need has been created for more nurses or substitutes for nurses. Meeting the public's increasing demand for quality health care that is both accessible and affordable has created a demand for health care providers and maximized the stress on every health care worker. As a result, the identification of which tasks are appropriate to nursing, which of these tasks can be delegated, and to whom they can be delegated is imperative. Delegation issues have become connected to issues of work overload, safety and quality of care, mix of staff, job security and turf, and nurses' job satisfaction. Delegation of non-nursing tasks also helps reduce health care costs by making more efficient use of nursing time and the facility's resources (Fisher, 2000).

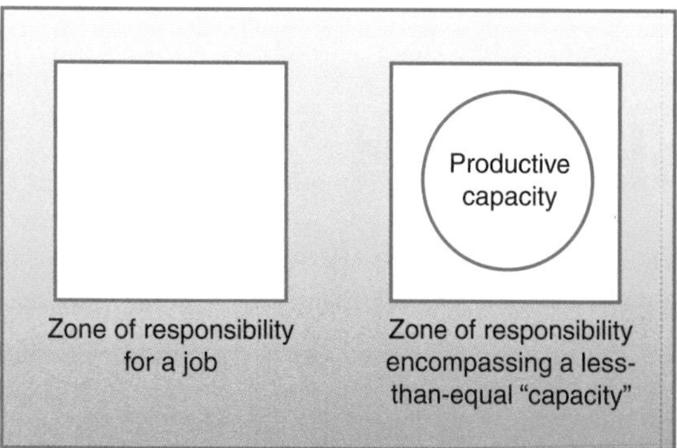

Figure 11.1
Zones of responsibility.

DEFINITIONS

The American Nurses Association (ANA) and the National Council of State Boards of Nursing (NCSBN) in their *Joint Statement on Nursing Delegation* (NCSBN, 2006) defined **delegation in nursing** as the process for a nurse to direct another person to perform nursing tasks and activities. The ANA described this as the nurse transferring responsibility, whereas the NCSBN called this the transferring of authority. The goal of delegation is workload distribution. It relies on trust. The **delegator** is the person—the RN or LPN/LVN—making the delegation. The **delegate** is the person receiving the delegation. **Supervision** is defined as the provision of guidance or oversight of a delegated nursing task. The availability of the supervising nurse occurs through various means of written and verbal communication. **Assignment** is the distribution of work that each staff member is responsible for during a given work period (NCSBN, 2006).

The ANA (1996) defined unlicensed assistive personnel (UAP) as individuals who are trained to function in an assistive role to the registered professional nurse in the provision of patient/client care activities as delegated by and under the supervision of the registered professional nurse. In the past, a nurse extender meant a nursing assistant or a corpsman. A nurse extender was an ancillary person trained to perform some basic client care tasks who may have been given a client assignment.

By definition, UAP work under RN/LPN/LVN supervision. The danger is that organizations may deploy them instead of RNs. For example, since 1975, the New York State Nurses Association has sponsored legislation known as the *Exempt Clause Repeal Bill.* Enactment of this bill would stop the dangerous and anachronistic custom of allowing unlicensed personnel to practice nursing including the administration of medications in state institutions under the jurisdiction of the Office of Mental Health (OMH) and the Office of Mental Retardation and Developmental Disabilities (OMRDD).

The Model Practice Act and Administrative Rules of the NCSBN (2006) provided for a Nursing Assistive Personnel Registry on which anyone who met all the requirements for certification was entitled to be listed. This included the certified nursing assistant (CNA), the certified nursing assistant II (CNA-II), and the medication assistant-certified (MA-C).

The Model Practice Act and Administrative Rules of the NCSBN (2006) goes on to spell out functions for the CNAs, CNA-IIs, and MA-Cs including the administration of medications with the proper training and when done under the supervision of a licensed nurse.

The basic distinction is whether the nurse extender performs direct client care. The definition of what UAP can and cannot do is not exclusive and is difficult to define. Alterations in the skill-mix percentage of RNs to UAP have been moving toward an increase in UAP and a decrease in RNs. Nurses argue that inadequate staffing ratios can create a potentially dangerous situation for client care and safety. In California, nurses have minimum nurse-client ratios in acute care hospitals that were passed in legislation. Staffing ratios are being considered in the U.S. House, U.S. Senate, Florida, Georgia, Hawaii, Illinois, Iowa, Missouri, New York, Oregon, Pennsylvania, Rhode Island, Vermont, and West Virginia (Department for Professional Employees, AFL-CIO, 2007; Global Insight, 2006).

Client care activities include all tasks and activities, mental and physical, necessary to care for clients and produce nursing and health outcomes. Nursing activities involve actions, tasks and direct

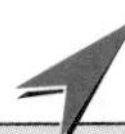

LEADING & MANAGING DEFINED

Delegation in Nursing

The process for a nurse to direct another person to perform nursing tasks and activities. Delegation involves the transfer of responsibility for the performance of a task from one person to a competent second person.

Delegator

The person making the delegation.

Delegate

The person receiving the delegation.

Supervision

The provision of guidance or oversight of a delegated nursing task; the availability of the supervising nurse will be through various means of written and verbal communication.

Assignment

The distribution of work that each staff member is responsible for during a given work period. Assignment occurs when a nurse directs an individual to do something the individual is already authorized to do (e.g., when an RN directs another RN to evaluate a patient complaining of chest pain, the second RN is already authorized to evaluate patients within the RN's scope of practice).

client contact, as well as the full scope of the nursing process. The act of delegating certain activities that are performed by nurses—but are not limited to them—does not create a situation in which nursing itself and the responsibility for it are delegated away. Core activities of the nursing process require specialized knowledge and judgment that only the nurse has.

BACKGROUND

Delegation of care originated from physician responsibilities being delegated to nurses. Nurses began to assume more and more tasks deemed as nursing care to the point that they could not complete them in the limited time frame. Thus phlebotomists, respiratory therapists, physical therapists, and UAP emerged to help provide more comprehensive care. The establishment of the health care team formed around these specialists needing to coordinate work. With this work structure, the need to delegate work arose.

The NCSBN has developed a number of tools relating to the roles of licensed nurses and assistive personnel that are found on their websites (www.ncsbn.org/contcaregrid.pdf; www.ncsbn.org/contcarepaper.pdf; www.ncsbn.org/340.htm). A document was published in 1995 to provide resources for boards of nursing, health policy makers, and health care providers about delegation and the roles of licensed and unlicensed health care workers (NCSBN, 1995). This work remains an important standardized framework for nursing delegation.

In a visual model format, the NCSBN (1998a) illustrated the plotting of RN, LPN/LVN, and UAP roles. This framework contains the two axes of client competency and self-care deficit. This selection of role-appropriate assignment to personnel is placed in the context of the client's needs. Consultation and coordination are identified as key RN roles. Companion documents include *The Continuum of Care Framework* (NCSBN, 1998b), which is a one-page table outlining and differentiating RN versus assistive roles, and a resource paper for regulatory agencies (NCSBN, 1998c).

The NCSBN (1997a; 1997b) developed a decision grid and an algorithm tool based on the delegation decision tree from the Ohio Board of Nursing. It gives specific assessment questions and indicates the path to follow in delegation decision making. This decision tree can be accessed at the NCSBN website (www.ncsbn.org/pdfs/delegationtree.pdf)

for easy review by students and nurses in practice. This caution should be noted: the tool must be altered to make it consistent with each state's nurse practice act and scope of practice.

In 2002, the NCSBN published results of their Practice and Professional Issues survey. Of the respondents, 78.9% of the RNs and 69.9% of the LPNs/LVNs reported providing supervision or direction to UAP. Most reported delegating basic care needs including bed making, baths, ambulation, and feeding. A surprising representation of 6.0% of the RNs and 13.9% of LPNs/LVNs surveyed were likely to delegate to UAP the administration of oral or topical medications.

PROCESS OF DELEGATION

Delegation is a decision-making process that requires skillful nurse judgment. The decision to delegate should incorporate critical thinking and sound clinical decision making. The process is to give a directive, set a time frame, and have periodic reviewing from the beginning of the task through its completion. In most cases, it is recommended that the nurse delegator and the delegate agree on the task, circumstances, and time frame and then arrange for feedback in which the delegate reports or the delegator evaluates progress toward completion of the task. One way to make certain that both delegator and delegate understand what the task is and how to complete it effectively is to follow up a verbal directive with written instructions so that each person can refer to them later. Figure 11.2 displays a sample delegation tracking form that can be generated by UAP to give to the nurse. As a vehicle for clear communication and verification of expectations and consensus, this form can be modified to be specific to each unit. The task should specify a time frame in which the entire task is to be completed.

Decisions to delegate need to be carefully and thoroughly evaluated. A reasonable first decision rule is to be able to delegate the care of clients whose care requirements are routine and standard. Once it is assessed that the person to be delegated to has the minimum competencies required for safe care and if the outcomes of care are relatively predictable, delegation is considered safe. If the client's reaction to illness and hospitalization is not threatening to his or her mental health or sense of self, it also is relatively safe to assume that this care can be delegated to UAP. For example, a client experiencing

Date __________

Task outcome __________

Task steps __________

Task location __________

Delegator __________

Delegate __________

Time frame __________

Decision responsibility/authority __________

Next communication __________

Other __________

Figure 11.2
Delegation tracking form.

an acute episode of hypertension would require the RN as opposed to UAP to monitor the vital signs. As for the LPN's/LVN's assignment, the nurse will delegate the care of clients who are not experiencing life-threatening situations.

In making a decision to delegate nursing tasks, the following five factors can be assessed (American Association of Critical Care Nurses [AACN], 2004):

1. Potential for Harm: The nurse must determine how much risk the activity carries for an individual patient.
2. Complexity of the Task: The more complex the activity, the less desirable it is to delegate. Only an RN should perform activities requiring complex psychomotor skills and expert nursing assessment and judgment.
3. Amount of Problem Solving and Innovation Required: If an uncomplicated activity requires special attention, adaptation, or an innovative approach for a particular patient, it should not be delegated.
4. Unpredictability of Outcome: When a patient's response to the activity is unknown or unpredictable (depending on how stable the patient is), it is not advisable to delegate that activity.
5. Level of Patient Interaction: Will delegation of a particular activity increase or decrease the amount of time the RN can spend with the patient and patient's family? Every time a nursing activity is delegated or one or more additional caregivers become involved, a patient's stress level may increase and the nurse's opportunity to develop a trusting relationship is diminished.

The NCSBN (1995) presented a format for the delegation decision-making process. The decision to delegate needs to be consistent with the nursing process. Thus the nurse needs to ensure appropriate assessment, nursing diagnosis, planning, implementation, and evaluation in a continuous process.

The over-arching determinant for the decision to delegate is the legal scope of delegation as set forth in the state's nurse practice act. Then the qualifications of both the delegator and the delegate are determined. When this baseline is in place, the licensed nurse enters the continuous process of delegation decision making. The situation is assessed, and a plan for specific task delegation is established, considering patient needs, available resources, and patient safety. The nurse needs to ensure accountability for the acts and process of delegation. This includes supervision of the performance of the entire task, any necessary intervention, and evaluation of the task performance and the delegation itself.

The joint ANA and NCSBN statement identifies nine principles of delegation specific to the RN, including:

- The RN may delegate elements of care but does not delegate the nursing process itself.
- The RN has the duty to answer for personal actions relating to the nursing process.
- The RN takes into account the knowledge and skill of any individual to whom the RN may delegate elements of care.

The decision of whether to delegate or assign is based on the RN's judgment concerning the condition of the patient, the competence of all members of the nursing team, and the degree of supervision that will be required of the RN if an element of care is delegated.

The RN uses critical thinking and professional judgment when following The Five Rights of Delegation:

1. Right Task (element of care)
2. Right Circumstance
3. Right Person
4. Right Direction/Communication
5. Right Supervision and Evaluation

When determining the *right task* (element of care) to delegate, the nurse will determine whether the element of care falls within the guidelines of established agency policies and procedures, the ANA Code of Ethics, and legal regulations for practice. The nurse then must consider whether the element of care can be delegated to any other staff members.

The *right circumstance* to perform the element of care indicates the delegate has the available resources, equipment, safe environment, and supervision to complete the task correctly. The *right person* will have the education and competency to perform the element of care. The right delegate will therefore be legally acceptable to complete the element of care.

The *right direction/communication* of delegated elements of care will be a clear, concise description of the task, including its objective, limits, and expectations. The nurse will allow for clarification without the fear of repercussions.

The *right supervision* of an element of care will include appropriate monitoring, intervention, evaluation, and feedback as deemed necessary. A process should be in place for the delegate to report to the RN both that the task was completed and the client's response.

In addition to the five "rights," three organizational principles are to be considered:

1. The RN acknowledges that there is a relational aspect to delegation and that communication is culturally appropriate and the person receiving the communication is treated respectfully.
2. Chief nursing officers are accountable for establishing systems to assess, monitor, verify, and communicate ongoing competence requirements in areas related to delegation, for both RNs and delegates.
3. RNs monitor organizational policies, procedures, and position descriptions to ensure that the nurse practice act is not violated, working with the state board of nursing if necessary.

The five "rights" can quickly help analyze whether a delegation decision will most likely result in a safe outcome. To facilitate the delegation process in a way that will ensure the client's personal health needs are addressed and the nurse's professional goals are achieved, effective communication techniques must be used (Marthaler, 2003). Box 11.1 outlines a personal checklist for the delegator to use for self-evaluation.

True delegation is real to the delegate. Delegators let delegates go on their own but only after instilling in them the highest standards of performance and adherence to a shared vision. The delegate then functions within the standards set by the delegator, who has given authority to do the job, make independent decisions, and be responsible for seeing that the job is done well. True delegation trust is earned over time. For the new nurse who basically has to prove his or her ability to delegate elements of care, this sometimes can take up to 2 years. Effective delegation requires that the delegate have the authority to accompany the responsibility. The delegator monitors the element of care completion and is alert for variances or other problems.

Box **11.1**

Delegator's Checklist

- ✓ Develop a good attitude.
- ✓ Decide what to delegate.
- ✓ Select the right person.
- ✓ Communicate responsibilities.
- ✓ Grant authority.
- ✓ Provide support.
- ✓ Monitor the delegation.
- ✓ Evaluate.

Data from Nelson, R. (1994). *Empowering employees through delegation*. Burr Ridge, IL: Richard D. Irwin.

The essence of the element of care being delegated is often overlooked. Recognition of the potential vulnerability of the client, and thus the presence of an inherently moral element to health care practice, has raised concerns in relation to proper moral regard and respect for clients (Niven & Scott, 2003). This means that nursing judgment about which elements of care are to be delegated requires consideration of the client's unique individual needs at that point in time. For example, obtaining vital signs on a client who is dying may be a reasonable delegation to UAP. However, because a nurse has spent much time explaining the process of the "do-not-resuscitate" status to the family, a trusting relationship has been established. The client's or family members' preferences for treatment/care need to be considered in delegating care activities.

The Joint Commission's 2007 Patient Safety Goal Requirement 2E, *Implement a standardized approach to "hand-off" communications* (The Joint

Commission, 2007), is applicable to delegation. Its provisions include the opportunity to ask and respond to questions. This assists in determining whether delegation can safely occur when a responsible delegator is not physically present. According to the Association of Operating Room Nurses (AORN) (2004), *off-site (indirect) delegation* is defined as direction provided through various means of written and verbal communications. The ANA refers to off-site supervision, and NCSBN refers to indirect supervision (NCSBN and ANA, 2006). For example, the nurse manager will make a list of assignments to be completed by UAP or the unit secretary—for example, check code cart, clean kitchen, clean break room, and restock personal protective equipment containers. The assigned duties for RNs will include who is in charge, who will be responsible to attend codes, or who will perform chart audits. The elements of care are assigned to reflect the ability, experience, and education of the individual delegate.

The ultimate responsibility and accountability rests with the RN because, in the end, the RN is accountable to his or her own superiors for fulfilling the responsibility to get the job done right and on time. Thus true delegation or off-site delegation means giving up some of the authority and holding onto the ultimate responsibility and accountability.

DELEGATION PITFALLS AND SOLUTIONS

Although it is in everyone's best interest to delegate, the process may be undermined from within the health care setting. Delegation suggests that work is being moved from one member of the primary health care team to another in a downward direction (Richards et al., 2000). As a result, the nurse most commonly delegates to UAP. The RN and UAP will naturally have psychological responses to delegation. The UAP sometimes resent the nurse delegating elements of care that could be completed by the nurse. On the other hand, the nurse may find it difficult to let go of control. When elements of care are delegated, strong feelings and reactions occur, including the nurse's desire to keep control. At times, the nurse reclaims some of the delegated responsibility. Nothing is more demoralizing for delegates than to discover that the delegator has undercut their responsibility. Nurses who are novice or insecure or need to feel indispensable are most likely to resist delegation or to "renege" on it later. Their motto is "If you want a job done right, you have to do it yourself." Box 11.2 displays reasons for reluctance to delegate.

Box 11.2

Delegation Reluctance

- The "I can do it better myself" fallacy trap
- Lack of ability to direct
- Lack of confidence in subordinates
- Lack of confidence in self
- Aversion to taking a risk
- Need to feel indispensable and difficulty letting go
- Fear of losing authority or personal satisfaction

Data from *Delegating* (videotape). (1981). Del Mar, CA: McGraw-Hill; and Poteet, G. (1989). Nursing administrators and delegation. *Nursing Administration Quarterly, 13*(3), 23-32.

When called on to delegate something important, nurses may suddenly discover that, for some reason, they do not trust their co-workers quite as much as they thought they did. How can work be delegated to people if they are not trusted? On the other hand, how can UAP earn the trust of the nurse who does not delegate to them? This is a real dilemma, facing both delegator and delegate. The absence of trust by the delegator is based on one of the most powerful of all feelings: fear. This fear is very real for the nurse, especially when it involves a loss of control and their license.

An emotional reality surrounds delegation. Delegation inevitably involves risk. Ignorance of the competencies or the scope of practice of health care team members can cause detrimental outcomes. Likewise, over-delegating elements of care also involves risk but, more important, is dangerous (e.g., allowing a nursing assistant in nursing school to start an intravenous line or asking an LPN/LVN to give discharge instructions because you are good friends and a favor is owed). Delegating an element of care that is completed incorrectly translates into potentially harming a patient and possibly incurring a lawsuit.

Conversely, successful delegation of a element of care may be threatening to a nurse's self-esteem or seen as a nurse's failure to personally accomplish work. This is a natural emotion (i.e., the fear that a delegate might surpass the nurse in ability or prestige), especially for individuals in a new role or job such as a new nurse manager or graduate nurse. The ability to delegate appropriately should be viewed as an achievement and be rewarded, not observed as a weakness or laziness.

In nursing, conventional wisdom and anecdotal experiences indicate how difficult it can be for nurses to delegate effectively. In fact, some nurses may find themselves unable to delegate. Historically, the RN was responsible for providing most of the direct client care, and total patient care delivery models are still in use. Nurses in critical care areas continue to care for patients in this manner. Nurses can become used to providing care themselves and may not learn how to delegate. Graduate nurses typically have had limited experience delegating in nursing school, and they have been delivering direct client care the majority of their time in the clinical arena. The schools of nursing are required to provide theory in delegation and management of patients but do not have requirements for application of these to vital competencies of patient care. The NCSBN (2002) noted that new graduate nurses do not feel their educational preparation adequately prepared them to supervise care provided by others. The NCLEX-RN® examination test plan effective 2007 includes test plan coverage of competencies related to delegation to assess the applied knowledge of new graduate nurses.

Under-delegation can be the result of a lack of motivation to delegate. Some nurses may find that they need to delegate, direct, and supervise others, yet they have no power over the rewards and disciplinary action that motivate cooperation. The new graduate nurse may have a tendency to under-delegate to seek recognition from co-workers that all of his or her tasks were completed by his or her own personal effort. Unfortunately, the new graduate may then be reprimanded for excessive overtime. Nurses may be reluctant to delegate because they feel that they need to complete the tasks themselves, lack the ability to direct, lack confidence in subordinates and self, have an aversion to taking a risk, have a fear of letting go, and have a fear of losing authority or personal job satisfaction (Poteet, 1989).

At times, delegates attempt to avoid delegation by fostering a myth that delegators are so indispensable that they need to do the work themselves. The delegates can actively foster the illusion of the delegator's indispensability. Sometimes this belief is genuine, but it may instead be a way for delegates to avoid being delegated to or accepting more responsibility. Delegates may fear criticism regarding mistakes because they lack confidence in their own abilities. Delegates' most common complaint is that they already have more work than they can handle, when in fact, the delegated elements of care are not extra work but a part of their job description. In addition, they may not have confidence in their own abilities. This can be a matter of reminding delegates that they do have the necessary skills and abilities, especially if they would push themselves a little. The delegator may feel that the delegates do have the job maturity, knowledge, and ability to handle the task, but the delegates may feel that positive incentives are not present. From the UAP perspective, why should they take on something extra or put in more effort if they perceive that they are not going to be rewarded? Box 11.3 outlines reasons why delegates avoid delegation responsibilities.

At times a nurse delegator can, in effect, never relinquish claim on authority by hovering after an element of care has been delegated. Hovering, or "breathing down somebody's neck," usually conveys a feeling of distrust. This behavior may lead to the delegate feeling that he or she really *does* lack ability. Delegation is not meant to intimidate or isolate the delegator or delegate. Having both individuals regard the goal of delegating as being to provide client-centered care in the most efficient way is the optimal delegation approach. Delegating appropriate tasks to the right person,

Box 11.3

Why Delegates Avoid Responsibilities

- Fear criticism for mistakes
- Lack necessary information and resources to do a good job
- Overwhelming workload
- Lack self-confidence regarding ability to successfully delegate
- Positive incentives may not be sufficient motivators
- Delegator's personality and preferences may interfere with the delegation process
- Easier to seek answers from the nurse than to decide on their own how to deal with problems

who can complete the task in an established time frame, will allow care to be completed in a timely manner. Useful strategies are to rotate duties to prevent burnout and capitalize on special expertise (e.g., when a nurse is "good" at starting IVs or caring for disoriented patients). Equally important, delegation can stimulate interest in a nursing career, maintain competencies, spark new interests, and prevent monotony.

Solutions to pitfalls of delegation are straightforward. When individuals are shown respect, they experience a sense of worthiness, of being seen and heard (Rushton, 2007). Licensed nurses and UAP experience an event as positive when they receive feedback and encouragement after delegation (Anthony et al., 2000). Recognizing the importance of the process of supervision and its implications for educational opportunities that focus on delegation competencies is essential for RNs. Peer staff and nurse managers can be consulted regarding delegating nursing activities to UAP or LPNs/LVNs to ensure accuracy. Detailed and specific activities need to be communicated to the delegate. By observing good performance, the RN will gain trust and confidence in UAP's abilities. In short, delegation gains empowerment over the care provided to clients. Ultimately, the chief nursing officer is accountable for delegation standard compliance.

LEGAL ASPECTS OF DELEGATION AND SUPERVISION

Nurses are accountable for following their state nurse practice act, standards of professional practice, policies of the health care organization, and ethical-legal models of behavior (Marthaler, 2003). Each state's governmental agency is the state board of nursing, the majority of whose governing board members are licensed practical/vocational and registered nurses who are empowered to license and/or regulate nursing practice (NCSBN, 2007). When this body interprets the law, the formal interpretations become administrative rules that have the force of law. State nurse practice acts and their official interpretations constitute a body of rules, codified within the legal regulatory system, that govern nursing practice and provide direction about delegation and supervision. The American Nurses Association (ANA) and each state's nurses association are the bodies that speak for the profession of nursing to define and guide the professional practice of nursing through definitions, standards of practice, and statements about delegation and supervision. Most state nurse practice acts contain language that allows registered nurses to delegate. The bottom line is that patients vary in needs, and those needs can be met by various providers of care. Ensuring that needs match the competency of the provider can ensure proper delegation and good patient care.

Standards of care are used to determine whether the minimum level of care has been delivered. The term *malpractice* refers to an improper performance of professional duties; a failure to meet the standards of care that result in harm to another person (Zerwekh & Claborn, 2003). This includes acts of delegation and supervision. When a nurse deviates from the internal standards of care of an organization, the nurse can be liable for malpractice or negligence.

The Iowa Board of Nursing (2003) defined *accountability* as being obligated to answer for one's acts, including the act of supervision. The RN is expected to recognize and understand the legal implications of accountability by knowing what accountability is and what it means in terms of nursing practice. Accountability includes acts of supervision, among other things. In a legal sense, *supervision* means personally observing a function or activity, providing leadership in the process of nursing care, delegating functions or activities while retaining the accountability, and evaluating or determining that nursing care being provided is adequate and delivered appropriately.

Delegation is considered to be part of the nurse's role. Nurses delegate, and they are delegated to. The nurse delegator is accountable to assess the situation and accountable for the decision to delegate. When a nurse delegates, the task must be performed in accordance with established standards of practice, policies, and procedures (NCSBN, 1995). The nurse is ultimately accountable for the appropriateness and supervision of the delegated tasks. Thus the nurse delegator may incur liability if found negligent in the process of delegating and supervising. The delegate is accountable for accepting the delegation and for the actions in carrying out the delegated tasks (Box 11.4). Therefore both the delegator and delegate share accountability. The nurse is accountable for supervision, follow-up, intervention, and corrective action in the event of an error. Assessment, evaluation, and nursing judgment should not be delegated; tasks and procedures may be delegated. Although others may suggest which acts to delegate, the individual nurse ultimately decides the appropriateness of delegation in a specific situation (NCSBN, 1995).

Delegating requires skillful written and verbal communication to avoid liability. If an activity is not documented, it is considered that it was not done. Clear documentation of assignments and additional clarification of the delegated tasks for each health care team member are required when delegating. Courts view written communication as an important reminder of "tasks" and attention to clients (Kraus & Cameron, 2004). The nurse's responsibility is to keep current with updates in the literature and guideline changes in the standards of care of delegation. The institution is responsible for informing nurses of all changes in policy through e-mail, memos, in-services, or staff meetings.

The legal issues associated with delegation include the following:

- The RN remains legally responsible for activities delegated.
- The RN is accountable for appropriateness of delegated task and its accurate completion.
- The organization for which the RN, UAP, and LPN/LVN work is liable for their negligence or malpractice when actions are within standard policy and practice.
- UAP cannot supervise other UAP.
- UAP cannot delegate to other UAP or nursing students.

The state administrative code also identifies nursing behavior that constitutes illegal conduct. This includes delegating nursing functions to others contrary to statute or state rules. Such nursing behavior is subject to licensure discipline. The state regulatory body can use any measure of discipline across the continuum, including revoking a license. In a legal sense, negligence or malpractice consists of failure of a professional person to act in accordance with the prevalent professional standards or failure to foresee possibilities and consequences that a professional person, having the necessary skill and training to act professionally,

Box 11.4

Who Has Accountability?

Delegator

- Own acts
- Acts of delegation
- Acts of supervision
- Assessment of the situation
- Follow-up
- Intervention
- Corrective active

Delegate

- Own acts
- Accepting the delegation
- Appropriate notification and reporting
- Accomplishing the task

should foresee. The nurse must perform at a level that exceeds or equals that of a reasonably prudent professional RN. Generally, practice issues are tested in courts of law. In this process, expert witnesses are used to interpret the standard of a reasonably prudent professional RN.

The nurse has an obligation or duty to act in the event of a breakdown in client care wherever in the chain that breakdown occurs. This means that the nurse is never permitted under law to passively observe substandard care. Delegation and supervision are key areas in which such issues may arise. The most common situation is of a fellow nurse or other health care provider demonstrably or clearly failing to provide the appropriate care to clients. Substandard care also may come about when a health care agency fails to exercise its corporate duty in providing sufficient numbers of RNs with appropriate delegation and supervision skills to ensure quality care. In the event the health care agency is compromising care, the nurse will initiate an assessment of how much client safety is being compromised. If there is clear actual or potential harm, the nurse must act directly. If the situation is ambiguous, such as an ethical issue, then the nurse must take some action appropriate to the circumstance. For example, this may be reported to the immediate superior, or the nurse may refuse to participate if that is appropriate.

Legal and ethical issues surround the tensions and trade-offs between quality and cost. For example, what constitutes an "unsafe" level of nurse staffing is not clear. Nurses face uncomfortable situations when deciding between labor budget pressures and staffing for clients' care needs. At what point does the nurse take action to report "unsafe" staffing levels? What action strategies are effective? How does the nurse who calls the fire department to report serious overcrowding of clients into hallways reconcile the duty to protect client safety with accusations of insubordination and potential job termination? Are there whistleblower protections? It is not uncommon for the nurse to find conflicts between an employer's expectations and the nursing standards of care, resulting in problems such as having insufficient time or staffing to adhere to the standards taught in nursing school or receiving poor evaluations for taking too long to render care (Martin & Cain, 2003).

Clearly, client safety and the obligation to do no harm are fundamental starting points. The nurse can analyze the situation and decide on a strategy. A framework for ethical analysis can be chosen to help clarify values and ethical choices. A legal analysis can be done to assess whether the elements of a malpractice claim appear to be in evidence: duty, breach of duty, proximate cause, and damages. Other assessments can be done by consulting organizational policies and standards, the state's nurse practice act and administrative rulings from the board of nursing, Code of Ethics For Nurses (ANA, 2001) and standards of practice, and standards and guidelines of specialty organizations. A clear legal duty to act is more urgent than is a question of ethics. Through reasoned investigation and analysis of the situation, the nurse then decides whether to act immediately, investigate further, document, report, or analyze the situation for future decision making. The standards of "reasonable," "prudent," and "good faith" form the foundations for legal and ethical decision-making strategies. Ultimately, the chief nursing officer is accountable for ensuring patient safety standards are met (NCSBN and ANA Joint Statement, 2006).

Nurses at all levels should be clear regarding their legal accountability when delegating. Questions regarding situations that may occur include these: What is my responsibility if a student errs or is negligent in caring for my client? What are the legal parameters of delegating to one of the UAP who has had only 2 weeks of training? What can I delegate and to whom?

LEADERSHIP AND MANAGEMENT IMPLICATIONS

Managers and administrators know the quality of care delivered to clients can be affected by the type of working relationships that exist between RNs and UAP (Potter & Grant, 2004). Delegation is a critical yet very difficult leadership and management skill. All nurses need to build a delegation competency.

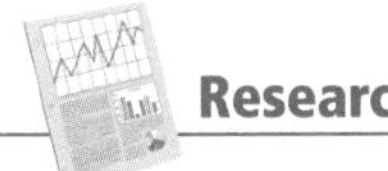

Research Note

Source: Rivers, F., Wertenberger, D., & Lindgren, K. (2006). U.S. Army professional filler system nursing personnel: Do they possess competency needed for deployment? *Military Medicine*, *171*(2), 144-149.

Purpose

The purpose of the study was to identify the perceived readiness of U.S. Army Professional Officer Filler Information System (PROFIS) personnel in the Great Plains Regional Command regarding nursing competency and readiness for deployment during combat missions or MOOTW. Soldiers were surveyed about perceived competency using the Readiness Estimate and Deployability Index (READI).

Discussion

Results illustrated a difference in perceived competency skills, compared with previous studies. The six dimensions of READI were lower in this research than in previous studies using the READI. Participants reported low competency for more than one half of the clinical competency skills, including caring for patients in hemorrhagic shock, implementing documentation in a field environment, reconstituting medications, performing in a code situation, implementing Advanced Cardiac Life Support protocols without a physician, caring for life-threatening injuries, and implementing triage categories. In operational nursing competencies, the participants indicated they had a low level of competency in obtaining a 12-lead electrocardiogram and low to moderate competency skills in deployable medical systems setup. The participants reported low readiness for dealing with death, dying, and carnage. Most thought that they had a low to moderate ability to adjust to crowded/mixed gender sleeping quarters and that they did not have enough opportunity to train with their deployment units. Based on the results of the study, these groups of PROFIS personnel tend to project a perceived feeling of not having the appropriate competency skills needed for deployment. These results support previous research findings regarding medical personnel and deployments.

As military personnel prepare for possible deployment, in view of the present world situation, these perceived feelings could greatly affect mission readiness. Family separation and the unknown greatly influence military deployments. Without the necessary confidence in their nursing skills, individuals could possibly experience even greater levels of stress and discord during deployments, which could affect the quality of care provided.

Application to Practice

Military nursing personnel must be trained to function efficiently for the next military deployment. If medical personnel are not trained effectively, then "many will die as lessons are relearned." Army nursing personnel are at risk of being unprepared without a conceptual model to guide professional practice and training. Individual readiness must be a priority for all nursing personnel, because nurses must sustain the health of soldiers to meet deployment missions. Readiness is fundamental to army nursing-readiness for deployment, readiness for the future of health care.

Nursing personnel must be trained to function efficiently. Nurses are at risk of being unprepared without a conceptual model to guide professional practice and training. Individual readiness must be a priority for all nursing personnel, because nurses must sustain the health of patients to meet patient safety standards.

Delegation means giving up some of the authority and holding onto the ultimate responsibility and accountability. Delegation benefits both nurses and organizations by gaining freedom, time, and greater efficiency from its effective implementation. Unfortunately, the amount of delegation by nurses varies (Richards et al., 2000). Delegation is directly related to leadership effectiveness and the use of leadership styles. It appears that leaders and managers may adopt one of two problem-solving

LEADERSHIP AND MANAGEMENT BEHAVIORS

Leadership Behaviors

- Enables followers to learn delegation and supervision skills
- Creates a positive work climate and teamwork
- Matches leadership style to readiness of followers and situation
- Is visible and available
- Communicates clearly
- Uses interpersonal relationship facilitation to aid group functioning
- Delegates
- Facilitates delegation and acceptance of responsibility

Management Behaviors

- Coaches subordinates to improve task maturity
- Performs careful assessments of abilities
- Is familiar with laws and regulations
- Makes assignments to match skills and abilities
- Monitors performance through supervision
- Documents
- Evaluates task accomplishment
- Provides training and education to develop delegation skills and understanding
- Disciplines employees
- Communicates clearly
- Delegates

Overlap Areas

- Facilitates delegation and acceptance of responsibility
- Communicates clearly
- Delegates

styles: adaptation or innovation. Adaptors generate ideas to solve problems. Innovators detach the problem, critically think about it, and search for a solution. The same may be true for styles of delegation. Individuals may adopt unique styles, and these styles may be a "fit" or a mismatch.

Leader behaviors for delegation and supervision include being around, being available, and helping the delegate through the task actions and decisions. Coaching actions of delegation are expected. Providing guidance and leadership in the development of the nurse's ability to delegate is an important aspect of RN skill building. Delegation is a managerial technique that helps people build skills and confidence. It is hard work and may not come naturally. Mentored guidance and leadership in building the skills related to delegation enhance individuals and build high-performing teams. This makes the facility accountable for delegation through the allocation of resources to allow for adequate staffing so registered nurses can delegate effectively.

Nursing practice in community health or home health care settings may include supervision and delegation of tasks off-site. The importance of the skills involved in assessing the competencies of UAP cannot be overestimated (McIntosh, 2003). Careful assessment, regular visits, and complete documentation are used when delegating in these settings (Barter & Furmidge, 1994).

Certain aspects of managerial work should never be delegated. These are discipline, praise, recognition, and morale issues. Sending others to do the manager's corrective directing is a counterproductive approach to a problem requiring attention. When a problem needs to be addressed in a direct, calm, unemotional, and fact-finding/clarifying approach, the manager is the best person to handle the situation. In addition, the manager should handle the discipline of employees. The direct managerial intervention of discipline maintains a climate within the work group, communicates a message, and shows discharge of duty. For example, if there is an area in which client care is not bringing about quality results or if there is some problem with regard to the delivery of client care, the manager needs to be directly active in the resolution of the problem. At the same time, praise

Practical Tips

Tip #1: Use Clear Communication

Be an open and honest delegator and delegate.

Tip #2: Practice to Standards

Familiarize nurses with national, state, and local practice standards.

Tip #3: Delegate According to Competency

Assess and maintain competencies of staff.

Tip #4: Stay Within the Scope of Practice

Delegate, assign, and make assignments within the scope of practice.

---

and recognition are powerful motivators if given by managers and supervisors.

As delegation and assigning nursing care evolves, potential problems can be assessed. The Institute for Healthcare Improvement (2008) recommended health care facilities use Failure Modes and Effects Analysis (FMEA). FMEA is a systematic, proactive method for evaluating a process to identify where and how care delivery might fail and to assess the relative impact of different failures in order to identify the parts of the process that are most in need of change. FMEA includes review of the following:

- Steps in the process
- Failure modes (What could go wrong?)
- Failure causes (Why would the failure happen?)
- Failure effects (What would be the consequences of each failure?)

Teams use FMEA to evaluate processes for possible failures and to prevent them by correcting the processes proactively rather than reacting to adverse events after failures have occurred. This emphasis on prevention may reduce risk of harm to both patients and staff. FMEA is particularly useful in evaluating a new process before implementation and in assessing the impact of a proposed change to an existing process. It is a formal strategy useful for continual improvements of care delegation processes.

The manager also needs to avoid delegation when there are morale issues. Morale, and its associated aspects of motivation and job satisfaction, should be addressed directly as a function of leadership and organizational management. Leadership style and the interpersonal and communication skills of the leader have a strong influence on employees' morale.

Open a continual dialogue among all nurses about the process of delegation and how to resolve related issues.

CURRENT ISSUES AND TRENDS

Delegation of care continues to evolve within health care teams and from the nurse to UAP. All jobs in the health care team have been expanded. At the same time, financial pressures related to reimbursement have hampered health care facilities' ability to generate sufficient funds to offset costs related to staffing patterns. Is delegation the result of expanded roles? Or was the expanded role the result of delegation?

Increasing demands for nursing care and not enough nurses to meet the demand have created troubled times and add constraints to the number of patients a nurse can care for (Hudspeth, 2007). According to the ANA, "Staffing should be based on achieving quality of patient care indices, meeting organizational outcomes, and ensuring that the quality of the nurse's work life is appropriate" (1999, p. 3). The Registered Nurse Safe Staffing Act of 2003 (ANA, 2003) is an example of how these issues are being addressed in legislation. Qualified foreign registered nurses are being sought to ease the shortage of RNs. In 2006, more than 13,000 first-time NCLEX-RN® examination candidates listed education codes from other countries. Starting in January of 2008, the NCLEX is being administered in South Korea, Hong Kong, Australia, Canada, Mexico, Germany, Taiwan, Japan, India, Manila, and the Philippines. The use of staffing agency or "traveler" nurses has become a significant budgetary problem but a solution to proper staffing. Delegation and supervision issues related to outsource or traveler staff take on a different character and urgency because these RNs are not part of the regular unit employees of the organization. Foreign nurses hold a nursing degree equivalent to a U.S. nursing degree and have had training to successfully complete the national licensure examination, thus indicating their capabilities to care for clients. Their unit orientation, familiarity with policies and procedures, and ability to know and reassess the competency of UAP and other team members may need to be customized and managed differently from that of regular unit employees. As the organization becomes more familiar with the agency or traveler nurse and competence has been established, delegation of tasks will become more extensive. The Bureau of Labor Statistics (2006) estimates that the United States will require 1.2 million new registered nurses by 2014 to meet the needs of the country—500,000 to replace those leaving practice and an additional 700,000 to meet growing demands for nursing services.

It is interesting to note that although cost containment produces downsizing and a dramatic increase in the use of UAP, a nursing shortage also tends to create pressure for the substitution of less-prepared personnel. The ANA's *Joint Statement on Maintaining Professional and Legal Standards During a Shortage of Nursing Personnel* (ANA, 1992) noted that during a time of RN shortage, there is a predictable trend to deregulate, remove, or reduce barriers to entry into the marketplace and substitute less-prepared persons for expediency purposes. Such shifts create serious allied issues related to delegation and supervision for RNs as they attempt to work in environments of fewer RNs and more non-RN personnel.

The end of the 1990s saw economic forces and health care costs come to an intersection. Changes in the health care system led to changes in the numbers and types of personnel who deliver direct care to clients (Potter & Grant, 2004). A decrease in the number of licensed caregivers and an increase in the number of UAP occurred. Hospitals had restructured, redesigned, and downsized RNs without paying attention to evidence-based practice changes or known effects on delegation, supervision, and client safety. While economic and efficiency concerns may prompt providers to utilize unlicensed assistive personnel, The American Nephrology Nurses' Association (ANNA) (2008) believed that the overall accountability and responsibility for nursing care rendered to patients and the coordination of patient care activities, including the provision of dialysis-related assessments and many specific interventions, rest with and are best accomplished by RNs who have been educated in the specialty of nephrology nursing. This "de-skilling" became visible in the 1996 settlement of a lawsuit in Ohio over the 1994 death of a client who underwent a hysterectomy and died because her caregivers were client care technicians, not RNs. The technicians missed the signs and symptoms of infection and shock (American Journal of Nursing [AJN], 1996a). Such reports sparked a round of legislative hearings and debate about regulating UAP by boards of nursing. The issues became contentious as nurses reported low morale, high workload stress, and a shifting of blame for unsafe care onto nurses who were labeled inflexible and not aware of how to delegate. Nurses insisted that mandated nurse-to-patient staffing ratios be enacted in laws. Hospital officials contended that these reports were exaggerated; nursing administrators opposed mandated staffing ratios (AJN, 1996b). These issues of the recent past set a precedent for future rounds of organizational cost-containment initiatives.

The escalating shortage of nurses, greater acuity of patient illnesses, technological advances, and increased complexity of therapies contribute to today's current chaotic and multifaceted health care according to the NCSB and ANA's *Joint Statement on Nursing Delegation* (2006). As health care becomes more complex, the knowledge and skill base of UAP is growing with the expansion of training opportunities, greater experiential learning, and opportunities to make more money (McIntosh et al., 2000). Delegation and supervision always will be intertwined with issues surrounding the use of nurse extenders and UAP. The Joint Commission (2004) stated that effective staffing has been linked to positive client outcomes and improved quality and safety of care. Concerns about declining quality of care and nurse staffing shortages led to legislation mandating minimum nurse-to-patient ratios in the state of California (Hodge et al., 2004).

Decisions about the use of UAP focus on what tasks they are to do and which ones belong only to the RN. Some guidelines include routine care needs, predictable outcomes, and nonthreatening illness states (Box 11.5). The nursing profession is challenged to find ways to balance the tension between professional judgment about care needs and the fiscal pressures of the organization.

Hiring UAP increases an organization's responsibility for screening, orientation, and training. The direct care RNs assume a major responsibility for supplementing minimally trained UAP and for supervising their delegated tasks (Barter & Furmidge, 1994). The ANA's position statement (1992) and the NCSBN's position paper (1995) recommended that nursing's bottom line remain "what is best for the client." The Institute of Medicine (IOM) (2003) released a report titled *Patient Safety: Achieving a New Standard for Care*, which noted, "to achieve an acceptable standard of patient safety… all health care settings [should] establish comprehensive patient safety programs operated by trained personnel within a culture of safety" (pp. 169-170). Thus staffing patterns and methods of care delivery should be scrutinized in terms of client outcomes and basic safety.

Delegation as a part of the RN's role occurs within the context of a care delivery system. The skill mix and care modality structure that best fit care delivery need vary over time and in specific settings and sites. Developing skills for managing role conflict, such as negotiation and delegation, is a useful strategy (Kleinman, 2004). Learning when and how to delegate is a key skill for developing effective nurse leaders and managers and for maintaining quality of care under conditions of rising client acuity, fiscal pressures, and shorter lengths of hospital stays (Hansten, 1991). Furthermore, the nurse ultimately decides and is accountable for appropriate and safe delegation, even when faced with employer pressure and staffing problems (NCSBN, 1990).

Box **11.5**

Delegation to UAP

Clients whose …

….care requirements are routine and standardized
….outcomes are predictable
….reaction to illness and hospitalization is not threatening to their mental health

Summary

- To delegate and assign is essential for every nurse in all health care delivery organizations.
- Delegation is the process for a nurse to direct another person to perform nursing tasks and activities.
- Supervision is the provision of guidance or oversight of a delegated nursing task and the availability of the supervising nurse through various means of written and verbal communication.
- Assignment is the distribution of work that each staff member is responsible for during a given work period.

- Delegation involves an assessment of competency.
- The delegation process involves selecting a capable person, explaining the task and outcomes, giving authority and means to do the task, and keeping in contact with the person delegated to.
- When strong feelings and reactions occur when delegation occurs, managers may be reluctant to delegate or subordinates may resist delegation.
- Delegation and supervision are part of the nurse's role.
- Laws and regulations influence delegation and supervision in nursing.
- The nurse ultimately must decide about appropriate and safe delegation.
- Delegation is related to leadership effectiveness.
- Delegation and supervision are issues surrounding the use of UAP.
- Client satisfaction and outcomes of care should be the same when delegation is used.
- State and health care facilities' policies for delegation should be reviewed regularly by the RNs, LPNs/LVNs, and UAP.

CASE STUDY

The beginning of the day shift when patients are to go for scheduled invasive procedures can be viewed as a very hectic beginning of the day. The night nurse had just finished admitting a patient who was scheduled for surgery within the hour. The consent had not been signed because the patient's daughter was her power of attorney. The patient going for surgery needed cefazolin (Ancef) 1 g, administered IV piggyback 30 minutes before surgery, as a preoperative medication. The surgery department had called to say "pre-op the patient."

Earlier in the week James and one of the UAP discussed how James would let her "do stuff" since she was in nursing school. She was thrilled with the anticipated experiences. Once surgery had called to pre-op the patient, James asked the unlicensed assistant to hang the piggyback as a big favor, since he still did not have the required paperwork completed for the patient to go to surgery. She hung the piggyback, and a few minutes later the patient put on the call light complaining of shortness of breath. The nurse went into the patient's room to find the patient in respiratory arrest. James notices that the piggyback was not hung on the correct patient, and the patient was allergic to the medication that was hung.

How could this happen when the student had been taught the 5 rights of medication administration? What should the nurse do?

PART III

CRITICAL THINKING EXERCISE

The staff on the oncology unit for the day shift (7 AM to 3:30 PM) for nine patients includes Sherry Trader, the charge nurse; James Fair, a recently hired staff nurse; and Julie Coggeshall, one of the UAP, who is in nursing school.

A 78-year-old woman admitted with the diagnosis of breast cancer is scheduled for a radical mastectomy at 8:30 AM. The patient is nonverbal to James, the nurse assigned to the patient. James tells the charge nurse that he has never prepared a patient who was to go to surgery for a mastectomy. The charge nurse indicates to James that the forms are no different from those for any other surgery.

1. What are the key issues to consider about when to delegate and assign care to this patient?
2. What are the problems presented in this case?
3. What are the possible solutions?
4. To whom and what tasks should be delegated to facilitate the patient's progression to surgery?

12

Power and Conflict

Kathleen B. Cox

CHAPTER OBJECTIVES

- Explain the importance of power to the nursing profession
- Describe the dimensions of power
- Differentiate between authority and influence and leadership and power
- Examine sources of individual, structural, and subunit power
- Identify strategies to establish the power base of the nursing profession
- Describe transitions in thinking about conflict
- Explore levels and types of conflict
- Examine components of stages of conflict
- Analyze the causes, core process, and effects of conflict
- Evaluate approaches used to manage conflict
- Exercise critical thinking to conceptualize and analyze possible solutions to a practice exercise

POWER

For many nurses, power has had a negative connotation. With major issues and challenges facing the health care delivery system in the United States and the nature of work in today's complex health care organizations, it is imperative that nurses accept the reality and legitimacy of power. Although the United States has one of the most sophisticated health care systems in the world, there are major issues related to costs, access, and quality. The United States spends more on health care than any other industrialized country. Total spending was $2.3 trillion in 2007, or $7600 per person. Total health care spending represented 16% of the gross domestic product (GDP) (Poisal et al., 2007). An estimated 43.7 million U.S. residents were uninsured when interviewed during the first 9 months of 2007, up from 43.6 million in 2006, according to the Centers for Disease Control and Prevention (Cohen et al., 2008). Finally, from 2004 through 2006, patient safety errors resulted in 238,337 potentially preventable deaths of U.S. Medicare patients and cost the Medicare program $8.8 billion (HealthGrades, 2008). Further, the *2007 National Healthcare Disparities Report* from the Agency for Healthcare Research and Quality (AHRQ) (2008) found that overall inequalities in health care quality and access among different racial, ethnic, and socioeconomic groups have not improved.

The chaos and uncertainty in the health care environment provide unlimited opportunities for the profession of nursing. Manojlovich (2007) noted that power is necessary to influence patients, physicians, and other health care professionals, as well as each other. Increasingly, nurse leaders recognize that understanding and acknowledging power and learning to seek and wield it appropriately are critical if nurses' efforts to shape their own practice and the broader health care environment are to be successful (Schira, 2004). Powerless nurses are ineffective nurses, and the consequences of nurses' lack of power have recently come to light (Manojlovich, 2007). Powerless nurses are less satisfied with their jobs, and more susceptible to burnout and depersonalization. Lack of nursing power may also contribute to poorer patient outcomes

(Manojlovich, 2007). As the largest health care profession, nursing must use power and influence as a legitimate tool to facilitate change in health care organizations and the health care system.

DEFINITIONS

Although power connotes strength and ability, the term *power* has different meanings. It can mean the ability to compel obedience, control, or dominate; or it can be a delegated right or privilege as occurs in the power to enact the staff nurse role. **Power** can be defined as the capability of acting or producing some sort of an effect, usually associated with the ability to influence the allocation of scarce resources. Other definitions identify power as the potential capacity to exert influence, characteristically backed by a means to coerce compliance. A key element of power is its aspect of being potential as well as actual.

The following are the three formal dimensions of power (Bacharach & Lawler, 1980):

1. The relational aspect
2. The dependence aspect
3. The sanctioning aspect

The **relational aspect of power** suggests that power is a property of a social relationship. Many definitions (Bierstedt, 1950; Blau, 1964; Kaplan, 1964; Mechanic, 1962) indicate that power has to do with relationships between two or more actors in which the behavior of one is affected by the other. Weber (1947) defined power as "the probability that one actor within a social relationship will be in a position to carry out his own will, despite resistance, and regardless of the basis on which this probability rests" (p. 52). Dahl (1957) also defined power as an interactive process and stated that "A has power over B to the extent that he can get B to do something B would not otherwise do" (pp. 202-203).

The second formal aspect, the **dependency aspect of power**, was addressed by Emerson (1957), who suggested that power resides implicitly in the other's dependency:

> Social relations commonly entail ties of mutual dependence between the parties. A depends on B if he aspires to goals or gratifications whose achievement is facilitated by appropriate actions on B's part. By virtue of mutual dependency, it is more or less imperative to each party that he be able to control or influence the other's conduct. At the same time, these ties of mutual dependence imply that each party is in a position, to some degree, to grant or deny, facilitate or hinder, the other's gratification. Thus, it would appear that the power to control or influence the other resides in control over the things he values, which may range all the way from oil resources to ego-support, depending on the relation in question. (p. 32)

Dependency is particularly evident in organizations that require interdependence of personnel

LEADING & MANAGING DEFINED

Power
The capability of acting or producing some sort of effect; the potential capacity to exert influence.

Relational Aspect of Power
Power is a property of a social relationship.

Dependency Aspect of Power
Power resides in the other's dependency on the powerful one.

Sanctioning Aspect of Power
Power is an active, direct manipulation of another's outcomes.

Empowerment
Giving individuals the authority, responsibility, and freedom to act on what they know and instilling the confidence to do so.

and subunits. Daft (2006) defined *interdependence* as the extent to which departments depend on each other for resources or materials to accomplish their task. The highest level of interdependence is reciprocal interdependence. Reciprocal interdependence exists when the output of operation A is the input to operation B, and the output of operation B is the input back again to operation A. Daft noted that hospitals are excellent examples of reciprocal interdependence because they provide coordinated services to patients.

The third formal aspect, the **sanctioning aspect of power,** is the active component of the power relationship, referring to the direct manipulations of the other's outcomes. Sanctions can consist of manipulations of rewards, punishments, or both. Sanctions are a significant part of the process through which parties actually affect one another. In summary, power is a property of a social relationship between two or more actors, in which one is dependent on the other. Sanctions are applied in the form of rewards, punishments, or both.

Empowerment

Empowerment is a corollary concept to power in groups and organizations. **Empowerment** is defined as giving individuals the authority, responsibility, and freedom to act on what they know and instilling in them belief and confidence in their own ability to achieve and succeed (Kramer & Schmalenberg, 1990). Thus empowerment has two meanings: the transfer of actual power and the inspiring of self-confidence. Both aspects enable others to act. Empowerment is a key leadership component.

Empowerment for nurses may consist of three components: a workplace that has the requisite structures to promote empowerment; a psychological belief in one's ability to be empowered; and acknowledgment that there is power in the relationships and caring that nurses provide. A more thorough understanding of these three components may help nurses become empowered and use their power for better patient care (Manojlovich, 2007).

Psychological empowerment is a psychological response to empowered work environments and consists of four components: meaning, competence, self-determination, and impact. Psychologically empowered employees feel that the requirements of the job are congruent with their own beliefs and values, which gives the job greater meaning. They are confident in their ability to perform the job, have control over their work, and have an impact on important organizational outcomes. Employees with low levels of psychological empowerment have less capacity to cope with organizational stressors and are more likely to respond passively. Laschinger and colleagues (2007) found that higher levels of structural empowerment were predictive of greater psychological empowerment, which in turn resulted in lower levels of emotional exhaustion and higher job satisfaction. Thus creating conditions that foster a sense of empowerment in managers is important to their well-being and retention.

Employee empowerment became a popular topic in the 1990s, especially in the business literature. With an emphasis on customer service and improving the bottom line through capitalizing on the creative and innovative energy of employees, businesses sought a strategic advantage. Empowerment programs were developed to improve productivity, lower costs, or raise customer satisfaction. However, growing evidence suggests that these empowerment programs fail to meet either managers' or employees' expectations, possibly because although empowerment programs promise employees power, they may not deliver on the promise (Hardy & Leiba-O'Sullivan, 1998).

Empowerment initiatives take two forms. First is the relational approach. The aim here is to improve performance by decentralizing power by delegating power, authority, and decision making. In theory, this reduces organizational barriers to getting the job done. Self-managing teams are one example (Hardy & Leiba-O'Sullivan, 1998).

The second empowerment strategy is the motivational approach. With this approach, there is less delegation of power and more emphasis on open communication and inspirational goal setting. The affective domain is emphasized, with feelings of ownership, responsibility, capability, commitment, and involvement. The goal is to improve employees' self-efficacy, ability to cope with adversity, and willingness to act independently and responsibly. Increasing self-efficacy and decreasing feelings of powerlessness have been linked to effective performance. Examples are training programs for group dynamics and group problem solving.

AUTHORITY AND INFLUENCE

Authority and influence are two major content dimensions of power (Bacharach & Lawler, 1980). There have been three conceptualizations of authority and influence: (1) some authors equate these terms; (2) others tend to equate power with influence and assert that authority is a special case of power; (3) still others view authority and influence as distinctly different dimensions of power. Several points of contrast are summarized in Table 12.1.

Influence Tactics

Kipnis and colleagues (1980) were among the first to investigate the influence behavior of managers. Content analysis led to the identification of 370 different forms of influence behavior, which were condensed into 14 categories. Subsequently, factor analysis brought about the following 8 forms of influence behavior:

1. *Assertiveness* means expressing one's own position to another without inhibiting the rights of others.
2. *Ingratiation* means trying to make the other person feel important—giving praise or sympathizing. Ingratiation is attempting to advance oneself by trying to make another person feel important.
3. *Rationality* means using logical and rational arguments, providing pertinent information, presenting reasons, and laying out an idea in a logical, structured way.
4. *Sanctions* are threats. Positive sanctions, or rewards, are addressed within motivation mechanisms.
5. *Exchange* means that to persuade, an exchange is offered; this is sometimes called "scratching each other's back."

Table 12.1

Authority and Influence Contrasted

Authority	Influence
Authority is the static, structural aspect of power in organizations.	Influence is the dynamic, tactical element.
Authority is the formal aspect of power.	Influence is the informal aspect.
Authority refers to the formally sanctioned right to make decisions.	Influence is not sanctioned by the organization and is, therefore, not a matter of organizational rights.
Authority implies involuntary submission by subordinates.	Influence implies voluntary submission and does not necessarily entail a superior-subordinate relationship.
Authority flows downward, and it is unidirectional.	Influence is multidirectional and can flow upward, downward, or horizontally.
The source of authority is solely structural.	The source of influence may be personal characteristics, expertise, or opportunity.
Authority is circumscribed.	The domain, scope, and legitimacy of influence are typically ambiguous.

6. *Upward appeal* means going to a higher authority—the childhood threat of "if you don't play by my rules, I am going to go tell Mom." Upward appeal simply means taking the appeal to a higher authority to arbitrate.
7. *Blocking* means deliberately keeping others from getting their way, threatening to stop working with them, ignoring them, not being friendly, or simply attempting to make sure others cannot accomplish their aims.
8. *Coalitions* are the result of a group of people getting together to speak or negotiate as one voice.

In their three-nation study of managerial influence styles, Kipnis and colleagues (1984) identified the most-to-least-popular strategies (Table 12.2).

Yukl and Falbe (1991) continued the work of Kipnis and colleagues (1980). They developed an instrument, the Influence Behavior Questionnaire (IBQ), to measure the influence behavior of managers. In later studies, the IBQ was developed further and psychometric tests were performed (Yukl et al., 1992; Yukl et al., 1993). The nine tactics cover a wide range of influence behavior relevant for managerial effectiveness or, in a broader sense, for getting things done in an organization. Influence tactics are identified in Table 12.3.

SOURCES OF POWER

Individual Sources of Power

Although multiple mechanisms of power have been identified, the most widely accepted power base classification is French and Raven's (1959) five sources of power. Their original conceptualization identified the following five power sources (Box 12.1):

1. Reward
2. Coercive
3. Expert
4. Referent
5. Legitimate

When reward power is used, people comply because doing so produces positive benefits. Coercive power depends on fear. An individual reacts to the fear of the negative consequences that might occur for failure to comply. Referent power is based on admiration for a person who has desirable resources or personal traits. Legitimate power represents the power a person receives as a result of his or her position in the formal organizational hierarchy. Expert power results from expertise, special skill, or knowledge. The problem with the French and Raven typology is that the list is not exhaustive and it ignores organizational sources of power. Figure 12.1 shows a combined conceptual framework for power that blends elements of multiple theories of power.

Table 12.2

Most-to-Least-Managerial Influence Strategies Used in All Countries

Strategy's Popularity	Managers Influencing Superiors	Managers Influencing Subordinates
Most popular ↑	Reason	Reason
	Coalition	Assertiveness
	Friendliness	Friendliness
	Bargaining	Evaluation
	Assertiveness	Bargaining
	Higher authority	Higher authority
↓ Least popular	Sanction	

Modified from Kipnis, D., Schmidt, S.M., Swaffin-Smith, C., & Wilkinson, I. (1984). Patterns of managerial influence: Shotgun managers, tacticians, and bystanders. *Organizational Dynamics, 12*(3), 58-67.

Table 12.3

Definitions of Influence Tactics

Tactic	Definition
Rational persuasion	The agent uses logical arguments and factual evidence to persuade the target that a proposal or request is viable and likely to result in the attainment of task objectives.
Inspiration appeals	The agent makes a request or proposal that arouses target enthusiasm by appealing to his or her values, ideals, and aspirations or by increasing target self-confidence.
Consultation	The agent seeks target participation in planning a strategy, activity, or change for which target support and assistance are desired, or the agent is willing to modify a proposal to deal with target concerns and suggestions.
Ingratiation	The agent uses praise, flattery, friendly behavior, or helpful behavior to get the target in a "good mood" or to think favorably of the agent before asking for something.
Personal appeals	The agent appeals to target feelings of loyalty and friendship toward him or her before asking for something.
Exchange	The agent offers an exchange of favors, indicates willingness to reciprocate at a later time, or promises a share of the benefits if the target helps to accomplish a task.
Coalition tactics	The agent seeks the aid of others to persuade the target to do something or uses the support of others as a reason for the target to agree as well.
Legitimating tactics	The agent seeks to establish the legitimacy of a request by claiming the authority or right to make it or by verifying that it is consistent with organizational policies, rules, practices, or traditions.
Pressure	The agent uses demands, threats, frequent checking, or persistent reminders to influence the target to do what the agent wants.

From Yukl, G., Falbe, C., & Joo, Y.Y. (1993). Patterns of influence behavior for managers. *Group and Organization Management, 18*(1), 5-28.

Other Sources of Power

Raven and Kruglanski (1975) and Hersey and colleagues (1979) identified two additional sources of power: (1) connection power; and (2) information power. A third type of power also has been identified: (3) group decision-making power (Liberatore et al., 1989). These three other sources of power are related to groups and organizations specifically, as opposed to French and Raven's (1959) original five sources of power, which relate more to an individual.

Within organizations, the power of connections comes from networking or knowing people and from being able to go across lines laterally to gather information. For example, this occurs when a nurse knows a colleague in another facility with whom to exchange information. For a nurse to know what

Box 12.1

French and Raven's Five Sources of Power

1. ***Reward power*** is giving something of value. For example, in nursing, rewards may be a pay raise, praise, a promotion, or a job on the day shift. Reward power is based on the ability to deliver desired rewards.
2. ***Coercive power*** is force against the will. For example, in nursing, coercive power can be the threat of firing, of disciplinary action, or other negative consequences. Coercive power is the power derived from an ability to threaten punishment and deliver penalties. It is a source of power used to apply pressure so that others will meet what is demanded.
3. ***Expert power*** means the use of expertise. It is knowledge, competence, communication, and personal power all combined in a reservoir of knowledge and experience. Expert power is a source of power held by those with some special knowledge, skill, or competence in a particular area. For example, the nurse with the greatest expertise in wound dressings will be sought out by other people in the work environment for this expertise. Expertise is an artful combination of skill and knowledge. It may be founded on depth of knowledge and/or psychomotor skill. In the use of knowledge and skill is power (i.e., because people need you or can benefit from your expertise, power exists). Therefore the use of expertise can be structured to accomplish or influence movement or action toward certain goals.
4. ***Referent power*** is a little more difficult to understand because it is subtle. It is the use of charisma to influence others. The followers of someone with referent power respond positively to the interpersonal communication and image of the charismatic person. In organizations, this translates into an informal leadership based on liking, charisma, or personal power. Referent power comes from the affinity other people have for someone. They admire the personal qualities, the problem-solving ability, the style, or the dedication the person brings to the work. Referent power can be viewed as an inspirational power, because people's admiration for someone allows that person to influence without having to offer rewards or threaten punishments. For example, in the political arena, occasionally there are charismatic political figures or orators. Their influence comes from their followers' liking or identification with them. An example in nursing is Florence Nightingale, who became a symbol of professional nursing. An emotional upsweep is felt by associating with a charismatic person. Referent power is a personal liking and identification experienced by others. Followers attribute referent power to a leader on the basis of the leader's personal characteristics and interpersonal appeal. Physical attractiveness may contribute to referent power.
5. ***Legitimate power*** means position power. It is the right to command within the organizational structure, based on the hierarchical position held. The President of the United States has power because of holding the position. Legitimate power is the most common source of power. It is what most often is called *authority.* The authority of position gives the person the right to act, order, and direct others. However, leadership and influence need not be confined to those with authority. Every person possesses the ability to tap different sources of power to use in a variety of situations.

Data from French, J., & Raven, B. (1959). The bases of social power. In D. Cartwright (Ed.), *Studies in social power* (pp. 150-167). Ann Arbor, MI: University of Michigan, Institute for Social Research.

effective nursing interventions are being used by other institutions helps the institution to be competitive and current. *Connection power* is one strategy to get information accurately and reliably. It also may be manifested as power based on having connections with powerful others. Connection power is based on another's perception that the influencer has access to powerful persons or groups.

Information is power. If information is given away, its power may be lost. This is especially true in situations that require negotiation. If information is used strategically, its possession can be a strong source of power. *Information power* is a source of power that can stem from any person in the organization. Kanter's (1977) research suggested that control of resources, especially information, is a

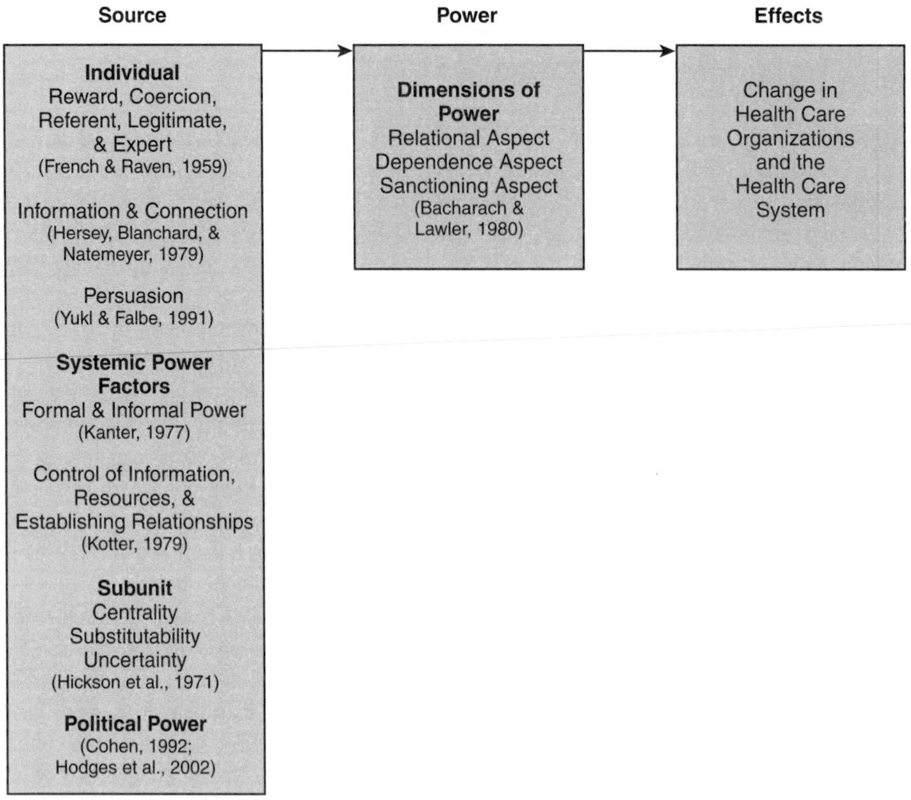

Figure 12.1
Conceptual framework for power.

major organizational power source. Information power is based on another's perception that the influencer either possesses or has access to information valuable to another.

Another source of power is derived from *group decision making*. This means that a creative synergy and force is created when a group comes together, makes decisions, and acts as a united front. For example, some professional groups have formed strong lobbies to influence state and national legislation. With more than 2.5 million licensed registered nurses in the United States, group decision making with resultant unity of action could be a powerful strategy for nurses to use to advance nursing's goals or policy agenda.

Persuasive power is an additional source of power identified by later researchers investigating French and Ravens' (1959) taxonomy. *Persuasive power* refers to skill in making rational appeals (Yukl & Falbe, 1991). Yukl and Falbe (1991) differentiated between position power and personal power. According to these authors, position power consists of legitimate, reward, coercive, and information power. Personal power consists of expert, referent, persuasive power.

In her structural theory of organizational behavior, Kanter (1977) asserted that "those with sufficient power are able to accomplish the tasks required to achieve organizational goals" (p. 166). Conditions in the work environment influence how much productive power is available to employees. According to Kanter, formal and informal systemic structures are the sources of workplace empowerment. Job discretion, recognition, and relevance to organizational goals are important dimensions of formal power. High levels of job discretion ensure that work is non-routinized and permit flexibility, adaptation, and creativity. Recognition reflects visibility of an employee's accomplishments among peers and supervisors. For example, an innovative staff development director or nurse manager whose techniques are reported in a respected nursing journal will enhance his or her influence in the hospital. Finally, relevance of job responsibilities and accomplishments to the organization's strategic plan or current problems is also important. A nurse who publishes will probably not accrue much power when the hospital's census is consistently low and Medicare reimbursement is down. The nurse may not be seen as contributing to the solution of pressing organizational problems. Another key systemic structure is informal power, which comes from the employee's network of interpersonal alliances or relationships within and outside an organization. Relationships with people at higher hierarchical levels confer approval, prestige, and backing, whereas peer networks provide reputation and "grapevine" information (Kanter, 1977).

In Kanter's model, individuals with high levels of formal and informal power have access to structures of productive power within an organization. These structures include lines of information, lines of support, and lines of resources/supply. The lines of information involve formal information that is necessary to carry out a job, as well as informal information that concerns the current state of affairs within an organization. Lines of support include positive feedback from superiors and important others, as well as support for job autonomy. Lines of resources address the ability to obtain the materials, money, and rewards necessary for achieving job demands. Access to opportunity for professional growth and movement in the organization completes the necessary tools for success at work. Kanter claimed that working in these conditions has a positive impact on employees (i.e., increased feelings of self-efficacy and job satisfaction, higher motivation, and less burnout). These empowering conditions create more productive work environments because employees are highly effective and more satisfied with their jobs, more committed to organizational goals, more likely to try out innovative approaches to work, and less likely to be stressed at work or to change jobs.

Kanter's theory has been tested extensively in nursing populations. These populations have been found to be only moderately empowered, with varying levels of access to information, support, opportunity, and resources (Laschinger & Havens, 1997; Laschinger, Finegan, Shamian, & Wilk, 2001). Higher levels of structural empowerment have been associated with higher levels of organizational commitment (Laschinger et al., 2000), greater participation in organizational decision making (Laschinger et al., 1997), higher levels of job autonomy (Sabiston & Laschinger 1995), higher levels of job satisfaction (Laschinger & Havens 1997; Laschinger, Finegan, & Shamian, 2001), and greater organizational trust (Laschinger et al., 2000). All these findings lend support to Kanter's theory.

Kotter (1979) maintained that the basic methods for acquiring and maintaining power are gaining control over tangible resources, obtaining information and control of information channels, and establishing favorable relationships. Basically, acquiring and maintaining power is an exercise in developing credibility by getting people to feel obligated in some way, building a good professional reputation through visible achievement, encouraging identification by trying to look and behave in ways that others respect, and finally, creating perceived dependence either for help or security. The keys to success at gaining power are as follows:

- Be sensitive to where power exists in the organization.
- Take calculated risks.
- Recognize that all actions can affect power, and avoid actions that will decrease it.
- Try to move up in the organizational hierarchy and toward positions that control a strategic contingency for the organization.

In summary, control of information and resources and development of support systems are common elements in both Kanter's and Kotter's theories.

THE POWER OF THE SUBUNIT

Subunit or horizontal power pertains to relationships across departments. Daft (2006) noted that although each department makes a unique contribution to organizational success, some contributions are greater than others. Pfeffer (1981) identified the following structural determinants of power within organizations:

- *Power is derived from dependence.* Simply stated, power comes from having something that someone else wants or needs and being in control of the performance or resource so that there are few, if any, alternative sources for obtaining what is desired.
- *Power is derived from providing resources.* Organizations require a continuing provision of resources such as personnel, money, customers, and technology in order to continue to function. Those subunits or individuals within the organization that can provide the most critical and difficult-to-obtain resources come to have power in organizations. Their power is derived from their ability to furnish those resources upon which the organization most depends.
- *Power is derived from coping with uncertainty.* Coping with uncertainty is a critical resource in the organization since it ensures organizational survival and adaptation to external constraints.
- *Power is derived from being irreplaceable.* Members must not only provide a critical resource for the organization but also prevent themselves from being readily replaced in that function. The degree of substitutability is not a fixed thing, however, so one might expect that various strategies will be employed by individuals and subunits who are interested in enhancing their power within the organization. Some of these might involve the availability of documentation, use of specialized language, centralization of knowledge, and maintenance of externally-based sources of expertise.
- *Power is derived from the ability to affect the decision process.* Because decisions are made in a sequential process, it is possible for an individual to acquire power because of his or her ability to affect the premises of basic values or objectives used in making any decision. A person can gain power by influencing the information about the alternatives being considered in the decision process.
- *Power is derived if there is a shared consensus within the organizational subunit.* If individuals within a subunit share a common perspective, set of values or definition of the situation, they are likely to act and speak in a consistent manner and present to the larger organization an easily articulated and understood position and perspective. Such a consensus can serve to enhance the power of the subunit among other organizational members.

The Strategic Contingencies Theory of intra-organization power proposed by Hickson and colleagues (1971) specified the conditions for the differentiation of power among organizational subunits. The Strategic Contingencies Theory of power relates the power of a subunit to its coping with uncertainty, substitutability, and centrality, through the control of strategic contingencies. *First*, according to Strategic Contingencies Theory, a unit will become powerful if it is able to control scarce resources that are important to the organization as a whole. *Second*, a unit will become powerful if it is able to control uncertainty. Organizations fear the unknown, because unanticipated events create havoc with financial commitments, long-range plans, and tomorrow's operations. Sources of uncertainty include a change in governmental policies, changes in supply and demand, and an unexpected downturn in the economy. *Third*, a unit will become powerful if its activities are central to the workflow of the organization. Subunits may influence the work of most other subunits. Centrality also exists when a subunit has an especially crucial impact on the quantity or quality of the organization's key product or service. A subunit's activities are more central when their impact is more immediate. Several studies in the management literature have provided support for

Practical Tips

Tip # 1: Handle Disruptive Conflict

If not handled productively, conflicts can be a disruptive rather than a constructive force.

Tip # 2: Manage Negativity

A first step in managing a conflict is to reverse the negative emotion associated with the conflict situation.

Tip # 3: Remember That Communication is Key

The key to resolving most conflict situations is good communication skills.

this theory (Crozier, 1964; Hinings et al., 1974; Salancik & Pfeffer, 1974). Dennis (1983) suggested that the nursing profession would do well to listen to and study the advice of Hinings and colleagues (1974): "For dominant power, take advantage of immediacy, reduce your substitutability, and then make a bid for a decisive area of uncertainty... but don't get involved in a network of interaction links before you can dominate it" (p. 56). In other words, find ways to help the organization decrease uncertainty, position yourself to be central rather than peripheral, and make your function indispensable or non-substitutable.

The Theory of Group Power within organizations was developed from a synthesis and reformulation of King's (1981) interacting systems framework and the Strategic Contingencies Theory of power (Hickson et al., 1971). Variables within the Strategic Contingencies Theory of power and their relationships were reformulated within King's framework. These variables are controlling the effects of environmental forces, position, resources, and role. Sieloff (2003) noted that although nursing groups are proposed to have a power capacity resulting from controlling the effects of environment forces, position, resources, and role, not all nursing groups have acted powerfully. Therefore four additional concepts were added to the theory as variables that intervened between a nursing group's power capacity and its ability to actualize that power capacity. These concepts are communication competency, goal/outcome competency, nurse leader's power competency, and power perspective. Every nursing group has a power capacity. The group has the potential to achieve its goals and become a more visible contributor to the progress of the organization. The value of the theory is that it provides nurse leaders at all levels with strategies that could be implemented to improve a nursing group's actualized power (Sieloff, 2003).

LEADERSHIP AND MANAGEMENT IMPLICATIONS

Robbins and Langton (1999) differentiated between power and leadership and indicated that the two concepts are closely intertwined. Leaders use power as a means of attaining group goals. Leaders achieve goals, and power is a means of facilitating goal achievement. One of the main differences between the two concepts relates to goal compatibility. Power requires dependence, but it does not require goal compatibility. On the other hand, leadership requires congruence between the goals of the leader and those being led. In addition, power focuses on intimidation, whereas leadership focuses on downward influence. Power maximizes the importance of lateral and upward influence, but leadership minimizes the importance of lateral and upward influence. Finally, power focuses on tactics for gaining compliance, whereas leadership research focuses on answers (Robbins & Langton, 1999).

Purpose

Ponte and colleagues' (2007) discussions with nurse leaders were guided by two specific aims: (1) to determine the characteristics of professional nursing power that practicing nurses believe are important at the individual level; and (2) to define strategies to help nurses attain power within their practice. Eleven nurse leaders, including a clinical nurse specialist, nurse manager, vice president, program manager, nurse scientist, dean, chief retention officer, and nurse faculty member, participated in the discussion. In the discussions, seven questions were posed, and the nurse leaders were asked to think about power in the broadest sense and to speak about what power means to them and how it is manifested in their practice and organization.

Discussion

Results of the discussions indicated that nurses who have developed a powerful nursing practice do the following:

- Acknowledge their unique role in the provision of patient- and family-centered care
- Commit to continuous learning through education, skill development, and evidence-based practice
- Demonstrate professional comportment and recognize the critical nature of presence
- Value collaboration and partner effectively with colleagues in nursing and other disciplines
- Actively position themselves to influence decisions and resource allocation
- Strive to develop an impeccable character; to be inspirational and compassionate, and to have a credible, sought-after perspective (the antithesis of power as a coercive strategy)
- Recognize that the role of the nurse leader is to pave the way for nurses' voices to be heard and to help novice nurses develop into powerful professionals
- Evaluate the power of nursing and the nursing department in organizations they enter by assessing the organization's mission and values and its commitment to enhancing the power of diverse perspectives

Application to Practice

Although the theoretical underpinnings that helped guide the methodology and analysis of findings were not presented, the results of the discussions provided insight into these nurse leaders' perceptions of power. As the authors noted, the results support existing literature on power and have implications for other group discussions that will assist nurse leaders to clarify what power means to them and to develop behaviors that enhance power. Finally, the report has implications for future qualitative studies in which the theoretical underpinnings are clearly identified.

POWER AND LEADERSHIP

Power and leadership are closely connected and highly intertwined concepts. This is because power is one of the vehicles by which a leader influences followers to take action. Nurses may be inclined to avoid an acknowledgment or analysis of power. However, to lead and manage, nurses need to acquire, possess, and use power.

Hersey and colleagues (2008) described the relationships among concepts of style of leadership, readiness level of followers, and power base use. They indicated that the readiness of the followers dictates which leadership style is likely to be successful and which power base would most successfully influence followers' behavior. Combining these concepts maximizes the leader's probability of success. Thus nurses should be able to use Situational Leadership® Theory to assess and predict style choice and power source use based on the situation and readiness of followers.

Readiness is the ability and willingness of individuals or groups to take responsibility for directing their own behavior in a situation. There appears to be a direct relationship between the level of readiness in individuals and groups and the power base type that has a high probability of effectiveness (Figure 12.2). Readiness is a task-specific concept. At the lowest level of readiness, coercive power is most appropriate. As people move to higher readiness levels, connection power, then reward, then

*Situational Leadership® is the registered trademark of the Center for Leadership Studies in Escondido, CA 92025. All rights reserved.

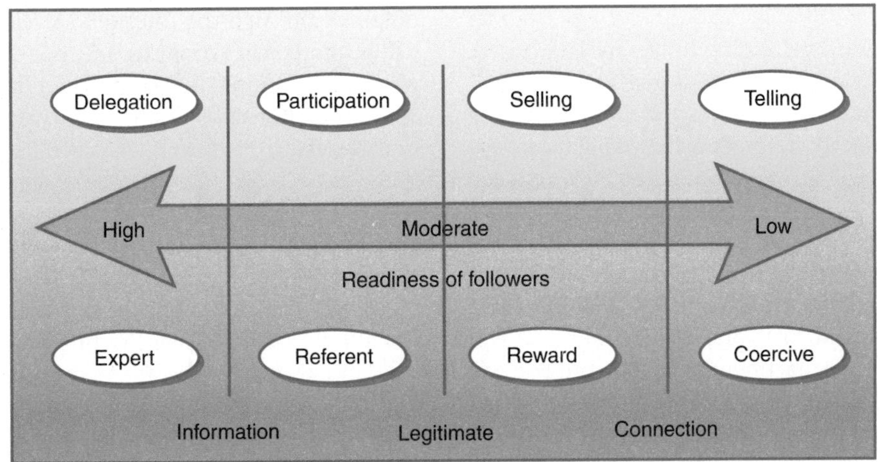

Figure 12.2
Power related to leadership. (Data from Hersey, P., Blanchard, K.H., & Johnson, D.E. [1996]. *Management of organizational behavior: Utilizing human resources* [7th ed.]. Upper Saddle River, NJ: Prentice-Hall.)

legitimate, then referent, then information, and finally, expert power impact the behavior of people. At the highest level, the followers have competence and confidence and they are most responsive to expert power (Hersey et al., 2008).

If power is the basic energy needed to initiate and sustain action, then power is a quality without which a leader cannot lead. Power is fundamental to leadership, in that leadership may be the wise use of power. This is especially true for transformative leadership (Bennis & Nanus, 1985). Power need is highly desirable in leaders and managers because power is necessary in influencing others. Assertiveness and self-confidence are associated with power and leadership. Leadership may be characterized as power in the service of others (Kouzes & Posner, 1987). For nurses, this may mean that they need to view power as an integral part of their professional roles in care management and client advocacy. Nursing leadership requires a willingness and ability to take on a power role and to expand the use of power bases.

All of these theories provide insight into the nature of power. Although the Strategic Contingencies Theory specified the conditions for the differentiation of power among organizational subunits, certainly the principles of uncertainty, centrality, and substitutability can be applied to increase the power of the nursing profession within organizations and also within the health care system. In addition, Sieloff's (2003) notion of leadership behaviors that foster nursing group power is also relevant.

Uncertainty

Nurses must demonstrate that they can cope with uncertainty. Examples of uncertainties include, but are not limited to, patient safety, the aging population, chronic diseases, bioterrorism, and technology, as well as access, costs, and quality of health care.

Quality of Care and Patient Safety

In November 1999, the Institute of Medicine (IOM) issued a comprehensive report on medical errors, *To Err Is Human: Building a Safer Health System* (Kohn et al., 2000). Speaking to the seriousness of the problem and issuing a call for action on the part of nurses and others, the report indicated that it is not acceptable for patients to be harmed by the health care system. Obviously, nurses who are directly involved with patients must play a key role in the assessment of organizational safety, creation of safer systems, and implementation and evaluation of those systems.

Aging Population

The population's increasing longevity is a source of uncertainty and a driving force for the development of improved services for the elderly. The number of elderly, defined as the population "age 65 and over," will grow by more than 50% between 2000 and 2020 and by an estimated 127% by 2050. Furthermore, the relative size of the elderly population is projected to increase from 12.6% of the population in 2000 to an estimated 16.5% in 2020. Between 2030 and 2050, one in five Americans will be elderly (U.S. Department of Health and Human Services, 2003). Nurses can increase power by demonstrating that they can maintain the health of the elderly and provide skilled nursing care in home and community settings.

Technology

The rapid growth in information technology has already affected health care delivery, and nurses need to be skilled in the use of computer technology. Developing expertise in new technology for diagnosis and treatment, as well as telemedicine, will enable nursing to become invaluable and indispensable.

Use of health care websites by consumers tripled in 2002 as individuals spent more time exploring their options before making health care decisions (Stokowski, 2004). However, many consumers will need assistance in understanding their options and making the decisions that are best for them. In a recent Harris poll, 92% of consumers indicated that they trusted the information nurses gave to them (Ulrich, 2001). Therefore nurses are well positioned to assume a central role as advisors and teachers.

The quality of consumer health information on the Internet is an important issue for nursing. The large volume of health information resources available on the Internet has great potential to improve health, but it is increasingly difficult to determine which resources are accurate or appropriate for users. Because of the potential for harm from misleading and inaccurate health information, the profession has a responsibility to ensure the availability and accuracy of information obtained through the Internet. Developing expertise in the use of computer technology is another way of becoming invaluable and indispensable and of demonstrating the ability to cope with uncertainty.

Chronic Disease

For millions of Americans, living with chronic disease is a way of life. Research is needed to determine best practices for care and management of chronic disease. To turn the tide on chronic disease, nurses need to be at the forefront of efforts to provide education for young and old clients on healthy lifestyles including diet, exercise, and stress management (Stokowski, 2004). Chronic diseases are the leading causes of death and disability in the United States. Chronic diseases account for 70% of all deaths in the United States, which is 1.7 million each year. These diseases also cause major limitations in daily living for almost 1 of 10 Americans or about 25 million people. Although chronic diseases are among the most common and costly health problems, they are also among the most preventable. Adopting healthy behaviors such as eating nutritious foods, being physically active, and avoiding tobacco use can prevent or control the devastating effects of these diseases (Centers for Disease Control and Prevention [CDC], 2008). By demonstrating the ability to handle this uncertainty, nursing can assume a central role in improving the care of the chronically ill.

Infectious Diseases and Bioterrorism

Recent years have seen the appearance of antibiotic-resistant infections, lethal strains of influenza, West Nile virus, severe acute respiratory syndrome (SARS), mad cow disease, and drug-resistant tuberculosis. In addition, the acquired immune deficiency syndrome (AIDS) virus continues to mutate and spread, and the threat of bioterrorism carries the risk for infecting millions with smallpox or anthrax. Rebmann (2006) pointed out that differentiation is needed between nursing bioterrorism preparedness and preparedness for other professions, organizational bioterrorism preparedness, and all-hazards preparedness. The author identified the defining attributes of bioterrorism preparedness for nursing as gaining knowledge, planning, practicing response behaviors, and evaluating knowledge level and content of response plan. Playing a vital role in the nation's bioterrorism preparedness and response is another way that the nursing profession can demonstrate the ability to cope with uncertainty and, therefore, establish power.

Cost and Access

In addition to coping with organizational uncertainties, the profession must be prepared to cope with uncertainties in the health care system. As noted earlier, access, cost, and quality are major uncertainties in the health care system. With health care costs and the number of uninsured increasing, nurse-managed health centers (NMHCs) could help meet the need for cost-effective quality care and for improving access. Currently over 250 NMHCs operate throughout the United States (National Nursing Centers Consortium, 2008). NMHCs are community-based health clinics that are managed by nurses in partnership with the communities they serve. Most are either independent nonprofits or academically based clinics affiliated with schools of nursing. NMHCs provide a full range of health services, including primary care, health promotion, and disease prevention, to low-income, underinsured, and uninsured clients. They record over 2.5 million client encounters annually and provide primary care to approximately 250,000 patients around the nation. This care is provided by nurse practitioners, clinical nurse specialists, registered nurses, health educators, community outreach workers, health care students, and collaborating physicians. NMHCs also act as important teaching and practice sites for nursing students and other health professionals. By providing accessible, high-quality, comprehensive primary care services to populations who have trouble accessing care, NMHCs reduce health disparities.

Although financial sustainability is the top issue facing these health centers, they offer another way of demonstrating nursing's ability to cope with uncertainty.

Centrality and Substitutability

Professional nurses have a high degree of centrality within health care organizations. They are critical to the operation of most health care organizations, and without nurses, many health care facilities would not be able to offer services. Nursing must maintain that power by becoming irreplaceable. Strong chief nurse executives with strong formal power are needed to create conditions within the organization and the health care system that make nurses difficult to replace. Thorman (2004) pointed out that it is critical that nurse leaders, including chief nurse executives and service line directors, be part of the institutional decision-making process about resource allocation, strategic direction, and planning for the future. Nagle (1999) cautioned that unless the value of registered nurses is established, other care providers will be substituted. In other words, the profession must demonstrate its economic value. Fortunately, research has demonstrated the relationship between staffing and patient outcomes. The Agency for Healthcare Research and Quality (AHRQ) published a systematic review of the literature on workforce characteristics (Kane et al., 2007). The AHRQ review identified 97 observational studies published between 1990 and 2006 and included 94 of these reports in a meta-analysis. This meta-analysis found strong and consistent evidence that higher registered nurse (RN) hours were related to lower patient mortality rates, lower rates of failure to rescue, and lower rates of hospital-acquired pneumonia. Results of the meta-analysis indicated that there was evidence that higher direct-care RN hours were related to shorter lengths of stay. Higher total nursing hours also were found to result in lower hospital mortality and failure-to-rescue rates and in shorter lengths of stay. Based on fewer studies, the review found evidence that the prevalence of baccalaureate-prepared RNs was related to lower hospital mortality rates, that higher RN job satisfaction and satisfaction with workplace autonomy were related to lower hospital mortality rates, and that higher rates of nurse turnover were related to higher rates of patient falls. The conclusion of the meta-analysis was that higher nurse staffing was associated with better patient outcomes but that the association was not necessarily causal.

 CONFLICT

The same turbulent health care environment that demands the use of power also creates the conditions that breed conflict. Health care in the United States has gone through dramatic changes in recent decades. Change increases conflict in organizations. Gerardi (2004) summarized the direct and indirect consequences of conflict. The direct costs include the following:

- Litigation costs that include attorneys' fees, expert testimony, deposition, lost work time, and document production
- Decreased managerial productivity as a result of time spent on resolving conflict
- Turnover costs
- Disability/stress claims
- Regulatory fines for noncompliance or loss of contracts or provider status with insurers and Medicare/Medicaid
- Costs associated with increase expenditures for patients with preventable poor or adverse outcomes
- Sabotage, theft, and damage to facilities

Indirect costs include the following:

- Loss of team morale, loss of motivation for organizational change, damaged workplace relationships, and unresolved tensions that lead to future conflicts
- Lost opportunities for pursuing capital purchases, expanding services, enhancing customer satisfaction programs, and developing staff and leaders
- Cost to reputation of an organization and of care professionals; negative publicity/media coverage
- Loss of strategic market positioning because of public disclosure of information regarding the dispute/bad public relations
- Increased incidence of disruptive behavior by staff and medical professionals
- Emotional costs including the turmoil for those involved in conflict

Health care organizations must find ways of managing conflict and developing effective working relationships to create healthy work environments. The effects of unresolved conflict on clinical outcomes, staff retention, and the financial health of the organization lead to many unnecessary costs that divert resources from clinical care (Gerardi, 2004).

Most people know when conflict exists because it is a part of everyday experience. Conflict is a part of life that arises because of the complexity of human relationships. Conflict has its origin in the fact that each person is unique and possesses a value system, philosophy, personality structure, preferences, and styles. Understanding how to maneuver around and manage conflict situations increases the ability to be more effective in both personal and professional roles.

DEFINITIONS

According to Kelly, a generally accepted definition of conflict does not exist (Kelly, 2006). **Conflict** is defined here as a clash or struggle that occurs when a real or perceived threat or difference exists in the desires, thoughts, attitudes, feelings, or behaviors of two or more parties (Deutsch, 1973). It exists as a tension or struggle arising from mutually exclusive or opposing actions, thoughts, opinions, or feelings. Conflict can be internal or external to an individual or group. It can be positive as well as negative.

Organizational conflict is defined as the struggle for scarce organizational resources (Coser, 1956). Values, goals, roles, or structural elements may be the specific locus of the struggle for scarce organizational resources. For example, two parties may be in opposition because of perceived differences in goals, a struggle over scarce resources, or interference in goal attainment. This opposition prevents cooperation (Deutsch, 1973). **Job conflict** is defined as a perceived opposition or antagonistic process at the individual-organization interface (Gardner, 1992). Conflict levels have an effect on productivity, morale, and teamwork in organizations

LEADING & MANAGING DEFINED

Conflict

A clash or struggle that occurs when a real or perceived threat or difference exists in the desires, thoughts, attitudes, feelings, or behaviors of two or more parties.

Organizational Conflict

The struggle for scarce organizational resources.

Job Conflict

A perceived opposition or antagonistic process at the individual-organization level.

Competitive Conflict

Rules-based conflict with the goal to win or beat an opponent.

Disruptive Conflict

Activity designed to attack, defeat, or eliminate an opponent through disruption.

Negotiation

A form of conflict resolution that uses bargaining and mediation strategies.

(Gardner, 1992). Conflict can serve to bind a group together, preserve a group by serving as a safety valve for hostility, integrate and stabilize a group, and promote growth through innovation, creativity, and change (Coser, 1956).

A review of the literature revealed several definitions of conflict. Social conflict is a struggle between opponents over values and claims to scarce status, power, and resources (Coser, 1956). According to Deutsch (1973), a conflict exists whenever incompatible activities occur or when one party is interfering, disrupting, obstructing, or in some other way making another party's actions less effective. The factors underlying conflict are threefold: (1) interdependence, (2) differences in goals, and (3) differences in perceptions. Conrad (1990) indicated that conflicts are communicative interactions among people who are interdependent and who perceive that their interests are incompatible, inconsistent, or in tension. Conflict is thus the interaction of interdependent people who perceive incompatible goals and interference from each other in achieving those goals (Folger et al., 1997). Wall and Callister (1995) defined conflict as a process in which one party perceives that its interests are being opposed or negatively affected by another party. Walton (1966) defined conflict as opposition processes in any of several forms (e.g., hostility, decreased communication, distrust, sabotage, verbal abuse, coercive tactics). Interpersonal conflict is a dynamic process that occurs between interdependent parties as they experience negative emotional reactions to perceived disagreements and interference with the attainment of their goals (Barki & Hartwick, 2001).

VIEWS OF CONFLICT

Robbins and Judge (2008) described transitions in conflict thought. The traditional view of conflict argued that conflict must be avoided because conflict indicated a malfunctioning within the group. This early approach assumed that all conflict was bad. Conflict was seen as a dysfunctional outcome resulting from poor communication, a lack of openness and trust between people, and the failure of managers to be responsive to their employees.

The human relations view argues that conflict is a natural and inevitable outcome in any group and that it need not be evil. Rather, it has the potential to be a positive force in determining group performance. Conflict was viewed as a natural occurrence in all groups and organizations. Because it was natural and inevitable, conflict should be accepted (Robbins & Judge, 2008).

The interactionist approach proposes that conflict can be a positive force in a group and explicitly argues that some conflict is absolutely necessary for a group to perform effectively. In the interactionist view, conflict is functional if it supports the goals of the group and improves its performance. Dysfunctional conflict, however, hinders group performance (Robbins & Judge, 2008).

Conflict can be competitive or disruptive. **Competitive conflict** is similar to games and sports, in which rules are followed and the goal is to win or beat an opponent. A **disruptive conflict** is some activity designed to attack, defeat, or eliminate an opponent. It is not based on rules jointly agreed to, and its objective is not focused on winning but, rather, on disrupting the opponent. The feelings and actions generated by competitive conflict focus on the positive; for disruptive conflict, feelings and actions focus on the negative (Filley, 1975).

Conflict is functional or constructive when it improves the quality of decisions, stimulates creativity and innovation, encourages interest and curiosity, provides a medium through which problems can be aired and tensions released, and fosters an environment of self-evaluation and change (Box 12.2). On the other hand, dysfunctional or destructive outcomes include a retarding of communication, reduction in group cohesiveness, and subordination of group goals to the primacy of infighting among members (Robbins, 2003). Extremely high or low levels of conflict hinder performance. An optimal level is high enough to prevent stagnation and stimulates creativity, releases tension, and initiates change. However, it is not so high as to be disruptive or counterproductive (Brown, 1983) (Figure 12.3).

Box 12.2

Effects of Conflict

Constructive Effects

- Improves decision quality
- Stimulates creativity
- Encourages interest
- Provides a forum to release tension
- Fosters change

Destructive Effects

- Constricts communication
- Decreases cohesiveness
- Explodes in fighting
- Hinders performance

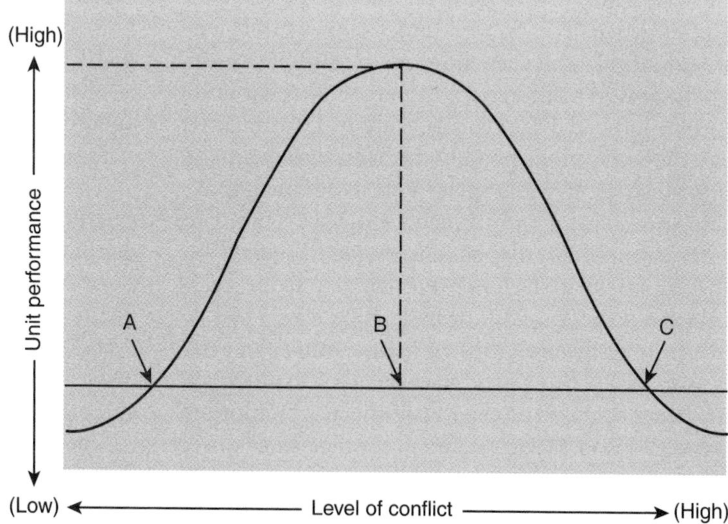

Figure 12.3
Conflict and unit performance. (From Brown, L.D. [1983]. *Managing conflict at organizational interfaces.* Reading, MA: Addison-Wesley Publishing.)

LEVELS OF CONFLICT

Thomas (1992) noted two broad types of conflict. The first refers to incompatible response tendencies within an individual, which Rahim and Bonoma (1979) referred to as *intrapersonal conflict* (Figure 12.4). *Intrapersonal conflict* means discord, tension, or stress inside, or internal to, an individual that results from unmet needs, expectations, or goals. Intrapersonal conflict is conflict that generates from within an individual (Rahim, 1983a, 1983b, 1983c). It often is manifested as a conflict over two competing roles. For example, a parent with a sick child who has to go to work faces a conflict: the need to take care of the sick child against the need to make a living. A nursing example occurs when the nurse determines that a client needs teaching or counseling but the organization's assignment system is set up in a way that does not provide an adequate amount of time. When other priorities compete, an internal or intrapersonal conflict of roles exists.

The second use refers to conflicts that occur between different individuals, groups, organizations, or other social units. Rahim and Bonoma (1979) identified these as interpersonal conflict, a category that includes intragroup conflict, intergroup conflict, and interorganizational conflict. *Interpersonal* means conflict emerging between two or more people, such as between two nurses, a doctor and a nurse, or a nurse manager and a staff nurse (Rahim & Bonoma, 1979). In this case, two people have a disagreement, conflict, or clash. Either their values or styles do not match, or there is a misunderstanding or miscommunication between them. Interpersonal conflict can be viewed as happening between two individuals or among individuals within a group. When it specifically involves multiple individuals within a group, interpersonal conflict is called *intragroup conflict*, which refers to disagreements or differences among the members of a group or its subgroups with regard to goals, functions, or activities of the group.

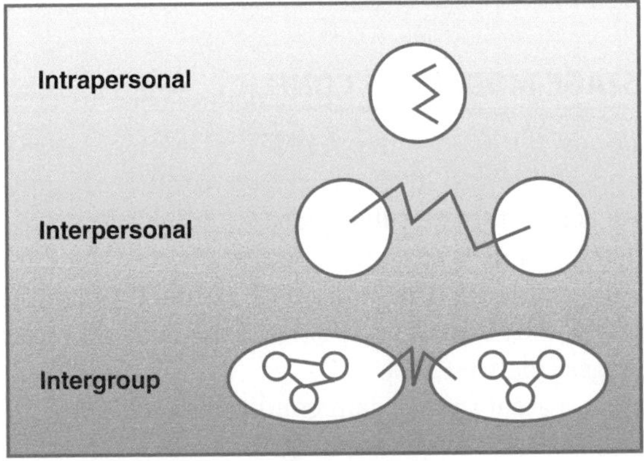

Figure 12.4
Types of conflict.

Intergroup conflict refers to disagreements or differences between the members of two or more groups or their representatives over authority, territory, and resources. Interorganizational conflict occurs across organizations (Rahim, 1983b; Rahim & Bonoma, 1979). It is conflict occurring between two distinct groups of people. For example, physicians and nurses may disagree about policies on third-party reimbursement for services, or lay midwives may seek to perform home deliveries without being prepared as licensed nurse midwives. Sometimes the conflict arises between departments or units as groups. For example, hospital nurses might find themselves in conflict with central purchasing if supplies are provided that do not meet nursing's needs or are defective.

TYPES OF CONFLICT

Three broad types of conflicts have been identified: relationship, task, and process. *Relationship conflict*, an awareness of interpersonal incompatibilities, includes affective components such as feeling tension and friction (Rahim & Bonoma, 1979). Relationship conflict involves personal issues such as dislike among group members and feelings such as annoyance, frustration, and irritation. This definition is consistent with past categorizations of conflict that distinguish between affective and cognitive conflict (Amason, 1996; Pinkley, 1990).

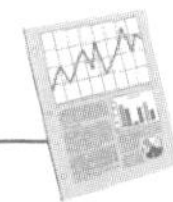

Research Note

Source: Cox, K.B. (2004). The intragroup conflict scale: Development and psychometric properties. *Journal of Nursing Measurement, 12*(2), 133-146.

Purpose

The intragroup conflict scale was developed to measure views of conflict, perceptions of behavior, and perceptions of affective states that occur in the core process of conflict. The scale was pilot tested with a sample of 184 staff nurses and was later used in a study of antecedents and effects of intragroup conflict in the nursing unit (n = 141). Data from the two studies were merged (n = 325).

Discussion

Using PCA with varimax rotation in the analysis of merged data, three factors that explained 69.2% of variance were extracted. Factor 1 reflects opposition processes and negative emotion; factor 2 reflects trust and freedom of expression; and factor 3 reflects views of conflict. Factor loadings ranged from 0.60 to 0.88 on factor 1, from 0.62 to 0.79 on factor 2, and from 0.69 to 0.80 on factor 3. Coefficient alpha for the three factors were 0.89 for factor 1, 0.88 for factor 2, and 0.79 for factor 3. Correlations with existing scales provided support for construct validity.

Application to Practice

The scale may be used to identify not only the presence of conflict in organizations but also the relationships between and among conflict and other concepts of interest to nursing administrators. As such, the scale may have the potential to contribute to the understanding of intragroup conflict in organizations.

Results of a meta-analysis revealed strong negative correlations between relationship conflict and team performance and also strong negative correlations between relationship conflict and team member satisfaction (DeDreu & Weingart, 2003).

Task conflict is an awareness of differences in viewpoints and opinions about a group task. Similar to cognitive conflict, it pertains to conflict about ideas and differences of opinion about the task (Amason & Sapienza, 1997). Task conflicts may coincide with animated discussions and personal excitement but, by definition, are void of the intense interpersonal negative emotions that are more commonly associated with relationship conflict.

Other studies have identified a third unique type of conflict, labeled *process conflict* (Jehn, 1995, 1997; Jehn et al., 1999). It is defined as an awareness of controversies about aspects of how task accomplishment will proceed. More specifically, process conflict pertains to issues of duty and resource delegation, such as who should do what and how much responsibility different people should have. For example, when group members disagree about who is responsible for completing a specific duty, they are experiencing process conflict.

STAGE MODELS OF CONFLICT

Pondy (1967), Filley (1975), Thomas (1976), and Robbins (2003) described conflict dynamics across a temporal sequence of stages or phases. These models provide significant insight into understanding the nature of conflict phenomena. Pondy's model consisted of the following four stages (Figure 12.5):

1. Latent (antecedent conditions)
2. Perception and feeling
3. Behavior manifestation (manifest)
4. Aftermath

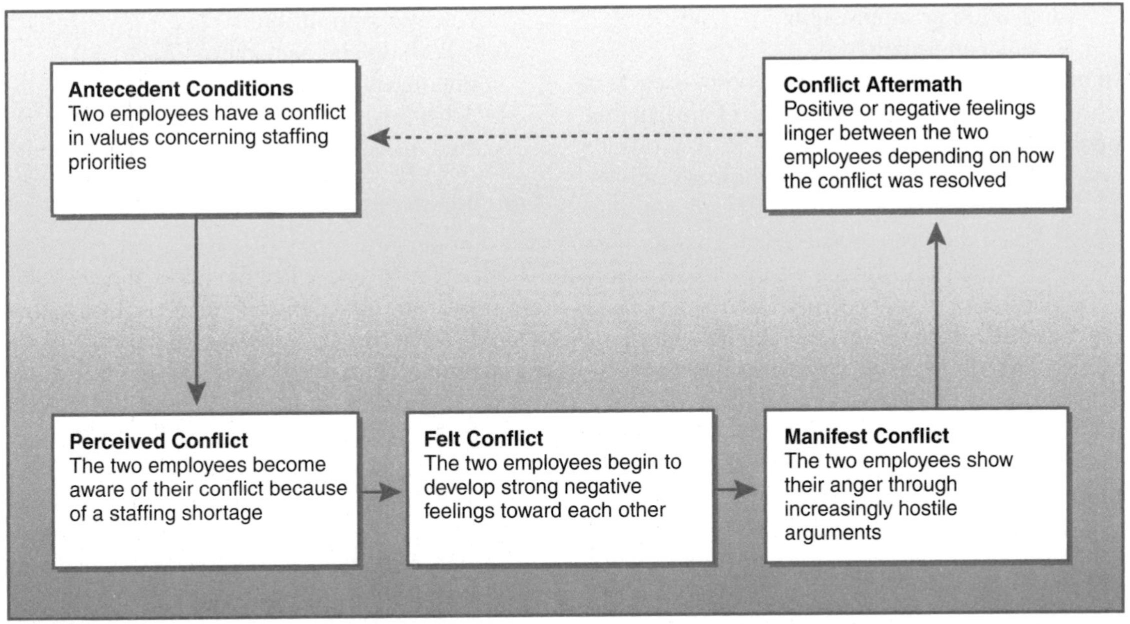

Figure 12.5
Pondy's stages of conflict. (Data from Pondy, L.R. [1967]. Organizational conflict: Concepts and models. *Administrative Science Quarterly, 12,* 296-320.)

The process begins with antecedent conditions such as unclear roles, competition for scarce resources, the quest for autonomy, or subunits with divergent goals. The process, depending on how it is handled, may be cyclical with the conflict aftermath becoming the antecedent conditions for a future conflict episode. The antecedent conditions form a background. This background leads to perceived conflict and then to felt conflict, which arises at an emotional level. One party senses that there is a problem and feels an emotional reaction beginning. These stages of perceived and felt conflict initiate manifest behavior. The conflict tension causes action. In this stage, the individual may verbalize negativity, attack another person, or try to change the situation or the environment as a way of reducing the tension.

At the stage of manifest behavior, visible evidence of conflict occurs. Subsequently, either the conflict is resolved or suppressed. For example, ventilating strong emotions by verbal expression may not resolve the problem but it calms an individual and suppresses the problem for a period of time. In the aftermath of this process, there will be new attitudes or feelings between the parties. These may be positive feelings because coping occurred and the individual felt positive and constructive in the resolution of the conflict. However, negative feelings may arise because of an inability to do anything to resolve the conflict or because the other person had more power. The negative feelings may fester. The memory of the conflict and feelings about how it was processed may linger and provide antecedent conditions for another cycle of conflict. Thus there is an aftermath to the conflict even if it is temporarily resolved. This is a residual effect from having had conflict or tension with which the individual invested psychological energy and emotion.

Filley's (1975) model is composed of the following six stages:

1. Antecedent conditions
2. Perceived conflict
3. Felt conflict
4. Manifest behavior

5. Resolution or suppression
6. Conflict aftermath

An emotional cycle of conflict was proposed as a process model of conflict by Thomas (1976). In this model, the conflict process begins as frustration, an affective-emotional trigger. Thomas's model (1976) bears a strong resemblance to Pondy's (1967). Frustration is one antecedent condition to conflict. Conceptualization is a form of cognition or perception of conflict. Frustration is an affective response, a form of felt conflict. Behavior and interaction both compare to Pondy's manifest conflict stage. Both models conclude with an outcome or aftermath conditions.

The Thomas (1976) process model depicted the following five major concepts (Figure 12.6):

1. Frustration
2. Conceptualization
3. Behavior
4. Others' reactions (interaction)
5. Outcome

The five stages of the Robbins and Judge (2008) model are as follows:

1. Potential opposition
2. Cognition and personalization
3. Intentions
4. Behavior
5. Functional or dysfunctional outcomes

Commonalities in the Stage Models

The models of Pondy (1967), Filley (1975), Thomas (1976), and Robbins and Judge (2008) are similar in that all indicate that conflict follows a predictable course. However, they differ in the number of identifiable stages or elements in a particular pattern. The following elements exist in all the models:

- Causes identified as conditions that occur before the conflict
- Core processes, including the perception that conflict exists, followed by some kind of affective state or emotional response
- Conflict behaviors, including a variety of behaviors from very subtle to violent
- Effect that includes outcomes such as resolution or aftermath consequences

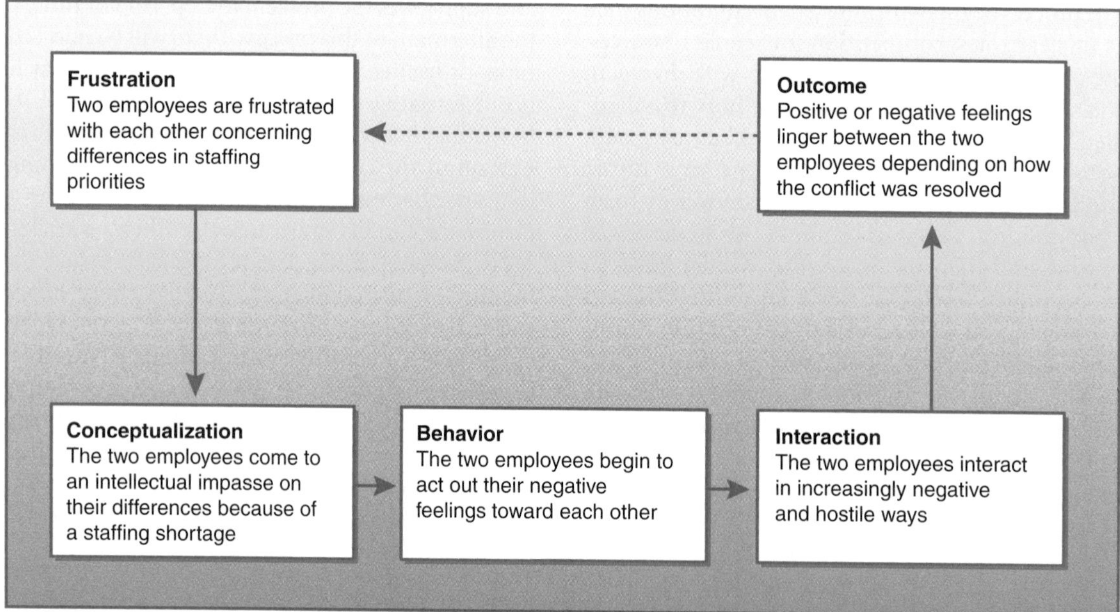

Figure 12.6
Thomas's conflict process events. (Data from Thomas, K.W. [1976]. Conflict and conflict management. In M.D. Dunnette [Ed.], *The handbook of industrial and organizational psychology* [pp. 889-935]. Chicago: Rand McNally.)

Cause, Core Process, Effect

Wall and Callister (1995) described a generic model of conflict, which is presented in Figure 12.7. As with any social process, there are causes and a core process that have effects. These effects in turn have an impact on the original cause. This conflict cycle takes place within a context (environment), and the cycle flows through numerous iterations. Wall and Callister indicated that the model is a general one that displays how the major pieces in the conflict puzzle fit together. The value of this model is that concepts from all other models may be subsumed under the major concepts of this generic model. In addition, the simplicity of the model facilitates the discussion of conflict according to cause, core process, and effect.

Causes of Conflict

According to Wall and Callister (1995), conditions that occur before conflict are identified as causes. Pondy (1967) identified the underlying sources of organizational conflict—competition for scarce resources, drives for autonomy, and divergence of subunit goals. In Filley's (1975) model, antecedent conditions include the following: ambiguous jurisdictions, conflict of interest, communication barriers, dependence of one party, differentiation in organization, association of the parties, need for consensus, behavior regulations, and unresolved prior conflicts. According to Rahim and Bonoma (1979), sources of intragroup conflict include leadership style, task structure, group composition and size, cohesiveness and groupthink, and external threats and their outcomes. Intergroup conflict is generated from system differentiation, task interdependence, scarce resources, jurisdictional ambiguity, and separation of knowledge from authority.

In a concept analysis of conflict in the work environment, Almost (2005) indicated that antecedents of conflict stem from individual characteristics, interpersonal factors, and organizational factors. Individual characteristics include differing opinions and values; demographic dissimilarity, which includes gender and educational differences; and generational diversity. Interpersonal factors include lack of trust, injustice or disrespect, and inadequate or poor communication. Finally, organizational factors include interdependence and changes due to restructuring.

PART III

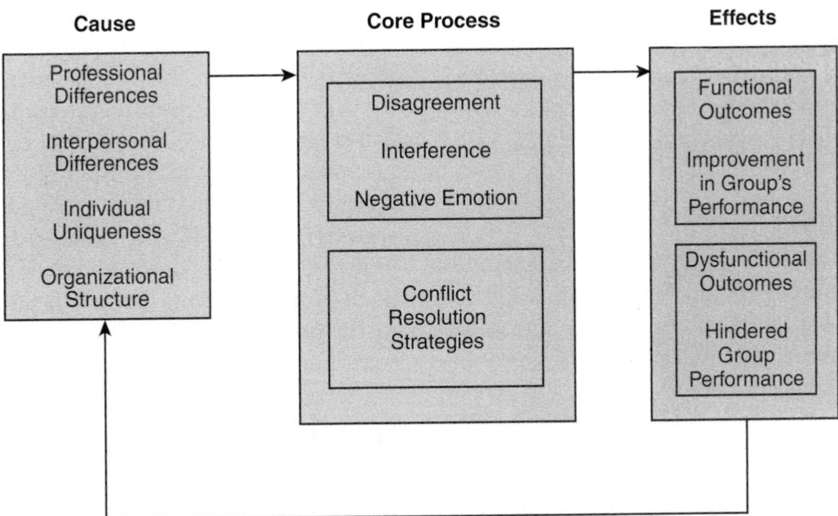

Figure 12.7
Conceptual framework for conflict. (Data from Wall, J.A., & Callister, R.R. [1995]. Conflict and its management. *Journal of Management, 21,* 515-558.)

The Core Process of Conflict

Although conflict has been defined in many different ways, disagreement, interference, and negative emotion are thought to underlie conflict situations (Barki & Hartwick, 2001). Disagreement, interference, and negative emotion can be viewed as reflecting cognitive, behavioral, and affective manifestations of interpersonal conflict. Disagreement is the most commonly discussed and assessed cognition in the literature. Although a number of different behaviors have been associated with and may be typical of conflict, they do not always indicate the existence of conflict. Conflict exists when the behavior of one party interferes with or opposes another party's attainment of its own interests, objectives, or goals. Finally, a number of affective states have been associated with conflict. However, it is the negative emotions such as fear, anger, anxiety, and frustration that have been used to characterize conflict. Barki and Hartwick (2001) proposed that interpersonal conflict exists only when disagreement, interference, and negative emotion are present in the situation.

In 2004, Barki and Hartwick conducted a comprehensive review of the literature in which two dimensions of conflict were identified. The first dimension identifies disagreement, interference, and negative emotion as three properties generally associated with a conflict situation. The second dimension identifies relationship and task content or task process as two targets of interpersonal conflict encountered in organizational settings. Barki and Hartwick's work has provided great insight into the core process of conflict.

Effects of Conflict

Almost (2005) noted that although conflict includes both positive and negative effects, more empirical evidence for negative outcomes was found than for positive outcomes in the concept analysis. The main effects of conflict are individual effects, interpersonal relationships, and organizational effects. Individual effects include job stress, job dissatisfaction, absenteeism, intent to leave, increased grievances, psychosomatic complaints, and negative emotions. Organizational effects include reduced coordination and collaboration and reduced productivity. Interpersonal relationships included both positive and negative outcomes. Positive outcomes include stronger relationships and team cohesiveness, whereas negative outcomes include negative perceptions of others, hostility, and avoidance.

Functional outcomes include increased group performance, improved quality of decisions, stimulation of creativity and innovation, encouragement of interest and curiosity, provision of a medium for problem solving, and creation of an environment for self-evaluation and changes. On the other hand, dysfunctional outcomes include development of discontent, reduced group effectiveness, retarded communication, reduced group cohesiveness, and infighting among group members, which then overcomes the focus on group goals (Robbins & Judge, 2008).

CONFLICT SCALES

Two conflict inventories are available to measure conflict. The Rahim Organizational Conflict Inventory-I (Rahim, 1983b, 1983c) is designed to measure three dimensions of conflict: intrapersonal, intragroup, and intergroup. The Perceived Conflict Scale (Gardner, 1992) contains four subscales of conflict: intrapersonal, interpersonal, intergroup/other departments, and intergroup/support services. This scale is designed to measure conflict in nursing. The scales can be used for objective measurement not only to determine how much conflict exists but also to determine the causes and effects of conflict and the relationship of conflict to other variables of interest to nursing administrators. Barki and Hartwick's (2004) proposed two dimensions have implications for the development of another instrument containing items that reflect these dimensions. An instrument that reflects the two dimensions could contribute to our understanding of conflict.

CONFLICT MANAGEMENT

There are many views about conflict management. Clearly, conflict is managed via the style and the strategy chosen by the conflict manager. Several conflict styles and strategies exist, meaning that individuals have choices. The ability to select among styles and strategies if something is not working provides flexibility for the person dealing with conflict.

Managing conflict relates to determining whether the level is too high or too low. Assessment of levels and sources is the first step in conflict assessment. The goal of conflict management is to stimulate growth and coping behavior but to avoid reaching the point at which conflict seems overwhelming. Conflict is an inherent element of change and is manifested in resistance to change. This indicates that nurses need to be alert to the predictability of resistance and conflict in any change process.

Personal styles and the interaction of styles contribute to conflict moments. The reality is that most people are more comfortable around people who are similar to them. If people are very different in terms of personality and styles, then how the styles interact contributes to conflict potential. Awareness of one's own style and the recognition of other people's styles contribute to effective management of conflict.

Multiple factors must be considered in conflict management. The important factors can form the basis for conflict management behaviors needed by nurses. These behaviors have been listed in a conflict management checklist (Box 12.3). The checklist can be used as a review or assessment for critically analyzing conflict situations.

Box 12.3

Conflict Management Checklist

- ✓ Identify the boundaries of the conflict, the areas of agreement and disagreement, and the extent of each person's aims.
- ✓ Understand the factors that limit the possibilities of managing the conflict constructively.
- ✓ Be aware of whether more than one issue is involved.
- ✓ Be open to the ideas, feelings, and attitudes expressed by the people involved.
- ✓ Be willing to accept outside help to mediate the conflict.

A companion tool is a series of systematic steps that have been recommended for nurses to use in handling conflict situations (Mallory, 1981) (Figure 12.8). The advantage of following a systematic approach to handling conflict is that the nurse becomes a better problem solver. This is especially important in conflict situations, which have a significant component of strong human emotions. The emotions may need to be defused before the content issues can be tackled.

Conflict Management Strategies

It is important to take action as soon as a conflict surfaces so that bad feelings will not linger and grow. Conflict in groups adds the complexity of multiple parties to the conflict situation. Usually the best place for a work group to clear the air is in a group meeting. During such meetings, issues can be defined and strategies worked out for managing the points of disagreement. Three overall frameworks or postures for conflict management are the defensive, compromise, and creative problem-solving modes.

The *defensive mode* produces feelings of winning in some and loss in others. Several conflict resolution strategies adopt a defensive mode. Sometimes if creative problem solving and compromise fail, this may be the only way to decrease some of the destructive effects of conflict. Or a defensive mode may be used initially to gain time to calm down or to think about how to proceed. Following are ways to defensively solve a conflict:

- *Separate the contending parties.* For example, people may be assigned to different shifts or teams or different days off and on.
- *Suppress the conflict.* For example, people may decide not to talk about their differences.
- *Restrict or isolate the conflict.* For example, the parties can agree to disagree about a conflict and move on to items that they do agree about.
- *Smooth it over or finesse it through an organizational change.* For example, sometimes it is possible to solve conflicts by restructuring around the issue.

PART III

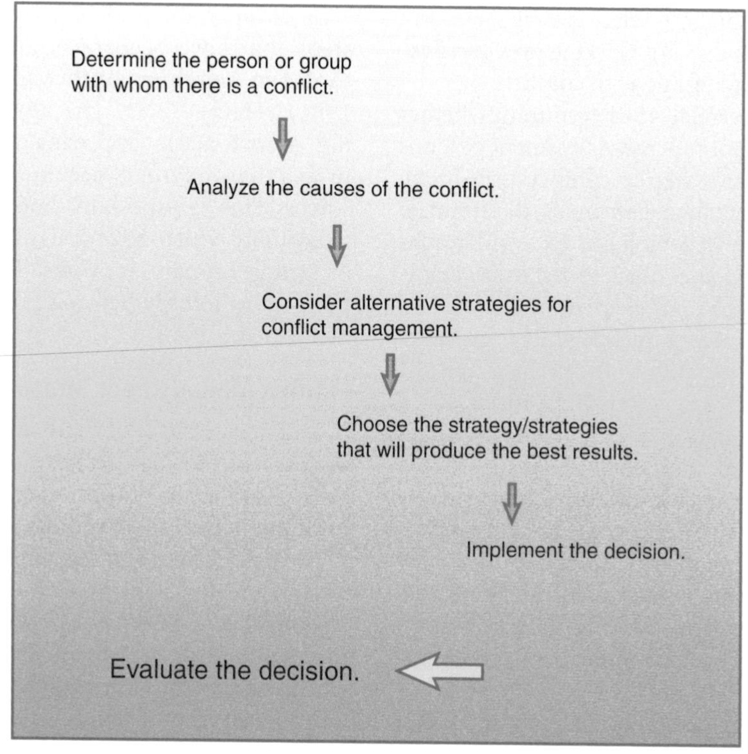

Figure 12.8
Handling conflict situations. (Data from Mallory, G. [1981]. Believe it or not: Conflict can be healthy once you understand it and learn to manage it. *Nursing, 11*[6], 97-101.)

- *Avoid the conflict to diminish the destructive effects.* For example, people can change the subject whenever the conflict arises or avoid the party or parties involved.

The second mode of conflict management is compromise. With a *compromise mode,* each party wins something and loses something. In the settlement, each side gives up a part of its demands. Thus each side may "go halfway" or "split the difference." A compromise comes about when both sides want harmony or an end to the conflict and are willing to give up something to settle the difference.

The third mode of conflict management is creative problem solving. Use of a *creative problem-solving mode* produces feelings of gain and no feelings of loss for all conflict participants. All parties work together collaboratively to arrive at a solution that satisfies everyone, and all parties feel that they win. Creative problem solving is the most effective mode of conflict management. As part of the creative problem-solving process, the following five steps for conflict management can be identified:

1. Initiate a discussion, timed sensitively and held in an environment conducive to private discussion.
2. Respect individual differences.
3. Be empathic with all involved parties.
4. Have an assertive dialogue that consists of separating facts from feelings, clearly defining the central issue, differentiating viewpoints, making sure that each person clearly states their intentions, framing the main issue based on common principles, and being an attentive listener consciously focused on what the other person is saying.

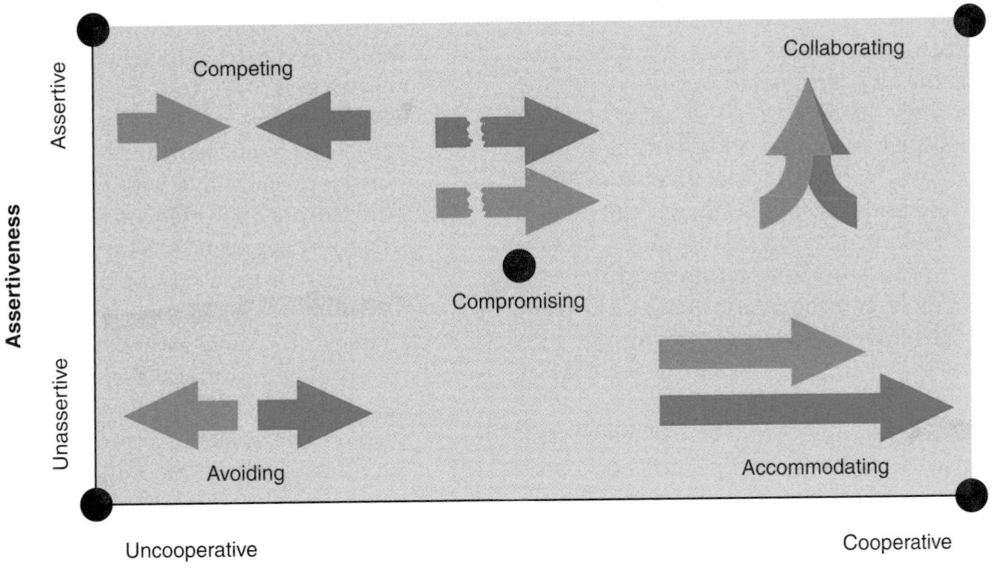

Figure 12.9
Dimensions of conflict handling intentions. (From Thomas, K. [1992]. Conflict and negotiation processes in organizations. In M.D. Dunnette & L.M. Hough [Eds.], *Handbook of industrial and organizational psychology* [2nd ed., vol. 3, p. 668]. Palo Alto, CA: Consulting Psychologists Press.)

5. Agree on a solution that balances the power and satisfies all parties, so that a consensus on a win-win solution is reached.

Conflict Handling Intentions

Blake and Mouton's (1964) five styles of handling interpersonal conflict are forcing, withdrawing, smoothing, sharing, and problem solving. Building on the Blake and Mouton model, Thomas (1976) reported that conflict has two dimensions, each representing an individual's intention with respect to a conflict situation (Figure 12.9). The dimensions are (1) assertiveness (satisfying one's own concerns) and (2) cooperativeness (attempting to satisfy another's concerns). When handling conflict, individuals vary in their degree of cooperation and assertiveness. The resulting behaviors are competing, collaborating, compromising, avoiding, and accommodating. *Competing* is an assertive strategy in which an individual's concerns are satisfied at the other's expense. *Collaborating* is an assertive, cooperative strategy in which individuals work together to find a mutually satisfying solution. *Compromising* incorporates both assertiveness and cooperating. In compromising, each individual involved in the conflict must give up something to resolve the situation. *Avoiding* is an unassertive, uncooperative strategy used when an individual postpones or sidesteps an issue. *Accommodating* is an unassertive, cooperative strategy used when an individual focuses on the concerns of the other while neglecting his own.

Conflict Resolution Strategies

Conflicts can be a source of chronic frustration, or they can lead to increased effectiveness in organizations and groups. It takes leadership and management to solve them creatively so that people exist more cooperatively with others. Leadership and management of conflict resolution have implications for work group morale and productivity. A fair proportion of a leader's or manager's time is spent on handling conflict.

Conflict management techniques stress the importance of communication, assertive dialogue, and empathy. Thus during conflict situations, the more that individuals look at the total situation and use positive communication techniques, the closer they will come to a successful resolution. Conflict resolution techniques have been identified, described, and categorized in a variety of ways by a variety of authors. Some terms have been used interchangeably, and some terms have similar but slightly different meanings. The following is an overall list for methods or strategies for conflict resolution (Figure 12.10):

- *Avoiding:* This is the strategy of avoiding conflict at all costs. Some people never acknowledge that a conflict exists. The individual's posture is "If I do not acknowledge there is a problem, then there is no problem." It is sometimes reflected in the phrase "leave well enough alone."
- *Withholding or withdrawing:* In this avoidance strategy, one party opts out of participation. He or she withdraws from the situation. This does not resolve the conflict. However, this strategy does give individuals a chance to calm down or to avoid a confrontation.
- *Smoothing over or reassuring:* This is the strategy of saying "Everything will be OK." By maintaining surface harmony, parties do not withdraw but simply attempt to make everyone feel good. It is similar to "smoothing ruffled feathers." Smoothing over or reassuring strategies use verbal communication to defuse strong emotions.

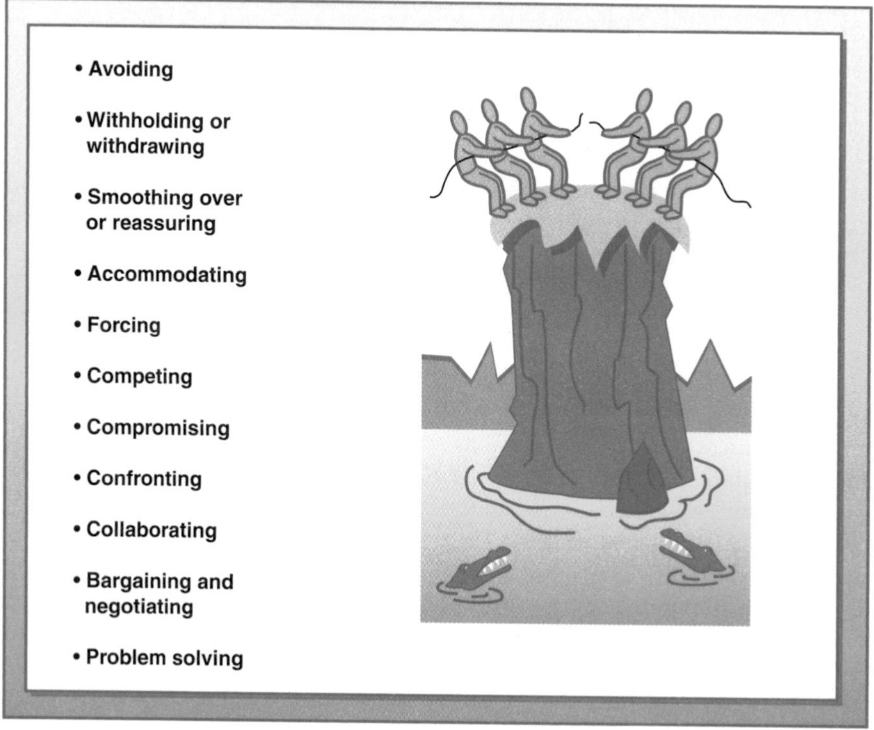

Figure 12.10
Strategies for conflict resolution. (Data from American Journal of Nursing [AJN]. [1987]. *Conflict management* [videotape]. New York: Author; Barton, A. [1991]. Conflict resolution by nurse managers. *Nursing Management, 22*[5], 83-86; Mallory, G. [1981]. Believe it or not: Conflict can be healthy once you understand it and learn to manage it. *Nursing, 11*[6], 97-101; Thomas, K. [1976]. Conflict and conflict management. In M.D. Dunnette (Ed.), *The handbook of industrial and organizational psychology* [pp. 889-935]. Chicago: Rand McNally.)

- *Accommodating:* This strategy is used when there is a large power differential. The more powerful party is accommodated to preserve harmony or build up social credits. This means that the party of lesser power gives up his or her position in deference to the more powerful party. Accommodation may be used when one party has a vested interest that is relatively unimportant to the other party. "Kill the enemy with kindness" is the related phrase.
- *Forcing:* This technique is a dominance move and an arbitrary way to manage conflict. An issue may be forced on the table by issuing orders or by putting it to a majority-rules vote. The hallmark phrase is "Let's vote on it." Forcing is an all-out power strategy to win while the other party loses.
- *Competing:* This is an assertive strategy in which one party's needs are satisfied at the other's expense. Competing is an all-out effort to win at any cost. It is sometimes reflected in the phrase "Might makes right." Competing strategies tend to follow rules and be similar to games and athletic contests. Applying for a job is a form of competition.
- *Compromising:* This strategy is called "splitting the difference." It is useful when goals or values are markedly different. It is a staple of conflict management.
- *Confronting:* This technique is called *assertive problem solving* and is focused on the issues. Individuals speak for themselves but in a way that decreases defensiveness and allows another person to hear the message. It is a staple of conflict management but requires courage. "I" messages are used; "you" messages are avoided.
- *Collaborating:* This is an assertive and cooperative strategy in which the parties work together to find a mutually satisfying solution. It is invoked with the phrase "Two heads are better than one."
- *Bargaining and negotiating:* These strategies are attempts to divide the rewards, power, or benefits so that everyone gets something. They involve both parties in a back-and-forth effort at some level of agreement. The process may be formal or informal.
- *Problem solving:* This strategy's goal is to try to find an acceptable, workable solution for all parties. It is designed to generate feelings of gain by all parties. The problem-solving process is employed to reach a mutually agreeable solution to the conflict.

Mediation is a conflict resolution process in which a neutral person facilitates communication, the development of understanding, and the generation of options for creative dispute resolution (Moore, 2003). Gerardi (2004) noted that mediation is a useful process to use when the goal of preserving the working relationship is as important as resolving the substantive problems. Although not all conflict situations require mediation, mediation techniques can be used to prevent escalation of conflicts. Effective techniques for improving collaboration and resolving conflicts include listening for understanding, reframing, elevating the definition of the problem, and creating clear agreements. Mediation techniques can be integrated into manager's practice to assist nurses in recognizing issues and addressing the actual needs of co-workers to prevent escalation of conflicts (Gerardi, 2004).

Face Negotiation Theory

Face negotiation is the focus of a theory developed by Ting-Toomey to describe and explain differences in responses to conflict on the basis of cultural backgrounds (Ting-Toomey, 1988; Ting-Toomey & Kurogi, 1998). This theory draws on the idea that *face* is a metaphor for our public identity, or self-image, and is an important element of social situations throughout the world. Specifically, face is "a projected image of one's self in a relational situation" (Ting-Toomey, 1988, p. 215). In the theory, *facework* refers to specific verbal and nonverbal messages that help maintain and restore face loss and uphold and honor face gain. All individuals want others to see them in a certain way, even though they may not be consciously aware of this desire.

Ting-Toomey (1988) originally considered face negotiation theory as a way to explain differences in conflict communication styles stemming from cultural preferences for individualism versus collectivism. She proposed that those in cultures best described as *collectivistic* would be more likely to seek to uphold "other-face," whereas those in *individualistic* cultures would more likely seek to uphold "self-face."

Face negotiation theory builds on the five-style dual-concern framework developed by Rahim (1983a) and is based on the degree to which a person is concerned with self-interest, as well as with the interests of others. The five styles are problem solving (also called *integrating, collaborating*, or *cooperating*), forcing (also called *competing* or *dominating*), avoiding (also called *suppressing* or *withdrawing*), yielding (also called *obliging, accommodating*, or *smoothing*), and compromising (Putnam & Poole, 1987; Rahim, 2001). The theory posits that collectivistic cultures favor the avoiding, yielding, and compromising styles; in contrast, individualistic cultures reputedly favor forcing and problem-solving styles (Ting-Toomey, 1988).

In 1998, the face negotiation theory was revised and the dimension of self-construal (self-image) was discussed in terms of the independent and interdependent self, or the degree to which people conceive of themselves as relatively autonomous from or connected to others (Ting-Toomey & Kurogi, 1998). The revised theory posits that the degree to which people see themselves as autonomous (independent; self-face) or connected to others (interdependent; other-face) is a better predictor of conflict interaction than their cultural or ethnic background. Ting-Toomey and Kurogi (1998) also added the concept of power to the theory to explain communicative differences based on the cultural dimension of power distance. In low-power distance cultures, differences in treatment based on status are less accepted. On the other hand, in high-power distance cultures, differences in treatment based on status are more accepted. The authors proposed that individuals of different status levels in low-power distance cultures are more likely to use the forcing style to resolve conflict, whereas in high-power distance cultures, those in lower-status roles may use styles such as yielding.

Cross-cultural empirical tests of the revised face negotiation theory supported much of the theory (Oetzel & Ting-Toomey, 2003; Oetzel et al., 2001). The 2001 study involved a cross-cultural comparison of four national cultures (Oetzel et al., 2001). The purpose of the study was to investigate face and facework during conflicts across four national cultures: China, Germany, Japan, and the United States. A questionnaire was administered to 768 participants in the four national cultures, in their respective languages, to measure 3 face concerns and 11 facework behaviors. The major findings of the study were as follows:

- Self-construals had the strongest effects on face concerns and facework, with independence positively associated with self-face and dominating facework and interdependence positively associated with other- and mutual-face and integrating and avoiding facework.
- Power distance had small, positive effects on all three face concerns and avoiding and dominating facework.
- Individualistic, small-power distance cultures had less other-face concern and avoiding facework and more dominating facework than collectivistic, large-power distance cultures.
- Germans had more self- and mutual-face concerns and used defending more than Americans.
- Chinese had more self-face concern and involved a third party more than Japanese.
- Relational closeness and status had only small effects on face concerns and facework behavior.

In the 2003 study of face-negotiation theory, Oetzel and Ting-Toomey tested the underlying assumption that face mediates the relationship between cultural or individual level variables and conflict styles. The sample included 768 participants and was drawn from the Oetzel and colleagues (2001) study. That previous study involved a cross-cultural comparison of the four national cultures, whereas the 2003 study tested the face-negotiation theory across all cultures.

The major findings of the 2003 study were as follows:

- Cultural individualism-collectivism had direct effects on conflict styles, as well as mediated effects through self-construal and face concerns.
- Independent self-construal was associated positively with self-face concern, and interdependent self-construal was associated positively with other-face concern.
- Self-face concern was associated positively with dominating conflict styles, and other-face concern was associated positively with avoiding and integrating conflict styles.
- Face concerns accounted for all of the total variance explained (100% of 19% total explained) in dominating, most of the total variance explained in integrating (70% of 20% total explained), and some of the total variance explained in avoiding (38% of 21% total explained) when considering face concerns, cultural individualism-collectivism, and self-construals.

Oetzel and Ting-Toomey (2003) noted that the findings empirically validated the face-negotiation theory (Ting-Toomey, 1988; Ting-Toomey & Kurogi, 1998). They concluded that this study provides a further step in understanding the complex nature of face and conflict behavior. The findings provide supportive evidence of the face-negotiation theory, especially that face concerns provide a mediating link between cultural values and conflict behavior. The authors also suggested that these findings are particularly significant given the relatively large sample size across four national cultures. Oetzel and Ting-Toomey (2003) pointed out that face-negotiation theory is a popular theoretical framework for research and practice, and their research further substantiates the usefulness of the theory. However, the authors noted that despite this support, future research is needed to better understand how face is negotiated in cross-cultural and intercultural conflicts to create more harmonious multicultural relationships. The theory has relevance for nursing, and future research efforts should be directed toward testing the theory with samples of nursing personnel.

Results of the studies indicated that nursing administrators need to be more attuned to face issues in the conflict dialogue process. The findings of the Oetzel and Ting-Toomey 2003 study demonstrated that display of other-face concern, which is maintaining the poise or pride of the other person and being sensitive to the other person's self-worth, can lead to a collaborative, win-win integrative approach or an avoiding approach. In contrast, individuals who are more concerned with maintaining self-pride or self-image during a conflict episode would devote effort to defending their conflict position to the neglect of other-face validation issue. In 2005, Ting-Toomey summarized face negotiation theory, its theoretical proposition, and research supporting the theory (Ting-Toomey, 2005). The theory clearly has implications for nursing research and nursing administration.

Conflict Resolution Outcomes

Whatever the conflict resolution style used, the individual must be aware of the outcome that results from the strategy selected. The outcomes of conflict are what actually happens as a result of the conflict management process. The three ways in which conflicts resolve are (1) win-lose, (2) lose-lose, and (3) win-win (Filley, 1975) (Box 12.4).

Box 12.4

Conflict Resolution Outcomes

Win-Lose

One party exerts dominance.

Lose-Lose

Neither side wins.

Win-Win

An attempt is made to meet the needs of both parties simultaneously.

Data from Filley, A.C. (1975). *Interpersonal conflict resolution.* Glenview, IL: Scott, Foresman; Filley, A., House, R., & Kerr, S. (1976). *Managerial process and organizational behavior.* Glenview, IL: Scott, Foresman.

A *win-lose* situation is one in which one party's views, ideas, or opinions predominate and the other side's are ignored. Putting something to a majority vote creates a win-lose situation in which the majority wins and the minority loses. A *lose-lose* situation is one in which the conflict deteriorates to the point at which both parties lose. Strategies of averaging, using bribes, using a third party to arbitrate, or trading may result in a lose-lose outcome. The *win-win* outcome is when each party gains something and the solution is acceptable to all parties. Problem solving, consensus building, and integrative decision making are techniques aimed toward a win-win outcome.

Managing clients or other nursing personnel places the nurse in many conflict resolution situations. The leader's role is to use positive communication techniques and alternatives to come to a resolution of conflicts. Many institutions have no officially sanctioned way to handle hostility among their members. Effective conflict management techniques establish a common etiquette to lessen conflict tension, increase mutual respect, engender confidence, and increase power through willing collaboration in the endeavors of the organization.

Filley (1975) described the win-win resolution as the optimum conflict management. Win-lose and lose-lose resolutions also occur, but effective managers should seek win-win resolutions. Win-win strategies focus on problem solving.

Negotiation is a fundamental form of conflict resolution. Negotiation includes bargaining power, distributive bargaining, integrative bargaining, and mediation. *Bargaining power* refers to another person's inducement to agree to terms. *Distributive bargaining* is what either side gains at the expense of the other. In *integrative bargaining*, the focus shifts to problem solving and negotiators reach a solution that enhances both parties and produces high joint benefits. *Mediation* is a process in which a third party encourages the two parties in conflict to acknowledge that they have injured the other but also are dependent on each other (Hampton et al., 1987).

Integrative bargaining tends to be more cooperative, and distributive bargaining tends to be more competitive. In general, integrative bargaining is superior to distributive bargaining. Fisher and colleagues (1992) proposed an alternative called *principled negotiation*. This approach calls for negotiators to use the following five fundamental principles to negotiate effectively with each other instead of against each other:

1. Separate the people from the problem.
2. Negotiate about interests, not positions.
3. Invent options for mutual gain.
4. Insist on objective decision criteria.
5. Know your **b**est **a**lternative **t**o a **n**egotiated **a**greement (BATNA).

Although there is no one best method of conflict resolution, competence in managing conflict is essential.

Conflict Resolution Inventories

Two instruments have been developed to measure conflict handling styles. In the Organizational Conflict Inventory-II, Rahim (1983b, 1983c) divided the handling of interpersonal conflict into the two dimensions of concern for self and concern for others, both in high and low degrees, to form a grid. Rahim then adapted Blake and Mouton's (1964) five types of handling interpersonal conflict (forcing, withdrawing, smoothing, compromising, and problem solving) into five styles of handling interpersonal conflict (avoiding, obliging, compromising, integrating, and dominating). The inventory measures the five identified styles.

Thomas and Kilmann (1974) also developed a style assessment and diagnosis inventory, called the *Thomas-Kilmann Conflict Mode Instrument (TKI)*. Their grid uses dimensions of assertiveness and cooperativeness on high to low degrees. The five styles are avoiding, accommodating, compromising, competing, and collaborating. This model blends a description of an individual's behavior on assertiveness and cooperativeness dimensions in situations in which the concerns of two people appear to be incompatible. The behaviors of individuals are thought to be a function of both personal predispositions and situational contingencies. Avoiding is low on both assertiveness and cooperativeness; collaborating is high on both aspects. Competing is high on assertiveness and low on cooperativeness; accommodating is low on assertiveness and high on cooperativeness. Compromising is in the middle. All modes have some use in specific situations (Barton, 1991).

Bartol and colleagues (2001) described the development of a scale designed to determine attitudes toward managing conflict. The authors indicated that the Bartol/McSweeney Conflict Management Scale is simple to use and suitable for nurses working in different settings. They pointed out that knowing one's predisposition toward conflict is the first step in creatively managing conflict.

Studies of Conflict Management in Nursing

Several studies used the TKI (Thomas & Kilmann, 1974) to measure staff nurses' and nurse administrators' ways of managing conflict. Hightower's (1986) investigation of hierarchical conflicts by 160 predominantly female (98%) nurse managers revealed that avoidance was the most frequently used conflict handling style, followed by compromise, collaboration, competition, and accommodation. Findings of Woodtli's (1987) study of 167 deans of baccalaureate nursing programs indicated that compromising was used most frequently. This was followed by collaborating, avoiding, accommodating, and competing. Cavanagh (1991) studied 145 staff nurses and 82 nurse managers in eight West Coast hospitals. Findings indicated that both staff nurses and nurse managers used avoidance as their major method of handling conflict. However, nurse managers used compromise almost as frequently as avoidance. Barton (1991) studied 69 nurse managers in a large, private, nonprofit teaching hospital in the Midwest. Findings of Barton's study indicated that compromising was the most frequently used conflict handling style followed by collaborating, avoiding, accommodating, and competing. In summary, avoiding and compromising were the most frequently used conflict handling intentions in nursing. It is interesting to note that none of the nurses used collaboration as their major conflict handling intention, and only the deans in Woodtli's study and nurse managers in Barton's study used collaboration with any frequency. Results of these studies have implications for including content on conflict resolution skills in all nursing curricula.

Sportsman and Hamilton (2007) conducted a study to determine prevalent conflict management styles chosen by students in nursing and to contrast these styles with those chosen by students in allied health professions. The associations among the level of professional health care education and the style chosen were also determined. A convenience sample of 126 university students completed the TKI. The difference was not significant between the prevalent conflict management styles chosen by graduate and undergraduate nursing students and those in allied health. Some of the students were already licensed in their discipline; others had not yet taken a licensing examination. Licensure and educational level were not associated with choice of styles. Women and men had similar preferences. The prevalent style for nursing students was compromise, followed by avoidance. The prevalent style for allied health students was avoidance, followed by compromise and accommodation. When compared with the TKI norms, slightly more than one half of all participants chose two or more conflict management styles, commonly avoidance and accommodation at the 75th percentile or above. Only 9.8% of the participants chose collaboration at that level.

LEADERSHIP AND MANAGEMENT IMPLICATIONS

Organizational Conflict

Thomas (1976) identified a "big picture" structural model of conflict that examines four factors that seem to influence the way conflict is handled in organizations: behavioral predispositions of individuals, social pressure in the environment, the organization's incentive structure, and rules and procedures. The different levels of power exist as a result of bureaucratic hierarchy and the resultant position power.

Organizational conflict is a form of interpersonal conflict that is generated from aspects of the institution, such as the style of management, rules, procedures, and communication channels. Conflicts that arise when an individual's needs and goals cannot be met within the system are generally organizational. Conflict may be necessary to groups and organizations. Conflict serves to unify and bind together a group by setting boundaries and strengthening a group's identity. Conflict may help stabilize a group by serving as a test of opposing interests within the group. Conflict may help integrate a group by distributing power. Conflict may be necessary for the growth of a group and its members. Conflict serves to stimulate creativity, innovation, and change (Coser, 1956).

Organizational leadership sets a tone for conflict and conflict management (Barton, 1991). This occurs because leaders and managers model behaviors of positive or negative conflict management and choose when and how to intervene in conflict situations. Choice of intervention style and timing of conflict management are functions of the individuals' behavioral predispositions and environmental pressure coupled with the organization's reward structure and coordination and control methods.

Specifically related to organizational conflict and the focus on groups in organizations, Pondy (1967) identified three strategies to use when attempting to resolve organizational conflicts—bargaining; using rules, procedures, and administrative control; and using a systems integrator. Bargaining might be useful when a conflict exists over scarce monetary resources. The administrative control approach might be helpful when clarification of role boundaries is needed. The systems integrator approach might be appropriate in a matrix structure or where there is a need to coordinate personnel in vertical and horizontal structures (Booth, 1993).

Sources of Conflict in Organizations

The sources of conflict frequently encountered in organizations are power, communication, goals, values, resources, roles, and personalities. Conflict

LEADERSHIP & MANAGEMENT **BEHAVIORS**

Leadership Behaviors

- Empowers followers
- Encourages the acquisition and use of power to accomplish group goals
- Models the constructive use of power
- Mentors and supports others
- Builds connections
- Enables group decision making
- Is visible and relates to others
- Demonstrates expertise
- Uses conflict constructively
- Enables followers to use power to manage conflicts
- Models constructive conflict resolution
- Encourages growth-producing conflict
- Mentors and supports followers in conflict management
- Builds conflict interventions
- Is visible in conflict situations
- Collaborates with others

Management Behaviors

- Uses power to obtain resources
- Manages power and conflict moments
- Negotiates from a power base
- Uses information strategically
- Gives rewards and punishments
- Exercises legitimate authority to accomplish work
- Plans for conflict management
- Organizes the environment to decrease frustration
- Directs subordinates in resolving conflicts
- Negotiates conflict resolutions
- Competes and bargains for scarce resources

Overlap Areas

- Uses power to achieve goals
- Uses power sources
- Manages conflicts
- Resolves conflicts

arises from a variety of sources. Power clashes lead to conflict. This happens if one person has more power than another. For example, in organizations, relationships exist between and among individuals with unequal power such as that between physicians and nurses.

Another source of conflict is the misunderstanding or breakdown of communication. Conflicts can be the result of clashes between deep-seated, sincere, but diametrically opposed views. Communication may be used to clarify opposing views. Because values are internalized, they are not easily changed but may be clarified by communication or become a barrier as a result of miscommunication. Conflict situations often arise suddenly with the awareness of conflict existing on an emotional level. Emotional intensity may be the first element communicated. The emotional reaction may include responses such as frustration or wanting to lash out with a strong verbal communication.

The roots or causes of conflict are many and varied. Other general sources of conflict that occur frequently in organizations are different goals, different ways to reach a goal, different values, overlapping or unclear designation of responsibility, lack of information, and personality conflicts. Irresolvable conflicts will need to be carefully managed within any work group to balance conflict levels. For example, nurses may thrive when the conflict level is sufficient to stimulate a clash of ideas that leads to creativity and innovation or growth. However, nurses may expend energy in nonproductive activity if the conflict level is too high or becomes destructive.

Conflict appears to be an inherent part of the work of nursing. Nurses are prime candidates for conflict because of the need to work collaboratively with people of varying social, ethnic, and educational backgrounds. Collaboration implies a distribution of power, yet nurses may be employed in a hierarchical system. When nurses work in groups, they work with a number of different colleagues and a variety of client types and personalities. These are complex interrelationships. Added to the complexity is the fact that multiple providers (e.g., physicians, nurses, nurse managers, ancillary personnel, the client, and the client's family) require coordination and communication to manage the care for any client.

Within health care, there is interdependence among members. This situation also provides conditions ripe for conflict to arise. Multiple care providers rely on one another to carry out portions of the work. For example, physicians depend on nurses to achieve certain client outcomes, nurses depend on physicians to achieve certain client outcomes, and both nurses and physicians depend on a variety of assistive or allied care workers to deliver the therapies or promote client outcomes. Nurses and physicians also depend on each other's expertise. For example, nurses need the physician to prescribe an analgesic if medication would be the appropriate intervention for pain. When physicians request certain therapies, they rely on nurses to assess and evaluate the client, coordinate the care, get the laboratory results ordered and processed, and see that therapy is delivered. The complexity of the interrelationships and the nature of interdependent work create conflict moments for nurses. This coincides with Kotter's (1979) ideas about dependency, power, and conflict in organizations. He viewed power as a mechanism to resolve conflict.

The source of a conflict can be interpersonal or organizational in nature. Furthermore, these categories often overlap. In some cases the conflict situation grows to involve multiple groups or pairs of groups.

Personal and organizational goals and values may clash over general policies. *General policy* refers to the course of action taken by an institution, department, or unit. Policies are the guidelines developed to handle specific issues. They are designed to give guidance about standardized ways to make decisions in recurring circumstances. However, professionals and other care providers may approach situations with diverse viewpoints about the "best" way to handle a specific problem. Disputes between nurses, physicians, and assistive personnel arise over methods and procedures involving specific diagnostic, therapeutic, clerical, or managerial routines. Clashes may result when a nurse's professional judgment as an autonomous professional intersects with standardized policies developed by the institution and designed to produce uniform behavior.

Resource allocation is an issue associated with the definition of organizational conflict. Cost-containment strategies have created conflict over scarce resources in organizations. Nurses often are placed in the center of this conflict. The scarcer the resources, the greater is the potential for conflict.

Power divisions occur across organizational and interpersonal lines to produce role conflicts. Role conflicts often manifest themselves in role overload and role ambiguity. Role overload is a common source of nursing conflict. It occurs when nurses are expected to perform the work of other employees or disciplines in addition to providing nursing care. The result of overload often is burnout. Another facet of role conflict, role ambiguity, occurs when the nurse's responsibility expands faster than is officially recognized. When roles are unclear, conflict can surface.

Another stress point for conflict in nursing occurs when the individual's needs intersect with the organization's needs and goals. Role stress and strain are a reality in the work existence of nurses. For example, other decision makers in the environment may hold one view about what the nurse's role should be, whereas nurses may have an entirely different view, and the two views may conflict. For instance, nurses consider a part of their role to be client advocacy. When an unfavorable outcome occurs, the nurse's client advocacy role may be placed in opposition to the institution's image or legal liability needs. Furthermore, nurses as individuals may need job security, practice autonomy, or pay equity. These needs may conflict with the organization's needs to hold down labor costs or control the practice decisions of its largest category of workers.

Sometimes conflict stems from individuals' attitudes, personalities, and personal behavior. *Personal behavior* refers to style, mannerisms, or work habits. Chronic lateness is an example of a personal behavior that frequently causes conflict. In all cases, it is important for leaders and managers to separate issues related to persons and personalities from issues arising from the actual problem or problems.

Whatever the cause, when a conflict occurs, an individual can expect that more information will be needed to process the conflict constructively. Similar to problem solving, conflict situations require information gathering and clear problem definition. However, the conflict may be difficult to define, especially if more than one causative factor contributes to the tension. Furthermore, the conflict may involve a covert, less obvious issue than what is presented on the surface. Conflicts often appear larger and more difficult to manage than what actually can be done about them. For example, intense or high levels of emotion are a part of conflict. Both the emotional and issues content of the conflict will need to be managed. By identifying both the areas of agreement and areas of disagreement and then defining the extent of each party's aims, a nurse leader or manager can begin the process of constructively reducing a seemingly overwhelming conflict to a manageable and functional one.

Clearly, if not handled productively, conflicts can be a disruptive rather than a creative force. Conflict involves energy. Within an organization, consistently avoiding or suppressing conflict is usually not effective because conflict can be the first process that occurs in an attempt to create changes or to innovate. If managed appropriately, conflict can motivate people to look at situations and others in new ways. It can lead to increased productivity and harmony. Modes of behavior such as aggressive, hurtful competition maximize the destructive effects of conflict. For nurses, the techniques of problem solving form a useful basis for handling conflict. However, nurses need to cultivate an understanding of conflict and an attitude of self-confidence in constructive conflict management.

A related issue for nurse leaders and managers is the need to address cross-cultural conflicts, especially between high- and low-context cultures. Intergenerational and other cultural issues are further discussed in Chapter 13.

When conflict does occur, there are several strategies to manage the conflict. *First*, the negative emotion associated with the conflict situation needs to be reversed. Strategies such as visualization, breathing techniques, exercise, and expressing thoughts in writing can help put the situation in the proper perspective and dissipate negative emotions. The situation can be viewed as a chance to learn, grow, and transform negative emotions (Adlersberg & Ottem, 2004).

Second, an appropriate approach to manage the situation needs to be carefully chosen. The choice of the most appropriate approach depends on a considered balancing of variables such as the situation itself, the time urgency needed to make the decision, the power and status of the players, the importance of the issue, and the maturity of the individuals involved in the conflict. Although most of us prefer certain approaches to others, the consistent use of one style may limit an individual's ability to manage conflict. With learning and experience, other approaches that are appropriate for the situation can be chosen.

Third, the key to resolving most conflict situations is good communication skills. Techniques such as active listening, open questions, paraphrasing, and clarifying inconsistencies should be used. The use of assertive statements that begin with "I" allows the expression of thoughts, feelings, and needs without attacking or blaming the other person (Adlersberg & Ottem, 2004).

Finally, the goal of conflict resolution is to create a win-win situation for all. Although it is not realistic to think that every conflict can be resolved in such an ideal fashion, win-win solutions are a worthy goal requiring hard work, creativity, and sound strategy.

CURRENT ISSUES AND TRENDS

POLITICAL POWER

With more than 2 million registered nurses in the nation, the nursing profession should be a tremendous force in political and public-policy debates. The reality offers the nursing profession a formidable power base that is largely untapped (Abood, 2007). Boswell and colleagues (2005) noted that, more than ever, nurses need to be involved personally and professionally in the political arena. Increasingly, decisions that influence nursing and health care are being made by politicians. All nurses are touched by the impact of policy and politics on health care and nursing practice, research, and education. Thus it is essential that nursing become involved in the political process. Barriers to political activism are thought to include heavy workloads, feelings of powerlessness, time constraints, gender issues, and lack of understanding of a complex political process (Boswell et al., 2005). In a recent article, Abood (2007) offered several strategies for effective action in the legislative arena—entering the legislative arena, understanding steps in the process, understanding the power players, understanding committees, and communicating with legislators.

Although today is an extremely turbulent time in health care, it is also a time of tremendous opportunity for the nursing profession. Nursing must accept the legitimacy of power and take advantage of the opportunity. Nursing curricula are an integral part of ensuring that nurses are capable of taking on a more active role in initiating and developing health policy processes (Whitehead, 2003). Including the concept of power in nursing curricula will better prepare nurses to participate in social and political decisions affecting health care. By creating dependency through becoming irreplaceable, demonstrating the ability to cope with uncertainty, and participating in the political process, the nursing profession will be able to establish its power base and use that power to facilitate change in health care organizations and the health care system.

As has always been the case, nurses derive their core power from being the health care providers whom the public most trusts. Caring generates power in relationships, and nurses can nurture this as a power source. Benner (1984) identified six types of power exercised by nurses (Box 12.5). Benner's (1984) six types of nursing practice–derived power can be compared to French and Raven's (1959) five sources of power for individuals. For instance, transformational and participative/affirmative nursing

Box 12.5

Power Exhibited by Nurses in Client Care

- *Transformational power:* the ability to assist clients to transform their self-image
- *Integrative power:* the ability to help clients return to normal lives
- *Advocacy power:* the ability to remove obstacles
- *Healing power:* the ability to create a healing climate and nurse-client relationship
- *Participative/affirmative power:* the ability to draw strength from a caring interaction with a client
- *Problem-solving power:* the ability, through caring, to be sensitive to cues and search for solutions to problems

Adapted from Benner, P. (1984). *From novice to expert: Excellence and power in clinical nursing practice.* Menlo Park, CA: Addison-Wesley.

practice power types would be similar to referent power. Integrative, advocacy, healing, and problem-solving types of power would be similar to expert power. French and Raven's (1959) legitimate, reward, and coercive power sources are more frequently applied to nurses as care managers than to nurses as care providers.

Individually, nurses can use power concepts to establish a power base and gain power in their work setting. For example, nurses can use information and expertise to construct powerful, persuasive arguments. Nurses can collect and analyze data that can be strategically used or controlled. They can be visible and persistent in goal pursuit. They can be creative and challenge the system to innovate. Nurses can use group power strategies such as networking, connecting, and collaborating to achieve professional goals.

Summary

- Power is a basic element in human relations and organizational behavior.
- Power is the capability to produce effects and allocate scarce resources.
- Power is the ability to exert influence over others by persuasion or coercion.
- Attitudes and values affect the use of power.
- Power is both personal and professional.
- French and Raven identified five sources of power.
- Three other power sources are connection, information, and group decision making.
- Perceptions and prestige are intertwined with power.
- Nurses derive power from nursing practice.
- Nurses can use a variety of sources of power and political strategies.
- Empowerment means developing a structure and environment in which people are motivated to excel.
- Conflict is a part of life and everyday experience.
- Conflict is a clash when threat or difference exists among people.
- Organizational conflict is a struggle for scarce resources.
- Conflict has both positive and negative aspects.
- Types of conflict include intrapersonal, interpersonal, and intergroup.
- Conflict can be competitive or disruptive.
- There are stages to the conflict process.
- There are many sources of conflict, but power clashes are at the root of conflict.
- Conflict is an occupational hazard for nurses.
- There is power in managing conflict.
- Nurses can follow a series of steps in handling conflict situations.
- There are three general strategies for conflict management.
- There are ten different conflict resolution techniques.
- Conflict outcomes are win-lose, lose-lose, or win-win.

CASE STUDY

After graduating from the University 3 years ago, Nurse Katie Gardner had been working as a public health nurse. She enjoyed her work, but after

3 years in the position, she decided to return to the hospital. As she stated, "I didn't want to lose the skills that I had acquired as a student." A year ago, she accepted a position on the evening shift in a surgical unit. After 3 months in the position, Katie was promoted to charge nurse on the evening shift. The nurse aides who were very capable caregivers had worked on the unit for years and quickly recognized Katie's inexperience. They complained bitterly about their assignments. They were continually argumentative and/or sarcastic. They often gave Katie the silent treatment and avoided eye contact. If asked to assist with an extra task on the unit, they were resistant, procrastinated, and made excuses about not having time. The evening supervisor and nurse manager did not offer much support. They indicated that good nurse aides were hard to find and Katie needed to learn to handle these employees. Katie was extremely discouraged and dreaded going to work. She was considering leaving the hospital. However, first she reviewed basic power and conflict theory. Perhaps communication strategies might work to address the issues.

1. What are the dimensions of power and conflict evident in this case study?
2. How is it possible to turn the situation around?
3. How can a win-win situation be created?
4. What power and conflict resolution strategies might be helpful?
5. Which communication techniques would be most constructive?
6. What are the disagreements, interference, and negative emotions involved in this situation?

CRITICAL THINKING EXERCISE

Nurse Katherine Trader had been the director of women's services for the past 10 years at a community hospital. She was well respected and had made many contributions to women's services. Her accomplishments included creating a variety of new programs for mothers and babies and designing and overseeing the construction of new birthing rooms for the obstetrical unit. Recently, the department was reorganized and it was decided that women's services would be divided into two departments. Nurse Trader was assigned to labor and delivery, the nursery, and the postpartum unit. A newly hired nurse who was a friend of the chief nursing officer (CNO) was assigned to the GYN unit and pediatrics. Although the new director had no prior management experience, those who interviewed her during the selection process were impressed with her credentials and experience and ultimately recommended that she be hired. Nurse Trader was unhappy with the reorganization but decided to do her best to make it work. She believed that the new arrangement was working until she noted that the new director was attempting to push her aside. The new director would communicate only via e-mail. Later, Nurse Trader learned that during meetings with the CNO, the new director would attempt to persuade the CNO that Nurse Trader was mismanaging her job. The new director also constantly complained to managers in other departments that Nurse Trader was not pulling her weight. On one occasion, Nurse Trader's subordinates asked her a question that she could not answer. The new director stated to the staff, "I can't believe she didn't know that." On another occasion after Nurse Trader instructed her staff to complete a task, the new director stated, "I wouldn't make you do something like that."

1. What are the dimensions of power and conflict evident in this case study?
2. How is it possible to turn the situation around?
3. How can a win-win situation be created?
4. What power and conflict resolution strategies might be helpful?
5. Which communication techniques would be most constructive?
6. What are the disagreements, interference, and negative emotions involved in this situation?

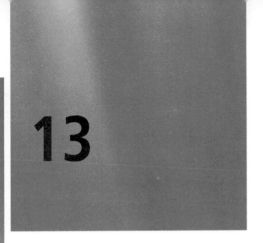

13 Workplace Diversity

G. Rumay Alexander

CHAPTER OBJECTIVES

- Develop an awareness of cultural diversity as it relates to personhood or the workplace
- Define cultural relativism, cultural competence, corporate culture, cultural diversity, fusion, race, world view, and symbolic violence
- Analyze cultural influences on health care and the working environment
- Recommend effective cultural competency strategies for the workplace
- Evaluate the impact of biases, stereotypes, and prejudices on nursing practice and provider interactions
- Demonstrate the impact and influence that data can have on strategic planning for the future
- Exercise critical thinking to conceptualize and analyze possible solutions to a practice exercise

The growing appreciation that we live in a global community not only has raised awareness of individuals in one culture to the values of those in other cultures but also has heightened an awareness of differing values in subcultures within local communities. The meltdown of the "melting pot" resulting from waves of immigration, the inability to keep pace with the demands for health care providers, and the subsequent recruitment of foreign nurses from Great Britain, Ireland, Canada, and the Philippines have had the unintended consequence of thrusting cultural diversity onto agendas that had resisted addressing the issue in spite of the fact that U.S. society has historically been characterized by its pluralism. It is no longer

Editor's note: After the 3rd edition of this book was published, I received a note from a Korean American second career nursing student who had lived in the United States for 21 years. She objected to the 3rd edition's statement that "*people of color* is a positive, politically correct term of inclusivity." This student's legitimate concern reflects the difficulty of finding acceptable terminology within and among different ethnic groups. The student's comments reemphasize the difficulty of communicating about this sensitive topic without the likelihood of offending. This is especially difficult in the construction of comments for larger audiences such as in talks to large groups and in text books.

As I responded to the student, "I have a Hispanic relative who is offended whenever someone talks about Latinos, Chicanos, etc. Her reaction is that they are just trouble makers. She is Hispanic and that is that. I have some friends who are African-American/black/people of color who do not care which term is used while others prefer a particular term and insist that other terms are racist. What I think this shows is the importance of respecting each individual's right to be thought of in the way that they find self-affirming. Once again this is easier on a one-to-one basis, but we must also strive to achieve it in all arenas."

Open discussion of the options available is certainly a step in the right direction. The editor appreciates the feedback from the aforementioned student, and in this 4th edition, the statement "*people of color* is a positive, politically correct term of inclusivity" has been removed. The phrases "candidates of color," "managers of color," and "executives of color" have been used when no other acceptable term seemed to apply.

Diane L. Huber

acceptable to presume that the current predominant Eurocentric culture in the United States is more right or more appropriate in all situations, nor is it to be expected as the majority view. This lack of acknowledgment however, has resulted in cultural diversity being intentionally ignored or benignly neglected or receiving rhetorical lip service in many sectors but noticeable in health care.

Being in touch with the realities of the changing nature of society is a fiduciary responsibility of organizations and is critical to the viability of institutions and professions such as nursing. Managing diversity in the workforce is a major business initiative that requires an intentional focus on the stewardship of differences—not on the ignoring of them. Any waste of talent is a loss of productivity, innovation, and wealth that organizations can ill afford. The advantages of strategically incorporating a fair and judicious workplace can bring tremendous yields, such as the following:

- Provide more supportive work environments, maximizing discretionary effort and consequently enhancing performance
- Improve retention of the best people, which directly affects costs of recruitment, selection, training, and start-up, as well as productivity and "brain drain"
- Fortify team effectiveness and take advantage of the wealth of skills available for the organization's maximum impact
- Capitalize on the likelihood that people from nontraditional environments, who often seem to push organizations to out-of-the-box thinking, can help address today's problems
- Capture the interest of more consumers and relate to more customers' needs, thereby increasing market share by means of a workforce that not only reflects the same market composition but also understands what only those who are members of the representative cultures can articulate
- Lay the groundwork and provide the appropriate contexts for future growth in business opportunities at a time when differences in race, culture, language, customs, and styles have become essential considerations.

The increased awareness of a global community over the past 30 years galvanized the following five major socioeconomic developments that have helped define American society and will continue to do so for the foreseeable future:

1. The emergence of a global economy
2. **Technoshrink**, which is the diffusion of information and telecommunications technology
3. The maturation of the Baby Boom generation
4. The continued rise of individualism at the cost of collective responsibility
5. The deterioration of principles of economic justice

All of these factors have special implications for the nursing profession.

The world population is expected to double by 2050, with 85% of the increase occurring in developing countries. The mean age of the global population is declining, with 50% of the world's current population younger than 20 years. Conversely, industrialized nations are "going gray," with a rising median age and a declining ratio of active workers to retired persons (Kotlikoff & Burns, 2004).

The demographic face of America is changing radically in the areas of age and ethnicity. Accompanying these seismic changes in demographics is a shift in "who is large and in charge." In less than a century, the United States will move from being "forever young" to "forever old." The largest part of this change will occur in the next 30 years as Baby Boomers retire (Health Resources and Service Administration [HRSA], 2003). In fact, by 2030 all 79 million Boomers will be at least 65 years of age. The gap between the number of working-age people and the children and seniors who depend on them will widen as Boomers age. There will be 72 young and elderly for every 100 people of working age by 2050, up from 59 in 2005. Experts expect this change to exact a fiscal toll that will shake the economy. All of the forces capable of enlarging the retired elderly population are in overdrive (Figure 13.1).

The distribution of the four major U.S. population groups (White, Black, Hispanic, and Asian American/Pacific Islander) is shifting as well. At the turn of the twentieth century, only one in eight Americans was non-White. According to a Pew

Percent of population in three age-groups: United States, 1950, 2000, and 2050

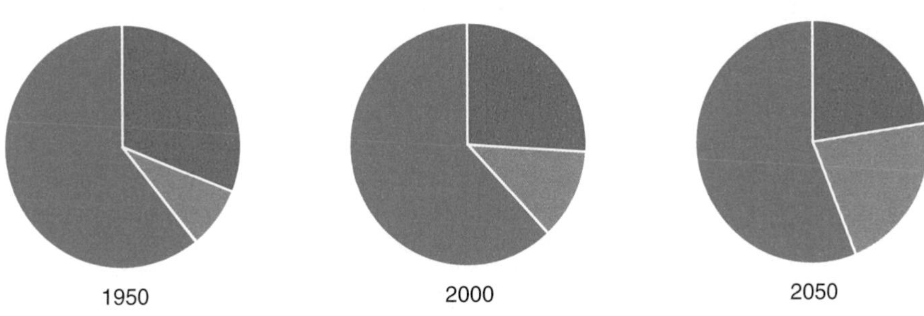

SOURCES: U.S. Census Bureau, 1950 and 2000 decennial censuses and 2050 middle series population projections.

Figure 13.1
Percentage of the population in three age-groups in the United States in 1950, 2000, and 2050. (Data from Centers for Disease Control and Prevention [CDC]. [2003]. *Health, United States, 2003 with chartbook on trends in the health of Americans.* Hyattsville, MD: Author. Retrieved November 25, 2008, from www.cdc.gov/nchs/data/hus/hus03.pdf.)

Research Center report (2008), the U.S. population will soar to 438 million by 2050, primarily driven by immigration. The number of people 65 years of age and older will increase to 19% while those 18 to 64 years of age will decline to 58% from 63%. Hispanics, already the largest minority group, will more than double their share of the population, from 14% in 2005 to 29%. Blacks will make up 13% of the population and Asians 9%. It has been projected that by 2050, nearly one in five Americans (19%) will have been born outside the United States. Whites who are not Hispanic will drop from 66% to 47%, making them a minority. An estimated one in three Americans will be Black, Hispanic/Latino, Native American, or Asian/Pacific Islander. In 2001, one in four Americans was non-White.

Adding to the demographic storm but in keeping with the reality of the changing lifestyle of many Americans and their offspring was a first-of-its-kind decision by the U.S. Census Bureau and the Federal government in 2000 to change the way in which the collection of racial and ethnic data would be compiled. Individuals were given the option of designating more than one race in addition to Hispanic ethnicity, and nearly 3% of the population exercised that option. Individuals could select any one of 15 different race categories plus three options for writing in a more specific race. This change, coupled with Hispanic ethnicity, brought an unintended consequence of yielding potentially up to 264 racial and ethnic combinations, thereby challenging the country's concept of what constitutes a minority.

The implications of increasing age and growing ethnicity are far reaching and include the following:

- More chronic illness
- Generational workforce issues
- Language and cultural challenges
- Stewardship of resources
- Ethical issues

Because ethnic minorities constitute a growing percentage of the working-age population, their representation in the professional health workforce will naturally rise but not necessarily in the same proportions as the overall population and thus not in the strategic places that impact the way we provide health care. The United States will rely increasingly on ethnic minority caregivers.

> *"Of all the forms of inequality, injustice in health care is the most shocking and inhumane."*
>
> *-Dr. Martin Luther King, Jr.*

DEFINITIONS

Cultural competency and cultural diversity are not two sides of the same coin, but they are intricately related. Equating diversity with inclusion has inhibited our ability to see it beyond race and gender. **Cultural diversity** refers to the variations among groups of people with respect to the habits, values, preferences, beliefs, taboos, and rules for behavior determined to be appropriate for individual and societal interaction. This refers not only to the idea that persons are unique but also to the notion that organizations are unique and possess a **corporate culture**, which is a way or manner in which business is conducted, often based on written and unwritten rules. Metaphors are often used to capture the nature of such cultures—for instance, a business or place of employment might be referred to as a *circus*, a *minefield*, a *roller coaster*, a *puzzle*, a *rat race*, or a *zoo*. In the context of **culture,** "values and beliefs" encompass what deserves attention, what gets rewarded, what things mean, and which reactions are acceptable in a given situation and which are not. An organization is defined by its actions and investments.

There are often disconnections between the values espoused and those that actually guide daily interaction—that is, between the *de jure* and *de facto* cultures. **Diversity,** stripped of its cultural and political baggage, is about differences that make a difference. A frequent mistake is to give the bulk of attention to race and gender in societal groupings in the definitions used to capture the meaning of inclusivity while giving only minor, if not negligible, attention to the other dimensions. The Human Genome Project provides evidence that all human beings share a genetic code that is over 99% identical. Yet when it comes to race, it is the social meanings and the assigned status with its political constructs that preoccupy many even to this day. Racism and its related elements of biases, stereotypes, and prejudices need to be understood as well. **Racism** is discrimination based on race or color. It is often accompanied by inferences of inferiority or subhumanism. It affects factors that, in turn, affect outcomes (Institute of Medicine [IOM], 2003) (Figure 13.2).

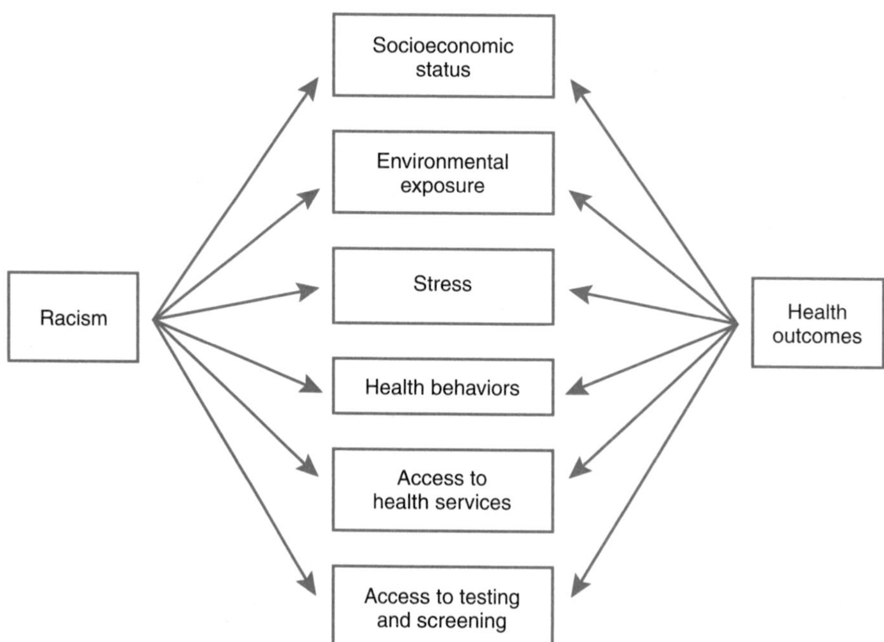

Figure 13.2
Racism as a precursor model. (From Institute of Medicine [IOM]. [2003]. *Unequal treatment: Confronting racial and ethnic disparities in health care*. Washington, DC: National Academies Press.)

Prejudice is an emotional categorical mode of mental functioning involving rigid prejudgment (stereotypes) and misjudgment of human acts. Prejudice that is operationalized at the organizational level is discrimination. Prejudices bring a mixture of exploitative gains such as economic advantage, social snobbery, or a feeling of superiority. The building blocks of prejudice are generalizations or preconceived notions about a group of people. They can be negative or positive, but seldom are they neutral. They provide a rationale for putting people in boxes, which keeps the real persons from being seen and known. **Stereotypes** are fixed and/or distorted views, whether positive or negative, toward all members of a group of people. Stereotypes that are a part of society encircle and cloud view points and perceptions, even though an individual may actively disagree or not consciously hold that stereotype.

LEADING & MANAGING **DEFINED**

Technoshrink

Diffusion of information and telecommunications technology.

Cultural Diversity

Variations among groups of people with respect to the habits, values, preferences, beliefs, taboos, thoughts, communications, actions, customs, and rules for behavior and among racial, ethnic, religious or social groups.

Corporate Culture

A way or manner of doing business.

Culture

Beliefs, behaviors, actions, values, communication, perceptions, traditions, and customs common to a population.

Diversity

Holding multiple perspectives without judgment.

Racism

Any type of action or attitude, individual or institutional, that prescribes and legitimizes a minority group's subordination by claiming that the minority is biogenetically or culturally inferior.

Prejudice

An emotional categorical mode of mental functioning involving rigid prejudgment and misjudgment of human acts.

Stereotypes

Fixed and/or distorted views, whether positive or negative, toward all members of a group of people.

Cultural Relativism

Maintaining a sense of objectivity and holding multiple perspectives without judgment.

Bias

A mental preference or inclination.

Cultural Competence

Having the capacity to function effectively as an individual and an organization within the context of the cultural beliefs, behaviors, and needs presented by consumers and their communities.

Ethnicity

Shared origins and shared culture.

Ethnocentrism

Interpretation of the beliefs and behavior of others in terms of one's own cultural values and traditions; belief that one's own culture is superior.

The concept of **cultural relativism** requires that individuals not judge but, rather, consider the actions, beliefs, or traits within their own cultural contexts to better understand them. It involves maintaining a sense of objectivity and an appreciation for the values of other cultures, not judging whether they are "good" or "bad" by external standards (Loustaunau & Sobo, 1997). Emotions have a way of manifesting themselves, and when the emotion is prejudice, the resulting manifestation is a **bias** or preference. Mix a strong preference or emotion with power and the means by which to use it and the stage is set for resultant acts such as disparity in health care outcomes because of a provider's views being influenced by his or her culture.

Providing care effectively to persons from a multiplicity of cultures is called *cultural competence.* **Cultural competence** includes recognizing the importance of integrating persons who are from a non-dominant group into the culture and considering their values in the process of organizational operations. There are many definitions for cultural competence, but transcending those definitions is the sense of a dynamic, evolving process. The Federal Civil Rights legislation and the 2001 National Standards for Culturally and Linguistically Appropriate Services (CLAS) in Health Care (Betancourt et al., 2002; Office of Minority Health, 2001) use an expanded definition of cultural competency (Center for the Health Professions, 2002):

> Cultural and linguistic competence is a set of congruent behaviors, attitudes, and policies that come together in a system, agency, or among professionals that enable effective work in cross-cultural situations. Culture refers to integrated patterns of human behavior that include the language, thoughts, communications, actions, customs, beliefs, values, and institutions of racial, ethnic, religious, or social groups. (p. 49)

Ethnicity is tied to notions of shared origins and shared culture. It should be acknowledged that cultural identities are simultaneously inclusive and exclusive. At times this works as an advantage on which to capitalize; at other times it is a disadvantage with challenges requiring attention.

Competence implies having the capacity to function effectively as an individual and an organization within the context of the cultural beliefs, behaviors, and needs presented by consumers and their communities (Center for the Health Professions, 2002).

BACKGROUND

What difference does difference make? Apparently a great deal, particularly in the workplace. With these changes come cultural factors that affect every facet of life—from the clothes we wear, the food we eat, the art forms and entertainment we prefer, and who marries whom to issues of education, housing, and census reporting. Also affected are how we think; how we look; our preference for doing things the way we do; and the systems in which we move, live, and experience our being. In an attempt to keep pace, health care institutions have joined with other business, social, educational, and economic endeavors to recognize the importance of workforce diversity. Differences in time orientation, communication patterns, value systems, perceptions of staff responsibilities or nursing roles, along with differences in educational preparation, are common sources of conflict. Eighty-five percent of the people fired in 2003 were fired because of relationship problems (Murphy Leadership Institute, 2004). Those who are different are often seen or labeled as the problem.

The need is growing to approach all relationships, whether with patients or colleagues, with full respect for the many dimensions of culture that, in varying degrees, exert a strong influence on any kind of encounter. Demographic changes mean there will be diverse approaches to work and diverse meaning to the work itself, which may affect who should do what work and why some interventions are done at all. For example, nurses from a socialized medicine system have difficulty seeing health care as a business. Yet the public now clearly demands value, accountability, and customization. Signals ignored, decisions deferred, and changes postponed all have an impact on the future. The aggregate consequences of choices, actions taken, and actions deferred also set a course for the evolving future.

In today's workplace, the ability to work with all health care personnel and their patients, including those who speak English as a second language or English as a new language, is a must. In fact, as of 2006, the Joint Commission on the Accreditation of Healthcare Organization's (JCAHO) Information Management Standard requires hospitals to collect information on patients' language and communication needs (JCAHO, 2005). Nurses can ill afford to ignore the fact that the place where health care professionals received their provider education or where they had prior work experiences has provided a filtered perspective. Nursing education outside of the United States is more focused on clinical skills and less on the psychosocial needs of patients or nursing theory. Such cross-cultural comparative perspectives influence behaviors in the workplace. From this awareness has emerged the understanding that the more each of us knows about these aspects of our patients' and co-workers' culture, the better able we will be to partner with colleagues in our day-to-day work. To understand, respect, and provide the best choices for the multitude of human responses to health and illness or the vicissitudes of life, the nurse must also recognize the multifaceted ways in which culture affects and morphs perspectives and outcomes.

CULTURAL AWARENESS

The diversity of our society is placing great demands on all of the world's systems. Cultural awareness is a crucial link to practicing empathy, understanding, valuing, and caring in health care and nursing care. Cultural awareness also involves recognizing the importance of integrating persons with other values in the process of organizational operations. Cross-cultural comparative perspectives influence health care practices whether prescribed or lived.

United States health care providers tend to impress, if not force, on people from cultures outside the United States, the Eurocentric concepts of patient autonomy, truth telling, informed consent, work rules of engagement, empowerment, and decision making. The expectations, attitudes, and behaviors of nurses are affected by their personal cultures as well as the culture of the nursing profession just as surely as the expectations, attitude, and behaviors of those with whom they come in contact, including their colleagues. For example, a staff meeting designed to plan for the future could be seen as a waste of time by those who, because of their generational influence or the locus of control dictated by their cultures, wish to spend company time working on issues and problems of the present. The Agency for Healthcare Research and Quality (AHRQ) (2003) has noted that cultural competence requires that organizations and their people value diversity, assess themselves, manage the dynamics of difference, acquire and institutionalize cultural knowledge, and adapt to diversity and the cultural contexts of the individuals and communities they serve. Without a sense of cultural competence, **ethnocentrism** can run amuck.

Assumptions about U.S. health care abound for those operating and navigating the health care system—whether they fit their culture or not. The most prevailing assumptions are as follows:

- Self-determination, autonomy, independence
- Right to know
- "I" make the decisions about my health care
- Moral obligations and medical ethics based on Judeo-Christian beliefs
- Health care providers have the "obligation to tell the truth"
- Duty to give all information to the competent patient (individual) or his or her surrogate
- The institution's written bill of rights for patients and staff are defined as individual rights rather than inclusive of other ways of viewing individuals within a group context
- Informed consent does not include family unless the individual is legally unable to make his or her own decision. In this situation, the individual chooses a family member or someone else or a legal protocol to procure a surrogate to make those decisions (Crow et al., 2000).

High Context and Low Context

The assumptions of high context and low context are a part of the health care context, which is always dynamic. The context dictates "where one is coming from" and how information or knowledge is communicated in human transactions or relationships, and it is culturally based. From a global perspective, the cultural context of the Western world is "low context." In low-context cultures, the explicit verbal or written message carries the meaning. Low-context cultures require extensive detailed explanations and information because they are making up for what is missing in a situation. In high-context cultures, often found in the non-Western world, that which is written or stated rarely carries the meaning. The meaning of the message is understood by reading between the lines for what is not written or stated. In high-context cultures, most of the meaning is assumed to exist by the nature of the situation (i.e., the context). Most nuclear families are high context, relying on high interpersonal interaction and subtle messages. Leaders from a low-context culture may have the power to define the rules of work and to determine what will be rewarded, who gets promoted, what benefits will be offered, and what values will define the organization. Therefore placing someone from a high-context workplace culture into a setting dominated by leaders from a low-context culture increases the likelihood of perceptions of inequity and workplace conflicts (Hall & Hall, 1990). Box 13.1 displays countries by low-context and high-context characteristics.

Box **13.1**

Low-Context and High-Context Cultural Differences

Low-Context (United States, Canada, England, Russia, Northwestern Europe)	High-Context (China, Japan, Arabia, Mexico, South America, Pacific Islands)
Very verbal	Less verbal or nonverbal
Individual	Group
Equality	Individual dignity
Democracy	Consensus
Personal freedom	Obligation to others
Fairness	Fate (karma, joss)
Achievement	Process/role
Innovation	Continuous improvement
Entrepreneurship	Communal
Competition	Cooperation

Cultural Competence

Cultural competence, to be properly understood, should be viewed as both a process and an outcome rather than a final point of destination. It involves an ongoing expansion and updating of an individual's understanding of different cultures. However, it is equally important to remember that culture shapes behavior but does not predict it. A person's identification with a culture does not necessarily mean that that person agrees with all the dominant beliefs in that culture. In fact, cultural diversity involves differences not only between cultures but also within cultures.

It is not only prudent but also wise for nurses to develop ways of working effectively in cross-cultural circumstances and exhibit respect for cultural difference. In today's world, culturally sensitive areas will arise in nursing practice such as gender differences, racial and ethnic differences, working in multicultural and interdisciplinary teams, and shifts in power. The nursing profession is projected to be one of the largest job growth areas among professions in the United States. New nursing job opportunities, along with replacement needs as projected retirements occur, provide a significant opportunity in nursing for increasing the presence of persons who can bring with them an understanding of the values of other cultures and an increase in the diversity of perspectives.

CURRENT ISSUES AND TRENDS

The basis for enhancing the work environment for all comes down to trust, respect, shared goals, affirmation of identity, and communications.

Recently the appearance of nooses in the workplace has surfaced feelings, which have gone underground in a politically correct world. Being "PC" should mean personal connections, not political correctness, because the world of work is all about relationships. With an increasingly diverse workforce, managers of every age are encouraged to emphasize the values of the organization before their personal values.

Race

There is an old saying, "*Sticks and stones may break my bones, but words will never hurt me.*" Life would be easier if that were true. But words *do* have meaning, power, impact, and influence. Nowhere is that more apparent than the use of the word or label "race" and all that is associated with it when this social construct is placed on the organizational table. Multi-racial designation is also a social construct, and now more than ever individuals are self-declaring the many facets of their heritage and lineage. Individuals can be Asian, Native American, or Black by experience or rearing influence. An example is Tiger Woods, who confuses America when he declares himself as Asian. Given our proclivity as humans to focus on the physical—those aspects that our eyes tell us are different—and given that people cannot disguise certain features, the dynamics of race continue to be fundamental to the understanding of the existence of health care disparities and the ever-present discrimination that occurs at every level. Race has always been a subtext in America. Like it or not, we live racially structured lives and, as expected, race affects work relationships.

The following excerpt, "10 Things Everyone Should Know about Race," was developed to accompany a three-part PBS series titled *RACE—The Power of an Illusion*. This piece outlines the current thinking that nudges us to question our notions of race.

> Our eyes tell us that people look different. No one has trouble distinguishing a Czech from a Chinese. But what do those differences mean? Are they biological? Has race always been with us? How does race affect people today?
>
> There's less—and more—to race than meets the eye (California Newsreel, 2003, p. 1)*:
>
> 1. **Race is a modern idea.** Ancient societies, like the Greeks, did not divide people according to physical distinctions, but according to religion, status, gender, class, even language. The English language did not even have the word "race" until it turned up in 1508 in a poem by William Dunbar referring to a line of kings.
> 2. **Race has no genetic basis.** Not one characteristic, trait or even one gene distinguishes all the members of one so-called race from all the members of another so-called race.
> 3. **Human subspecies don't exist.** Unlike many animals, modern humans simply have not been around long enough or isolated enough to evolve into separate subspecies or races. Despite surface appearances, we are among the most similar of all species.
> 4. **Skin color really is only skin deep.** Most traits are inherited independently from one another. The genes influencing skin color have nothing to do with the genes influencing hair form, height, blood type, musical talent, athletic ability or forms of intelligence. Knowing one trait, like skin color, does not necessarily tell you anything else about him or her.
> 5. **Most variation is within, not between, "races."** Of the small amount of total human variation, 85% exists within any local population, be they Italians, Kurds, Koreans or Cherokees. About 94% can be found within any continent. That means two random Koreans may be as genetically different as a Korean and an Italian.
> 6. **Slavery predates race.** Throughout much of human history, societies have enslaved others, often as a result of conquest or war, even debt, but not because of physical characteristics or a belief in natural inferiority. Due to a unique

**RACE—The Power of an Illusion* was produced by California Newsreel in association with the Independent Television Service (ITVS). Major funding was provided by The Ford Foundation and the Corporation for Public Broadcasting Diversity Fund. It is available on videocassette and DVD from California Newsreel (www.newsreel.org).

set of historical circumstances, ours was the first slave system where all the slaves shared similar physical characteristics.

7. **Race and freedom evolved together.** The U.S. was founded on the radical new principle that "All men are created equal." But our early economy was based largely on slavery. How could this anomaly be rationalized? The new idea of race helped explain why some people could be denied the rights and freedoms that others took for granted.
8. **Race justified social inequalities as natural.** As the race idea evolved, white superiority became "common sense" in white America. It rationalized not only slavery but also the extermination of Indians, exclusion of Asian immigrants, and the taking of Mexican lands by a nation that otherwise professed a deep belief in liberty and equality. Racial practices became institutionalized within American government, laws, and society.
9. **Race is not biological, but racism is still real.** Race is a powerful social idea that gives people different access to opportunities and resources. Our government and social institutions disproportionately, albeit often invisibly, channel wealth, power, and resources to the "unmarked" race—white people. This affects everyone, whether we are aware of it or not.
10. **Colorblindness will not end racism.** Pretending race does not exist is not the same as creating equality. Race is more than stereotypes and individual prejudice. To combat racism, we need to identify and remedy social policies and institutional practices that advantage some groups at the expense of others.

Culture is a kind of knowledge that all of us in society use and act on. It provides a basis for self-evaluation of our "learned humanity." Nurses have an obligation to fulfill their social contract with society and, above all, to do no harm to those in their care. This means nurses must be prepared to the best of their ability to care for all those in their communities of practice and to work effectively with providers from other cultures and subcultures. Nursing school curricula, policies, practices, and continuing education offerings need to be revised for this to occur. Curriculum is enormously powerful. It defines what is real and what is unreal, what counts and what is unimportant, who or what is normal and natural versus who or what is abnormal and deviant. It determines where the margins or peripheries are and who occupies them. It has the power to teach us what to see and thereby the power to render people, places, things, and even entire cultures invisible. Nursing education's embrace of the "caring paradigm" functions in a manner that makes it very difficult for nurses to discuss, let alone, recognize the racism that still permeates programs (Campinha-Bacote et al., 1996).

Multicultural Teams

Diversity is a basic component of a strong team. Valuing team members creates synergistic relationships, which translate into a higher quality of production. Ignoring diversity inhibits full participation and may even disrupt the workings of an effective team. Because much of the diversity of individuals is far below the surface, it may be difficult to recognize that there is a clash of cultures that is causing a team not to gel. In fact, relationships may be significantly damaged before anyone realizes that the conflicts that the team experience are not about what the team members say they are about. Recent research (Brett et al., 2006) has identified four categories of challenge that arise from differing styles of communication in multicultural teams that can jeopardize important projects:

- Direct versus indirect communication
- Trouble with accents and fluency
- Differing attitudes toward hierarchy and authority
- Conflicting norms for decision making

Of note are some words of caution. Individuals who cannot articulate their thoughts or feelings may be wrongly judged as less intelligent. Such logic can devalue those team members and subject them to disrespect, ridicule, and ostracism. Proceed with caution about communication style preferences, decision making, and organizational structure. Individuals from Western cultures such as the United States prefer direct forms of communications, such as asking questions, giving opinions freely, and making eye contact; they tend to judge those who do not do so as dishonest and not trustworthy. Westerners also prefer flat hierarchal structures, but our colleagues from egalitarian cultures are uncomfortable on flat teams. Furthermore, an approach called *fusion* is getting serious attention from political scientists and government officials. It seems that today, more than ever, multicultural populations want to protect their cultures rather than integrate or assimilate. An awareness of cultural mismatches is the first step in being proactive in the approach to managing multicultural teams or, equally important, being a good team member.

Generational Workforce Diversity

A growing challenge in nursing leadership is the management of generational workforce diversity. Sociologists categorize generational groups into what they call *cohorts* (Alexander, 2001). These cohorts are members of a generation who are linked through shared life experiences in their formative years. As each new cohort matures, it is influenced by what sociologists call *generational markers.* Individuals are all products of their environment. Generational markers are events that affect all members of the generation in one way or another. Thus being aware of generational differences is essential for every organization's leadership in managing a multi-age workforce. Each generation possesses unique characteristics and often deems the values and behaviors of another as character flaws instead of cultural differences (Table 13.1). Each generation must discover its mission.

The Baby Boomers, born between 1946 and 1964, are occupying the leadership chairs of many executive suites, including those in health care organizations. Boomers present a striking contrast and replace members of the previous generation, those born between 1925 and 1945, often referred to as the *Mature Generation* or the *Silent Generation.* Members of the Silent Generation grew up in a period of strong military and political leaders, a time when respect for authority was expected, conformity was the characteristic most treasured and exhibited, and children were to be seen but not heard.

Boomers, historically the second largest generation in the workforce, have dominated U.S. society for many years. Beginning in January of 1996 and continuing for the next 18 years, a Baby Boomer will turn 50 every 18 seconds, and their preferences in every facet of American life are affected by their sheer numbers alone (U.S. Census Bureau, 1996). Efficiency, teamwork, quality, and service have thrived under their leadership. Boomers grew up in a period of unprecedented economic growth during which the United States had virtually no strong economic competitors. They grew up thinking they were special and that they could ignore or break rules and still be successful. They love convenience and brought true meaning to "charge it" when it comes to debt management. Financial security will remain a central issue for many. Consequently, many Boomers will work past the age of retirement. They have questioned traditional authority structures, blurred gender roles, and made vigorous attempts to push systems toward their ideas of perfection. During the Vietnam War,

Table **13.1**

Generational Characteristics

Matures	Baby Boomers	Generation X	Millennials
Hard work	Personal fulfillment	Uncertainty	What's next?
Duty	Optimism	Personal focus	On my terms
Sacrifice	Crusading causes	Live for today	Just show up
Thriftiness	Buy now/pay later	Save, save, save	Earn to spend
Work fast	Work efficiently	Eliminate the task	Do exactly what's asked

Data from Center for Generational Studies, Aurora, CO.

the Civil Rights confrontations, and Watergate, Baby Boomers saw clearly the vulnerability of authority, and they have been reluctant to accept formal authority since. Their preference is for a more participative and less authoritarian workplace.

Support for such a workplace environment comes also from members of Generation X (X'ers), born between 1965 and 1980, who share with Boomers an aversion to authority but with a decided preference for a balanced life. X'ers are the first generation of latchkey kids; as such, they found the need to be resourceful at an early age. Their childhood years have been marked with economic uncertainty, and thus they are skeptical of traditional practices and beliefs. In their view, employment contracts are agreements that either side can cancel at will, which means that placing their future in the hands of employers makes them extremely uneasy and is thus highly unlikely. The length of time spent with an organization is less relevant to X'ers than how to protect themselves from the capriciousness of business challenges (Wendover, 2002). Trust imposes its own constraints and has its own rules.

Both the youngest group in the workplace and the largest group in U.S. history are the Millennial workers, those born between 1981 and 1999. This group is known by several other monikers, including *Generation Y, Generation Why?, Nexters,* and the *Internet Generation.* The common marker of their developmental years is technology. This group is the most demographically diverse generation in this country's history. These workers have astonishing multitasking skills. They also tend to have a positive outlook and a desire to improve the world.

Many believe that Millennials are shallow on basic skills; but because they grew up with computers, they can create solutions that other generations could not have imagined. Technology guides their every move. They are problem solvers who grew up in a flourishing economy. Millennials matured in a world in which shortcuts, manipulation of rules, and situational ethics seem to have reigned. They got the message somehow that the final word is not the final word. They do not live to work; they work to live. Thus they have a different set of expectations about the world of work. Most enjoy the liberty of working on their own in a style that favors their work ethic. Millennials have learned that their presence is in demand. To thrive, they need clear definitions of outcomes, resources to do what needs to be done, and a deadline.

Nurses recognize that cultural diversity, awareness, and unconditional positive regard for people are critical core concepts (Habayeb, 1995). Yet, somehow, cultural diversity is not seen as a powerful variable in how nurses communicate and interpret behaviors or mediate conflict among themselves. There can be a direct impact on how problems, assessments, diagnoses, and intervention strategies are determined. As global trends in mobility, migration, cultural identity importance, and changing roles increase, the need for awareness is greater (Leininger, 1997). Shifts in the site of care to the community, a rise in moral/ethical issues in health care, and a desire by many, but not all, consumers to control and regulate their own health care—along with a concomitant desire to make it better for others—have created a necessity to know and respect diverse perspectives (Galanti, 1999; Gazmararian et al., 1999).

Attracting a Culturally Diverse Workforce

Reaching for cultural competence in the health care workplace requires not only that institutions strive for a greater understanding of the values represented by divergent clients but also that efforts be increased to diversify the makeup of nursing and other health care professions. The Pew Health Professions Commission report (1998) spoke directly to this need:

> Not only would renewed commitment to diversity be the fairest way to accommodate all potential medical practitioners, it would be in the best interest of those parts of the population that bear the greatest burdens of poor health. Students that come from medically underserved communities have demonstrated a much greater willingness to return to them to practice. By knowing the language and cultural mores of the population they serve, they offer a more complete and effective kind of care.

Workplace diversity is an issue for both the workforce and the clients. The institutions that take the initiative to strive for cultural competence can engender respect for the similarities and differences that both employees and clients bring to the health care endeavor. Success with cultural competence concerning employees will improve understanding for culturally diverse clients. In turn, success with culturally diverse clients will help an institution recruit and maintain a culturally diverse workforce. The inevitable conflict that can occur when persons with diverse value sets work together will decrease as success is achieved in cultural competence in interpersonal relationships.

Cultural diversity in the workplace has both advantages and challenges. The synergy of diverse viewpoints can improve nursing's knowledge base and care strategies. Yet the differences among people can give rise to communication gaps and conflict. The same issues of communication, interpersonal space, social proscriptions, time sense, and other variations in beliefs and behaviors that are important when interacting with clients need to be balanced and smoothed in work groups and teams. The nurse care manager can employ cultural competence principles in leading and managing work groups. Strategies of respect for differences, exploring beyond the comfort zone, withholding judgment of others, emphasizing the positive, and practicing good communication techniques are strategies for success (Grossman & Taylor, 1995).

Efforts to pursue cultural competence must incorporate the broad base of diversity. The American Association of Colleges of Nursing (AACN) has reiterated the importance of intensifying efforts to increase diversity in programs that prepare nurses (AACN, 2008).

Diversity initiatives in the nursing profession will have a marked opportunity in the coming years since the outlook for growth in nursing jobs is bright. The U.S. Bureau of Labor Statistics (BLS) (Hecker, 2004) projected that nursing, the largest health care occupation, will grow faster than the average for all other occupations. In fact, in 2004, registered nurses ranked number-1 of the 10 occupations with the largest projected job growth in the years 2002 to 2012. This top-10 list is used in career guidance and may have an impact on nursing school enrollments.

Each nurse lives and works within a meld of cultural aspects and values. This includes influences from race, community, ethnicity, lifestyle, and professional and organizational cultures. The nursing leadership and management challenge is to effectively manage diversity.

LEADERSHIP AND MANAGEMENT IMPLICATIONS

Differences per se do not create tensions in the workplace; the judgments people make about one another do. The goal of leadership is to get divergent points of view working for the common good, with the outcome being accomplishing what needs to be done (Alexander, 2002). It would behoove leaders to consider the knowledge about generations

PART III

LEADERSHIP & MANAGEMENT BEHAVIORS

Leadership Behaviors

- Envisions holistic care, including cultural competence
- Influences others to be culturally sensitive
- Inspires trust and confidence among culturally diverse people
- Leads others toward cultural competence

Management Behaviors

- Coordinates care to include cultural assessment and planning
- Integrates cultural diversity into the workplace
- Plans cultural sensitivity training
- Organizes teams that include culturally diverse workers

Overlap Areas

- Plans for cultural diversity issues
- Motivates others toward culturally competent communication

and cultural parameters when putting people together to accomplish the goals of the organization and when choosing communications, messages, and the best modality to fit the recipient.

Data suggest that it will be many years before the profiles of health professionals reflect the population as a whole (Health Resources and Services Administration [HRSA], 2002). This underscores the need for all health care providers in a given community to be culturally competent. Advocates argue that increased representation of minorities in the health workforce not only will increase equity but also will improve the efficiency of the health care delivery system (American Hospital Association [AHA], 2002). The nurse care manager can employ cultural competence principles in leading and managing work groups (Davidhizer et al., 1998).

A related issue is the recruitment of foreign-born registered nurses into the United States to alleviate the current nurse shortage. Although this strategy may be part of the solution to the U.S. shortage, it has ethical ramifications. Given a global shortage of RNs, is this practice ethical? What preparations are made to increase cultural sensitivity once foreign-born RNs arrive?

Estimates from the 2000 Sample Survey of Registered Nurses (HRSA, 2001) indicated that approximately 86.6% of RNs were non-Hispanic White, 4.9% were non-Hispanic Black, 3.5% were Asian; 2% were Hispanic; 0.5% were American Indian or Alaskan Native; 0.2% were Native Hawaiian or Pacific Islander, and 1.2% were of two or more racial backgrounds. The Bureau of Health Professions (BHP) of the U.S. Department of Health and Human Services (USDHH) reported that African Americans and Hispanics are underrepresented in the registered nurse workforce relative to their proportion in the overall population (Section 3.3.2). Under-representation of racial/ethnic groups in the workforce may inhibit recruitment into the profession because of a lack of role models. The key is being sensitive to differences. These statistics point to the need for nursing to fuel strong cultural competence initiatives. The focus needs to be on both culturally competent client care practices and a culturally competent workplace environment. Lack of understanding of cultural practices may result not only in longer hospital stays, noncompliance issues, loss of meaningful, more readmissions to health care facilities, and more ER visit but also in the loss of meaningful provider-to-provider communications (AHA, 2003).

Strategies for Cultural Competence

Learning and showing respect for differences, exploring beyond the comfort zone, withholding judgment of others, emphasizing the positive, and practicing good communication techniques are strategies for success (Grossman & Taylor, 1995). Leaders are urged to develop a human resources strategic plan that outlines how the organization will recruit and retain a diverse staff that reflects the community. Much time and concern are being focused on the supply of workers in the future. A favored formula is known as "½ × 2 × 3"—meaning half as many people work twice as hard and are paid, on average, twice as well, yet produce three times as much. This formula makes it poignantly clear that understanding the workforce is not only wise but also urgent. Cultural competency standards should be incorporated into all aspects of the institutional strategic plan for such areas as patient care, patient education, staff training, and community outreach. Sharing data and providing cultural competency education are needed at board or trustee level to inform and enlighten those who are making major institutional decisions.

Managers are challenged to examine policies and practices in every phase of the organization within the context of generational differences. Recruiting techniques, communications, human resource policies, and benefit plans must be tailored to these varying groups (who have varying needs) and the values they embrace. In a global economy, the workforce continues to change, challenging generational and racial/ethnic stereotypes.

Cultural differences in ways of doing things are learned and transmitted via cultural environments. Because cultural differences are learned, cultural sensitivity and competence, regardless of the setting, also can be learned. A few suggestions are as follows:

- Know your own culture, values, and biases.
- Listen and observe.

- Emphasize the corporate values up front.
- Develop the ability to be a teacher and a learner at the same time.
- Hold up your end of the bargain. Follow through with commitments.
- Give clear directions, provide support and resources, and always give a deadline of completion for projects.
- Delegate the outcomes instead of the individual tasks.
- Give the big picture. Give examples of how to make tenure and success work in a win-win situation for all involved.
- Consider the rules and procedures you implement within the workplace. Be sure they are clear, but expect them to be interpreted in ways you had not anticipated.
- Manage your expectations. Be open to ideas and comments.
- Provide straightforward steps for decision making.
- Be courageous, and correct behavior. Take action, document, and follow through.
- Manage according to values and attitudes of the individual's generation.
- Provide the opportunity to grow.

The Sullivan Report "Missing in Action" and the Institute of Medicine's (IOM) "Unequal Treatment" speak to the fact that inequities also extend into the educational system and impact on future nurse supply issues. Recruitment into nursing is often built on a strong background in science, and increasing minority recruitment will be aided by minorities having access to preparation in the sciences and similar mental training for increasing processing skills and abstract levels of thinking. If non-privileged students are not prepared in science, mathematics, and other skills that equip them for college, then the disparities in the workplace will continue. The issue of minority performance in science is a preparation problem, not an achievement problem. *Science Highlights 2000*, published by the National Assessment of Educational Progress (NAEP) (Dantley, 2004), provided a current picture of student performance in science by racial/ethnic subgroups. According to this report, science performance at the national level is disaggregated into three content areas—earth science, life science, and physical science for grades 4, 8, and 12—and based on three ability levels: low, middle, and high performance. Examination of the most recent high school NAEP data revealed that all percentile scores are declining for each ability level, with the middle, or 50th, percentile decreasing the most. Accordingly, Black high school students performed the lowest in each science area.

Optimal health requires a safe community, a safe home, adequate food and clothing, and access to quality education. Policy decisions at the federal and state levels play a great role in the optimal health equation. Politics determine which schools are funded and which are underfunded, as well as which nurses to hire and which to ignore. Legislators decide how much money to commit to state universities, thus implicitly deciding who can attend based on tuition rates and other constraints. The terms and conditions of education, affirmative action, rising tuition costs, lack of financial aid, and other issues need attention. The best social program is a quality education for all.

Other strategies include incorporating diversity into mission statements, career development and management programs for minority groups (often using mentoring, examining recruitment and retention practices, community involvement and outreach, diversity dialogue groups, and targeted education and training programs). Building competence in problem solving and intervention techniques can be augmented by practice exercises. Exercises such as analysis of body language can help in understanding cultural differences, as follows (ISCOPES, 2003):

- **Silence:** You may view silence as awkward; however, other cultures are quite comfortable with periods of silence.
- **Distance:** The most comfortable physical distance between you and another person varies from culture to culture. The typical American generally prefers to be about an arm's length distance away from another

Practical Tips

Tip #1: Avoid Unquestioned Assumptions

Make every attempt to bring out and examine all assumptions before making decisions. Unquestioned assumptions often result in misinterpretation between generations.

Tip #2: Understand That Values Vary

Foreign-born populations do not fall into the same categories and values as their American counterparts of the same age or generational cohort. They are more apt to focus on survival.

Tip #3: Set Clear Rules

Having rules of engagement set by all team members at the beginning of any project will minimize friction, conflict, misunderstandings, and disrespectful acts.

Tip #4: Understand the Need for Cultural Analysis

Culture is not static. Take time to assess and analyze the culture you work in to be better able to spread positive cultural sensitivity.

person. Hispanics usually prefer closer proximity than most Americans. Allow the other person to establish the proper distance for the interaction.

- **Eye Contact:** The amount of eye contact that is comfortable varies with each culture. Many Americans are brought up to look people straight in the eye. However, some cultures have been taught not to make eye contact. Staring is considered impolite in some groups. However, if you avoid eye contact or break eye contact too frequently, it may be misinterpreted by the participant as disinterest. Sitting next to someone, rather than directly across from them, will reduce eye contact.
- **Facial Expression:** Expression of emotion between people of different cultures varies from very expressive, as with Hispanics, to total non-expressiveness, as with Asians. Many Americans have a tendency to regard people who are more expressive as immature and those with less expression as unfeeling.
- **Body Language:** The position, gestures, and motion of the body can be interpreted differently depending on the culture. The use of hands is a common vehicle for nonverbal expression. A firm handshake may be a positive gesture of goodwill in the Anglo-American culture, but some other cultures prefer only a light touch. Many cultures use handshakes more frequently than do most Americans, some even as a greeting between husband and wife. Standing with hands on hips may imply anger to some participants. Pointing or beckoning with a finger may appear disrespectful to some cultures. Conservative use of body language is wise when you are uncertain as to what is appropriate within a cultural group. Observing actions and interactions may give you direction. Being open with participants and asking general questions about body language can also help.

Cultural competence practice exercises often use vignettes or case studies. Some examples are presented in the Case Study in this chapter.

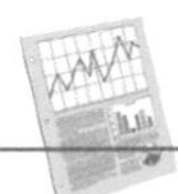

Research Note

Source: American College of Healthcare Executives (ACHE). (2003). *A race/ethnic comparison of career attainments in health care management: 2002.* Chicago: Author. Retrieved June 10, 2004, from www.ache.org/pubs/research/research.cfm

Purpose

The purpose of this cross-sectional study of White, Black, Asian, and Hispanic health care executives was to determine whether race/ethnic disparities in health care management careers still exist and whether they have narrowed since 1997.

Discussion

A 1992 joint study by the American College of Healthcare Executives, an international professional society of health care executives, and the National Association of Health Services Executives, whose membership is predominantly Black, compared the career attainments of their members. The study found that, although Blacks and Whites had similar educational backgrounds and years of experience in the field, Blacks held fewer top management positions, less often worked in hospitals, earned 13% less, and were less satisfied in their jobs.

In 1997, the study was replicated and included White, Black, Asian, and Hispanic health care executives. That research showed that disparities in the proportions of top-level management positions continued to exist between White women and minority women but that there were no significant differences in the proportion of top positions held by male managers in the various race/ethnic groups. Other measures of career attainment continued to show disparities between Whites and minorities: Whites were more often employed in hospitals and, in general, expressed higher levels of satisfaction with various aspects of their jobs. While the earnings gap grew between White and Black women, it narrowed between White and Black men. Other minority executives' earnings fell between the White and Black averages.

The findings of the third study show that minorities continue to lag behind Whites in several areas, including job satisfaction, winning senior-level jobs, and median total compensation.

Application to Practice

Although the field has progressed in promoting racial and gender diversity in health care management during the past 30 years, evidence shows there is still a long way to go.

Suggested recommendations, which, it is hoped, are important steps toward leveling the playing field, were as follows:

- Establish flexible hiring criteria that allow for judgment relative to talent and potential, and avoid limiting positions to those with precise prior experience.
- Identify internal candidates of color who exhibit leadership attributes to assume senior-level executive positions. Through such systematic succession planning, organizations will develop a diverse talent pool to draw from as senior leadership positions become available.
- Promote executives of color to senior-level positions, especially in organizations serving predominantly minority communities.
- Urge senior executives to speak out and advocate for diversity in the organization's leadership team.
- Encourage senior managers to promote managers of color by following guidelines for succession if these have been established; conducting candid, periodic evaluations of such managers; and providing counselors to help bridge cultural differences between minorities and Whites on the management team.

Summary

- Managing diversity is about acknowledging differences.
- Factors of a global economy, diffusion of information, generational issues, the rise of individualism, and the deterioration of economic justice all affect nursing and society.
- The distribution of major U.S. population groups is shifting.
- Cultural diversity refers to variations among groups of people with respect to habits, values, preferences, beliefs, taboos, and rules for behavior.
- Racism is related to biases, stereotypes, and prejudices.
- Cultural relativism requires that individuals consider their own cultural contexts.
- Cultural and linguistic competence is a set of congruent behaviors, attitudes, and policies that enable effective working together.
- Generational cohorts exist and may clash in the workplace.
- Symbolic violence in the workplace creates both safety and respect issues.
- U.S. health care providers need to explore the differences between high-context and low-context cultures.
- Welcoming environments support the recruitment and retention of a diverse nurse pool.
- Health disparities describe differences in the burden of disease and other adverse health conditions that exist among specific populations.
- Racial and ethnic disparities arise from patient-related and system-related factors.
- The nursing workforce does not match the profile of the population in terms of diversity.
- Nurses and nursing leaders need to manage diversity effectively.

Case Study

Case 1

"I have had it with the 27-year-old twit I now work for," Charlie said to his wife. "I walked into her office today to discuss the system analysis she wanted me to do, but she had that tribal music going and I couldn't understand half of what she was saying. When I asked her to turn it off, she did. But she looked at me like I was senile. I was working for this company when she was in diapers.

Then there's that tongue stud in her mouth. How can you talk when that thing's banging around on your teeth? She may be a bright kid, but she doesn't have a clue how to work with us."

1. What can Charlie do to foster his relationship with his supervisor?
2. What parameters would you set around his supervisor's management style?
3. Now reverse the situation. How do you think the 27-year-old supervisor views the aging Boomer Charlie? What parameters would you set around Charlie's interpersonal interactions at work?

Case 2

In a disagreement between two employees, one Black and the other a Filipina, a few heated words were exchanged. Wanting to avoid an escalation of the conflict, the Filipina employee walked away. The Black employee, on the other hand, valuing direct confrontation of conflict and wanting to settle the problem, followed her co-worker, trying to talk to her. This only caused more anxiety and panic for the Filipina woman, who had been taught to value harmony and smooth interpersonal relationships. Thus she continued to refuse to discuss it. When the Black woman persisted, the Filipina turned and threatened her co-worker, telling her if she came any closer, she would hit her. The result was a grievance in which both employees reported being physically threatened by the other.

1. What perceptions of each employee can be explained by cultural differences?
2. How could this conflict have been avoided or defused?
3. Why is dealing with conflict important?

CRITICAL THINKING EXERCISE

Example 1

A female college student from another country sought health care for menstrual pain after arriving in the United States. She went to a physician to obtain a prescription for medication to ease the pain. The physician decided that the woman should have a Pap smear. Being unmarried, the patient could not agree to this for religious prohibition reasons. She tried to explain the situation to both the doctor and the nurse, but neither realized the cultural/religious issue nor seemed to understand the patient's inability to comply. The nurse told the woman, "Whatever your reasons are, you should have the Pap smear first as a diagnostic procedure." The woman refused, left the clinic, and did not return.

Example 2

Ramadan is the holy month of fasting and prayer in the Muslim religious tradition. During Ramadan, Muslims refrain from food and drink from early morning until early evening. Although pregnant women, children under the age of 14, and those who are ill are exempt from the fast, many Muslims will not take medications during the hours when they are fasting. Muslim patients who normally take medication, such as those with diabetes, can benefit from guidance that would help them alter their medication schedules in keeping with their fast.

Questions

1. What is the problem in each example?
2. Whose problem is it?
3. What should the nurse do in each case?
4. How can the nurse be culturally competent in each case?

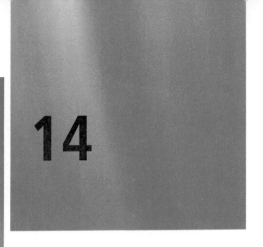

14 The Health Care System

Thomas R. Clancy

CHAPTER OBJECTIVES

- Define and describe the U.S. health care system
- Trace the historical background of changes to the U.S. health care system over time
- Identify organizations, agencies, and components related to the health care system
- Analyze relevant challenges and trends
- Exercise critical thinking to conceptualize and analyze possible solutions to a practice experience

The health care system in the United States has evolved into a unique patchwork of diverse components. It is not a true "system" in the strict sense of the word. There is no central oversight agency to coordinate operations to achieve efficiency or fairness. Rather, the U.S. health care system is fragmented and complex, composed of a multitude of players with different objectives, some of whom may be functioning in isolation from or in conflict with others. It operates under a complicated variety of rules and regulations. Utilization of health care services varies widely by geographical region, with much of the variation attributable to differences in resources and capacity to provide care. Considered as a whole, it is also a large employer with a huge economic impact nationally, at the state level, and in many local communities. Although citizens of other countries frequently look to the U.S. health care system for its health professions educational programs and some tout it as the best in the world, its access and quality vary.

DEFINITIONS

Basic health and medical care is a pervasive social need. Taken as a whole, the collective subsystems of health care form a unique system. In a broad sense, the health care delivery system refers to the major components of the system and the process that enables individuals to receive health care (Shi & Singh, 2001). The **health care system** is defined as all of the structures, organizations, and services designed to deliver professional health and wellness services to consumers.

Traditionally, U.S. health care has been organized around the physician and the acute care hospital. A triad of client, nurse, and physician became the basis of health care delivery, although not all members had equal status. Today, health care is increasingly more complex and care frequently is delivered by a multidisciplinary team of providers across a continuum of care. Nursing personnel constitute the largest group of health care providers in the United States. They are the health care personnel who both deliver and coordinate care for clients. Therefore nurses are poised to be the care providers most prepared for population health and care coordination roles. As health care becomes coordinated and integrated across settings and sites, nurses will need to better understand the larger health care system.

LEADING & MANAGING DEFINED

Health Care System

All structures, organizations, and services designed to deliver professional health and wellness services to consumers.

Medicare

The national health insurance program for persons ages 65 years and older, some disabled persons, and persons with end-stage renal disease.

Medicaid

A joint federal and state program designed to pay for medical long-term care assistance for individuals and families with low incomes and limited resources.

EVOLUTION OF THE HEALTH CARE SYSTEM

Today's health care system is much different from health care in the early history of this country. It has been transformed from a relatively weak and minor enterprise into a vast and sprawling empire. Advancements in science played an important part in this transformation, but social and other factors, including the growing involvement of government, were instrumental as well.

Government plays a pervasive role in the financing and delivery of services in the U.S. health care system (Feldstein, 1994), and its influence is exercised at the federal, state, and local levels. This pervasiveness was not always the case, however; the government's role has evolved over time (Litman, 1997). Justification of the role of government in health care is often made along the lines that health care is not like other goods. It truly can be a matter of life and death, and the absence of personal health and medical knowledge forces many people to rely on advice from the non–health care sources. Furthermore, it is known that private enterprise may not have the incentive to adequately address the health issues that society deems necessary. For example, it may make sense from a business perspective to focus only on areas in which money can be made. This, unfortunately, might preclude access to costly life-saving services or pharmaceuticals. Funding for medical education and research, which can be viewed as public goods, would also likely be significantly less without government participation. On the other hand, the involvement of government in the health care system at multiple levels sometimes leads to confusing, conflicting, and cumbersome regulations. In fact, regulatory paperwork now requires at least 30 minutes for every hour of patient care provided in hospitals and, in many cases, much more (American Hospital Association [AHA], 2002).

First 150 Years

As eloquently described in *The Social Transformation of American Medicine* (Starr, 1982), in the early stages of this country the family was the locus of most care for the sick. Many held the belief that ordinary people were capable of treating illness. In fact, guides to domestic medicine were popular and used to spread medical knowledge. Early hospitals were primarily charitable organizations. The people who used them tended to be poor, without access to family, or in need of isolation. Because of the spread of infection, early hospitals were also places that people were well advised to avoid.

Advances in medical knowledge and technological progress during the latter half of the nineteenth century led to greater reliance on hospitals as locations for the delivery of care and the dissemination of new knowledge. Important factors in this development included the ability to control pain through drugs such as morphine; to anesthetize patients with ether, chloroform, or other options; and to control the spread of infection with antiseptic procedures. Also instrumental were the establishment of laboratories and the use of x-rays to facilitate diagnosis. Eventually, hospitals became regarded as necessary for the delivery of care because of the superior services they could provide. This success enabled hospitals to attract paying patients, which encouraged the growth of health insurance.

Although health insurance was already in existence, the beginning of modern private health insurance can be attributed to the creation of a Blue Cross plan in 1929, whereby an arrangement for hospital services was struck between a group of teachers and the Baylor Hospital in Dallas, Texas (Whitted, 1999). Coverage for physician services came about later with the establishment of Blue Shield plans. The growth and development of hospitals also facilitated increases in both the number and specialization of the health care system's workforce. By 1929, the number of hospitals had grown to 6665, up from only 178 in 1872 (Raffel & Barsukiewicz, 2002; Shi & Singh, 2001).

The skill set of early doctors varied widely since there were no significant barriers to becoming a doctor and most were trained under an apprenticeship system (Raffel & Barsukiewicz, 2002). For instance, of the 3500 to 4000 doctors at the time of the American Revolution, only about 400 had formal medical training. Many people counted being a doctor as among their multiple occupations. The first medical school in this country was chartered in Philadelphia in 1765. Medical schools multiplied after the War of 1812, growing to 42 schools by 1850, but many were of dubious quality (Starr, 1982). The Association of American Medical Colleges, organized in 1876, sought to improve the quality of medical education. In 1891, it supported a 3-year training period and, in 1894, was persuaded to support a 4-year curriculum. By 1900, there were 160 medical schools, although the American Medical Association, which was founded in 1847, deemed only 82 acceptable, 46 doubtful, and 32 unacceptable (Raffel & Barsukiewicz, 2002).

The Carnegie Foundation for the Advancement of Teaching was invited by the American Medical Association to conduct an independent assessment of the nation's medical schools. Abraham Flexner performed the work on behalf of the Foundation. His report of 1910 had a profound effect on modern medicine. The Flexner Report concluded that there was an oversupply of poorly trained physicians produced by a number of educationally deficient medical schools. By 1915, the number of medical schools had decreased by 36, or by slightly more than one-third, although some of this decrease was the result of mergers. Flexner had actually recommended a greater decrease, but state legislatures frequently sought to keep at least one medical school in their state. Changes brought about as a result of the Flexner Report led to significant improvements in the physician education process (Raffel & Barsukiewicz, 2002; Starr, 1982).

Like physicians' abilities, the abilities of early nurses also varied widely. Physicians gave lectures to nurses intermittently during the early and mid-1800s, but this did not constitute formal courses of instruction. Private duty nursing was the main form of employment for early nurses. In the 1870s, the formation of nursing schools in Connecticut, Massachusetts, and New York marked the beginning of formal training of nurses in the United States. Growth of hospital training schools for nurses followed, with student nurses providing a low-cost source of labor. By 1900, there were more than 400 schools of nursing and more than 1700 by 1920. Quality concerns existed, however, and shortly after the 1926 creation of the Committee on the Grading of Nursing Schools, the Committee produced a report concluding that there were too many inadequately prepared nurses and that improvements were necessary. Enhancements to educational programs were made in the 1930s, including changes in coursework and a shift of focus in the primary function of nursing schools as places to educate nurses, not simply to provide services to hospitalized patients. After the 1930s, hospital staff nursing replaced private duty nursing as the major form of nursing employment (Kalisch & Kalisch, 2004; Schorr & Kennedy, 1999).

Rise of the Modern System

In answer to a shortage of hospital beds, due in part to a standstill in civilian construction during World War II, the Hill-Burton Act of 1946 was passed to create a federal-state matching program to fund the construction of hospitals. This program proved extremely successful, and the number of nonfederal, short-term general and specialty hospitals grew from 4444 with 473,000 beds in 1946 to 5407 hospitals and 639,000 beds by 1960 (AHA, 2004a). The expansion of acute bed capacity under Hill-Burton enabled hospital utilization to increase. Admissions alone jumped from 13.7 million in 1946 to 23.0 million in 1960. This contributed to a need for more health care providers, as did factors such as greater expectations from a more affluent public and pressures from underserved areas.

The 1959 publication of the Surgeon General's Consultant Group on Medical Education report (the Bane report), which predicted a physician shortage of 40,000 by 1975, played an important role in expanding the physician supply (Blumenthal, 2004). The Health Professions Educational Assistance Act of 1963 provided federal funds for construction and modernization of medical and health science schools and inducements to expand enrollments. Medical school enrollments, for example, grew from 32,000 in 1963 to over 50,000 by 1973 (Jolly & Hudley, 1998), and new technicians, paraprofessionals, and allied health occupations began to arise around this time (Thomas, 2003). The Nurse Training Acts of 1964 and 1971 are examples of legislation passed during this period that specifically provided federal funds for nursing education (Sultz & Young, 2004).

With increases in buildings and human resources necessary to deliver health care addressed, facilitating patient access represented the next challenge. Employer-based health insurance did exist, but it was more available in larger, urban-based companies than in rural parts of the country (Geyman, 2002). For most people, the only way to obtain and keep health insurance was to work for an employer who provided it. Although not comprehensive in nature, Titles 18 and 19 of the Social Security Act created the Medicare and Medicaid programs, respectively, in 1965. **Medicare** was designed as a federal program to provide access to health care for the elderly, and **Medicaid** was designed as a combination federal/state program to provide access to health care for the poor. Medicaid's dual-program status has resulted in each state customizing the program to fit its needs within general parameters established by the federal government, whereas Medicare is more uniform. Both programs have grown substantially since their inception, and their escalating costs are significant challenges to be addressed. In fact, Medicaid expenditures are now approximately 21% of all state spending (National Governors Association, 2004), and in 2003, Medicare spending totaled \$6880 per enrollee, or about \$272 billion (Medicare Payment Advisory Commission [MedPAC], 2004). Table 14.1 provides a list of terms related to the health care system.

The increasing complexity of hospitals and the environment in which they operated resulted in the need for more of a business orientation, and professional administrators began to arise as leaders. Nurses and physicians had previously occupied this role. Government became increasingly concerned about cost control and accountability as it expanded its involvement in health care. In the 1970s, health system agencies and certificates of need (CON) were implemented as strategies to alleviate these concerns. These initiatives sought to address cost and accountability issues through planning and regulating the supply of services. After it was clear that they failed to stem rising costs, prospective payment was introduced in the Medicare program in 1983 with the implementation of diagnosis-related groups (DRGs).

The idea behind DRGs was to encourage efficiency in the inpatient hospital setting by fixing payment for categories of similar patients in advance. Before the implementation of DRGs, hospitals received cost-based reimbursement, whereby the more they did, the greater the reimbursement, so there were few incentives to control costs. The implementation of DRGs also helped facilitate a shift in the delivery of care from the inpatient to

Table 14.1

Glossary of Acronyms Related to the Health Care System

Acronym	Full Name
AHA	American Hospital Association
AHRQ	Agency for Healthcare Research and Quality
BBA	Balanced Budget Act of 1997
BBRA	Balanced Budget Refinement Act of 1999
BIPA	Benefits Improvement Protection Act of 2000
CDC	Centers for Disease Control and Prevention
COGME	Council on Graduate Medical Education
USDHHS	U.S. Department of Health and Human Services
DRGs	Diagnosis-Related Groups
EMTALA	Emergency Medical Treatment and Active Labor Act
ERISA	Employee Retirement Income Security Act
GAO	General Accounting Office
HEDIS	Health Plan Employer Data and Information Set
HIPAA	Health Insurance Portability and Accountability Act of 1996
HMO	Health Maintenance Organization
HRSA	Health Resources and Services Administration
JCAHO/TJC	Joint Commission on Accreditation of Healthcare Organizations/ The Joint Commission
MedPAC	Medicare Payment Advisory Commission
MMA	Medicare Prescription Drug Improvement and Modernization Act of 2003; Medicare Modernization Act
NCQA	National Committee for Quality Assurance
NIH	National Institutes of Health
OECD	Organization for Economic Cooperation and Development
PhRMA	Pharmaceutical Research and Manufacturers of America
PPO	Preferred Provider Organization

the outpatient setting. The concept of fixing payment for like categories of care was subsequently adopted by other payers and even expanded to the outpatient side. However, this strategy is still vulnerable to increases in volume or enhanced coding of the health problems used to assign a DRG.

In 2008, the Centers for Medicare & Medicaid Services (CMS) unveiled plans to create 745 new severity-adjusted DRGs (Medicare Severity DRGs [MS-DRGs]) to replace the 538 existing ones. The MS-DRGs base payments on cost rather than charges to better reflect the severity of a patient's condition. The agency believes this payment track would more accurately reflect the costs of caring for a patient and reduce incentives to "cherry-pick" the healthiest and more profitable patients.

The MS-DRGs are an update of the original prospective payment system but could have far-reaching impacts, For example, CMS claims the reimbursement levels for hospitals overall should increase by $3.3 billion, or an average of 3.3%, to more than 3500 acute-care hospitals provided they report quality data to the agency. However, the American Hospital Association (AHA) argues that the proposed rule would result in a $5 billion reduction to hospital payments because of changes to the standard payment rate (Lubell, 2007).

Managed care systems, such as health maintenance organizations (HMOs) and preferred provider organizations (PPOs), were yet another development in the quest to contain costs. Managed care represents a shift in the power relationship between payers and providers. Managed care refers to linkages between the financing and delivery of services in such a way as to permit payers to exercise control over the delivery of services. Common elements include provider panels, limited choice, gatekeeping, risk sharing, and quality management and utilization review (Sultz & Young, 2004). The premise is that costs can be controlled by constraining beneficiary choice of providers while supplying providers with an incentive for efficient practice. Managed care has been successful in stemming the rise of health care costs, although public reaction to gate keeping and restrictive networks has been negative in many cases. The number of people enrolled in HMOs actually peaked in 1999 at 81.3 million and dropped to 76.1 million in 2002 (National Center for Health Statistics [NCHS], 2003). Still, all but 5% of employees covered by employer health benefits in 2003 were enrolled in some form of managed care (Sultz & Young, 2004).

Patients were not the only group to react to managed care. Providers also expressed concerns and many sought "any willing provider" laws to prohibit closed panels that would have denied them business. Individual states' ability to address concerns across the spectrum of managed care plans was limited, however, by the Employee Retirement Income Security Act (ERISA) of 1974. Although ERISA was intended primarily to keep employees from losing their pensions and to free employers from differing state regulations, it also had the effect of limiting the ability of states to regulate health plans covered by ERISA. This latter provision preempted a state's ability to mandate benefits for managed care plans covered by ERISA and necessitated, for example, federal action to address coverage limitations related to areas such as postnatal hospitalization (Mariner, 1996).

The Balanced Budget Act of 1997 (BBA) was a major reform that called for savings in excess of $125 billion in Medicare and Medicaid spending over 5 years. Among the many changes, including the creation of Medicare+ Choice plans, which offered broader choices to Medicare beneficiaries, were reductions in Medicare and Medicaid payments to providers. Teaching hospitals were particularly hard-hit, experiencing both care-related payment changes and cuts in medical education payments (Dickler & Shaw, 2000). When Congress created the prospective payment system for Medicare in 1983, it included graduate medical education payments that increased with the number of trainees. Although the number of U.S. medical school graduates increased only modestly in the years since DRGs were implemented, the number of trainees in hospitals increased significantly as a result of an influx of international medical school graduates (Blumenthal, 2004). The BBA capped the number of residency positions eligible for federal support at each hospital and phased in a reduction of indirect medical education payments.

Several pieces of legislation—including the Balanced Budget Refinement Act of 1999 (BBRA); the Medicare, Medicaid, and State Children's Health Insurance Program Benefits Improvement and Protection Act of 2000 (BIPA); and the Medicare Prescription Drug, Improvement, and Modernization Act of 2003 (Medicare Modernization Act [MMA])—helped restore some funding that had been cut by BBA and expand access to health insurance for children. The MMA bill also contained language that significantly changed the Medicare program by calling for the creation of a prescription drug benefit for Medicare beneficiaries. An interim prescription drug discount card program began June 1, 2004, and is the first step toward realizing this benefit. Implementation of the Medicare drug benefit in 2006 increased Medicare's share of total national prescription drug spending from 2% in 2005 to 18% in 2006 (Kaiser Family Foundation, 2008). Highly controversial during debate, the MMA has received even greater attention since its passage and the revelation that its projected costs are $534 billion over the next 10 years, rather than the approximately $400 billion Congress was told.

In summary, the evolution of the modern health care system has been described as encompassing four phases. The institutionalization of health care phase occurred from about 1850 to 1900, with the establishment of large hospitals and the clustering and coordination of services and personnel. The second phase, occurring from 1900 to World War II, was associated with the introduction of the scientific method into medicine and the subsequent recognition of medicine as having a solid scientific base. The third phase, from World War II until the 1980s, is characterized by the growing interest in the social and organizational structure of health care with the growing involvement of the federal government and the increased attention toward financing. Finally, the fourth and current phase is described as an era of limited resources, restrictions on growth, and reorganization of the methods of financing and delivery of care (Torrens, 2002).

COMPONENTS OF THE HEALTH CARE SYSTEM

Health care has been defined as "the total societal effort, undertaken in the private and public sectors, focused on pursuing health" (Longest et al., 2000, p. 4). The U.S. health care system is composed of a diverse collection of organizations and individuals that address specific needs in ways that are sometimes separate, coordinated, or overlapping. These needs include such tasks as the production and delivery of services and supplies, financing, and oversight. A broad continuum of health care services exists over which components may interact, including preventive care, primary care, specialized care, chronic care, long-term care, subacute care, acute care, rehabilitative care, and end-of-life care (Shi & Singh, 2001). Patients can become involved with the health care system at any of these points. Because changes in one component can affect others, it is important to be aware of environmental trends.

Providers

There are more than 200 occupations and professions among the health care workforce (Sultz & Young, 2004), encompassing a diverse range of provider roles, including physicians, nurses, dentists, pharmacists, and allied health professions, such as physical and occupational therapists, laboratory technologists, and dietitians. Different services tend to be rendered by these providers, depending on their training and scope of practice. One can also classify providers by type of organization, such as community health centers, hospitals, or nursing homes. The major characteristics differentiating institutional providers include services offered (e.g., primary, secondary, tertiary, or quaternary), length of direct service provision (i.e., short-term, long-term), ownership (i.e., public, private), financial provisions (i.e., for-profit, not-for-profit), teaching status, geographical location, and accreditation and licensure status (Brooks, 2003).

Physicians

Physicians are the highest-paid professionals in the United States (Weinberg, 2004) and occupy the dominant role in the provider hierarchy. This is related to their training and knowledge, as well as requirements that care be delivered under their orders (Raffel & Barsukiewicz, 2002). They are independent practitioners who hold primarily a Doctor of Medicine (MD) or a Doctor of Osteopathy (DO) degree. Although graduates from foreign countries also practice here, most U.S. physicians received their degree from one of this country's 126 allopathic medical schools or 20 colleges of osteopathic medicine. The number of allopathic medical school graduates remained relatively stable each year between 1995 and 2001 at approximately 15,800, whereas the number of osteopathic medical graduates increased from approximately 1800 to 2600 (NCHS, 2003). Approximately 25% of the physicians in the United States are international medical graduates, and this represents a growing trend (McMahon, 2004). The number of physicians per 1000 population grew from 2.4 in 1990 to 2.8 in 2000. This ratio was equal to the median of the industrialized countries that are members of the Organization for Economic Cooperation and Development (OECD) in 1990 but is lower than the 3.1 median reported for 2000 (Anderson et al., 2003).

Earning a degree does not constitute the final step in the process before a physician can receive a permanent license. Although state laws vary, the minimum requirement is at least a 1-year graduate medical education experience, and many states require more. Most physicians complete residencies lasting several years, specializing in areas including, but not limited to, anesthesiology, dermatology, emergency medicine, family practice, general surgery, internal medicine, neurology, obstetrics-gynecology, ophthalmology, orthopedics, pathology, pediatrics, psychiatry, radiology, and urology. The National Resident Matching Program is a computerized service used to match residency positions with physicians, based on the interests of both parties. Most physicians in the United States are specialists rather than primary care physicians. A growing number are becoming hospitalists, which is a relatively new role in which they care for the patients of office-based physicians when these patients require inpatient hospital care.

Hospitalists represent one of the fastest growing specialties in American hospitals today. Nearly 78% of hospitalists are trained in internal medicine and focus their practice strictly on acute care, hospitalized patients. Hospitalist programs developed as a result of the following (Wachter & Goldman, 1996):

- Limitations on resident duty hours imposed by the Accreditation Council for Graduate Medical Education (ACGME) and the American Osteopathic Association (AOA). This reduced inpatient coverage by as much as 25% in academic and community-based hospitals participating in residency programs.
- Economic pressures on primary care physicians to increase office practice productivity. These physicians found treating more office patients in lieu of maintaining a hospital-based practice more financially feasible. This resulted in many primary care physicians giving up their hospital-based practices.
- Ongoing pressure on hospitals to reduce length of stay, reduce cost, and maintain on-site coverage 24 hours a day, 7 days a week.

Nurses

Nurses are the largest group of health care professionals. Most work in hospitals, although opportunities exist in a number of settings such as physician offices, nursing homes, schools, insurance and pharmaceutical companies, occupational health or home health care, or as independent practitioners (Raffel & Barsukiewicz, 2002). Approximately 90% of registered nurses are female (Weinberg, 2004). The nursing workforce is aging, with most nurses in the 35- to 49-year-old age-range. Projections are for nearly half of the nursing workforce to be older than 50 years by 2010 (Buerhaus et al., 2003). Differences exist with respect to the means by which registered nurses enter the field. Hospital diploma, associate degree, and baccalaureate degree programs constitute the major pathways, with diploma programs on the decline and the profession's preference for baccalaureate preparation. Only 2310 nurses graduated from diploma programs in 2001, compared with 41,567 from associate degree programs and 24,832 from baccalaureate programs (NCHS, 2003). Master's and doctoral level preparation also exist. The doctorate of nursing practice (DNP) is a new addition to many nursing programs. The DNP prepares nurses for leadership as advanced practice nurses, clinical experts, health care executives, policy experts, and informaticians. Licensed practical nurses/licensed vocational nurses, certified nurse midwives, certified registered nurse anesthetists, and advanced registered nurse practitioners are additional nursing-related designations.

Hospitals

Hospitals represent one of the most recognizable components of the health care system. The total number of hospitals in the United States in 2002 was 5794. These hospitals contained some 976,000 beds, admitted more than 36 million patients, and provided more than 640 million outpatient visits. The majority of these were general, community hospitals. Only 323 hospitals (5.6%) had more than 500 beds, and only 375 hospitals (6.5%) had between 6 and 24 beds. The largest percentage of hospitals had 100 to 199 beds (23.9%), followed by 23.2% with 50 to 99 beds, 18.0% with 25 to 49 beds, 12.3% with 200 to 299 beds, 7.0% with 300 to 399 beds, and 3.5% with 400 to 499 beds. Hospitals employ more than 4.6 million full-time equivalent personnel, including 99,829 physicians and dentists, 1,073,468 registered nurses, and 155,863 licensed practical nurses/licensed vocational nurses (AHA, 2004a).

Insurers and Payers

Insurers and third-party payers represent yet another component involved in the U.S. health care system. They are important in facilitating access to and payment for services. Unlike countries with a single-payer system, multiple payers are common in the United States. Commercial insurers, Blue Cross/Blue Shield plans, Medicare, and Medicaid are examples, as are businesses that choose to self-insure. According to America's Health Insurance Plans (AHIP), as of 2009 nearly 1300 member companies are providing health insurance coverage to more than 200 million Americans (AHIP, 2009). Insurance companies are regulated by the states, although self-insured plans are exempt from state regulation under ERISA. In 2002, approximately 85% of the U.S. population was covered by private or government health insurance, with slightly more than a quarter of the population enrolled in an HMO (U.S. Census Bureau, 2003, Chart 151). Private payers accounted for 54% of spending on personal health care in 2002, which can be broken down as private insurance accounting for 35%, out-of-pocket spending 14%, and other private payments accounting for 5%. Public spending on health included Medicare at 17%, Medicaid and the State Children's Health Insurance Program spending at 16%, with other public spending accounting for 12% (MedPAC, 2004).

Education and Research

Although payment and delivery are important components, without organizations and individuals involved in education and research, the human resources and skills necessary for the health care system would not exist. Medical, nursing, and allied health provider schools and programs are a needed part of the educational system. They also contribute to the knowledge base. Academic health centers are the principal sites for educating and training health personnel, as well as important sites for research (Sultz & Young, 2004). A disproportionate amount of indigent care is also provided in this setting.

Funding from and research by public and private foundations and government agencies are also imperative for the advancement of the field. The magnitude of government funding on research has expanded over time, even though the total percentage of dollars expended on health research and development by the federal government has been declining. It is estimated that approximately 6 cents of every health dollar spent in 2002 was for research. Of this approximately $92 billion, 54% came from industry, 34% came from the federal government, and 12% came from other sources (Thompson & Propst, 2004). The Pharmaceutical Research and Manufacturers of America (PhRMA) (2004) reported that its members alone spent an estimated $33.2 billion on research for new disease treatments in 2003.

One of the primary ways in which government is involved in the funding of research is through the National Institutes of Health (NIH). The NIH is part of the U.S. Department of Health and Human Services. It both conducts and supports medical research using a competitive peer review process. The NIH's budget doubled over the course of 5 years in the mid-2000s. With a 2004 budget of approximately $28 billion, more than 80% of the budget is competitively awarded to external investigators. A portion is also dedicated for internal scientists conducting research, primarily on the NIH campus in Bethesda, Maryland. The NIH has promulgated a "roadmap" to provide a framework for the priorities that NIH will address and to hasten the movement of discoveries from the bench to the bedside. The three themes of the "roadmap" are (1) new pathways to discovery, (2) research teams of the future, and (3) reengineering the clinical research enterprise (National Institutes of Health [NIH], 2004).

Suppliers

Suppliers also make up a significant piece of the health care system. A huge assortment of medical supplies and products must be continuously provided in a timely fashion, along with routine items such as paper, pens, and food. New diagnostic, therapeutic, and monitoring technologies must also be developed, installed, and maintained. The pharmaceutical industry, in particular, is a major supplier in the health care system, with the distribution and development of new, more-effective drugs a key goal. Information technology suppliers are also playing an increasingly important role.

Supply management is critical for health care providers. If a provider holds too much inventory, there are implications for cash flow and storage costs, as well as obsolescence. Too little inventory can result in shortages of critical items. Arrangements are often made with suppliers for maintaining just-in-time inventories. Providers also seek to join group purchasing organizations to enhance their buying power.

Professional Associations

Professional associations exist in almost every field. They are organized to promote a profession's mission to society, to provide collective action, and to enhance and protect the interests of its members. Local, state, and national chapters may exist. A professional association may engage in a number of activities, including, but not limited to, promoting the field, developing standards, communicating news, providing educational programming, honoring achievements, and lobbying on behalf of the profession. Several health-related groups are among the most powerful lobbyists in Washington, D.C. Among them are the American Medical Association, the American Hospital Association, the Health Insurance Association of America (which merged with the American Association of Health Plans in October 2003 to form America's Health Insurance Plans), and the Pharmaceutical Research and Manufacturers Association (Birnbaum, 2001). The American Dental Association, American Public Health Association, and the American Nurses Association also play important roles.

Regulatory Bodies

A number of entities at the national, state, and local level are involved in the regulation of the health care system. Congress, as well as state legislatures and local officials, pass laws governing the operation of the health care system. As might be suspected, these laws cover a broad spectrum, from what constitutes the practice of a particular occupation to how health insurance plans may operate. Numerous health occupations are subject to regulation via licensure, certification, or registration. Health facilities, health products, and educational institutions are regulated as well. The regulations are made and enforced by various licensing boards and state and federal agencies, including the Centers for Medicare and Medicaid Services, the Office of the Inspector General, the Food and Drug Administration, and the Occupational Safety and Health Administration, to name a few. Although many regulatory bodies have a government connection, private entities such as The Joint Commission (TJC), formerly called the *Joint Commission on the Accreditation of Healthcare Organizations (JCAHO)*, and the National Committee for Quality Assurance (NCQA) also play significant roles.

The TJC is an independent, not-for-profit organization that engages in the accreditation of various health care organizations, including home care organizations, ambulatory care organizations, assisted living facilities, long-term care facilities, clinical laboratories, and hospitals. More than 16,000 organizations are accredited by TJC including more than 4700 hospitals. Accreditation is voluntarily sought for many purposes, including fulfillment of state licensure requirements and certain third-party payer requirements, including Medicare certification requirements (TJC, 2009).

The NCQA is another private, not-for-profit organization. Among the reasons managed care plans voluntarily seek NCQA accreditation is to demonstrate compliance with state requirements. More than half the states recognize NCQA accreditation as meeting this purpose (National Committee for Quality Assurance [NCQA], 2003a).

LEADERSHIP AND MANAGEMENT IMPLICATIONS

Health care forecasters predict that soon the principal point of care delivery will no longer be at the acute care hospital. Care will move toward being community-based. As the health care delivery system is reconfigured in this dramatic way, the roles and functions of the nurse will undergo a simultaneous dramatic change. A de-emphasis on acute medical care will increase the demand for nursing skills.

The complexity of the nursing role is increasing with technological advancements and the greater overall acuity of hospitalized patients as more care delivery shifts to the ambulatory setting. Accepted standards of practice are changing such that health care teams are becoming more involved in treatment decisions and health care providers other than physicians, such as physician assistants and nurse practitioners, are assuming greater roles. There is also an increasing movement toward the practice of evidence-based medicine and health care. Nurses are contributing to the outcomes research on which that is based. In addition, the growing emphasis on prevention and management of chronic conditions has implications for the skill sets nurses require, including the ability to educate patients under conditions of multiculturalism and short interaction times.

The need for coordination of care internally within a setting, as well as across settings, serves as an important reason for nurses to know how the health care system functions. Horizontal and vertical integration provide increased opportunities for managing a continuum of care, and the nursing profession plays important roles across this continuum. However, the complexity of the health care system is rapidly becoming a problem in and of itself. The frequency of uncertain and unexpected events in health care today is symptomatic of many complex systems.

LEADERSHIP & MANAGEMENT BEHAVIORS

Leadership Behaviors

- Understands the health care system
- Is knowledgeable about health care economics and finance
- Provides planning and direction for salary equity and workforce skill mix
- Guides the organization's human resources policies
- Fosters creativity and innovation

Management Behaviors

- Understands the health care system
- Is knowledgeable about health care costs/charges
- Administers the salary structure and position control plan
- Implements human resources policies
- Manages resources and reduces costs

Overlap Areas

- Understands the system
- Understands the impact of economic and health care policies on nursing service delivery

Complex Adaptive System Behavior

A complex system is characterized by multiple entities (e.g., health care providers, departments, equipment) interacting in a rich social network that is highly connected to both the internal and external environment. Complex systems are ubiquitous and have been studied extensively in multiple fields including the physical, biological, and social sciences.

Complex adaptive systems (CASs) are special cases of *complex systems,* the key difference being that a CAS can learn and adapt over time. Such adaptation can actually change the structure of the system. Hospitals, for example, are complex adaptive systems (Clancy, 2008).

Characteristics of Complex Adaptive Systems

It is useful to examine complex adaptive systems' characteristics:

- Feedback results when a response feeds back on its source of stimulus and alters behavior. Feedback can result in networks of information brokers and create preferential attachment (the larger a node, the more connections it receives; the more connections it receives, the larger it becomes). Human memory also serves as a source of feedback and can create non-linear (amplification or moderation) behavior. For example, delays in medication administration tend to grow at an exponential rate with staffing shortages.
- Autonomous agents have the capacity to make independent decisions. Humans are autonomous agents and can make choices. This enables adaptation. For example, health care organizations readily adapt to technological change by adopting new services.
- Improbable events occur more frequently in complex systems because information becomes trapped in feedback loops and then suddenly presents itself. These improbable events are often interpreted as "outliers" when, in fact, they are part of a very complicated but deterministic process.
- Complex systems are unstable. This instability results from preferential attachment, which is a form of feedback. Preferential attachment leads to the formation of hubs (e.g., a computer hub) that dominate a network. If one of these hubs breaks down, the entire network is susceptible to crashing.
- Complex system behavior is not normally distributed. Because the constituent parts of a complex system are not independent of each other, their behavior does not form a normal or bell-shaped curve. This results in more frequent, large deviations in behavior. For example, adverse drug events occur at a much higher rate than would be predicted by a normal distribution.

These anticipated changes in the U.S. health care delivery system appear to offer exciting opportunities for the value of nursing to more fully emerge and be recognized. Because nurses manage and coordinate the environment in which all providers deliver client care, as well as directly provide some of that care, managed care programs rely heavily on the expertise and actions of nurses. As health care delivery changes to emphasize primary care, nursing is poised to become a mainstay of the health care delivery system. Nurses in advanced practice have a special set of abilities to offer the health care system. New roles for nurse practitioners (NPs), such as primary care and case and disease management jobs, capitalize on nurses' skills. This trend is being identified as the "age of the nurse."

Leadership in nursing means knowing the group's goals and how to get to the "preferred future." Innovation in the form of fostering creativity and implementing new ideas is a key strategy. Nurses have the skills to focus on the care of special populations, such as the elderly, and on community and preventive population-based services. Nursing will need to make strides in solving internal problems such as diverse educational levels and in generating research to demonstrate effectiveness. Clearly, however, nurses' unique preparation in leadership and management ability and coordination and integration roles appear to be a good "fit" with the direction of change in health care.

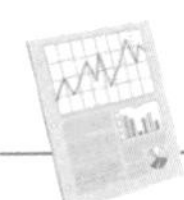

Research Note

Source: Johnson, N. (2007). *Two's company, three is complexity.* Oxford, UK; Oneworld.

Purpose

The purpose of this book was to provide a fundamental understanding of complex systems theory and its applications. Research efforts are focused on predicting future behavior from historical patterns or trends. For example, during highly turbulent times, complex system behavior can be predicted through trended patterns. An analogy in health care is the rate of admissions to a nursing unit. Research has shown that the probability of an upward trend in admissions (turbulence) continuing is greater than the probability of admissions declining.

Discussion

The application of predictive models would be useful in the following complex hospital processes: (1) staffing a nursing unit; (2) patient safety, falls, and medical errors; (3) implementation of information technology such as clinical decision support or provider order entry; and (4) implementation of a new professional practice model.

Application to Practice

The accuracy of predictive modeling in health care processes has been enabled by increases in computational power. Moore's Law, a common heuristic used in the field of computer science, estimates that computational power doubles every 18 months. Theory in complex system behavior is being studied through virtual experiments. For example, agent-based modeling creates virtual organizations in which complex system behavior can be simulated and then later applied to real systems. The financial markets are already using this methodology to predict stock market trends. Application of these methods is just beginning to infuse into health care, specifically in the area of staffing and patient safety.

CURRENT ISSUES AND TRENDS

The health care system is facing many challenges. Costs are high and increasing, new technologies continue to drive up costs, too many people lack access to health care, and aging Baby Boomers will increase health care demand at a time when human resources may not be sufficient. Quality is inconsistent, error rates are too high, and not enough attention is directed toward prevention. In addition to health care, providers must also contend with issues related to homeland security and information privacy.

Financial Issues

Health care spending in the United States has grown from $1.6 trillion in 2002 to $2.1 trillion in 2006. Rising at the rate of almost 7% (twice the rate of inflation) and making up about 17% of the gross domestic product (GDP), total spending was $2.4 trillion in 2007, or $7900 per person (National Coalition on Health Care, 2009). Hospitals accounted for 31% of the total amount of spending, and professional services to physicians and clinical services accounted for 21%. Although Congress has attempted to reign in Medicare costs, spending rose 19% in 2006 to a total of $403 billion (Dobias, 2007) and was $426 billion in 2007 (Kaiser Family Foundation, 2008).

The economic and social impact of the U.S. health care system on communities, states, and the nation as a whole is huge. Even disregarding the benefit of improved health status, the ripple effect of spending on employees, supplies, buildings, and equipment helps support the economy and generate taxes. In addition, spending by patients and visitors also contributes to the economy. The Association of American Medical Colleges, which represents the nation's 126 accredited allopathic medical schools and some 400 major teaching hospitals and their faculty, has estimated the combined economic impact of its member institutions in 2002 totaled more than $326 billion (Tripp Umbach Healthcare Consulting, Inc., 2003). Nationally, each hospital job supports approximately two additional jobs, and hospitals directly or indirectly support one of every nine jobs in the United States (AHA, 2004b).

Increases in per capita health care spending still provide employers with an incentive to reduce costs through health plan design changes and greater employee cost sharing (Hewitt Associates, 2004). In an attempt to control premiums for employers while meeting patient desires for flexibility in access, health plans are developing products that shift more financial responsibility to patients and are enhancing their management of high-using patients. Disease management programs, focusing on conditions such as asthma, diabetes, and hypertension, along with intensive case management of high users of health care, are examples of approaches being considered (Draper & Claxton, 2004). Instituting tiered copayments within HMO networks is also gaining momentum as HMOs seek to permit choice while encouraging prudent behavior (Steinbrook, 2004).

Health care spending is, and historically has been, highly concentrated on a small percentage of people. The top 1% of the population accounted for 27% of aggregate expenditures in 1996, with the top 5% accounting for 55%, and the top 50% of the population accounting for 97%. The lower 50% of the population collectively accounted for only about 3% of total health expenditures. It is interesting to note that the majority of people in the top 1% are not elderly nor do they consider themselves to be in fair or poor health (Berk & Monheit, 2001). The top 10% most costly beneficiaries in fee-for-service Medicare accounted for nearly two thirds (63%) of the total Medicare spending in 2005 (Kaiser Family Foundation, 2008). During the last year of their lives, the nearly 5% of Medicare beneficiaries who die each year account for approximately one quarter of Medicare outlays (MedPAC, 2004).

The rising cost of medical malpractice insurance is also a growing challenge to the health care system. Many health care providers are experiencing decreased availability of malpractice insurance and higher prices for the options that exist. Physicians in Illinois, Pennsylvania, Nevada, New Jersey, New York, and West Virginia, among other states, have walked off the job or threatened to do so (Haugh, 2003), and some hospitals are no longer providing normal newborn care. Some providers are also choosing to retire or relocate to areas where malpractice insurance is more available and affordable. Although losses on malpractice claims appear to be the largest driver of increased premium costs, falling investment income for insurers has also contributed (General Accounting Office [GAO], 2003). Arguments have been advanced that the increases in the frequency of claims and size of payouts are attributable to increased public awareness of medical errors, lower levels of trust in the health care system, advances in medical innovation and intensity, rising patient expectations, and increasing reluctance of attorneys to settle cases for amounts that sufficed in the past (Studdert et al., 2004). One consequence of this challenge is the increasing adoption of defensive medicine practices, such as declining high-risk cases or ordering extra tests.

Technology is also a major driver of increasing health care costs. Types of medical technology include those related to diagnosis (MRI), survival (intensive care units), illness management (pacemaker), cure (organ transplant), prevention (vaccines), and systems management (information systems) (Longest et al., 2000). Spending more for technology does not guarantee health improvements for a population (Blank, 1997). While new technologies may replace older versions and improve efficiency, it is not uncommon for a new technology to be provided in addition to, rather than in place of, an older technology. Nor is it uncommon for a new technology to result in more services being provided, particularly as patients demand the latest and providers seek to distinguish themselves from competitors, which increases costs overall.

Some advances in technology require highly trained technicians to operate them and/or necessitate special construction to house them. Although greater knowledge of the cost-effectiveness of a new technology is useful, the advances being made in many areas, such as robotic surgery, are undeniably impressive. Relative to other countries, the availability of advanced medical technology in the United States is fairly high. For example, compared with other OECD industrialized countries, the United States had 8.1 MRI units per million population in 2000 compared with the median of 4.7, and the United States had 13.6 CT scanners per million population compared with the median of 12.2 (Anderson et al., 2003).

Pharmaceuticals, with price increases many times the rate of inflation, present a particular financial strain on those without prescription drug coverage. Prices among the top 30 brand-name drugs dispensed to senior citizens rose, on average, by 4.3 times the rate of inflation from January 2003 to January 2004 (Families USA, 2004a).

The fragmentation of the health care system contributes to the difficulty in sharing information among providers. Uneven information system distribution and lack of coordination contribute to the challenge. It is estimated that 20% of laboratory tests and x-ray studies are performed because prior results are unavailable and that net efficiency gains of more than $131 billion per year could be achieved through greater information technology use in health care. On April 27, 2004, a presidential executive order created the position of a national health information technology coordinator within the Department of Health and Human Services to coordinate efforts toward a national health information infrastructure (Fyffe, 2004).

Efforts continued in 2006 when the American Medical Informatics Association (AMIA) sponsored a broad initiative to improve clinical decision support (CDS) capabilities and increase use of CDS throughout the U.S. health sector. The immediate goal of AMIA is to ensure that *optimal, usable,* and *effective* clinical decision support is *widely available* to providers, patients, and individuals *where and when they need it* to make health care decisions. The ultimate goal of these activities is to improve the quality of health care services and to improve health in the United States (Osheroff et al., 2006).

Improving quality through clinical integration remains a significant challenge in hospitals today. Characteristics of clinical and financial integration include the following:

- Ability to track a patient's health status through different settings without gaps in continuity of care
- Elimination of duplicative clinical and administrative tasks
- Successful interoperability of both hospital and physician private practice information technology
- Shared value in joint venturing between hospital- and physician-based practices; includes reduced competition among physician-owned and hospital-based specialty facilities (e.g., ambulatory surgery centers, diagnostic imaging centers)
- One unique patient medical record that can be shared by multiple providers across all levels of care
- Reduction of medical errors as a result of better coordination among providers
- Alignment of strategic goals among all providers, whether independent or employed

Clinical integration of services begins by aligning incentives for both hospitals and private physician practices. For example, provider order entry systems have been shown to reduce medication errors through clinical decision support and alerts. However, keyboard entry of orders by physicians can take longer than traditional paper-based orders. This impacts physician productivity and creates resistance to system adoption. Ironically, federal laws are often the key barriers to more widespread clinical integration. Physician self-referral (Stark Laws), Medicare anti-kickback laws, Internal Revenue System tax-exempt laws, and antitrust law (Sherman Act) all limit financial relationships among hospitals and physicians. As a result, joint care initiatives can be impeded, making it difficult for doctors and hospitals to improve care coordination across settings.

Government agencies have begun to realize the effects of federal law on clinical integration. For example, legislation has allowed hospitals and private physicians to share in the cost of an electronic health record that integrates both entities' medical records. This enables the seamless transmission of information among various levels of care (Taylor, 2008).

Access

The view of many in the United States that health care is "a right" remains in conflict with the reality of access. The United States is rare among the industrialized countries of the world in that it does not guarantee access to health care. Instead, most people in the United States tend to obtain health insurance through an employer or a spouse or parent who is employed and has access to health insurance, although the percentage of workers covered by employee-based health insurance has been declining. Nearly 175 million Americans are covered by employer-based insurance (Gabel et al., 2003), and there are tax and competitive reasons why many employers provide access to this benefit. Not all employers are financially able or willing to provide access to health insurance for their employees, however, and even when an employer offers health insurance, many employees still cannot afford it. For those who have health insurance through their employer or their spouse's employer, the loss of a job, a change in jobs, a divorce, or the death of the spouse may result in a disruption in their health insurance coverage. Furthermore, not all health insurance is the same; high copayments, high deductibles, or coverage limitations, such as those for mental health services, may impinge on access to care. A market for individual insurance exists but tends to be expensive. Consequently, many people cannot afford health insurance.

Government programs such as Medicare, Medicaid, and the State Children's Health Insurance Program were designed to address the lack of affordable health insurance, although not all people without health insurance qualify for these programs. The number of people served by Medicare and Medicaid combined is approximately 80 million. The costs of these programs continue to grow. Estimates were that approximately 82 million Americans were without health insurance for all or part of 2002 and 2003 (Families USA, 2004b), and many more are underinsured. During 2007 and 2008, 86.7 million people, or one out of every three Americans under the age of 65, was uninsured for some period of time (Families USA, 2009). Hospitals have started to consider possible modifications to their billing and collection practices for those with a limited ability to pay in order to lessen such patients' financial burden.

A consequence of being without insurance is poorer health (Institute of Medicine [IOM], 2004a). Uninsured people are more likely to go without needed care and to be in worse condition when they do present for care. Differences exist by race with respect to lack of health insurance. For example, working Hispanic and Black adults are more likely to be uninsured than working White adults (States Health Access Data Assistance Center, 2004). Hospital emergency rooms often serve as the safety net for the uninsured. The Emergency Medical Treatment and Active Labor Act (EMTALA), passed as part of the Consolidated Omnibus Budget Reconciliation Act of 1986, ensured that people who present to an emergency room will be seen. Care delivered in the emergency room setting, however, tends to be the most expensive.

Access to care is also shifting from a traditional acute care model to a decentralized model in which a hospital is supported by several disease-focused ambulatory centers. These centers may include freestanding ambulatory surgery, diagnostic imaging, and urgent care centers. Decentralized care models support the development of regional networks in which various health care facilities work collaboratively to focus on an entire continuum of care. For example, the treatment of acute myocardial infarction may require coordination of freestanding clinics, hospitals, and emergency services to minimize transport to a cardiac catheterization laboratory.

Workforce

A sizable number of people are employed in the health sector. In 2002, more than 4.6 million people were employed in ambulatory health care settings, such as offices of physicians, dentists, and other health practitioners, as well as in medical and diagnostic laboratories and home health care services. Another 4.2 million were employed in hospitals, and 2.7 million were employed in nursing and residential care facilities (U.S. Census Bureau, 2003, Chart 160). When considered by occupation, these totals included approximately 825,000 physicians, 180,000 dentists, and 2.3 million registered nurses employed in 2002 (U.S. Census Bureau, 2003, Chart 615). Of course, the health sector can be thought of in broader terms than this. The numbers grow substantially when considering people employed in the insurance, pharmaceutical, and medical supply professions, for example.

Workforce shortages represent a cyclical challenge in the U.S. health care system. When key players are in short supply, access to and quality of care may be compromised and costs may increase. The aging of the U.S. population is anticipated to have important implications for the health care workforce. Assuming constant consumption and productivity over time, the aging population is anticipated to increase demand for physicians from 2.8 per thousand in 2000 to 3.1 in 2020, and the demand for full-time equivalent nurses from 7.0 to 7.5. Concerns also exist that many in the aging health workforce itself may be retiring as demand grows and thus it may be difficult to attract sufficient numbers of new health workers (National Center for Health Workforce Analysis, 2003). For example, the number of physicians older than 65 years has almost tripled in the past 25 years. The number of nurses in their 60s will grow from 217,538 in 2004 to 373,573, in 2010. Between 2010 and 2015, 35% of nurses plan to retire (Runy, 2008). Clearly, this is a serious problem.

Shortages of nurses are nothing new, although the nursing shortage that began in 1998 lasted longer than most. A number of factors likely contributed to the shortage and relate to economic, workplace, social, and demographic forces (Buerhaus et al., 2003). Multiple strategies have been attempted to alleviate this shortage, including increasing wages, enhancing recruitment and retention programs through signing bonuses and work environment improvements, using agency nurses, hiring foreign nurses, and recruiting more men and women into nursing through scholarship and loan repayment programs and accelerated degree programs. Despite these measures, women have more career options than ever before, hospital environments and nursing work shifts are often unattractive, pay rates are flat over time, and the lack of nursing faculty has limited enrollment gains that otherwise could have occurred. Without substantial change, the difficulty in filling nursing positions may continue. The National Center for Health Workforce Analysis, using a baseline scenario, indicated that a 41% increase in the demand for full-time equivalent registered nurses will occur between 2000 and 2020 (National Center for Health Workforce Analysis, 2003).

Although predictions of physician supply were tending toward a projected surplus, Cooper and colleagues (2002) estimated that demand for physicians will exceed supply by 200,000 in 2020. Analyses undertaken for the Council on Graduate Medical Education (COGME) by Salsberg have also predicted a physician shortage, but in the range of 85,000 by 2020 (Blumenthal, 2004). In 2004, the COGME report concluded that a significant shortage of physicians over the next 15 years is likely and medical school capacity should increase (Council on Graduate Medical Education [COGME], 2004). Major professional associations such as the Association of American Medical Colleges and the American Medical Association are no longer projecting surpluses, although neither of these organizations has endorsed the shortage estimates. The costs of educating a surplus of physicians must be weighed against the price of a shortage. The challenge of addressing this country's future physician needs is complicated by the lag time typically associated with policy change and implementation, in addition to the long production cycle to produce each new physician.

Quality, Safety, and Satisfaction

The use of and expenditures for health care services vary widely across the United States. It may surprise some that this is not necessarily explained by differences in medical diagnosis. Rather, researchers have attributed much of the variation to differences in the resources and capacity of an area to provide health care, implying in some cases that supply drives demand (GAO, 2004). States with higher Medicare spending have actually been found to have lower-quality care, with the additional spending occurring on expensive care that does not change health outcomes (Baicker & Chandra, 2004).

Per capita spending for health care in the United States is higher than in other industrialized nations (Anderson et al., 2003), but arguments can be made that this has not necessarily resulted in the best health results. Many countries have longer life expectancies at birth than does the United States (NCHS, 2003). Japan, Sweden, Canada, France, Australia, Spain, Finland, the Netherlands, the United Kingdom, Denmark, and Belgium have all been reported to have higher average rankings on health indicators in various studies of industrialized countries. The United States' low ranking on infant mortality is frequently among several measures cited to support this conclusion. Possible explanations regarding these findings are complex and need further study. Among the explanations proposed are differences in public behavior, income inequality, primary care infrastructure, effects from the health system itself, and combinations of these factors (Starfield, 2000).

Various takes on the public's perspective of the U.S. health care system have been reported. Lavizzo-Mourey (2003) asserted that an overwhelming percentage would assign a grade of D, citing an enormous and growing gap between expectations and the quality being delivered. The first annual National Healthcare Quality Report acknowledged that "high quality health care is not yet a universal reality" and that "greater improvement is possible" (U.S. Department of Health and Human Services [USDHHS], 2003). The Joint Canada/U.S. Survey of Health, however, found Americans were generally satisfied with the quality of health care received and were more likely than Canadians to report the quality of their health care services was excellent (Sanmartin et al., 2004). According to the Joint Survey, approximately 42% of Americans rated the quality of care they received as excellent and 47% rated it as good. Only 2% of Americans thought the quality of care they received was poor. More than 53% of Americans also reported that they were very satisfied with any health service received, 37% were somewhat satisfied, and 4% were neither satisfied nor dissatisfied. Less than 2% were very dissatisfied with the care received (Sanmartin et al., 2004).

There are severe financial and human consequences of the inconsistency of performance of the health care system. Approximately 1000 needless deaths occur each week because of failures to deliver appropriate care. In addition, more than $11 billion in lost productivity could be avoided if best practices were adopted (NCQA, 2003b). Patient safety events associated with hospitalized children have alone been estimated to have contributed to more than $1 billion in additional hospital charges in 2000 (Miller & Zhan, 2004).

A growing consensus is emerging today that the U.S. health care system fails to deliver its potential benefits and, in fact, harms too frequently (IOM, 2001). It has been estimated that as many as 98,000 hospitalized Americans die each year as a result of errors in their care (IOM, 2000). Much of the blame has been directed at the outmoded systems of work. New information technologies are seen as a critical component for moving the country toward care that is evidence-based, patient-centered, and systems-oriented so that the best knowledge can be applied across providers and settings.

Created in June of 1998, the Committee on the Quality of Health Care in America was charged with devising a strategy to improve quality of the

U.S. health care system over the next decade. It proposed that all health care organizations, professional groups, and public and private purchasers should pursue six major aims—that health care be safe, effective, patient-centered, timely, efficient, and equitable (IOM, 2001). Educational aspects related to quality improvement are also being addressed. The Committee on Health Professions Education has developed a new vision for clinical education. This vision includes five core competencies and indicates that "all health professionals should be educated to deliver patient-centered care as members of an interdisciplinary team, emphasizing evidence-based practice, quality improvement approaches, and informatics" (IOM, 2004b, p. 3).

Posting of quality and cost data on websites for consumers is a growing phenomenon. *U.S. News and World Report* has provided ratings of top hospitals and medical specialties for years, and the National Committee on Quality Assurance's (NCQA, 2003b) Health Plan Employer Data and Information Set (HEDIS) has been in existence for some time. More sources of quality information are becoming available every day. For example, HealthGrades.com was founded in 1999 and the Leapfrog group launched a national quality and safety measurement and reporting effort in 2000. Insurance companies and employers are joining the trend. Concerns exist, however, on the part of providers as to the validity of some of the information presented (Lee et al., 2004). Controversy continues about whether process or outcomes data are better measures. Donabedian argued that the most direct route to assessing quality of care is by examination of the process, with assessment of the structure and the outcome being less direct methods (Donabedian, 1980).

In 2003, a national voluntary effort known as *The Quality Initiative* to compile public information on hospital quality was announced. The Medicare Prescription Drug, Improvement, and Modernization Act of 2003 actually required hospitals to submit data for a set of 10 quality indicators established by the Secretary of Health and Human Services to avoid a deduction in their Medicare market basket percentage increase.

In an effort to control costs and improve quality, the Centers for Medicare and Medicaid Services (CMS) is in the process of implementing a number of demonstration projects whose focus is on aligning quality and financial incentives. Hospitals will be invited to participate in a demonstration project aimed at gain-sharing. Under the demonstration project, hospitals would pass on a portion of their savings to participating physicians when improvements result from efficiencies and quality (Firshein et al., 2007).

Pay-for-performance (P4P) demonstration projects were initiated by CMS in 2005. Under these programs, a percentage of the hospital's base operating payments for each discharge or DRG payment is contingent on the hospital's actual performance on a specific set of measures. Those measures include both clinical and process outcomes. Results on P4P have been mixed. In a survey of 75 P4P sponsors including government agencies, health plans, and purchaser coalitions in 2006, 75% indicated that the programs improved quality, clinical outcomes, and patient satisfaction. However, a report by the Robert Wood Johnson Foundation in 2007 indicated that the contribution of P4P to quality improvement efforts was difficult to interpret (Firshein et al., 2007).

CMS is also embarking on a significant change in policy by recommending that hospitals be denied payments for certain hospital-acquired conditions. These conditions include infections not documented on admission, objects left in patients during surgery, and air embolisms caused by medical error. In addition, for eight selected conditions, the CMS will no longer allow elevation to a higher-paying DRG unless the conditions were present on admission. Three of these conditions include infections.

Practical Tips

Tip #1: Knowledge Is Needed

Understand the health care system in order to affect health policy.

Tip #2: Form Coalitions in Nursing

Foster nurse coalitions to capitalize on the power of nurses being the largest group of health care professionals.

Tip #3: Emphasize Local Activism

Work within your local health care delivery system to create positive, magnet work environments that help attract and retain RNs in a time of nurse shortage.

Population Changes and Care Demands

The population of the United States is aging. During the course of the past century, an increase of more than 12 years occurred in the median age as the population went from one half being younger than 22.9 years in 1988 to one half being younger than 35.3 years in 2000. The size of the population older than 65 years increased more than tenfold during this period, and rapid growth in this age bracket is expected to continue once the leading edge of the Baby Boom generation reaches 65 years in 2011 (Hobbs & Stoops, 2002). This has implications for the U.S. health care system in general, because care needs for this age-group are higher than for younger people and providers with expertise in caring for the elderly will be in demand. It also has implications for the Medicare and Medicaid programs in particular, because many in this age-group will be eligible for services covered by these programs. As the ratio of active workers to beneficiaries is expected to decline from approximately 4.0 today to 2.4 by 2030 (MedPAC, 2004), questions are being raised about whether the funding support for the Medicare program from the payroll and income taxes paid by active workers will be sufficient.

Three broad categories are commonly used to classify medical care: preventive, curative, and restorative (Shi & Singh, 2001). Nearly 95% of U.S. health care expenditures go to direct medical services, whereas only about 5% are allocated to prevention and health promotion (USDHHS, 2003). The call to establish a greater preventive orientation in the health care system is increasing with the rise in chronic conditions. These conditions affect almost half of the U.S. population, are the leading cause of illness, disability and death, and account for the majority of health care expenditures (IOM, 2001). Half of the deaths in the United States in 2000 were attributed to a number of preventable behaviors and exposures. Among the most common of these were tobacco (associated with 18.1% of the total U.S. deaths in 2000), poor diet and physical inactivity (associated with 16.6%), and alcohol consumption (associated with 3.5%) (Mokdad et al., 2004).

The use of complementary and alternative medicine is growing in the United States. Marketing initiatives to promote products and dissatisfaction with conventional medicine are among several proposed explanations for this growth. The National Center for Complementary and Alternative Medicine (NCCAM) defined complementary and alternative medicine as "a group of diverse medical and health care systems, practices and products that are not presently considered to be part of conventional medicine" (NCCAM, 2004, p. 1). What is considered to be complementary or alternative medicine changes over time as proven therapies are adopted into conventional medicine and new therapies are developed. Complementary medicine is used in conjunction with conventional medicine, whereas alternative medicine is used in place of it.

In 2002, when the definition included prayer for health reasons, nearly two thirds of adults reported using complementary or alternative medicine. When prayer was excluded, approximately one third of adults reported using complementary or alternative medicine. About one fourth of adult users tried complementary and alternative medicine on the recommendation of a conventional medical provider, with women tending to use these therapies more frequently than men. Besides prayer for health, use of natural products, deep-breathing exercises, meditation, and chiropractic care were among the most common therapies used. The use of complementary and alternative medicine is not without risk, however, since many of its therapies are untested or have the potential to interact with concurrent conventional therapies (Barnes et al., 2004), especially if all therapies and medicines are not disclosed to the health care provider.

The patient's role in relation to health professionals is changing from one primarily of submission and compliance to one of being a partner in the decision-making team. Not only has the Internet facilitated patient knowledge about various diseases and treatments but also direct-to-consumer marketing has educated them to some extent. Pharmaceutical company direct-to-consumer marketing was only $151 million in 1993 (Findlay, 2001) but increased to $2.6 billion in 2002 and continues to grow (Zaneski, 2004).

Privacy

The Health Insurance Portability and Accountability Act (HIPAA) of 1996 significantly changed the health care system. Among the areas addressed by this legislation was the portability of health insurance, enabling people to change jobs without fear of being denied coverage for preexisting health conditions as long as certain conditions were met. Before this, a phenomenon known as "job lock" often caused people to remain with an employer to retain coverage for an existing health condition.

Probably the most widely recognized change brought about by HIPAA was greater privacy protection for health information. HIPAA required the U.S. Department of Health and Human Services (USDHHS) to develop a national set of privacy rules (absent action by Congress), which the USDHHS did (Frank-Stromborg, 2004). The standards established represent a national, federal base of privacy protections, with state laws permitted to provide additional protections. Health care providers are required to protect the privacy of health information and to provide patients with a privacy notice describing various rights, including the right to inspect and amend information, to request restrictions on the release of their information, and to obtain an accounting of disclosures of their protected health information. Business associate agreements governing the sharing of health information with external parties were also required to be developed. Civil and criminal penalties may be imposed on providers who violate the privacy provisions. This has led to costly educational and training efforts and redesign of systems to enhance compliance.

A survey by the American Health Information Management Association found that 91% of respondents thought their institutions were at least 85% compliant with HIPAA privacy requirements nearly a year after the April 14, 2003, implementation date. The area most frequently identified as problematic was accounting for release of protected information (American Health Information Management Association, 2004). Concerns have also been identified relative to the impact on research on human subjects because of factors such as increased time and money required for redacting identifiable information, negative impacts on subject recruitment, and impaired ability to collaborate (Ehringhaus, 2004).

Homeland Security

Although not the first acts of terrorism on U.S. soil, the tragic events of September 11, 2001, which resulted in the destruction of the World Trade Center towers in New York and damage to the Pentagon in Virginia, served as a wakeup call to most Americans that the world was changing. A new cabinet-level position, Secretary of the Department of Homeland Security (DHS), was created in recognition of the country's vulnerabilities. More than $8.2 billion in grants have subsequently been provided to states and localities by DHS to enhance preparedness since its creation (Department of Homeland Security [DHS], 2004). First-responder training and the creation of teams of medical professionals to respond to disasters are two examples of developments.

Concerns have mounted about possible physical, cyber, chemical, biological, or radiological incidents, and emerging new epidemics such as severe acute respiratory syndrome (SARS) have raised questions about the health system's preparedness to respond. Improvements are being sought in a number of areas. Curricular enhancement in health professions schools and continuing education of practitioners are part of the plan, as is integration of hospitals, emergency medical services, public health, and others when responding to emergencies. Improved collaboration and communication, enhanced planning and disaster training, and infrastructure upgrades such as improvements in disease reporting, surveillance systems, and laboratory capacity are under way as well.

The Agency for Healthcare Research and Quality (AHRQ) is playing a key role in supporting preparedness research and is particularly interested in "surge capacity" to meet large-scale needs in a timely manner. Among the potential strategies to increase hospital surge capacity are discharging patients early, using outpatient areas and hallways for bed space, and partnering with other health care facilities, local schools, and armories (Agency for Healthcare Research and Quality [AHRQ], 2004). Challenges with rallying and rotating sufficient staff, managing crowds of worried people well, and securing necessary supplies are but a few of the additional issues that must be addressed. It is anticipated that bioterrorism will remain a high-profile issue and that ongoing dedicated funds for building and maintaining preparedness capacity will be required (Staiti et al., 2003).

Growing Complexity

The evolution of U.S. health care services over the past 150 years has resulted in what is likely one of the most complex organizational systems in the world. A complex organizational system can be defined as having multiple entities (people, organizations, and artifacts), a rich social network, feedback, and autonomous decision makers. Characteristics of complex social systems are nonlinear behavior (a small stimulus can result in exponential behavior or visa versa), self-organization (system parts increase order without central control), emergence (unexpected or novel system behavior that cannot be predicted from the constituent parts), and adaptation (the organization continuously adapts to changes in the environment).

The growing complexity of the U.S. health care system will result in more difficulty predicting the outcomes of policy changes at all levels of the system. This is because system parts (providers, payers, and suppliers) are not independent of each other and their interaction can produce multiple outcomes. For example, the quest for transparency of clinical performance metrics to the public has resulted in a plethora of new regulations required of hospitals. These include The Joint Commission's and CMS' National Patient Safety Goals, Core Measures, and Surgical Care Improvement Project. The manner in which hospitals collect, encode, transfer, store, and review the data elements used in the calculations of clinical performance varies considerably. This can result in significant variation in hospitals for similar clinical performance metrics, more as a result of their ability to correctly interpret coding guidelines than as a reflection of quality. This can be disastrous for hospitals, especially if there is a lag in reporting data. The unintended consequence of this process is that a hospital's first indication of a clinical performance problem is a posting on a public website. In other words, the public often knows the results before the hospital does.

Given the growing organizational complexity of the U.S. health care system, health care facilities will need to become "contingency minded." Unexpected events will occur more frequently and with greater speed. The ubiquity of information resulting from growth in technology and the Intranet is accelerating change. Health care facilities that have the capacity to quickly adapt and take advantage of unplanned opportunities will benefit most.

CONCLUSIONS

The U.S. health care system continues to evolve in response to a number of social, political, economic, scientific, and environmental issues, among other factors. The specialist-driven biomedical model has been the prevailing paradigm over much of the history of the health care system in this country. Although this system lacks a single central point of coordination for its diverse conglomeration of entities, some degree of interaction does occur among components and quality health care is frequently provided, although with acknowledged gaps and weaknesses.

The growing costs of the U.S. health care system represent a burden to many, including the federal government, state governments, employers, and patients. Americans are enchanted with medical technology, however, and have not been inclined to explicitly ration care as is done in other countries. In truth, though, a lack of health insurance serves to ration care for many. Among the numerous other ethical concerns that exist within the U.S. health care system are the allocation of scarce resources such as organs for transplantation, emerging capabilities to genetically alter humans, and potential advancements involving stem cells.

Cost challenges and the increased attention on quality provide opportunities for work redesign. This is particularly true given shortages of various health professionals and growth in tiered benefit plans in which high costs without substantiated additional benefit diminish attractiveness. Nurses, as key members of the delivery system, are in an excellent position to assist in addressing these concerns. However, in such an environment, nurses may feel caught between patient expectations and payer constraints while trying to provide quality care. Although much success has been achieved during the U.S. health care system's brief history, many challenges and opportunities remain. Understanding the system is a first step for nurses on the road to greater effectiveness in health care delivery.

Summary

- The U.S. health care system is fragmented and complex.
- The U.S. health care system has evolved over the past 150 years into a major enterprise.
- Government plays a major role in the financing and delivery of health care services.
- Components of the health care delivery system include providers, hospitals, payers, education, research, suppliers, professional associations, and regulatory bodies.
- Nurses have key skills for population-based health and illness care coordination.
- There are many issues facing the U.S. health care system.
- Understanding the health care system aids nurses' effectiveness in care delivery.
- The complexity of hospital processes is becoming a problem in and of itself.

CASE STUDY

St. Mary's is a 400-bed community hospital located in a large Midwestern city. As part of its 5-year strategic plan, St. Mary's plans to transition from a paper-based medical record to an electronic medical record (EHR). To make this change, St. Mary's will have to install and integrate a suite of clinical software applications. These include the following:

- Computerized clinical documentation and care planning
- Bar-coded medication administration
- Computerized provider order entry systems
- Clinical decision support

The total cost to implement the entire suite of applications over 5 years is estimated at $25 million. Is this a justifiable expense? How will the hospital raise the funding? Do the software applications really benefit nursing?

CRITICAL THINKING EXERCISE

As the nurse informaticist for St. Mary's Hospital, you are responsible for identifying how the various clinical applications will improve care and lower cost. Consider the following questions in addressing this issue:

1. What specific processes will be impacted? Provide examples of how an EHR can improve patient safety and clinical outcomes.
2. Which stakeholders in the hospital system will be most affected by the change and why? Will these changes be positive or negative?
3. How will the EHR reduce hospital expenses?
4. How do you measure the financial impact of reduced medical errors and improved clinical outcomes?
5. How will providers' workflow change after implementation of the clinical applications?
6. How will you measure whether you have achieved your initial strategic objectives?

15

Health Policy, Health, and Nursing

Katherine R. Jones

CHAPTER OBJECTIVES

- Define and describe policy, public policy, and politics
- Define and describe health policy
- Review the policy-making process
- Compare selected policy formulation models
- Examine interest group strategies
- Describe the legislative process
- Describe and compare policy analysis models
- Define evidence-based policy making
- Exercise critical thinking to conceptualize and analyze possible solutions to a practice exercise

Policy influences nurses throughout their careers. After graduation from nursing school, regulatory policies dictate that the graduate must pass a licensing examination to use the initials *RN* and to practice as a registered nurse. On the job, nurses must comply with institutional policies that spell out such things as dress code, overtime and floating requirements, minimum staffing levels, and performance review criteria and procedures. Thus nurses are influenced by policies at the state and national level (e.g., prescriptive authority, Medicare reimbursement for nurse practitioners) and at the local level (e.g., institutional policies at the worksite). Nurses also have a role in influencing policy via political action. This may involve participating in political action committees (PACs), providing information to legislative staff members, or holding elected office. In addition, nurses may prepare and submit policy briefs or present testimony on specific health, nursing, or other relevant topics. Nurses and nursing organizations are increasingly visible and vocal in the policy arena. To prepare nurses for these activities, nursing school curricula at all levels have added competencies specific to policy concepts and activities. Learning activities include both didactic (how to prepare testimony) and experiential (meeting with elected representatives) assignments.

As members of their professional associations, nurses may contribute money to PACs as well as contribute to the creation of policy agendas. If nurses desire greater involvement in policy, they may serve in a governmental relations capacity (e.g., as lobbyists) or work on a political campaign to help elect officials with specific political beliefs. At the local level, many nurses play important policy roles as they serve on boards of directors of nonprofit agencies and hospitals. Finally, nurses may run for office themselves and develop a political agenda that includes health and nursing issues; or they may become policy analysts for an organization or association, evaluating the impact of proposed or newly created policies on various stakeholder groups. In short, given the pervasiveness of policy influences on their everyday lives, nurses should be well informed about policy and the policy-making process.

As nursing has matured as a profession, nurses have become more aware of the need for activism in health policy and politics at all levels. As the largest health care provider group, it is appropriate and advisable for nurses to be a visible and vocal presence in the debate about health policy directions. As individuals, nurses hold personal perspectives as consumers of health care, for both themselves and their families/significant others. As citizens of the United States, nurses exercise their voices when they vote. As a professional group, nurses are integral to the delivery of health care services. As such, nurses form a special-interest lobbying group, with identifiable skills and abilities, and special but not always singular interests in health care issues. In summary, to have an influence over legislation, regulations, and other health policy decisions, nurses organize, lobby, testify, coordinate grassroots activities, serve on legislative staffs, contribute to PACs, and become elected officials or policy analysts. Involvement in policy and politics is an essential nursing activity, because if nurses are not visible and active, others will make decisions affecting nursing and health issues that are important to nursing.

Cohen and colleagues (1996) identified the following four stages of political development for the nursing profession:

1. Buy-in: Recognizing the importance of activism
2. Self-interest: Developing and using political expertise to further the profession's self-interests
3. Political sophistication: Moving beyond self-interest, recognizing the need for activism on behalf of the public
4. Leading the way: Providing true leadership on broad health care interests

Nursing is certainly either approaching or has actually reached stage 4 of political development, providing leadership in areas of national and international importance.

DEFINITIONS

Because the terms *policy* and *politics* carry different meanings, it is important to distinguish between these two concepts. **Policy** is the formulation of value statements, the "shoulds" and "oughts" of larger and more important issues (Milstead, 2008). Policy can be defined as a goal, program, proposal (Milstead, 2008), direction, decision, law, or standard (Block, 2008; Milstead, 2008). Policy encompasses the choices that a society, segment of society, or organization makes regarding its goals and priorities and the way it allocates its resources to attain these goals (Mason et al., 2007). Policy decisions are, therefore, meant to direct or influence the actions, behaviors, or decisions of others (Longest, 1997). Public policies are authoritative decisions made in the legislative, executive, and judicial branches of government (Longest, 2002) that are intended to direct or influence the actions, behaviors, or decisions of others (Longest, 1998). Processes to create public policy include enactment of legislation and associated rules and regulations; administrative decisions including interpretative guidelines for rules and regulations; and judicial decisions that interpret the law (Hanley & Falk, 2007). More simply, public policy encompasses anything a government chooses to do or not to do (Dye, 1992).

The two major types of public policy are *regulatory* and *allocative* (Longest, 2001). Regulatory policies are designed to influence the actions, behaviors, and decisions of others through directive approaches for the purpose of ensuring that public objectives are met (Longest, 2001). Allocative policies, on the other hand, are designed to provide net benefits to some distinct group or class at the expense of others to ensure that public objectives are met (Longest, 1998, 2001). Policies are generated at institutional levels (e.g., personnel policies in a long-term care facility) and at local, state, and national levels (e.g., public health sanitation policies, meat inspection rules). Institutional policies are developed by a discrete employer to govern its operations; such policies specify what the institution's goals are and how it will operate, how the institution will treat its employees, and how employees will work (Mason et al., 2007). Organizational policies are promulgated by professional organizations or other official entities and function as position statements, guidelines, or rules (Mason et al., 2007).

Politics, on the other hand, is the process of influencing the allocation of scarce resources

(Mason et al., 2007) or the use of power for change. Policy permeates all organizations including worksites, legislatures, professional groups, and families (Kelly, 2003). Politics operates within the context of competition and conflicting values and is a fundamental aspect of operating where multiple interest groups compete for scarce resources (Mason et al., 2007). Nurses become involved with political activities in four different spheres of influence: workplace, government, organizations, and the larger community (Mason et al., 2007).

Health policy consists of those public and private policies directly related to health care service delivery and reimbursement (Hanley & Falk, 2007). Health policies typically address the quality of services, the cost of services, and/or access to these services (Fawcett, 2007). Health policy decisions usually influence a category of providers (physicians, nurses, pharmacists), organizations (hospitals, clinics, managed care organizations, health plans, medical schools), or care recipients (the elderly, children, the poor, the chronically ill; those who are HIV-positive) (Longest, 2001). Examples within these categories include policies related to prescriptive authority for nurses, pay-for-performance plans for providers, and the State Children's Health Insurance Program (SCHIP) for children. Health policies include (1) health-related decisions made by legislators that are codified in the statutory language enacted in legislatures (i.e., laws); (2) rules and regulations designed to implement legislation or to operate government and its various health-related programs; and (3) judicial decisions related to health (Longest, 1998). The federal, state, and local levels of government all are involved in formulating health policy and making decisions to promote the health of individual citizens (Hanley & Falk, 2007). Health policy can be general (Employee Retirement Income Security Act (ERISA)—employer-sponsored health plans exempted from state insurance regulations) or specific (all teenage girls required to obtain the human papillomavirus vaccination). Health policy decisions set an overall tone for how a society decides to solve recurring issues in the health care needs of the people.

PUBLIC POLICY MAKING

Policy making goes on in many settings. It is an activity that has been described as complex, multidimensional, dynamic, nonlinear, and cyclical (Block, 2008; Mason et al., 2007). Public policy is developed through the acts of government or governmental agencies, such as by national commissions, by legislation, by the judicial system, by state and local governments, in the private sector, and by regulatory agencies. In some countries, a centralized ministry of health is the major health policy agency. In the United States, health care policy making is highly pluralistic, with policy decisions occurring at multiple levels of society (McLaughlin & McLaughlin, 2008). This decentralization creates complexity, but it also provides multiple opportunities for nurses and others to influence the policy process (getting a proposal on the policy agenda, influencing legislative action, shaping the rules and regulations implementing the new law).

Policy making depends on both values and analysis. This is because policy choices arise from

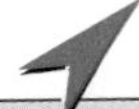

LEADING & MANAGING DEFINED

Policy

A plan, direction, or action goal.

Politics

The process of influencing the allocation of scarce resources or the use of power for change.

Health Policy

The entire set of public policies that are related to or influence health and illness.

both personal (ideological) values and as a result of formal analyses. Within the health policy arena are numerous and recurring conflicts over values. One long-standing debate centers on how to address the problem of growing numbers of uninsured in the United States and thus promote greater access to needed health care services. One option is to expand existing public programs, such as the SCHIP, to include pregnant women and low-income adults without children, as well as families at higher income levels. Opponents believe that this violates the original intent of the SCHIP program, crowds out private insurance coverage, and needlessly expands a government program. Instead, these groups advocate for tax credits or subsidies to help these individuals purchase health insurance in the private markets.

Four approaches to public policy making have been identified (Hanley & Falk, 2007):

- Rational Model: Policy makers define the problem, rank order goals, generate and examine alternatives, and select the policy alternative that most closely achieves policy goals (Dye, 1992).
- Incremental Model: Policy proposals begin with the status quo; limited changes reflect turf, goals, and politics of political subsystems.
- Kingdon's Policy Streams Model: Problem streams, policy streams, and political streams coalesce when the window of opportunity opens (Kingdon, 2003).
- Stage-Sequential Model: Systems-based model views the policy process as a sequential series of stages in which a number of functions occurs (Anderson, 1990; Ripley, 1996).

Academicians believe that formal analyses based on the rational model should be conducted to provide input into policy-making decisions. For example, detailed economic analyses or predictive modeling may be done to predict cost or program outcomes. But it is important to keep in mind that the selection of which analyses to perform and how to interpret the results also reflect the decision makers' values and perspectives (Dunn, 1994).

Cost-effectiveness analysis (CEA) is one evaluation strategy used to inform decision makers about how much health improvement can be achieved per dollar invested in a specific policy alternative (Allred et al., 1998). CEA has also has been proposed as an appropriate strategy for making resource allocation decisions in the delivery of care and for improving clinical care overall (Stone, 1998). CEA uses a decision analysis technique derived from operations research and game theory to evaluate the outcomes and costs of health interventions. A CEA cost-effectiveness ratio is calculated, with the health outcome measured in health units and cost of treatment measured in dollars. In this rational model of decision making, a policy problem is identified and then alternative policy options are proposed, modeled, and analyzed. The CEA is believed to be an objective approach to determining which policies should be followed or which programs should be funded (Buerhaus, 1998; Stone, 1998). However, CEA is not often the basis for making policy decisions in the United States—the political process is.

Policy makers in the public sector face the challenge of deciding how to allocate public resources. These resources are limited, so one desired policy objective can be achieved only at the expense of another worthy objective. At the state level, this means that enhanced funding for prisons and tourism may come at the expense of funding for higher education and programs to promote the arts. At the federal level, higher expenditures for defense and Social Security may translate into lower or flat budgets for highways and biomedical research. Moreover, specific policy choices will result in some winners and some losers in terms of achieved benefits. For example, the Medicare Part D drug benefit helped some Medicare beneficiaries without prior coverage pay for their prescribed medications, but at the same time the new law led to higher out-of-pocket costs for many who had existing supplemental policies with a drug benefit, as well as for those whose drug costs were covered under Medicaid.

Public policies may take one of several different forms. Laws are perhaps the best known form of public policy. They have had extensive impact on the health care field. For example, the

Health Insurance Portability and Accountability Act of 1996 (HIPAA), which is administered by the Centers for Medicare and Medicaid Services (CMS), has multiple unrelated provisions. The health insurance reform aspect of the Act provides for the portability of health insurance coverage and may be extremely important at times of job loss. The administrative simplification component of the Act calls for national standards for electronic health care transactions; national identifiers for providers, health plans, and employers; and security and privacy of health data. These new requirements have had a major impact on health care providers, as well as researchers and educators.

Rules and regulations are another aspect of policy. These are established to guide the implementation of laws (Longest, 2001). Such rule making may generate hundreds or thousands of pages of text. Operational decisions by agencies within the executive branch also represent policies (Longest, 2001). CMS is in the process of implementing rules related to pay-for-performance reimbursement for providers and denying reimbursement for the costs associated with certain facility-related complications such as health care–acquired pressure ulcers and catheter-related infections. Policies may be derived also from judicial decisions. Several courts ruled on Congress's attempts to ban partial-birth abortions, overturning the legislation and, in effect, allowing existing policies to stay in place. However, the shifting majority on the U.S. Supreme Court (liberal to moderate to conservative) now supports this type of restriction on abortions. This illustrates the important point that policy is never static—changing times often present the opportunity to revisit any policy issue and to change existing laws and regulations.

FACTORS DRIVING PUBLIC POLICY MAKING

Market Failures

Public policy making occurs when the marketplace fails to allocate resources efficiently. In a freely competitive market, the following five conditions are said to exist (Longest, 1997, 2001):

1. Both buyers and sellers of services or products have sufficient information to make informed choices.
2. A large number of buyers and sellers participate in the market; no one buyer or seller dominates the market.
3. More sellers of the service or product can easily enter the market.
4. Each seller's products or services can be substituted for those of competitors.
5. The quantity of products or services available in the market does not unduly influence the balance of power toward either buyers or sellers.

To address market failures, the government has a choice of the following actions:

- Do nothing.
- Attempt to improve the working of the market.
- Require people to behave in specified ways.
- Provide incentives that influence the decisions of individuals and organizations.
- Engage directly in the provision of goods and services.

Health Policy and Market Failure

In the United States, it has long been presumed that private markets (capitalism) best determine the production and consumption of goods and services, including those produced by the health care system (Longest, 1997). However, private markets sometimes fail to achieve desirable social objectives, and the government may choose to intervene to correct or address the market failure using one or more of the strategies described above. The health care industry is one example of a situation in which markets cannot function effectively to allocate goods and services. Longest (1997) has described how the health care marketplace violates the assumptions of a freely competitive market: consumers in general do not have the information necessary to make informed decisions but, instead, must rely on information and guidance provided by the supplier of those services; sellers of health care services do not easily enter the market but are, instead, confronted by an extensive array of regulations and certification and licensing requirements; and health insurance is said to alter consumer decisions to obtain health care services because the buyer is shielded from the actual costs of purchasing those services. This latter point is less true today, as a result of ever-increasing levels of deductibles and co-payments in addition to required cost-sharing on escalating health insurance premiums. Regardless, to address these and other market failures, the government generates policies relevant to the health care marketplace. The policies have ranged from "do nothing" to direct engagement in the provision of goods and services. For example, as a nation, the United States has done little toward establishing a comprehensive long-term care service delivery and financing program. On the other hand, the government provides comprehensive health care services directly to the nation's veterans through the national Veterans Health Administration health care system.

PUBLIC POLICY-MAKING PROCESS

Public policies are made within the public policy-making framework (Longest, 2001). The public policy-making process is dominated by three major players: interest groups that are affected by or concerned with a particular policy area; the executive agency that has administrative responsibility over the related policy area; and the congressional committees and subcommittees that have legislative authority in these policy areas (Block, 2008). These three players have been termed the "Iron Triangle" because of their lock on policy development (Kronenfeld et al., 1984).

Interest Group Politics

Interest Groups and Lobbying

Most problems get placed on the policy agenda through the efforts of organized interest groups. In general, organizations have a significant advantage over individuals in the political marketplace (Longest, 2002). Organizations have more resources and usually have more concentrated interests. An interest group is an organization of people with similar policy goals who enter the political process to try to achieve those goals (Lineberry et al., 1995). According to Weissert and Weissert (2002), interest groups are individuals who organize themselves around some common interest and who seek to influence public policy; in addition, they may show policy makers problems with their policy proposals and make suggestions for improvement (i.e., educating others about their views and concerns). Lobbyists for interest groups send unsolicited information, provide specific data at the request of congressional offices, attend meetings, meet with legislative staff members, and orchestrate phone and letter campaigns. They may also conduct media campaigns to influence public sentiment and provide candidates with money. Through combining and concentrating their resources and forming coalitions, interest groups can have a large impact in political markets (Longest, 2002). Some of the most effective interest groups, based on their size and resources, are the American Medical Association (AMA), American Hospital Association (AHA), American Association for Retired Persons (AARP), American Association of Health Plans (AAHP), and the Pharmaceutical Research and Manufacturers of America (PhRMA). In nursing, the American Nurses Association (ANA) has been an increasingly active and effective interest group, but the ANA does not speak alone for nurses. The American Association of Nurse Anesthetists (AANA), American College of Nurse Midwives (ACNM), American Association of Colleges of Nursing (AACN), National League for Nursing (NLN), American Organization of Nurse Executives (AONE), and other nursing groups are also active. However, the presence of so many nursing interest groups may serve to fragment the profession and its potential overall influence in public policy making.

The American Nurses Association is increasingly active in the political arena. A current focus of these efforts is embodied in the Safe Staffing Campaign *(www.safestaffingsaveslives.org/)*, which fights for safe staffing legislation. As described on the ANA website, this initiative supports establishment of nurse-patient ratios that are set by nurses in the workplace, based on unit-by-unit circumstances and needs. At the federal level, ANA worked with Senator Daniel Inouye (D-HI) and Representative Lois Capps (D-CA) during the 108th session of Congress to develop and introduce the Registered Nurse Safe Staffing Act, which holds hospitals accountable for the development and implementation of valid, reliable nurse staffing plans based on each unit's unique characteristics and needs. This bill (S73/HR4138) was reintroduced for the 110th Congress, with Inouye, Capps, and Representative Ginny Brown-Waite (R-FL) as lead sponsors. This bill has not yet passed. At the state level, ANA works in coordination with constituent member (state) associations to implement a nationwide state legislative agenda that focuses on issues important to nurses, including valid and reliable nurse staffing systems. So far, nine states plus the District of Columbia have enacted legislation and/or adopted regulations addressing nurse staffing. Finally, ANA also pursues legal action in support of the safe staffing initiative. For example, ANA filed suit to prevent the U.S. Department of Health and Human Services (USDHHS) from allowing The Joint Commission (TJC) to use its own minimum standards for nurse staffing in its accreditation process. ANA sought a court order to require that USDHHS ensures that TJC uses standards that are at least equivalent to USDHHS standards. These actions are pending and are part of ANA's ongoing efforts to establish safe nurse staffing laws nationwide via their Nationwide State Legislative Agenda.

Box 15.1 provides a list of many of the health-related interest groups. Longest (1997) described four major strategies that interest groups use to influence the public policy-making process: lobbying, electioneering, litigation, and influencing public opinion. In addition, a fifth strategy of coalition building is a major interest group strategy.

Box 15.1

Health Care Interest Groups

- American Academy of Pediatrics
- American Association for Homes and Services for the Aging
- American Association of Colleges of Nurses
- American Association of Health Plans
- American Association of Nurse Anesthetists
- American Association of Retired Persons
- American Cancer Society
- American College of Healthcare Executives
- American College of Nurse Midwives
- American College of Surgeons
- American Dental Association
- American Federation of Home Health Agencies
- American Health Care Association
- American Heart Association
- American Hospital Association
- American Medical Association
- American Nurses Association
- Association of American Medical Colleges
- Association of University Programs in Health Administration
- BlueCross BlueShield Association
- Group Health Association of America
- Health Insurance Association of America
- Hospice Association of America
- National Association for Home Care
- National Association of Medical Equipment Suppliers
- National Association of Pediatric Nurse Practitioners
- National Association of Public Hospitals
- National Association of Social Workers
- National Council for Senior Citizens
- National League for Nursing
- National Student Nurse Association
- Pharmaceutical Research and Manufacturers of America

Lobbying

Interest groups attempt to influence the views of individual representatives and senators or key members of the executive branch on specific issues. The exertion of influence in public policy making is the process by which people work to persuade others to follow their advice, suggestions, or orders (Keys & Case, 1990). Interest groups hire lobbyists (also called *governmental relations officers* or *specialists*), who communicate with policy makers for the purpose of influencing their decisions to be more favorable to, or consistent with, the preferences of those doing the lobbying (Buchholz, 1994). Some interest groups are more effective than others. Milio (1984) identified the following guidelines for effectively influencing policy: organize; do your homework; frame your arguments to appeal to the specific audience you want to persuade; concentrate your finite organizational energies; act in a timely fashion at the right points in the policy-making process; and always obtain or develop the best data available on your policy position.

Electioneering

The strategy of electioneering involves working to elect or retain in office policy makers who are sympathetic to the interests of the group's members (Longest, 1997). One very popular way to do this is to direct money into PACs. Another approach is direct involvement with political campaigns, including fund raising, participation in phone banks, and canvassing neighborhoods. In the 2005-2006 election cycle, ANA-PAC endorsed 112 candidates for federal office—ANA's highest seal of approval. Of the 112, 100 won, yielding an 89% win rate *(www.nursingworld.org/MainMenuCategories/ANAPoliticalPower/ANAPAC/EndorsementProcess.aspz)*.

Litigation

This strategy involves the use of lawsuits to challenge existing policies, stimulate new policies, or alter specific aspects of the implementation of policies (Longest, 1997). Litigation may be used at both the state and federal levels; this is an increasingly popular way to exert influence in the policy arena. One example is the case brought by the California Hospital Association to challenge the implementation of the newly legislated minimum staffing ratios in California hospitals. Another is the lawsuit filed in October 2007 against the California Department of Education by the ANA and its state affiliate ANA/California to stop the school system from allowing unlicensed volunteer school personnel to administer insulin to students *(www.safestaffingsaveslives.org/WhatisANADoing/LegalAction.aspx)*.

Shaping Public Opinion

Policy makers are influenced by public opinion, so interest groups may be able to achieve their objectives by helping shape these opinions. This may be accomplished by running television or newspaper advertisements. The Harry and Louise campaign, for example, was effective in turning public opinion against Clinton's Health Care Reform Plan in the 1993-1994 time frame. Related to a specific health care issue, media campaigns about the negative consequences of second-hand smoke were influential in many states passing legislation to ban smoking in pubic and sometimes private settings.

Coalition Building

A fifth strategy is coalition building. Achieving substantial changes within an organization may require collective, not individual, action (Kelly, 2003). Coalitions are groups of individuals or organizations that join together around a common goal. According to Wakefield (2008), enlisting the support of others who share the same goals or interests often results in achieving desired goals. In legislative politics, nursing organizations use coalition building when dealing with state legislatures and congress (Kelly, 2003). To build and maintain effective coalitions requires leadership, membership, and resources (Bowers-Lanier, 2007). The leader must be motivational and possess excellent organizational skills; members are required to learn how to function effectively in a new membership role; and resources are needed to accomplish the required work.

Policy Development

Health policies are created within the dynamic public policy-making process that takes place at the federal, state, and local levels of government. Health policies are also created in the private sector. For example, health plans have policies related to the required procedures for accessing medical specialists; hospitals have policies related to mandatory overtime or floating staff to other units. These policies, similar to those in the public sector, are also authoritative decisions that influence the actions, behaviors, or decisions of others (Longest, 2002). The development of any kind of policy is a process that reflects the values of the individuals or groups supporting that policy position. These individuals or groups identify a problem for which a policy solution is sought. Block (2008) outlined six phases of public policy making: (1) agenda setting; (2) policy formulation; (3) policy adoption; (4) policy implementation; (5) policy assessment; and (6) policy modification. Longest (1997, 2002) collapsed some of these steps and identified the following three interconnected phases of the public policy-making process (Figure 15.1):

1. *Formulation phase:* Incorporates activities associated with agenda setting and the subsequent development and adoption of the legislation
2. *Implementation phase:* Incorporates activities associated with rule making and policy operation; mobilization of human and financial resources to comply with the policy (Longest, 2002)
3. *Modification phase:* As a result of policy assessment, addresses whether the implemented policy is in compliance with its statutory requirements and achieving its objectives in regard to the policy problem (Dunn, 1994)

It is important, however, to recognize that the policy process is not necessarily sequential or logical (Milstead, 2008).

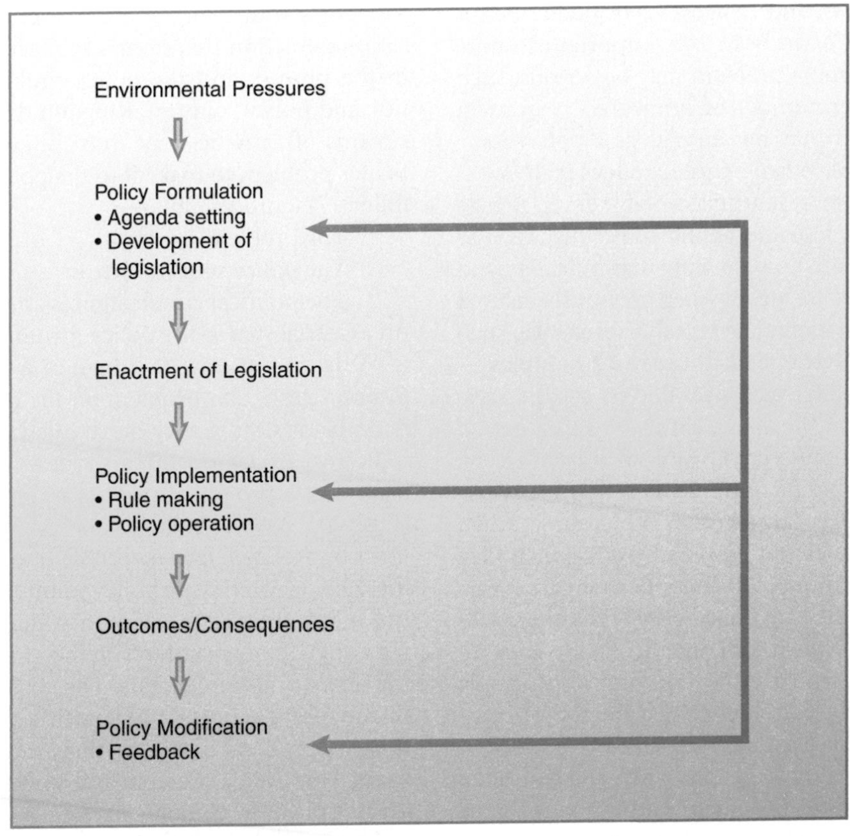

Figure 15.1
Public policy-making process. (Modified from Longest, B.B. Jr. [2002]. *Health policy making in the United States* [3rd ed.]. Chicago: Health Administration Press.)

Policy Formulation Phase

Policy formulation is the initial and perhaps most crucial phase of public policy making. Agenda setting is concerned with identifying a societal problem and bringing it to the attention of government (Milstead, 2008). To get on the policy agenda, an issue must successfully compete with a multitude of other issues trying to get on the agenda. Success depends on overall appeal of the issue, amount of political support it has garnered, and perceptions of viability of the proposed policy solutions (Kingdon, 2003; Longest, 1998). A window of opportunity is created for a policy issue to emerge when problems, possible solutions, and political circumstances come together in a favorable configuration (Furlong, 2008). Kingdon (2003) described this as a *confluence of problem streams,* and Longest (2002) described it as the *saliency of an issue.* It is important to note that even though a problem may be serious, such as the growing number of uninsured persons in this country, it may not emerge as a policy issue to be addressed. When a problem does reach what is considered to be an unacceptable level, it may finally emerge into the public consciousness. For example, data are now showing that mortality and morbidity rates are higher when previously insured individuals no longer have health insurance, such as when early retirement causes loss of employer-sponsored health insurance. Recent studies have also shown that the U.S. health status as a nation lags behind countries with universal health care. Problems tend to be noticed when they are widespread and affect large numbers of people, when they affect a small but powerful group, when they attract the attention of the nation via media coverage, or when they are linked closely to other well-accepted policy issues (Longest, 2002). Lack of health insurance may be kept off the policy agenda by the opposing forces, concerned about the potential costs of policy solutions, dislike for larger government and "socialized medicine," and threats to the profits of powerful interest groups such as the drug companies and hospital supply corporations. When a problem comes to the forefront, possible alternative policies to address the problem are generated. Differences or conflict may arise over the criteria to be used in evaluating alternative solutions to the problem. Policy making is delayed because of the time it takes to critique and debate the relative merits of competing alternatives. There may be disagreements over the relative merits of each alternative, implementation issues, feasibility issues due to costs or other resource requirements, and political considerations (Longest, 2002).

Thus policy making is more of a political process than a rational decision-making process. The preferences and influences of interest groups, coalitions, political bargaining, vote trading, and ideological biases may come into play at any point in the public policy-making process.

Kingdon Model of Policy Formulation

Kingdon's framework (2003) described the constant interaction that occurs between participants in the process and the policy problem, its politics, and policy solution. Kingdon described three streams of activities that must line up for a particular problem to make it to the policy agenda, as follows (Figure 15.2):

1. The problem stream
2. The policy solution stream
3. The political circumstances stream

An essential step in the policy formulation process is to figure out how to convince a policy maker to put a particular problem on the policy agenda. A problem stream may be revealed by systematic indicators of a problem, a sudden crisis, or feedback that a program is not working as intended (Furlong, 2008). At least one possible solution must be available for any problem to be placed on the agenda. Alternative policy solutions come from the many subsystems of policy making, including congressional staff, researchers, interest group members, and bureaucrats. The goal, as described in Kingdon's model, is to match a possible solution to a problem that is floating around the policy space. However, a problem and a possible solution are not the only elements necessary for generating policy development. There also must be the political will to make it happen. The political stream considers other factors in the environment that

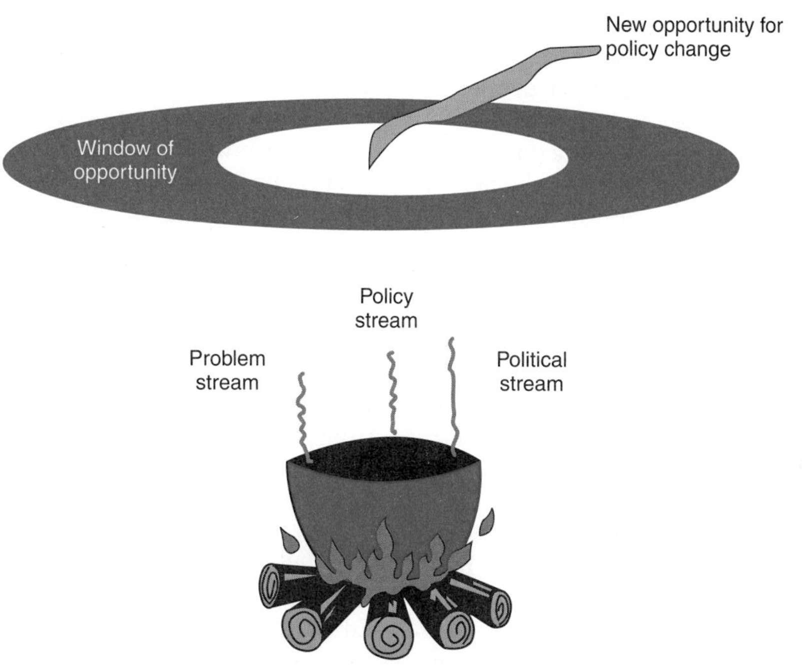

Figure 15.2
A depiction of how Kingdon's model of public policy formation might look.

influence the policy agenda, such as the economy, size of the federal deficit, public attitudes and opinions, positions of key political leaders, changes in administration, and the presence of other competing items on the policy agenda (Longest, 1997). The coupling of problems and policy streams allows for the creation of policy change only when the political stream is favorable as well; this "window of opportunity" occurs on an infrequent basis.

Policy proposals that receive serious consideration must meet several criteria, including technical feasibility, fit with the dominant values and the national priorities of the day, and budget feasibility (Kingdon, 2003). A recent example of the confluence of a policy problem and solution with a positive political stream was the passage of the Medicare Prescription Drug, Improvement, and Modernization Act of 2003. Pressure to do something about the high cost of prescription medicine and lack of a drug benefit in the Medicare program was mounting. The media reported stories of elderly individuals doing without food or heat to pay for their prescription medications. States were setting up programs that were not consistent with the ideology of the federal administration (e.g., state-level negotiation with drug companies to lower drug prices; importation of drugs from Canada). Possible policy solutions at the federal level included adding a new benefit to the current Medicare program (expanded government entitlement) or using a private sector approach. Choosing the latter, the new legislation has created a government-subsidized prescription benefit as part of Medicare but opens the program to price competition through a premium support model. CMS was tasked with implementing this complex law. The program is now in the policy assessment and policy modification phases.

Stage-Sequential Model of Policy Formulation

The stage-sequential model is another model explaining public policy making. In this model, the policy process is viewed as a series of stages in which a number of functional activities occur

(Anderson, 1990; Ripley, 1985, 1996). A group's policy problem is first identified and placed on the policy agenda. Next, a policy is developed, adopted, implemented, and evaluated. The stages are dynamic and cyclical and include a policy evaluation and oversight stage to identify whether the program is functioning well or might require revision or even generation of an entirely new policy. The specific steps in the stage-sequential model are as follows:

- *Stage 1:* Identification of the policy problem (e.g., the problem might be identified as safety and quality issues in hospitals; the problem could then be restated as a policy problem or issue—that of inadequate numbers of RNs staffing hospital units).
- *Stage 2:* Policy formulation (e.g., the establishment of laws requiring hospitals to meet minimum staffing ratios for RNs, as done in California).
- *Stage 3:* Program implementation (e.g., the California Department of Health was charged with establishing the minimum staffing ratios for different types of units within hospitals).
- *Stage 4:* Policy evaluation (e.g., the implementation, performance, and impact of the policy solution [minimum staffing ratios] are evaluated to determine how well the new policy is meeting its stated goals and objectives). Issues to be explored include whether sufficient numbers of RNs are available to meet the mandated ratios in all hospitals; whether substitution is occurring (RNs for other health professions categories); and whether patient safety and quality of care have improved as a result of having more nurses at the bedside.

The process itself is dynamic and cyclical rather than linear. The stages often are not clear-cut, with implementation and evaluation sometimes being done in tandem and with proposals moving back and forth among the stages (Hanley & Falk, 2007) rather than proceeding from Stage 1 to Stage 4.

Legislative Process

The policy formulation phase concludes with the development of legislation. Formal enactment of legislation bridges the policy-making process into the next phase of policy implementation.

At the federal level, bills are introduced in the U.S. House of Representatives or the Senate and then assigned to a committee with jurisdiction over the substance of the bill. A number of committees in the House and Senate are involved with health legislation. In the House, a health-related bill is usually considered by the Energy and Commerce Committee or its Subcommittee on Health and Environment, the Ways and Means Committee or its Subcommittee on Health, the Committee on Veteran's Affairs, the Committee on Education and Labor, or the Select Committee on Aging. In the Senate, a bill may be heard by the Health, Education, Labor and Pensions Committee or its Subcommittee on Public Health, the Senate Finance Committee or its Subcommittee on Health Care, the Committee on Finance, the Committee on Labor and Human Resources, the Committee on Veteran's Affairs, or the Select Committee on Indian Affairs. Appropriations are decided by the Appropriations Subcommittee on Labor, Health, and Human Services, Education, and Related Agencies in both the Senate and the House.

There are three types of committees in Congress, as follows (Wakefield, 2008):

1. Oversight committees that monitor issues related to the committee focus
2. Appropriation committees that allocate funding on a fiscal-year basis to support specific programs (The appropriations levels cannot exceed the ceilings established by the authorizing legislation, but they can, and often do, fund at a significantly lower level.)
3. Authorization committees that establish or change federal programs and set limits on the amount of federal funding that can be spent to implement a particular program

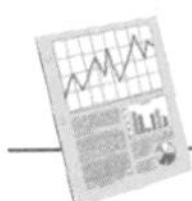

Research Note

Source: Odom-Forren, J., & Hahn, E.J. (2006). Mandatory reporting of health care–associated infections: Kingdon's multiple streams approach. *Policy, Politics, & Nursing Practice, 7*(1), 64-72.

Purpose

Odom-Forren and Hahn use Kingdon's Multiple Streams Framework for policy analysis to examine the process of Kentucky's mandatory health care–associated infections (HAI) reporting bill within the national context. The problem stream was characterized as infections that patients acquire during treatment for a medical condition. The importance of HAI has emerged nationally within the larger context of patient safety. The magnitude of the problem was supported by alarming statistics: 2 million infections, 90,000 deaths, and $4.5 billion in costs annually. Patients with HAI were reported to have increased suffering, higher costs, longer lengths of stay, and more life-threatening complications. Advocates of mandatory reporting believe that public disclosure will serve as an incentive to hospitals and clinicians to improve infection practices.

Discussion

Groups that have served to focus attention on this issue included consumer groups (CU), credentialing agencies (TJC), and regulatory agencies (CMS), in addition to personal stories of horrible experiences with HAIs. The alternative options contained in the policy stream include information flow via confidential, voluntary reporting to agencies that already collect the data (i.e., CDC); non-public mandatory reporting to a state agency; advocacy for national legislation for mandatory reporting; and limited mandatory reporting (exclusion of ambulatory surgery centers). The political stream has been described as incorporating public mood, pressure group campaigns, and changes within government (Kingdon, 2003). The national mood was strongly in favor of more public disclosure. Constituents at the state level in particular were said to contact their elected representatives to support mandatory infection reporting by hospitals. The IOM, ANA, and APIC were among the proponents of mandatory reporting, while the most vocal opponent was the Kentucky Hospital Association. A national consensus conference was held in 2005 to address the benefits of mandatory public reporting and included the APIC, CDC, AHA, CU, NQF, and SHEA. The AHA at this time was said to realize that objections to public disclosure might be perceived as attempts to stonewall or obfuscate.

Application to Practice

The authors concluded that a window of opportunity had opened for mandatory reporting of HAI nationally because of increased public awareness of the problem, the significance of the problem, the coalescing of professional organizations, governmental agency involvement in dealing with HAI in a public manner, CDC dissemination of guidelines for states debating public reporting, media involvement and interest, and consumer group involvement and interest. However, public reporting legislation did not get passed in Kentucky because of more pressing issues including the state budget, nursing groups focused on prescriptive authority for narcotics, limited support by other professional associations, lack of media coverage, and lack of a strong coalition supporting the bill statewide. This article demonstrates how nurses can use policy models to analyze the various factors surrounding a policy issue.

AHA, American Hospital Association; *ANA,* American Nurses Association; *APIC,* Association for Professionals in Infection Control and Epidemiology, Inc.; *CDC,* Centers for Disease Control and Prevention; *CMS,* Centers for Medicare & Medicaid Services; *CU,* Consumers Union; *IOM,* Institute of Medicine; *NQF,* National Quality Forum; *SHEA,* Society for Healthcare Epidemiology of America; *TJC,* The Joint Commission.

The chair of the authorization committee determines which bills will be considered by the committee during a legislative session. During the deliberations, hearings are held and oral or written testimony presented. After the hearings, a bill is next "reported out" or sent to the floor of the House or Senate for a vote. Both chambers must act on a bill before it can become a law. Successful bills are sent to conference committees composed of members from both the House and Senate to negotiate any differences in the respective bills. Finally, the negotiated final version of the bill is reported out for a final vote by both chambers and, if passed, forwarded on to the President for signature and enactment into law or vetoed. Re-authorization of programs occurs every 3 to 5 years.

Policy Implementation Phase

After a law is enacted, the focus shifts from the policy formulation phase to the policy implementation phase. Policy implementation is the process of putting a policy into effect to accomplish its intended goals and objectives. The new policy may direct change in the actions or behaviors of individuals or organizations, or it may rearrange existing behavior patterns to comply with the policy decision (Wilken, 1999). Enacted laws seldom contain enough explicit language to guide their implementation completely (Longest, 1998). Executive agencies must therefore create the rules and regulations that they think are necessary for a newly enacted program to become functional (Hanley & Falk, 2007). Often, there are mismatches between legislative intent and the resulting bureaucratic outcomes (Smart, 2008). Implementation of a policy may consist of modifying policy objectives to correspond with available resources or mobilizing new resources to achieve the original objectives (Wilken, 1999). Regardless of which mechanism occurs, the policy is changed to some degree during the implementation phase (Mazmanian & Sabatier, 1983).

The organization or agency that is responsible for implementing the new law must publish in the *Federal Register* a Notice of Proposed Rule Making (NPRM) (Longest, 2002). Once the rule is drafted, the public can review and comment on the proposed rules for implementing the law. This often results in changes in the proposed rules and is one of the most active points of involvement for individuals and organizations seeking to influence the policy-making process (Longest, 1997). Rules and regulations established through the formal rule-making process have legal standing and are, in effect, policies. These policies are codified in the Code of Federal Regulations (CFR) and are available to the public to read and review (Longest, 2002).

Stages of implementation proceed in the following order: passage of basic statutes; policy decisions of implementing agencies; compliance of target groups with those policy decisions; intended or unintended consequences or outcomes; revisions or attempted revisions in the basic statute (Mazmanian and Sabatier, 1983; Wilken, 1999). Because of the continued involvement of different interest groups, it is important to constantly monitor the implementation of a new program or law (Longest, 1998). The following three issues are critical to address (Mazmanian and Sabatier, 1983; Wilken, 1999):

1. To what extent are the policy results or outcomes consistent with the officially stated objectives?
2. To what extent have the original objectives been modified during the implementation process?
3. What principal factors have affected the degree of change and modifications that have occurred in the new program?

Policies must be effectively implemented to have a chance of achieving their intended effect (Longest, 1997). Although laws are implemented primarily in the executive branch of government within departments such as USDHHS, Labor, Education, and Commerce, the legislative branch does maintain oversight responsibility of policy implementation through funding appropriations, hearings, and agencies such as the General Accounting Office (GAO) and Congressional Budget Office (CBO) (Longest, 1997). Wilken (2008) has concluded that policy implementation is inherently unpredictable.

During this phase, various forces will try to change the policy, including interest groups, opposition parties, affected individuals and organizations, and the bureaucracy that has the responsibility for implementation (Wilken, 2008). More important, however, members of the nursing community, from individual nurses to national nursing organizations, can also affect implementation of new policy programs and laws (Wilken, 1999). This may be a particularly important area in which nurses can strategically affect the benefit of patients, nurses, and/or society.

The operations phase of policy implementation involves the actual conduct and running of programs. Such policy implementation can be studied from either a top-down or bottom-up perspective (Wilken, 2008). Success or failure is judged against the specific policy goals. The analysis focuses on examining who participates in the new program, for what reasons, and with what effect. From the bottom-up perspective, analysts look at the individuals (frontline personnel; street-level bureaucrats) who are interacting directly with the consumers (Wilken, 2008). Problems with implementation are usually blamed on vague rules that provide insufficient guidance or on inadequate resources to fully implement the program. As a result, the implementers may alter the program because of perceived problems with the policy. From the top-down perspective, implementation issues are usually blamed on those individuals charged with implementing the new program or policies. Managers may be accused of being incompetent or of not having a clear understanding of program intent.

Thus two aspects are important to consider in policy implementation: (1) the policy itself; and (2) the characteristics and capabilities of the organization and individuals charged with its implementation (Longest, 1998). Clearly written laws with well-articulated goals are easier to implement than laws with vague or conflicting objectives. Also, policy implementation is easier when there is a good fit between the implementing organization and the goals/objectives of the policy (Longest, 1998).

Policy Modification Phase

In this phase of the public policy-making process, individuals and organizations provide feedback to the policy makers and policy implementers regarding the impact of the new law or program. Actual experiences in the implementation phase are presented to the lawmakers, the courts, or the legislative branch. Portions of the new programs might be struck down or modified, or the entire bill may be vacated, as happened with Medicare Catastrophic Coverage. The Medicare Catastrophic Coverage Act, passed in 1988, was a major reform initiative, but it was short-lived. Angry senior citizens were quick to let their congressional representatives know their displeasure with the law, and it was repealed in 1989. In short, policy modification is an important phase of the policy-making process. Individuals will seek changes that provide more benefits or protect existing ones; those who are affected negatively by a policy will seek to modify it and reduce the negative consequences; those who formulate or implement policies will seek changes when the policies fail to measure up to their preferences and objectives (Longest, 2002). Longest (2002) pointed out that the policy modification phase makes the public policy-making process both dynamic and continuously evolving. In addition, some policies are made obsolete because of biological, social, cultural, demographic, ecological, economic, ethical, legal, psychological, and technological changes and advances (Longest, 1997).

ALLOCATIVE AND REGULATORY HEALTH POLICIES

Health policy is a subset of public policy. It includes those public policies that are related to or influence health and illness. Health policies generally affect either a group of individuals or certain types of organizations. A complex and large number of decisions go into health policy formulation. Health policies emerge in the forms of laws, rules and regulations, judicial decisions, resource allocations, and broad "macro" policies such as global health care budgets.

Health policy is important to nursing in multiple ways, from the regulation of practice to the structure of the practice environment and professional practices (Algase et al., 2004). Health policy decision making influences what nurses and other clinicians can do in practice and determines what professional services will be reimbursed by government and third-party payers and for how much (Algase et al., 2004).

As noted earlier, health policies fall within two broad categories: allocative and regulatory (Block, 2008). Allocative policies are designed to provide benefits to one group of individuals or organizations at the expense of others in order to meet specific policy objectives (Longest, 2002). Some allocative policies are meant to address imbalances in supply and demand of certain products or services. An example is the passage of the Nurse Faculty Loan Program, meant to increase the supply of nurse faculty in the future. Other allocative policies are used to ensure that certain segments of the population have access to health care services (Longest, 1997). The funding of graduate medical education programs under the Medicare program is an example of an allocative policy. Given the expense of medical education, it was believed that a sufficient supply of physicians would not be produced without this public subsidy of medical education. Regulatory policies, on the other hand, are meant to influence the actions, behaviors, and decisions of others through a directive approach. State practice acts that dictate what activities are within a health professional's scope of practice are an example of a regulatory policy. Longest (1997) has identified the following five categories of regulatory health policies:

1. Market-entry restrictions
2. Rate or price-setting controls on health service providers
3. Quality controls on the provision of health services
4. Market-preserving controls
5. Social regulation

The first four types of health policies are focused on economic issues; the fifth, however, seeks to achieve socially desired ends (Longest, 1997). Market-entry regulations include the state policies related to licensing of practitioners or organizations, including advanced practice nursing certification and prescriptive authority. Rate-setting regulations include the Medicare program's imposition of the prospective payment system (PPS) using diagnosis-related groups (DRGs) and the resource-based relative value scale (RBRVS) payment system for physicians under Medicare. Regulations related to quality controls include the safety and efficacy standards that must be met before a new drug is approved by the FDA. Another example is the requirement by CMS for public reporting of performance data by both nursing homes and home health agencies (Nursing Home Compare and Home Health Compare). Market-preserving regulations are those that seek to retain competitiveness among providers and organizations by restricting the formation of monopolies through enforcement of the Sherman Antitrust Act, the Clayton Act, and the Robinson-Patman Act (Longest, 2001). Socially desirable regulations include rules for workplace safety (Occupational Safety and Health Administration [OSHA]) and rules that prevent age and sex discrimination in hiring (Longest, 2002).

UNINTENDED CONSEQUENCES OF PUBLIC POLICY

Analysis may reveal that policies intended to have one outcome may have unintended consequences that totally overwhelm the intended outcomes. An example of this is what happened as a result of a state Medicaid drug cost-containment policy for the chronically mentally ill (Soumerai, 2003). The intent of the policy was to reduce Medicaid expenditures for drugs used to manage chronic mental illness. In New Hampshire, the state Medicaid program introduced a drug-payment "cap" that set a limit of three reimbursable medications a person could receive per month. A structured policy analysis revealed that the drug cap did indeed reduce the use of prescription drugs among the elderly and mentally ill but at the same time increased hospital and nursing home admissions, partial hospitalizations, distribution of psychoactive medications by community mental health centers, and use of emergency mental health services. The analysis showed that vulnerable populations are likely to experience adverse effects from hastily applied drug cost-containment policies and that the resulting compensatory measures may create more expenses than the policy removes (Soumerai, 2003).

POLICY ANALYSIS

Policy analysis is a subfield of political science that seeks to understand and build up knowledge of the whole process of public policy (Hudson & Lowe, 2004). More specifically, policy analysis is the systematic study of the content and anticipated or actual effects of existing or proposed policies. Policy analysis is concerned with determining which of various alternative policies will achieve a given set of goals in light of the relations between the policies and the goals. It is concerned primarily with explanations rather than with prescriptions (Block, 2008). Policy analysis is carried out by individuals from multiple disciplinary backgrounds and professional groups (Block, 2008), including nursing. Policy analysis is methodologically diverse, using both qualitative and quantitative methods, including case studies, survey research, statistical analysis, and model building.

Health policy analysis is the process of assessing and choosing among spending and resource alternatives that affect the health care system, public health system, or health of the general public. Health policy analysis involves the following steps, mirroring the general policy analysis process:

1. Identifying or framing the problem
2. Identifying who is affected (stakeholders)
3. Identifying and comparing the potential impact of different options for dealing with the problem
4. Choosing among alternative options
5. Implementing the chosen option(s)
6. Evaluating the impact

Stakeholders can include government, private health care providers, industry groups, professional associations, industry and trade associations, advocacy groups, and consumers.

It has been pointed out that standardized assessment of major health policy changes in the United States does not occur (Grudzen & Brook, 2007), resulting in a sort of "social experimentation" (Daniels & Sabin, 2002; Rosenthal & Daniels, 2006) with a lack of accountability for the results. Wharam and Daniels (2007) have proposed a framework for moving toward more accountability in health policy implementation, calling for evidence that benefits of proposed policy change exceed the harm. They describe the four essential elements of a system that maximizes effectiveness and ethical characteristics of health policy reform: (1) review to ensure policy's fundamental precepts are ethical; (2) targeted pilot projects or timely retrospective assessments to address benefits and harms to stakeholders; (3) studies to determine if unintended consequences can be satisfactorily minimized; (4) feedback systems to maintain acceptable outcomes after policy implementation. *Outcome domains* are defined as health outcomes (chronic illness control), access to care, and income spent on health care.

LEADERSHIP AND MANAGEMENT IMPLICATIONS

Power

The ability to influence in any realm, including policy making, requires power. Power comes from the Latin word *potere,* meaning "to be able." Power is the ability to influence others in an effort to achieve goals (Kelly, 2003). Sources of power (French & Raven, 1959; Longest, 1997) include the following:

- *Legitimate or positional power* is derived from an individual's position in a social system or in an organization, or status within a group; also called *formal power* or *authority* (Longest, 2002). Executives and union leaders tend to have more power than supervisors or rank-and-file employees.
- *Reward power and coercive power* is based on an individual's ability to reward compliance

or to punish noncompliance, with the preferred decisions, actions, and behaviors that are sought from others (Longest, 1997). Reward and coercive powers are derived from the ability to provide or withhold from any person something of value to that person. For example, supervisors and managers usually have the power to determine pay increases and nominate individuals for promotion.

- *Expert power* is derived from possessing expertise, knowledge, skills, or information that is valued or needed by others (Longest, 1997). Expert power might include the ability to solve problems or perform critical tasks. It may also be vested in trusted advisers or associates. In the health care field, physicians are often viewed as the professional group possessing expertise related to health care issues.
- *Referent power* refers to a circumstance in which persons, organizations, or interest groups engender admiration, loyalty, and emulation from others to such an extent that they gain the power to exert influence as a result (Longest, 2002). This is also called *charismatic power.* Some recent examples include the ability of the actor Michael J. Fox to garner support for increased funding for Parkinson's disease research and Christopher Reeves for spinal cord injury. Nurses have referent power to some extent because of their position of trust with the general public.

Hersey and colleagues (2008) added two other sources of power to this list: (1) information power—when one individual has special information that another individual desires; and (2) connection power—granted to those perceived to have privileged connections with individuals or organizations. Power is translated into influence through interpersonal and political skills (Longest, 1997). Nurses as a group tend to have fewer resources and less cohesion than other powerful groups in health care. Nurses on the whole also tend to lack prowess in the public arena and visibility in the political process; as a group, nurses generally lack the knowledge, skills, and sophistication to influence health policy (Algase et al., 2004). However, this has been changing in recent years as the associations representing nurses become more politically active and engage the services of experienced and effective lobbyists.

LEADERSHIP & MANAGEMENT BEHAVIORS

Leadership Behaviors

- Envisions directions for health policy initiatives
- Communicates about health policy issues
- Acts to influence health policy and legislation
- Enables followers to influence health policy
- Lobbies influential decision makers
- Models supportive networking for information and influence
- Drafts legislation
- Encourages followers to be politically aware and active

Management Behaviors

- Communicates about health policy needs
- Gives testimony
- Writes letters to support a policy direction
- Negotiates for scarce resources
- Implements laws and regulations affecting nursing practice

Overlap Areas

- Communicates about health policies
- Takes action to influence and acquire scarce resources

Becoming Active in Policy

Longest (2004) has stated that successful management of health care organizations requires managers to become "policy competent." This refers to understanding policy environments, responding to an organization's policy environment, and shaping an organization's policy environment. The discipline of nursing has identified the importance of policy advocacy as a strategy to enhance population health, as well as the need for nurses to become more knowledgeable about the policy process (International Council of Nurses [ICN], 2001). The ICN has published guidelines for shaping effective health policy and identified nurses' essential roles in influencing health policy and understanding the policy process (Reutter & Duncan, 2002). Several authors have gone further and called for nurses to expand their policy focus from health policy to complex social problems such as poverty, homelessness, and violence (Morgan & Marsh, 1998; Reutter, 2000; Reutter & Williamson, 2000). The American Nurses Association's Social Policy Statement (Cohen & Milone-Nuzzo, 2001) asserted that social policies are under the purview of nursing care and research.

Public policy is a process as well as a product, requiring choices about valuing aspects of life (Malone, 1999; Stone, 1997). Specific skills and knowledge are required for policy work (Reutter & Duncan, 2002). Critical elements of the policy process include problem framing and definition, creation of policy agendas, policy instruments and their implementation, policy network and community analyses, and evaluation of policy impacts (Reutter & Duncan, 2002). Nurses must be aware that political, economic, and social contexts determine which policy problems, agendas, and strategies are enacted. Cramer (2002) found that greater participation of nurses in political activity occurred when individuals possessed the values of political interest, political information, personal efficacy, and civic skills. She believed that instilling these values is a deliberate process that begins early in a nurse's education and continues through graduation. She suggested that professional associations partner with schools to ensure a future cadre of nurses who possess at least a minimum level of information and interest in policy and the political process.

To become politically active and participate in public policy making, the practicing nurse can do the following:

- Establish a base of contact with elected officials, community leaders, and public policy makers.
- Work with professional associations—keep eyes and ears open to activities that bear upon legislative priorities.
- Become members of grassroots networks, to stay informed and work within a framework for participation in public policy process.

To prepare nurses to become politically active and effective, schools can do the following:

- Provide educational preparation in policy advocacy.
- Require course work in sociology, economics, political science, and policy.
- Assign students to monitor and report on state and national legislation potentially affecting nurses or patients.
- Encourage or require students and faculty members to attend a Legislative Day at their state capital.

It is also crucial that nurse researchers translate their findings into policy-relevant recommendations (Jones et al., 1997). To use research and data to influence policy and policy making, reports of nursing research should consider the following questions (Wakefield, 2001):

- Is the linkage between the topic and specific public policies or programs explicit?
- Is the topic related to a current or emerging health policy concern?
- Is the research framed in the context of health care access, costs, and/or quality?
- Are populations important to policy makers identified?
- Is the language understandable to policy makers and the general public?

- Do research reports include policy-relevant content in the literature review and in the discussion of findings?
- Can the manuscript content be used at all stages of the policy-making process?
- Is the content useful to advocacy groups?

Decisions are made that influence the context in which care is delivered and affect the occupation and practice of nursing. These decisions may restrict or enable payment for care services or affect rules governing licensure and the work environment. The decisions are made with or without nursing's involvement and goals. Therefore nurses will be drawn into politics and need to refine their political skills and power bases. It is vital that nurses become involved in both politics and health policy. Nurses reflect a long and distinguished tradition in health promotion, wellness, and public health advocacy. They remind the public that health care is more than medically focused disease treatment and surgery. For example, nurses have taken the leadership to pressure state legislatures to pass motorcycle helmet laws for the purpose of primary prevention of head injuries and have been very active in anti-smoking campaigns at the state level.

Nurses also can take a leadership role at the local, state, and federal levels of health policy activities. For example, nurses can use their expertise to develop white papers and policy analysis data for key decision makers. Nurses can vote, lobby, campaign, and protest as activism methods to influence health care policy. Nurses can be locally active in communities by being involved on boards and commissions and by communicating about health policy issues. Buresh and Gordon's (2000) book is an excellent resource guide.

At the individual level, nurses' leadership and management roles in client care management involve the use of influence at multiple levels. Nurses need to take the responsibility to keep informed about health policy and political issues within the organization, as well as external to the organization. Awareness may be triggered and enhanced by sources such as professional organizations' position papers, professional journals, newspapers and other public media, and networking with colleagues in person or electronically. Nurses may contact their elected representatives for information or to express an opinion. Clearly, nurses need to stay informed and aware of health policy issues. They need to communicate their positions to others and to support and lobby in conjunction with others as a group strategic action team. By taking these leadership actions, nurses can influence others to make changes needed to positively affect health care policy and politics.

CURRENT ISSUES AND TRENDS

Current Policy Issues

Several issues are currently at the top of the nursing policy agenda. The nursing shortage, including the shortage of nurse faculty members, is of high concern, because it relates to patient safety and quality of care. State legislators are taking the nursing shortage very seriously (Cooksey et al., 2004). In 2002, the shortage was ranked as a "high priority" by 39 states and a "priority" by another 7 states (National Conference of State Legislatures [NCSL], 2001). Some states have reported substantial growth in total applicant pools in nursing schools as a result of different recruitment initiatives; yet not all of these applicants can be accommodated because of faculty shortages and insufficient numbers of new clinical educational sites. The shortage of nurse faculty members has made it onto the national policy agenda. Two major programs have been established to increase the supply of qualified nursing faculty. As part of the Nurse Reinvestment Act of 2002 (PL107-205) the Nurse Faculty Loan Program (NFLP) has been initiated. The institution (nursing school) must enter into an agreement with the USDHHS Health Resources and Services Administration (HRSA) to establish and operate the NFLP fund. The fund must provide for loans made to students enrolled full time in an eligible advanced degree program in nursing (masters or doctorate) at the school. Loan recipients must complete the educational program and, after graduation, may cancel up to 85% of the loan while serving as full-time nurse faculty at a school of nursing. In addition, the U.S. Department of Education has expanded the Graduate Assistance in Areas of National Need (GAANN) program to include nursing students. This program provides fellowships to assist graduate students with excellent records who demonstrate financial need and plan to pursue the highest degree available in their course of study in a field designated as an area of national need. Grants are awarded to programs and institutions to sustain and enhance capacity for teaching and research in areas of national need.

Nursing Organizations' Policy Agenda

Most, if not all, professional nursing associations develop an annual list of policy issues pertinent to their association members. These associations typically have on their professional staffs one or more governmental relations experts, who monitor state and federal policy initiatives that could affect their association members either positively or negatively. For example, the Association of Operating Room Nurses (AORN) publishes its legislative and regulatory priorities in its official journal and on its website. Every year, AORN leadership develops and recommends legislative priorities at both the state and national levels. The AORN Board of Directors reviews and approves the list, which then steers the organization's public policy activities. The four priorities for 2008 were listed as follows on their website:

1. Preserving the role of registered nurses as circulators in the operating room
2. Preserving and protecting the perioperative RNs scope of practice
3. Seeking financial reimbursement for the RNFA (registered nurse first assistant)
4. Supporting workplace safety and patient safety initiatives.

In addition, the organization monitors legislative initiatives affecting perioperative nursing at the state level. The current list is categorized according to workplace safety issues (safe patient handling, whistleblower protection, nurse staffing in health care facilities) and patient safety issues (infection reporting, error/adverse event reporting).

Of interest to nurse managers and executives are the policy agenda and initiatives carried out by the American Organization of Nurse Executives (AONE). The AONE has a grassroots network of 49 state chapters, which keep abreast of the latest legislative, regulatory, or practice issues affecting nursing. The AONE also provides chapter leadership with up-to-date information; allows access to current information from government and private sources through a leader Listserv; sponsors quarterly chapter calls to enable networking across chapters; and has partnered with the AHA to form the AONE/AHAPAC, which lobbies Capital Hill leaders on relevant issues. The AONE 2008 legislative agenda identifies priorities within the broad categories of education and leadership development; public policy and advocacy; information technology; international nurses; access and coverage; and reimbursement policy. Specific activities to support nurse executive interests included advocacy for an increase to the FY2009 federal appropriation for the Nurse Education Act; foster and promote a climate for patient safety and quality outcomes that is evidence-based and not legislated mandates or ratios; collaborate with quality partners such as TJC, National Quality Forum (NQF), and the federal government to ensure that proposed regulatory changes achieve desired results; support legislative efforts that promote the migration of international nurses to the United States; and support efforts to secure federal status for nurse-managed centers. As these two examples demonstrate, legislative priorities may be narrowly defined or broad; nursing organizations often join with other organizations with similar policy interests; and positions on specific policy issues may differ across nursing organizations.

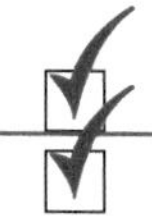

Practical Tips

Tip # 1: Be Current

Keep up-to-date with policy developments and issues.

Tip # 2: Disseminate Widely

Write and publish in professional and popular journals and magazines.

Tip # 3: Join Forces

Join special interest associations.

Tip # 4: Persuade Stakeholders

Make well-prepared presentations to key stakeholders.

Tip # 5: Network

Know and use key positions and nursing networks.

Tip # 6: Form Alliances

Identify and work with nurses in influential positions outside nursing.

Tip # 7: Communicate

Communicate your position through appropriate strategies.

Modified from International Council of Nurses (ICN). (2001). *Guidelines on shaping effective health policy.* Geneva, Switzerland: Author.

There is a strong linkage between health policy and health. All health care professionals, therefore, have a vested interest in understanding the health care policy-making process (Longest, 2001). Nurses' political development has been described as moving through four stages. The first was "buy-in," through beginning participation in politics and policy. The second was "self-interest," or the leading of collective efforts for nursing's self-interest. The third was "political sophistication," by participating in coalitions targeted to broader health issues. Nursing is now said to be moving to the fourth stage of "leading the way," which is characterized by taking the lead in mobilizing constituencies to action related to issues outside of nursing (Cohen et al., 1996; Leavitt et al., 2007). For nurses, a higher degree of political competence would translate into a greater ability to assess the influence of public policy on nursing practice and a greater ability to exert influence in the public policy-making process (Longest, 1997, 2001). Essential competencies in this domain of practice include knowing how and where to exert influence by knowing how public policies are formulated, implemented, and modified (Longest, 1997). As described by Kingdon (2003), nurses can influence health policy in the formulation phase by helping define the problems that are placed on the policy agenda; in the implementation phase by monitoring the rules and regulations that guide the implementation of new laws and providing formal comments on proposed rules and regulations; and in the modification phase by providing data related to the intended and unintended consequences of a policy. Development of political competency needs to occur as part of the basic educational preparation of nurses. Also, specialization in health policy making at the graduate level is needed, especially through interdisciplinary training programs.

Summary

- Nurses need to be visible and vocal in public policy and health policy debates.
- Policy is the formulation of value statements.
- Politics is the influencing of the allocation of scarce resources.
- Health policies are a set of public policies influencing health and illness.
- The public policy-making process follows stages of formulation, implementation, and modification.
- The Kingdon and stage-sequential models are two policy formulation models.
- There are four strategies used by interest groups.
- Health policies may be allocative or regulatory.
- Nurses have a leadership and management role in public and health policy.

CASE STUDY

Nurse Diane Kiplinger has always been politically active. She has volunteered in numerous presidential campaigns and has been the local county Republican Party chair. She has been active with the League of Women Voters. Now a pressing nursing and health care issue is on the forefront: mental health parity. Nurse Kiplinger knows just what to do. She begins networking with state and local nursing groups to build support. She starts outreach efforts to align with other interest groups. She enlists faculty and students from the nearby university to write letters, develop fact sheets and position papers, and hold seminars. She hosts gatherings with legislators and organized media events, using Buresh and Gordon's (2000) book as a guide. When the tragic death of a child occurs as a result of a lack of mental health funding, she works with the distraught parents to lobby for Medicaid reforms and other insurance legislation. As a result, mental health parity becomes a state health policy agenda issue and a compromise bill is enacted.

CRITICAL THINKING EXERCISE

Nurse Kelly Murrell works with the organ donation team of the tertiary care hospital. She has been active in efforts to increase public knowledge about signing donor cards and the need for organ donation. Currently, there is debate over whether the allocation priority of organs should go to the local area where the organ is donated or to the person at the top of the national list of the most ill transplant-eligible patients. The issue is controversial, confounded with stakeholder interests, and emotionally charged. Nurse Murrell feels the decision will directly affect her patients and the viability of this transplant program. However, in the past, Nurse Murrell has thought that politics do not belong in health care delivery and has concentrated only on quality clinical care and consumer education.

1. What is (are) the problem(s)?
2. Why is (are) it (they) a problem(s)?
3. What should Nurse Murrell do?
4. What public policy issues are involved?
5. What politics are involved?
6. What health policy issues are involved?
7. What actions can Nurse Murrell take to affect public health policy?

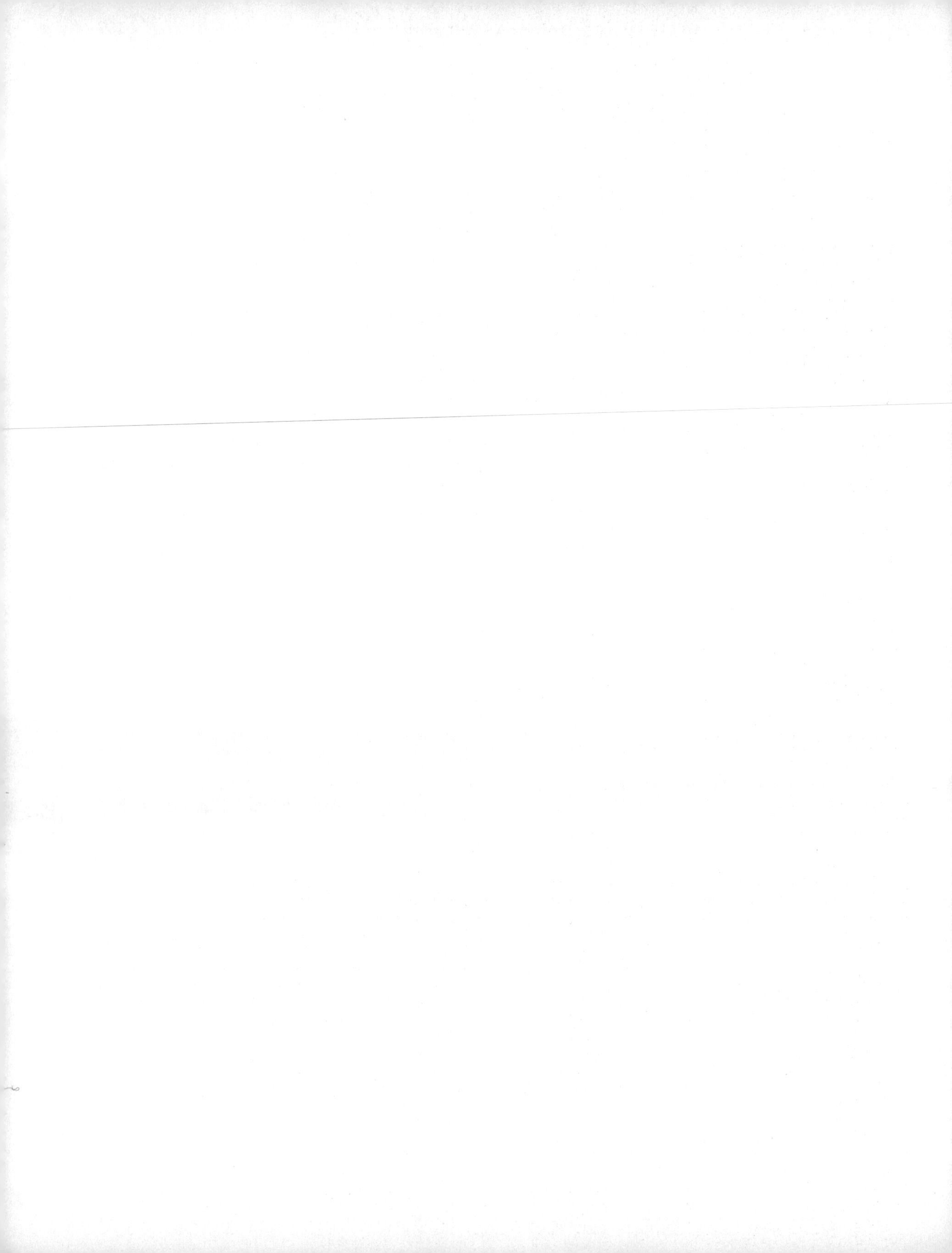

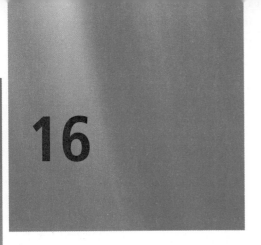

Evidence-Based Practice: Strategies for Nursing Leaders

Laura Cullen Cindy Jean Dawson Kathleen Williams

CHAPTER OBJECTIVES

- Define evidence-based practice
- Outline strategies for building an evidence-based practice culture in an organization
- Discuss the role of nurse leaders in promoting evidence-based practice
- Illustrate use of the Iowa Model of Evidence-Based Practice to Promote Quality Care when implementing evidence-based practice changes
- Describe effective strategies to use when implementing an evidence-based practice change
- Describe how nursing leaders can articulate the business case for evidence-based practice in discussions with governing boards
- Describe current trends in evidence-based practice
- Exercise critical thinking to conceptualize and analyze possible solutions to a practice exercise

Nursing has a long history of using research to improve practice, beginning with Florence Nightingale's work, reemphasized with research utilization efforts, and progressing to the current trend in using best evidence in guiding patient care. There is now a rising expectation by consumers as well as in regulatory standards that evidence-based knowledge be used in health care. Despite national and international policy and research agendas, provision of evidence-based care does not meet expectations, with provision of recommended care occurring little more than half the time (Asch et al., 2006; Clark, 2005; Mangione-Smith et al., 2007; McGlynn et al., 2003; McInerny et al., 2005; Peterson et al., 2006; Shrank et al., 2006; Zuckerman et al., 2004) and a continuing gap that exists between the conduct and application of research findings. Using the evidence-based practice (EBP) process to answer clinical and operational questions can be challenging.

Nurses in leadership positions have responsibility for building and expanding use of evidence-based practices in care delivery to improve patient and organizational outcomes. A number of models are available to provide direction for the EBP process for individual projects. Implementing evidence-based practice initiatives as an organizational program requires additional strategies for success. Less information is available to guide nurse executives in building evidence-based practice programs within health care organizations. Given this challenge, a building-block approach is outlined to provide guidance. The use of evidence-based practice has grown, yet the science of translation research on which evidence-based practice work is based is still developing. The application of evidence-based practice is the responsibility of every nursing leader, especially in the nurse manager role. This chapter outlines successful strategies used to expand an evidence-based practice program.

DEFINITIONS

An understanding of evidence-based practice and related concepts such as implementing practice change requires requisite knowledge of a variety of terms. **Evidence-based practice** is a process of shared decision making in a partnership between patients and providers that involves the integration of research and other best evidence with clinical expertise and patient values and preferences in making health care decisions (Cullen, 2007; McCormack et al., under development; Sackett et al., 2000; Titler, 2002). Evidence-based practice involves a process similar to research utilization. The process of using research findings as a basis for practice is known as **research utilization.** Research utilization encompasses critique of research studies, synthesis of findings, a determination of the applicability of findings, review for application with implementation of scientific findings in practice, an evaluation of the practice change, and dissemination of results to expand scientific knowledge.

The use of the term **best practice** is popular but unclear. Clarity in definition and use remains elusive as "best practice" and "evidence-based practice" are sometimes used interchangeably. Common use of the term is to describe innovative practices that are recognized by peer organizations and that contribute to meeting quality or fiscal goals (American Society for Quality; Australian Government Department of Veteran Affairs, Guideline for the Provision of Community Nursing Care). To promote understanding, it is recommended that the extent of evidence use in "best practices" initiatives be identified when the term is used.

Translational research is the scientific investigation of methods and variables that influence the rate and extent of adoption of evidence-based practices by individuals and organizations to improve clinical and operational decision making in the delivery of health care services. This includes testing the effect of interventions aimed at promoting the rate and extent of adoption of evidence-based practices by nurses, physicians, and other health care providers and describing organizational, unit, and individual variables that affect the use of evidence in clinical and operational decision making (Titler, 2004; Titler & Everett, 2001). *Translation science* is often used interchangeably with *implementation science.* **Implementation science** includes scientific investigations that support movement of evidence-based, effective health care approaches from clinical knowledge into routine use, testing strategies to promote uptake and use of innovations, and explicating factors that promote and hinder use of scientific knowledge in health care delivery (Greenhalgh et al., 2005; Rubenstein & Pugh, 2006; Titler, 2007). The terms *translational research* and *implementation science* are often used interchangeably.

Organizational context refers to the health system environment in which the proposed evidence-based practice is to be implemented. The core elements that help describe the organizational context include the prevailing culture of the system (e.g., patient-centered); the nature of human relationships in the system, including the leadership styles that are operational (e.g., team work, clear role delineation); and the organization's approach to routine monitoring of performance of systems and services within the organization (Kitson et al., 1998).

Translational research has provided guidance about effective strategies for implementing evidence-based practice. **Academic detailing or educational outreach** is the use of a marketing strategy that uses presentations by a trained person who meets one-on-one with practitioners in their setting to provide information about the evidence-based practice. This may include feedback on the provider's performance. The detailer may be from inside or outside the provider's organization, and the information maybe tailored to address site-specific barriers (Avorn & Soumerai, 1983; Davies et al., 1995; Jiang et al., 1997; O'Brien et al., 2007; Pippalla et al.,1995; Sohn et al., 2004; Titler, 2002). The terms *academic detailing* and *educational outreach* are used interchangeably.

Informal leaders who influence peers by evaluating innovations for use in certain settings and promoting clinicians' use of evidence in clinical decision making are referred to as **opinion leaders.**

Opinion leaders are likeable, trustworthy, informative, and influential (Doumit et al., 2007; Majumdar et al., 2007).

Performance gap assessment is a strategy of demonstrating an opportunity for improvement at baseline and outlining current practice related to specific indicators (Oxman et al., 1995; Schoenbaum et al., 1995). This data-driven strategy is used early in the implementation to garner commitment for practice changes.

Reinfusion is a planned and systematic process used to promote integration of the evidence-based practice into daily practice after initial pilot implementation and evaluation. Project integration will take several months and is facilitated by using **audit and feedback** of results from monitoring of care processes and outcomes through the quality improvement process. Audit and feedback is most effective when feedback is actionable providing direction for subsequent improvements (Hysong et al., 2006).

LEADING & MANAGING DEFINED

Evidence-Based Practice
The integration of research and other best evidence with clinical expertise and patient values in health care decision making.

Research Utilization
The use of research findings as a basis for practice.

Best Practice
Clarity in definition of best practice remains elusive; the goal of best practice is to provide useful interventions in clinical practice. The extent that "best practices" are evidence-based is unclear.

Translational Research
The scientific investigation of methods and variables that influence use of evidence-based practices to improve decision making in the delivery of health care services.

Implementation Science
The scientific investigation of strategies supporting adoption of evidence-based practice recommendations.

Organizational Context
The health system environment in which the proposed evidence-based practice is to be implemented.

Academic Detailing or Educational Outreach
Structured presentations designed to influence provider adoption of a recommended practice.

Opinion Leaders
Informal leaders promoting clinicians' use of evidence in clinical decision making.

Performance Gap Assessment
The strategy of demonstrating an opportunity for improvement at baseline and outlining current practice related to specific indicators.

Reinfusion
A planned and systematic process used to promote integration of the evidence-based practice into daily practice after initial pilot implementation and evaluation.

Audit and feedback
Monitoring of key indicators and outcomes with active reporting of results back to clinician-users to promote adoption of a recommended practice.

Practice Guideline
A systematically developed standard, designed to assist both provider and patient in making decisions about appropriate health care for specific clinical circumstances.

Systematic Review
The structured and systematic combination of findings from research into powerful and clinically useful reports to guide practice.

A **practice guideline** is a statement designed to assist providers and clients in making decisions about appropriate health care for specific clinical circumstances (Sackett et al., 2000). Guidelines are systematically developed, link the evidence with health outcomes (benefits and harms), and continue to require subjective judgments when making decisions for use (Woolf & Atkins, 2001). Guidelines are developed with the intent to influence practitioner behavior by making clear practice recommendations.

A rigorous scientific process used to combine findings from research (usually randomized controlled trials) into a powerful and clinically useful report to guide practice is known as a **systematic review.** Components of a systematic review include the question being reviewed, search strategies and yields, selection (inclusion or exclusion) criteria, review/appraisal methods, study descriptions, synthesis method (e.g., meta-analysis), results, and implications (Titler, 2002). Rigor used in development varies considerably among reports.

The best process to use when addressing clinical issues depends on the question at hand and the extent of research or other evidence available on the topic. Several processes may be used to improve care, from quality/performance improvement to evidence-based practice or the conduct of research. For questions that can be addressed through quality improvement, improvements can be brought to the patient care level quickly and efficiently. Clinical questions with little or no research that include patient risk may be good questions to answer by conducting research.

The shift from research utilization to evidence-based practice reflects the realization that not all clinical questions have been answered through research; thus other forms of evidence (e.g., lower rigor research, case studies, expert opinion) may be required to guide practice. An emphasis on use of evidence-based practice includes the application of the best available evidence and also represents a desire to improve patient outcomes with a consideration for patient values and preferences when making patient care decisions. Evidence-based practice is a broader, scientific process for improving health care quality by building on what is learned from quality improvement, research utilization, and the conduct of research.

MODELS

Evidence-based practice work in nursing has led to the development of several models to guide nursing practice (Goode & Piedalue, 1999; Kitson et al., 1998; Logan et al., 1999; Rosswurm & Larrabee, 1999; Rycroft-Malone et al., 2002; Stetler, 2001; Stevens, 2004; Titler et al., 2001). The challenge for clinicians is to successfully implement practice changes using a model as a guide during implementation. It has been said that invention is hard but implementation is much more difficult, meaning that creating guidelines is hard but implementing the recommendations is even harder (Berwick, 2003).

The Diffusion of Innovations Model (Rogers, 2003) has been adapted to support the hard work of implementing practice change in health care (Dobbins et al., 2002; Greenhalgh et al., 2005; Titler & Everett, 2001). Evidence-based practice models have been used successfully to improve adoption of evidence-based practice recommendations (Bowman et al., 2005; Cullen et al., 2005; Hogan & Logan, 2004; Logan et al., 1999; Madsen et al., 2005; Stebral & Steelman, 2006). One strategy to promote coordination of efforts is to adopt one evidence-based practice model for use across the organization and multidisciplinary initiatives. Evidence-based practice models tend to follow a basic problem-solving process and can be used parallel to other quality improvement processes (e.g., Six Sigma). Senior leadership support for evidence-based practice can be leveraged by outlining the similarities between evidence-based practice and existing quality improvement processes and structures.

IMPLEMENTING EVIDENCE-BASED PRACTICE CHANGES

Implementation of evidence-based practice changes can be challenging in complex health care settings. Despite the research supporting use of effective strategies for implementing evidence-based practice changes, the use of ineffective implementation strategies persists (Bloom, 2005). In fact, Bloom (2005) stated that use of these ineffective implementation strategies results in "reduced patient care quality and raises costs for all, the worst of both worlds" (p. 380). Education is an essential first step to develop an understanding of why and how the evidence-based practice is done, but education alone will not result in use of practice guidelines (Cooke et al., 2004; Cullen, 2006; Cullen & Titler, 2004; Green et al., 2007; Marinopoulos et al., 2007; O'Brien et al., 2001; Wells et al., 2007). In addition to education, multifaceted interactive interventions are needed to communicate the practice change to clinicians (Dobbins et al., 2002; Greenhalgh et al., 2005; Marinopoulos et al., 2007; O'Brien et al., 2001; Titler, 2008; Titler & Everett, 2001).

One model, the Translational Research Model (Figure 16.1) has been used to guide implementation strategies in a series of multi-site experimental studies funded by the Agency for Healthcare Research and Quality (PI Titler, RO1 HS10482 and PI Titler, 2 RO1 HS010482) and the National

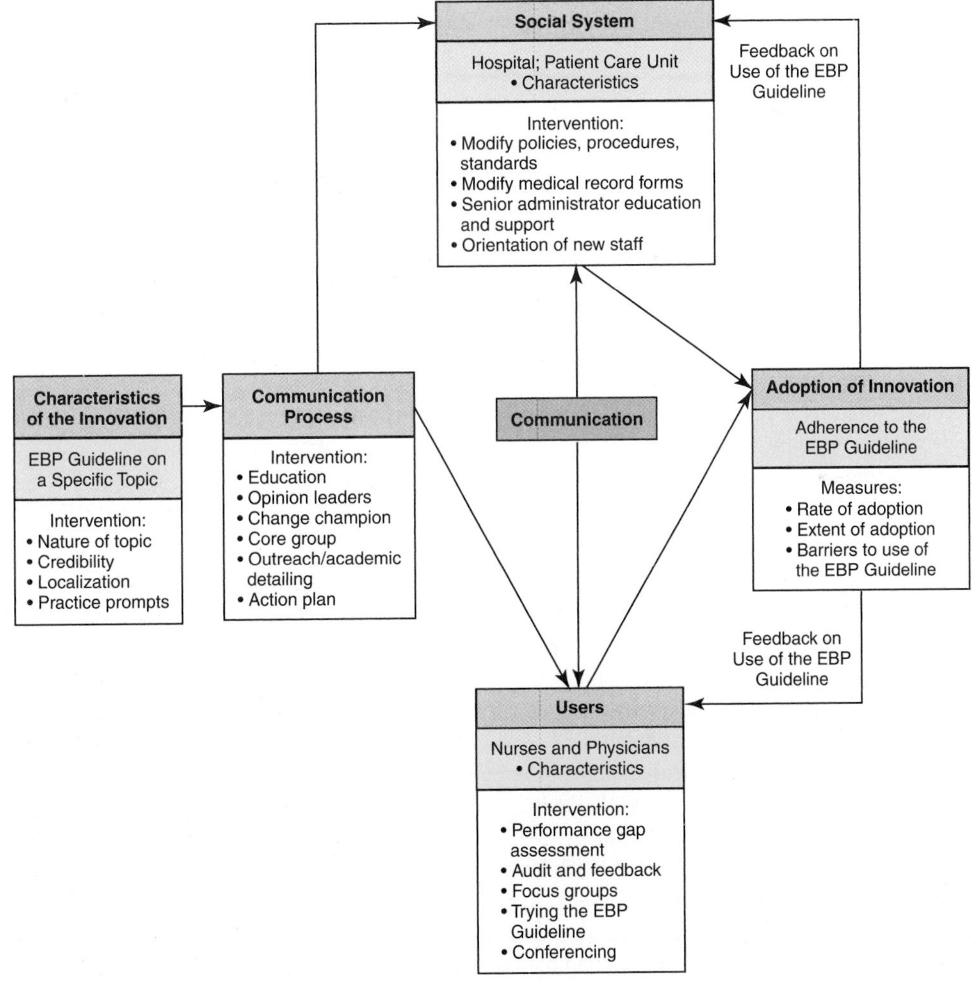

Figure 16.1
Translational Research Model. *EBP,* European best practice. (Reproduced with permission from Marita G. Titler, PhD, RN, FAAN [Titler & Everett, 2001].)

PART IV

Cancer Institute (PI Herr, R01-CA115363-01). Use of the Translational Research Model (Titler & Everett, 2001) has been effective in promoting adoption of evidence-based practices. Multiple interactive and reinforcing strategies, as outlined in the model, promote adoption of evidence-based practice recommendations. Strategies to capture a busy clinician's attention (Cullen, 2006) are important to include in the project implementation plan. Academic detailing or educational outreach is one such implementation strategy that is effective in promoting adoption of evidence-based practice recommendations (O'Brien et al., 2007). Academic detailing involves a multifaceted approach to discussions with practitioners (Box 16.1). Use of academic detailing has been shown to be an effective way to communicate with practitioners.

When done by an opinion leader, academic detailing with a performance gap assessment is a highly effective example of using multifaceted interactive strategies in promoting adoption of evidence-based practice. In practice, this approach can be used to garner consen-

Box 16.1

Strategies for Using Academic Detailing or Educational Outreach

As Outlined in the Literature*

- Meet one-on-one with practitioners
- Meet in/near the work setting
- Use two-way communication to increase involvement in educational interactions
- Establish the messenger's credibility and lack of conflict of interest
- Define the specific problems and objectives
- Provide information specific to the evidence-based practice topic using brief (e.g., 10-15 minutes) graphic materials to sustain interest
- Give both sides of controversial issues (for "inoculation" vs. counter-argument)
- Troubleshoot implementation challenges
- Concentrate on a few key messages (include alternatives that are being discouraged)
- Provide positive feedback about key indicators that are specific to the practitioner or team
- Provide reminders, reinforcement, and rewards to sustain improvements

Adapted for Use in Practice

- Clearly articulate the goal (e.g., stroke certification to improve patient care and patient outcomes)
- Reaffirm the team's support for reaching that goal (e.g., recognition for previous support and commitment)
- Identify one key indicator (e.g., swallow screening) from the practice recommendations to address in achieving the goal
- Report the performance gap data demonstrating an opportunity for improvement (e.g., percent of swallow screens completed within 24 hours of admission)
- Outline the evidence for the issue, including the extent of existing research supporting the practice recommendation and gaps in current knowledge (e.g., limited evidence about elevating the head of bed for bedside swallow screening in selected stroke patients)
- Identify current strategies in place to meet the indicator goal (e.g., physician orders on admission, nursing assessment within 24 hours of admission, referral as indicated)
- Admit to the challenges in meeting the goal (e.g., busy workloads; timely differential diagnosis for type of stroke)
- Outline the unattractive alternatives to meeting the goal (e.g., nasogastric tube placement for oral intake; delayed administration of oral medications)

Box 16.1

Strategies for Using Academic Detailing or Educational Outreach—cont'd

- State the desire to make the change systematic and with minimal impact on workload (e.g., preprinted orders to make the process easy for the clinicians)
- Brainstorm to identify innovative approaches to achieve the goal (e.g., location of preprinted orders within the documentation system)
- Develop an action plan with next steps, division of responsibility, and timeline, and again recognize efforts toward the goal and reiterate group decisions (e.g., stroke certification)

*Source: Soumerai S.B., & Avorn J. (1990). Principles of educational outreach ("academic detailing") to improve clinical decision making. *Journal of the American Medical Association, 263*(4), 549-556.

sus from a multidisciplinary team by leading discussions using these strategies. A recent systematic review has synthesized the research on academic detailing (O'Brien et al., 2007; see the Research Note on p. 374).

Clinicians tend to buy into the need for the practice change when there is a strong evidence base, the topic addresses an identified need, data demonstrate an opportunity for practice improvement within the clinical area, and the practice change offers a relative advantage. Localizing or adapting practice recommendations to fit the local setting and culture is an essential step in the process and often the role of the opinion leader and team of local experts (Doumit et al., 2007; Titler, 2002). Once the practice has been adapted and is ready for piloting, additional planning is needed for implementation and evaluation. Development of a fluid action plan can be highly effective in keeping the team on task and collectively moving forward (Schimizu & Shimanouchi, 2006). Additional strategies for implementation address both the clinician users and the organizational system (see Figure 16.1) (Titler & Everett, 2001). A case example demonstrates the effectiveness of a staff nurse–led team, using an evidence-based practice model to address a clinically relevant issue for the patients and setting.

CASE STUDY OF AN EVIDENCE-BASED PRACTICE PROJECT

The project *Stapedectomy: Development of a Patient Education Brochure—An Evidence-Based Approach* (Williams, 2006) used the Iowa Model of Evidence-Based Practice to Promote Quality Care (Titler et al., 2001). Stapedectomy is an elective procedure for otosclerosis offering the patient an improved quality of life by improving hearing. Otosclerosis is two times more common in females, with middle-aged women the highest risk population (Andresen et al., 2008). The project was triggered by an interest in expanding use of evidence-based care and a lack of standardization in care delivery for these patients in one large academic medical center in the Midwest. The project purpose was to validate conventional postoperative restrictions and patient education after middle ear surgery. The project was accepted for development through the *Evidence-Based Practice Staff Nurse Internship* (Cullen & Titler, 2004), thus receiving organizational support and establishing the project as an organizational priority. A multidisciplinary team was formed, including a staff nurse as project director.

Synthesis of the Evidence

A literature search and evaluation of the evidence showed a dearth of research and guidelines and a lack of consensus among otologists on postoperative restrictions after middle ear surgery (Harrill et al., 1996). The range in postoperative restrictions includes the following:

- Water precautions ranging from 2 to 4 weeks
- Avoiding nose blowing from 1 to 2 weeks
- Limiting heavy lifting and strenuous activity from 2 to 4 weeks
- Avoiding air travel from no restrictions to 6 months

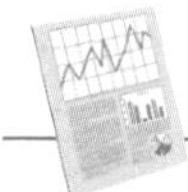

Research Note

Source: O'Brien, M.A., Rogers, S., Jamtvedt, G., Oxman, A.D., Odgaard-Jensen, J., Kristoffersen, D.T., et al. (2007). Educational outreach visits: Effects on professional practice and health care outcomes. *Cochrane Database of Systematic Reviews*, (*Issue 4*), Art. No. CD000409. DOI: 10.1002/14651858.CD000409.pub2.

Purpose

The purpose was to develop a systematic review describing the impact of academic detailing as an intervention to improve health care practices and outcomes. Databases searched to identify potential studies for inclusion included the Cochrane Effective Practice and Organization of Care (EPOC) registry, and MEDLINE and CINAHL up to March 2007. Two reviewers critiqued potential studies, extracting data using a checklist developed by EPOC and assessing the quality of the studies independently, including only randomized controlled trials. Main results are based on inclusion of 69 studies involving over 15,000 health professionals. Studies were categorized by their targeted impact on behavior into two groups—prescribing and other behavior.

Discussion

Academic detailing has been most widely tested using pharmaceutical representatives influencing physician prescribing in primary care. In 29 trials, the behaviors addressed were prescribing practices, and in 17 of these trials, the goal of the intervention was to decrease inappropriate prescribing. In 29 trials, the behavior addressed management of a variety of common problems encountered in primary care (e.g., managing risk for cardiovascular disease, asthma, or diabetes). In 11 trials, the behaviors were preventive services (e.g., smoking cessation counseling). Many trials used a social marketing theoretical framework and most used academic detailing in combination with other implementation strategies. Inconsistent application of academic detailing makes direct comparison somewhat difficult. Individual visits, instead of group sessions, appeared to have a greater impact. The effect of combined interventions (i.e., academic detailing plus other implementation strategies) was greater than use of academic detailing as a single intervention, but this was not statistically significant and these findings remain controversial among translation scientists. Measuring a downstream impact on patient outcomes is the ultimate goal, but testing has not been sufficient and demonstrating this impact is difficult and inconsistent. Cost savings associated with use of academic detailing to improve provision of appropriate care have also been generally positive but inconsistently demonstrated.

Application to Practice

A number of interventions to promote adoption of evidence-based practices have been tested. Numerous randomized control studies are evaluating use of the academic detailing intervention to promote use of evidence-based practice guidelines. Use of academic detailing individually or in combination with other implementation strategies is effective in changing practitioner behavior in the majority of cases, but the extent of the impact varies. The technique used in academic detailing involves a number of components (see Box 16.1).

A growing body of research is identifying strategies that promote adoption of evidence-based practice changes. Multiple, interactive, and repetitive strategies are necessary to promote adoption of evidence-based practices to improve patient care and outcomes. Interventions for implementing evidence-based practice can be effective by communicating the practice change to clinicians-users in a way that fits within the organizational context.

Practical Tips

Tip #1: Envision

Create a vision and strategic plan for the next 3 years for your unit or organization.

Tip #2: Build Capacity

Build organizational capacity for evidence-based practice through a building-blocks approach (e.g., develop educational offerings, build evidence-based practice responsibilities into job descriptions, include evidence-based practice on agendas, ask "what is the evidence" when making clinical and operational decisions).

Tip #3: Motivate

Commit to evidence-based care delivery and generate interest and enthusiasm of staff nurses (e.g., create opportunities for staff nurse–directed projects and highlight successes).

Tip #4: Measure

Measure and report project outcomes and the business case for evidence-based practice to senior leaders and the governing board.

The literature search identified that there were several adverse patient outcomes, from tinnitus, noise intolerance, sound distortion, dizziness/vertigo, to taste disturbance (House et al., 2001; Lundman et al., 1999; Ramsey et al., 1997; Sakagami et al., 2003). Sufficient research evidence to provide clear recommendations for specific precautions or for duration of precautions was lacking. Critiquing the evidence was essential and forced the project director and team to refocus the project purpose to the development of a patient education brochure for patients diagnosed with otosclerosis using evidence-based patient education (Williams, 2006).

Piloting

Using the Iowa Model of Evidence-Based Practice to Promote Quality Care (Titler et al., 2001), the team selected the desired patient outcome and collected baseline data for the pilot. The desired outcome was increased patient satisfaction with preoperative education before stapedectomy. The project director collaborated with the internal data management department, Office of Clinical Quality and Safety Performance Improvement (CQSPI), and developed a questionnaire for those patients undergoing stapedectomy for otosclerosis. The questionnaire addressed patient satisfaction with preparation for the procedure. A second questionnaire was administered to patients post-stapedectomy and was specific to surgical outcomes. The questionnaire captured the patient's perceptions of hearing quality, noise sensitivity, taste changes, recovery time, and pain. Results from the questionnaires guided the team in the development of written education materials for patients undergoing stapedectomy. Patient queries helped identify desirable information to include in the brochure's section concerning postoperative experiences. Important content identified was information about postoperative dizziness, sensitivity to noise, taste changes, driving after surgery, and time to return to work. As the chair of the nursing department's patient education committee, the advanced practice nurse on the team assisted in preparation of the written material. As the project objective shifted to focus on patients undergoing stapedectomy, an additional review of the literature was performed that concerned creating, writing, and designing evidence-based patient education materials. Reader literacy and material readability were considered throughout the process. The newly developed brochure readability showed 23% passive sentences, grade level according to Flesch-Kincaid was 6.6, words per sentence were 12.4, and Flesch-Kincaid reading ease was 69.1 (standard is 60 to 70). All measurements are consistent with Aldridge's (2004) strategies to improve the readability of education materials. Two brochures were developed with identical information but different designs and font size. Patients provided input about preference during the implementation stage.

Implementation

To promote adoption of the practice change, the project director shared the new brochure with nursing staff, posted it on the unit, and provided the majority of patient education before stapedectomy. As the opinion leader and clinical expert, the project director implemented the practice change by incorporating the brochure as she educated patients on stapedectomy. The brochure explained and listed the patient's hearing levels before and after the procedure, the middle ear anatomy and disease process of otosclerosis, specifics about the procedure, success rates, risks, restrictions, and a designated area for patients to jot down questions to be addressed during subsequent clinic visits. The project director's introduction of the evidence-based practice brochure rapidly resulted in adoption.

The usefulness and quality of the patient education brochure was validated before implementation (Burns & Grove, 2005). A survey given to patients before the development of the educational brochure showed that patients had concerns and questions about the procedure that had not been answered (e.g., a description of the procedure, success rates, noise intolerance, vertigo, taste changes, hearing, driving after surgery, and returning to work). The team agreed that improved written material was needed to address the patient feedback. The project director piloted the new education materials and resurveyed patients' satisfaction with stapedectomy preparation. Implementation of this project was simple. Using Roger's Diffusion of Innovations Model (Rogers, 2003) and the Translation Research Model (Titler & Everett, 2001), key physicians, nursing staff, and audiologists supported the change. Physicians were pleased with the additional written information that confirmed verbal counseling. Nursing staff agreed that the additional information could potentially reduce triage calls and improve patient knowledge of potential risks and outcomes. This could ultimately result in cost savings to the organization by reduction in return visits to providers and increased patient safety.

Evaluation

The pilot results demonstrated improved patient satisfaction. Feedback on the brochure design showed that patients desired the smaller-font brochure with the additional space for diagrams and space for writing questions for the return visit to providers. Areas showing improvement in satisfaction were increased knowledge and understanding, reduced anxiety and fear, and increased cooperation and compliance. For example, patients reported that they strongly agree that the information was easy to understand (pretest = 55%; post test = 80%) and remember (pretest = 46%; post test = 80%). Patients indicated they felt more prepared the day of their surgery (strongly agree: pretest= 64%; post test = 80%). Patients reported an improved understanding of what would happen during surgery (strongly agree: pretest = 36%; post test = 60%) and during their recovery (strongly agree: pretest = 55%; post test = 70%). The success of this project in the care of the patient undergoing a stapedectomy has stimulated similar projects, using the same process for other groups. The team effort by health care providers and patients produced valued written education materials and a tested process to replicate.

ORGANIZATIONAL CONTEXT

The case study demonstrates ready adoption in a clinic. As seen in this clinic, the organizational culture will impact adoption of evidence-based practices and patient outcomes (Boström et al., 2007; Brewer, 2006; Cummings et al., 2007; Titler, 2004; Titler & Everett, 2001; Wallin et al., 2006). Organizational systems must be designed to support the incorporation of evidence-based practices into clinical practice if adoption is to occur. A "fix-the-system" approach is now commonly used in quality improvement, but practice change will be better facilitated when documentation, policies and procedures, and education include the essential components from the practice guideline. Regardless of whether paper or automated systems are used, documentation systems are designed to support clinical practice and must capture the essential elements of the guideline that practitioners are expected to perform. The documentation system can serve as a "trigger" to assess important risk factors (e.g., risk for falling, risk for pressure ulcer development), patient conditions (e.g., pain intensity, duration, or location), and outcomes of care (e.g., development of pressure ulcers or oral mucositis). Automated documentation systems may also provide the opportunity for decision support to assist clinicians in the implementation of evidence-based practice guidelines.

The need for education regarding a practice change is fundamental. The organization can support use of evidence-based practices by incorporating education about the practice guideline into orientation for new hires, competency review for current employees, and education for senior leadership. Education is a necessary first step but is insufficient alone to create a practice change (Green et al., 2007; Marinopoulos et al., 2007; O'Brien et al., 2001). Educational strategies must capture the attention of busy clinicians (Cullen, 2006). An additional strategy is to incorporate the practice change into organizational policies and procedures. The policy and procedure committee membership can include clinical experts representing varied clinical services; these experts can provide an excellent critique of a new policy or procedure and make recommendations so policies link practices with the evidence and support the adaptation of guidelines for use within their organization.

The quality improvement committee also can support evidence-based practice. The quality improvement committee has standardized forms, a reporting system, and an established process for use of the results to continuously improve practice until the practice reaches the established goal and becomes integrated. Using the quality improvement system for reporting evidence-based practice changes provides efficient communication within the existing organizational infrastructure. The quality improvement process also supports ongoing planning, monitoring, and reinfusion of the expected care delivery, supporting successful adoption and integration of evidence-based practices.

Successes need to be celebrated along the way. Celebrations help build a culture that supports and expects the use of evidence in practice. The celebration should include formal recognition from high-level organizational leaders, visibility for the team and project champions, accessibility to practitioners within the organization, and a clear articulation of the benefits of the evidence-based practice project. Celebrations provide the opportunity to put practitioners in the spotlight for doing great work. Recognition can clearly articulate the benefits to and commitment of the organization. Celebrating successes will promote buy-in and commitment to the evidence-based practice process and will strengthen the foundation for future projects.

ORGANIZATIONAL INFRASTRUCTURE

Strategies for implementing evidence-based practices occur at both the project/clinical level, as illustrated in the case study, and also at the organizational level. Titler and colleagues (2002) stated that integrating evidence-based practice at the organization or social system level can be accomplished through a building-block approach and that leadership efforts can focus on the following:

> ...four major building blocks: (1) incorporating evidence-based practice terminology into the mission, vision, strategic plan, and performance appraisals of staff; (2) integrating the work of evidence-based practice into the governance structure of nursing departments and the health care system; (3) demonstrating the value of evidence-based practice through administrative behaviors of the chief nurse executive; and (4) establishing explicit expectations about evidence-based practice for nursing leaders (e.g., nurse managers and advanced practice nurses) who create a culture that values clinical inquiry. (p. 26)

Development of a mission and vision statement inclusive of evidence-based practice provides a foundation for this work at all levels of the organization and begins the process of building a culture in which evidence-based health care practices are the expected norm (Newhouse, 2007; Reeleder et al., 2006; Titler et al., 2002; Vaughn et al., 2002). The vision statement can stretch the current boundaries of evidence-based practice and promote work that leads staff to "reach" for a higher standard. An example of a vision statement might be that the organization will develop a center of excellence for evidence-based practice and be seen as a leader in use of evidence-based practices in care delivery. To support the vision, an infrastructure for evidence-based practice is needed as another building block. The infrastructure should take advantage of the expertise currently available and not be added work in an already busy workplace (Newhouse, 2007). Performance appraisals based on job descriptions with evidence-based practice components across all job classifications promote positive reinforcement and priority setting in the busy work environment. Additional expertise can be developed through collaborations with a practice network (Table 16.1), local nursing faculty, or hiring a nurse researcher (Hagedorn et al., 2006; Reeleder et al., 2006; Shirey, 2006; Shortell, 2004; Udod & Care, 2004; Zwarenstein & Reeves, 2006).

A committee with expertise in the research and quality improvement processes likely will have the requisite skills to facilitate evidence-based practice. In many organizations, the clinical practice committee may have the right membership to develop expertise in the evidence-based practice processes. Critical skills include critique and synthesis of the evidence, development of an implementation and evaluation plan, statistical analysis for quality improvement, and reporting of results (Cullen et al., 2005; Newhouse, 2007). The right committee or council will differ in each organization but

Table **16.1**

Collaborating Networks Supporting Evidence-Based Practice

Networking Opportunity	Information and Website
National Nursing Practice Network	www.nnpnetwork.org/ University of Iowa Hospitals and Clinics
Arizona Consortium for the Advancement of Evidence-Based Practice	http://nursing.asu.edu/caep/azcaep/index.htm Arizona State University
Contact, Help, Advice and Information Networks (CHAINs)	http://chain.ulcc.ac.uk/chain/index.html National Health Services, United Kingdom
Interest groups in Registered Nurses' Association of Ontario	www.rnao.org/Page.asp?PageID=751&SiteNodeID=113 Registered Nurses' Association of Ontario; Ontario, Canada

should reflect the expertise and functions needed to promote evidence-based practices.

The value of evidence-based practice must be "lived" through the behaviors of nursing leadership. Action steps for building a culture that values evidence-based practice can be included in the departmental strategic plan (Cullen et al., 2005; Newhouse, 2007; Reeleder et al., 2006; Titler et al., 2002; Vaughn et al., 2002). Discussion during committee meetings can stimulate interest in and use of evidence-based practice; including an evidence-based practice item on each agenda is a key strategy. Accountability is outlined in committee functions (Cullen et al., 2005; Titler et al., 2002). An organizational culture that promotes use of evidence values nurses questioning their practice, provides education about evidence-based practice, adopts an evidence-based practice model, and recognizes and rewards the work (Pepler et al., 2006). Recruiting and hiring nurses with interest in evidence-based practice also will help build the desired culture. Orientation can contain basic evidence-based practice concepts and protocols, with new staff learning from colleagues who can share experiences from evidence-based practice project teams on their unit. This provides recognition for the work done, sets the expectation that evidence-based practice is important in clinical care, and demonstrates that nurses have authority over their practice. Evidence-based practice must be alive in daily practice, not just "pulled off the shelf" when organizational leaders appear in the clinical area. Another building block involves the use of evidence-based practice components in performance appraisals for all roles. Leadership is needed across all organizational levels and roles when implementing evidence-based changes (Davies et al., 2006; Wallin et al., 2005).

LEADERSHIP ROLES IN PROMOTING PRACTICE

Many roles are essential and complementary in the work of evidence-based practice. From the chief nurse executive through nurse managers, advanced practice nurses, and staff nurses, everyone has a role in evidence-based practice work. Nurse executives have organizational responsible for creating a culture in which clinicians expect evidence-based practice, creating the capacity to accomplish evidence-based practice, and developing and sustaining a vision inclusive of evidence-based practice—all important building blocks for evidence-based practice. Innovative organizations with responsive leadership that support staff will promote use of evidence-based care (Estabrooks et al., 2007). Allocating resources and time has been demonstrated to be important to promote evidence-based health care (Boström et al., 2007; Cullen, 2007; Fleuren et al., 2004; Gifford, 2006; Gifford et al., 2007; McCormack et al., under development; Nagy et al., 2001; Pepler et al., 2006; Udod & Care, 2004).

Senior leaders also have a responsibility to articulate the business case for evidence-based practice to governing boards. Communication with boards has been identified as one of the Institute for Healthcare Improvement's (IHI) "protecting 5 million lives from harm" campaign *(www.ihi.org/IHI/Programs/Campaign/)*. The goal of the IHI initiative is to increase the reporting and discussion about quality improvement initiatives at board meetings. Key messages to share with board members include reporting the linkages between evidence-based practice and the organization's mission, values, strategic plan, and committee's functional responsibility within the organizational and nursing infrastructure. Reporting of project results is essential to garner continued support and recognition for the program. Using the existing reporting mechanisms to report about evidence-based practice project results can capitalize on existing structures and processes. Project results will then reach senior leadership to garner support in future decision making. Additional direct reporting of project results to senior leaders can be used to supplement the reporting rolled up within quality improvement. When a staff nurse–led project resulted in an estimated $1.9 million cost savings (Cullen et al., 2005), the program director shared project results with the CEO, which led to acquisition of additional resources for project implementation and program development.

Reports will best capture attention when addressing three to five talking points or take-away messages with clear links to organizational priorities and infrastructure. Reporting anticipated outcomes can be helpful early in the process. Project outcomes that target patients and families, staff, and fiscal results are valued by the organization and need to be considered in evaluation planning. Project outcomes targeting key initiatives would include patient satisfaction and other Center for Medicare & Medicaid Services (CMS) reportable measures (e.g., care for heart failure patients, practices preventing surgical site infections, pressure ulcer prevention). Cost savings or cost avoidance may not be achieved with every project but should be calculated whenever possible. A large volume of cost data is available in the literature and can be used to calculate estimated cost savings. For example, data demonstrate that each decubitus ulcer adds $735/case, having a total impact of $16.4 million in the United States in 2002 (Zhan et al., 2006). Postoperative sepsis adds $8881/case and has a total impact in the United States of $59.2 million (Zhan et al., 2006). These incidents and costs continue to exist despite an extensive body of research around prevention and treatment of both conditions. If an evidence-based practice project reduced only 10 cases of postoperative sepsis in 1 year, an estimated cost savings for that organization would be $88,810, not even including the patient and family experience, which would be an additional highly valued outcome. Reporting program and project results, linked within the organizational infrastructure, and capturing important outcomes assist the governing board in seeing the connection between these activities and the overall organizational mission. Nursing leaders have a responsibility to clearly articulate evidence-based practice work in a way that will be heard by decision makers.

The strategies discussed in building an organizational infrastructure for evidence-based practice are effective in developing the culture, building the capacity, and sustaining the vision at both the organizational and unit level. The nurse manager is responsible, parallel to the nurse executive, for developing the unit culture. Developing a positive unit culture is at least as important for promoting evidence-based practice as the organizational culture and will impact patient outcomes (Zohar et al., 2007). Managers' use of participatory leadership that is responsive to and supportive of staff will promote evidence-based care by staff nurses (Boström et al., 2007; Cummings et al., 2007; Wallin et al., 2006). The nurse manager sets the expectations for the unit, discusses the importance of the work of evidence-based practice with the unit nurses and other disciplines, encourages and responds to new ideas, promotes staff questioning practice, supports the team with time to work on the project, is a project cheerleader, tracks progress, facilitates moving the project through appropriate committees, and allocates resources as needed. By encouraging nurses to attend and present at conferences, stimulating inquiry and participating in research, nurses on their unit will increase use of evidence-based practice changes (Boström et al., 2007; Cummings et al., 2007; Pepler et al., 2006). The nurse manager's commitment to improvement and performance feedback is critical to project success and can significantly affect project outcomes (Wallin et al., 2006; Wallin et al., 2005).

The advanced practice nurse partners with project team leaders and plays an important role in project development. Capitalizing on their existing knowledge and skills will facilitate use of research findings in practice (Newhouse, 2007; Pepler et al., 2006). Advanced practice nurses can function as opinion leaders and facilitators (Cullen & Titler, 2004; Wallin et al., 2003). They have the ability to take on the most challenging steps in the process, leading a team, identifying potential roadblocks, facilitating problem solving during implementation and evaluation, reporting results, and providing expertise throughout the evidence-based practice process. Critique and synthesis of the evidence, development of an evaluation plan, and analysis of results are steps that utilize this expertise. Strong skills are needed for the facilitator to keep a team focused and moving forward. These nurses may also act as mentors for the team and the project director (Cullen & Titler, 2004). The path to improving care can be bumpy, and teams will need encouragement to address the barriers and sustain the commitment and momentum all the way to completion.

Staff nurses are ideally positioned to identify important and clinically relevant topics to develop into evidence-based practice projects. As bedside clinicians, they are the key to quality and use of evidence-based practices. Staff nurses can function as change champions and core group members within their current functions. The staff nurse also can function as an opinion leader or even project director (Cullen & Titler, 2004). Integration of practice changes through the evidence-based practice process can be complex, and facilitating actual change is a difficult challenge.

Use of a bottom-up approach (what is important to nurses at the bedside) for topic selection by staff nurses can facilitate adoption of the practice change. Clinicians will "pull" the practice change into their care instead of having the change "pushed" down from above or outside the organization (Kirchhoff, 2004). Programs are needed to help staff nurses integrate evidence-based practice change into care delivery (Cooke et al., 2004; Cullen & Titler, 2004; Hinds et al., 2000; Lacey, 1995; Newman et al., 2000; Tranmer et al., 1995; Wells et al., 2007). When staff nurses receive sufficient support, they are effective at integrating evidence-based practice changes into care delivery and find the experience to be empowering (Cooke et al., 2004; Cullen & Titler, 2004; Wells et al., 2007). Staff nurses are expert clinicians who have the skills to collaborate and problem solve, finding many creative solutions. They are critical to providing quality care through implementation of evidence-based practices.

One important role that will keep the project moving forward is that of the project director. The project director is responsible for establishing meeting schedules and timelines with the group, running the meetings, maintaining the action plan, delegating work assignments, and overseeing the process and progress. The focus of the project director must always be on moving the project forward, despite challenges, as a key strategy for success. The project director may orchestrate discussions for identifying potential challenges, addressing those that cannot be avoided but continuing to move forward despite distractions. Staff nurses can function as project directors if they are given sufficient support and mentorship (Cullen & Titler, 2004). Staff nurses and nursing leaders work together with complementary skills and expertise to address challenges and issues inherent in evidence-based practice.

CASE STUDY OF STRATEGIES USED BY A NURSE MANAGER

Development of the stapedectomy evidence-based education project required a collaborative team effort. The nurse manager had a pivotal role in the project's success. The nurse manager's responsibilities begin before the start of any evidence-based practice project. The otolaryngology-head and neck surgery clinic of one large, academic medical center in the Midwest is a unit with a vision, culture, and capacity for evidence-based practice (Cullen et al., 2005). The unit vision is patient-centered care in an ambulatory setting. Innovation is an expectation with a team approach. The positive unit culture is exemplified in the number of pilot projects, research studies, product trials, value analysis, and evidence-based practice projects in which the unit participates. The environment fosters the ability to create opportunities for change (Cullen et al., 2005). The nurse manager, working with administration, continues to build capacity by generating staff interest in evidence-based practice. The nurse manager challenges all staff nurses to propose evidence-based practice projects to improve patient care by validating practice or change practice based on the evidence. Staff nurses have an expectation to be involved with clinical research, attending and presenting at regional and national nursing meetings, obtaining certification in the specialty, and participating in unit initiatives. Creating an environment of enthusiasm for evidence-based practice is the goal.

An announcement went out with a call for applications to the *Evidence-Based Practice Staff Nurse Internship* (Cullen & Titler, 2004). Nurses were encouraged to submit ideas for an evidence-based practice project from clinical questions in their subspecialty, otorhinolaryngology practice. The best projects were considered for the organization's internship program. The staff nurse proposing the stapedectomy project was chosen. The nurse demonstrated positive attributes and was energetic, willing to change, and a team player. The project was meaningful with clear potential for success.

Significant time is required to complete an evidence-based practice project. Time was scheduled for the project director to work on the project. Non–patient care time dedicated to the project sends a message of support and commitment to the staff (Cullen et al., 2005). As needed, managers would assume patient care to ensure that the nurse attended all the internship classes. The project director relied on assistance from the manager to schedule meetings, take minutes, and provide follow-up on issues. The nurse manager kept supervisors and other stakeholders in the loop as planning for implementation approached. Developing unit champions can be useful. The project director was the change champion for the stapedectomy project. She served as a role model, clinical expert, change communicator, and leader. The implementation of the project was a success.

Fortunately, implementation went smoothly; however, a plan was in place if challenges arose. The plan was to use the "tag, flag, and nag method for effective follow-up and project integration" (Cullen et al., 2005, p. 134): (1) "tag" the nurses who are successful with change and recognize efforts; (2) "flag" staff who appear more resistant for one-to-one meetings to discuss the importance of the project; (3) "nag" staff members who are clearly noncompliant. Change champions can be encouraged to assist with intervention because often they are more successful peer to peer. The resistant staff members need special attention by management to either comply or seek another area of employment (Cullen et al., 2005).

As the evidence-based practice project rolled out, the nurse manager informed all the players, set the date, planned schedules, educated, and would have potentially hired additional staff to support the start-up. Education takes place anywhere and anytime. The most effective place for giving and receiving information is at the bedside. Meeting informally for questions before and after implementation was key.

The project evaluation is ongoing. Peer review is effective with impromptu discussions throughout the change. Approaches to a positive outcome include making the project fun, providing practice prompts (e.g., pocket cards, posters, screen savers, clipboard covers), monthly reminders of progress, and catchy theme-song logos. Strategies for success are effective communication, recognition, staff participation, time given to complete the project, team approach, and keeping management in the loop. Recognition is invaluable. Managers who provide frequent and positive recognition are more effective. Formal recognition both internally in the organization and externally in journals and newspapers is encouraged. The stapedectomy project has been presented locally and nationally at nursing conferences. Evidence-based practice has added an exciting dimension to otolaryngology-head and neck nursing clinical practice. With the internship and project complete, more projects are planned to keep the momentum going.

LEADERSHIP AND MANAGEMENT IMPLICATIONS

Regardless of job title, all nurses have a role in making evidence-based practice changes successful. A multifaceted approach is needed when integrating evidence-based practice at the project or organizational level. Change is difficult. Combining strategies to build on existing strengths should be considered. For example, educational offerings may already exist in familiar formats (e.g., posters, in-services); adding new approaches can stimulate interest (e.g., executive summaries, resource manuals, selected research references). Identifying those nurses and physicians who are innovative and influential among their peers to function as opinion leaders is important. A performance gap assessment can motivate participation. Academic detailing, along with audit and feedback, should be included throughout implementation. Simple

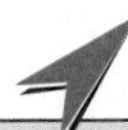

LEADERSHIP & MANAGEMENT BEHAVIORS

Leadership Behaviors

- Inspires evidence-based practice focus and challenges all practice interventions regarding evidence base
- Enables the identification and use of evidence-based knowledge to drive practice and improve outcomes
- Describes a vision for both client and systems outcomes based on evidence
- Enables evidence-based practice using organizational systems to support care delivery based on evidence (e.g., computerized documentation)
- Removes barriers to use of evidence in practice
- Articulates the value of evidence-based practice

Management Behaviors

- Identifies outcomes of care and service based on evidence
- Evaluates the consistency, quantity, and quality of evidence base for practice
- Manages the process of practice based on evidence
- Analyzes variances
- Takes corrective action when variances occur

Overlap Areas

- Determines evidence base for management and practice
- Leads and manages implementation of innovations

solutions should be sought first; creativity becomes important when addressing barriers. Staff nurses can often bring fresh approaches to address challenges.

A building-block approach should be considered when developing the organizational culture and capacity for evidence-based practice. Evidence-based practice should be incorporated into strategic documents, including the mission statement, vision, strategic plan, job descriptions, performance appraisals, and committee functions. Leadership that demonstrates and expects evidence-based practice will promote its use in clinical and operational decision making. Dialogue must be conducted during important meetings about use of evidence for decision making. Prioritizing and holding leaders and clinicians accountable for the work are essential. The use of multiple, interactive strategies will promote adoption of evidence-based practice at all levels in the organization.

CURRENT ISSUES AND TRENDS

Senior leaders have responsibility for developing an organizational culture promoting evidence-based health care. The organizational context consists of elements that include culture and climate, interactive human relationships, and the measurement and evaluation processes specific to the organization (Titler, 2004). There is a growing recognition of the importance of organizational context on the rate, extent, and sustainability of evidence-based health care practices (Dopson et al., 2002; Ferlie & Shortell, 2001; Rogers, 2003; Scott-Findlay & Golden-Biddle, 2005; Titler, 2002), yet research is still needed. Research to better understand and measure organizational context was rated the top priority by a leading group of translation scientists (Titler, 2005). The organizational context is a result of organizational, unit, and individual characteristics (Greenhalgh et al., 2005), resulting in a complex and dynamic context that is unique to each practice setting. Additional research is needed to better understand the role organizational context plays in impacting adoption of evidence-based practice and effective strategies to impact the organizational context, thus encouraging adoption of evidence-based care delivery. Many organizations have effectively promoted adoption of evidence-based practices and have developed well-established paths to follow within their system; however, practice organizations are overwhelmed with the volume of change continually bombarding them. Research is needed to better understand how organizations can benefit from the efficiency of scale in using the well-established path for successful adoption and how to balance the shear volume of change.

Leadership is essential in developing an organizational culture promoting innovation and evidence-based practice. Leadership is one important contextual factor impacting an organization's ability to consistently use evidence to inform practice (Aarons, 2006; Davies et al., 2006; Fleuren et al., 2004; Vaughn et al., 2002; World Health Organization, 2007). An exhaustive body of research on barriers consistently finds that leadership support is essential for success (Fink et al., 2005; Funk et al., 1991a, 1991b; Hutchinson & Johnston, 2006; Ring et al., 2005) and leaders have a responsibility to provide resources, structures, and processes (Fink et al., 2005; Hutchinson & Johnston, 2006; Pravikoff et al., 2005). A better understanding of specific leadership strategies is needed. More research testing leadership strategies and articulating the most effective organizational context and infrastructures would move understanding forward.

More research is also needed to describe effective networks and collaborative models. Shirey (2006) described regional collaborations, centered around several centers with expertise in evidence-based practice in the United States. To date, this model has not materialized but others have. The National Nursing Practice Network® (NNPN) was developed at the University of Iowa Hospitals and Clinics *(www.nnpnetwork.org)*. The NNPN has committed to the promotion and implementation of evidence-based practice through a collaborative model designed to promote shared learning and participation with nearly 50 member organizations. Specialty organizations also have a long history of supported collaboration around clinical issues amenable to research and improving quality care. International efforts have also supported adoption of evidence-based practice recommendations. The National Guideline Clearinghouse™, sponsored by the Agency for Healthcare Research and Quality, provides a large repository for international guidelines, offering free access to guideline summaries and links to access full reports *(www.guideline.gov)*. Sigma Theta Tau International, the nursing honor society, has supported international collaboration, educational offerings, and resources through its leadership and commitment to evidence-based care, meeting the needs of its clinician members *(www.nursingsociety.org)*. In addition to the Registered Nurses' Association of Ontario (RNAO) in Ontario, Canada, the Joanna Briggs Institute in Adelaide, Australia, provides a growing library of guidelines and additional resources *(www.rnao.org* and *www.joannabriggs.edu.au)*. Each of these organizations offers a unique model supporting dissemination of evidence-based information for adoption in practice.

CONCLUSION

Nursing has a long history of valuing provision of the best care and using the best evidence for care improvements. Despite the many years of work, there are many challenges to using evidence-based care in the current health care environment. Nurses in leadership positions have responsibility for supporting evidence-based clinical care as well as evidence-based operational decision making. Two models outline the process for updating clinical practices that are also applicable when addressing operational issues. Implementation is one of the most challenging steps in the evidence-based practice process. Multiple reinforcing and interactive strategies are needed to facilitate implementation. Effective, evidence-based implementation strategies can be combined to create a highly influential implementation plan.

Nursing leaders can build a strong program supporting evidence-based care delivery using a building-block approach. Building on the organization's vision, mission, and value for high-quality care provides a foundation for success. Nurse leaders must connect their evidence-based initiatives to the organization's vision, mission, values, and infrastructure to garner support and resources for provision of the best care delivery. Implementing evidence-based practices is best accomplished by understanding the interplay between organizational and unit factors that are supported through the organizational infrastructure. The infrastructure supporting evidence-based practice is essential for creating the desired organizational and unit culture and capacity. Communicating the business case for evidence-based practice will help nurses articulate their impact in a way that will be heard by senior leaders. Leadership is a vital ingredient to success. Complementary skills are needed within all nursing roles to create effective evidence-based practice teams. Every nurse has a responsibility to support evidence-based care delivery to improve outcomes for our patients and their families, staff, and the organization.

Summary

- Nurses use the evidence-based practice process to answer clinically relevant questions.
- Not all clinical questions have been answered by research, so other forms of evidence may be needed.
- Evidence-based practice emphasizes use of the best available evidence.
- Evidence-based practice involves integration of best evidence with clinical expertise and patient values in decision making.
- Rogers' Diffusion of Innovations Model is often used as a framework for evidence-based practice changes.
- An innovation is communicated to clinician-users through channels over time within a social system.
- Multiple interactive strategies are needed for communicating the practice change to clinician-users within the context of the organization.
- Nurses have leadership roles in evidence-based practice at all levels.
- Evidence-based practice is a priority in nursing.
- Organizational infrastructures can effectively support evidence-based care delivery.
- Use of a building-blocks approach supports expanding evidence-based practice initiatives and programs.
- Current issues include a need for research to better understand leadership and organizational strategies to promote evidence-based practice, how to capitalize on opportunities for collaboration, and expanded use of resources internationally.

CASE STUDY

A member of your general surgery unit staff approaches you with a practice question. This senior nurse wants to know whether bowel sounds are a good indicator for return of gastrointestinal (GI) motility for her patients after surgery. As a nurse manager, you recognize this as an opportunity to build an evidence-based practice project for your unit. The following benefits are anticipated:

- Improving care
- Empowering staff nurses
- Developing a new unit culture that uses evidence in daily practice

What Are Your Next Steps?

You recognize that you will need a strong team, a review of the evidence, an implementation plan, and an evaluation method. Partnering with experts in the organization will best match the skills and expertise needed. The staff nurse raising the question is the unit quality improvement coordinator. She is already an opinion leader and is ideally suited to lead a team; you are committed to helping her. The team develops an action plan and divides responsibility for the project. Team members tackle each of the following: reviewing the literature, developing a survey of current nursing practice within the hospital, notifying physicians of the practice review, developing a physician practice survey, developing an educational poster based on the literature review, and developing strategies for implementing a potential practice change.

An early obstacle occurs when you cannot find any research on auscultation of bowel sounds. This is a good time to add a team member who can tackle the search for, critique of, and synthesis of the evidence. The nursing survey is revised and sent to a national group of experts to determine current practice trends. Certified wound, ostomy, and continence nurse practitioners are identified as appropriate experts to provide the team with the necessary guidance. Simultaneously, the physician's practice survey is sent to general surgeons within the organization. A secondary analysis of basic science research, a small body of other literature, and the surveys indicate that bowel sound assessment is not the best indicator of return of GI motility following abdominal surgery. A change in practice is needed.

A traditional practice, such as bowel sound assessment, can be difficult to change. Multiple interventions are needed. The team decides to use multiple strategies for implementation: opinion leaders, change champions, audit-feedback, educational posters, a resource manual, practice prompts, and documentation changes. Processes and outcomes are reviewed through the evaluation process. The team reviews nursing knowledge, compliance with documentation of return of GI motility, nurses' perception of facilitators of the practice change, and rates of bowel obstruction and paralytic ileus. The data suggest that nursing documentation of return of flatus improves (60%; pre-group; 88%; post-group) and that documentation of first bowel movement also improves (60%; pre-group; 88%; post-group) and could be better, so a task force works with the nursing informatics group to revise the documentation process. Bowel obstruction rates are lower in the post-group (0%;) than in the pre-group (4%;), and paralytic ileus rates decrease from 12.5%; in the pre-group to 0%; in the post-group, creating some confidence that eliminating bowel assessment is not causing any patient harm.

This project was successful in many ways; yet like so many EBP projects, additional work is needed. The unit quality improvement coordinator will now complete reinfusion and integration through the unit's quality improvement efforts. A fundamental practice question has been answered, and patient care improvements continue through the EBP process (Madsen et al., 2005).

CRITICAL THINKING EXERCISE

Nurse Melissa Miller works in the surgical intensive care unit at a Midwest tertiary care facility. Often her critical care patients have altered airways including tracheostomy. Tracheostomy care is a nursing intervention that frequently challenges a nursing staff. A review of ICU tracheostomy care policies and procedures reveals nursing care based on literature that is 10 to 15 years old. Before her transfer to the intensive care unit, Nurse Miller worked on an otolaryngology unit with patients undergoing tracheostomy during major resections for head and neck cancer. Despite the specialty focus on the upper airway, tracheostomy care varied. An example of the practice variation is the controversy about instillation of saline before tracheal suctioning (Hudak & Bond-Domb, 1996). Nurse Miller wants to take the lead in developing a clinical practice guideline for tracheostomy care. What process does she follow?

1. What is the advantage and definition of a clinical practice guideline?
2. What is the evidence base for pursuing a standardized clinical practice guideline for tracheostomy care?
3. Who should be identified as the stakeholders?
4. What patients should be targeted?
5. What change/process steps need to be taken using the Iowa Model of Evidence-based Practice to Promote Quality Care?
6. What is the problem?
7. Why is the problem pertinent to the organization?
8. What are the key issues?
9. What is the first step?
10. How can the nurse identify practice variation?
11. What evidence is needed to guide practice?
12. How does a nurse implement the new guideline?
13. Who needs education and competency assurance?
14. What outcomes should be measured?
15. How are these outcomes measured?
16. Who can assist with ongoing compliance with the practice change?

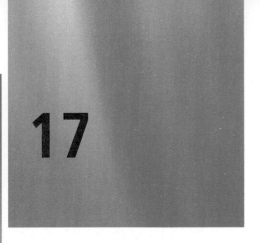

17 Mission Statements, Policies, and Procedures

Diane L. Huber

CHAPTER OBJECTIVES

- Define and describe organizational mission statements, policies, and procedures
- Determine the product of nursing care
- Compare the two dimensions of a social system
- Associate strategic planning with organizational mission statements
- Distinguish among types of organizational purpose statements
- Differentiate policies and procedures
- Relate organizational philosophy to nursing practice
- Exercise critical thinking to conceptualize and analyze possible solutions to a practice exercise

The provision and management of nursing care to clients are complex endeavors that usually are embedded within the context of an organization. Understanding organizations and how they function is important to nurses who are employed by those organizations because practical implications for the work nurses do arise as a result of the managerial structure imposed by an organization. An organizational structure can be both efficient and effective. However, this situation does not occur by chance. Without specific direction, day-to-day operations fall apart. Thoughtful operational documents form the backbone for managerial planning and direction.

Within an organization there is an established framework for management. For each organization, a characteristic collective of power and authority is vested in the managerial hierarchy. This legitimated authority, given by position, is used with the management process, management skills, and whatever resources are available to meet the organization's goals. The elements of management and the resources available combine to form the basic framework for the management and functioning of an organization. Organizations have a mission—to produce a product or service. This goal will be expressed in mission statements and carried through into policies and procedures, all documents that form the basis for guiding standard operations. These documents are generally gathered into an overall strategic plan.

Strategic plans are a collection of written descriptions of organizational values, goals, and vision. They collectively form a conceptual description of an organization and display the framework for an organization's beliefs, intent, desired future, planning, and operations. Underlying mission statements are explicit values that drive organizations and people. Some common themes in health care mission statements are the provision of quality care, customer satisfaction, and continuous improvement.

Mission, values, and vision are the glue that holds an organization together. They describe what the organization is trying to do, how to go about it, and where it is headed. This helps keep an organization on track and provides yardsticks with which to measure present performance. Groups can be brought to crisis by conflicts over basic issues of mission, values, and vision. Without these agreements in place, no organization is truly viable (Adams, 2004). Following are some thoughts about mission, vision, and values:

The mission of the United States is one of benevolent assimilation.

-President William McKinley

If your job is to fix trucks, the bottom line is how many trucks you fix. The combat army has a totally different ethic: Accomplish your mission and take care of your men.

-Col. Harry Summers, U.S. Army

Where there is no vision, the people perish.

-Proverbs 29:18

Your vision will become clear only when you can look into your own heart... Who looks outside, dreams; who looks inside, awakes.

-Carl Jung

The very essence of leadership is that you have a vision.

-Rev. Theodore M. Hesburgh, C.S.C.

If you don't know where you're going, any path will get you there.

-Synopsis of Alice and the Cheshire Cat from Lewis Carroll's Alice's Adventures in Wonderland

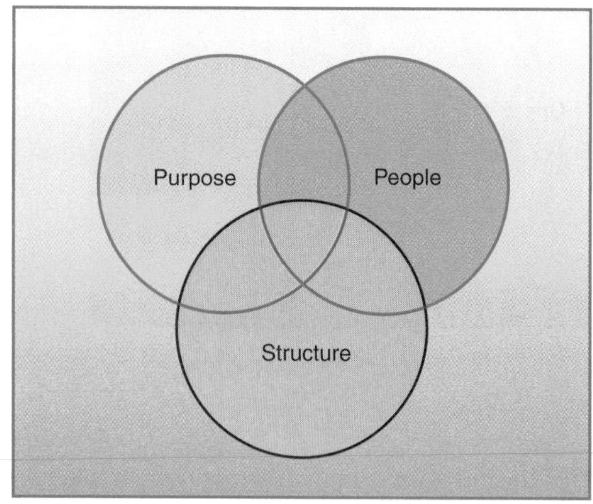

Figure 17.1
Components of an organization.

Mission, vision, and values statements can be mere words on a page, or they can be "living documents" that unify an organization around a purpose. The process of development of these statements needs to begin with bringing members into basic agreement and alignment around the statements.

DEFINITIONS

An **organization** is a group of people with specific responsibilities who act together for the achievement of a specific purpose determined by the organization. An organization usually is thought of as an institution, such as a hospital or manufacturing company. All organizations have a purpose, structure, and some collection of people (Figure 17.1). The actual character or nature of any organization is highly variable, depending on the purpose, structure, and collection of people that form the organization.

BACKGROUND

Business management theory has contributed ideas about how to organize a business so that it makes money and runs efficiently. Theories based on business firms do not always apply directly to nursing because nursing is a service industry. Drucker (1973), a prominent business management theorist, said that service institutions are more complex than either businesses or governmental agencies. In a service industry such as nursing, the two key aspects of effectiveness are quality and cost control. Furthermore, service agencies such as hospitals rely on professional staff to accomplish their mission. Thus the relationship of professionals to their employing institutions affects organizational effectiveness in health care. Nurses work primarily in groups, thus making work group functioning and the interactions among people important for effectiveness and mission accomplishment in nursing.

As a service industry, health care has a product. The basic product of health care is client care service, such as disease treatment or health promotion. Health may be the ultimate outcome to be achieved. An interesting question is whether the product of nursing is the same as the product of health care. Quality care is one ideal product of health care. Kramer and Schmalenberg (1988a, 1988b) said that the product of a hospital is a quality, accessible, cost-effective service called *client care.* In hospitals, 90% of client care is delivered by nurses. If the product is "quality care," valid

LEADING & MANAGING DEFINED

Organization

A group of persons with specific responsibilities who are acting together for the achievement of a specific purpose determined by the organization.

Philosophy

An explanation of the systems of beliefs that determine how a mission or a purpose is to be achieved.

Policy

A guideline that has been formalized.

Procedure

A description of how to carry out an activity.

and reliable measurement is needed to ensure that "quality care" is delivered and received. The idea has been posed that nursing is not a service composed of tasks but, rather, a business with a product of enhanced client outcomes and contained costs (Zander, 1992). This idea takes Drucker's conceptualization and merges ideas about a service industry with ideas about traditional for-profit businesses. For nursing, the product is derived from the use of expertise to solve problems for clients. Similarly, the product of nursing administration relates to the use of expertise to solve problems for nurses within systems of care.

Organizations are designed to accomplish goals and can be understood as social systems. The Getzels and Guba model (Getzels, 1958) indicated that there are two dimensions to a social system. One part is the environment of the organization. An institution has certain role expectations, a culture, an ethos, and values. If an organization has certain goals—for example, quality client care and cost containment—then individuals have a role in the system with certain expectations related to achieving the goals.

The other part of the social system is the individual person, who has a personality and certain needs. For example, the needs may be for power, achievement, or affiliation. The individual's personality and needs disposition will interact with the institution's need for goal achievement. Somewhere in that dynamic interaction, the behavior seen in organizations is manifested as a result. Sometimes organizations appear to be in total chaos; sometimes they run smoothly and efficiently. The manifested result depends on the dynamic interaction between the organization, with its need to achieve goals, and individual employees, with their own personalities and unique drives and desires (Getzels, 1958) (Figure 17.2). In a study of role behaviors, activities, and knowledge domains in case management (Park & Huber, 2009), the Getzels model was modified to examine work setting and professional discipline for the importance of activities and knowledge. Both organizations and employees have a set of values, personality, and culture. Thus nurses can examine their personal and group "fit" with any organization as one criterion for effectiveness.

For nurses as professional employees, the question is "Whom do they serve?" Do they serve the needs of the organization as a business—with pressures for efficiency, mass production, and cost containment? Or do they serve the needs of the client—who may want teaching and counseling time, rehabilitation time, home care planning coordination, and individualized but time-consuming care? An underlying dynamic tension between bureaucratic and professional values, called "reality shock," is identified as a problem for nurses (Kramer, 1974). This parallels the organizational-individual tensions that arise in social systems. The behavior of any nurse in a health care organization can be seen as a dynamic interaction and an outcome of the nurse interacting with the specific social system in which the nursing care delivery is embedded.

An examination of organizational mission statements such as the philosophy, goals, and objectives statements promotes a greater understanding of the

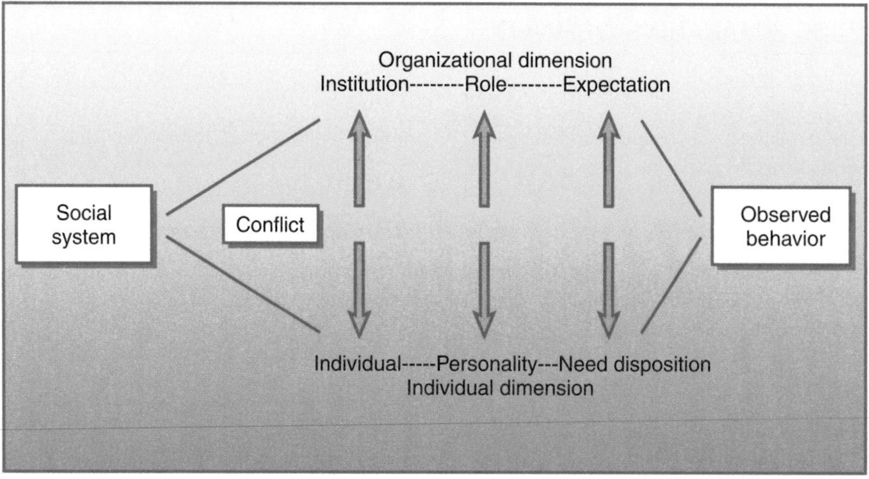

Figure 17.2
Social system and behavior. (Data from Getzels, J. [1958]. Administration as a social process. In A. Halpin [Ed.], *Administrative theory in education* [pp. 150-165]. Chicago: University of Chicago Press.)

specific institution and may promote more effective organizational participation by nurses. To begin to learn how the organization runs, the first step is to examine the philosophy, structure, and policies. The functional aspects of organizations include the culture, philosophy, purposes, objectives, policies, and procedures related to the work environment. They are key aspects of managerial planning.

ORGANIZATIONAL MISSION STATEMENTS

Strategic Planning

Strategic plans are deliberative organizational documents developed to identify, gain consensus about, and communicate where an organization is going, over what timeframe, how it will get there, and how it will decide whether it got there (McNamara, 2008a). The focus for a strategic plan often is the entire organization because these documents need to be unifying and integrated tools for the entire organization. Strategic plans may be developed for specific products, services, or programs, but these would need to be integrated with the total organizational plan. Often a business plan is used instead. Key to all strategic planning efforts is concentrated attention on the clarity of the meaning of words and on gaining consensus about the final result to develop a sense of ownership in the plan.

Factors such as leadership, culture, complexity, size, and internal expertise will have an impact on which model or approach is chosen for strategic planning. Some examples of types of strategic planning models are goals-based, issues-based, organic, and scenario planning (McNamara, 2008a). For example, issues-based strategic planning would start by exploring the issues facing the organization, then identifying strategies for those issues, and then moving to action plans. The most common form of strategic planning is the goals-based form. This starts with a focus on the organization's mission, followed by vision and values statements. Next, goals are identified, and strategies to achieve the goals, action plans to identify who is responsible and accountable, and time frames are detailed. The time line (e.g., 1 year, 5 years) into the future and the length of the strategic plan vary. The benefits of strategic planning include the ability to "clearly define the purpose of the organization and to establish realistic goals and objectives consistent with that mission in a defined time frame within the organization's capacity for implementation" (McNamara, 2008a, p. 3). This may require an outside facilitator.

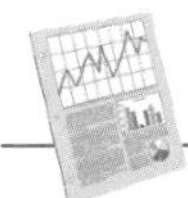

Research Note

Source: Drenkard, K.N. (2001). Creating a future worth experiencing: Nursing strategic planning in an integrated healthcare delivery system. *Journal of Nursing Administration, 31*(7/8), 364-376.

Purpose

The nurse executive team of a large not-for-profit integrated health care delivery system needed a strategy in order to have nursing care viewed as a competitive advantage in meeting the system's core values of caring for and about people, community responsibility, and innovation. This article describes the planning process, tools, methodology used, and lessons learned.

Discussion

Strategy was seen as a solution to pressing nursing work environment pressures and problems. The strategic planning process was based on an eight-step business planning model. The methodology used a transformational leadership assessment tool, quality planning methods, and large group intervention to engage nurses in implementation strategies. Systems theory formed the foundation for thinking about the process and the application of the results to multiple levels of the organization. Detailed information is given about the following: getting started; the strategic planning process of assessment of the current state, creation of a vision, gap analysis, priority setting using quality tools, engagement of nursing in planning, baseline measurement and target selling; refinement of implementation plans and evaluation of outcomes; application at the unit level; and lessons learned.

Application to Practice

The strategic planning journey is clearly and explicitly detailed in this exemplar on strategic planning. The description is rich in detail and visual displays. Other organizations and nurse executives can use this article as a guide and roadmap to replicate the best parts and avoid or anticipate pitfalls.

Mission Statements

Using a goals-based strategic planning method, the first step is to develop a mission statement. The mission of any organization is its purpose, function, and reason it exists. Organizations exist to do something such as produce a product or deliver a service. The founders' intentions for what they wanted to achieve by starting this organization need to be reexamined and refreshed periodically to keep the organization dynamic (Adams, 2004). For a health care organization, the mission relates to health care services—for example, client care, teaching, and research. For a nursing department's purpose, constraints include the organization's purpose, the state nurse practice act and other legal parameters, the context of the local community, and the directives of regulating agencies. The mission statement should be short, concise, and clear. The mission of the nursing department should mesh with the mission of the institution.

In developing a mission statement, factors such as the organization's products, services, markets, values, public image, and activities for survival need to be considered (McNamara, 2008b). In addition, the intent of the organization's founders and its history are useful to review. Often employees are unaware of historical background. Because the mission statement needs to describe the overall purpose of the organization, the wording needs to be carefully crafted. It needs to be derived by a process that respects the organization's culture. The statement needs to have sufficient description to clearly identify the purpose and scope and suggest some order of priorities (McNamara, 2008b).

Vision Statements

Vision statements are designed to address the preferred future of the organization. They draw on the mission, beliefs, and environment of the organization and are positive and inspiring. Vision statements are crafted to describe the most desirable state at some future point in time. Often, one step in planning is a gap analysis of the difference between the current state and the vision (Drenkard, 2001). The advantage of vision statements are that they transcend bounded thinking; identify direction; challenge and motivate; promote loyalty, focus, and commitment; and encourage creativity. Vision statements are designed to rise above fatigue, tradition, routine, and complacency. Visioning is setting a high-level direction through turbulent times and creating a compelling picture of a desirable future state. Imagery and stories may be used to sustain the vision. Vision statements need to be vivid enough to keep the organization moving forward.

Values Statements

Core values are strongly held beliefs and priorities that guide organizational decision making. Core values are things that do not change. They are anchors or fundamentals that relate to mission and purpose and hold constant, whereas operations and business strategies change. Values drive how people truly act in organizations. They are the bridge to align how people actually behave with preferred behaviors (McNamara, 2008b). Adams (2004) stated, "Articulating values provides everyone with guiding lights, ways of choosing among competing priorities, and guidelines about how people will work together" (p. 2).

One way that core values are expressed are through lists or values statements as part of a strategic plan. Another way to express values as statements is to compose a statement of philosophy. Some organizations have philosophy statements, and others use a mix of mission, vision, and values statements as a proxy for their philosophy. Both individuals and organizations can compose a statement of philosophy. For an individual, this would be an expression of personal and professional values, vision, and mission. Although difficult to do, writing a personal professional statement of philosophy is an exercise in clarity and communication.

A statement of **philosophy** is defined as an explanation of the systems of beliefs that determine how a mission or a purpose is to be achieved. An organization's philosophy states the beliefs, concepts, and principles of an organization. It serves as a guide for and an explanation of actions (Poteet & Hill, 1988). The philosophy is abstract: it describes an ideal state and gives direction to achieving the purpose. It may begin with "We believe that… ." For example, the system of beliefs, or philosophy, might be stated in any of the following ways:

- We believe that everyone has a right to the highest quality of client care.
- We believe that we have an obligation to render quality client care at a cost-effective price.
- We believe that any person who walks through the door should receive care, regardless of his or her ability to pay.

The philosophy has implications for a nurse's practice role. If an organization's stated mission includes client care, teaching, and research, then all employees will be expected to be involved in all three aspects of the mission. Part of the nurse's job will be to teach students and be involved in research. The nursing department's philosophy should be congruent with the organization's philosophy. The three vital components that form the core of a nursing department philosophy are the client, the nurse, and nursing practice (Poteet & Hill, 1988).

The organization's philosophy is important to assess as it relates to one's personal philosophy. For example, a potential employee on a job search might compare his or her own philosophy, both of nursing practice and of management, with the philosophy of an organization in which he or she might secure employment. Is there a match? For example, hospitals owned by religious organizations may prefer to hire people who share this same religious faith. If the nurse is not of that religious faith or if he or she has a prejudice or a lack of knowledge about that religious faith, it is advisable to assess personal fit with that particular organization. If some part of the philosophy is personally distasteful, it can have implications for functioning within the practice environment. For example, a specific religious tradition may still be pervasive within the organizational culture, even though the stated philosophy may say that the organization provides care to people of all faiths. That may be bothersome. One example occurs when an organization that is owned and run by a religious group opens each administrative meeting with a prayer. Another example occurs when a nurse believes in providing the total scope of public health services to clients but the organization is run by for-profit principles that dictate the provision of only those services that make a profit. Taking a job in an organization suggests an implicit agreement to cooperate with the organization's values while at work.

Action Planning

Strategic planning efforts proceed from a focus on mission, vision, and values to the identification of major strategic goals and specific action plans. Establishing goals is an analytical process of deciding what the organization wants to achieve. According to Nickols (2000), actions and decisions are multidimensional in that many different kinds of effects might be sought and created. Furthermore, interventions in complex systems may have a ripple effect when unintended and unforeseen results occur. Nickols recommended using a goals grid: four squares that map out answers to two "Do we want it?" questions and two "Do we have it?" questions. The two "Do we want it?" questions are as follows:

1. What do you want that you do not have (trying to achieve)?
2. What do you want that you already have (trying to preserve)?

The following are two "Do we have it?" questions:

1. What do you not have that you do not want (trying to avoid)?
2. What do you have now that you do not want (trying to eliminate)?

The goals grid is a useful method for analyzing goals and objectives clearly, in an organized fashion and from four perspectives. Consciously thinking this through is an effort to improve performance efficiency and effectiveness by focusing on goals.

In the early phase of goal identification, often an environmental analysis is conducted. One common method is called *SWOT analysis* (strengths, weaknesses, opportunities, and threats). Strengths are positive and internal, weaknesses are negative and internal, opportunities are positive and external, and threats are negative and external factors of the organization's environment. Critical issues are identified and analyzed by a SWOT analysis. This allows the organization to pinpoint and focus in on the critical few issues that have the most impact. As a result of issues analyses, the organization can then set major goals to be achieved.

Sometimes groups doing strategic planning become tired, bored, or overwhelmed at this point. However, there is one more key phase to accomplish: action planning. Each major goal needs to have objectives, responsibilities, and timelines specified for tracking and evaluation purposes. Without careful action planning and diligent managerial follow-up monitoring, the strategic plan is in danger of drifting away, being ignored, or "collecting dust on a shelf" (McNamara, 2008a, p. 10). Communicating and monitoring the plan are key managerial activities. Managers are aided in this effort by the use of spreadsheet formats and clearly specified objectives to guide actions, decisions, and revisions.

Objectives

Objectives are written, behavior-specific statements of desired outcomes. *Objectives* are defined as the identified outcomes directing activity toward achieving the purpose of the organization or unit (Trexler, 1987). Organizations use written, behavior-specific objectives so that each employee knows what the organization is trying to achieve. Objectives are the fundamental strategy of an institution, and the objectives of each work unit are used for establishing priorities, strategies, plans, work assignments, and the allocation of resources (Drucker, 1973; Trexler, 1987). Objectives need to be specific, realistic, attainable, and challenging; they must fit with the organization's goals and emphasize the work of greatest importance.

Policies and Procedures

Policies and procedures are two functional elements of an organization that are extensions of the mission statements. Both are written rules derived from the mission statement. Together they determine the nursing systems of the work unit and the department of nursing. The purpose of policies and procedures is to provide some order and stability so that the unit functions in a coordinated manner within the larger structure of nursing and the institution. Organizations need to integrate the behaviors of employees to avoid random chaos and maintain some order, function, and structure. These plans are often referred to as *standard operating policies and procedures.* They guide personnel in decision making.

Policies

A **policy** is a guideline that has been formalized. It directs the action for thinking about and solving recurring problems related to the objectives of the organization.

There will be specific times when it is not clear who is supposed to do something, under what circumstances it should be done, or what should be done about unusual circumstances. For example, often there are controversies about the dress code because of disagreements about the definition of what is "appropriate." This occurs, for example, when the dress code says, "Nurses will come to work dressed in appropriate attire."

Policies direct decision making and serve as guides to increase the likelihood of consistency in decisions and actions. Policies should be written, understandable, and general in nature to cover all employees. If written, they should be readily available in the same form to all employees. Policies should be reviewed during employee orientation because they indicate the organization's intentions for goal achievement.

After institutional approval, policies need to be collected in a manual or computerized database that is indexed, classified, and easily retrievable. Policies so organized can be easily replaced with revised ones, which often become necessary in light of new environmental circumstances. Policy formulation in any organization is an ongoing core process. Hospitals will have a standing committee for the review of policies as a part of the organizational structure. Policies establish broad limits on and provide direction to decision making; yet they permit some initiative and individuality for unique circumstances.

Policies can be implied, or unwritten, if they are essentially established by patterns of decisions that have been made. In this situation, the informal policies represent an interpretation of observed behavior. For example, the organization may expect caring treatment for all clients. This expectation may not be written as a policy of the organization. However, by the decisions and disciplinary actions that occur, an employee can infer that there is a policy that will be enforced even though it is not written. However, the vast majority of policies are and should be written. Informal and unwritten policies are less desirable because they can lead to systematic bias or unfairness in their application and enforcement (Box 17.1).

Some general areas in nursing require policy formulation. These are areas in which there is confusion about the locus of responsibility and in which lack of guidance might result in the neglect, malpractice, or "mal-performance" of an act necessary to the client's welfare. For example, clear

Box 17.1
Policies

- Serve as guides
- Help coordinate plans
- Control performance
- Increase consistency of action
- Should be written
- Usually are general in nature
- Refer to all employees

policies need to be in place about medication error reporting and follow-up. In those areas in which it is important that all persons adhere to the same pattern of decision making given a certain circumstance, a policy is necessary so that it can be used as a guideline. Also, areas pertaining to the protection of clients' or families' rights should have written policies. For example, the use of restraints to manage difficult clients came under scrutiny as the Omnibus Budget Reconciliation Act of 1987 (OBRA) pushed restraint-reduction strategies and created policy revisions. Another example is the need for policies related to "do not resuscitate" and end-of-life care (Wilson, 1996). Areas involving matters of personnel management and welfare, such as vacation leave, should have written policies. In such cases, the lack of a uniform policy would be considered unfair. Many conflicts arise about the scheduling of vacations: How many people can be off at any one time? How long in advance must a vacation request be made? How is the priority for granting requests to be determined (e.g., by seniority or by order of request)? The policy is the guideline for determining specific decisions.

Procedures

Procedures are step-by-step directions and methods for actions to follow in common situations. **Procedures** are descriptions of how to carry out an activity. They are usually written in sufficient detail to provide the information required by all persons engaging in the activity. This means that procedures should include a statement of purpose and identify who is to perform the activity. Procedures should include the steps necessary and the list of supplies and equipment needed. A procedure is a more specific guide to action than a policy statement. Procedures usually are departmental or divisionally specific, so they will vary across an institution. They may be very detailed as to how to perform a specific procedure on a specific unit. They help achieve regularity. They are a ready reference for all personnel (Box 17.2).

The similarities between policies and procedures are that both are a means for accomplishing goals and objectives. Both are necessary for the smooth functioning of any work group or organization. The difference between a policy and a procedure is that a policy is a general guideline for decision making about actions, whereas a procedure gives directions for actions. For example, policies about the use of restraints to manage difficult clients would indicate when such restraint use is appropriate. Procedures would cover how to apply specific devices.

A policy is a more general guide for decision making; a procedure is more like a cookbook recipe or a how-to guide giving specific directions about how to perform a certain act or function. There are legal implications to the application of policies and procedures. For example, the nurse may be held liable for failing to follow written policies and procedures. Thus it is important for nurses to be informed about the policies and procedures governing practice in an institution.

Box 17.2

Procedures

- Provide step-by-step methods
- Are written in detail
- Provide guidelines for commonly occurring events
- Provide a ready reference
- Guide performance of an activity
- Should include the following:
  - A statement of purpose
  - Identification of who performs activity
  - Steps in the procedure
  - A list of supplies and equipment needed

LEADERSHIP AND MANAGEMENT IMPLICATIONS

Change and competition in health care create circumstances that may drive the need to create or revise an organization's or a department of nursing's strategic plan, vision statement, or statement of philosophy. The philosophy should be a dynamic and vital values statement. Graham and colleagues (1987) described how to implement a new or changed philosophy. They used a marketing-based

LEADERSHIP & MANAGEMENT BEHAVIORS

Leadership Behaviors

- Inspires a vision that is reflected in a philosophy
- Enables followers to accomplish the purpose
- Motivates followers to achieve objectives
- Influences the group to develop the philosophy creatively
- Provides personal consideration
- Guides the development of policies and procedures

Management Behaviors

- Ensures that the nursing department philosophy is meshed with the organization's philosophy
- Measures outcomes
- Reviews and revises policies and procedures
- Directs subordinates to achieve objectives
- Monitors purpose and objectives
- Implements the "philosophy in action"

Overlap Areas

- Develops a philosophy, purpose, and objectives
- Develops policies and procedures

perspective to transform a traditional philosophy statement into a positioning statement. They articulated a vision and provided a framework for planning to thrive, rather than merely survive, in times of change. This implies that a philosophy may be different from the vision in an organization. Both statements may be required. Graham and colleagues (1987) set a goal of having a philosophy statement that was "unique, concise, measurable, and easy to remember" (p. 15). To accomplish this through group work, a marketing strategy called *positioning* was used as a basis for discussion and communication. A positioning statement about four areas of excellence was developed and integrated into all aspects of the organizational documents and nursing care processes.

Clearly, both the strategic plan and the philosophy need to be reviewed periodically and may need to be revised completely if major changes occur. This is especially true in the case of a merger (Appenzeller, 1993). Normally, the philosophy guides actions. However, in times of rapid change, revision may be required so that the strategic plan and the philosophy reflect current practices.

Periodic review is necessary to keep pace with what is or should be occurring in the work environment. With rapid change, it may be easy to overlook the philosophy and mission statements. If the philosophy needs to be revised, who does this? Commitment to a strategic plan or philosophy of nursing is fostered by input from all members and by the participation of the group in its formulation. In one facility, this process included task force selection, preparation of the task force, review of strategies to develop a philosophy, details of the process used, and presentation of the resulting document (Cody, 1990).

One implication for leadership and management is the relationship of organizational documents such as strategic plans and goals with the leader's/manager's responsibility to create a productive work environment. Brown-Stewart (1987) discussed "thinly disguised contempt," or the translation of managerial decisions into the work environment. The reality of effectiveness in a managerial role is that managers can have a tremendous impact on the work environment by virtue of their basic personality, problem-solving and decision-making strategies, and managerial and leadership style. When the organization's environment promotes contempt, it may affect the availability of competent nurses. Specifically, through the strategic construction of a philosophy and culture, leaders and managers affect the morale and job satisfaction of the nurses. This can be done by a focus on core values.

Behaviors that reflect a lack of concern for people and contempt for employees create barriers to developing excellence in organizations. Brown-Stewart (1987) listed the following four ways in which contempt for people is demonstrated:

1. Telling clients what they want instead of responding to the clients' perceived needs
2. Casting aspersions on or depersonalizing clients
3. Habitual lack of courtesy
4. Contempt for employees

The concept of "thinly disguised contempt" is closely related to the idea of a "philosophy in action." Although written mission statements exist, the implementation of these documents comes through people, especially in managerial decision making and resource allocation. According to Brown-Stewart (1987), some examples of contempt behaviors are a consumptive, as opposed to investment, attitude toward employees; lack of orientation; ambiguity of mission, values, and job requirements; lack of adequate proximate employee parking areas; preferential treatment of physicians; ignoring the client's family; lack of attention to the client's comfort; inadequate amount and inappropriate mix of nursing staff on duty; failure to communicate; and insensitivity when creating an inconvenience. Some issues such as parking may be difficult to resolve. However, organizational decisions will reflect valuing/nonvaluing to employees. Thus the leadership and management style becomes important at the interface of mission and values with culture and philosophy and any individual nurse in a work environment.

One result of organizational philosophies and cultures that create barriers to quality nursing practice is that nurses manifest a sense of job dissatisfaction, feelings of frustration or powerlessness, a sense of not being a part of the decision-making process, and a feeling that supervisors are not empathetic. Because nurses as professionals work primarily as employees, tension in the relationship with the work environment results in a concern about job satisfaction, commitment, and turnover. Literature on job satisfaction in nursing is extensive. The research on social integration, for example, indicates that nurses feel happy and more satisfied if they are part of a cohesive work group. Thus the philosophy and mission statements may need to be examined to see whether they support work-group cohesion. For example, leaders and managers can operationalize values that promote positive resolution of conflict in work groups. Resources can be allocated to work-group functioning. Philosophy statements can speak directly to valuing a positive work climate.

It is important to look at the factors in the environment that might impede the functioning of nursing and that therefore could make nurses dissatisfied, unhappy, or at risk for a high degree of turnover. Nurses feel strongly about needing job autonomy and having control over their practice. They feel that they need autonomy to meet legal requirements and client care needs adequately. Generally, nurses want improvements in pay, image, and working conditions (Minnick et al., 1989). These are the three areas in which nurses seek substantial changes. The issues related to working conditions include shift work and rotation, floating, the number of weekends worked, job security, workload, the amount of recognition for the actual work done, the level of legal liability carried, and a sense of autonomy. If nurses are vested with the responsibility to carry out complex client care, then they feel the urgency to be free from interference as they make basic decisions about client care that are necessary to affect outcomes.

Healthy Work Environment

Nurse leaders and managers can create and maintain an environment that facilitates the practice of the professional nurse. Leadership is required to bring about a good environment. Three elements form the basis for the creation of a positive professional work environment: fun, hope, and trouble. Nurses can use these elements to support each other, stimulate creativity, and work together successfully (McCloskey, 1991). Another aspect of leadership and management in times of change is the creation of a healthy work environment as a nursing administration core value. Striving for a healthy work environment is a conscious choice. Respect is a hallmark criterion. Elements for constructing such an environment include acknowledgment of the reality of the present environment, clear behavioral expectations and standards, systems and structures to ensure that organizational changes are enduring,

Practical Tips

Tip #1: Personal Philosophy

Compose your own personal philosophy. What do you believe? Why? What are your core values? What is your personal philosophy of nursing? Consider using the goals grid.

Tip #2: Compare Personal and Workplace Philosophies

Acquire the philosophy (or mission/vision) statement from your place of work. Do you agree with it? How does it compare with your personal statement?

Tip #3: Dialog with Peers

Form an informal group of your peers. Talk about what the philosophy, values, and mission are for your group. How does this translate into everyday actions? Are fun, hope, and trouble part of your work life? How?

and a means to continually assess the health of the work environment.

Leaders have both the opportunity and the responsibility to preserve concepts of dignity, integrity, honesty, and compassion in the working environment of nursing. In the University of Minnesota Health System, a document listing the characteristics of a healthy work environment was developed and disseminated to describe expectations for the key components of open communication, trust, and mutual respect in effective working relationships. Kreitzer and colleagues (1997) offered this example: "In a healthy work environment: I am viewed as an asset, people call me by name, my contributions and talents are acknowledged and recognized, communication is open, direct and honest" (p. 38).

Nurses are a key and critical component of the functioning of a health care organization. In today's environment, clients come to a hospital for nursing care. As care delivery shifts toward home and community settings, clients still seek nursing care because of needing the assessment, education, and evaluation skills of nurses. Thus keeping a happy, stable, and satisfied nursing workforce is an organizational pressure for hospitals and other health care organizations delivering nursing services. This can be formally expressed as a positive core value in strategic plans.

Caring and Advocacy

Caring is one fundamental philosophical principle of nursing. It has been described as the essence of nursing, and the visibility of caring as an important nursing concept is growing (Pepin, 1992). *Caring* has been interpreted as meaning that persons, events, projects, and things matter to an individual (Benner & Wrubel, 1988). Caring in nursing is seen as related to attention and concern for the client; responsibility for the client; and regard, fondness, or attachment to the client (Gaut, 1983). Swanson (1991) offered the following definition of caring: "a nurturing way of relating to a valued other toward whom one feels a personal sense of commitment and responsibility" (p. 162). The five categories or processes of caring are knowing, being with, doing for, enabling, and maintaining belief (Swanson, 1991).

As the basis or essence of nursing practice, caring can be seen to be a crucial component of nursing department and unit mission, vision, values, and philosophy statements. It then should be explicit in the written documents and obvious in the "philosophy in action." Perhaps, however, not all organizations value caring. If caring is valued by an organization, this will be reflected in decisions, resource allocations, types of power used, handling of conflict, recognition of nurses as professionals, and strategies chosen to motivate nurses. Thus the philosophy of the institution provides a glimpse at the concept of caring and its intersection with leadership and management. If it is a cherished value, then the concept of caring will be incorporated into leadership styles. For example, does caring about employees come through in the day-to-day work situation? Caring can be manifested in resource decisions about personnel, equipment, and supplies. How do organizations respond to a nursing shortage? What strategies are used when there is a need to reduce the size of the workforce? In some organizations, the philosophy includes a "culture of yes," which embodies a "can-do" ethic. Nurses can examine the written philosophy and the obvious decision patterns to see whether caring is valued and promoted in the organization.

Patient *advocacy* also is a fundamental philosophical principle of nursing. This core value emphasizes the protection of patients' rights. Patient advocacy is assumed to be an inherent part of clinical practice. Because advocacy is so embedded in nursing practice, it may be invisible and difficult to describe (Foley et al., 2002). Advocacy was initially incorporated into nursing practice when nurses developed a sense of service more to their patients than to physicians. This central role of advocacy was formalized in the 1970s when language changes occurred and the code of ethics published by the American Nurses Association included a definition of patient advocacy (Foley et al., 2002). Research into nurses' advocacy experiences has revealed that learning about advocacy may be haphazard and situationally dependent. Nurses reported that advocacy was part of who they were, that they learned advocacy by watching other nurse-patient interactions, and that they felt more confident in difficult situations that required intervention on behalf of patients when they had strong advocacy skills (Foley et al., 2002).

CURRENT ISSUES AND TRENDS

In times of change, organizational strategic plans, philosophies, policies, and vision statements also may undergo change. What would happen if nurses were the supervisors of physicians—that is, if physicians were employees and the nurses actually managed the work flow? There have been a few organizations in which nurses have admitting privileges and physicians do not. Across the country, alternative systems of care delivery are being tested and some of those systems are focused on community-based and nurse-managed centers. There is a persuasive argument that advanced practice nurses are cost-effective providers of primary care. In an era of fiscal constraint, nurses have an opportunity to redefine and reposition their roles within the health care delivery system. Strategic plans may need to change in response.

Positive job motivation is an important element in the functioning of human service organizations. It could be assumed that job satisfaction should follow from an environment in which each person's expertise is acknowledged and respected and nurses go home at the end of their shift feeling good about their work. Thus the influence of philosophy and values on organizational culture may be more visible if it is practiced as well as being written.

Summary

- An organization is a group acting to achieve a goal.
- The two dimensions of a social system are the environment and the individual.
- Behavior in organizations is a function of the dynamic interaction of these two dimensions.
- Service industries, such as nursing and health care, emphasize quality and cost control.
- Strategic plans are developed to clearly communicate the organization's purpose and direction.
- The main parts of a strategic plan are the vision, values, and mission statements and the action plans using goals and objectives statements.
- Policies and procedures are two functional elements of an organization that flow from the mission statements and help guide decision making and performance.
- Organizational philosophies affect nursing practice through elements related to culture, job satisfaction, and turnover.
- Strategic plans may need to be revised as circumstances change.

CASE STUDY

The executive director (ED) of StayAtHome, a not-for-profit home health care agency, had a problem. He thought that the agency was drifting along aimlessly. The most recent Board of Directors' meeting also had been challenging. He had been intensely questioned by the Board members about financial and performance outcomes, despite the fact that the agency was operating in the black. Action was needed. Determined to turn the situation around, the ED began to ask each Board member to help him to better understand the concerns. Then he did the same thing with each of his staff. He began to see how the various stakeholders held widely differing philosophies. It was time to do an in-depth revisiting of the organization's vision, values, and mission statements and the goals and objectives statements. A strategic planning facilitator was hired, and a strategic planning retreat was held in which Nickols' (2000) goal grid was used to frame the dialog.

CRITICAL THINKING EXERCISE

Nurse Manager Anthony Gardner finds himself in the nurse executive's office. Nurse Gardner has a problem with a staff nurse who was seen yelling at two nursing assistants in the middle of a crowded area. Nurse Gardner is asked to discuss what happened. Nurse Gardner says the staff nurse was irritated by the nursing assistants' loitering and yelled at them to get back to work. Nurse Gardner says he is too busy to spend all his time supervising nurses who have no sense of teamwork. The nurse executive carefully explains that a staff opinion survey has uncovered that a significant proportion of the staff reported experiencing abuse or confrontation in the workplace, leading to conflict, tension, and stress. A major component of the reported abuse on this unit was "being yelled at." The nurse executive explained that the hospital has embarked on a new "healthy work environment" initiative and that written behavioral expectations and standards exist. The nurse executive gives a copy of these standards and the "respect, communicate, and take responsibility" philosophy to Nurse Gardner.

1. Is there a problem?
2. What is the problem?
3. Whose problem is it?
4. What should the nurse manager do?
5. What interactions should have occurred before this point?
6. Whose values are in operation in this situation? Is there a clash of values?
7. If so, how should they be resolved?
8. Are there any legal considerations?

The ED took some time to carefully think through the situation and analyze the organization's status. He realized that goals were unclear and unfocused. Many questions arose, and the ED's objectives seemed to conflict with statements made by board members.

To engineer a solution, the ED hit upon a plan: he would prepare an exercise to clarify goals and objectives. First, the ED worked through the following questions:

1. What are you trying to achieve?
2. What are you trying to preserve?
3. What are you trying to avoid?
4. What are you trying to eliminate?

Next, he plotted these on the goals grid (Nickols, 2000). Then he formulated objectives for each of the goals in the four quadrants.

Armed with his initial goals grid exercise, the ED prepared materials (blank forms and the four questions) for the next board meeting. He called the president of the board to discuss the exercise and what he hoped to gain from it. They both agreed that the board would do the exercise "cold" and then compare their results with the ED's.

The exercise was well received at the next board meeting. It generated a lively discussion. Consensus around goals was reached, and further work on specific objectives was delegated to committees. The board decided to hire a consultant to plan and implement formal strategic planning for the agency.

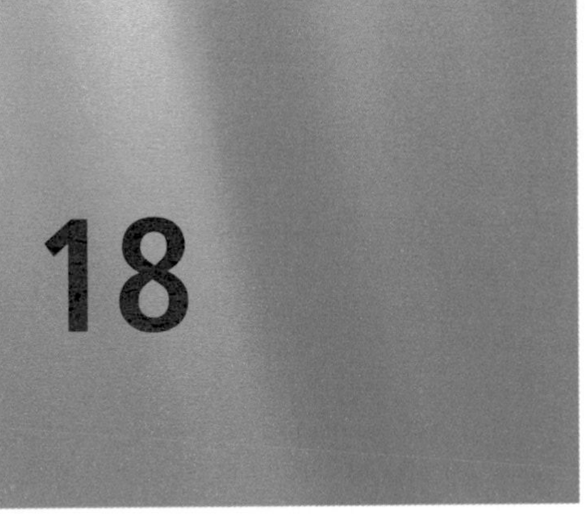

18 Organizational Structure

Raquel Meyer

CHAPTER OBJECTIVES

- Explain objective, subjective, and postmodern perspectives on organizations
- Review major theories of organizations as social systems
- Describe key organizational design concepts: division and coordination of labor, organizational forms, hierarchy, organizational shapes, and power
- Identify current trends in health care and the impact on organizational structure
- Discuss implications for nursing leadership and management
- Exercise critical thinking to conceptualize and analyze possible solutions to a practice exercise

Structure refers to the arrangement of the parts within a larger whole. *Organizations* are groupings that consolidate smaller elements into a larger, systematized whole. When membership in an organization comprises humans, organizations are essentially social structures that rely on human activity. An organization meaningfully coordinates group activity toward a shared goal because collective efforts are often necessary to manage large-scale work processes and outcomes efficiently and effectively. Many types of organizations are necessary to deliver nursing and health care services to diverse populations across sectors and geography. In health care, obvious organizational goals might be safety and quality of care, cost reduction, and increased efficiency.

Organizational social structure is defined as the ways in which work is divided and coordinated among members and the resulting network of relationships, roles, and work groups (e.g., units, departments). The social structure of an organization influences the flow of information, resources, and power among its members. Whether as employees or as independent practitioners, nurses work for, or interact with, organizations. How nurses' roles interface with the structure of the organization influences the accomplishment of organizational goals. Research examples throughout this chapter highlight associations between the organizational structures in which nurses work and clinical, nurse, and organizational outcomes.

ORGANIZATION THEORY

There are many ways to understand organizations, and each understanding reflects different assumptions and tensions regarding the nature and dynamics of organizations. The history of organization theory has been shaped by multiple disciplines including management, engineering, psychology, sociology, and anthropology. Although this has created a rich and varied understanding of organizations, the field of organization theory is highly fragmented and contested in terms of approaches to and assumptions about the phenomenon of "organization" (Clegg & Hardy, 1999). Objectivism, subjectivism, and postmodernism reflect three broad perspectives regarding the nature of reality and the nature of knowledge with respect to the concept of "organization" (Hatch & Cunliffe, 2006). These perspectives are reviewed briefly with attention to the meanings of social structure, management, and power.

Objective Perspective

When approached as an objective entity, an organization exists as an external reality, independent of its social actors. Organizations are viewed as logical and predictable objects with identifiable and scientifically measurable characteristics (e.g., size) that can be predicted, observed, or manipulated (Hatch & Cunliffe, 2006). The purpose is to uncover laws that enhance the generalizability of knowledge. Social structure is a consequence of the division and coordination of labor, which results in a formal set of interrelated and interdependent roles and work groups. Management determines the formal relationships and standardizes the behaviors of individuals and groups in order to align organizational functioning with internal demands (e.g., technology) and external demands (e.g., market conditions, regulatory standards) (Reed, 1992). Typically, power is conceptualized as a resource to be allocated among roles and groups. Modernist theories related to bureaucracy and systems, as well as the schools of scientific management and human relations, have focused on improvements to efficiency, motivation, and performance in the achievement of collective goals (Reed, 1992). These theoretical approaches, which focus on the formal aspects of organizations, are examined in detail in this chapter.

Subjective Perspective

In contrast to objectivism, a subjective approach to the phenomenon of organization asserts that an organization cannot exist independent of its social actors. The organization is a social reality that can be known only through human experience, relationships, and shared meanings and symbols (Hatch & Cunliffe, 2006). Because knowledge is considered to be relative, open to interpretation, and context dependent, the purpose of inquiries is to uncover collective meanings that resonate with the experiences of those involved (Hatch & Cunliffe, 2006). Social structure therefore arises from and is continuously transformed through social interaction, which is played out against a backdrop of formal rules and material resources directed by management (Reed, 1992). Power is reflected in the struggle between social actors who proactively and self-consciously shape organizational arrangements and secure scarce resources to serve their interests (Hatch & Cunliffe, 2006; Reed, 1992).

The subjective perspective focuses on the informal aspects of organization and on the freedom of individuals to make choices and to influence organizational life. Symbolic-interpretive theorists are interested in "how the everyday practices of organizational members construct the very patterns of organizing that guide their actions" (Hatch & Cunliffe, 2006, p. 126). Examples of daily social practices include routines (e.g., care maps), improvisation, and communities of practice. For example, instead of viewing routines as mechanisms to standardize the behavior of individuals (i.e., an objective approach), a subjective approach might examine the changing nature of routines as members selectively modify, adapt, and retain practices in response to varying contexts and conditions (Feldman & Pentland, 2003). In a community of practice, learning occurs through voluntary social interaction whereby practitioners committed to a common interest self-organize informally to build ongoing relationships, partake in joint activities, and share resources (Wenger, 2008). An example in nursing would be an informal group of staff nurses who routinely have lunch together and who come to rely on this activity as a source of knowledge related to patient care in terms of problem solving, information exchange, and networking (Wenger, 2008).

Postmodern Perspective

Departing from the polarization between objectivism and subjectivism, the postmodern view challenges the meanings and interpretations associated with the concept of organization. The basic premise is that the world is known through language.

Because language is continually reconstructed and context dependent, knowledge is essentially a power play (Hatch & Cunliffe, 2006). Notions of order and structure are the subject of scrutiny. Organizations may be thought of as disorderly entities characterized by conflicts and misunderstandings (Reed, 1992). Managerial practices and structures within organizations are seen to legitimize the interests of those in power (Hatch & Cunliffe, 2006; Reed, 1992). Even Weber (1978) cautioned that bureaucracies were essentially domination structures that shape the form and purpose of social action through a system of rational rules and norms. Those who control bureaucracies therefore exert significant power over social action. Thus the postmodern organization is understood both as an arena in which power struggles between dominant and subordinate groups play out and as a text to be rewritten to free its members from exploitative and controlling influences (Hatch & Cunliffe, 2006; Reed, 1992).

For instance, postmodernists challenge the assumption that social structure results from the division and coordination of work among roles and groups. Clegg (1990) suggested that excessive fragmentation of work results in a disjointed and confusing experience for workers who become dependent on more powerful members in the hierarchy to make sense of work flow and goals. To counter this excess control over member actions, he proposed the idea of **differentiation** whereby people self-manage and coordinate their own activities. Other examples of postmodern approaches to organization include feminist critiques of bureaucracies (e.g., Eisenstein, 1995) and anti-administration theory (Farmer, 1997).

KEY THEORIES OF ORGANIZATIONS AS SOCIAL SYSTEMS

In the field of organizational design, the organization is typically approached as a social system from the objective perspective. Different theories within this tradition have contributed to our understanding of organizational social structure (Table 18.1). However, these theories have also been critiqued for rationalizing social action, for favoring efficiency and productivity over other values (e.g., equity, justice), and for adopting an elitist view of management (Hatch & Cunliffe, 2006; O'Connor, 1999; Scott, 1992).

Bureaucratic Theory

Although often criticized for its oppressive qualities and administrative burden, the concept of bureaucracy may be better understood when placed within a historical context. Theorist Max Weber (1864-1920) was a German lawyer, professor, and political activist who noted the push of industrialism toward mass production and technical efficiency (Prins, 2000). Weber sought to explain, from a historical perspective, how the bureaucratic structure of large organizations differed from and improved upon other forms of societal functioning (e.g., feudalism). He viewed bureaucracy as a social leveling mechanism founded on impartial and merit-based selection (i.e., legal authority), rather than a social ordering determined by kinship (i.e., traditional authority) or personality (i.e., charismatic authority) (Weber, 1978). However, Weber warned of the potential dehumanizing effects of bureaucracies that emphasized purely economic results (i.e., formal rationality) at the expense of other important social values such as social justice and equality (i.e., substantive rationality) (Weber, 1978). Weber's descriptions of authority and rationality are foundational concepts in the study of organizations. His interpretation of hierarchy and its relevance to health care organizations are explored later in the chapter.

Scientific Management School

Arising from the experiences and ideas of business leaders and engineers in the manufacturing industries, the scientific management school sought to determine the single best way to structure an organization (Donaldson, 1996). A well-known theorist in this field is Frederick W. Taylor (1856-1915), an engineer who authored *The Principles of Scientific Management* in 1914 (Prins, 2000). Along with colleagues, Taylor's vision was to improve labor relations and the low industrial standards that plagued the American manufacturing industry

Table 18.1

Comparison of Theories of Organization as Social System

	Context	View of Organization	Goal of Management	View of Managers	View of Workers	Exemplar Theory
Bureaucratic Theory	Rise of industrialism	– Closed system – Stable entity – Formalized structure	Enforce legal, rule-bound functioning to achieve technical and economic efficiency	Impartial and qualified decision makers	Obedient and status seeking	Bureaucracy (Weber, 1978)
Scientific Management School	Early twentieth century manufacturing industry	– Closed system – Stable and predictable entity – Formalized structure	Apply scientific methods and monetary incentives to plan, control, and evaluate work flow and outputs	Impersonal and goal oriented	Reliable, predictable, and economically motivated	Principles of Scientific Management (Taylor, 2003)
Classical Management Theory	Early twentieth century manufacturing industry	– Closed system – Stable and predictable entity – Formalized structure	Apply administrative principles to divide and coordinate work activities	Specialists in planning, coordination, and supervision	Skilled and specialized technicians	Theory of Organization (Gulick, 1937)
Human Relations School	Post–World War I—Increasing activism and unionism	– Closed system – Behavioral structure	Enact leadership skills to empower workers and gain their cooperation to improve performance	Democratic leaders and open communicators	Socially and psychologically motivated	Participative Decision Making (Likert, 1961)
Open System Theory	Post–World War II	– Open and adaptive system dependent on environment – System of interdependent activities – Organization as a process	Integrate system functioning to balance stability, flexibility, growth, and survival	Internal and external boundary spanners	Semi-autonomous agents	Contingency Theory (Lawrence & Lorsch, 1967)

through the application of technical solutions (e.g., time and motion studies) (Prins, 2000). He proposed that "THE principal object of management should be to secure the maximum prosperity for the employer, coupled with the maximum prosperity for each employé...for each employé (this) means not only higher wages than are usually received by men of his class, but, of more importance still, it also means the development of each man to...the highest grade of work for which his natural abilities fit him" (Taylor, 2003, p. 235). The goal was to enhance organizational performance in a milieu of improved cooperation between management and labor by matching the work performed with the worker's skills and with economic incentives. However, the experiments and engineering techniques associated with this approach were ultimately criticized for reducing the worker to a mere input in the production process (Prins, 2000). The application of scientific principles to improve the task performance and productivity of workers reflected a bottom-up approach to organizational design (Scott, 1992). In nursing, efforts to redesign nursing jobs or to measure nursing workload often rely on this tradition.

Classical Management Theory

In contrast, classical theorists such as Fayol, Urwick, and Gulick evolved a top-down approach to organizational design. Based on experience as company executives, these practitioners identified principles of administration and management functions that could be applied in the design of organizations. Key concepts such as differentiation, coordination, scalar principle, centralization, formalization, specialization, and span of control became central to the study of organizational structure. These concepts, which describe the formal aspects of an organization's social structure and their application to health care organizations, are examined in relation to nursing later in the chapter.

Human Relations School

Theorists in the human relations school emphasized the informal, rather than formal, aspects of organization social structure. The disciplines of industrial psychology and industrial relations founded this approach, which now persists as the field of organizational behavior (O'Connor, 1999). The social and psychological needs and relationships of workers and groups were thought to be important to work productivity. Improved cooperation between management and workers was proposed to enhance performance and to reduce industrial strife (O'Connor, 1999). The famous Hawthorne experiments were influential in this school of thought. Initial interpretations of the Hawthorne experiments suggested that psychological factors influenced worker motivation because improved worker productivity was observed when researchers gave special attention to workers, regardless of changes to physical surroundings (Scott, 1992). Concepts such as job enlargement and job rotation were promoted to offset the alienation workers experienced because of excessive **formalization** and division of work processes (Scott, 1992). Formalization is the extent to which the organization uses explicit rules, procedures, job descriptions, and communications to prescribe roles and role interactions, govern activities, and standardize behaviors (Hatch & Cunliffe, 2006; Scott, 1992).

Streams of study included leadership behavior, small group dynamics, participative decision making, morale, motivation, and other worker characteristics and behaviors (Scott, 1992). However, research has not adequately demonstrated links between these concepts and improved productivity (Scott, 1992). In nursing, this school of thought is reflected in efforts to meet the professional development needs of nurses, to enhance nurse autonomy and empowerment, and to involve nurses in decision-making processes to improve organizational functioning.

Open System Theory

The open system theory approach emphasizes the dynamic interaction and interdependence of the organization with its external environment and its internal subsystems. For example, contingency theory posits that there is no single right way to structure an organization. Effective

LEADING & MANAGING DEFINED

Differentiation

Division of labor by function, occupation, rank, subunit, or spatial location (Blau, 1970).

Formalization

Extent to which the organization uses explicit rules, procedures, job descriptions, and communications to prescribe roles and role interactions, to govern activities, and to standardize behaviors (Hatch & Cunliffe, 2006; Scott, 1992).

Specialization

Extent to which work is divided and assigned to positions and divisions (Scott, 1992; Hatch & Cunliffe, 2006).

Size

A quantitative measure of personnel, physical capacity, volume of inputs or outputs, or discretionary resources of an organization (Kimberly, 1976).

Coordination

Integration of different parts of an organization to carry out a collective set of tasks at the organizational or work-group levels (Van de Ven et al., 1976).

Integration by Program

The coordination of work around the delivery of particular products or services (Charnes & Tewksbury, 1993).

Centralization

The extent to which decision-making authority is concentrated in the top level of the hierarchy (i.e., centralized) versus spread down through the hierarchy (i.e., decentralized) (Carter & Cullen, 1984).

Hierarchical Centralization

Extent to which decision-making authority is vested at the top levels of the hierarchy versus extended down through the hierarchy (Scott, 1992).

Span of Control

Number of personnel reporting directly to an individual manager (Meyer, 2008).

Scalar Principle

The creation of levels of authority in a hierarchy (Scott, 1992).

organizational performance depends on the fit between structure and multiple contingency factors such as technology, size, and strategy (Donaldson, 1996). Because contingencies vary according to the organization's environment, the system is perceived as adapting to its environment. Mark and colleagues (1996) applied contingency theory to the evaluation of nursing care delivery system outcomes. Key variables included environment (e.g., organizational size, skill mix), technology (e.g., stability of patient acuity, diversity of patient conditions), structure (e.g., degree of centralization), and effectiveness (e.g., patient and administrative outcomes). The basic premise was that, to perform effectively and produce quality outcomes, an organization must structure its nursing units to complement the environment and technology.

Technology is a core concept in contingency theory and refers to the work performed. Technology can be examined in terms of task uncertainty (i.e., repetitive nature of the task), diversity (i.e., number of different components), and interdependence (i.e., degree to which work processes are interrelated) (Scott, 1992). Highly repetitive and distinct tasks are amenable to mass production technologies (e.g., manufacturing industry). In contrast, highly uncertain and interdependent tasks require discretion, improvisation, and more intense coordination structures

Practical Tips

Tip # 1: Scan the Environment

Effective scanning of political, social, economic, labor market, and population health trends in the external environment informs the types and feasibility of revisions needed to your organizational structure, mission, and strategic objectives.

Tip # 2: Assess Stakeholders

Assessing stakeholder values, expectations, and power allows you to address conflicting objectives and uncover needs that may influence how the organization is structured. In addition to internal stakeholders (e.g., medicine, finance), developing strong relationships with external stakeholders will enable you to engage in meaningful negotiations around service accountabilities, shared resources and responsibilities, and outcomes.

Tip # 3: Align Resources and Outcomes with Values

Ethical leadership calls for a fit between structural outcomes and organizational values. Effective structures not only contribute to fiscal and efficiency priorities but also influence the extent to which your organization can uphold its core values. For example, if your organization is committed to interprofessional practice, you may wish to consider how well the organizational form, coordination mechanisms, and empowerment structures support team activities and integration.

across team-driven networks (Donaldson, 1996; Scott, 1992). The work performed by health care professionals is often considered to be highly uncertain, diverse, interdependent, and reliant on group coordination. For example, in a study of hospital joint replacements, teams with high levels of shared knowledge and goals and mutual respect positively influenced patient-assessed quality of care despite shortened lengths of stay (Gittell, 2004). In this study, task uncertainty was intensified by time constraints (i.e., shorter length of stay), task diversity was reflected by the multidisciplinary roles, task interdependence resulted as multidisciplinary work was performed concurrently, and the coordination device was teamwork.

Theories of networks are also applied to organizational structure. Social network analysis, which builds on a systems view of organizations, examines and interprets the structures and patterns of the formal and informal relationships among members of the organization (Tichy et al., 1979). Early theories of social network analysis focused on the observable properties of networks, including the type of exchanges (e.g., affect, power, information, services), the nature of the links (e.g., strength, reciprocity, expectations), and the structural characteristics (e.g., size, density, clustering, openness, stability) (Tichy et al., 1979). Data about these properties can be graphed to illustrate the social behavior of the organization's members. However, less manifest aspects of social networks, including the value, economic or otherwise, that actors derive from social networks (i.e., social utility) can also be studied (Balkundi & Kilduff, 2006). In nursing, for instance, social network analysis has been used to explore the social and geographical ties of senior nurse executives and physicians in the United Kingdom in relation to profession, gender, age, rank, location, and frequency of contact (West & Barron, 2005).

KEY ORGANIZATIONAL DESIGN CONCEPTS

Division and Coordination of Labor

A formal organization that employs people to achieve predetermined goals divides the work among its members by assigning tasks and delegating responsibilities to positions and work units. Structure is a by-product of the basic need to divide the labor into the specific tasks to be performed and a consequent need to coordinate these tasks to accomplish the activity or goal. The structure of an organization can be defined as the "total of the ways in which its labor is divided into distinct tasks and then its coordination is achieved among these tasks" (Mintzberg, 1983, p. 2).

The division (or differentiation) of work by occupation or by function is a form of **specialization**. Specialization is the extent to which work is divided and assigned to positions and divisions (Scott, 1992; Hatch & Cunliffe, 2006). As occupations and functions multiply in number, an organization increases in complexity and **size** (Katz & Kahn, 1978). Size is a quantitative measure of personnel, physical capacity, volume of inputs or outputs, or discretionary resources of an organization (Kimberly, 1976).

The advantages of specialization include improved work performance and a critical mass of experts (Charnes & Tewksbury, 1993). In health care, specialist roles have emerged to address the increasing complexities of care and technology. For example, occupations such as social work, physiotherapy, occupational therapy, and respiratory therapy represent specialized areas of knowledge that subdivide care with the aim of improving efficiency and outcomes. Within nursing, specialist roles have also evolved to address specific facets of practice. Advanced practice roles such as clinical nurse educators, nurse practitioners, and nurse anesthetists represent specialized areas of nursing knowledge. Organizations may also differentiate work units by function to serve distinct client populations. For instance, rather than a single, general intensive care unit, an organization may establish several intensive care units by medical specialty (e.g., cardiovascular, neurosurgical, neonatal). At the work-group level, nursing care delivery models (e.g., team, primary, or total nursing care models) reflect different ways of dividing and coordinating the work among a team of nurses caring for clients.

Subdividing work creates breaks in work flow. Organizations address this challenge by integrating work processes across roles and subunits using coordination devices (Katz & Kahn, 1978). **Coordination** (or integration) involves bringing together and connecting the smaller elements of an organization to achieve a set of collective tasks (Van de Ven et al., 1976). Coordination is especially necessary when resources must be shared or the work performed by different work groups or roles is interdependent (Charnes & Tewksbury, 1993). Although coordination mechanisms can improve efficiency, performance, and conflict resolution, their misuse can also result in information overload and communication breakdowns (Van de Ven et al., 1976).

At the work-group level, coordination involves programming and feedback devices (March & Simon, 1958). In health care, common programming devices used to control work processes are the following:

- Standardization of worker skills coordinates work indirectly by specifying the kind of training or education required to perform the work. In nursing, the standardization of worker skills occurs for advanced practice nurses when a master's degree is required or certification is mandated.
- Standardization of work processes coordinates work by pre-specifying or programming content before the work is undertaken. In nursing, standardization of work processes occurs when nurses use routines such as clinical pathways or best practice guidelines.
- Hierarchical referral may occur when exceptions or unanticipated events arise (Galbraith, 1974). In nursing, hierarchical referral happens when a nurse coordinates the resolution of an exceptional or non-routine clinical situation with a nurse specialist or physician.

- Standardization of work outputs coordinates work, before the work is undertaken, through the specification of the results, product, or performance desired or expected. In nursing, work outputs are standardized when care is specified as outcomes objectives or care is managed for outcomes achievement.
- Standardization of communication methods coordinates work by providing a uniform infrastructure of information to facilitate exchange among those involved in common work processes (Venkatraman, 1994). In nursing, standardization of information is achieved through electronic health records, which allow nurses and other care providers direct and simultaneous access to client information in a consistent format (Gittell & Weiss, 2004).

Feedback mechanisms entail the transfer of information in an adaptive and reciprocal manner to foster the exchange of information (Mintzberg, 1983; Gittell, 2002):

- Mutual adjustment coordinates work by using simple informal communication. In nursing, mutual adjustment occurs when one nurse consults another nurse about practice issues, such as how to interpret a policy, or when nurses, physicians, and allied health professionals participate in patient rounds.
- Direct supervision coordinates work through the use of a supervisor taking responsibility for the instruction and monitoring of the work of others. In nursing, direct supervision takes place when a nurse supervises the work of unlicensed assistive personnel.
- Boundary spanning roles coordinate work by managing relationships as well as the bidirectional flow of information and materials across functional divisions (Gittell, 2003). In nursing, case managers exemplify a boundary spanning role because these roles manage relationships, exchange information, and negotiate resources with internal and external parties to facilitate care across occupations, services, sectors, funding agencies, and locations.

The types of coordination that are used depend on the degree of stability and predictability of the work situation (March & Simon, 1958) and the size of the work unit (Van de Ven et al., 1976). For example, acute health care settings are typically characterized as highly uncertain and interdependent work situations. Patient health needs, acuity, and care trajectories are often highly variable and unpredictable. To ensure comprehensive care, nurses coordinate patient care activities with the work of others in a reciprocal manner because the work performed is highly interdependent. Traditionally, programming devices are thought to be effective under stable and predictable conditions (March & Simon, 1958) and with larger work units (Van de Ven et al., 1976). However, as conditions become increasingly uncertain and variable, as in health care, coordination by feedback is more likely to be used (March & Simon, 1958). Recent research suggests that both programming and feedback devices improve health care team performance (Gittell, 2002). This is because standardized routines and care paths may enhance, rather than replace, the interactions among health care providers, particularly in situations of increasing uncertainty (Gittell, 2002).

At the organizational level, the coordination and division of labor influences size and the degree of organizational centralization and formalization. As organizations grow in size, work units are increasingly subdivided to ensure tasks are accomplished; however, this process slows as organizations become very large, because the gains achieved by subdividing work occur at the expense of the coordination mechanisms necessary to unify system functioning across subunits (Blau, 1970). The need to balance the division of labor with the coordination of subunits and roles eventually constrains organizational size (Blau, 1970). At the organizational level, coordination is often measured by the degree of centralization and formalization. Health care organizations tend to be decentralized and less formalized because professionals are employed to manage highly uncertain work (Scott, 1992). However, as organizations grow and as the work becomes increasingly complex, specialized,

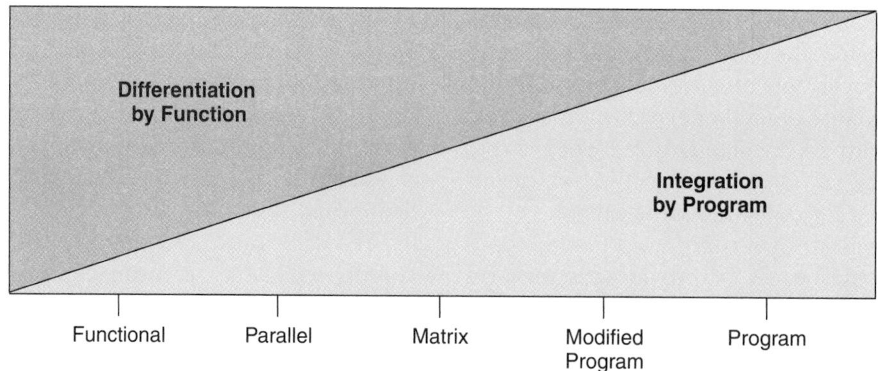

Figure 18.1
Continuum of organizational configurations. (Adapted from Charnes, M., & Tewksbury, L. [1993]. *Collaborative management in health care: Implementing the integrative organization* [p. 28, Figure 2.1]. San Francisco: Jossey-Bass. This material is used by permission of John Wiley & Sons.)

and interdependent, there is a pull toward greater centralization and formalization (Scott, 1992).

Organizational Forms

The division and coordination of labor lead to varied organizational forms. As illustrated by the sloping triangles in Figure 18.1, organizational forms reflect a trade-off between differentiation by function and integration by program. *Differentiation by function* refers to the division of work by occupation. **Integration by program** means the coordination of work around the delivery of particular products or services. Five basic organizational forms can be situated along a differentiation-integration continuum (Charnes & Tewksbury, 1993).

Functional and program forms represent extreme examples of differentiation and integration. This chapter describes these two configurations, and the Research Note extends the discussion by comparing these forms in the hospital sector (Young et al., 2004). Parallel and modified program forms that offset the limitations associated with functional and program forms are then explained. Finally, the matrix form, which represents the most balanced form, is described. In reality, organizations are not usually found in these pure forms but, rather, reflect hybrids of the forms described as follows.

Functional Form

At the extreme left end of the continuum, dividing the work by occupation leads to a functional organization whereby health professions and non-professional services are arranged according to the type of work performed. The emphasis is on the personnel inputs to the organization (Figure 18.2). Examples are nursing, respiratory therapy, admitting, and environmental services. Within each functional department, management develops specific structures, policies, procedures, and human resource practices. In this type of organizational form, professionals report directly to a discipline-specific supervisor (e.g., nurses would report to a nurse manager). Members of a functional group (e.g., nursing) are likely to interact more frequently, develop social relationships, receive supervision and evaluations from within the group, and conform to professional standards (Charnes & Tewksbury, 1993).

By dividing personnel according to the type of work performed, organizations can capitalize on the expertise, experience, efficiency, and professional standards that each discipline offers (Charnes & Tewksbury, 1993). Other benefits include cost reduction through shared resources and enhanced monitoring of cost, performance, and quality (Charnes & Tewksbury, 1993). Professional development, identity, advocacy, and career advancement are also promoted (Charnes & Tewksbury, 1993). Disadvantages of the functional form are its potential to overemphasize professional silos, to discourage informal relationships across disciplines, and to fragment

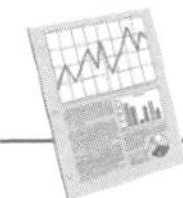

Research Note

Source: Young, G.J., Charnes, M.P., & Heeren, T.C. (2004). Product-line management in professional organizations: An empirical test of competing theoretical perspectives. *Academy of Management Journal, 47*(5), 723-734.

Purpose

This article compared the influence of functional and program organizational forms on performance and professional staff outcomes in general hospitals.

Discussion

Although the concept of organizational form has been empirically evaluated in manufacturing contexts, the extent of its relationship to outcomes in professional organizations has not been examined. The workforces of professional organizations such as hospitals are composed of highly educated personnel (e.g., nurses, social workers) who exercise significant discretion in the coordination and execution of their own work activities. In this study of hospitals, the two organizational forms observed were functional and program. The functional form arranges positions according to occupations whereby health care providers report through a traditional hierarchy to a manager of departments for their respective clinical discipline. The program form groups positions by service whereby professionals report to a manager outside of the traditional discipline-based hierarchy.

This observational, cross-sectional correlational study sampled 11 U.S. general hospitals. Site visits and interviews were used to classify the 44 participating clinical areas, of which 32 were functional forms and 12 were program forms. A response rate of 55% resulted in 1171 health care providers surveys, of which 90% were completed by nurses. Nurses, social workers, pharmacists, and therapists rated their perceptions of service quality, clinical innovation, opportunities for professional development, and job satisfaction. Program forms were significantly associated with less professional development opportunities and with lower job satisfaction. However, associations were not observed between program form and perceived performance outcomes and between functional form and either performance and staff outcomes.

Application to Practice

Program management forms are used pervasively in health care, as organizations have shifted toward patient-centered models of care that streamline services according to disease or clinical populations, rather than by occupation. In this study, no clear advantages to either organizational form were observed. However, job dissatisfaction and lack of professional development opportunities in program forms may generate management challenges related to staff turnover and outmoded professional skills and knowledge. Lower job satisfaction in program forms may indicate a poor fit between expectations for professional autonomy and the administrative control necessary to coordinate the varied work activities of many disciplines. The results of this study suggest that nurse leaders and hospital administrators managing program forms need to ensure adequate educational resources are made available to the various disciplines to support professional development. Further research is needed to link organizational forms across health care settings to objective outcome measures, as well as to patient outcomes.

care delivery (Charnes & Tewksbury, 1993). Coordination of activities becomes challenging because group members have functionally based differences in work goals, thought worlds, and status (Gittell, 2003). Because the work of nursing is highly interdependent with other professional and non-professional work, nurse leaders in functional forms may use coordination mechanisms and leadership behaviors to span the boundaries between disciplines to facilitate the flow and

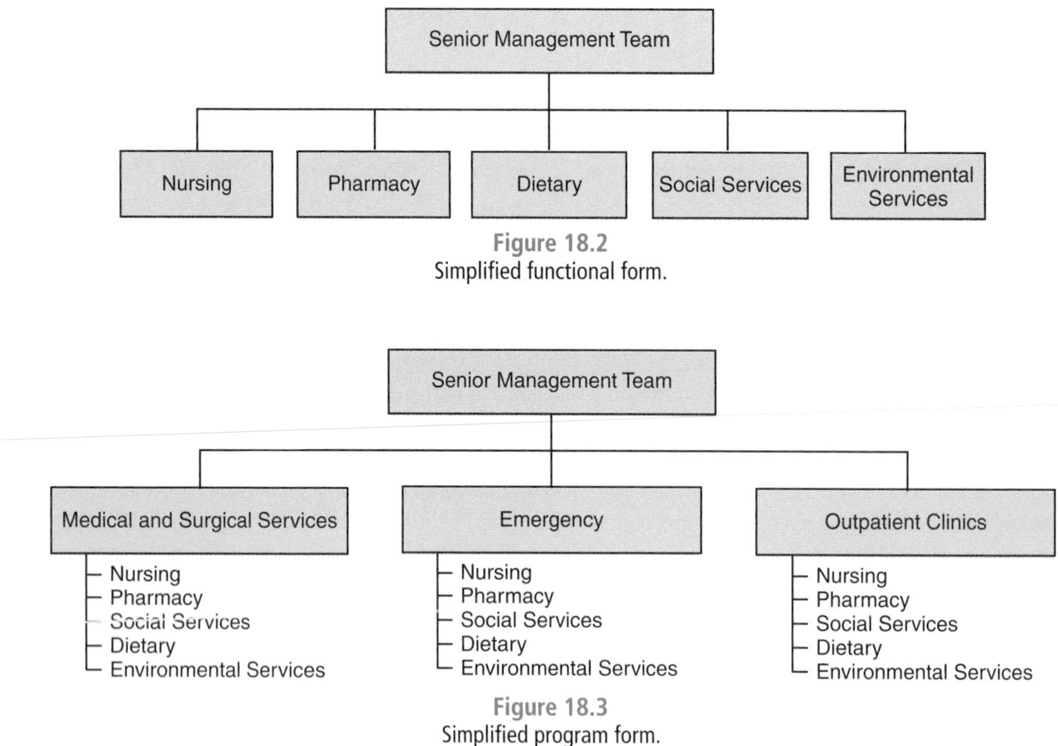

Figure 18.2
Simplified functional form.

Figure 18.3
Simplified program form.

exchange of information, resources, and work activities. Although prevalent in health care in the 1980s, functional forms have gradually been replaced by program or matrix forms to enhance client centeredness.

Program Form

At the extreme right end of the continuum, program organizations emphasize integration of the work by consumer, service, or geography (Charnes & Tewksbury, 1993; Hatch & Cunliffe, 2006). The emphasis is on the outputs of the organization (Figure 18.3). In health care, programs may be managed according to consumer health needs (e.g., diabetes, cancer), consumer age (e.g., elderly, neonates, women), services (e.g., addictions, rehabilitation), medical specialty (e.g., neurosciences, endocrinology), or geography (e.g., catchment areas). Although the corporate structure is shared, each program tends to operate as a semi-autonomous unit with its own management team composed of medical, administrative, and nursing representatives (Charnes & Tewksbury, 1993; Leatt et al., 1994). Professionals who work in program organizations may not report to a discipline-specific supervisor.

Program designs can optimize service delivery because local experts with accountability for costs, outcomes, and staffing control resources and can make timely operational decisions (Leatt et al., 1994). Patients can access integrated services from an array of health professionals with specific clinical expertise. With the program form, there is a push toward a multidisciplinary team approach (Leatt et al., 1994). However, clients who require access to more than one program may find it difficult to coordinate services among different programs. Integration by program occurs at the expense of decreased coordination among programs (Charnes & Tewksbury, 1993). Although organizational relationships with medical staff are enhanced when programs are grouped by medical specialty (Charnes & Tewksbury, 1993), health care professionals may be isolated from their colleagues in other programs. With respect to nursing for instance, no organization-wide mechanisms would exist to systematically handle professional nursing issues in terms of standards, resources, or professional advocacy. Because each program operates independently, processes, and procedures are likely to be duplicated and programs may compete for resources or develop goals that diverge from the corporate mission (Leatt et al., 1994).

Parallel Form

To address the challenges of purely functional forms, new mechanisms in the parallel form assist in coordinating across functional departments (Charnes & Tewksbury, 1993). These mechanisms can include teams, specialists, task forces, liaison roles, and standing committees. For example, rather than each functional department separately establishing procedures to hire staff, a specialized human resource department may be created to deal with recruitment and employment issues across the organization. Another example is a rapid response team in a hospital that is composed of intensive care physicians and nurses and respiratory therapists. This team assists staff throughout the hospital in detecting and managing imminent patient deterioration and in resuscitating compromised patients. Likewise in home care, nurses with particular expertise such as wound care or palliation might be responsible for referrals across multiple districts. Task forces bring together members from various divisions in an organization to address a concern. For example, developing and implementing critical pathways, evidence-based practices, disease management initiatives, case management projects, or outcomes management efforts generally require an interdisciplinary team of specialists. These types of mechanisms foster collaboration and cross-fertilization of knowledge across divisions and can reinforce consistency in clinical and management practices by standardizing procedures.

Modified Program Form

To offset the fragmentation and isolation of functions in pure program structures, organizations maintain the program structure and develop integrative mechanisms to unify functions and occupations across programs (Charnes & Tewksbury, 1993). For example, a nurse executive could address professional nursing issues related to standards, educational resources, and research activities across the organization. Unlike his or her counterpart in a functional nursing department who has line authority, a nurse executive in a modified program would not directly control operations, finances, or personnel issues (known as *staff authority*). A nurse executive with staff authority must use personal influence and leadership skills to effect change.

Matrix Form

In a pure matrix form, people and work are organized along both functional and program dimensions (Charnes & Tewksbury, 1993). Essentially, the program form overlays the functional form (Figure 18.4). Although some employees may have dual reporting relationships, staff members are evaluated by both supervisors (Charnes & Tewksbury, 1993). The budget and decision making are shared between functional and program divisions. A matrix configuration has the flexibility to adapt to change and to deliver services innovatively and efficiently by drawing on a varied talent pool (Hatch & Cunliffe, 2006). In contrast, innovation in program forms is costly because additional cross-coordination may be required across functional divisions or specialists may need to be hired for each program (Hatch & Cunliffe, 2006). However, true matrix forms are rarely seen and are difficult to maintain because the additional management infrastructure is costly and dual reporting relationships may be ambiguous and lead to conflict (Charnes & Tewksbury, 1993). Success requires well-educated workers who can handle a multifaceted communication and authority web. Nurses in matrix organizations need strong interpersonal and teamwork skills to negotiate these complex environments.

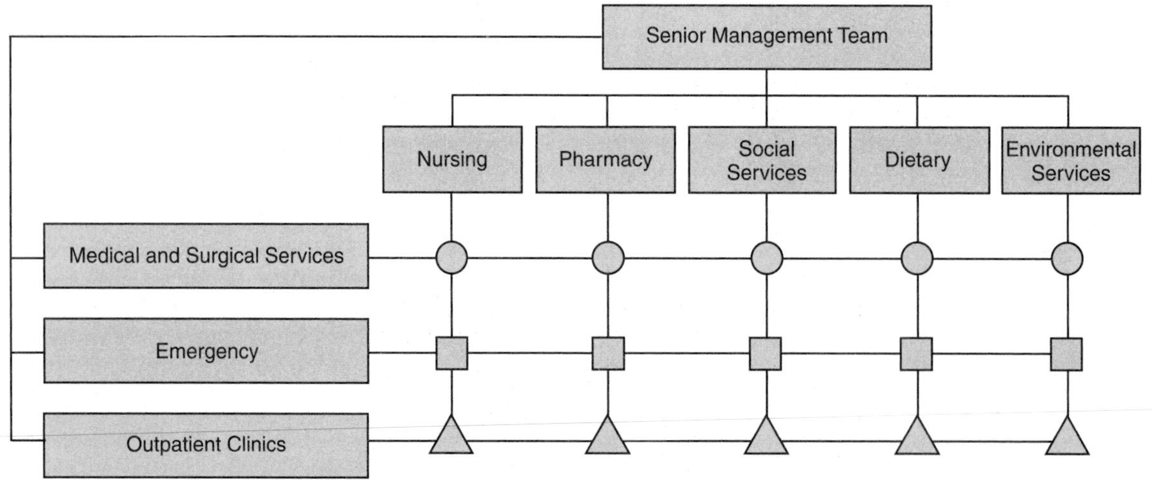

For example, team members for Outpatient Clinics (△) are drawn from different functions.

Figure 18.4
Simplified matrix form.

Hierarchy

In bureaucratic and classical management theory, hierarchy is the structure of authority in an organization (Gulick, 1937; Weber, 1978). Authority is equated with the enforcement of regulations, which brings about a governing order among the formal social relationships of organizational members (Weber, 1978). Authority is vested in positions, rather than in persons, and creates an impartial mechanism whereby the supra-ordinate position directs the actions and the norms expected of subordinate positions (Weber, 1978). Centralization is a multidimensional concept frequently associated with authority and hierarchy. **Centralization** refers to the extent to which decision-making authority is concentrated in the top level of the hierarchy (i.e., centralized) versus spread down through the hierarchy (i.e., decentralized) (Carter & Cullen, 1984). **Hierarchical centralization** can vary according to the decision type (Carter & Cullen, 1984). Hierarchical centralization is the extent to which decision-making authority is vested at the top levels of the hierarchy versus extended down through the hierarchy (Scott, 1992).

Corporate strategy is likely to be decided by top executives, whereas procedural work decisions may be devolved to work units or employees. For instance, a nurse executive could be required to centralize some budgetary decisions, whereas others could be devolved to lower levels in the hierarchy. A specific example would be the need to centralize a component of professional development expenditures required by union contracts (e.g., organization-wide funding for nursing certification) in contrast to decisions at the work unit level to fund nurses to attend ad hoc specialty conferences. Participation is an alternate dimension of centralization that refers to the scope of involvement and influence of organizational members in decision making (Carter & Cullen, 1984). In a study of Belgian hospitals, nurses who perceived that their work decisions were tightly controlled by a supervisor (i.e., high hierarchical centralization) and that they had little influence on program decisions (i.e., low participative centralization) reported lower job satisfaction (Willem et al., 2007).

In addition, hierarchy creates a reporting structure whereby formal lines of communication, in conjunction with role descriptions, delineate the responsibilities and accountability of each position for work processes and outcomes. Organizational positions are traditionally described in terms of staff and line positions (Gulick, 1937). Staff positions are outside the direct hierarchical authority chain. These positions provide expertise and knowledge to support the line positions in meeting the organization's goals. A nursing example of a staff position is a clinical nurse specialist (CNS) who is hired for knowledge development and expert consultation for selected patient groups. Line positions are in the direct line of hierarchical authority from top to bottom in an organization. These positions are central to controlling or generating the product or service of the organization. Line positions include vice presidents, directors, managers, and frontline nurses because these positions are authorized either to supervise production processes or to produce the organization's output. In nursing, although frontline nurses are commonly referred to as "staff" nurses, these nurses hold line positions that deliver services to care recipients.

Hierarchy also enables organizations to assign responsibilities based on the complexity and skill requirements of the work and to ensure individual accountability (Jaques, 1990). Responsibility is the allocation and acceptance of a task. Responsibility is the obligation to take on and accomplish work and to secure the desired results. A manager assigns or delegates responsibility to a subordinate, and thus responsibility flows down the organizational chain. In accepting the obligation of an assigned task, the staff person is accepting responsibility to accomplish the task. Accountability is the liability for task performance and is determined in a retrospective analysis of what occurred. The assignment of responsibility and the granting of authority create accountability. Accountability flows upward or outward: from staff to manager or from provider to client. Reporting relationships are important to create channels of appeal (Weber, 1978) and to ensure employees are held accountable for the work assigned (Jaques, 1990). In turn, managers require the necessary authority to ensure the completion of work (Gulick, 1937; Jaques, 1990). The manager represents the organization at the point of contact with staff, and thus the reporting relationship is also a mechanism by which staff can access organizational resources to identify and solve complex problems (Blau, 1968). Ideally, managers also apply their leadership skills to reporting relationships to release the energy and talents of people in ways that add value to the work performed (Jaques, 1990). Examples of "value added" include improved employee productivity, organizational commitment, and organizational citizenship behaviors.

ORGANIZATIONAL CHARTS

Hierarchy reflects the formal structure of the organization, which can be identified on an organizational chart. An organizational chart is a visual display of the organization's positions and the intentional relationships among positions. The organizational chart reflects the various positions and the formal relationships between and among the positions and, by extension, the people who are a part of the organization. The organizational chart generally presents the line positions, linked together by solid lines to show the flow of authority. Administrative roles are generally shown in vertical and horizontal dimensions. Staff positions or advisory bodies may be depicted on the chart with dotted lines to show consultative relationships. Organizational charts help with administrative control, policy making and planning, and the evaluation of the organization's strengths and weaknesses. Charts are used to orient personnel because relationships and expected patterns of interaction within the formal organization are made clear. For example, an organizational chart of a matrix structure may show dotted lines for the project or interdisciplinary team relationships. Dotted lines mean that a relationship to the position or the group would form for a project. In the process of applying for a job, obtaining the employer's organizational chart will help understand the relative positioning of individuals within the organization and how the organization is structured—or at least how decision makers believe it is structured.

In addition to a formal structure, organizations are characterized by an informal structure. The informal structure is simply the network or pattern of social relationships and friendship circles that are outside the formal structure. It is an interconnected web of relationships that operate in and around the formally designated lines of communication. The informal structure does not appear on the formal organizational chart.

ORGANIZATIONAL SHAPES

The shape of an organization structure can be described as relatively tall or flat. Several structural factors influence the shape of an organization. The formal reporting relationships among positions, which ensure the assignment of responsibility, authority, and accountability, result in hierarchical levels. The **span of control** of managers, which is the number of employees reporting directly to a management position, also influences organizational shape (Meyer, 2008). For instance, when managers on average have fewer direct-report staff, the organizational shape is relatively taller. Another structural factor involves decisions about the number of management layers in the hierarchy (i.e., **scalar principle**). Increased layers of management help the organization cope with increasing work complexity and extended time lines (Jaques, 1990). A tall organization structure assumes a pyramidal shape with multiple management layers (Figure 18.5). In contrast, a flat organization structure has minimal management layers (Figure 18.6). Advantages and disadvantages associated with tall and flat organizational shapes are summarized in Table 18.2. However, a narrow focus

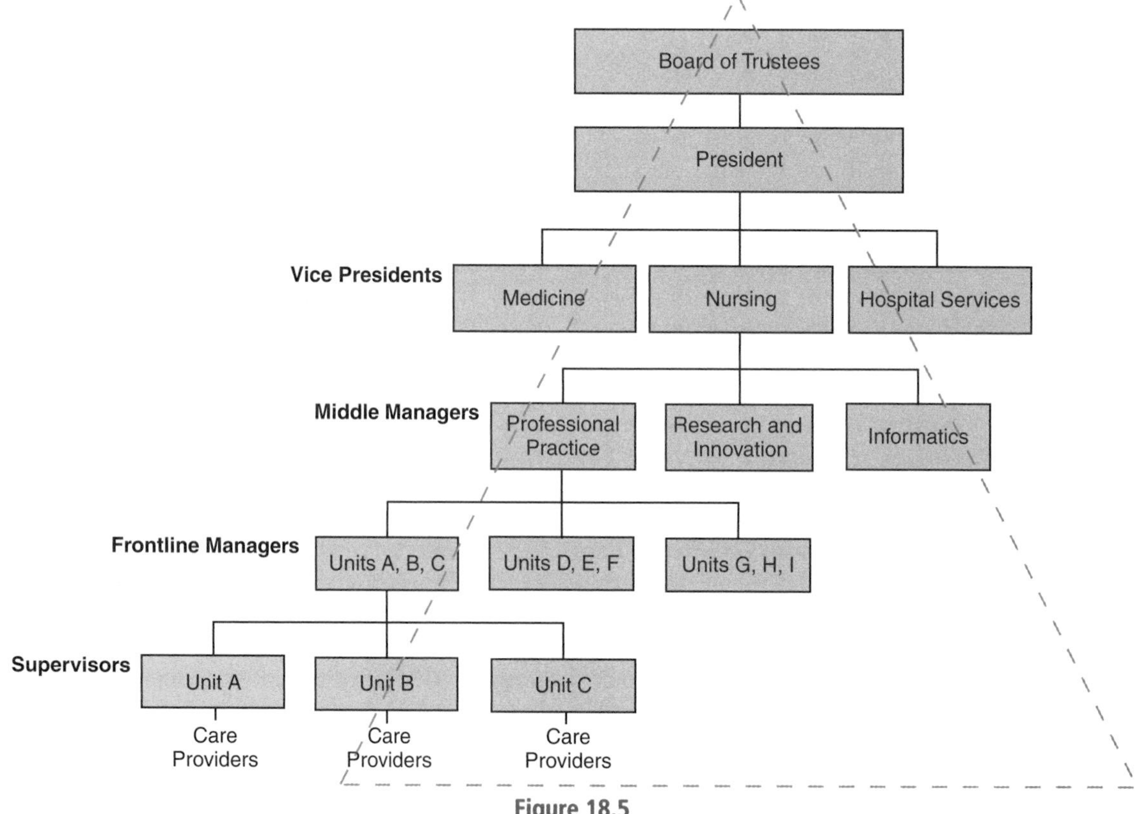

Figure 18.5
Simplified tall organizational structure.

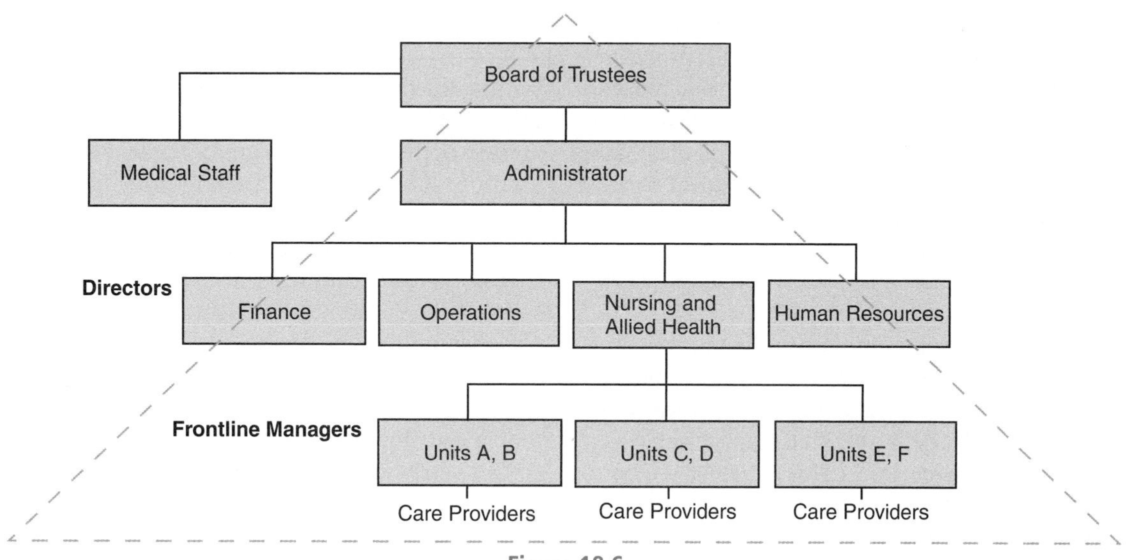

Figure 18.6
Simplified flat organizational structure.

Table 18.2

Comparison of Flat and Tall Organization Structures

	Tall Organization	Flat Organization
Advantages	Increased access to managers and organizational resources Greater supervisory capability Layers of skill to deal with varying degrees of work complexity Layers of accountability for work completion Layers of responsibility to address short-term, medium-term, and long-term issues and planning	Fewer divisions facilitate streamlining of goals, problem-solving, and resource use Greater hierarchical decentralization; potential for greater staff autonomy through increased delegation Greater innovation Enhanced responsiveness to consumers at point of service Less cross-coordination required Less costly management infrastructure
Disadvantages	More hierarchical centralization; potential to micro-manage staff activities Slowed vertical decision making and distorted communication Less innovation Difficult way-finding for consumers Greater cross-coordination required Costly management infrastructure	Decreased access to managers and organizational resources Decreased supervisory capability Overextension of managers Vertical communication delays

on the hierarchical structure of an organization without attention to the people and processes within the organization, or the outcomes achieved, can be misleading. For instance, factors that can potentially offset the effects of tall organizations include the competence and leadership of members, the use of merit-based rewards, the effectiveness of reporting relationships, and the sharing of information and authority (Ashkenas, 1999; Jaques, 1990).

Span of management refers to the number and ordering of management positions and resources relative to other personnel and can be measured at organizational, departmental, managerial, work group, or employee levels (Meyer, 2008). There are many competing theoretical arguments about factors influencing the span of management, and decisions about the amount, type, and distribution of nursing management resources within health care organizations are influenced by a multitude of factors at the consumer, nurse, work group, manager, organizational, and regional levels (Table 18.3) (Meyer, 2008). A key controversy about the span of control of nurse managers relates to supervisory responsibilities. On the one hand, wider spans of control for managers are proposed because nurses and other health care professionals are experts committed to professional codes of ethics and regulated standards, therefore requiring less direct supervision (Meier & Bohte, 2003). On the other hand, narrow spans of control are deemed necessary because (1) nurses require managerial support and access to organizational resources and information to coordinate complex work processes to achieve positive outcomes (Blau, 1968; Laschinger et al., 1999), and (2) the introduction of unregulated workers into health care settings has required more direct, hands-on supervision to ensure that care standards and organizational expectations are met. This counter-argument suggests that the span of control of frontline nurse managers should factor in the needs of staff for manager support and supervision. In nursing, relationships between the span of control of frontline managers and nurse and patient outcomes have been investigated.

POWER

Within the objective perspective, power has been conceptualized as a resource. Kanter's (1977) theory of the structural determinants of behavior in organizations has been investigated in nursing systems (Laschinger, 1996). For Kanter, power refers to "the ability to get things done, to mobilize resources" (p. 166). It is not the power to control or dominate others. When power is shared, rather than monopolized, employees are empowered and the organization is more likely to benefit. More activity can be accomplished by organizational members, and the capacity for effective action is increased. Kanter (1977) described three work empowerment structures: opportunity, power, and proportion. The structure of *opportunity* refers to expectations and future prospects (i.e., opportunities for growth, mobility, job enrichment). The structure of *power* stems from access to information, support, and resources. The structure of *proportion* denotes the social composition of the organization's workforce (e.g., gender, minorities). Empowered work environments are those in which all employees have access to opportunities to learn and grow and to information, support, and resources necessary for the job. Indeed, frontline nurses' job-related empowerment has been positively associated with various nurse outcomes, including organizational commitment (Laschinger & Finegan, 2005; Young-Ritchie et al., 2007); intent to remain in the organization (Nedd, 2006); and interactional justice, respect, trust in management, and job satisfaction (Laschinger & Finegan, 2005). Nurses who occupy positions at higher levels in the nursing hierarchy report increasingly greater degrees of empowerment (Laschinger, 1996). Thus nurses in management positions are likely to perceive greater access to opportunity and power structures than frontline nurses.

In Kanter's (1977) study, effective leaders were seen as both competent and powerful. Sensitivity with subordinates was secondary to having upward credibility within the organization; leaders to whom others listened, who accessed resources, and who produced results within the

Table 18.3

Factors Influencing the Span of Management in Healthcare

Level	Factors
Region	Funding and administration models, health care system structures and cultures; degree of reform; cross-border service use; health care worker mobility[e]; population growth; geography; sectors[d]; technology[a]
Organization	Size; stage of development; degree of decentralization of support services (e.g., human resources, finances)[a]; culture[a,h]
Manager	Organizational level[e]; scope of responsibilities[a,b,e,h]; mix of assigned areas[b]; profession[b,e]; leadership[c,f]; skills[a,d,e]; education[a,e,h]; experience[a]; budget[b,g]; reporting demands[g]; support roles[a,b,h]; diversity of staff functions[a,g]
Work Group	Care delivery models[a,h,i]; professional and skill mixes[a,g,h]; staffing stability[g]; unit type and size[b,h]; occupancy rates[a,g,h]; task interdependence[a]; distance or location[a,b,h]
Employee	Profession and need for supervision[a,i]; education[a]; experience[h]; work stability[h]; complexity[a]
Health Care Consumers	Acuity; care complexity and duration; immediacy of decisions; degree of coordination[a]

Reproduced from Meyer, R.M. (2008). Span of management: Concept analysis. *Journal of Advanced Nursing, 63*(1), 104-112. This material is used by permission of Blackwell Publishing.
[a]Alidina & Funke-Furber, 1988.
[b]Altaffer, 1998.
[c]Doran et al., 2004.
[d]Filerman, 2003.
[e]Mahon & Young, 2006.
[f]McCutcheon, 2004.
[g]Morash et al., 2005.
[h]Pabst, 1993.
[i]Redman & Jones, 1998.

broader organization were perceived to be effective. Kanter (1977) proposed that effective leadership evolves from both formal and informal sources of power in the organization. Formal power is derived from work that is relevant to pressing organizational issues and that provides opportunities to perform extraordinary and highly visible activities; informal power comes from relationships and alliances with people in the organization.

Kanter (1977) also theorized that "power begets power" (p. 168). Research indicates that nurses who are managed by empowered leaders also are empowered (Laschinger, 1996). For example, front-line nurses in organizations in which chief nurse executives had line authority reported significantly greater global empowerment with respect to resources than their counterparts in organizations in which chief nurse executives had staff authority (Matthews et al., 2006). The authors suggested that the formal power accessible to nurse executives with line authority enabled them to secure the staffing resources necessary for frontline nurses to provide high quality of care. Considered overall, the research suggests that empowerment structures positively impact both nurses and managers and can inform the design of the organizational structures in which nurses work.

LEADERSHIP AND MANAGEMENT IMPLICATIONS

The global and local challenges for nursing within organizations and across systems are numerous. Leaders and managers can influence the structure in which goals are accomplished. In fact, determining the structure is a key responsibility of leaders and managers in planning an organization that is conducive to high-quality nursing care. As environments and technologies evolve, the management team may need to rethink and redesign the organization and work-group structures to better match the changing conditions and to achieve the desired outcomes. In nursing, determining the structure is a planning and organizing aspect of the management process that can be informed by evidence and theory from the management field. According to the Institute of Medicine (2004), just as clinicians are compelled to seek, evaluate, and apply empirical evidence, so too should managers incorporate management research in their practice.

Leaders and managers may be involved in revising or changing organizational structures. *Restructuring* means revising or modifying the structure to reshape it or switch to another structural form. Restructuring efforts have typically been geared toward fixing existing operational processes. Lean, decentralized, self-governing organizations that empower first-line caregivers are the preferred structures. Reengineering is a radical redesign of business processes (Hammer & Champy, 1993; Moss et al., 1994). To begin anew, processes are analyzed from the point of view of the consumer, as well as the requirement to achieve greater cost containment, quality, service, and speed. User-friendly processes, efficiency, and economy are key ideas. Job redesign focuses on who does what tasks and on maximizing flexibility, cross-training, and productivity (Curtin, 1994).

Changes to organization structure afford opportunities to empower nurses. Strategies include maximizing nurses' scope of practice, creating autonomous and visible nursing roles relevant to organizational priorities, providing more leadership opportunities for nurses at all levels, and clinical laddering (Registered Nurses' Association of Ontario [RNAO], 2006). Fiscal and material resources can also be deployed to empower nurses by facilitating access to knowledge development opportunities (e.g., courses, conferences) and by providing adequate resources for job completion (e.g., staffing). A decentralized, participative structure can be promoted through coordination mechanisms that involve nurses in councils and task forces (e.g., related to clinical practice or nurse retention) and in information exchange (e.g., newsletters, open forums, web technologies).

A transparent and participative approach to the development of programming devices to standardize work processes (e.g., care maps, electronic health records) can be used to build shared goals for interdisciplinary teams. Organizations can also deliberately foster informal coordination mechanisms to enhance the relational and functional networks in which work is accomplished (Galbraith et al., 2002). For example, physical co-location, communal space, communities of practice, rotational job assignments, electronic chat groups, and interdisciplinary training programs can foster spontaneous interactions and relationships across functional, professional, and geographical silos, resulting in knowledge sharing, problem solving, and innovation (Galbraith et al., 2002).

Hierarchical reporting relationships can be greatly enhanced by transformational leaders who establish trust with nurses by communicating role and behavior expectations, by giving constructive performance feedback, and by recognizing and rewarding successes (RNAO, 2006). When workers fall outside organizational lines of authority (e.g., outsourced services, nursing agencies), managers and leaders require skill in negotiating standards and performance outcomes, in resolving problems across organizational boundaries, and in building relationships and shared goals to overcome differing alliances (Porter-O'Grady, 2003).

In more highly matrixed organizations, nurse managers and leaders must network with interdisciplinary stakeholders within and across programs and support services. Success for leaders with line authority requires strong relational skills, credibility, an ability to link resource use to outcomes using a business model, and an in-depth understanding of the needs of clients and staff (Lorenz, 2008). The trends toward increased outsourcing, decreased reliance on traditional in-patient services for revenues, and increased specialization of health services require an entrepreneurial skill set and innovative leadership roles to build business partnerships and alliances and to foster change at the point of service delivery (Porter-O'Grady, 2007). In the context of nurse and manager shortages, organizations need to recruit and deploy management resources in line with objectives by re-evaluating the number of management layers and the span of control of individual positions, as well as by developing a nursing leadership succession plan. To be supportive of nursing staff, nurse managers need access to the support and information of senior management and peers, professional development and mentorship, an office easily accessible to staff, administrative support, and a strong and shared organizational culture (Kramer et al., 2007).

CURRENT ISSUES AND TRENDS

During the 1990s, health care systems in many developed countries were subjected to restructuring, decentralization, specialization, and performance management, resulting in the de-layering of management structures in an effort to contain

LEADERSHIP & MANAGEMENT BEHAVIORS

Leadership Behaviors

- Inspires a shared vision of an ideal or desired structure
- Prompts and motivates the group to restructure when necessary
- Ensures nursing representation and involvement in decision making across the structure
- Enables staff to function within the structure
- Uses relational skills to engage internal and external stakeholders

Management Behaviors

- Collaborates in the development of an organizational chart
- Critically evaluates and integrates research into structural design and evaluation
- Scans the environment and plans for restructuring to match environmental conditions
- Plans the structure and decides on line and staff positions
- Decides on number and types of positions and related duties
- Negotiates standards, performance expectations, and deliverables for external contracts
- Monitors accountability and deliverables
- Provides authority to match responsibility
- Implements and evaluates structure for effectiveness and desired outcomes
- Monitors stresses and strains created by structure

Overlap Areas

- Influences people to work within a structure or across structures
- Plans and develops the structure
- Makes decisions about the management structure
- Generates an empowering environment at all levels within the structure

costs and achieve outcomes (Canadian Nursing Advisory Committee, 2002; Mahon & Young, 2006). Those managers remaining in the system faced expanded roles. Instead of a traditional head nurse role responsible for patient care on a single unit, the role of the nurse manager typically grew to encompass the management of finances, operations, and human resources across multiple clinical areas and services in program management structures with regulated and unregulated multidisciplinary staff (Duffield & Franks, 2001; McGillis Hall & Donner, 1997; Shaffer, 2003).

The twenty-first century has ushered in significant concerns related to the global community and public safety. These issues are intensified by calls for transparency, accountability, and public reporting in the management of health care services, which in turn, have increased demands on the internal structures and external boundaries of organizations. There is a trend toward planning and coordinating efforts across organizations and jurisdictions, which has been mirrored in the field of organization theory. The focus has shifted from "intra-organizational" to "inter-organizational" phenomena (e.g., clusters, networks, international strategic alliances) (Clegg & Hardy, 1999).

At a global level, increasing shortages of nurses and other health care professionals has engendered a call for developed countries to create self-sufficient and sustainable nursing workforces by increasing domestic supply (Little & Buchan, 2007). This requires jurisdictional planning and coordinated activities and investments across health systems and organizations. At the organizational level, employers need to attract and retain nurses through changes to work conditions and structures (e.g., creating full-time positions, re-dividing work to remove non-nursing tasks, supplying adequate staffing and material resources to accomplish the work) (Little & Buchan, 2007). These strategies are necessary to stabilize the nursing workforce within organizations and to ensure that nursing intellectual capital, the knowledge, skills, and competence that nurses possess (Covell, 2008), are retained in the organization.

At a societal level, preparedness for disasters, bioterrorism, and pandemics has required health care organizations, communities, and jurisdictions to pool resources and coordinate activities along the external boundaries of organizational structures. In addition, the movement toward clinical integration across settings to provide seamless care and to better manage chronic illness has generated significant boundary and inter-organizational work. Clinical integration is a delivery mechanism whereby hospitals and physicians share responsibility and information about care recipients across settings for a single care episode or longer (Taylor, 2008). However, clinical integration efforts continue to be challenged by significant legal, financial, regulatory, and leadership issues across jurisdictional and organizational boundaries (Taylor, 2008; Thielst, 2007). Traditional institutional health care services have decreased in intensity and duration and shifted to outpatient or community-based formats (Porter-O'Grady, 2007). An associated consequence has been the compression of nursing care because of shortened lengths of stay and increased patient acuity, as well as the outsourcing of support services (Birch et al., 2003; Porter-O'Grady, 2007).

Increased awareness and disclosure about medical errors and preventable adverse events have encouraged organizations to address consumer safety through risk reduction and the development of cultures of safety (Academy of Canadian Nurse Executives & Association of Canadian Academic Healthcare Organizations, 2005; Leape & Berwick, 2005). To address safety, new coordination mechanisms and safety standards are based on the science of human factors engineering, which takes a systems approach to understanding and preventing critical incidents (Hoffman et al., 2006). A systems approach considers how adverse events occur in relation to management, organization, and regulatory factors such as policies and procedures, information technology, staffing practices, and physical structures (Hoffman et al., 2006). Recall that policies, procedures, and information systems are coordination devices. For instance, safety risks may be reduced when nurses standardize care through the use of evidence-based care maps. Organizations are also compelled to collaborate in the development and sharing of safety innovations. The Center for Quality Improvement and Safety in the United States (Leape & Berwick, 2005) and the Canadian Patient Safety Institute in Canada are examples of how safety innovations can be widely shared and standardized across organizations.

Summary

- Health care organizations must structure to achieve efficiency, accountability, and quality outcomes.
- Objective, subjective, and postmodern theoretical perspectives highlight the varied assumptions about the purpose, social structure, management, and power within organizations.
- Organizational design theories approach the organization as a social system amenable to measurement, prediction, and manipulation.
- Contingency theory proposes that there is no one right way to structure; structure is influenced by multiple factors (e.g., technology, size, strategy, environment).
- The social structure of an organization is essentially a network of relationships that divides and coordinates the work, resulting in different organization forms.
- Organizational shape is influenced by hierarchy and the distribution of managerial resources in terms of span of control and the scalar principle.
- Decision-making authority can be centralized or decentralized within the hierarchy and may vary according to whether the decision is clinical or corporate in nature.
- Empowered work environments ensure that all employees have access to career growth opportunities, as well as the information, support, and resources necessary for the job.

CASE STUDY

Bed Turnaround

Between 11 AM and 8 PM, as many as 17 patients will be discharged and new patients will be admitted on a medical-surgical unit with 34 beds. The responsibility for patient transport and housekeeping duties belongs to the support associate (SA). The SA is pulled away from cleaning a room four or five times per room to transport patients for discharge or to and from ancillary testing. Meanwhile, new admissions are held in the emergency department or outpatient center, awaiting a clean bed. Often, a centralized housekeeping team is STAT-paged to clean the room.

Further analysis identifies that the lack of trust between departments in this facility often results in sending out "spies" to "truly assess" bed status. Lack of teamwork exists between the SAs and housekeeping personnel. The average bed turnaround time from the point of patient discharge to the bed being ready for occupancy is 82 minutes.

As a result, a multidisciplinary team is formed to identify options for reducing bed turnaround time and to evaluate the SA role. Team members consist of an administration representative, the medical-surgical unit manager, three SAs, two housekeeping personnel, a unit clerk, the housewide bed coordinator, and one registered nurse (RN).

Through the work of this team, the reporting relationship of the unit-based housekeeper responsible for cleaning the common areas (e.g., nurses' station, waiting rooms, and hallways) is changed to a matrix reporting structure in which the housekeeper reports directly to the Director of Environmental Services but also has a dotted-line relationship to the individual department director. In addition, a centralized support associate STAT team is initiated to work from 1 PM to 11:30 PM Monday through Friday and 7 AM to 3 PM on Saturdays. Dispatch of the STAT team is delegated to the charge RN via a beeper versus going through the centralized Environmental Services Department. On the off-shift, the STAT

SA team reports to and is dispatched by the off-shift supervisor. Finally, one SA per unit is assigned to perform strictly discharge room cleaning, which eliminates transport interruptions. As a result of these structure and role changes, the time from discharge of a patient to the time a bed is ready is decreased 53%.

Bed Turnaround Process

Indicator	Baseline July/August/ September 2008	February 2009
Discharge of patient to bed ready	82 minutes	38 minutes

CRITICAL THINKING EXERCISE

Nurse Caitlin Schultz recently transferred from a director role in an inpatient nursing unit to assume the director role of another department. The previous department director had established a council for recruitment and retention. Composed of three registered nurses and two social workers, this team established a program to fund flowers for any staff member experiencing a family death, wedding, or birth; organized holiday activities at the department level; and assisted the director in recognizing staff members during Nurses' Week.

As part of the annual Nurses' Week celebration, each nursing employee was recognized at the department level with an awards luncheon, attended many different scheduled events, and received a tote bag with the hospital's logo. Within 1 month of starting the new role, the director attended the first Recruitment & Retention Council meeting, at which the team was discussing preparation for the upcoming week by recognizing one of the nursing specialties practiced in their department.

Staff discussions centered on how to obtain more money from the budget to buy yet another gift for only RN staff members. As the conversation continued, the director became concerned that the focus of the team was centered on recognizing only the RNs (as accomplished during Nurses' Week activities) versus focusing on the work and contributions of the entire department as it pertained to that particular specialty.

1. Is there a problem?
2. What is the problem?
3. How can the director's authority, responsibility, and accountability be explained?
4. What elements of organizational structure could be helpful in this situation? Which could be barriers?
5. What options are there to refocus the team?
6. What problems and decisions face the staff nurses?
7. What challenges face the director?

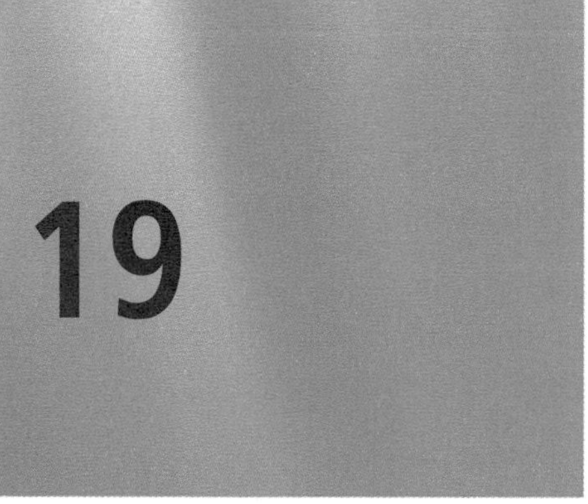

Decentralization and Shared Governance

Claudia DiSabatino Smith

CHAPTER OBJECTIVES

- Define and differentiate centralization and decentralization
- Describe examples of centralization and decentralization
- Define and describe shared governance
- Describe one shared governance model
- Evaluate problems associated with implementation of shared governance
- Explore research related to shared governance
- Analyze and identify possible solutions to a case study via critical thinking methods
- Exercise critical thinking to conceptualize and analyze possible solutions to a practice exercise

The growing disparity between the supply and demand of registered nurses poses new challenges for nursing and health care administrators. The preliminary findings of the 2004 National Sample Survey of Registered Nurses indicated that the number of licensed RNs increased only 7.9% (U.S. Department of Health and Human Services [USDHHS], 2005) since 2000, when the previous survey was conducted. In addition to fewer people entering and staying in nursing, the nursing workforce is aging. Approximately 40% of the U.S. nurse workforce is projected to be older than 50 years by the year 2010 (USDHHS, 2005; U.S. General Accounting Office, 2001). Factors that are leading to an impending crisis in health care include the shrinking nursing workforce, the aging population, the coming of age of the Baby Boomer generation, and the increased need for health care services for the aging population. The call for the provision of safe, reliable, high-quality patient care in an affordable, efficient, portable, and transparent system has become a critical issue (Bush, 2006). The widely documented global nursing shortage has been characterized as more complex and of greater magnitude than any past nursing shortages (American Nurses Association, 2002; Robert Wood Johnson Foundation, 2002) and continues to impact the provision of quality patient care. Research studies that link nurse-patient staffing ratios to patient outcomes (Aiken et al., 2002) paint an even bleaker picture in view of the nursing shortage and the renewed focus on patient safety (Institute of Medicine [IOM], 2004; The Joint Commission [TJC], 2007). In response to the technical and social transformation, maturing technology, and more educated patients, health care systems are reconfiguring clinical care and service delivery to more mobile, fast-paced, consumer-driven models. Such changes provide additional convenience for patients and less need for inpatient nursing staff to care for uncomplicated patients, but they do not lessen the need for nurses to provide highly technical care to complex patients with multiple co-morbidities.

Recommendations to improve the nursing shortage include the implementation of measures found in Magnet™-designated hospitals that appear to improve nurse retention through increased job satisfaction (Hatcher et al., 2006). The implementation of such strategies empowers nurses, leading to increased professional autonomy and active participation in decision making on issues of nursing practice and the work environment (Tourangeau et al., 2006). One such strategy is the reconfiguration of traditional hierarchical organizational structures that include multiple levels of managers, which have historically contributed to nurses' frustration with their lack autonomy and decision-making authority. The traditional organizational structure is no longer adequate to support a professional practice model of nursing because of the increasing numbers of nurses who have pursued advanced nursing education. Implementing a shared governance model is one means of empowering nurses to make decisions at the point of care regarding patient care and the practice environment.

DEFINITIONS

Shared governance is a model of organizational decision making premised on a decentralized organizational structure in which staff nurses are empowered through autonomy and accountability. Although it requires an organizational philosophy of belief in the value of shared power and decision making, shared governance is discussed as an aspect of an organization's power structure. Terms related to the concept of shared governance include *centralization, decentralization, horizontal decentralization, organizational chart, selective decentralization, synergy, span of control, and vertical decentralization.*

MANAGEMENT CENTRALIZATION AND DECENTRALIZATION

Hospitals are organized and their work is structured around a guiding philosophy. The philosophy serves as the institutional framework that shapes the direction of the acquisition of knowledge and skills and is the pivotal factor in the course of the long-term development of the institution.

LEADING & MANAGING DEFINED

Shared Governance

An accountability-based model of shared decision making that leads to the empowerment and autonomy of professional nurses; through shared decision making, nurses at the point of service have control over their nursing practice, peer issues, education, quality, and work environment.

Organizational Chart

Visual representation of the framework that demonstrates horizontal and vertical reporting relationships within an organization.

Selective Decentralization

A concentration of power for decision making that resides in functional divisions within the organization; examples include a central sterile processing department, central pharmacy, central human relations department.

Centralization

The extent to which power and authority for decision making rests in top levels of the organization.

Decentralization

The extent to which power and authority for decision making are systematically dispersed to middle and lower levels of the organization; examples include vertical decentralization, horizontal decentralization, and selective decentralization.

Span of Control

The number of subordinates who report to one manager.

Synergy

A condition that exists when parts of an organization interact to produce a joint effect that is greater than the sum of the parts acting alone; the concept that the whole is greater than the sum of its parts (e.g., 1 + 1 = 3).

Organizations that invest in knowledge that increases the productivity of human capital or improves the tacit knowledge of their professional staff are likely to experience productivity increases that are consistent with the growth of the economy (North, 1990). The mission statement, core values, and vision are the instruments that give voice to the organization's philosophy. Likewise, the **organizational chart** is a visual representation of the horizontal and vertical reporting structure of the organization. The organizational chart visually illustrates the chain of command, the span of control for managers, and its operating relationships. Figure 19.1 illustrates an example. At a glance, the chart permits the trained observer to make a statement about the organizational philosophy of the organization—whether the authority is primarily centralized or decentralized (Straub & Attner, 1994).

Centralization and decentralization can be viewed as organizational philosophies about power distribution that pertain to the hierarchical level of decision-making authority in the institution. Institutions organize and structure themselves by defining departmental function and authority relationships to achieve a more coordinated effort. An institution's organizational philosophy drives plans and decisions about who reports to whom, as well as who does what. Executives may use **selective decentralization** where power for decision making is concentrated in the functional areas of staffing, purchasing, and operations. Alternatively, they may choose to set limits on purchases at each level of the organization by dollar amounts. A well-organized institution can plan, implement, and evaluate strategies much more effectively than a poorly organized institution.

Centralization and **decentralization** are relative terms when applied to the operating philosophy of institutions. In institutions in which the executive leader retains more decision-making authority, the operation takes on a more centralized philosophy. Centralized authority allows for rigid control over decision making and power in the institution. However, as institutions have evolved into more complex global operations, it has become extremely difficult for chief executives to manage the information overload that occurs in a highly

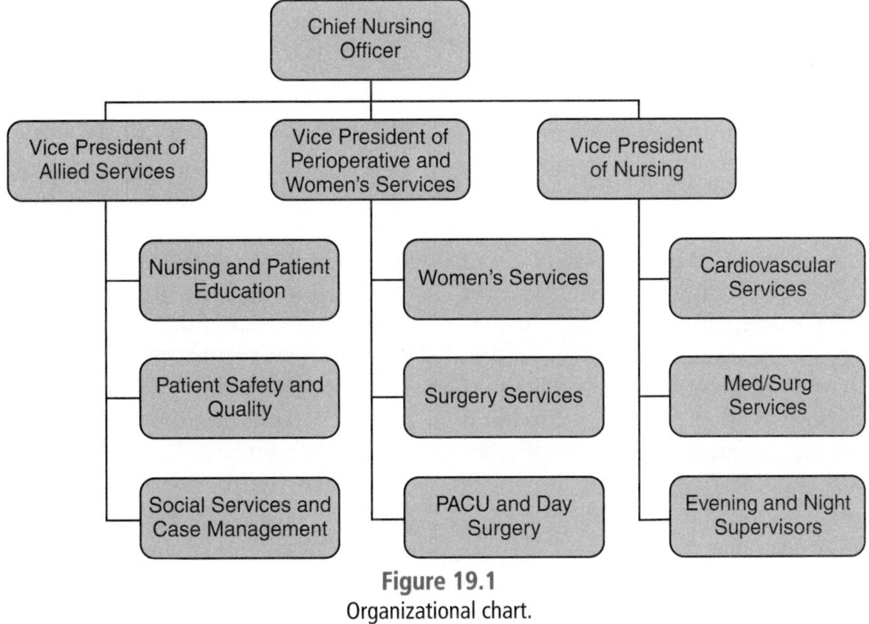

Figure 19.1
Organizational chart.

centralized structure, as well as to stay abreast of new developments. Information asymmetry occurs, bringing about the need for hierarchical development. *Information asymmetry* refers to an imbalance in the level of knowledge about a specific topic or area. An institution with centralized decision making is demonstrated in the following scenario:

> Mary Jones is the nursing director of 2 Main, a medical nursing unit in General Hospital. As such, Nurse Jones interviews nursing applicants to fill the open nursing positions on 2 Main. At the conclusion of the interviews, she offers hiring recommendations to the chief nursing officer (CNO), Sherry Smith. Nurse Smith reviews the file of each applicant interviewed and listens to the recommendation of the nursing director. Nurse Smith usually is in accord with the recommendation of the nursing director, but she holds the final word in the matter. Once the CNO's approval is gained, the nursing director is free to contact the applicant and offer the approved candidate the open position.

Although this is a somewhat simplistic example, the reader should note that the retention of decision-making authority is maintained at the nurse executive level.

In an organization with a more decentralized philosophy, decision-making authority rests in levels closer to the point of service in the organizational framework, rather than in the executive levels of the organizational chart. Institutions with decentralized decision making encourage and facilitate greater innovation, more input, and faster response times. Decisions are made closer to the point of service/care, rather than the information passing up through the chain of command to an executive who is far removed from the situation. "Decision-making that is decentralized and collaborative is an essential component in care environments that support excellence in patient care" (Golanowski et al., 2007, p. 342). However, administrators must ensure that point-of-service nurses have the necessary skills to feel confident in making such decisions. It is important for nurses to have knowledge, expertise, decision-making skills (Golanowski et al., 2007), and conflict resolution and communication techniques to feel comfortable enough to practice autonomously and make effective decisions. In the following scenario, the involvement of empowered professional staff nurses in making a hiring decision that directly impacts them in their workplace is featured:

> Charlotte Black is the nursing director of 4 East, a medical nursing unit in City Hospital. With three staff nurse positions vacant, she posts the openings and selects three staff nurses from her unit to serve as the selection committee who will interview candidates for the positions. Based on the needs of the nursing unit and the availability of nursing applicants who match those needs, Nurse Black screens the files of the applicants. She passes the files of those nurses who meet the requirements for the positions to the selection committee, who then schedules interviews with the applicants. Once the selection committee has interviewed each candidate, it decides on the best candidate for each position. The committee's recommendations, along with the rationale for its choices, are discussed with Nurse Black. Nurse Black meets with the candidates recommended by the selection committee, interviews them, and makes the job offers.

This scenario clearly illustrates a more decentralized organizational philosophy. In this scenario, the CNO does not take an active role in the hiring process of staff nurses. The decision is made based on the input of the staff nurses who will be working side-by-side with the applicant. It is important to note that, although the two examples are extremes that would appear on opposite ends of a continuum, many institutions exhibit varying degrees of centralization or decentralization.

Smaller institutions commonly use a more centralized structure, with more involvement by the CNO in day-to-day matters. As institutions become larger and take on more complicated organizational structures, it is not feasible for the CNO to be involved in all of the smaller-scale decisions.

In the health care arena, in which specialized knowledge abounds, information asymmetry occurs between central leaders and those in the specialty care areas. For example, nurses in the cardiac catheterization laboratory are highly specialized; they are better able to make knowledgeable decisions regarding care of a patient who has a cardiac catheterization than is the CNO or the vice-president of patient care. This represents a clear example of information asymmetry. Information asymmetry is one of the theoretical justifications that lead to the development of hierarchies (Miller, 1992).

Hierarchies develop when decision making is delegated from the top of the organizational level downward to lower operational levels, where specialized knowledge resides. The degree of decentralization may vary from minimal, in which decisions rest in the hands of one or a few leaders, perhaps at the vice-presidential level, to maximal, in which many employees who are at the point of service on the organizational framework are empowered to make decisions. Managers who delegate authority to subordinates find that they can devote more time to planning and evaluating strategies. A philosophy of centralized decision making results in a narrower span of control and more levels of management. An organization with a philosophy of decentralized decision making generally means that the **span of control** should be larger for each manager. When subordinates are empowered to make decisions, fewer levels of management will be required because the staff learn to manage and make decisions about problems at the point of service, or operational level. However, this necessitates that staff are empowered and educated in decision-making skills. One effect of decentralization is that staff members are more vulnerable because fewer people are available to provide functional supervision, to complete quality monitoring, and to carry out unit-specific responsibilities that were previously part of the role of the assistant manager. This situation presents a challenge for nurses in executive positions (Beyers, 1999) and for nurse managers who are saddled with more of the responsibilities that were previously handled by both upper-level administrators and subordinate assistant nurse managers.

Relinquishing decision-making authority to those with the necessary specialized information to make effective decisions allows managers the time to implement strategies to communicate the institutional plan to all employees. Institutions that employ a more decentralized organizational philosophy, emphasize planning and evaluation, and communicate clear goals and objectives to their employees are more likely to develop synergy within the institution. Synergy relates to an increase in effectiveness or achievement that is produced as a result of combined action or cooperation. **Synergy** results when departments or divisions of an institution work together to accomplish a common goal and, in the process, produce a much greater output than each individual department would have attained if working alone (David, 1987).

Nurses provide a unique clinical perspective to policy development and strategic planning. Nurses, like nurse administrators, focus on the design and management of patient care. Facilitating patients' movement through the maze of the health care system has emerged as one of the primary roles of the nurse. The decade of the 1990s, with its emphasis on organizational redesign and systems thinking, brought about significant and long-needed change. The vision of a seamless continuity of care that focuses on the welfare of the patient and family was finally recognized as an urgent need. Although bureaucracy and notions of power continued to be seen as areas of conflict, redesign efforts have focused on open communication across disciplines and shared decision making. The traditional view of organizational barriers within hierarchies, caused by the "silo" effect within disciplines, has been replaced by a more contemporary valuing of multi-disciplinary delivery of care.

SHARED GOVERNANCE

Shared governance has been described as a management strategy to transform the role of nurses from one that was "devalued and subservient to meaningful and autonomous" (Ludemann &

Brown, 1989, p. 49). "Shared governance is more than just a nursing practice framework; it is a partnership between nursing management and clinical staff" (Frith & Montgomery, 2006, p. 274). Advocates of shared governance argue that it is a strategy for leaders to improve patient outcomes through the engagement of knowledgeable, empowered nurses who make decisions and provide quality patient care at the point of service (Porter-O'Grady et al., 1997). Work relationships are based on partnership, accountability, equity, and ownership (Porter-O'Grady et al., 1997) and result in improved quality of care, increased job satisfaction, and commitment to the organization (Porter-O'Grady, 2001; Prince, 1997). Research suggests that registered nurses who are empowered to make decisions about nursing practice and the workplace through shared governance have higher levels of job satisfaction and are more likely to remain in the organization (McClure & Hinshaw, 2002). Shared governance exemplifies decentralized decision making.

Kanter's theory of organizational empowerment (Kanter, 1993) provides the theoretical underpinnings for shared governance. Her theory asserts that social structures in the workplace have a larger impact on attitudes and behaviors than individual personalities. Kanter suggested that avenues of power provide for the sources of structural empowerment in an organization. Avenues of power include access to information, access to resources required to do the job, having the opportunity to learn and grow, and being supported. In addition, she suggested that the informal job factors that influence empowerment are the alliances that workers have with superiors, peers, and subordinates. Workplaces that are structurally empowering provide many of the opportunities for involvement, commitment, and transparency within the institution that shared governance offers. Empowered workers are more likely to have increased feelings of respect for and trust in management and organizational justice, which relates to one's commitment to an organization (Moore & Hutchison, 2007), which may impact retention.

Decentralization and shared governance were strategies first introduced in the late 1970s and employed in the 1980s to address the acute challenges of the nursing shortage, nurse turnover, and nurse retention. The idea was to empower staff nurses by involving them in client care decision making and in some organizational decision making (Jones et al., 1993). This was seen as a radical departure from the traditional hierarchical hospital management structure in which nurses had little authority, little voice in governance, and low control within the organization (Hess, 1994). The situation in the health care market of the first decade of the new millennium is not unlike that of the early 1980s. Aside from the burgeoning nurse shortage and an aging population of both patients and health care workers, there are more career choices available for females, a lack of qualified nursing faculty, and little real change in the hierarchical management style of hospitals. Questions have been raised in the literature as to whether the implementation of shared governance represented a true change in hospital management style or merely served as a cosmetic Band-Aid.

Described as an accountability-based model, shared governance is a vehicle through which nurses actively engage in making decisions regarding nursing practice, quality of patient care, education, nursing peer issues, and issues in the work environment. Shared governance promotes involvement, investment, participation, sharing of power, interdependence, cooperation, horizontal relationships, autonomy, and accountability for nursing decisions. Nursing effectiveness is enhanced through the sense of ownership that comes with more active involvement in the leadership of the organization. Professional practice environments, known for their improved patient outcomes, are characterized by institutions in which nurses have a high level of autonomy, strong leadership, support from administration, and control over their practice, all of which are results of shared governance (Tourangeau et al., 2006). Shared governance is not a theory, a conceptual framework, an organizational principle, or a structure; shared governance is a concept that leads to the empowerment of nurses

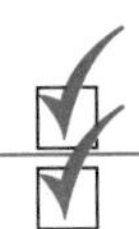

Practical Tips

Tip #1: Ask the Experts

When making decisions, gather information and input from the people closest to the point of service. Nurses at the point of service offer feedback that is based on reality—how things really are—instead of giving information based on how things should be.

Tip #2: Ask the Experts Early

Seek information from point-of-service experts early in the information-seeking process, not as an afterthought. This validates the importance of their feedback for point-of-service experts and avoids wasting time addressing issues that are not the root of the real problem.

Tip #3: Do Not Make Value Judgments on Expert Feedback

Listen openly to feedback from experts. Ask questions to drill down to the core of the problem. Avoid making quick value judgments. Take some time to think about the feedback. Reassemble the group if necessary to ascertain further information and additional thoughts of the group after further consideration.

Tip #4: Do Not Seek Feedback from Experts If You Have Already Made Your Decision

Inviting point-of-service experts to offer feedback serves to empower nurses. However, it can damage leader-staff nurse relationship if the manager/leader ignores feedback in making the decision, the decision is already made and staff feedback was simply a formality, or no decision is made.

and, ultimately, to professional autonomy (Porter-O'Grady, 2003b). It is a journey rather than a single event in time (Porter-O'Grady, 2001; Thompson et al., 2004). Shared governance is seen as a strategy for fostering professional nursing practice through empowerment of nurses.

Empowerment refers to a process whereby nurses recognize that they have legitimate power and authority to make decisions regarding their practice. There is no transfer of power, but merely a change from an external to an internal locus of control. Authority is not given or taken away. Clinicians at the point of service are given the opportunity to be an integral part of the decision-making process, but even more important, they act on the opportunity and are responsible for implementing changes to improve patient care quality and the quality of the work environment. Accountability takes the place of responsibility in clinical practice (Porter-O'Grady, 2001). Empowerment is accomplished through the journey toward shared governance.

The shared governance journey begins with the education of health care executives but must also include education of administrators, managers, and staff nurses. Research suggests that in order for behavioral change to be sustained in an organization, a supporting structure must be in place (Argyris, 1994). The challenge for administrators is not in creating the structure that supports shared governance but, rather, in developing a culture that supports, encourages, and maintains it. Creating the structure is the easy part of the implementation of shared governance (Brooks, 2004). Perhaps the greater challenge for administrators is justification of the cost in terms of personal time and effort and financial commitment. Evidence supports the value of shared governance in nursing practice (George et al., 2002), but a paucity of direct evidence exists regarding the financial cost and benefits of its implementation (Brooks, 2004; Hess, 2004). The literature reveals indirect cost savings that have been attributed to the implementation of shared governance. Such cost savings have been evidenced in the areas of recruitment and orientation, the utilization of registry nurses, and the number of management staff positions (DeBaca et al., 1993). Furthermore, longitudinal research in the area of financial costs and cost benefits, including the return on investment of shared governance implementation, is warranted (Herrin, 2004).

Shared governance is a dynamic process, one that is constantly changing. It changes as the organization changes, as personnel change, and as the times change. "Because shared governance is a continuum, people need to be met where they are on their journey and coached to progress to the next point" (Moore & Hutchison, 2007, p. 565). Education must be continually available to employees in institutions that practice shared governance. Programs are needed to instruct new employees and newly elected unit representatives, to continually develop leadership behaviors in nursing staff, and to support and guide nurse managers. Educational programs should include consensus building and conflict resolution; planning and conducting effective meetings; successful communication techniques and skills; collecting, aggregating, and displaying meaningful data; and strategies for successful problem solving. Nurse managers are key in determining the degree of shared decision making that will actually occur at the unit level. Those managers who are willing to relinquish control and grant staff members the opportunity to undertake the leadership role for unit activities are likely to find additional time for coaching and mentoring, as well as for planning and strategizing. Meanwhile, it is the nurse manager who fosters the development of leadership behaviors in staff nurses, which ultimately leads to the empowerment and autonomy of the nursing staff.

When governance is restricted to the level of the nursing unit, staff autonomy and participative decision making may increase without affecting the overall organizational structure (Hess, 1994). Shared governance in nursing does not exist unless the authority and accountability for decisions that define and regulate nursing practice and those shared with management are solidified with actual decision-making structures and processes (Maas & Specht, 1990). If an institution employs a shared governance model in which patient care quality is truly the primary focus and point-of-service clinical staff members are empowered as knowledge workers and decision makers, this should be reflected in both the organizational chart and resource allocations. One example of such an organizational chart is depicted in Figure 19.1.

One obstacle to the implementation of shared governance is the different levels of knowledge that registered nurses bring to the health care setting as a result of the variety of basic educational programs of nursing. Traditionally, nurses have worked in strong, hierarchical institutions with centralized decision making and clear authority structures, rigid approval mechanisms, and extensive policies and procedures. This presents another obstacle in that such conditions constrain peer-based, lateral, and collegial dialogue. As a result, nurses may not have depth of experience in attending committee meetings, setting agendas, developing consensus, dealing with conflict, and conducting meetings. Additional obstacles to shared governance include inadequate time for education and buy-in by the nursing staff, staff apathy, and insufficient incentives (Golanowski et al., 2007). Finally, nurse leaders and managers who rule autocratically present an obstacle to the implementation of shared governance. For the long-time nurse manager, this radical departure from the traditional autocratic management style presents a whole new paradigm, along with the challenges and uncertainty that accompany it.

In institutions that practice shared governance, the focus shifts from the skill and expertise with which the nurse manager manages the nursing unit to the skill and innovation of the clinical nursing staff. Staff nurses are viewed as knowledge workers (Drucker, 1999). The responsibility for unit outcomes rests with the whole team, not the individual nurse manager. The clinical credibility of the patient care unit's staff nurses impacts the relationships, communications, collegiality, and ability to collaborate with other health care professionals. The nurse manager's role shifts to one of mentoring, coaching, facilitating, enabling, and supporting the staff personnel. The nurse manager builds a culture of trust and respect as he or she role-models adaptation to change, all the while creating an environment in which the care of the patient and family is the central focus. Key elements for successful implementation of shared governance include a client focus, participation in decision making, consensus management, free expression, individual accountability, proper timing, and a sense of cohesion through a common language (Herrick, 1998). Further, the institution that espouses a shared governance philosophy needs to continually focus on recruiting leaders who understand and support the concept of the right people making the right decision at the right location (Golanowski et al., 2007), while continually supporting leaders, managers, and nursing staff with the education and tools to encourage active participation, accountability, and effective decision making.

The degree of nurse participation in decision making varies with shared governance models and may range from minimal or informal participation to true sharing of authority and accountability. In his earlier work, Porter-O'Grady (1987) described three approaches to shared governance in nursing: the *councilor model, congressional model,* and *administrative model.* Ten years later, Porter-O'Grady and colleagues (1997) expanded the focus to include shared governance of whole-systems using the councilor model. The councilor model structures staff and manages governance through the use of committees or councils of elected representatives. Each council is responsible for certain functions and has clearly defined authority. Primary councils within nursing include practice, quality improvement, education, and management. The congressional model is designed much like the U.S. representative form of government, with elected representatives using the democratic process for decision making. The administrative model has two separate tracks—one with a clinical focus and the other with a management focus. Figure 19.2 displays the councilor model as it is defined in one large teaching hospital in a metropolitan area.

For successful implementation of the shared governance concept, a supporting structure must be designed to fit the individual operating philosophy of the institution or health system. Regardless of the structure, implementation of the shared governance concept establishes the expectation for staff nurse participation and the acceptance of personal accountability. With the emergence of multidisciplinary teams and new health care systems, nurses will need to reevaluate the models of shared governance to make way for developing partnerships, but additional analyses may be necessary as health care reform and revised payment mechanisms drive changes in the health care delivery systems.

As integrated networks form "new organizations," lateral and relational designs are emerging to support community-based health care delivery. These organizations are challenged to create delivery systems that promise a seamless continuum of care. Clinical accountability and personal "buy-in" by staff nurses become issues of higher importance as partnerships of multidisciplinary players provide service in multi-site care environments. Shared governance, with its emphasis on mutual respect and accountability, can form the basis for an integrated delivery care system, something that is referred to as *whole-systems shared governance* (Porter-O'Grady et al., 1997). This affords nurses the opportunity to take a leadership role in integrated care networks, based on experiences with decentralization and shared governance.

LEADERSHIP AND MANAGEMENT IMPLICATIONS

Shared governance continues to be one of the many "best practice" options in the nurse leader's toolbox (Herrin, 2004). Although not a new

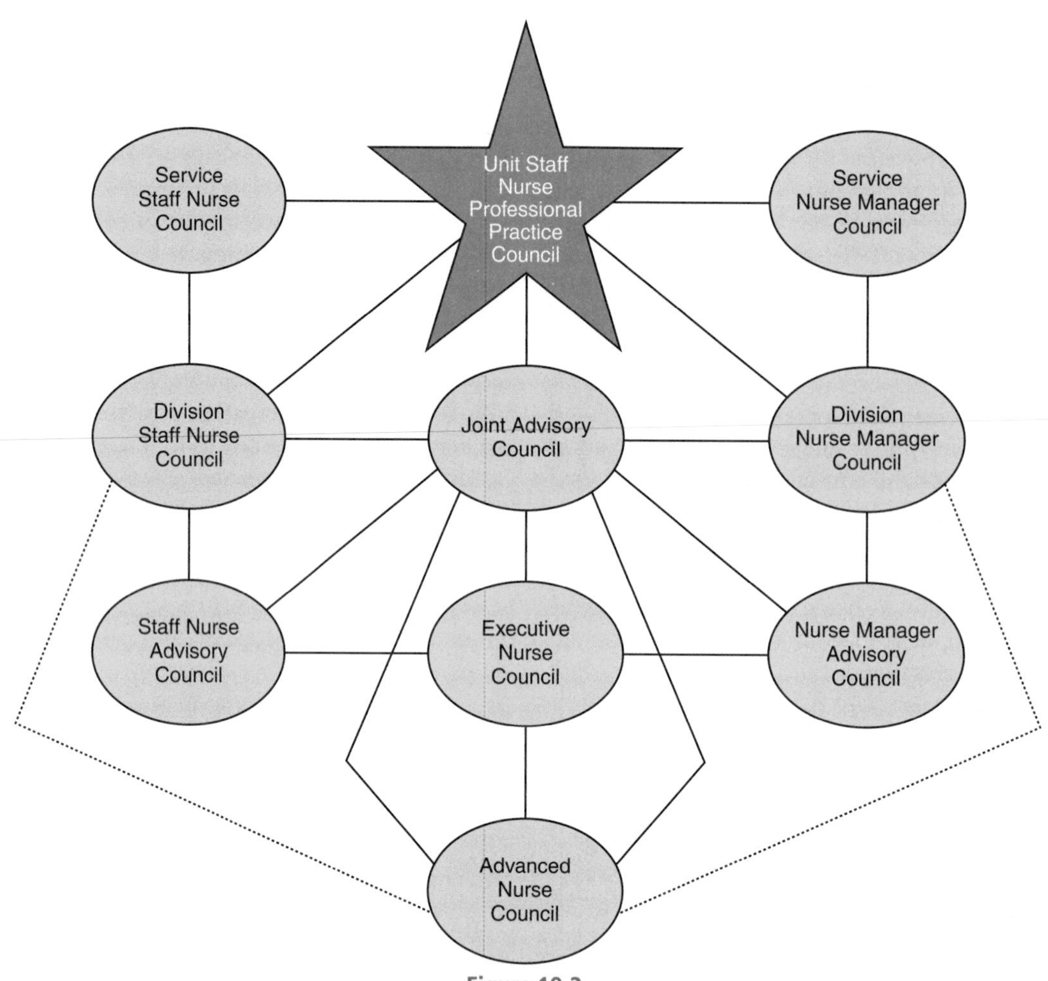

Figure 19.2
Councilor model of shared leadership. (Courtesy St. Luke's Episcopal Hospital, [2000]. Houston, TX: Author.)

concept to the nursing profession, it remains an illusive dream to some and an exhaustive process to others. Shared governance requires slow, gradual development, role-modeling and mentoring by nurse leaders, and continual coaching, nurturing, and education for nursing staff and management. However, institutions that are successful in implementing and maintaining a shared governance culture see evidence of nurses who exude empowerment, autonomy, and commitment to the institution through improved staff nurse retention.

New evidence affirms the need to improve workplace partnerships between nurses and their employing institutions (IOM, 2004) to ensure the future success of health care. Implementation of shared governance is one strategy to create a culture in which individual professional accountability and autonomy are respected and encouraged. By employing the attributes of accountability, partnership, equity, and ownership (Porter-O'Grady, 2003b), a bond is forged between the nurse and the employing organization. Nurses who enter into such bonds are more committed to the institution and less likely to depart. Evidence suggests that feelings of accountability and ownership by staff lead to improved organizational (Finkler

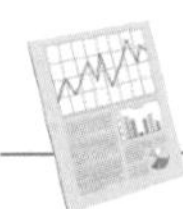

Research Note

Source: George, V., Burke, L.J., Rodgers, B., Duthie, N., Hoffmann, M.L., Koceja, V., et al. (2002). Developing staff nurse shared leadership behavior in professional nursing practice. *Nursing Administration Quarterly, 26*(3), 44-59.

Purpose

The purpose of this research was to demonstrate that implementation of a shared leadership concept educational program in an organized delivery system increases staff use of leadership behaviors, creates professional nursing practice autonomy, and improves patient outcomes. An educational program was offered to professional nurses who wanted to assume greater leadership accountability in the clinical practice environment. Classes consisted of four 8-hour-day modules delivered over a 2-month period to enable participants to practice the concepts on the nursing units. On day 1, the nurses completed a self-assessment with the *Leadership Practices Inventory—Individual Contributor: Self (LPI-IC: Self)* (Kouzes & Posner, 1993). They also distributed the *Leadership Practices Inventory—Individual Contributor: Observer (LPI-IC: Observer)* (Kouzes & Posner, 1993) to five colleagues who work with them in the clinical setting and who would give honest, constructive feedback on the nurse's frequency of leadership behavior use. On the final day, the nurses received a summary comparing the observer feedback with their personal self-assessment.

Discussion

Three studies were conducted between 1995 and 1999 to investigate the process and outcomes of participation in the shared leadership concepts program (SLCP). The first study examined the difference between pre-program and post-program self-perceptions of leadership behavior of nurses who participated in the SLCP and those who did not participate. The second study compared the pre-program and 6-month post-program changes in leadership behavior and professional nursing practice autonomy. The third study described nurses' perceptions of the processes and outcomes associated with their development and continued use of leadership behaviors in the clinical setting after participation in the SLCP.

Application to Practice

In Study 1, there was a statistically significant increase in leadership behaviors between pre-program and post-program for the group who attended the SLCP. In Study 2, the nurses showed statistically significant increases in all five self-reported leadership behaviors (i.e., challenging, inspiring, enabling, modeling, and encouraging) and nursing professional practice autonomy. Neither of the two studies established linkages with patient outcomes. In Study 3, improvements in patient outcomes were documented and were linked to increased use of leadership behaviors. The studies demonstrated that a shared leadership development educational program and the development of a supportive milieu are effective in improving leadership behaviors in the clinical setting and the respective patient outcomes.

et al., 1994; Westrope et al., 1995) and patient outcomes (Aiken et al., 1997; Green & Jordan, 2004; Herrin, 2004; Porter-O'Grady, 2003b). Institutions that implement strategies like "the 14 Forces of Magnetism" demonstrated in Magnet™-designated hospitals realized improved patient outcomes and improved nurse retention (McClure & Hinshaw, 2002). The 14 Forces of Magnetism from the Magnet Recognition Program® addressed each of the following areas (McClure and Hinshaw, 2002):

- Quality of nursing leadership
- Organizational structure
- Management style

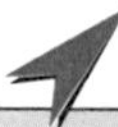

LEADERSHIP & MANAGEMENT BEHAVIORS

Leadership Behaviors

- Integrates work effort
- Facilitates communication
- Coordinates plans and actions
- Envisions an empowered decision-making environment
- Enables participation
- Liaisons with group members and outside the group

Management Behaviors

- Coaches individual employees
- Teaches others how to handle conflict
- Collaborates with staff
- Consults across units
- Creates a participative governance environment
- Communicates widely
- Coordinates work activities

Overlap Areas

- Communicates
- Coordinates activity
- Enables participation in decision making

- Personnel policies and programs
- Professional models of care
- Quality of care
- Quality improvement
- Consultation and resources
- Autonomy
- Community and the hospital
- Nurses as teachers
- Image of nursing
- Interdisciplinary relationships
- Professional development

The implementation of shared governance has far-reaching implications for nurse leaders in today's health care environment in which the focus on health care delivery systems is to provide patient care safely, efficaciously, and efficiently. Involving professionals in the governance of the organizations in which they work is considered pivotal to ensure positive outcomes for costs, coordination of care, and satisfaction (Havens, 1998). Although costs of implementing shared leadership remain uncertain, savings incurred through treatment efficiency, decreased lengths of hospital stay, reduced nurse turnover, and less orientation time cannot be overlooked. Nurses benefit from a renewed sense of commitment to the organization, empowerment, increasing autonomy, and education and training in conflict resolution, collaboration, and decision-making processes. Organizational benefits include increased commitment of staff to the organization; accountability of the nurse; a new level of professional autonomy; a more efficient model for point-of-service decision making; more expert involvement at the point of service; a more assured, confident patient advocate; and improved financial outcomes. Patients benefit from a more efficient model of health care service, more committed health care professionals, quicker responses at the point of service, and a more assured, confident patient advocate.

Nurse leaders stand to realize numerous organizational gains as professional nurses embrace the quest for empowerment and professional autonomy. However, the journey to shared governance is slow and arduous as staff nurses are groomed for opportunities of ownership and accountability and taught how to manage these responsibilities. Guiding counsel from the nursing profession's most nurturing leaders is needed to support both staff nurses and nurse managers as they cope with the change from a hierarchical system to one of shared leadership. Mentoring by clinically credible role models will be an important facet of the transformation toward shared governance.

The goal is to transfer leadership wisdom not only to aspiring leaders but also to all employees.

Along this journey, expert leaders provide tools for employees to do their jobs well and to help them feel successful (Porter-O'Grady & Malloch, 2002).

CURRENT ISSUES AND TRENDS

Shared governance continues to be a viable alternative for many health care organizations and systems. Although a relatively recent innovation, it is recognized as the prime example of a decentralized organizational model. There are as many variations and degrees of shared governance as there are cultures within organizations. Although the concept has been a topic of interest since the early 1970s, the number of average-size health care systems using this accountability-based model continues to be small compared with the number of traditional hierarchical organizational structures.

Models of shared decision making, such as shared governance, make sense in an environment in which workers are valued, supported, and respected. Leaders who capitalize on those principles possess the ability to use synergy to transform the workplace by partnering with the staff who function at the point of service. Visionary leaders encourage expert workers at the point of service to question long-time practices to establish new, more efficient practice models. Such leaders encourage "out of the box" thinking and make allowances for occasional failures. Leaders who cling to traditional management styles instead of embracing an entirely different set of leadership skills may find that their organizations cannot compete successfully in the fast-paced, consumer-driven, technologically advanced health care market. Whatever defines the contextual framework of success in the past can be temptingly easy to use as the measure of current success, resulting in the wrong measure for the right issue (e.g., staffing ratios, more staff, keeping patients longer, more money) (Porter-O'Grady, 2003a).

Both leaders and workers should anticipate continued change. Successful change enhances and improves the worker and the workplace. One strategy employed by proactive leaders to ease the staff's difficulty in accepting change is through small discussion groups in which the popular book *Who Moved My Cheese?* (Johnson, 1998) is read and discussed. Such strategies have been demonstrated to assist staff members to cognitively reframe the idea of change.

The critical nature of the current and forthcoming nursing shortage encourages nursing leaders to consider the 14 Forces of Magnetism (McClure & Hinshaw, 2002) as elemental in developing an organizational culture of excellence, which is critical in their effort to recruit and retain professional nurses. Decentralization of the nursing hierarchy using methodologies such as shared governance is found in most hospitals and health systems that have received Magnet™ designation. Studies demonstrate that Magnet™-designated hospital systems have improved recruitment and retention of professional nursing staff, patient outcomes, and patient satisfaction. Nurses in these systems also report higher role autonomy and greater job satisfaction, as well as higher decision-making abilities and control over practice (Scott et al., 1999). Nurses who have grown in clinical skill and knowledge and developed professionally over years of experience in such a culture of excellence take much knowledge with them as they approach retirement.

The challenge facing tomorrow's nursing leaders will be to design models of care that make use of the knowledge and expertise, the decision-making prowess, and conflict-resolution skill of the aging nurse. In a shared governance culture, the answers to this and other challenging patient care issues may be found in the nurses who provide care at the point of service. It is up to forward-thinking nurse leaders to pose the question and be open to new ideas.

Summary

- Decision-making power is a key element of organizational structure.
- Centralization is the extent to which power and authority for decision making rests at the top of an organizational structure.

- Decentralization is the extent to which power and authority for decision making are systematically dispersed to middle and lower levels of the organization.
- Vertical decentralization is distribution of authority down the chain of command, or line of authority flowing from the top of the organization to the bottom.
- Horizontal decentralization is the flow of power outside the line of authority by which non-management personnel are able to affect decision processes.
- Selective decentralization refers to a concentration of power that resides in functional divisions of an organization.
- *Centralization* and *decentralization* are relative terms on opposite ends of a continuum that indicate levels of decision-making power and authority.
- Shared governance is an accountability-based model of shared decision making that affords professional nurses at the point of service control over their nursing practice.
- Shared governance is a process that leads to the empowerment of professional nurses in the clinical setting.
- Different levels of shared governance exist within health care institutions, just as different cultures exist within different institutions.
- As accountability for nursing practice increases, so do feelings of empowerment and professional autonomy in professional nursing staff.
- Research suggests that hospitals with shared governance have improved nurse retention and improved patient outcomes.
- Some form of decentralization and, specifically, shared governance is evidenced in Magnet™-designated hospitals.
- Obstacles to implementation of shared governance include the varied levels of skill and knowledge of nurses; lack of nurse experience and education about collaboration, conducting effective meetings, decision making, and conflict resolution; and the large number of traditional autocratic nurse leaders and managers.
- Three operating models of shared governance have been identified as councilor, congressional, and administrative. The councilor model is the most common and contemporary.

CASE STUDY

The purpose of this case study is to consider one example of implementing change in a large academic teaching hospital in Houston, Texas, that has had shared governance in place in the department of nursing since 1987. The case study describes an actual scenario that took place in 2007 as related by C. Bishop, RN, chairman of the Staff Nurse Professional Practice Council at St. Luke's Episcopal Hospital.

Ms. Karen Myers, RN, MSN, CNAA-BC, is the senior vice president of patient care and chief nursing officer of St. Luke's Episcopal Hospital, a 700-bed teaching hospital in a large metropolitan area known as the Texas Medical Center of Houston, Texas. Ms. Myers is well respected among her peers and subordinates. She is seen to be a no-nonsense, "tells it like it is" leader. She reports to the executive vice president, who directly reports to the president/chief executive officer of the health system. Ms. Myers has two vice presidents, six directors, and one manager who report directly to her. She has regularly scheduled meetings with each of her direct reports. She encourages them to meet regularly with personnel who report to them. She has an approachable personality, such that nurses who know her throughout the hospital call her by her first name when they see her in the halls or the cafeteria. In meetings in which medical staff are in attendance, she is addressed formally as Ms. Myers.

1. Based on the information presented thus far, can you determine what type of organizational structure is in place? Centralized or decentralized? Explain.
2. What factors do you look for when determining whether an institution has a centralized or decentralized organizational structure?

Late in 2007, St. Luke's Episcopal Hospital, in its commitment to patient safety, implemented many nursing documentation changes in an effort to improve documentation accuracy. New regulations from the Centers for Medicare and Medicare Services for restraint use and documentation necessitated new policies and a new documentation tool. Revised standards from The Joint Commission made it necessary to revise several documentation forms. Because the ICUs document with a paper documentation system and the rest of the hospital uses computerized documentation, changes must be made in both documentation formats. A few of the revised forms were the medication history and medication reconciliation form, a patient screen and referral form, pre-procedure checklists, and a universal transfer form. Revisions in computer documentation were made for the minimum assessment standards, the patient/family education screen, patient goals, and the patient history screen. Each of the revisions was initiated in the appropriate committee and then approved by representatives on each council in the Shared Leadership structure. The Staff Nurse Professional Practice Council (SNPPC) comprises one staff nurse from each patient care unit; the Nurse Manager Council (NMC) consists of all nurse managers; and the Executive Nurse Council (ENC) consists of key nursing administrators from every service within the nursing division, as well as the chairman of both the NMC and the SNPPC. Documentation revisions were ultimately approved and implemented by the hospital Forms Committee. The documentation revisions occurred over a short period, and many of the nursing staff complained to their SNPPC representatives that they were overwhelmed by the number of changes and the short period in which they were initiated. In one of the monthly meetings of the SNPPC, the staff nurses' concerns were discussed. The SNPPC decided to put together a documentation guide to assist staff nurses with the many recent documentation changes. The SNPPC chairman presented the idea to the ENC, where it was unanimously approved. "Do The Write Thing" is an artfully designed binder that presented all of the new changes in documentation in a catchy, colorful, easy-to-read format. One copy of "Do The Write Thing" was distributed to each SNPPC representative for use on each patient care unit. Effectiveness of the SNPPC project was measured by the staff nurses' success in using the forms and articulating to The Joint Commission accreditation team the care provided to the patient as documented on the new forms.

1. Based on the additional information given in the case study, how would you classify Ms. Myer's organizational style? Centralized or decentralized? Explain.
2. How does an institution with shared governance differ from an institution without shared governance?
3. What key factors in the case study help you determine whether this is an example of shared governance, participative management, or autocratic rule?
4. Identify some leadership behaviors that develop in professional nurses as a result of practicing in a shared governance environment.
5. Describe some ways that registered nurses may be involved in governance of the nursing unit when shared governance is fully functioning.

Reference: St. Luke's Episcopal Hospital. (2007). *Shared leadership* (NURSAD-007/IP/500). Houston, TX: Author.

CRITICAL THINKING EXERCISE

Esther Brown complains bitterly as she sees the new schedule posted in the nurses' lounge. Once again she is scheduled to work on the days that she requested to be off. As Dorothy Troy reads on the bulletin board that she has been assigned to do unit-based chart reviews for the next 3 months, she also voices her complaints: "The nurse manager didn't even ask me; she just assigned me! I've never even done it before!" Several staff nurses also are disgruntled because of unresolved issues on the nursing unit. Nursing staff are regularly absent from work, necessitating the use of registry nurses to maintain adequate staffing ratios. The continuity of patient care is suffering. Patients complain regularly that staff members do not answer their call lights promptly. Physicians complain to administration that they can never find a nurse when they need one. And, when they do find a nurse, the nurse can never tell the physicians anything about their patients. The nurse manager is frustrated, exhausted, and discouraged. She laments that she wants to do a good job but just can't get everything done.

1. What are the areas of concern in this scenario?
2. What should Nurse Brown do?
3. What should Nurse Troy do?
4. What strategies would you offer to the nurse manager to improve the situation on the unit?
5. Does this unit represent an example of centralized or decentralized decision making? Explain.

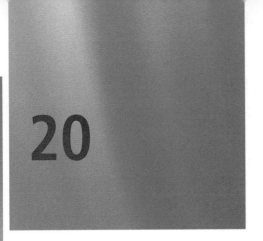

20 Models of Care Delivery

Amy London Deutschendorf

CHAPTER OBJECTIVES

- Determine the differences between professional practice models and care delivery models
- Associate models of care delivery with organizational structure and process variables
- Define and describe the required elements of effective patient care delivery systems
- Classify and define traditional, current, and evolving nursing care models
- Analyze the advantages and disadvantages of each care delivery system
- Evaluate trends shaping the development and use of care delivery systems in the United States
- Describe nursing leadership roles in the development and implementation of care delivery models
- Exercise critical thinking to conceptualize and analyze possible solutions to a practice exercise

The goals of successful patient care delivery include high-quality and low-cost care and the achievement of patient clinical outcomes and satisfaction levels. The ability to reach these objectives depends on the organization's approach to the matching of human and material resources with patient characteristics and health care needs.

The assignment of nursing and multidisciplinary staff to clients needing care is a basic activity of health care systems to achieve these goals. According to the American Nurses Association (ANA), assignment is defined as "The transfer of responsibility for the performance of a task from one individual to another while retaining accountability for the outcome" (ANA, 2005, p. 1). The assignment must be within that individual's scope of practice. An element of assignment is delegation, which can be defined as the "transfer of responsibility for the performance of the activity from one individual to another while retaining accountability for the outcome" (ANA, 1997, p. 1). Both assignment and delegation are methods used by managers to deliver patient care within the structure of the health care system. The determination of the structure and method by which assignments are made is a managerial responsibility. Although this is part of a process of developing a model of nursing care delivery, it reflects a unidimensional framework that does not consider the structural and contextual factors that make up a model for professional group practice in a complex health care environment (Anthony et al., 2004). The historical methods of providing patient care based on industrial-age concepts of organization, linear processes, and roles aligned with distinct and separate departments are not workable in the current information age (Wiggins, 2006). Pure nursing care delivery models, mainly reflecting the care of the patient by registered nurses on a discrete unit (Minnick et al., 2007), are characteristic of the "siloed" approaches of the industrial age.

Nursing leaders are the primary designers and stewards of systems for the provision of client care and the betterment of the organization (Morjikian et al., 2007). Nurses, as the major providers of care, develop and implement patient plans of care in collaboration with the multidisciplinary health care team within the framework of the care delivery model. The model of care delivery has a direct relationship to the allocation of control over decisions about client care. It is the means through which nurse managers delegate effectively and thereby free up and manage time as a scarce resource. Manthey (1989) said that the type of care delivery system or care model determines whether professional practice exists among the nursing staff on a particular unit because delivery systems define control over nursing decision making. This means that autonomy over practice decisions is determined largely by the care model and the resultant nurse decision-making latitude. The type of care delivery system used has implications for job satisfaction, the character of professional practice, and the amount of authority that is actually transferred to the staff.

The determination of a nursing care model or system of care delivery depends on the identification of organizational structures, patient care processes, and health care provider roles that are necessary to achieve care goals. Examples of structure and process criteria are found in Box 20.1. Trends in the health care environment strongly influence organizational structure. Examples of these trends are found in the "Current Issues and Trends" section of this chapter. Organizational structure and process variables may inhibit or facilitate the work of nurses (Neidlinger & Miller, 1990) and multidisciplinary providers and have been closely correlated with quality outcomes (Aiken & Patrician, 2000). Only after critical evaluation of these variables within the context of the current health care environment can a model to deliver care be conceived.

Box 20.1

Examples of Structure and Process Criteria

Organizational Structure

- Governance
- Teaching status
- Aggregated units
- Technology level
- Case mix
- Operating budget
- Nursing hours/day
- Skill mix
- Nurse-to-patient ratio
- Use of temporary staff members
- Workload
- Nursing education/experience
- Support for professional development
- Continuing education
- Expert resources

Organizational Processes

- Care delivery model
- Care planning
- Patient assessment/monitoring
- Documentation
- Policies/procedures
- Support personnel
- Supplies
- Patient education
- Implementation of physician orders
- Patient/family communication
- Symptom management
- Staff communication
- Medication administration

Data from the Advisory Board Company. (1999). Understanding the impact of changes in nurse staffing: A review of recent outcomes studies. *Nursing Watch 4*, 1-15. Reprinted from Deutschendorf, A.L. (2003). From past paradigms to future frontiers: Unique care delivery models to facilitate nursing work and quality outcomes. *Journal of Nursing Administration, 33*(1), 52-59.

DEFINITIONS

There is confusion over the differences between the terms *professional practice models* and *models of care delivery* (Wolf & Greenhouse, 2007). These concepts are often used interchangeably, yet their meanings are quite different. Professional practice models refer to the conceptual framework and philosophy under which the method of delivery of nursing care is a component. Examples of professional practice models include Relationship-Based Care (Koloroutis, 2004), the Synergy Model, (Hardin & Kaplow, 2005), and Watson's Caring Model (Watson & Foster, 2003). Hoffart and Woods (1996) described five subsystems in a professional nursing practice model:

Box 20.2

Elements of Nursing Care Delivery

The fundamental elements of any nursing care delivery system are as follows:

- Clinical decision making
- Work allocation
- Communication
- Management
- Coordination

Data from Manthey, M. (1990). Definitions and basic elements of a patient care delivery system with an emphasis on primary nursing. In G. Mayer, M. Madden, & E. Lawrenz (Eds.), *Patient care delivery models* (pp. 201-211). Rockville, MD: Aspen.

- Professional values
- Professional relationships
- A care delivery model
- Management or governance
- Professional recognition and rewards

Models of care delivery are the operational mechanisms by which care is actually provided to patients and families (Person, 2004). The basic elements of any care delivery systems are identified as nurse/patient relationship and clinical decision making, work allocation and patient assignments, interdisciplinary communication, and the leadership or management of the environment of care (Manthey, 1991; Person, 2004) (Box 20.2). Coordination is a critical component that must be considered to manage task interdependencies upon which process and clinical outcomes rely. Relational coordination (Gittell et al., 2000) is described as the management of the multiple dimensions of communications and relationships between and among health care providers that are necessary to provide quality and efficient care.

Care delivery models must address both *direct patient care functions* and *indirect patient care functions* (Deutschendorf, 2003) (Box 20.3). Direct patient care functions are facilitated by and depend on management (Fox et al., 1999) or indirect functions. For example, the client care assignment system is an aspect of operations included in indirect patient care functions. It is how the work is distributed. Using human resource decisions such as staffing and skill mix, a framework for the deployment of nursing staff and other interdisciplinary providers and their assignment to client care can be determined. Although the nurse manager is ultimately accountable for the achievement of direct and indirect patient care functions, the scope of responsibility necessitates appropriate delegation and assignment to competent unit staff. Delegation and assignment of management functions are vital to developing and maintaining professional nursing practice.

Box 20.3

Direct and Indirect Patient Care Functions

Direct Patient Care Functions

- Assessment
- Monitoring
- Prioritizing goals
- Care coordination
- Therapeutic interventions
- Evaluation
- Communication
- Patient education

Indirect Patient Care Functions

- Clinical practice
- Education/research
- Leadership
- Operations
- Personnel management
- Quality improvement
- System coordination
- Other

Data from Fox, R.T., Fox, D.H., & Wells, P.J. (1999). Performance of first-line management functions on productivity of hospital unit personnel. *Journal of Nursing Administration, 29*(9), 12-18. Reprinted from Deutschendorf, A.L. (2003). From past paradigms to future frontiers: Unique care delivery models to facilitate nursing work and quality outcomes. *Journal of Nursing Administration, 33*(1), 52-59.

LEADING & MANAGING DEFINED

Care Delivery Model

A method of organizing and delivering care to patients and families to achieve desired outcomes.

Private Duty Nursing

One nurse to one client.

Group Nursing

Private duty nurses in group practice.

Total Patient Care

One-shift responsibility for a client.

Functional Nursing

Assignment by functions or tasks.

Team Nursing

Care to a group of clients by a mixed-staff team.

Modular Nursing

Construction of geographical modules to facilitate team nursing.

Primary Nursing

24-hour accountability by a nurse for specific clients from hospital admission through discharge.

Case Management

"A collaborative process of assessment, planning, facilitation and advocacy for options and services to meet an individual's health needs through communication and available resources to promote quality cost-effective outcomes" (CMSA, 2002, p. 5).

Managed Care

"The systematic integration and coordination of the financing and delivery of health care" (Grimaldi, 1996, p. 6).

Structured Care Methodologies

Standardized interdisciplinary tools based on evidence to facilitate quality outcomes and reduce practice variation; may include protocols, order sets, clinical pathways, and practice guidelines.

Current and Evolving Types

Mixed models emphasizing outcomes management, integrated and multidisciplinary professional practice, and spanning the health care continuum.

The professional practice model can be thought of as a link between the problems presented by client populations, the purposes of professional occupations, and the purposes of health care organizations. For any practice model, the degree of integration of the nursing care given to a client, the degree of continuity in assignment of nursing personnel caring for a client, and the type of coordination used to plan and organize the client's care need to be consistent with general client characteristics, available nursing resources, and the organizational support available to nursing (Mark, 1992).

BACKGROUND

Executive leadership is responsible for making decisions about and designing strategies to create a climate and environmental context. Organizational environments exert a strong influence over patient care delivery, either positive or negative. Nursing care delivery can be seen as the dynamic balance between routine resource management and the structure, process, and content of practice. One outcome is that the system for distribution of nursing personnel must ensure that staff members of the right skill mix

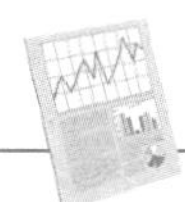

Research Note

Source: Minnick, A.F., Mion, L.C., Johnson, M.E., & Catrambone, C. (2007). How unit level nursing responsibilities are structured in U.S. hospitals. *Journal of Nursing Administration, 37*(10), 452-458.

Purpose

There is a lack of consistent evidenced-based definitions regarding the elements of nursing care models and their influence on outcomes of care. The purpose of this article was to describe the prevalence of standard nursing care models in acute and intensive care units, as well as the assignment of non–unit-based personnel resources. Standard nursing care models included team, functional, primary, total patient care, patient-focused care, and case management. Forty acute care, non-federal hospitals were selected from six different metropolitan areas, which encompassed 56 intensive care units (ICUs) and 80 adult medical and surgical units. Average daily census for each hospital was at least 99 patients. The selection of hospitals was representative of all U.S. geographical regions and included at least one large academic medical center. Data collection was achieved through staff and leadership structured interviews related to staffing deployment, roles, and care delivery models. Definitions of the elements of each patient care delivery model were identified through a comprehensive literature review.

Discussion

None of the elements of traditional care delivery models were fully implemented on any unit and were inconsistent intra-organizationally as well. Although many nurses reported that they used a primary care model, the defined elements of primary care were not evident. Although the ICUs were more likely to identify a "primary nurse," there was a wide variation in consistent nursing/patient assignments across both ICUs and adult acute care units. Nursing personnel such as nursing assistants and licensed practical nurses/licensed vocational nurses (LPNs/LVNs) might be assigned to patients rather than tasks. Non-unit supportive personnel were not designated to specific units and were not considered to be part of unit staffing. Case management was inconsistently implemented across units in the same organization.

Application to Practice

Although nursing care models are well-defined in the literature, implementation of these models including their defined elements is varied and incomplete. Nursing administrators need to understand how the sporadic use of nursing personnel, such as case managers or LPNs/LVNs on one unit but not another will impact the work of the RN who may have to assume additional responsibilities. This study revealed the prevalence of inconsistent practices of patient care assignments, roles, and responsibilities intra-institutionally as well as inter-institutionally. Future research focused on the understanding of how nursing and non-unit providers are deployed will be key in developing patient care delivery models that will result in positive clinical outcomes.

and numbers are promptly deployed so that clients are cared for in an appropriate and timely manner. Studies have demonstrated the impact of skill mix and nurse staffing on patient outcomes (Aiken et al., 2002; Kane et al., 2007; Needleman et al., 2001), further clarifying the need for appropriate role and resource deployment. The four strategic decisions to make are a philosophy of resource utilization, a choice of delivery system, common and individual practice expectations, and a development of the role of the RN (Manthey, 1991). These four strategic decisions may be made at different levels in any organization. If these decisions are made only by the chief nurse executive, then shared governance and decentralization do not exist.

Both older and newer systems and models of patient care delivery are in use. The complexity of the health care environment strongly influences organizational decisions regarding patient care. Fiscal responsibility, accountability to the consumer, and quality and safety outcomes are priorities in an environment of increasing health care costs and health care errors. The development of new models is characterized by changes in the health care climate, including costs, consumer expectations, patient characteristics, and new medical information and technology (Wolf & Greenhouse, 2007). Although all models have their advantages and disadvantages, there is no one right way to structure patient care. The appropriate **care delivery model** is the one that maximizes existing resources while meeting the objectives of direct and indirect patient care functions (Deutschendorf, 2003). In addition, pieces of older systems often are incorporated into new delivery models as they are developed. Therefore it is important to understand the variety of models available, both old and new. Pure nursing models (effective in less complex times) have yielded to collaborative practice and interdisciplinary approaches with the proliferation of health care provider roles, expedited care processes, and increased severity of illness.

TRADITIONAL TYPES OF NURSING CARE DELIVERY SYSTEMS

Historians mark the emergence of modern nursing from the time of Florence Nightingale's work in the Crimea. She instituted reforms centering on hygiene, cleanliness, and nutrition. Nightingale believed that nursing care of patients included spiritual well-being as well as the environment (Tiedeman & Lookinland, 2004). The Nightingale model was transported to the United States, and nursing practice evolved from there over the course of the twentieth century (Kalisch & Kalisch, 1978). The evolution of nursing models of care has resulted from the impact of economic, social, and political agendas over the past 80 years (Tiedeman & Lookinland, 2004).

The nursing models of care in the history of American nursing include the following (Lee, 1993; Tiedeman & Lookinland, 2004):

1. Private duty
2. Functional
3. Team
4. Primary
5. Case management

Of these, functional, team, primary, and case management were and are currently associated with hospital nursing practice. Private duty and case management were associated with public health, home health care, and community health but have been adapted to the inpatient setting. Private duty, later called *case* or *case management,* was the original way nursing care was delivered; it later became the foundation for public health nursing and community service delivery.

Private Duty Nursing

Private duty nursing, sometimes called *case nursing,* is the oldest care model in the United States. Private duty nursing is defined as one nurse caring for one client. In this model, complete and total care is provided by one nurse but the nurse carries only one client assignment. Originally, when the nurse went into the home, the nurse did the cooking, cleaning, bathing of wounds, and organizing of the household functions, basically functioning as a home manager. In American nursing practice, private duty was the original way that graduate nurses found employment, although some had administrative positions in hospitals and some worked in public health (Reverby, 1987). A form of hospital case nursing evolved between 1900 and the 1930s. When the Great Depression hit, most families were too poor to afford private duty nurses and so nurses were without jobs. Hospitals then began to employ graduate nurses.

Reverby (1987) noted that during the depression years, a great transformation from private duty to hospital staffing took place in nursing. As the graduate nurses who had been doing private duty moved into the hospital, they wanted to retain the type of care model to which they had become accustomed. Private duty, the idea that one nurse does the total care of one client, was transplanted into hospital settings for as long as nurses were paid by clients. When nurses became employees of hospitals, the kind of client care that private duty allowed was not possible within the organizational structure of hospital staff nursing. The organization of work in hospitals was task-focused, not client-focused (Reverby, 1987).

The advantage of private duty nursing was that the nurse's focus was entirely on one client's needs. This fostered closeness in the nurse-client relationship and increased RN and client satisfaction with care delivery. The disadvantage was that private duty is a costly model because of its low efficiency. Furthermore, job security was tenuous and irregular (Lee, 1993; Reverby, 1987). Other disadvantages were that nurses had little job mobility and were relatively isolated from colleagues.

Two main variations to the basic pattern of private duty nursing developed: group nursing and total patient care. Group nursing was an early alternative model that combined private duty concepts with hospital staff nursing. Total patient care was a hospital care model characterized by 8-hour shift accountability.

Group nursing was a care model proposed in the 1930s by Janet Geister, then the executive director of the American Nurses Association (ANA). Defined as nursing group practice, the idea of group nursing in hospitals was similar to divisional private duty in which several clients shared a private nurse. The plan was to reorganize private duty from individual to group practice, both inside and outside the hospital. Thus the registry of private duty nurses would be transformed into a group practice and linked to a community's public health nursing service. Facing political pressure, the plan died. Hospitals also experimented with a group nursing care modality, described as being halfway between a private duty arrangement and graduate nurse hospital staff nursing. Under this plan, clients were grouped together in a special unit in which several clients shared a private nurse. Thus three nurses could do 8-hour shifts for two clients instead of four nurses being needed for 12-hour shifts. The hospital paid the nurses' wages but charged the clients directly as a surcharge on the hospital bill. The advantages included shorter hours for nurses, order and regularity in hospital staffing, steady employment for nurses, slightly cheaper rates for clients, and responsibility for the total care of several clients for the nurse. Nurses obtained the autonomy and care delivery method of private duty without its isolation and uncertainty. Nurses were members of the hospital's staff, yet their time was specifically allocated only to a set number of clients who paid for this service directly. However, economic and political pressures for more efficiency, productivity, and service cut off the adoption of this system in hospitals (Reverby, 1987). It is interesting to note the parallels between group nursing and what eventually came to be the way physicians organized themselves.

Total patient care has been defined as a case method for organizing nursing care in which nurses are responsible for total care of a client for the hours in which that specific nurse is present (Glandon et al., 1989; Hegyvary, 1977). Examples initially occurred in intensive care, hospice care, and home health care. The term *total patient care* has come to mean the assignment of each client to a nurse who plans and delivers care during a work shift (McCloskey et al., 1991; Minnick et al., 2007). Total patient care reemerged in the mid-1990s as a prevalent care delivery system after reengineering and restructuring occurred. The term has become confused with team or primary nursing care delivery systems. Total patient care has been described as a "form of primary nursing" (Reverby, 1987); however, the accountability for patient care coordination throughout the acute episode does not happen. The advantages are the intensity of focus with shift-only responsibility. Significant disadvantages are lack of communication and continuity of care for the client over time. Models of total patient care have contributed to task- and shift-based care that diverts attention from achievement of future patient goals (Bower, 2004).

Functional Nursing

Functional nursing emerged as a care model in the 1940s. In this model, the division of labor is assigned according to specific tasks and technical aspects of the job. It has been defined as work allocation by functions or tasks, such as passing medicine, changing dressings, giving baths, or taking vital signs (McCloskey et al., 1991). Under functional nursing, the nurse identifies the tasks to be done for a shift. The work is divided and assigned to personnel, who focus on completing the assigned task. Tasks are divided based on the complexity of judgment and technical knowledge and a variety of workers other than RNs to complete the assignment. Functional nursing has the advantage of being efficient for taking care of the tasks related to handling a large number of clients and using workers with varying skill levels (Tiedeman & Lookinland, 2004). Because the division of labor is clearly delineated, administrative efficiency is maximized.

Functional nursing was the norm in U.S. hospitals from the late 1800s through the end of World War II. Factors such as increases in client acuity, greater complexity of care delivery, and expansion of the number of paying clients increased demand for hospital nursing services. As hospitals searched for ways to improve efficiency and service yet control labor costs, the functional division of tasks was instituted to get the work done. Cyclical shortages of nursing labor, exacerbated during times of war, accelerated staffing shortages and the demands of work. This organization of work, combined with frequent understaffing, forced nurses to be task-oriented rather than client-oriented. It was a major reason why graduate nurses disliked staff nursing as compared with private duty (Reverby, 1987).

In the early 1900s, business and industry concepts of "scientific management" emphasized efficiency. The efficiency was gained by breaking down a work process into its component task steps and then analyzing and timing the steps, establishing standards, and determining the best way to perform each task. Thus managerial control over the planning and execution of work could be established. Assembly lines in factories were one result. Functional nursing was developed as a result of this concern for task analysis and proper division of the nursing workload. Under this model, there might be a "temperature nurse," a "medication nurse," a nurse for the right side of the ward, and a nurse for the left side of the ward (Kalisch & Kalisch, 1978; Reverby, 1987). Functional nursing was not oriented to individualized and holistic client care but, rather, facilitated a fragmented approach to patient care. One advantage was that there was little confusion about roles and duties. When applied to nursing, this method was efficient and inexpensive but nurses and clients hated it. Client satisfaction dropped under this kind of care delivery system. Clients felt that they could not identify who was their nurse caregiver.

Team Nursing

Team nursing is a care model that uses a group of people led by a knowledgeable nurse. It is a delivery approach that provides care to a group of clients by coordinating a team of RNs, licensed practical nurses/licensed vocational nurses (LPNs/LVNs), and aides under the supervision of one nurse, called the *team leader* (Glandon et al., 1989; Hegyvary, 1977). Team nursing has been defined as the assignment of a group of clients to a small group of workers under the direction of a team leader. Each team member provides most of the care to his or her assigned clients, although some tasks (e.g., medications) may be assigned separately (McCloskey et al., 1991).

Team nursing is designed to make use of each member's capabilities to meet the nursing needs of his or her group of clients. It is a delegation of care to a designated team of staff members. The staff members have various levels of expertise, but they are formed into a team. The nurse leader takes into account the level of expertise and then divides the assignments accordingly so that the clients who are assigned to a team of caregivers have their needs appropriately met. Team nursing developed in the early 1950s in response to a shortage of RNs and in reaction to the dissatisfaction with functional nursing.

The advantages of team nursing are that each member's particular capabilities can be used to the maximum. This model supports group productivity and the growth of team members. Communication is vital. A sense of contribution via the team can be fostered. Oversight for novice nurses and temporary personnel can be facilitated. However, it takes a skilled RN to be a team leader. Furthermore, an RN team member may not be functioning up to his or her full potential because of being assigned an ancillary role, which creates some underutilization of the RN personnel.

One variation of team nursing is **modular nursing.** Modular nursing is based on the existence of specific facilities and on actual structural and spatial changes to enable hospital nurses to stay near the bedside. Structural modules based on client acuity are clustered in larger districts based on geography. Nurses are stationed near their clients, and a wider range of responsibility is delegated to them. Open design and convenient access architecture provide for decentralization of care delivery based on the spatial arrangement of the unit and enhanced communication (Magargal, 1987). The development of an innovative new care delivery system needs to be in synchrony with the philosophy of care (Guild et al., 1994). The essential features of modular nursing are as follows (Anderson & Hughes, 1993):

- A module consists of a group of nurses and a group of clients.
- Clients are grouped by spatial or floor-plan clustering.
- Nurse/client assignment is standardized.
- Modular care-planning rounds occur regularly.
- A unit-based modular committee is established.

In one facility, decentralizing nursing activity to three modular substations for a 50-bed unit allowed for a reduction in RN skill mix from 63% to 46% (Abts et al., 1994).

Functional nursing was a precursor of team nursing. Both models emphasized efficiency and care delivery with a limited number of RNs. However, team nursing corrected some deficiencies in care fragmentation and regimentation that were a problem with functional nursing.

Primary Nursing

Primary nursing began in the 1970s as a way to overcome the discontent with functional and team nursing's emphasis on tasks and discrete functions that directed nurses' attention away from holistic care of the client. This matched a societal trend toward accountability, as well as nursing's rising level of professionalism. Primary nursing is an approach in which a nurse has responsibility and accountability for the continuous guidance of specific clients from hospital admission through discharge. Thus the primary nurse provides for the total nursing process for the client during a period of hospitalization (Glandon et al., 1989; Hegyvary, 1977). Primary nursing has been defined as the assignment in a hospital of each client to a primary nurse who plans, delivers, and monitors care under a 24-hour responsibility from admission to discharge (McCloskey et al., 1991). The hallmark of the primary nursing concept is the 24-hour accountability element. Autonomy, authority, and accountability in the primary nurse's role are basic to primary nursing. When the nurse is not actually taking care of clients, an associate delivers the care. However, the primary nurse makes the care and treatment coordination decisions, supervising the entire stay, 24 hours per day, for the length of the hospital stay. This increases continuity of care and consistency in assignments. Primary nursing does not mean that the primary nurse takes care of clients 24 hours a day. Rather, the 24-hour accountability is for the supervision and delegation of client care. Primary nursing has been called the first formal professional model in hospital nursing (Zander, 1992).

The advantages of primary nursing include a focus on the client's needs, greater nurse autonomy, and greater continuity of care. Primary nursing eventually came to be associated with all-RN staffing but has moved away from that position. Problems in the implementation of primary nursing have included the wide variation in its operationalization and implementation. The result has been confusion and lack of a structure to enable primary nurse autonomy. Under cost-containment pressure, an all-RN staff is difficult to justify. Total accountability may create burnout, and a poorly prepared RN may feel threatened by primary nursing.

Research conducted to compare team nursing with primary nursing care models has found higher quality of nursing care, higher levels of nurse satisfaction, increased continuity of care, improved nurse retention, and positive client outcomes with primary nursing. Levels of client satisfaction were equal and cost comparisons were inconclusive between the two models (Gardner, 1991; Lang & Clinton, 1984; Lee, 1993).

Private duty was a precursor of primary nursing (Poulin, 1985). Both care delivery models emphasized the closeness of the nurse-client relationship, but primary nursing was more cost-effective. Primary nursing was a care model that evolved in reaction to the desire of RNs to return to more direct and active care instead of supervision of ancillary workers as in the team nursing care model. This approach promoted greater RN professional authority, accountability, autonomy, and continuity of care. Initially, an all-RN staff was thought to be needed. Compatible support systems were needed for a primary nursing care model to be effective. Primary nursing is highly sensitive to human resource distribution, skill mix, staff competency levels, and client care needs. However, as budget constraints, shortened lengths of stay, increased client severity, and pressures for cost containment in hospitals grew in the late 1980s and early 1990s, it was difficult to maintain primary nursing care models (Cohen & Cesta, 2005).

Case Management

Case management as a nursing model of care evolved in the late 1980s. It has been defined as both a process and a care delivery model. Case management has developed as a method to *manage care*. **Managed care** is care coordination that is organized to achieve specific client outcomes, given fiscal and other resource constraints. Managed care has been described as "the systematic integration and coordination of the financing and delivery of health care" (Grimaldi, 1996, p. 6).

Practical Tips

Tip #1: Understand Your Unit's Outcomes

Patient satisfaction with care, communication, and discharge plans is a strong indicator that care delivery has been effective. If your patient satisfaction scores are not what you would like, investigate the experiences that patients are having on your unit. Nurses are frequently frustrated when there is a conflict between what is expected of them and what work is left to be accomplished. If your nurses are unhappy, it is important to understand if processes of care are inefficient and ineffective. Evaluation of events such as "near misses," falls, and sentinel events is essential to know whether the method of care delivery on your unit is meeting the needs of patients.

Tip #2: Assess Communication Strategies

Assess how multidisciplinary communication regarding the plan of care is occurring on your unit. If your nurses are consistently surprised when discharge orders are written, communication probably needs improvement. Try establishing daily multidisciplinary "rapid" rounds mandating the participation of staff nurse and key providers on the health care team. Other methods are daily "huddles" and "tuck-in" rounds, both of which help the bedside nurse plan care for the patient. Helping nurses participate in rounds with meaningful information is a powerful professional development tool.

The Case Management Society of America (CMSA) is the professional organization representing case managers in practice. It is a multidisciplinary organization. The CMSA definition of case management is "a collaborative process of assessment, planning, facilitation and advocacy for options and services to meet an individual's health needs through communication and available resources to promote quality cost-effective outcomes" (CMSA, 2002, p. 5).

In nursing, the ANA first defined nursing case management as a system of health assessment, planning, service procurement, service delivery, service coordination, and monitoring through which the multiple service needs of clients are met (American Nurses Association [ANA], 1988; Zander, 1990). Hospital acute care case management today is an attempt to reconfigure the delivery of hospital care away from previous care models. Case management and care coordination have been the care delivery models used for years by public health and community health nurses (Mikulencak, 1993). In these settings, case management has been client-needs centered, rather than shift-, unit-, or system-centered. Case management can occur inside or outside the hospital only, extend across the health care continuum, or be linked to a population focus (Lee, 1993; Lyon, 1993).

Case management in acute care hospital nursing is a system of client care delivery that focuses on the achievement of client outcomes within effective and appropriate time frames and resources. Case management has components of health services delivery, coordination, and monitoring through which multiple service needs of clients are met. Hospital-based acute care nursing case management is focused on an entire episode of illness, crossing all settings in which the client receives care. Care is directed by a case manager, who is not always a nurse, and can be unit- or population-focused.

Case management is frequently associated with the use of **structured care methodologies** (SCMs). SCMs are streamlined interdisciplinary tools used to "identify best practices, facilitate standardization of care, and provide a mechanism for variance tracking, quality enhancement, outcomes measurement, and outcomes research" (Cole & Houston, 1999, p. 53). Examples of SCMs are critical pathways, evidenced-based algorithms, protocols, standards of care, order sets, and clinical practice guidelines. The use of best evidence is considered the gold standard to reduce practice variation in an environment focused on patient outcomes. Critical paths outline time and the sequence of events for an episode-of-care delivery. Resources appropriate in amount and sequence to a specific case type and individual client are managed for length of stay, critical events and timing, and anticipated outcomes. A *critical path* is a written plan that identifies key, critical, or predictable incidents that must occur at set times to achieve client outcomes within an appropriate length of stay in a hospital setting. The critical path is a tracking system for health outcomes, complications, activity, and teaching/learning (Fuszard, 1988).

In the face of strong economic external forces, acute care hospitals turned to case management to help reduce provider practice variation and to ensure the appropriateness of care. Case management was seen as a way to incorporate and build on the strengths of earlier care models yet provide a professional practice model for nurses through autonomous decision making and collaborative practice. The risk with case management models is that incorporation into unit care delivery may not occur. Care goals for the patient, as determined by the case manager, may not be communicated to the bedside nurse. The case manager becomes the care coordinator and decision maker for care planning, and the unit nursing staff may become more focused on technical tasks. Converting case managers from a service-based approach to a unit-based model may not only improve efficiencies but also enhance integration into the patient care delivery model, improving communication and collaboration with the multidisciplinary health care team (Zander & Warren, 2005).

CURRENT MODELS

Nursing shortages and health care reform have had a strong impact on the creation of **current and evolving types** of patient care delivery models. Nurse staffing models were retooled in the late 1980s as a result of a severe nursing shortage and in an attempt to complement the work of the professional nurse with the use of nursing extenders (Eastaugh & Regan-Donavan, 1990; Lookinland et al., 2005; Powers et al., 1990). In an era of managed care, fiscal restraint became a driver for restructuring, reengineering, and redesign. Nurses were perceived as more "costly than cost-effective" as a result of their 24-hour responsibility for patient care and contribution to the overall labor budget (Hall, 1997). Many of the resulting structures for patient care were staff mix models, in which nurses are partnered with a variety of "extenders" or multiskilled workers. Outcome studies have clearly demonstrated the negative impact of "substitution models" in which extenders have not been used to complement nurses but, rather, served as replacements, thereby increasing RN-to-patient ratios (Aiken et al., 2002; Needleman et al., 2001). Unruh (2003) found that it was not the ratio of skilled to unskilled workers that influenced patient outcomes but, rather, the RNs' hours of care. It has not been determined which models are the most effective to fully utilize professional nursing skills in patient care while optimizing tasks that can be safely delegated (Duffy et al., 2007; Jennings, 2008; Lookinland et al., 2005).

Many of the models that evolved in the 1990s are identified in the literature as mixed models, or some form of second-generation primary nursing or professional practice models that emphasize outcomes management, collaboration, the use of a variety of caregivers with variable competency and preparation, and integrated practice (Bard et al., 1994; Jones-Schenk & Hartley, 1993; Lengacher et al., 1993; Parkman & Loveridge, 1994; Wolf et al., 1994; Zander, 1992). Concepts of accountability, cost containment, effectiveness, seamless continuum of care, integration, multidisciplinary collaboration, new roles, alteration in skill mix, and new assignment systems are key components. All seek to reconfigure nursing's work within resource constraints, care needs, and current ideas about professional nursing practice.

Patient-focused or patient-centered care emerged as one method of patient care delivery to meet the needs of organizations that were reengineered to be more competitive and cost-effective. Patient-centered care is defined as "the redesign of patient care in the acute care setting so that hospital resources and personnel are organized around the patient's health care needs" (Maehling, 1995, p. 62). It is part of a redesign effort to realign the structure and processes involved in delivering care to center around the patient to improve efficiency and resource use. Patients are aggregated according to care requirements or similar service demands (as opposed to similar diagnoses). Protocols or pathways form a central point of focus. Key factors in the implementation of a patient-focused model are the cross-training and multi-skilling of team members for task performance and increased flexibility (Higginbotham, 1999). With a patient-focused approach, there is an ongoing process to seek out and determine what is important to the person receiving care. This approach adopts the perspective of the person receiving care and strives to establish mutual goals between patient and provider to meet unique needs. To reach this complexity challenge, horizontal structures with an emphasis on relationships and effective working partnership are built (Comack et al., 1999).

More recently, patient-focused care teams have been configured that are made up of RNs, LPNs/LVNs, respiratory therapists, housekeepers, dietitians, and nursing technicians, with the RN as the leader of the team. The advantage of patient-focused care redesigns is that they center systems and services closer to the patient. This strong customer focus may increase patient satisfaction and conserve resources. However, implicit in these redesign efforts is a series of significant work group and culture changes affecting the financial operations and cost structure of hospitals. It also requires a commitment for initial allocation of resources to achieve ultimate financial and clinical outcomes. There are also concerns related

Table **20.1**

Roles Associated with Direct Patient Care Functions

Direct Patient Care Roles	Functions
Registered nurse (RN)	Complex care, critical thinking, leadership, delegation, oversight, teaching, care coordination, independent decision making
Licensed practical nurse (LPN)	Assistance, collaboration, intervention, data collection, some patient education
Unlicensed assistive personnel (UAP)	Defined skills, activities of daily living, limited scope of competency, complementary rather than substitution
Unit secretary	Physician orders, supplies, clerical, phone, laboratory/diagnostic results
Ancillary services (e.g., social worker, respiratory therapist, nutritionist, physical therapist)	Focused care based on intensity and professional scope
Case manager	Clinical care coordination, discharge planning, outcome management

From Deutschendorf, A.L. (2003). From past paradigms to future frontiers: Unique care delivery models to facilitate nursing work and quality outcomes. *Journal of Nursing Administration, 33*(1), 52-59.

to appropriate delegation, acceptance of assignments, and follow-up accountability (Duffy et al., 2007). Outcome studies on the implementation of patient-focused care vary in terms of provider and patient satisfaction, costs, and clinical outcomes (Barry-Walker, 2000; Seago, 1999).

Because the acute care environment is multifaceted around multiple levels of care, patient types, diseases, and providers, a single organizational model for patient care delivery may be unrealistic. Deutschendorf (2003) proposed the development of unit-based models that incorporate an evaluation of structure and process criteria that influence direct and indirect patient care functions to determine an appropriate model. Nursing units that have a large percentage of novice nurses in an environment of increased activity and severity of illness may benefit from a modified "team" approach to ensure appropriate oversight and continuity of care. Care provider roles that support direct and indirect patient care functions are evaluated and potentially realigned as appropriate. Tables 20.1 and 20.2 display examples of both direct and indirect patient care function-related roles.

INNOVATIVE AND FUTURE MODELS

The increase of health care errors, brought to our attention with the pivotal Institute of Medicine's (IOM) report *To Err Is Human: Building a Safer Health System* (Kohn et al., 2000), is a symptom of care delivery process and structures that have become dysfunctional, disorganized, and inappropriate as the health care environment has become increasingly complex. The IOM's 2001 report *Crossing the Quality Chasm: A New Health System for the 21st Century* described the need for sweeping change and redesign of patient care delivery systems to foster innovation and improve the delivery of care. It called for a comprehensive strategy and action plan that included high-functioning interdisciplinary teams that delivered safe, effective, patient-centered, timely,

Table 20.2

Roles Associated with Indirect or Management Patient Care Functions

Indirect Patient Care Roles	Functions
Assistant manager	Staffing scheduling, evaluation, clinical resource provision
Charge nurse	Unit care coordination, problem solving, communication
Secretary	Clerical support, record keeping, supplies
Clinical nurse specialist	Practice consultation, education, episodic case management, performance improvement
Educational specialist	Staff development, orientation, adult learning, broad-based program education/implementation, preceptor and charge nurse development
Advanced level nurses/professional practice teams	Performance improvement application into education and practice at unit level, unit resource, unit development of practice and education standards

From Deutschendorf, A.L. (2003). From past paradigms to future frontiers: Unique care delivery models to facilitate nursing work and quality outcomes. *Journal of Nursing Administration, 33*(1), 52-59.

efficient, and equitable health care. Despite the dramatic activity from the public and private sectors and regulatory agencies demanding the demonstration of safety and quality outcomes, most hospitals and health systems have made only incremental changes toward the kind of patient care redesign called for by the IOM (Kimball et al., 2007). Previous practice models that were either "nursing" or "medical" are single-discipline–focused in an environment in which there are many structures of rationality and points of view. The focus on the hospital as the "hub" of all health care activity must be shifted to encompass the primary care environment as well (Vlasses & Smeltzer, 2007). Emphasis on continuity of care through transitions of care with seamless communication and care coordination is a theme that must be addressed with future models to ensure quality and safety outcomes.

In 2005, Partners HealthCare in Boston collaborated with Health Workforce Solutions to identify innovative models of patient care delivery that met the following criteria (Kimball et al., 2007):

- Primarily adult patients were served.
- Nurses served as primary caregivers.
- Acute care hospitals were involved.
- Technology, support systems, and new roles were integrated.
- Quality, efficiency, and financial outcomes were improved.

Their research identified 10 models meeting the stated criteria. All of them had common elements, which included an empowered RN role, heightened concentration on the patient and family, methods for smoothing patient transitions and handoffs across levels of care, optimizing technology, and outcomes management through performance measurement (Kimball et al., 2007).

The "12-bed hospital" is designed to improve communication and continuity through the development of 12- to 16-bed units creating a feeling of a small hospital within a large one. A registered nurse functions as the patient care facilitator (PCF) for each unit and assumes 24/7 accountability for individualized patient care. The PCF is the primary point of contact for the interdisciplinary team, as well as the patient and family. The PCF mentors and educates new staff members and is responsible for achieving performance measures identified through a dashboard of quality, financial, and efficiency indicators. Initial outcome studies have suggested that patient satisfaction is improved, length of stay is shortened, and patient safety measures have reduced the number of falls with injury and the number of pressure ulcers (Kimball et al., 2007; Smith & Dabbs, 2007).

The Partnership Care Delivery Model is conceived as a multidisciplinary model of care that is patient- and family-centered, with all of the disciplines participating in collaborative practice. The term "partnership" implies that all disciplines are equally accountable for patient outcomes of care. The key components of this model include daily multidisciplinary rounds, partnerships with patients and families, education and support, and a systems approach to care delivery (Wiggins, 2006).

The Transistional Care Model incorporates the role of advanced practice nurses (APNs) to provide comprehensive care coordination and home follow-up of high-risk elders (Kimball et al., 2007). The APN in collaboration with physicians and other members of the health care team coordinates care during the patient's hospitalization, including discharge planning and the alignment of resources to facilitate post-discharge outcomes such as the reduction of readmissions and emergency department use. The APN not only provides a comprehensive assessment of the patient's health care status and development of plan of care in the acute care setting but also follows the patient into the home setting to ensure the continuation of the patient care plan. Outcomes achieved as a result of the implementation of the Transitional Care Model include decreases in time to discharge and total hospital readmissions, decreased total health care costs, and increased patient and physician satisfaction.

The Medical Home Model was originally conceived by the American Academy of Pediatrics as a method to care for children with chronic diseases. The current model has been developed as a collaborative effort among several professional physician organizations to provide patient-centered care that is focused on prevention, health promotion, and coordinated care across the life span (Vlasses & Smeltzer, 2007). This model refocuses patient care from the hospital to the primary care setting. The interdisciplinary team is responsible for coordinating care across all levels of care and includes the provision of comprehensive health care services. Continuity and coordination across specialties, access to services, and patient responsibility for decision making are key components of this model. These models are being testing for efficacy and efficiency (Vlasses & Smeltzer, 2007).

Fundamentally, a care delivery systems is the way clients' needs are matched to health care resources to achieve positive clinical outcomes. Through many complex relationships, the care delivery model influences the quality of nursing care provided and its cost. A number of nursing care models have been developed, and there is evidence of evolutionary changes and repeating cycles (Barnum, 1990). Traditionally, care delivery was provided within a pure nursing framework. Over time, nursing care delivery methods were changed and adapted to better fit external forces and the balance of the needs of clients and the needs of employing organizations. With these changes came variations in assignment systems, skill mix, and the role of the nurse. Nursing care delivery has become more complex as integration with other provider disciplines is essential to meet the client's needs through the entire continuum of care. Future trends point to greater integration and multidisciplinary team collaboration models for service delivery as health care reform drives changes in the organizations within the health care industry.

LEADERSHIP AND MANAGEMENT IMPLICATIONS

The current health care environment is dynamic and continues to change at a rapid pace. Health care costs continue to rise, and safety outcomes have not dramatically improved since the initial IOM report *To Err is Human* (Altman et al., 2004; Leape & Berwick, 2005). For nursing to ensure its status in health care, nursing leaders and managers must have a broad vision to facilitate the design of care delivery models that meet the objectives of cost containment, patient satisfaction, quality, and safety outcomes over the course of the care cycle (Vlasses & Smeltzer, 2007). Nursing leaders are in the perfect position to lead the changes essential in care delivery redesign.

Nursing, as a major percentage of the health care labor force, must be able to demonstrate its effectiveness in producing financial as well as clinical outcomes. Nurse leaders are responsible for creating the formal business plan, which includes quantitative analysis of costs and benefits with revenue and expense calculations (Morjikian et al., 2007). It is critical that caregiver costs, roles, and activities be clearly understood. Although outcome studies in recent years have clearly linked professional staffing ratios to clinical outcomes (Unruh, 2008), including patient morbidity and mortality, the focus on nursing recruitment and retention to alleviate the most recent nursing shortage has resulted in increased costs. Nursing salaries have increased, as well as monies spent for temporary nurses used to achieve adequate staffing ratios. Exploring ways to maximize nursing hours without increasing numbers of nurses should be a priority (Lambrinos et al., 2004). Staff mix models employing both professional nurses and unlicensed personnel must be carefully constructed to ensure communication and coordination of care (Hall & Doran, 2004). Nurse retention significantly lowers costs associated with turnover (up to two times a nurse's salary) and is associated with nursing satisfaction (Atencio et al., 2003). Multiple studies have demonstrated the relationship of nursing satisfaction to work environment, leadership, and perceptions of autonomy, which include the method in which care is delivered.

The kind of sweeping change that is called for by today's health care consumer necessitates nursing leaders who are not only champions for the change

LEADERSHIP & MANAGEMENT BEHAVIORS

Leadership Behaviors

- Envisions an effective and professional care delivery system
- Creates a business model for change
- Considers structure and process variables that impede and facilitate care delivery
- Models stewardship for the organization
- Enables professionals to deliver quality and cost-effective care
- Communicates with internal and external customers
- Mentors and engages staff in change processes
- Influences shared decision making about care models
- Balances tensions from competing stakeholders
- Delegates

Management Behaviors

- Plans a care delivery modality
- Organizes staff for client care assignments
- Communicates clearly
- Delegates assignments
- Monitors resource utilization
- Evaluates the effectiveness of care delivery
- Makes care delivery system adjustments as needed
- Implements care delivery system changes

Overlap Areas

- Develops a care modality
- Communicates
- Delegates

process but also experts in change management (Vlasses & Smeltzer, 2007). External and internal communication strategies are paramount to successful change outcome (Morjikian et al., 2007). Understanding stakeholder investment and managing the frequency and accuracy of information dissemination are key strategies. It is essential to engage all members of the interdisciplinary health care team in care delivery redesign, respectfully regarding context and points of view. Staff nurses undergoing changes in roles and care delivery models may have feelings of uncertainty, distrust, role ambiguity, and powerlessness (Ingersoll et al., 1999) unless they are fully engaged in the process. Staff nurses who perceived their managers as powerful in the organization were more likely to perceive their own ability to influence change (Ingersoll et al., 1999). Nurses' involvement in decision making enhances their feelings of autonomy. The effective nursing leader must ensure consistent and frequent communication about changes while enlisting input from the bedside caregivers. Preserving and developing professional nursing roles are vital in the creation of interdisciplinary models (O'Rourke, 2003). Mentoring staff to participate in the creation of new care delivery methods is an aspect of effective leadership.

Although there appears to be no one right model of care, nurses will be involved in the planning for care delivery, tinkering with improvements in the current model, exploring new models developed by others, or attempting to develop their own new model of care delivery. The leadership and management challenge is to balance risk taking and adoption of innovations with the pragmatic necessity to be systematic, evaluative, and realistic. Knowing and understanding organizational culture and formal and informal networks for getting things accomplished and having complete knowledge of the origin and purpose of policies, practices, and procedures are critical for nursing leaders to be seen as leaders in care delivery redesign (Morjikian et al., 2007). The central components of practice that need to be considered in the construction of a patient care delivery model are the direct and indirect patient care functions; provider roles and responsibilities; competencies and experience; fiscal accountability and changes in reimbursement; patient characteristics, severity, and clinical service intensity; evidenced-based practice; and new medical information and technology (Deutschendorf, 2003; Wolf & Greenhouse, 2007). Nurses' autonomy and job satisfaction are affected by the work environment and the structure of the care model used. Leadership is needed to strike a balance between nurses' needs and preferences and those of clients, physicians, and organizations.

CURRENT ISSUES AND TRENDS

Influential Trends

A number of social, technological, environmental, economic, and political trends have shaped and influenced the type of nursing care delivery systems in use in U.S. hospitals. From 1900 to 1950, the following trends were influential (Lee, 1993):

- The status of women and expectations of altruism
- The apprenticeship model of nursing education
- Advances in health care scientific knowledge
- Transfer of equipment-based technologies from physicians to nurses
- Task analysis and division of labor
- Hospital control of nursing education
- Patient location by disease diagnosis
- Cyclical nurse shortages precipitated by epidemics, war, and the peak of the efficiency movement in nursing care delivery
- The Great Depression
- The strike as a negotiation strategy
- Passage of state registration laws
- Upgrading of nursing education standards
- Unsatisfactory working conditions in hospitals and inadequate salaries for nurses

From 1950 until the late 1980s, general health care trends continued to encourage the professionalism of nursing practice. General trends that were influential included the following (Lee, 1993):

- Changes in demographics, social mores, and lifestyle patterns

- Advances in professional self-regulation and nursing knowledge
- Changes in the role of the nurse and in nursing education
- Swings in the organization of hospital nursing care delivery from functional (before the 1950s) to team (early 1950s) to primary nursing (1970s) to case management (late 1980s)
- Participatory management and shared governance
- Cycles of nurse staffing shortages
- Increasing hospital patient acuities
- Political activism, advocacy, legislation, and regulation
- Rise of consumer concern about cost, quality, and access
- Health care reform movement and legislation
- Expansion of hospital and health care service
- Mergers and integration
- Emerging role of advanced practice nurses
- The rise of nursing centers and nurse-run clinics
- Beginning shifts in emphasis to community health care and primary prevention
- Changing professional opportunities for women

The nurse shortage in the late 1980s resulted in increased nursing salaries and an exploration of alternative approaches to patient care delivery, including the expanded use of nurse extenders. At the same time, the escalation of health care costs resulted in shifts in the health care industry, including restructured reimbursement and finance mechanisms. The federal prospective payment system and managed care emerged as methods to control spiraling health care costs and limited hospital services to the acutely ill (Gerardi, 2005). Efficiency and effectiveness became paramount in determining care delivery. As the hospital work environment became increasingly stressful and alternative professional opportunities for women increased, a severe nurse shortage developed in the late 1990s. The following trends emerged in the 1990s and have influenced the current state of nursing practice (Deutschendorf, 2003):

- Increased severity of illness and complexity of care
- Fewer patient admissions
- Decreased lengths of stay
- Rapid patient turnover
- Objective of acute care as "stabilization and transition"
- Renewed focus on productivity and efficiency
- Changes in the focus of health care delivery from episodic acute care to a continuum of health care services, including prevention, ambulatory care, and chronic illness care
- An aging patient population living with chronic illness
- Focus on patient function rather than cure
- Proliferation of new medical information and technology
- Consumer and regulatory demand for competency and quality outcomes
- Evidenced-based medicine and practice
- Restructuring and reengineering care delivery models
- Rising consumer expectations
- New communication and computing technologies
- An aging nurse population
- Work ethic changes emphasizing personal versus professional role and time over money

As a result of the rapid environmental changes, often the processes of care became incoherent and chaotic. The current health care environment is characterized by the following (Deutschendorf, 2003; Minnick et al., 2007; Ritter-Teitel, 2002; Wolf & Greenhouse, 2007):

- Undefined care delivery models
- Multiple providers per patient
- Ineffective communication strategies and handoffs among providers and along transitions of care
- An erosion of safety and quality outcomes
- Nursing and other health care provider shortages
- Changes in staffing patterns, staff/patient ratios, and skill mix
- Emphasis on task completion

- Underutilization of professional nursing and lack of system supports for nursing
- Loss of expert resources such as advanced practice nurses
- Decreased patient exposure and lack of continuity because of 12-hour shifts and patient turnover
- Application of nursing process (assessment, planning, intervention, and continued evaluation) not geared to rapidly changing patient conditions
- Increased requirements for clinical and multidisciplinary documentation
- Determination of evidenced-based nursing practice
- Emerging interdisciplinary and collaborative practice models over patient care transitions
- Focus on quality and safety outcomes

The challenges for patient care in the future are massive. The work environment of the nurse is dramatically different now from any other time. Cost containment and demands for quality and safety outcomes will continue to drive systems of patient care delivery. The need for structures to incorporate real-time interdisciplinary communication and care planning over all care transitions is essential to improve patient safety outcomes. The "age of information" will test the ability of the system to integrate discovery into safe practice. Even though studies (Aiken et al., 2002) have demonstrated the relationship between nurse-to-patient ratios and patient outcomes in ICUs and have resulted in increased focus on the nurse's work environment and value, dramatic evaluation must occur to create a vision for health care delivery models of the future. Professional nursing has an opportunity and an obligation to participate in shaping future models that address the changes in patient populations, as well as clinical and financial trends. The American Organization of Nurse Executives (AONE) has created a strategy focused on the future development of care delivery models based on the complexities of the current and future health care milieu (Haase-Herrick & Herrin, 2007). Guiding principles address the following: nursing work as knowledge and caring, patient/client-directed care, access to new medical information and technology, "critical synthesis" of knowledge, understanding the relationships of care, and management of care throughout the continuum (Haase-Herrick & Herrin, 2007). Operationalization of the guiding principles can occur only after careful examination and creation of supporting organizational structures and processes.

Both recurring themes and new evolutionary issues can be seen in a review of trends affecting care delivery systems. Clearly, forces and pressures outside of professional nursing work to influence care models. It is not known which is the best model for each patient care setting, and research evidence to support specific inpatient nursing care models is seriously limited (Jennings, 2008). The evaluation of new patient care delivery systems must include specific quality, financial, and patient satisfaction outcomes. Nurses are urged to examine their client populations, come to grips with the business aspects of health care, and remain vigilant in analyzing emerging economic and clinical trends in order to be active participants in the creation of patient care delivery models of the future.

Summary

- Goals of patient care delivery include the provision of high-quality and low-cost care to achieve clinical outcomes and patient satisfaction.
- Assignment and delegation are methods used by organizations to provide patient care within the context of patient care delivery.
- Organizational structure and processes influence the determination of the care delivery model.
- Professional practice is a structural variable that influences the selection of care delivery models.
- A nursing care model is a method of organizing and delivering nursing care.
- Types of nursing care models are private duty, functional, team, primary, case management, and evolving.
- Private duty means one RN to one client.

- Total patient care is responsibility for all aspects of patient care for a designated shift.
- Functional nursing is assignment to tasks.
- Team nursing is the care of a group of clients by a skill-mixed team.
- Primary nursing is 24-hour accountability by an RN for specific clients over a hospital stay.
- Case management is the coordination and monitoring of services across the continuum of health care.
- Evolving care models focus on clinical effectiveness, resource management, professional practice, multidisciplinary collaboration, and continuity across the health care spectrum.
- Social, technological, environmental, economic, and political trends have shaped and influenced nursing care delivery systems.

Case Study

Overview

Memorial Medical Center was a 400-bed teaching hospital. The care delivery model for all areas was total patient care, with RNs of different experiences having shift responsibility for a group of seven to eight patients on medical and surgical floors. The third floor was a general medical unit with 72 beds. Patient diagnoses included cardiovascular (with telemetry monitoring), renal, pulmonary, oncology, and gastrointestinal diagnoses. An interim patient care manager had responsibility for the unit. Charge nurses were responsible for daily operations and frequently had patient assignments. Novice nurses accounted for 30% of the staff. Certified nursing assistants were occasionally assigned to a nurse but were more likely to be assigned tasks. Their responsibilities included basic custodial care and did not include simple technical skills. They were frequently assigned as "sitters," thus removing them from direct patient care.

There were many patient and physician complaints regarding the nursing care provided. Reporting of significant incidents and "near misses" had increased. The nursing director for the area conducted a comprehensive assessment of patient care to determine whether changes in the method of care delivery were needed.

Findings

It was found that patient care delivery at Memorial Medical Center was fragmented, with functions being performed among multiple caregivers with little communication. It was believed that staff did not have the opportunity to develop skills and expertise in specialty areas because of the scope of patient problems. Nursing assessments and reassessments were not timely or complete, and evidence of nursing care planning was limited in clinical documentation. Nurses were frequently unaware of the patient's diagnosis and medical plan of care. Nursing tasks were the focus of care, and evidence of critical thinking for decision making was lacking, especially among novice nurses. Care coordination was performed by the case manager but was not communicated to the point-of-care nurse. Discharge planning was usually not considered at time of admission and frequently delayed discharge. Communication of the plan of care from shift to shift and from caregiver to caregiver was inadequate because of a lack of continuity (with 12-hour shifts), problem identification, and prioritization. Multidisciplinary communication between providers (including physicians and nurses) was sporadic and incomplete. Nurses were not comfortable with delegation of tasks to the certified nurse assistants (CNAs) and frequently assumed non-nursing functions. There was no mechanism of oversight or support for novice or temporary nursing staff.

Care Delivery Redesign

The nursing director and the nursing vice president agreed that care delivery redesign was necessary to meet the objectives of quality patient care. The nursing director began by forming a team of multidisciplinary care providers and nursing staff who worked on the third floor. The group was surveyed as to their perceptions of patient care processes on the unit. Objectives for the redesign were constructed based on feedback from the staff, as well as a review of the literature. Staff members expressed anxiety regarding changes, but all agreed that transformation was necessary to improve the quality of care and working conditions.

It was determined that the third floor of Memorial Medical Center should be split into two separate units to maximize exposure to, and "knowing" of, specific patient populations. Patients were aggregated based on intensity of service, acuity, and diagnosis (cardiovascular/pulmonary and oncology/renal, with telemetry available on the cardiovascular unit). Staff members were assigned permanently on each unit based on preference but with an understanding that rotation to the sister unit was available after 6 months.

Because many members of the staff were inexperienced and temporary nurses were used to fill vacancies, it was decided to implement a modular approach to care delivery. A module consisted of 16 to 20 patients with an experienced nurse partnered with novice or agency nurses and 1 or 2 CNAs. Complete intershift report was taken by the module members, facilitating communication and continuity if one staff member was off the unit or not scheduled the following day. Daily multidisciplinary care-planning rounds, facilitated by nursing, were established for all patients and included participation from all members of the interdisciplinary team. The practice of hourly rounding and focused assessments was instituted to improve monitoring and surveillance of rapidly changing patient conditions.

A new level of CNA was established to increase simple skills that could be performed. This competency was validated in a skills lab. Skills were defined that could provide the most benefit to nurses and the least risk to patients (e.g., performance of electrocardiograms [ECGs]). Nurses and CNAs attended team-building workshops to facilitate understanding of delegation responsibilities and roles. A unit secretary position was approved for all shifts to assume clerical responsibilities for patient care.

The patient care manager remained responsible for both areas; however, a permanent charge nurse position without direct patient care responsibility was established on each unit.

Evaluation

Process, quality, safety, and financial outcome indicators were established before redesign. Because clinical outcomes must follow successful implementation of processes, it was decided to measure process indicators for 6 months and then quality indicators at 6 months, 1 year, 18 months, and 2 years. At the end of the first year, nursing satisfaction and perceptions of quality care delivery were improved, including facilitation of assessment, monitoring, achievement of care goals, organization of care, delegation, patient teaching, documentation, and continuity. Agency usage was down, and attrition of new graduates was reduced by 20%. Patient satisfaction scores were beginning to demonstrate improvement with regard to pain management, discharge preparation, and meeting of care needs. Although the incidence of pressure ulcers remained constant, the number of patient falls was reduced.

It was demonstrated that careful and deliberate planning with the participation of stakeholders and end-users can result in a successful project. Care delivery models can be established that maximize existing resources, ensure multidisciplinary collaboration, provide oversight and mentoring of staff, and ultimately result in improved patient quality outcomes.

CRITICAL THINKING EXERCISE

Nurse Manager Lisa Beach has just assumed responsibility for a 32-bed surgical/orthopedic unit that includes trauma patients. She has a vacancy rate of 20%, which is filled with per diem and hospital pool nurses. The activity on the unit is great, with a patient turnover of up to one third for a 24-hour period. Patient acuity is high, as is service intensity. Most of the patients require some type of posthospital care, including acute rehabilitation, skilled nursing, and home care. Nurse Manager Beach is concerned about recent increases in the average length of stay on the unit and about patient/family complaints. Nurses have complained about workload, even though the average nurse-to-patient ratio is 1:6 to 1:7. She has decided that process redesign is in order and has obtained permission from her nursing director to explore care delivery model alternatives for implementation.

1. What should the first step be in planning for a new care delivery model?
2. How can Nurse Manager Beach engage the staff in this change?
3. What care delivery models would be appropriate to meet the objectives of direct patient care functions on this unit?
4. What are the direct and indirect patient care functions that are not currently being performed?
5. What roles might be needed to support direct and indirect patient care functions on this unit?
6. How would the nurse manager evaluate implementation of a new model of care delivery?

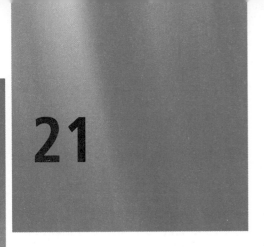

Case Management

Diane L. Huber

CHAPTER OBJECTIVES

- Substantiate the importance of case management
- Define and describe managed care and case management
- Differentiate case management from managed care
- Trace the history of case management
- Compare differences in definitions and models of case management
- Analyze the development of case management in nursing
- Outline the main service components in case management models
- Analyze nursing role changes under case management and managed care
- Exercise critical thinking to conceptualize and analyze possible solutions to a practice exercise

Case management (CM) is an intervention strategy used by multiple health care providers and systems to advocate for clients, coordinate health care delivery, and facilitate outcomes of both cost and quality. Arising out of pressures for cost containment, and later valued for quality control in the midst of alarming medical errors, CM came to be seen by health plans, and later hospitals, as a major solution to serious problems of mission and margin.

Case management is a multi-interdisciplinary provider intervention that crosses settings and sites of care. Previously used as a strategy in social services, rehabilitation, and public health, by the 1990s CM was a popular way to address coordination of care for the ill and the poor and for managing catastrophic injury or illness. Case managers were deployed to decrease fragmentation, reduce expense by streamlining care, and control costs by linking, advocating, coordinating, negotiating, educating, and monitoring. As CM became more popular, case managers' employment settings shifted to hospitals.

Registered nurses (RNs) have emerged as the large majority of case managers, especially in hospitals, in part because of the function of determining medical necessity for health care payment and because of care coordination for complex medical discharge planning needs (Park et al., 2009; Zander, 2002). Zander called CM "the nursing process applied at a system level" (2002, p. 58). This is because CM services by nurses are designed to produce a balance between the demands of the mission (quality health care) and the operational margin (costs and resources). Case management has grown in conjunction with the experience of risk by payers and providers (Zander, 2002).

Case management has garnered considerable attention in health care. It has been suggested that the processes associated with CM have the potential to save money, improve effectiveness, and maintain or improve the quality of care (Lu et al., 2008). However, a diversity of CM approaches exists. For example, "case management may describe a patient care delivery system, a professional practice model, a group of activities that a nurse performs within an organizational setting, or a separate service provided by private practitioners" (Goodwin, 1994, p. 29). The term *case management* can be specific to an institution, refer to services rendered to a population or community, or be a separate service provided by independent case managers or health insurance companies (Goodwin, 1994). Models have been implemented in many settings, including acute care, long-term care, and community health care (Huber, 2005; Zander, 2002). Case management is a central component of integrating and coordinating care across the health care continuum. It is focused on the individual recipient of services.

Case management is an approach to managing care and service delivery that is designed to coordinate care, decrease costs, and promote access to appropriate and needed services. Case management has a heritage more than a century old but has gained wide implementation and popularity as systems of managed health care have emerged. Managed health care, more simply called *managed care,* has gained momentum and evolved as a response to national concern over rising health care costs and expenditures, increasing care fragmentation, and lack of continuity and access under fee-for-service reimbursement. By the end of the 1990s, health maintenance organizations (HMOs) had become the most predominant form of health care coverage among U.S. businesses with more than 100 employees (Beilman et al, 1998; Coleman, 1999; Tahan, 1998). Case management is a major strategy used by managed care reimbursement systems.

Internal and external pressures on the health care delivery system have been intensifying, including a shortage of RNs and the aging of "Baby Boomers." A convergence of cost, quality, and access demands has created a complex and volatile environment. Complexity arises from the simultaneous balancing of needs for quality, productivity, and flexibility. Health care providers are directed to manage both clinical care outcomes and associated resources by providing cost-efficient and cost-effective health care services and being accountable for the value of services relative to the costs of those services. Specifically, the pressure on nurses is to balance quality of care with client advocacy. Thus nurses need to demonstrate and document the effect of nursing care on client outcomes and on the efficiency and price competitiveness of provided services. The benefits achieved need to exceed the costs incurred. Furthermore, nurses need to demonstrate that they can provide services more cost-effectively than other providers (Hicks et al., 1992). The mounting pressures on the health care delivery system since the mid-1980s have provided an impetus for the explosive growth of case management as both an economically important strategy for controlling costs and an opportunity for health care services improvement during economic hard times.

Like health care, CM as a professional practice role is in transition. For example, the Case Management Society of America (CMSA), the organization representing case managers, was founded in 1990. Since then it has grown to an international nonprofit organization dedicated to the support and development of the profession of case management. It has over 70 affiliated and prospective chapters and more than 11,000 individual members (CMSA, 2008a). It has promulgated the following:

- Standards of Practice (CMSA, 2002; in revision for 2009)
- Ethical Statement on Case Management Practice
- Support of a certification program through the Commission for Case Manager Certification (CCMC), which is an independent separate entity
- State of the Science papers on adherence and patient participation

In 1997, CMSA formed an Education Committee and the Council for Case Management Accountability (formerly called *Center for Case Management Accountability*) to establish evidence-based standards of practice (CMSA, 2008a). Subsequent State of the Science papers have been issued on patient adherence and patient involvement and empowerment (CMSA, 2008b).

Because a major role of case managers is to manage risk and coordinate care, case managers are in demand. The case management industry is playing an increasingly important role in managed care and cost-containment environment. The number of case managers rose from an estimated 5,000 to

10,000 in 1985 to a total in the range of 50,000 to 100,000 in 1995—a tenfold increase in 10 years (Chan et al., 1999). The estimate in 2004 was that more than 100,000 case managers practice in the United States (Commission for Case Manager Certification [CCMC], 2004). These case managers come from diverse training backgrounds, disciplines, and practice settings, including nursing, social work, occupational health, and rehabilitation counseling. In the CCMC's 2004 roles and functions research, of 3957 case managers, 92.6% (n = 3665) were RNs, 3.7% (n = 146) were social workers, and 3.7% (n = 146) were rehabilitation counselors by profession (Park et al., 2009; Tahan, Downey, & Huber, 2006; Tahan & Huber, 2006; Tahan, Huber, & Downey, 2006). CCMC has certified more than 27,000 individuals as case managers (CCMC, 2004).

DEFINITIONS

Managed Care

Managed care is defined as follows (MedicineNet.com, 2008):

> Any system that manages healthcare delivery with the aim of controlling costs. Managed care systems typically rely on a primary care physician who acts as a gatekeeper through whom the patient has to go to obtain other health services such as specialty medical care, surgery, or physical therapy. (p. 1)

Managed care is one form of health care reimbursement strategies. The generic term *managed care* has been applied to a wide variety of organizational structures, prepayment arrangements, negotiated discounts, and agreements for prior authorization and audit of performance, all designed to lower costs and maximize the value of received services and the resources used. The three most commonly associated managed care–related organizational structures are health maintenance organizations (HMOs), preferred provider organizations (PPOs), and privately managed indemnity health insurance plans. Some interpretations of the term *managed care* carry the connotation of financial arrangements that place restrictions on providers and consumers to influence price, site of care delivery, or use of health care services (Hicks et al., 1992). Utilization review and gatekeeper functions are emphasized. What is managed in managed care are the financial aspects. Managed care organizations (MCOs are now the predominant form of health insurance coverage, covering about 160 million enrollees. Of MCOs, PPOs are the most common form (61%), with HMOs following (21%) (Lu et al., 2008).

In the nursing literature, the term *managed care* was first used to describe the process of managing and coordinating care delivery in hospitals. It was defined as a clinical system that organizes and sequences the process of caregiving at the client-provider level. The objective is to better achieve cost and quality outcomes (Zander, 1991). Managed care serves to restructure the tools and systems used in client care. It is based on a process of anticipating and describing care requirements in advance and then comparing

PART IV

LEADING & MANAGING DEFINED

Managed Care

"Any system that manages healthcare delivery with the aim of controlling costs. Managed care systems typically rely on a primary care physician who acts as a gatekeeper through whom the patient has to go to obtain other health services such as specialty medical care, surgery, or physical therapy" (MedicineNet.com, 2008, p. 1).

Case Management

A collaborative process of assessment, planning, facilitation, and advocacy for options and services to meet an individual's health needs through communication and available resources to promote high-quality, cost-effective outcomes (CMSA, 2002).

actual occurrences with the anticipated path. Managed care was seen as project management at the provider-client level and as a unit-based care that is organized to achieve specific client outcomes, given fiscal and other resource constraints. Resources appropriate in amount and sequence to a specific case type and individual client are managed for length of stay, critical events and timing, and anticipated outcomes (Hampton, 1993; Zander, 1992).

Confusion has arisen over the variability in the definitions of the terms associated with managed care and case management. Definitions are fluid because of the evolving and volatile nature of the health care industry. "With health care changing by the nanosecond and managed care entities growing, mixing and mutating even more quickly, the words used to describe, distinguish and categorize various entities and activities are confusing even the most sophisticated professionals" (Grimaldi, 1996, p. 5). However, managed care has now come to refer to a reimbursement strategy of arrangements and organizations, such as HMOs, that incorporate mechanisms aimed at resource allocation and utilization management designed to eliminate waste, fragmentation, and duplication in order to drive down costs.

Managed care refers to a system that provides the structure and focus for managing the use, cost, quality, and effectiveness of health services. Managed care is the umbrella under which case management may be one cost-containment strategy. However, in some instances CM has evolved into meaning a separate hospital professional nursing care delivery model that is unit-based and focused on support for standardized patterns of care and length of hospitalization. Case management differs from managed care in that the focus for delivery of care is based on an entire hospitalization for a targeted diagnosis-related group (DRG) and is not geographically confined to the patient's unit. It implies consistency of coordinator or provider across health care settings. Both managed care and case management employ critical paths, case management care plans, and variance analysis.

Case Management

Multiple disciplines lay claim to CM. **Case management** is a term that refers to client-focused strategies concentrating on the coordination and integration of health services for clients with complex or costly health problems. CM has a strong interdisciplinary component. There have been a variety of definitions of CM, often reflecting the perspective of a specific discipline. As the professional organization representing case managers, CMSA's definition comprises the generally accepted description of CM (CMSA, 2002):

> Case management is a collaborative process of assessment, planning, facilitation and advocacy for options and services to meet an individual's health needs through communication and available resources to promote quality cost-effective outcomes. (p. 5)

Definitions of CM vary according to multidisciplinary perspectives. For example, both nursing and social work have their own definitions. The American Nurses Association (ANA) first defined case management in 1988 in a way similar to the New England Medical Center's definition of acute care nursing CM. Case management, as a general concept, was defined as a system of health assessment, planning, service procurement, service delivery, service coordination, and monitoring through which the multiple service needs of clients are met (ANA, 1988; Zander, 1990). The current definition by ANA and the American Nurses Credentialing Center (ANCC) is the following (ANCC, 2009):

> Nurse case managers actively participate with their clients to identify and facilitate options and services, providing and coordinating comprehensive care to meet patient/client health needs, with the goal of decreasing fragmentation and duplication of care, and enhancing quality, cost-effective clinical outcomes. Nursing case management is a dynamic and systematic collaborative approach to provide and coordinate health care services to a defined population. Nurse case managers continually evaluate each individual's health plan and specific challenges and then seek to over-

come obstacles that affect outcomes. A nurse case manager uses a framework that includes interaction, assessment, planning, implementation, and evaluation. Outcomes are evaluated to determine if additional actions such as reassessment or revision to a plan of care are required to meet client's health needs. To facilitate patient outcomes, the nurse case manager may fulfill the roles of advocate, collaborator, facilitator, risk manager, educator, mentor, liaison, negotiator, consultant, coordinator, evaluator, and/or researcher. (p. 1)

From the social work perspective, CM was defined as a specialized practice designed to coordinate the services needed to sustain the most vulnerable populations that are at the greatest risk (Raiff & Shore, 1993). According to the National Association of Social Workers (NASW), social work CM is defined as follows (NASW, 2008):

> ... a method of providing services whereby a professional social worker assesses the needs of the client and the client's family, when appropriate, and arranges, coordinates, monitors, evaluates, and advocates for a package of multiple services to meet the specific client's complex needs. (p. 3)

Despite the variety of definitions, the general meaning of CM is any method of linking, managing, or organizing services to meet client needs. CCMC (2008a,b) has defined CM as the following:

> Case management is a collaborative process that assesses, plans, implements, coordinates, monitors, and evaluates the options and services required to meet the client's health and human services needs. It is characterized by advocacy, communication, and resource management and promotes quality and cost-effective interventions and outcomes. (2008b, p. 3)

Thus CM entails the coordination and sequencing of care. It helps tighten the plan of care and link direct caregivers and services across facility and service boundaries.

Acute care hospital nursing CM is a system in which the accountability for the care management of clients in a specific DRG category, disease group, or other population over an entire hospitalization is assigned to an RN. The nurse case manager coordinates care across the continuum of services. Hospital nursing CM usually is targeted at high-risk, high-volume, and/or high-cost populations. Although all clients need to have their care coordinated, CM functions best to coordinate health care services for high-risk populations across community, acute, and long-term care settings (Simpson, 1993). Zander (1991) defined CM as a matrix model at the clinician-provider level in acute care.

Case management in acute care nursing is an attempt to reconfigure the delivery of hospital care into a more integrated system management care modality. Case management and care coordination have been the care delivery modalities employed by public health and community health nurses (Mikulencak, 1993). In these settings, CM has been centered on client needs rather than being shift- or unit-centered. Case management can occur in the hospital only, extend across the health care continuum, or be linked to a population.

CM is described as a system of client care delivery that focuses on the achievement of client outcomes within effective and appropriate time frames and resources. It is a system of health services delivery, coordination, and monitoring through which multiple service needs of clients are met. CM operates at the intersection of organizational systems and the delivery of clinical care. It is focused on an entire chronic or catastrophic condition or conditions, crossing all settings in which the client receives care. New services across the continuum of health care are incorporated as needed. Care is directed by a case manager, often a nurse, and focuses on a multidisciplinary team effort.

A term related to CM is *disease management*, which is defined as a comprehensive, integrated approach to care and reimbursement based on a disease's natural course. Disease management programs contain a series of clinical processes and services across the health care continuum that rely on informatics to identify and manage a medical or chronic condition in a particular at-risk population to improve care, promote wellness, and manage or reduce costs (Ward & Rieve, 1997). Such disease state CM programs are population-based approaches to the identification and management of chronic conditions. Health status is assessed, plans of care are developed, and data are collected to evaluate the effectiveness of the program (Levitt et al., 1998). These programs are focused on the group level of aggregation and may be community-focused or population health–focused.

Critical Pathways

A *critical pathway* is a written plan that identifies key, critical, or predictable incidents that must occur at set times to achieve client outcomes within an appropriate time frame, such as a length of stay in a hospital setting. A critical pathway has been defined as an "outline or diagram that documents the process of diagnoses or treatment deemed appropriate for a condition based on practice guidelines" (MediLexicon, 2008, p. 1). Critical pathways are tools used to help providers identify, measure, and analyze care processes and desired patient outcomes (Renholm et al., 2002). They detail essential care steps and describe the expected progress. They include time-dependent functions and organize and integrate provider interventions in a multidisciplinary format and across multiple settings or levels of care (Cesta & Tahan, 2003). Providing an overview of the whole process, critical pathways are best practice tools that identify and document the standardized, interdisciplinary processes that need to occur for a patient to move toward a desired outcome in a defined period of time. Elements include all providers' assessments and interventions, laboratory and other diagnostic tests, treatments, consultations, activity level, patient and family education, discharge planning, and desired outcomes (Renholm et al., 2002). Critical pathways have been described as protocols of interdisciplinary treatments, based on professional standards of practice and placed in order on a decision tree (Simpson, 1993).

Critical pathways are called by a variety of names, such as *critical path, coordinated care path, clinical pathway, clinical protocol, care track, care step,* or *evidence-based practice protocols.* They are case management tools that map out the plan of care and guide and document care within a framework that reflects the research, experience, and consensus priorities of a multidisciplinary group of providers actively engaged in providing care to the target population. Critical pathways are cause-and-effect visual grids or paths to direct care toward goals. They show key incidents and expected behaviors. Critical pathway elements include an index of problems, a timeline, a variance record, and the path or grid. Critical pathways are one form of structured care methodologies, or streamlined interdisciplinary tools, that identify best practices and facilitate standardization of care (Cole & Houston, 1999).

A critical pathway is a document that organizes the sequence of events for an episode of care. Both processes and outcomes are incorporated. Some see critical paths as creating a cookbook approach to care delivery. However, critical paths do organize and sequence the usual path of client care and form a standard of care. Variances are noted and analyzed. The process of developing and using critical paths encourages both critical thinking and accountability. Critical paths can be used to educate, prepare, and orient care providers and to negotiate expectations and care roles with clients. Critical paths can and should be individualized to each client. They are major tools of outcomes management and coordination of care delivery.

Benchmarking and evidence-based practice are used in constructing and evaluating critical pathways. Benchmarks form a frame of reference against which an institution can compare itself relative to others. Benchmarking is a useful strategy for helping to understand internal processes and performance levels. Benchmarks help identify performance gaps. Consensus benchmarks can be established by professional societies, health systems, national databases, or texts and manuals (Cesta & Tahan, 2003).

Critical pathways display expected outcomes. A difference between what was expected and what actually occurred is called a *variance.* A variance is a deviation from a standard. Variances can be either positive or negative. Sources of variance include client- and family-related, systems-related, or provider-related factors. A process needs to be in place to document, collect, and analyze variances for trends and opportunities for cost reduction and quality improvement (Cesta & Tahan, 2003). A literature review revealed that the use of critical pathways has a positive impact on patient care outcomes (Renholm et al., 2002).

BACKGROUND

Case Management Models

A variety of case management models have arisen; some are nursing models, and others are non-nursing models. The core elements center around a case manager who coordinates and monitors the care given to clients by multiple health care providers and services in an attempt to decrease service fragmentation and improve the quality of care (Rheaume et al., 1994). Weil and Karls (1985) identified eight main service components common to all case management models (Box 21.1).

CM exists in many contexts and settings, including insurance-based programs, employer-based programs, workers' compensation programs, social services programs, independent CM practice, for-profit CM companies, medical practice, nursing practice, public health nursing and home health care agencies, maternal-child settings, and mental health settings.

Box **21.1**

Service Components of Management Models

1. Client identification and outreach
2. Individual assessment and diagnosis
3. Service planning and resource identification
4. Linking clients to needed services
5. Service implementation and coordination
6. Monitoring service delivery
7. Advocacy
8. Evaluation

Data from Weil, M., & Karls, J.M. (1985). *Case management in human service practice: A systematic approach to mobilizing resources for clients.* San Francisco: Jossey-Bass.

CM programs incorporate assessment and problem identification; planning; procurement, delivery, and coordination of services; and monitoring to ensure that the multiple services needs of the client are met. These are clinical systems that focus on the achievement of client outcomes, within effective and appropriate time frames and resources, or the entire episode of illness, crossing all settings in which the client receives care. The case manager's role is as a practitioner who actively coordinates the client's care. CM is by definition a *process*. It expands on components of the nursing process to respond to the needs of clients along the care continuum and across multiple settings.

Using patient-focused strategies to coordinate care, CM becomes a system or design for moving a recipient through the health care system. A model of CM will be designed for a large, rather generic target group or population (e.g., hospitalized, long-term care, chronic care, rehabilitation) or for a specified "expanse" on the health care continuum (e.g., an episode in one setting, in one organization, or for the whole continuum). A model of CM will specify the standards for care and resource use, relationships, and responsibilities in a more general sense. The nurse may or may not be a direct care provider.

Several organizing frameworks or methods of classification have been considered in grouping CM models. Because of the variability in how CM programs are set up, classification into model types helps describe and better compare them. The following are common ways of describing CM models:

- Organizational versus practice models
- External versus internal case management models
- Episodic versus continuity models
- Provider versus purchaser models
- Hospital-based CM versus community-based models
- Case management programs that cross the continuum of care

Using these distinctions, CM models can be understood in terms of perspective (e.g., organization or providers), scope (e.g., services inside an organization), and time (e.g., one episode or across time and settings).

In the literature, many types of CM models and labels are found. There are multiple discipline–related models and one generally accepted overarching general model. Two factors are common across all CM models: the core component is coordination of care, and the core principle is advocacy. In addition to coordination of care, advocacy, brokering of services, and resource management, there are fairly common process elements in CM models regardless of the specific discipline. These models are typically tailored to fit unique target groups, vulnerable populations, settings, or other factors found in the discipline.

Nursing and health care models tend to focus on the management of health/illness or disease or the rehabilitation needs of an individual or population. These models are sometimes called *medical models, medical-social models, acute care nursing CM models,* or *disease management models.* In the nursing literature, there has been some confusion about whether CM is a care delivery model or an intervention that entails a process. In both nursing and social work, there is a differentiation between CM designed to *deliver* services and CM designed to *coordinate* the provision of services (Ridgely & Willenbring, 1992).

There are two basic CM models identified in the nursing literature: the New England Medical Center model of acute care nursing case management and the community-based model of Carondelet St. Mary's.

The New England Medical Center model is an extension of primary nursing methodology called *nursing CM* and is focused on the acute care hospital episode (Zander, 1990, 1991, 1992, 1994, 2002). This model exemplifies organization-specific models; it is hospital-based CM. It is best known for structuring the episode of care. In the mid-1980s, this model was introduced at the New England Medical Center, using principles of planning and concurrent management from engineering and other fields to extend primary nursing into outcomes management. The goal was to balance cost, process, and outcomes. The New England Medical Center model is a client-centered approach instituted during episodes of acute illness. It focuses on outcomes, resource utilization, and nursing accountability (Clark, 1996). Written, standardized documents such as case management plans, timelines, and critical paths were developed and evolved into CareMap® tools that formed the basis for a comprehensive hospital case management system at the New England Medical Center. The complete CareMap® system includes the following:

- Variance analysis
- Use of an outcome-time focus in all multidisciplinary communication
- Case consultation and health care team meetings for clients at more-than-acceptable variance
- Continuous quality improvement

The New England Medical Center model defined CM as a care delivery model called *nursing CM.*

Carondelet St. Mary's Community Nursing Network, or the Arizona Model (Forbes, 1999), used professional nurse case managers (bachelor's and master's level), organized as a nursing HMO, at the hub of a network to broker services. This model type is known as a *beyond-the-walls, medical-social, across-the-continuum of care model.* It is best known for its innovative work in moving beyond the episode of care and into the continuum. This hospital-to-community model used case managers to follow the movement of high-risk clients from acute care to community to long-term care settings. Case managers are responsible for clients with chronic health problems, and the relationship is long-term (Clark, 1996).

There are four models in social work: brokerage, primary therapist, interdisciplinary team, and comprehensive. Social casework emphasizes the development of new resources, linkages to existing service agencies, coordination of care, advocacy, and teaching. Casework typically includes increasing the individual's self-reliance and independence, as well as coordinating and integrating care (Ridgely & Willenbring, 1992). The emphasis is on vulnerable populations.

The brokerage model emphasizes the case manager's traditional linkage function. Clients are linked to a network of providers and service coverage

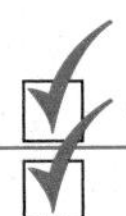

Practical Tips

Tip # 1: Reflective Practice

Using the definition of care coordination, reflect on your own practice and work group. Identify at least one example of lack of care coordination. Would case management principles help? How?

Tip # 2: Use Informatics Capabilities

Review your informatics (IT) system. Identify one way in which IT software programs could help better coordinate care.

Tip # 3: Link to Other Disciplines

Form an ad hoc liaison with social services and pharmacy to discuss improvements to discharge planning.

using assessment and referral and ensuring the availability of service activities (Raiff & Shore, 1993). The brokerage approach is sometimes described as a generalist approach. The case manager is a professional responsible for an individual client or a set of clients. The generalist carries out all CM functions and provides the basic direct service, coordination, and advocacy necessary in all CM programs (Weil & Karls, 1985). The primary goal is to increase the likelihood that clients will receive the right services, in proper sequence, and in a timely fashion. To achieve this, the case manager plans a comprehensive service package and negotiates through barriers that prevent clients from accessing needed services. Cost savings may or may not be an explicit goal, but such savings may be expected because the case manager facilitates better access to cost-effective alternatives, achieves better coordination and less duplication of services across agencies, reduces utilization of more expensive and less effective sites of care or services, and diverts clients from admissions (Ridgely & Willenbring, 1992).

In the primary therapist model, the case manager's relationship to the client is primarily therapeutic, and CM functions are undertaken as a part of, or an extension of, therapeutic intervention. The client has one person to relate to about treatment, service access, and case coordination. However, the therapist may feel that CM is a secondary activity to therapeutic work (Weil & Karls, 1985).

The interdisciplinary team model uses a specialized interdisciplinary team in which each member has a specific responsibility for service activities in his or her area of expertise. In combination, the activities of these specialized case managers constitute a complete CM process. The team might divide responsibilities by activity, such as intake, service linkage, and case monitoring (Weil & Karls, 1985). Team structures vary considerably. In some, all case managers on the team are interchangeable and serve the total group of clients. Other programs consist of multidisciplinary teams in which each professional provides specific services to the clients assigned to the team. In other cases, individual case managers carry individual caseloads but provide backup assistance to each other. Despite being called "teams," the specific configuration actually may be critical to the program's success (Ridgely & Willenbring, 1992).

The comprehensive service center model is used in service centers that provide comprehensive services, including social and emotional support, vocational training, and residential facilities. This type of program is often rehabilitative (Weil & Karls, 1985) and is seen in areas such as developmental disabilities and long-term physical disabilities. A personal strengths model may be used to help clients focus on and achieve goals (Huber, 2005).

Other models of CM in health care include independent practice or private case management. Private CM covers those services contracted for by individuals or families or those subcontracted for by other groups. This approach arose because of the concern over rising health care costs and the confusion that accompanies the choices consumers must make. The case manager has three main functions: coordination, advocacy, and counseling (Clark, 1996). Some examples include entrepreneurial or small independent case managers and practices in for-profit, large, national CM companies.

Long-term care, rehabilitation, occupational health, workers' compensation, pharmacy, and medical case management models exist. Many medical models fall within disease management programs.

Insurance models include brokerage, gatekeeper, catastrophic, HMO types, and governmental models. The brokerage model within insurance companies includes an emphasis on linkage with no provision of direct services. It is similar to the broker in other social work models except for a strong emphasis on conserving benefits utilization.

Gatekeeper (managed care) models manage access to services and promote the use of cost-effective alternatives to expensive services (Ridgely & Willenbring, 1992). They can produce cost savings by managing care, including substituting less costly, more appropriate services and sometimes simply by not authorizing higher-cost services. Rather than facilitating access, gatekeepers must restrict access to control utilization and, thereby, costs. The ability of these case managers to create savings depends on the availability of appropriate cost-effective alternatives, case manager authority within the care system, and case manager ability to control financing for the care they deem appropriate (Ridgely & Willenbring, 1992). The case manager functions much like a purchasing agent (Clark, 1996).

Focused on catastrophic diseases or events such as acquired immunodeficiency syndrome (AIDS) or brain injuries, catastrophic CM is often used with workers' compensation cases and life-care planning. It is designed to manage and maximize insurance and health care benefits, which may be capped at a lifetime maximum. Early warning strategies are adopted to detect the potential for high-cost cases and to deal with both clients and service providers proactively to optimize and economize the health services used (Cline, 1990).

In HMO (managed care) models, prospective or capitated reimbursement systems put providers at financial risk. This creates pressure on providers to control total costs, provide and promote prevention-oriented services, and substitute lower-cost services, preferably without sacrificing quality. One example of managed care models is integrated health care, defined as a network of organizations that provides or arranges to provide a coordinated continuum of services to a defined population and is held accountable for the population's health status (Shortell et al., 1993). Federal, state, and local government agencies also manage and reimburse care via programs such as Medicare, Medicaid, and workers' compensation.

Few interdisciplinary models exist. The following two were described in the literature:

1. One model for acute care case management for nurses and social workers has been described (Dzyacky, 1998). It is a program designed to integrate utilization management functions with discharge planning and separate the practice of social work from discharge planning activities. Discharge planning tasks were divided into two categories—simple and complex. Case facilitator nurses became responsible for simple discharge planning cases; social workers handled the complex category.
2. One model for nurse–social worker collaboration in managed care also has been presented (Hawkins et al., 1998). Called the *Biopsychosocial Individual and Systems Intervention Model,* it is derived from a combination of interdisciplinary collaboration models at the organizational and administrative levels and a case management intervention approach for individuals and small systems levels. Nurses and social workers are

assumed to collaborate as equal partners in interdisciplinary team case management using a trans-disciplinary model.

The one general, overarching model that is becoming widely accepted as the generic case management model is Wagner's Chronic Care Model (Improving Chronic Illness Care, 2008; Wagner, 1998; Wagner et al., 2001). The Chronic Care Model addresses concerns about how to manage chronic illnesses. The six elements of the health care system that encourage quality chronic illness care are the community, the health system, self-management support, delivery system design, decision support, and clinical information systems. The specific concepts related to the six elements are patient safety, cultural competency, care coordination, community policies, and case management. Chronic disease/illness care is important because almost one half of all Americans (133 million people) live with a chronic condition. Almost one half of these have multiple conditions to deal with. This order of magnitude has generated great interest in strategies to be proactive and focused on keeping people as healthy as possible (Improving Chronic Illness Care, 2008). Case management is an attractive strategy because it is aimed at care coordination and decreased system-related fragmentation.

History of Case Management

Different disciplines practice case management; thus the history of its development varies according to the perspective of the specific discipline reporting it. The social work perspective is that the roots of CM grow from social work's historical tradition and the work of Mary Richmond in the era of the early settlement houses and charity organization societies (Raiff & Shore, 1993). This was a social casework concept at the turn of the twentieth century. Since the 1970s there has been a resurgence in CM as a result of shifts in the locus and financing of health care and human services and problems with service fragmentation and inaccessibility.

The insurance companies' perspective is that CM arose in insurance companies because of the need to manage catastrophic and high-cost cases. For example, Liberty Mutual is often credited with having pioneered the concept of in-house case management/rehabilitation programs in insurance companies in 1943 as a cost-containment measure for workers' compensation. This concept was expanded in 1966 by the Insurance Company of North America (now CIGNA) when it started an in-house program incorporating vocational rehabilitation and CM that later became the company *Intracorp*. Some view George Welch of CIGNA as the true father of modern CM, as demonstrated in the following perspective (Siefker et al., 1998):

> Case management as part of the insurance industry or other third-party payer systems seems to have had two somewhat separate origins: the worker's compensation system and the accident and health insurance system. (p. 3)

The history of CM in nursing began with private duty nursing, the oldest care modality in U.S. nursing. With the rise of the early settlement houses, coordination of health care services for immigrants and the poor was a concern. This was the beginning of public and human services in the United States. Both nurses and social workers were key initiators. The Henry Street Settlement was founded in 1895 by two nurses (identified as social workers), Lillian Wald and Mary Brewster. In 1902, Lillian Wald founded the first school of nursing. By 1900, visiting nurse services were established to provide comprehensive community services and case coordination (Tahan, 1998).

Community service coordination, a forerunner of CM, began at the turn of the twentieth century in public health programs. The Visiting Nurse Service was one of the first community health programs. Providing service coordination has always been a focus of public health nursing. Service coordination has since evolved into CM, but case management considerably expands on coordination of community services. The concept of a continuum of care was used after World War II to describe the extended community services needed for mental health clients. The term *case management* first appeared in the early 1970s in social welfare literature, followed by a use in the nursing literature. The 1981 Omnibus Budget Reconciliation Act plus

Medicare prospective reimbursement encouraged comprehensive, coordinated services. As a result of changing reimbursement structures, insurers have been focused on programs to contain the rising costs of health care. Case management emerged in the fields of psychiatry and social work in the 1920s, was used by visiting nurses in the 1930s, developed and flourished in acute care in the 1980s, and was found in all settings in the 1990s (Cesta & Tahan, 2003).

In nursing, CM historically has been the care delivery model associated with public health and community health nursing. Thus it was operational in settings outside hospitals and operated without the umbrella of managed care. In these settings, CM focused on accountability of process and outcomes of care delivery. Traditional CM principles also were operational in several care models that evolved over time. CM also was used in social service agencies, community mental health services, rehabilitation settings, and long-term care.

In the 1960s, contemporaneous with government legislation enacting Medicare and Medicaid coverage, the insurance industry began to evolve CM models (Siefker et al., 1998). This pre-emergence decade set the stage for a series of dramatic evolutionary changes in CM each decade since the 1960s.

Many trace the "rise" of CM models to the 1970s. Certainly the past 35 years or so have brought about an amazing growth and change. The effects have been dramatic. In the 1970s, as the federal government began to analyze actuarial data on health care costs, expenditures, and projections, CM became a useful strategy in health maintenance organizations (HMOs), long-term care demonstration grants, and social work efforts to manage the deinstitutionalization of the chronically mentally ill. The 1970s saw the rise of both solo providers of CM services (independent companies) and large national CM companies. Models of catastrophic CM and workers' compensation predominated, and the certification as certified rehabilitation counselor (CRC) began.

The 1980s saw a decade of rapid spread and wild growth in CM models. With the advent of DRGs and prospective payment mechanisms, CM came to be seen as one answer to cost stabilization and cost predictability. It spread into models of social health maintenance organizations and other insurance settings. Independent CM companies grew and thrived. The certified disability management specialist (CDMS) certification was begun, and the New England Medical Center's nursing CM (acute care) model was developed and disseminated into hospital-based CM.

The decade of the 1990s was a time of reevaluation. Rapid growth leveled off, and hospitals began downsizing their number of RNs. However, interest that had been sparked in the 1980s carried over into the 1990s as health care providers, payers, employers, health plans, and professional organizations struggled to integrate CM practice and identify the knowledge base. Two groups merged to form the professional organization representing CM practice: the Case Management Society of America (CMSA). The Commission for Case Manager Certification (CCMC) was established and offered the certified case manager (CCM) credential. A proliferation of other certifications, usually within provider disciplines, occurred. CMSA developed and published standards of practice (SOP) for CM in 1995 and updated this in 2002. The SOP document is under revision for 2009. Both CMSA and CCMC adopted the same consensus definition of CM, although CMSA modified its definition in 2002. The managed care technique of utilization management became more closely aligned with CM. Models of CM also proliferated, usually within hospitals and the acute care sector, but without standardization. Jobs for case managers began to shift into acute care, the insurance industry, and large private companies. Organizational accreditation for CM programs was introduced by the Commission on Accreditation of Rehabilitation Facilities (CARF) and the Utilization Review Accreditation Commission (URAC). Rigorous research results began to emerge to demonstrate the value of CM models. CM models came under scrutiny for their value and cost-effectiveness. Interest arose in using CM principles and applying them to populations with chronic diseases, which was the pre-emergence phase of disease management.

THE CASE MANAGEMENT PROCESS

Sometimes called *care management, outcomes management,* or *clinical resource management,* CM has elements related to access, decision support, and outcomes achievement. Increasingly, the element of organizational compliance has become associated with CM. Other CM functions are access, utilization review and management, discharge planning or transition management, episode tracking and continuous quality improvement, health prevention and disease management, and contracting. These functions may be standalone or combined in various ways, especially in hospitals in which the functions of utilization review and discharge planning can be balanced (Birmingham, 2007).

According to the CMSA's *Standards of Practice for Case Management* (2002), the key functions of a case manager are assessment, planning, facilitation, and advocacy. Collaboration with the client and with those involved in the client's care is essential. Specialized skill and knowledge are needed in positive relationship building; effective communication; negotiation; knowledge of contractual and risk arrangements; ability to affect change, perform evaluation, plan and organize, and promote autonomy; and knowledge about funding sources, health care services, human behavior, health care financing, and clinical standards and outcomes. The process of CM begins with the identification of individuals with high-cost, complex care needs who can benefit from CM services. The case management intervention begins with first contact with the client and/or family and continues as an ongoing relationship until termination.

Assessment

To develop a plan of care, a comprehensive assessment of health needs is done. Tools such as surveys or questionnaires, assessment batteries, telephone assessment strategies, or electronic communication may be used. Interviews of the client and/or family, physician and other providers, and other health care team members are important. Assessment needs to cover health behaviors, cultural influences, and belief and values systems and must include identification of potential barriers, negotiating realistic goals, and searching for alternatives (CMSA, 2002).

Planning

To maximize the client's health status and achieve goals and outcomes, planning is done with the client, family, health care providers, payers, and the community. The plan of care needs to be evidence-based and individualized. The goal of planning is to derive an action plan that is appropriate, fiscally responsible, high-quality, evidence-based, and feasible. Contingency plans need to be in place for variances. Reevaluation should be ongoing (CMSA, 2002).

Facilitation

Facilitation uses strategies of communication and coordination and the involvement of the client and family throughout the CM process. Facilitation also is focused on linking parts of the service delivery system and streamlining care delivery. Coordination and education are key strategies (CMSA, 2002).

Advocacy

Case management advocacy is a function related to client empowerment, autonomy, and self-determination. Advocacy actions are supportive and educative and represent the client's best interests. Representing the client's best interest includes advocating for early referral, necessary funding, appropriate treatment, and timely coordination of services. When conflicts arise, the case manager advocates for the needs of the client (CMSA, 2002).

The CM process is represented by the activities that case managers perform. The CCMC (2008) has identified eight essential activities with direct client contact that constitute CM: (1) assessment, (2) planning, (3) implementation, (4) coordination, (5) monitoring, (6) evaluation, (7) outcomes, and (8) general activities of care delivery. Research to identify case manager roles and functions has been done by the CCMC (Park et al., 2009; Tahan, Downey, & Huber, 2006; Tahan & Huber, 2006; Tahan, Huber, & Downey, 2006).

CASE MANAGEMENT IMPLEMENTATION

"Nursing case management will continue to evolve as a strong method to provide decision support to and procurement and evaluation of resources for patients, families, physicians, and organizations" (Zander, 2002, p. 58). In hospitals, CM has become a popular and effective means to decrease length of stay and secure important outcomes. In managed care arenas, CM has been identified as a major strategy for cost containment that also folds in quality control.

Persuasive arguments exist for implementing CM: "The success of case management in increasing the use of community-based services among a variety of chronically ill and medically fragile populations and in decreasing the frequency and length of stay of hospitalization is well documented" (Erkel, 1993, p. 27). Despite this assertion, one research synthesis of 18 studies of inpatient CM published between 1988 and 1995 revealed inconsistent findings across studies. The author concluded that there were not enough data to conclusively endorse CM programs (Cook, 1998). However, one randomized, controlled clinical trial in primary care clinics in a group model HMO compared diabetes control in clients receiving nurse CM and clients receiving usual care; significant results for improved glycemic control were found with nurse CM (Aubert et al., 1998). It appears that nurse CM can be significantly more effective in helping certain client groups attain positive outcomes and should be implemented where indicated. Close follow-up, continuous reinforcement, and systematic treatment adjustments helped adult clients with diabetes.

Four basic principles guide nursing CM:

1. Coordination and integration of a continuum of holistic care
2. Promotion and preservation of health through periods of transition and risk
3. Conservation and allocation of scarce resources
4. Provision of follow-up care that tracks and guides service delivery over the long term and across episodes and settings

Thus the nurse case manager remains in a relationship with clients over time and across boundaries. The nursing concept of discharge is replaced by accompaniment as the nurse follows the client, acting to connect and coordinate a broad continuum of sites and services (Hinitz-Satterfield et al., 1993). Nurses "accompany" clients in a cognitive and communication sense. Only in certain models will nurses literally provide care across the continuum.

Coordination and continuity are the keys to managing care over the health care continuum and across organizational boundaries. Thus care must be managed carefully within each area or unit and between health care areas. Case management focuses on provider continuity; managed care focuses on the continuity of the plan. Both must be integrated into the care delivery system using a systems perspective (Falk & Bower, 1994).

The unit or area is the most basic locus at which to begin the coordination of care. In nursing, the care delivery system functions to coordinate care at the unit level. Coordination and continuity can be shift-based or unit-based. If the existing care delivery system does not accomplish goals of coordinating care, then a unit-based role with accountability for coordinating care across time will need to be developed (Falk & Bower, 1994).

Despite widespread dissemination of CM as a provider intervention and system strategy, some problem areas remain. These include the confusion over definitions and identification of exactly what CM is. Organizations also have struggled with whether and how to internally combine or separate CM and related functions. With an emphasis on financial viability or "margin," CM programs have been analyzed and challenged to justify the allocation of scarce resources to them.

Controversies exist in the field regarding methods and measurements to assess the value of CM. The two basic outcomes categories to be captured are clinical outcomes and financial outcomes. For clinical outcomes, CMSA (Braden, 2002) identified the following six direct outcomes of CM:

1. Patient knowledge
2. Patient involvement
3. Patient participation in care
4. Patient empowerment
5. Patient adherence
6. Coordination of care

Thus changes (improvement) in a key indicator such as patient knowledge can be a direct measure of the clinical effectiveness of a CM intervention. When the outcome of improved patient knowledge is linked by research evidence about improved patient knowledge reducing chronic relapse or use of health care resources, then the effectiveness of CM is further strengthened.

Proving financial gain has been somewhat more problematic for CM. In some areas such as diabetes, congestive heart failure, and mental health, CM has acknowledged acceptance. In other areas such as substance abuse treatment, financial benefit has been difficult to demonstrate. This is partly because CM is an intensive one-on-one service delivered by expert providers. In adding on a service cost, CM programs do not result in the same dramatic savings as reducing a day of hospital care or eliminating a procedure or treatment. The Centers for Medicare & Medicaid Services (CMS) have noted this dilemma, as follows (CMS, 2003):

> In the past, we have conducted several demonstrations of case management for chronic illnesses, including the national channeling demonstration and the Alzheimer's Disease demonstration. The evaluations of these demonstrations found that none of them showed sufficient savings to cover the additional costs of case management.
>
> There are several possible reasons for the lack of positive results. First, the most appropriate individuals were not always targeted and enrolled into the demonstration. In many cases, the sites enrolled patients with less severe, and therefore less costly conditions, making it more difficult to achieve cost savings by avoiding normal utilization patterns of acute or long-term medical care. The disease management demonstration Web site *www.cms.hhs.gov/healthplans/research/DMDemo.asp* contains additional information about these demonstrations.
>
> We are currently conducting other demonstrations that test either case or disease management. In one demonstration, Lovelace Health Systems in Albuquerque, New Mexico was chosen to operate demonstrations of intensive case management services for high-risk patients with congestive heart failure and diabetes to improve the clinical outcomes, quality of life, and satisfaction with services. The other is a larger scale demonstration involving 15 sites authorized by the Balanced Budget Act (BBA) of 1997 (Pub. L. 105-33, enacted on August 5, 1997) to evaluate methods such as case management and disease management that improve the quality of care for beneficiaries with a chronic illness. The coordinated care demonstration was designed based on the findings of a review of best practices for coordinating care in the private sector. More information about the Coordinated Care Demonstration can be found on our Web site *www.cms.hhs.gov/healthplans/research/coorcare.asp*. (pp. 9675-9676)

Fortunately, research is beginning to emerge and be identified to substantiate savings from CM interventions. Peer-reviewed research studies on effectiveness include Allen and colleagues (2002), Fitzgerald and colleagues (1994), Goodwin and colleagues (2003), Laramee and colleagues (2003), Norris and colleagues (2002), Riegel and colleagues (2002), Sesperez and colleagues (2001), and Weiman (1995).

DEVELOPMENT OF CASE MANAGEMENT PROGRAMS

Case management programs are structured around roles and functions of case managers. The case manager's role balances the aspects of provider, care coordinator, and financial manager. Frequently identified case manager roles are advocate, facilitator, provider, liaison, coordinator, collaborator, broker, educator, negotiator, evaluator, communicator, risk manager, mentor, consultant, and researcher. Case management functions are often identified as care coordination, facilitation and brokerage, education, advocacy, discharge planning, resource management, and outcomes management.

For provider-based case managers, a CM program can be built based on CMSA's *Standards of Practice for Case Management* (2002). The practice components identified in the standards document can be used as the foundation for establishing a step-by-step process. Following the standards as an outline emphasizes comprehensiveness and professional practice (Birmingham, 1996). Job descriptions also can be revised or composed to reflect the CMSA's *Standards of Practice.*

CM programs are developed using a number of situation-specific elements. Two initial assessments are helpful: assessment of the organization and assessment of client populations. The organizational assessment focuses on identification of resources, whereas the client population assessment focuses on how care is experienced by clients and the characteristics of client populations served by the organizations. (Box 21.2 lists related assessment questions.) If CM is used for specific client populations, priority would go to clients who demonstrate the following (Falk & Bower, 1994):

- Have a high rate of recidivism or frequent emergency department encounters
- Have unpredictable needs for care
- Have significant complications, co-morbidities, or variances in usual care patterns
- Fall into high-risk profiles
- Are high-cost

The general process for the development of a case management program can be synthesized as follows:

1. Assess the organization and the client population served. This assessment provides a baseline for implementation.
2. Identify high-volume or high-risk case types. This assessment will indicate priority areas for care coordination.
3. Determine the usual client care problems, issues, or difficulties related to the high-volume or high-risk case types. Determine desired goals.
4. Form an interdisciplinary care team of the interrelated care providers who will be involved with the case types.
5. Develop and design a multidisciplinary critical pathway for each selected case type. The path should outline and specify measurable clinical outcomes, key professional care processes, and exact corresponding timelines as based on practice patterns, professional standards of care, and length-of-stay parameters. The input and involvement of the client and each provider group, in relation to achieving client outcomes, should be clearly specified. The pathway would mark the occurrence of routine treatments, tests, consults, client activities, medications, diet, educational interventions, and discharge planning. Variance from the path triggers analysis and intervention.
6. Develop a pilot program or trial site.
7. Evaluate the pilot program and consider system-wide implementation. Review the pilot program's articulation with the existing mode of nursing care delivery.

Tahan (1996) mapped out a 10-step process for developing CM programs: (1) design the format, (2) select the target population, (3) organize the interdisciplinary team, (4) educate the team, (5) examine the current process, (6) review the

Box 21.2

Case Management Assessment Questions

Organizational Assessment

- What clinical and support services are needed?
- When in the client experience are services most appropriately provided?
- How should services be provided?
- Where are services best delivered?
- Who are the most appropriate providers?
- Where and by whom are services best managed?

Client Assessment

- What are the major client populations served by the organizations—by volume, diagnosis, cost, payer mix, and high-intensity/resource use outliers?
- What is the service path followed by client populations—by entry point, internal flow, discharge, and recidivism?
- What groups of clients fall into high-risk categories—by volume?
- What clients are at risk for less-than-desired outcomes—by morbidity, mortality, infection rates, falls, and clinical outcomes?

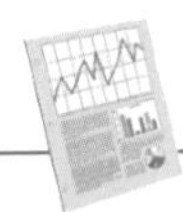

Research Note

Source: Harrison, J.P., Nolin, J., & Suero, E. (2004). The effect of case management on U.S. hospitals. *Nursing Economic$, 22*(2), 64-70.

Purpose

Case management (CM) has been shown to be an effective strategy in acute care, long-term care, and outpatient settings with diverse populations and conditions. Well-designed programs are important for effective use of hospital resources and reduction of costs. Demonstrated benefits have been shown for increasing quality of care, patient and family satisfaction, patient adherence, and increased quality of life. The purpose of this research was to evaluate which characteristics distinguish between hospitals with and without CM models. Do they have unique market characteristics, more efficient management, or greater profitability? Hospital CM programs (n = 2725) and hospitals without (n = 1714) as drawn from the American Hospital Association annual survey were analyzed on 11 variables. The Area Resource File and the Centers for Medicare & Medicaid Services' (CMS) Minimum Data Set also were sources of data. Data were analyzed for mean differences, correlations, and by multivariate logistic regression to identify significant relationships.

Discussion

Hospitals with CM programs were more likely to be located in markets with higher incomes and fewer elderly, have higher return on assets and occupancy rates, have lower operating expenses per discharge, be larger, have more clinical services, and have more enrolled capitated lives. Of these, the percentage of elderly, HMO penetration, return on assets, and number of clinical services were related most significantly to hospitals with CM programs. Thus the profile of hospitals with CM programs is as follows: likely to be found in efficient, complex hospitals with a variety of services in a market with high HMO penetration and a smaller Medicare population.

Application to Practice

Case management programs are more prevalent in larger, more complex hospitals, and CM may be critical to coordination of care across services and to improving operational efficiency as a competitive advantage to HMOs. There was a strong positive relationship between CM and an increasing return on assets. Hospitals without CM need to consider using CM as a strategy to improve efficiency and profitability. As size and complexity of a hospital increase, CM becomes more important. Successful coordination of chronic care across the continuum is a key strategy for financial profitability for hospitals.

literature, (7) establish the length of the plan, (8) develop the content, (9) conduct a pilot study, and (10) standardize the plan. This process emphasizes the interdisciplinary team approaches needed and highlights the importance of preparing people and the organization to facilitate success.

Some research is beginning to emerge that evaluates CM programs (see Research Note). Harrison and colleagues (2004) found a link between hospital profitability and the existence of CM programs. Larger hospitals with high clinical complexity and a growing managed care population tended to benefit the most from full CM programs.

LEADERSHIP AND MANAGEMENT IMPLICATIONS

All nursing roles contain a component of management. This may range from basic clinical care management to executive leadership of an organization. McClure (1991) has noted that nurses have two roles: (1) caregiver and (2) care coordinator. Nurses in management positions in an organizational hierarchy are organization managers and coordination specialists who integrate units and systems. Management of client care by nurses makes them clinical managers. The shift to managed care in integrated health systems has highlighted CM as a key strategy for nursing practice management and empowerment of nurses. It also has made multidisciplinary collaboration an imperative.

Future effectiveness is thought to be based on decisions about what types of organizational structures and nursing care delivery systems best enable nurse-managed client care and best support nurses in practice. One related question is, How much management structure does a nurse require to be effective? One assessment is the extent to which a nurse provides client care or manages the care of clients. Case management is one specific approach to redesigning care delivery for client care improvement. This may mean that some traditional management practices and habits will need to be changed or discarded. Case management has come to be a part of care delivery management that emphasizes the expertise of nurses.

Mark (1992) advocated an approach to determining the organization of practice that starts with clients at the core of care delivery systems. Then the goals, roles, and activities valued by nursing staff, medical staff, critical support services, and other stakeholders can be explored. A new practice model and structure can then be created to be consistent with client characteristics, nursing resources, and available organizational support. Various practice models incorporate dimensions of the following:

- Degree of integration of nursing care given to a client
- Degree of continuity of assignment of nurses to clients
- Type of coordination used to plan and organize care

As nursing care delivery systems evolve, the configuration of these dimensions will need to be addressed and evaluated. Nurse leaders can examine the state of health care management in their organizations and develop strategies to implement coordination of care models to best meet client, organizational, societal, and professional priorities (Kelly, 1992). Given the interdisciplinary nature of CM, model development and success may require a "buy in" by other health care disciplines and other organizational stakeholders. Physicians and hospital administrators are crucial stakeholders for the success of CM programs.

Another leadership and management implication is the human resources deployment of personnel for CM. Who should be a case manager? What roles and functions should case managers be assigned? How much secretarial/clerical support is needed? How will case managers be organized? Given the decision to implement a CM program, leaders and managers will need to make these personnel and systems decisions. In addition, appropriate credentialing for the job is a consideration. Certification

LEADERSHIP & MANAGEMENT BEHAVIORS

Leadership Behaviors

- Enables nurses to coordinate care
- Creates a vision of high-quality and cost-effective care delivery
- Communicates care management concepts
- Integrates clinical nursing practice
- Evaluates care delivery systems
- Influences policy and organizational systems
- Inspires a multidisciplinary team

Management Behaviors

- Develops critical paths
- Tracks variances
- Integrates clinical nursing practice
- Communicates care management needs
- Organizes nursing care delivery
- Directs others in coordinating care
- Evaluates care coordination
- Influences employees to implement managed care

Overlap Areas

- Integrates clinical nursing practice
- Communicates
- Evaluates care delivery

typically is an official credential of an individual granted by a nationally recognized agency based on eligibility and passing a national examination. It affirms an advanced degree of competence and is a peer review process (Cesta & Tahan, 2003). Individual certification, as a mark of professional achievement, is more rigorous than a certificate of attendance or merit and differentiated from accreditation, which is a review of an agency or program. Some accreditation bodies are granting "certification" to programs. This essentially is a certificate of achievement or quality designation.

CURRENT ISSUES AND TRENDS

"Effective and efficient patient management is important in all health care environments because it influences clinical and financial outcomes as well as capacity" (Bower, 2004, p. 39). Case management is a premier strategy to manage patient care within and across settings. This is a major concern in both nursing and health care. Case management operates at the nexus of care coordination of systems and between and among parts of the health care delivery system.

CM as a process and intervention strategy continues to grow and develop. Trends and issues in CM reflect its complexity and centrality to health care delivery systems.

The first decade of the 2000s has included standardization and precision in CM models. Certification and accreditation are becoming imperatives for case managers and their programs. Multi-interdisciplinary team models are becoming the norm. Automated systems are required for documentation and population health management because they efficiently integrate, identify, risk stratify, capture, and report care trends and alert providers to variance in outcomes. Value and return on investment are imperatives for CM models. Because chronic diseases are on the rise and consume a significant segment of financial resources, disease management programs for populations with chronic diseases also are blossoming and becoming more sophisticated.

Top trends in CM include establishing definitions; shifting case management roles, job functions, and employment settings; and demonstrating outcomes and financial return on investment. Patient safety and other consumer issues have resulted in greater consumer communication and education. Chronic care management is gaining momentum and may accelerate the integration of CM and disease management. Outcomes research is growing and needs to expand. Nurses are employed by hospitals as case managers; thus the nurse shortage has had an impact on CM. Education for CM needs to be addressed, as well as the confusion around certificates, certification, and continuing education. Multidisciplinary teams are becoming the norm for CM. Relationships with physicians need to be collaborative and collegial. There is a trend toward increasing legislation and rules and regulations in CM practice. Interest in legal and ethical issues in CM practice continues to grow.

CM is growing as a role and a job for nurses. As organizations struggle with definitions, models, and organizational arrangement choices, nurses will increasingly have opportunities and challenges related to implementing CM roles and functions.

In the shift of nursing care delivery systems toward CM, the balance between nurses' roles may shift. Some of the primary caregiving component may be exchanged for care coordination roles. This is the movement away from service provision and into service coordination as the central component of nurses' practice. CM has undergone radical, rapid change during the past 20 years. Initially, case managers concentrated on catastrophic cases. However, the emphasis now is shifting to focus on population segments, either those specifically at risk or entire populations. Requirements for a broader focus and new technologies for tracking large groups of people have assisted this evolution (Howe, 1999).

Continued pressure for cost-effective health care has pushed payers such as Medicare into managed care arrangements. Managed care organizations use CM as one strategy to control costs. The nurse case manager is pivotal to overseeing critical paths and facilitating interventions and coordination activities; advanced registered nurse practitioners (ARNPs) have been used in some models. There is opportunity in the strategic economic importance of the CM process. CMSA has been advocating for changes in the Current Procedural Terminology (CPT) codes to incorporate codes related to case management services and to secure reimbursement for these codes. Six new codes were added in 2008 related to telephone evaluation and case management.

Summary

- Cost, quality, and access pressures in health care have provided an impetus for CM and managed care.
- Managed care is a clinical system that organizes and sequences caregiving by providers.
- CM is a system of health assessment and service coordination.
- A critical path is a written plan that identifies key incidents needed to achieve client outcomes.
- *Managed care* is a broader term than *case management.*
- CM is a nursing care model historically associated with community health nursing but now adapted to acute care hospitals.
- There are a variety of CM models.
- In developing CM programs, both the organization and client populations should be assessed.
- One of nursing's two main roles is care coordinator.
- Organizational structures and nursing care delivery systems need to mesh to support nurses and clients.

CASE STUDY

The conference room was packed. Tension filled the air. No one wanted to speak up or "tip their hand" by stating a position. The group was gathered to address a serious issue: what to do about the exponential rise in obesity-related health care costs. First, there was the practical matter of illness, disability, and expense associated with the physical and organ-systems damage as a result of nutrition and weight-bearing issues. Then there was the genuine concern for shortened life span or decreased quality of life.

However, the pall hanging over the group was an unspoken concern for being labeled as discriminatory toward overweight people. The challenge for the group leader was to initiate a balanced dialogue that moved the group into strategy and action.

The group leader began with a review of the data on incidence and prevalence, local population statistics, the evidence base for health effects, cost figures, and recent media attention on this issue. This generated a lively discussion. Many problems and issues were identified. The next step was to identify a desired action plan. Was it better to implement a CM program for targeted individuals identified as high-risk/high-cost or to implement a disease management program for the entire population?

CRITICAL THINKING EXERCISE

Nurse Christopher Huber works at a community mental health center. The incidence of clients exhibiting problems with dual diagnoses (mental illness plus substance abuse) has been rising. Getting authorization for third-party payment remains a major challenge. Nurse Huber suspects that the incidence and prevalence of dual diagnosis are greater than appear to be recognized. Little program coordination exists to handle such complex cases. Furthermore, there appears to be a link between dual diagnoses, homelessness, and crime. Nurse Huber has heard that some funding may be available or possible through government payment sources for "case management." He wonders whether CM is effective for clients with dual diagnoses.

1. What is the problem?
2. Whose problem is it?
3. What should Nurse Huber do first?
4. What approach to care coordination should Nurse Huber take?
5. What other resources might Nurse Huber enlist?
6. How can Nurse Huber develop an interdisciplinary approach?

Population Health Management

Diane L. Huber

CHAPTER OBJECTIVES

- Identify disease management and population-based care management forces
- Define and describe disease management and population-based care management
- Discuss distinguishing features of disease management
- Outline the process of population-based program planning
- Illustrate population-based risk assessment
- Integrate chronic conditions care with disease management
- Examine current trends in disease management and population-based care
- Exercise critical thinking to conceptualize and analyze possible solutions to a practice exercise

Disease management (DM) is an important and effective intervention designed to coordinate care and services delivery for better outcomes and lower costs. It is one of three initiatives that are used in the realm of coordination of care: case management (CM), DM, and population health management (PHM). First is CM, which basically involves an intensive focus on an individual patient in relation to one or more health conditions. Case management is often triggered by complex, high-cost, or high-volume conditions. The second initiative is DM, which moves up a level of aggregation. DM generally involves an intensive focus on a disease or health condition of a population group, which is subsequently applied to individuals. It often is used to address chronic conditions. The third initiative, which moves up yet another level of aggregation, is PHM. PHM is a community-based population strategy, such as devising health strategies for all adolescents in a school system or all elders in a community. DM, then, is a population-based strategy for the management of groups needing specialized health care services. Some combine DM and PHM under the category of PHM. For this chapter, CM, DM, and PHM are discussed and differentiated.

Two major forces have triggered the rise and proliferation of DM programs: (1) the proliferation of managed care systems as a prevailing form of organized health care delivery (the influence of health plans), and (2) the national attention generated by the Institute of Medicine's (IOM) (2004) health care quality initiative, *Crossing the Quality Chasm: The IOM Health Care Quality Initiative.* Health plans led the charge to address the care coordination and service integration needs of clusters of members who had identifiable health conditions, generally chronic in nature. In 1996, the IOM launched an ongoing effort focused on the assessment and improvement of the United States' quality of health care. Now in its third phase, the IOM's 2001 document, *Crossing the Quality Chasm: A New Health System for the 21st Century,* highlighted the need for profound changes in the environment of care, including revamping practices that fragment the care system. The report identified the coordination of care across patient conditions, services, and settings over time as a major organizational challenge yet a key dimension of patient-centered care.

Certain diseases manifest in clinical conditions that need careful, extended management to achieve the greatest possible health or quality of life and avoid potentially large costs. In an acute care, episodic-based care and reimbursement system, care coordination is too often ignored by providers.

Disease management programs were developed and implemented largely as managed care health plan initiatives. They have evolved into proven and effective strategies to make groups of individuals healthier while saving scarce health care coverage dollars (Lipold, 2002). The federal government's Centers for Medicare & Medicaid Services (CMS, 2004) has taken notice of DM programs, sponsored DM demonstration projects, and encouraged contracting with DM vendors for outsourced medical management programs (Lewis, 2004) because DM has been found to be effective in select populations.

Disease management efforts usually target people with chronic conditions for which long-term management, patient education, and close monitoring of symptoms can minimize or prevent complications and acute exacerbations. Reducing emergency department visits and hospitalizations saves money and is better for the health of people. Thus DM programs aim to help individuals cope with chronic conditions in a way that reduces detrimental clinical and functional effects and the need for and cost of medical care (Johnson, 2003).

It is widely recognized that health care delivery can and must be improved. Clearly, the pressures to provide access to care, maintain a high level of quality, and control expenditures are converging on a traditionally fragmented and acute care–focused system. Projections are that sociodemographic and economic tidal waves are set to converge into a "perfect storm" of crisis over health care in the near future. These tidal waves include the aging of the U.S. population, the effect of the maturing of the Baby Boom generation, high pharmaceutical costs, advancing medical technology, dramatic increases in chronic health conditions, and U.S. government budget deficits. The solutions are not easy or obvious. However, DM is one major innovative strategy that is being closely watched, carefully analyzed, and undergoing research testing to determine its potential to improve health outcomes across multiple populations while lowering costs and improving patient satisfaction with care delivery (Huber, 2005).

The community has become a more viable focus for health care services. Social and economic pressures demand that health care organizations focus on ways to provide cost-effective, population-based care. Hall (1998) stated, "In a capitated, managed-care environment, health care organizations contract to provide the entire continuum of care to a given population at a per capita rate" (p. 40). Thus viability rests on the ability to respond appropriately to the needs of a specific population group. This requires accurate identification of the population's needs along with subsequent development of essential, relevant, and cost-effective programs that provide planned interventions and create aggregate change (Hall, 1998).

DEFINITIONS

Disease Management

To better understand **disease management (DM),** the term needs to be defined and differentiated from similar terms. Although there are various definitions of DM, the standardized definition is the one developed by the Disease Management Association of America (DMAA; now called *DMAA: The Care Continuum Alliance; www.dmaa.org*), the professional trade organization of the DM community. The definition of DM promulgated by DMAA is as follows (DMAA, 2008a):

> Disease management is a system of coordinated health care interventions and communications for populations with conditions in which patient self-care efforts are significant. Disease management:
>
> - Supports the physician or practitioner/patient relationship and plan of care,
> - Emphasizes prevention of exacerbations and complications utilizing evidence-based practice guidelines and patient empowerment strategies, and
> - Evaluates clinical, humanistic, and economic outcomes on an going [sic] basis with the goal of improving overall health. (p. 1)

LEADING & MANAGING DEFINED

Disease Management

A comprehensive, integrated approach to care and reimbursement based on a disease's natural course.

Population-Based Care Management

The integration and coordination of health services to a specified population.

Population

A collection of individuals who have in common one or more personal or environmental characteristics (Williams, 1996).

Community

A locally based entity, composed of systems of formal organizations reflecting societal institutions, informal groups, and aggregates (Schuster & Goeppinger, 1996).

It is seductive to think of DM as the medical management of a disease. At least two major characteristics that distinguish DM programs would be overlooked by viewing this strategy as the medical management of a disease. First, this would imply that DM fell within the domain of physician practice. DMAA has stressed the multidisciplinary nature of DM, although medical care is a central component. Clearly, the management effort in DM programs is aimed at a population or group, and it is targeted at health, not just the cure of diseases. Second, this would imply that only biophysiological diseases were of concern. This connotation would leave out behavioral health domains and other conditions such as obesity or high-risk pregnancies. Although discrete and specific diseases are a large segment of DM efforts, it is important to revisit the definitions and note the emphasis on populations and conditions. Some advocate the use of "population health management" (PHM) as a substitute for "disease management" because it is more specific to the breadth of disease management efforts. Zitter (1997) noted that population-based care was based on DM principles. The Chronic Care Model (Improving Chronic Illness Care, 2008; Wagner, 1998) best displays a PHM conceptualization of chronic DM.

The following six components of any DM program have been identified by DMAA:

1. Population identification processes
2. Evidence-based practice guidelines
3. Collaborative practice models to include physician and support-service providers
4. Patient self-management education (may include primary prevention, behavior modification programs, and compliance/surveillance)
5. Process and outcomes measurement, evaluation, and management
6. Routine reporting/feedback loop (may include communication with patient, physician, health plan and ancillary providers, and practice profiling)

According to DMAA (2008a), "Full Service Disease Management Programs must include all six components. Programs consisting of fewer components are disease management support services" (p. 1).

These components have been reformulated into a flow schematic model by Wilson and MacDowell (2003) in which population selection and evidence-based guidelines flow to providers and patients, which flow to measures and evaluation, which has a feedback loop to providers and patients. The DMAA components have been formulated into an evaluation checklist in Table 22.1.

Table 22.1

Checklist to Evaluate Disease Management Programs

Component	Present (yes); Absent (no)	Specific Method or Metric Used
Population identification and selection		
Risk assessment		
Risk stratification		
Use of evidence-based practice guidelines		
Type of practice model		
Collaborative mechanism		
Single-discipline predominates (identify)		
Patient self-management		
Education		
Primary prevention		
Behavior modification		
Lifestyle change motivation		
Telephone contact		
Health advocates		
Compliance/adherence		
Surveillance		
Process, outcomes management		
Process identification and measurement		
Process evaluation		
Outcomes identification and measurement		
Outcomes evaluation		
Process and outcomes management		
Feedback loop		
Communication to:		
Patient		
Physician		
Health plan		
Ancillary providers		
Practice profiling		

From Coggeshall Press. (2008). *Care for the total population.* Coralville, IA: Author.

Related Definitions

To better understand the concept of DM, several related definitions are presented. The first major distinction is between CM and DM.

Case Management Defined

Two major definitions of CM emerge from among a variety of definitions in the field. The first is the definition established by the Case Management Society of America (CMSA), the major professional association representing case management practice. This is considered to be the generally accepted standardized definition. CMSA's definition of CM is as follows (CMSA, 2002):

> Case management is a collaborative process of assessment, planning, facilitation, and advocacy for options and services to meet an individual's health needs through communication and available resources to promote quality cost-effective outcomes. (p. 1)

The definition by the Commission for Case Manager Certification (CCMC) remains the consensus definition adopted by a consortium of CM groups and first issued in 1995. The CCMC definition of CM is as follows (CCMC, 2008):

> Case management is a collaborative process that assesses, plans, implements, coordinates, monitors, and evaluates the options and services required to meet the client's health and human services needs. It is characterized by advocacy, communication, and resource management and promotes quality and cost-effective interventions and outcomes. (p. 3)

Other CM definitions exist. Most are discipline-specific and promulgated by professional organizations representing provider disciplines such as nursing, pharmacy, or social work. Of note is an attempt to formulate a "consumer friendly" definition of CM by the Case Management Leadership Coalition (CMLC). This definition is "Case managers work with people to get the health care and other community services they need, when they need them, and for the best value" (CMSA, 2004, p. 37).

Differentiation of Case Management and Disease Management

It is not immediately clear or obvious how CM and DM are the same or different. This has caused some confusion in the field. CM and DM are distinct and separate strategies, but a considerable area of overlap exists because both are interventions designed to coordinate care for better outcomes and lowered costs. Thus CM and DM might be thought of as looking at two sides of the same coin. Figure 22.1 displays this visually.

Case management generally involves work with an intensive focus on coordinating the care of the individual client in relationship to one or more diseases or health conditions. Disease management generally involves intensive focus on a disease or health condition in relationship primarily to a population group, with application subsequently to individuals. DM is more population-based than client-centered and more proactive in approach than episodic (Huston, 2001).

Thus CM and DM are two different strategies, employed at two different levels of aggregation. The focus (individual versus group, episode versus continuum) varies. However, both are critical interventions for coordination of care and integration of systems.

Other Related Definitions

Concepts of the continuum of care and population health are related to understanding DM. These terms are each defined next.

Continuum of Care

A continuum of care is a linkage of health services across health care delivery settings and sites of care. In one view of the continuum of care, Aurora Health Care (2004) listed prevention and early detection, family and community services, primary and specialty care, pharmacies, behavioral health care, emergency care, hospital care, rehabilitation, home care, long-term care, and end-of-life care as components of its continuum of care. From a systems integration perspective, Aikman and colleagues (1998) divided the continuum of care into community care and acute care, with community care on either

Case Management	***...two sides of the same coin...*** **Disease Management**
Assessment	Population identification processes
	Evidence-based practice guidelines
Planning	Collaborative practice models to include physician and support-service providers
Facilitation	Patient self-management education (may include primary prevention, behavior modification programs, and compliance/surveillance)
	Process and outcomes measurement, evaluation, and management
Advocacy	Routine reporting/feedback loop (may include communication with patient, physician, health plan and ancillary providers, and practice profiling)

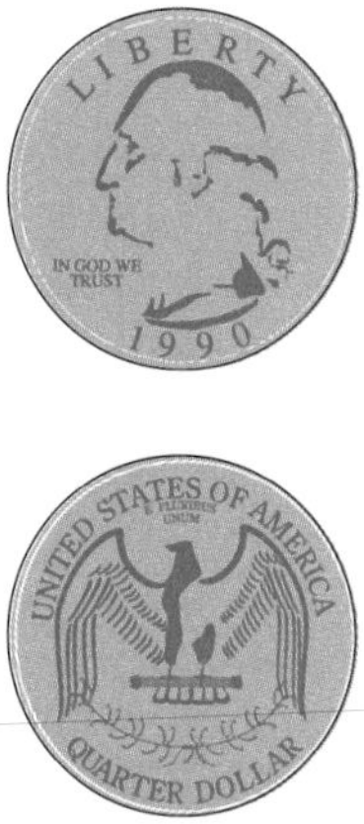

Figure 22.1
Differentiation of case management and disease management. (From Coggeshall Press. [2008]. *Care for the total population.* Coralville, IA: Author.)

side of acute care in three overlapping circles. The continuum contained health promotion/illness prevention, public health, primary care, diagnostics/drugs, ambulatory care, acute inpatient, rehabilitative/chronic, long-term care, home services, and palliative care segments.

Both DM and CM programs will vary according to the specific characteristics of the setting of service delivery, the target population, and the scope of the continuum of care. The setting may be acute care, long-term care, community health, or other settings. The target population may be a specific medical disease, chronic condition, age cohort, insurance group members, catchment area, or other group. The continuum of care may be conceived of as within a facility, across the life span, across specific transitions, or other defined episode or time span. Clarity in the specification of what the continuum of care encompasses is important for understanding and comparing disease and case management programs.

Population Health Improvement

As the field of DM grows and evolves, it has begun to merge with the concept of population health improvement. DMAA changed its name in 2007 to *DMAA: The Care Continuum Alliance* and now advocates a Population Health Improvement Model. They explain it as follows (DMAA, 2008b):

> The population health improvement model highlights three components: the central care delivery and leadership roles of the primary care physician; the critical importance of patient activation, involvement and personal responsibility; and the patient focus and capacity expansion of care coordination provided through wellness, disease and chronic care management programs. The convergence of these roles, resources and capabilities in the population health improvement model ensures higher levels of quality and satisfaction with care delivery. Further, coordination and integration are important tools to address health care workforce shortages, individual access to coverage and care, and affordability of care. (p. 1)

DMAA has identified the key components of the population health improvement model as follows (DMAA, 2008b):

- Population identification strategies and processes;
- Comprehensive needs assessments that assess physical, psychological, economic, and environmental needs;

- Proactive health promotion programs that increase awareness of the health risks associated with certain personal behaviors and lifestyles;
- Patient-centric health management goals and education which may include primary prevention, behavior modification programs, and support for concordance between the patient and the primary care provider;
- Self-management interventions aimed at influencing the targeted population to make behavioral changes;
- Routine reporting and feedback loops which may include communications with patient, physicians, health plan and ancillary providers;
- Evaluation of clinical, humanistic, and economic outcomes on an ongoing basis with the goal of improving overall population health. (p. 1)

An important feature of DMAA's population health improvement model is its identification of outcomes. The five outcomes are as follows (DMAA, 2008b):

> Accountable measurement of progress toward optimized population health should include:
> - Various clinical indicators, including process and outcomes measures;
> - Assessment of patient satisfaction with health care;
> - Functional status and quality of life;
> - Economic and healthcare utilization indicators; and
> - Impact on known population health disparities. (p. 2)

Health Canada noted that using a population health approach signals a shift in thinking to a broader view of health as a capacity or resource, not merely the absence of disease, as follows (Health Canada, 2004):

> Population health is an approach to health that aims to improve the health of the entire population and to reduce health inequities among population groups. In order to reach these objectives, it looks at and acts upon the broad range of factors and conditions that have a strong influence on our health. (p. 1)

Income, education, the environment, and biology are examples of broader factors that impact health.

Population-based care management is defined as the integration and coordination of health services to a specified population. Population-based health care is focused on aggregates and communities. The basic definition of a **population** is a "collection of individuals who have in common one or more personal or environmental characteristics" (Williams, 1996, p. 25). Also called an *aggregate,* the members of a community who are defined in terms of geography, special interest, disease state, or another common characteristic are a population. The research-related term is *target population.* In community health, population-focused practice is directed toward care for defined populations or subpopulations as opposed to care for individual clients (Williams, 1996).

A **community** is defined as "a locally-based entity, composed of systems of formal organizations reflecting societal institutions, informal groups, and aggregates. These components are interdependent, and their function is to meet a wide variety of collective needs" (Schuster & Goeppinger, 1996, p. 290). The term *community* can include groups of diverse or similar people living in one geographical location; an interactive link of families, friends, and organizations; or systems or groups bound by shared needs and interests (Carroll, 2004). The concept of community includes dimensions of people, place, and function. The community is considered to be the client when the nursing focus is on the collective or common good rather than on the health of an individual. Thus community-oriented nursing practice is directed toward healthy change for the whole community's benefit. The unit of service may be individuals, families, groups, aggregates, institutions, or communities, but the purpose is to affect the entire community (Schuster & Goeppinger, 1996). Thus the term *community* denotes a local entity, whereas the term *population* refers to an aggregate with any common characteristic (not necessarily tied to a place).

The term *community health* involves meeting the collective needs of a group by identifying problems and managing interactions both within the community and between the community and the larger society. Risk factors, health status indicators, functional ability levels, health promotion, health outcomes, and prevention of identified chronic diseases are the focus of data gathering, program planning, and implementation processes and activities. Community participation and partnership are key concepts because active participation in a decision-making process induces a vested interest in the success of any effort to improve the health of a community. Community partnership is a basic tenet of community-oriented approaches. For nurses, the concept of community as client directs the nursing focus to the collective or common good instead of individual health. Population-based care draws on partnership and community as client concepts. These community health concepts also foster culturally competent health care services (Schuster & Goeppinger, 1996).

BACKGROUND

Chronic health conditions pose a formidable challenge to the health care delivery system. The management of chronic conditions is a particular burden for health care payers and employers. Chronic disease creates two particular difficulties for businesses. First, these conditions in the workforce lead to diminished productivity. Second, these conditions result in a greater portion of the business's revenue being diverted into health care expenditures (Javors et al., 2003). Further effects impact the health care delivery system, society, and individuals' functioning and activities. Of particular concern is the increasing trend of chronic illness in relatively younger people (Javors et al., 2003).

Population and health trends are tracked by governmental agencies such as the U.S. Census Bureau, Centers for Disease Control and Prevention (CDC), Bureau of Labor Statistics (BLS), and Health Resources and Services Administration (HRSA), as well as private foundations and organizations. Table 22.2 provides information about these agencies. Clearly, health and health care delivery systems data are continually in flux. However, the available statistics are impressive.

Table 22.2

U.S. Agencies Tracking Population and Health Trends

Agency	Website Address
U.S. Census Bureau	www.census.gov
Centers for Disease Control and Prevention (CDC)	www.cdc.gov
Bureau of Labor Statistics (BLS)	www.bls.gov
Health Resources and Services Administration (HRSA)	www.hrsa.gov

By 2003, approximately $1 trillion was spent per year on health care and about 75% of direct health care expenditures went to treating chronic diseases and their complications, many of which are preventable (Javors et al., 2003). Almost 50% of all Americans reported having one or more chronic diseases. By 2010, the estimates are for 120 million people will have one or more chronic diseases, resulting in $582 billion in costs (Nobel & Norman, 2003). As Baby Boomers, a group including 28% of the total U.S. population in 2000 (U.S. Census Bureau, 2001), age in the next decade, chronic disease numbers are projected to rapidly rise. Costs are a considerable pressure, since, on average, individuals with chronic conditions cost 3.5 times as much to serve as others and they account for a large proportion of services (80% of all bed days and 69% of hospital admissions) (Nobel & Norman, 2003).

According to the CDC (Centers for Disease Control and Prevention [CDC], 2008, p.1):

> Chronic diseases—such as heart disease, cancer, and diabetes—are the leading causes of death and disability in the United States. Chronic diseases account for 70% of all deaths in the U.S., which

> is 1.7 million each year. These diseases also cause major limitations in daily living for almost 1 out of 10 Americans or about 25 million people. Although chronic diseases are among the most common and costly health problems, they are also among the most preventable. Adopting healthy behaviors such as eating nutritious foods, being physically active, and avoiding tobacco use can prevent or control the devastating effects of these diseases.

The chronic conditions that pose a particular economic burden but can be helped by DM are characterized by high prevalence, high expense, relatively standardized treatment guidelines, and a significant role played by the member's behavior on the progression of the condition (Cousins & Liu, 2003).

Other forces of change sweeping in DM programs include the following (Ho, 2003):

- High health care cost trends
- Weak economy and soft labor market
- Increase in consumerism
- Heightened demand for increased quality and patient safety
- Up to 300% variance in provider costs and quality

Thus DM has arisen as a major strategy to address these concerns. It has demonstrated effectiveness in mental health (Ziguras & Stuart, 2000) and Medicare (Martin et al., 2004) populations. Attractive features include effective population management, coordination of care for chronic conditions, consistency of care for at-risk populations, customization of care support, encouragement of adherence to treatment, and proactive interventions.

Disease Management Programs

DM programs offered by health plans can be developed in-house or purchased either from a vendor or another organization such as a hospital. In a stratified random sample of 65 health plans, all of which were members of the American Association of Health Plans (AAHP), 64% of the diabetes DM programs were developed in-house, 27% were purchased from a vendor, and 9% were purchased from other sources (Welch et al., 2002). Employers also contract directly with DM providers. It has been estimated that about 200 DM-related service programs are available from health plans, hospitals, pharmacy benefit management and pharmaceutical companies, and companies specializing in DM (Lipold, 2002).

Proactive outreach is a major strategy of DM programs. Nursing outreach programs are the core element. Personal communications (usually via telephone) between an expert nurse and the health plan participant build a personal relationship, help identify knowledge deficits and counseling needs, facilitate close monitoring and progress toward goals, enhance treatment adherence, and promote clinical and cost stabilization.

The personal nurse, functioning as a personal health advisor, establishes a single point of contact and coordination of care and service for patients having health problems and promotes a trusting relationship. Whether employed by a health plan or a contracted outside vendor, the DM provided by nurses functioning as personal health advisors and advocates is central to effective outcomes.

The core of the DM concept is to comprehensively integrate care and reimbursement based on a disease or health condition's natural course. Both clinical and nonclinical interventions are timed to occur where and when they are most likely to have the greatest impact. This sequencing and targeting ideally prevents occurrences or exacerbations, decreases the use of expensive resources, and creates positive health outcomes through the use of prevention and proactive CM strategies. Chronic conditions are the focus, and systematic ways of delivering health care interventions to patients with similar characteristics are the methods used (Zitter, 1997). DM models focus on the identification, standardization, and coordination of services across the continuum of care and for populations with the same or similar health care needs.

Disease Management Models

DMAA has not offered a conceptual model of DM beyond its definition. However, two useful models, one for CM and one for DM, visually illustrate concepts related to PHM across the continuum of care. The CM model (Coggeshall Press, 2008) (Figure 22.2) depicts CM following traditional

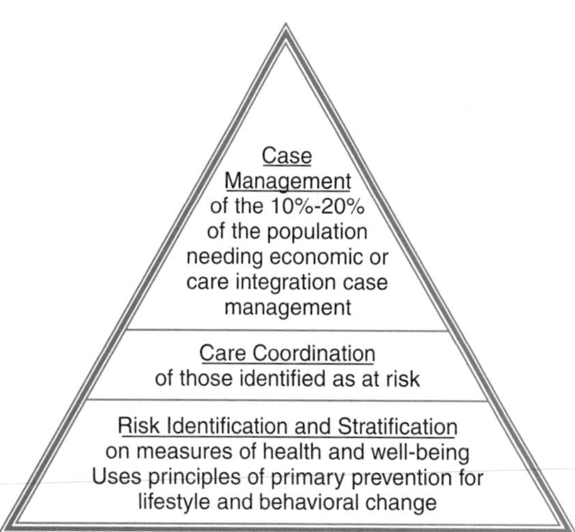
Case Management
of the 10%-20% of the population needing economic or care integration case management
Care Coordination
of those identified as at risk
Risk Identification and Stratification
on measures of health and well-being
Uses principles of primary prevention for lifestyle and behavioral change

Figure 22.2
Case management model. (From Coggeshall Press. [2008]. *Case Management Model.* Coralville, IA: Author.)

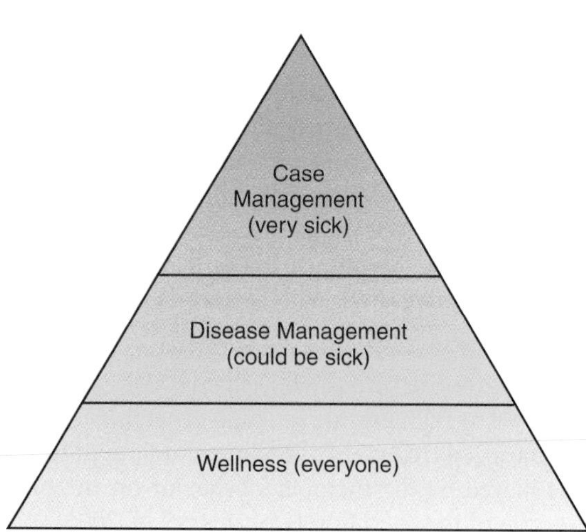

Figure 22.3
Levels of intervention. (From Coggeshall Press. [2008]. *Care for the total population.* Coralville, IA: Author.)

public health concepts and incorporating concepts of the Pareto Law (2008). The DM translation of the Pareto Law is that 80% of the CM target population would be able to follow a standardized DM care program but 20% would vary or "fall off the path." Intensive resources would then be targeted to the 20%. The pyramid shows a base of strategies applied to all members, with gradual narrowing and focusing of interventions for greater precision and conservation of resources. Applied to DM, the pyramid visual can be drawn simply as wellness, DM, and CM (Figure 22.3). A model integrating both DM and CM is depicted in Figure 22.4. The entire population (base of the triangle) would be targeted for prevention and assessed for risk identification and stratification. Care coordination and DM would be used for those individuals identified as at-risk. Then case management would be applied as an intervention for the 10% to 20% of the population projected to need intensive intervention, surveillance, and follow-up for complex care needs.

The second model was reported in the literature (Ho, 2003) as PacifiCare Health System's approach to DM. Using the same pyramid visual, segments started at the base with preventive health management (e.g., screening, education), followed by acute episode management, DM, special population care, and catastrophic care management of complex cases. Such conceptual models assist with understanding and communicating the array of programs and the level at which each is targeted. The coverage of the continuum of care is evident.

A related model that addresses aspects of chronic care is called the *Chronic Care Model.* This model identifies the essential elements of a health care system and community that encourage high-quality chronic disease care. The six basic elements are (1) the community, (2) the health system, (3) self-management support, (4) delivery system design, (5) decision support, and (6) clinical information systems. Developed by the staff of the MacColl Institute for Healthcare Innovation and supported by the Robert Wood Johnson Foundation, the model can be applied to a variety of chronic illnesses, health care settings, and target populations. The model is being tested by the Improving Chronic Illness Care program. Themes of care coordination and CM fall under the basic elements (Improving Chronic Illness Care, 2008; Wagner, 1998).

History

The genesis of the rise of DM occurred in the late 1980s and into the 1990s in the U.S. health care

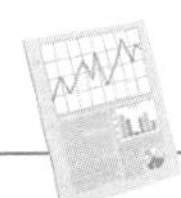

Research Note

Source: Patel, P.H., Welsh, C., & Foggs, M.B. (2004). Improved asthma outcomes using a coordinated care approach in a large medical group. *Disease Management, 7*(2), 102-111.

Purpose

Asthma affects more than 14 million people with costs at $11.3 billion per year. The purpose of this study was to discuss the development of a multidisciplinary asthma disease management (DM) program in one large medical group practice in an urban area and evaluate its outcomes as of 2001. Population data were analyzed from an administrative claims database (n = 3486) at baseline of 1 year (1998-1999) and compared with the follow-up time frame (1999-2000). A medical record audit was conducted to examine recorded adherence with asthma guidelines and documentation. The DM intervention was the development of the patient registry, systematic assessment of asthma control using the Asthma Therapy Assessment Questionnaire, nurse case management, and physician education.

Discussion

At baseline, disease control problems were frequent and 34% of adult respondents reported missing work because of asthma. Documentation needs for written treatment plans were uncovered. Beneficial results from the program included improved medical record documentation and patient education. Emergency department (ED) visits and hospitalization as related to asthma showed statistically significant decreases. The authors suggested that the greatest determinant of the overall success of the program was a realization that improving patient outcomes is a shared goal of the entire system. This led to the redesign of care processes to improve coordination and continuity of care.

Application to Practice

This DM program was comprehensive and involved an important clinical process redesign using patient and provider education and a case management (CM) strategy. The program was successful and sustainable based on significant improvement in several essential processes of care and in ED and hospitalization events. These results support the replication of similar programs in other organizations.

delivery system. Nested within the general evolution of CM practice, managed care organizations and health plans began to look closely at DM after initial CM programs had been launched. Further refinements in program quality and cost savings were desired. With some experience in CM to draw upon, the unique challenges of chronic conditions occurring on a large scale needed to be addressed. In pharmaceutical companies, DM emerged as a way to encourage medication adherence.

DM programs became evident in the 1990s with selected visible exemplars. Programs grew and spread rapidly. Todd and Nash's book *Disease Management: A Systems Approach to Improving Patient Outcomes* was published in 1997. In 1999, DMAA was organized. The years since then have seen the growth and increased sophistication of these broader DM programs for populations with chronic conditions. In a stratified random sample survey of 65 health plans in 2000, Welch and colleagues (2002) found that the prevalence of DM programs in health plans increased considerably between 1996 and 2000. Prevalence rates increased from 45% to 83% for diabetes, from 50% to 77% for asthma, and from 14% to 57% for congestive heart failure. These were thought to be conservative estimates. Other estimates are that revenues in the DM industry grew from $77 million in 1997 to $350 million in 1999, and that in 1999, 56% of employers, 67% of HMOs, and 64% of point-of-service (POS) plans offered DM to their beneficiaries (Berger et al., 2001). In 2000, health

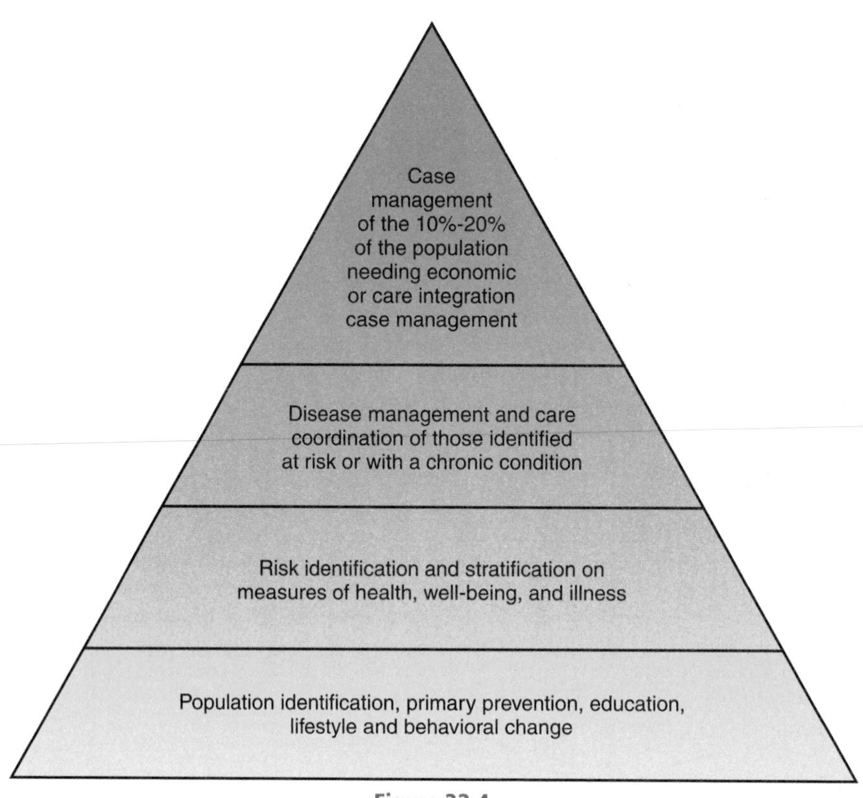

Figure 22.4
Integrated model. (From Coggeshall Press. [2008]. *Care for the total population.* Coralville, IA: Author.)

plans spent about $360 million on DM, and the figures for 2002 were expected to be about $510 million (Nobel & Norman, 2003). Projections for 2003 were for $725 million in revenue (Cousins & Liu, 2003), and the continual increase in health care spending continues to trend upward.

Todd and Nash (1997) described four generations in the history of DM. This view identified DM as an evolving phenomenon that is progressing in sophistication. The first generation was distinguished by enhanced services. One or more services outside the usual medical care were added to help address illness care. These developments often were prompted by quality report card or accreditation requirements.

The second generation saw the targeting of the sickest patients because they are the highest risk for generating costs. Outreach, education, and proactive, ongoing follow-up to reduce costly acute care episodes are featured.

The third generation saw the true integration of care and a true population-based focus. Risk identification and stratification occur. All important elements of care are addressed for the population using evidence-based protocols. Treatment is centrally coordinated, and health outcomes and costs are tracked.

The fourth generation is projected to contain a true health management model that focuses on optimizing health through wellness and prevention. Lifelong health education and strong incentives for healthy lifestyle behaviors will be featured. Resources will be allocated based on who is most likely to respond and benefit. DM programs are moving into the third generation and are looking to the future fourth generation.

POPULATION-BASED PROGRAM PLANNING

Both DM and PHM tend to occur within organized programs. Nurses need to have skills and knowledge in health care program planning to best showcase their unique contribution to DM.

Health care program planning emerged in the early 1980s. It began as a key aspect of health education and health promotion endeavors. Early models contained operational planning, program development, and strategic planning. In the late 1980s, business plans became more common as tools for both new ventures and health care program development. Now, program planning also needs to address the evidence base for practice and outcomes evaluation criteria. Programs also must be evaluated for their potential and relative worth in terms of cost, quality, and value (Hall, 1998).

A comprehensive program plan enables an assessment of the potential for success before allocating resources, provides a plan to streamline and facilitate implementation, identifies all needed resources, and outlines a way to obtain reliable and valid evaluation data. An integrated population-based program planning model contains the following four components (Hall, 1998):

1. Contextual analysis
2. Implementation plan
3. Budget
4. Evaluation plan

A program outline would discuss the problem, state the need, identify assumptions, and present objectives and standards (Hall, 1998).

Community-focused or population-based care delivery planning follows the nursing process. The six basic steps are as follows (Schuster & Goeppinger, 1996):

1. Establishing the contract partnership
2. Assessing
3. Determining the nursing diagnosis of the problem
4. Planning
5. Implementing interventions
6. Evaluating interventions and outcomes

Assessment involves gathering data, developing a composite database, and interpreting the data. Data gathering usually involves obtaining existing data about the demography of a community. Data such as population characteristic distributions of age, gender, socioeconomic status, and race; vital statistics such as morbidity and mortality; disease incidence and prevalence; community institutions and resources distribution; and health care provider characteristics and distribution are gathered (Schuster & Goeppinger, 1996). Because of the influence of managed care reimbursement, the top few employers in the community might also be determined, since the health care needs and policies of the largest groups of insured individuals will have an influence on community health needs and resources.

Population and community health status may be profiled by vital statistics such as births and deaths, the incidence and prevalence of the leading causes of mortality and morbidity, health risk profiles of selected aggregates, and functional ability levels. The structure of community health may be profiled by the number and location of health facilities such as hospitals and nursing homes, the health-related planning groups, health workforce types and numbers, and health resources utilization patterns. Data may be gathered by existing databases, surveys, interviews of key informants, or published reports. The five key methods of collecting data are (1) informant interviews, (2) participant observation, (3) windshield surveys (the drive-by equivalent of simple observation), (4) secondary analysis of existing data, and (5) surveys (Schuster & Goeppinger, 1996).

After data gathering and assessment, a nursing diagnosis of the problem is generated. A modification of the nursing diagnosis format can be used. The three parts are "risk of," "among," and "related to." Each part is filled in to identify the problem clearly. The planning phase is then begun. It consists of problem analysis, problem prioritization, goals and objectives determination, and intervention activity development. Problem analysis may

Practical Tips

Tip # 1: Locate Your Population Members

Think of ways to identify populations of interest within the scope of your practice. Then identify one way to access a registry of patients' names or contact information.

Tip # 2: Use Large Databases

Partner with a health statistician in an insurance company to run epidemiological variables from claims data.

Tip # 3: Teach Others About DM

Prepare a background overview presentation on predictive modeling and return on investment (ROI). Present this to your work group.

---

use a matrix or spreadsheet to map and identify direct and indirect precursors and consequences; relationships among problems, precursors, and consequences; and supportive data. Origins and impacts of the problem, points for intervention actions, and parties with an interest in the problem and solution need to be identified (Schuster & Goeppinger, 1996).

The problems identified as part of the assessment need to be ranked to determine relative importance. Priorities are established by using predetermined criteria. The following six criteria are recommended (Schuster & Goeppinger, 1996):

1. Community awareness of the problem
2. Community motivation to resolve it
3. The nurse's ability to influence problem solution
4. Availability of relevant expertise
5. Severity of consequences
6. Speed with which resolution can be achieved

Goals and objectives for high-priority problems need to be established in precise, clear, behaviorally stated, incremental, and measurable terms. A search for the evidence base for any recommended interventions needs to be done. If standardized evidence-based protocols exist, these should be used. Intervention activities also can be mapped on a spreadsheet, along with a probability rating of the likelihood that the activity will foster achievement of the objective and be implemented. Interventions are then implemented and evaluated. Evaluation criteria include successful intervention implementation, meeting of partnership objectives, problem resolution, participant satisfaction, and development of community strengths. Evaluation of both costs and effectiveness is important. The process includes a feedback loop to renegotiate the partnership if needed (Schuster & Goeppinger, 1996).

POPULATION-BASED RISK ASSESSMENT

The aggregate health care costs of chronic conditions increase yearly as individuals grow older. Older individuals tend to have chronic conditions that require complex care. It is estimated that one third to one half of all health care spending is consumed by the elderly. With the shift in demographic trends toward increasing numbers of elderly, there is a shift in the need for preventive care and chronic illness management services (Coleman, 1999). To meet this challenge, managed care organizations have created infrastructures of population-based risk assessment, demand management (self-management and decision support systems such as call centers), DM, and CM.

Illustrating the continuum of care as spanning the well and worried well (self-directed care and primary care), the acutely ill (secondary and tertiary care), and the chronically ill (tertiary care and long-term care), Coleman (1999) identified the corresponding infrastructure. Demand management spans the entire continuum. Case management and DM cover primary care through long-term care and focus on acute and chronic conditions. Case management is identified as valuable for high-volume, high-risk conditions and those who have catastrophic illnesses.

To be effective at individual and population-based care management, both case and DM programs need to identify, assess, and define the populations to be served early in the program planning effort. After the population has been defined, individuals within the population need to be selected and assessed for the appropriateness of case or disease management as an intervention. Profile characteristics may be age, number of chronic illnesses, or number of medications. Sometimes a survey such as a health assessment questionnaire is used to screen for high-risk indicators (Aliotta, 1996).

Population-based risk identification is an innovation that helps determine the best use of staff and clinical resources while also identifying the long-term health needs of groups and populations. Risk identification can be comprehensive when it spans health promotion, wellness, chronic disease, illness, and disability. It can be specific when identifying persons at risk for high-cost, high-intensity, or long-term health care needs. Levels of risk are primary (prevention), secondary (early detection), and tertiary (management of an episode of care) (Burgess, 1999).

A more detailed model of population care management contains these six levels: population needs assessment, identification of health services, targeted health planning, wellness and prevention, care management, and case management (Qudah & Brannon, 1996). Population-based risk identification leads to referring individuals into CM and DM programs. "Disease management is largely an ambulatory care program" (Goldstein, 1998, p. 102). Extended CM often is targeted at persons with complex conditions, multiple diagnoses, or extended-term care requirements. Cost-effectively managing populations requires careful risk identification and then the application of population-based principles and care strategies.

Zitter (1997) outlined the following six key success factors for the development and implementation of any DM program:

1. Understanding the course of the disease
2. Targeting patients likely to benefit from the intervention
3. Focusing on prevention and resolution
4. Increasing patient adherence through education
5. Providing full care continuity
6. Establishing integrated data management systems

The selection of a specific DM program for initiation and implementation can be guided by an analysis of the environment and potential target populations. Nobel and Norman (2003) identified the following four modules used by effective DM programs:

1. Candidate identification and stratification
2. Enrollee recruitment
3. The intervention itself
4. Evaluation

Each module contributes an important link in the process, and the four combine to form a process loop. Timely access to critical information is needed in each of the four modules.

Gillespie outlined the following seven criteria useful in the selection of a condition as a candidate for implementing a DM program (Gillespie, 2002):

1. Availability of treatment guidelines with consensus about the appropriateness and effectiveness of care
2. Generally recognized problems in therapy that are well documented in the medical literature
3. Large practice variation and a variety of drug treatment modalities
4. Large number of patients with the disease whose therapy could be improved
5. Preventable acute events that are often associated with the chronic disease (e.g., an emergency department or urgent care visit)
6. Outcomes that can be defined and measured in standardized and objective ways and that

can be modified by application of appropriate therapy (e.g., decreased number of emergency department visits or hospitalizations)

7. The potential for cost savings within a short period (less than 2 years) (p. 226)

In a stratified random sample survey of 65 health plans in 2000, Welch and colleagues (2002) found that virtually all DM programs exhibited the following characteristics:

- Used evidence-based guidelines
- Identified the population with a disease
- Stratified the population by risk
- Matched the intervention with the need
- Educated patients in self-management
- Evaluated the program's process and outcomes

LEADERSHIP AND MANAGEMENT IMPLICATIONS

Managing the Continuum of Care

Nurses need to focus on managing the continuum of care as a basis of nursing practice. Collaboration and communication are essential elements of coordination and integration across a "seamless" continuum of care: "Continuity of patient care involves a series of coordinating linkages across time, settings, providers, and consumers of health care. Communication is a core task in coordinating patient care" (Anderson & Helms, 1998, p. 255). Continuity of care, as a care management strategy, often requires that clients be tracked through multiple organizations or settings of care. The communication of client data and care needs is fundamental to continuity of care. Therefore coordination of care involves communication across boundaries. This need is increased with the multiple and complex elements of chronic illness management and decreased hospital inpatient stays (Anderson & Helms, 1998). Individual nurses may not see immediate opportunities in their jobs for true continuity of care. However, as the emphasis on DM and PHM accelerates, nurses have a leadership role and opportunity to use their skills creatively with DM and PHM perspectives. The principles and protocols of CM, DM, and PHM hold value for advanced registered nurse practitioners (ARNPs). These three care management strategies can provide the organization and administration frameworks useful for doctor of nursing practice (DNP) students and graduates as they manage their specialty populations.

One critical application of managing the continuum of care is the facilitation and management of interdisciplinary and interorganizational communication for continuity of care. This is an imperative

LEADERSHIP & MANAGEMENT BEHAVIORS

Leadership Behaviors

- Envisions improved health services for populations
- Encourages interdisciplinary and interorganizational coordination
- Inspires nurses to develop population-based health care plans
- Creates linkages across care settings
- Enables providers to work together to coordinate care delivery

Management Behaviors

- Plans for coordination of population health care
- Organizes interdisciplinary teams
- Directs critical pathways and other population-based care plans
- Manages interorganizational linkages across the continuum of care
- Controls provider actions for coordinated outcomes

Overlap Areas

- Leads population-based care planning
- Motivates providers to coordinate care for populations and communities

because information transfer is necessary for planning and planning is necessary for continuity of care. Information exchange problems and gaps were found in a study of CM and interorganizational referral communication between a hospital and a home health agency within one health care system (Anderson & Helms, 1998; Anderson & Tredway, 1999). The need for barrier reduction in interorganizational communication is an urgent continuity-of-care need. Resources need to be redirected toward reducing obstacles and facilitating data and information transfer to improve the health of individuals and to manage population health care better.

Three major strategies of DM programs are (1) the use of an interdisciplinary team, (2) outcomes evaluation to measure results, and (3) the application of information management technologies. These three core techniques are used with a population health focus to improve overall health outcomes.

Included in the DMAA definition of DM components is that collaborative practice models include physicians and all support service providers. Provider disciplines have become areas characterized as "silos" that prevent integrated care. The interdisciplinary team needs to form and collaborate on the total plan of care, with each discipline integrating its expertise. For medical conditions, physicians, nurses, pharmacists, dietitians, social workers, and any other allied health professional with specific expertise need to be incorporated into the team. Communication among and between team members is the key to a successful program.

CURRENT ISSUES AND TRENDS

DM is an established health care trend. The viability of health care organizations may depend on how an organization responds to the needs of specific population bases (Hall, 1998). A current trend is for the development of integrated population-based programs. For example, a children's home-based asthma management and prevention service was developed for a military clinic in the southeastern United States (Hall, 1998). The University of Virginia School of Nursing developed a nurse-managed primary care clinic to serve low-income elderly and disabled housing authority residents (Glick et al., 1996). The Visiting Nurse Service of New York has had a Community Nursing Organization Medicare demonstration project to deliver community-focused nursing CM services to elderly clients (Storfjell et al., 1997). Nurses' roles include integrating, coordinating, and advocating for individuals, families, and groups to improve continuity and enhance appropriate service use. The disease manager's role is to screen for risks, monitor risk factors over time, and initiate both preventive and treatment measures.

Research results are being reported about population health-related care delivery. For example, Bryan and colleagues (1997) investigated the learning needs of hospital-based nurses preparing to change from acute care to community-based care. A national Delphi study was done to determine competencies for nursing leadership in public health. The results showed four areas of needed competency: (1) political competency, (2) business acumen, (3) program leadership, and (4) management capability (Misener et al., 1997). Outcomes for community health practice have been studied (Alexander & Kroposki, 1999), and a useful measure of population health status has been analyzed (Kindig, 1999). The effects of CM on the context of nursing practice have also been studied (Lynn & Kelly, 1997). Evidence-based guidelines for public health nursing practice have been explored and developed (Strohschein et al., 1999). These research projects are beginning to lay a foundation for evidence-based practice in DM and PHM by showing that DM and PHM are viable programs to address cost and quality issues.

Another current trend is the identification of patient adherence as a driver of disease cost and the need for intervention with clients to foster adherence (Aliotta, 1996, 1999). *Adherence* is the extent to which the client continues a negotiated treatment. *Maintenance* is the extent to which a client continues health behavior without supervision. This compliance/adherence engagement is critical because the ultimate benefit of a treatment plan depends on the extent to which the client implements it. Adherence may directly improve outcomes. For example, poor adherence has been implicated in drug-resistant strains of tuberculosis. Aliotta (1999) stated, "Current best evidence suggests a strong potential for establishing linkages between adherence and better outcomes in the area of chronic illness" (p. 82). Nurses have the skills to deliver adherence interventions.

Information management technologies are critical at every stage of a DM program. Nobel and Norman (2003) divided the information management arena into information gathering, information integration and analysis, and information deployment. Effective programs need timely access to clinical, administrative, financial, and logistical information flows. Once acquired, these large databases need to be analyzed to identify opportunities for effective interventions to enhance the management of care and services. Deployment of information is reflected in strategies of notification, alerts, reports, and assessment of trends and the impact of interventions. A variety of information management technologies are emerging, such as biometric and handheld devices that can collect and distribute information (Nobel & Norman, 2003).

Technological innovations in informatics have made possible the rapid analysis of large databases. In turn, statistical analyses have become more sophisticated. Currently, claims databases are the primary sources used for data mining and profiling for DM, although related databases such as pharmacy and nursing care are being linked or merged with claims databases for more robust disease profiling and prediction. Two important applications of information management technologies in DM are predictive modeling and calculation of return on investment (ROI). Predictive modeling is the use of statistics to calculate expected costs based on variables such as demographics, diagnoses, pharmacy claims, and survey data (Kramer, 2004). Predictive models have been used in other industries, such as credit card companies and retailers, for years. Applied to DM, predictive models would be able to analyze data to answer questions such as, How much of a cost trend is being driven by age and how much by illness? Which complications and co-morbidities drive costs (Kramer, 2004)?

Calculation of ROI is being attempted in CM (Smith et al., 2003) and DM. ROI is one method used to describe the impact of case or disease management. It is a dollar calculation of the value of cost savings produced by the case or disease manager in exchange for what is spent on the program. It is a desirable benchmark given cost pressures. Although no standardized formula yet exists, there is beginning convergence on the inclusion of hard and soft savings criteria (Smith et al., 2003).

Summary

- Disease management is an innovative strategy for managing chronic conditions.
- Progress needs to be made in health care coordination of chronic conditions and in population health.
- Managed care and the Institute of Medicine are two forces that have emphasized DM and care coordination.
- DM programs have six components for comprehensive care.
- Population-based health care focuses on aggregates and communities.
- A population is a collection of individuals who have a characteristic in common.
- Population-based care management is the integration and coordination of health services to a population.
- DM programs offer coordination, consistency, and customization.
- Community participation and partnership are key elements.
- There are four components of population-based program planning.
- The six steps of population-based care planning follow the nursing process.
- Population-based risk assessment is a part of chronic illness management and resource management.
- Care for a population is depicted as a triangle.

- DM programs use evidence-based guidelines and risk stratification.
- Nurses need to manage the continuum of care and have the skills to address advocacy and adherence.
- Collaboration and communication are essential to care coordination.

CASE STUDY

The disease manager (DM) for Big Insurance Company (BIC) is reviewing today's printout from the predictive modeling analysis of pharmacy claims for attention deficit/hyperactivity disorder (ADHD) drugs. Several trends pop out. Of concern is the alarming jump (83% increase) in the number of prescriptions filled for ADHD drugs from 1999 to 2003 and suggestions that ADHD is overdiagnosed. Along with this are concerns of cost (average cost of a 30-day prescription for the popular nonstimulant medication was $108) and therapy adherence. The ADHD drugs are expensive, have side effects, and often are not accompanied by the recommended adjunctive behavioral therapy or dose-to-side-effects adjustment.

The DM then reviews individual claims profiles and selects those with erratic prescription refills. She begins to call individual families for interviews to determine the scope of factors related to adherence. She reaches the mother of Linda, a 15-year-old girl diagnosed with ADHD by a clinical counselor. She was placed on one of the common ADHD drugs, which she does not like to take. Her father is an elementary school teacher, and her mother is a factory worker. The mother relates that Linda is taking her medications "pretty much" and that she needs to take them. She reports no problems except her occasional forgetting to take the drugs. When asked about behavioral therapy, the mother states that Linda's participation in extracurricular events takes up her time so they don't have her doing any therapy sessions. The DM obtains the mother's permission to talk to Linda and arranges a time when Linda can talk to her privately.

The DM calls Linda at the appointed time. She asks Linda to describe her experience of ADHD, the diagnosis, and how things have been going. Linda tells her that she hates taking the medicine and dislikes its side effects. She says that her father complains about the cost and that when she did not want to take her medicine, her father told her to take it once a week so her mother would still think she was taking it. The DM begins a list of pro and con adherence factors in her database. An evidence-based treatment plan will be needed.

CRITICAL THINKING EXERCISE

Nurse Gloria Davis just got her dream job as a case manager for diabetes care in a large integrated delivery system. Nurse Davis is deeply committed to high-quality client care. She has structured an excellent teaching program that is administered through the ambulatory clinics. She has instituted population data collection using the SF-36 and Diabetes Quality of Life tools. Nurse Davis has begun to collect trend data on HbA_{1c} values and frequency of blood glucose instability or complications. The next outcome to measure is client satisfaction. Nurse Davis assumes that client satisfaction is related to compliance with treatment. The first step is a small focus group. In the focus group meeting, Nurse Davis discovers that client interactions with a health care provider are becoming more impersonal. The clients have fewer choices about to whom and where they can go for services, must get complicated authorizations, need to fill out more forms, have to listen to more recorded messages, and are waiting longer for appointments. On clinic days they wait a long time to see their provider only briefly. The process of coming in for care actually makes many of these clients feel worse.

1. What is the problem?
2. Why is it a problem?
3. What are the key issues?
4. What should Nurse Davis do first?
5. How should Nurse Davis handle this situation?
6. What problem-solving style should Nurse Davis use?
7. What leadership and management strategies might be useful?

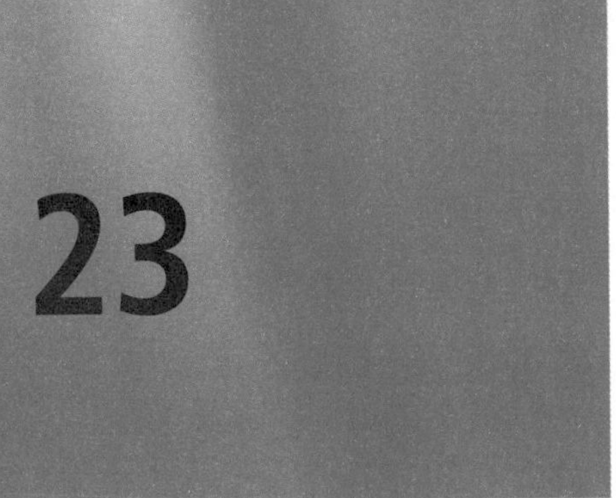

Patient Acuity

Kathy Craig

CHAPTER OBJECTIVES

- Define patient acuity
- Trace the development of patient classification systems
- Critique patient classification systems
- Discuss the interaction between patient classification systems and acuity
- Examine indicators of acuity
- Evaluate research related to acuity and patient classification systems
- Exercise critical thinking to conceptualize and analyze possible solutions to a practice exercise

The patients, clients, and cases that nurses manage and provide care for differ with respect to how intensively and extensively they require nursing services. Acuity matters in the work of nurses. However, measuring acuity is complicated. Beginning attempts were called **patient classification systems (PCS).** Whether crude or sophisticated, PCS attempt to quantify patients' needs for care to match these to the corresponding activities and efforts nurses will need to contribute in service delivery. The two core PCS elements are time and activities.

The interest in the concept of acuity, the rating of complexity in patients' conditions or clients' cases, is undergoing resurgence. In the beginning of PCS in the 1960s, PCS were used to characterize the degree of illness and risk of physiological collapse that patients displayed, usually in hospital settings and in 8-hour or shift-by-shift intervals of change. Traditional PCS are nurse classifications of patient acuity ("acuity PCS"), which are now computer aided and detailed. The earliest PCS are reflections of the disease staging used in medical practice, in which staging classifications identified severity of disease from an epidemiological standpoint with the medical perspective of the individual as the unit of analysis.

In contrast, modern acuity PCS address the individual's severity of illness from a holistic wellness standpoint. From this perspective, acuity PCS include the individual patient's adjustment to illness, at whatever particular stage the patient's disease might be. Nursing PCS incorporate symptomatology from every cause such as secondary and co-morbid conditions, as well as the primary disease. Modern acuity PCS also incorporate elements of self-care, mobility, psychosocial coping, adherence, and personal caregiver support as fundamental elements of overall or holistic acuity. As a common feature of acuity PCS, these pertinent data are synthesized through various methods into an acuity factor, scale, or score. This PCS acuity factor arises organically from the components of each individual's health status and life situation. In this respect, holistic acuity reaches beyond patient acuity to indicate the complexity of the intensity of the nurse's care that is required for maximal self-sufficiency, stability, and safety relative to the specific individual patient.

Acuity PCS are most applicable if they are tailored to the professional discipline, such as nursing, social work, or rehabilitation therapist, that is practicing case management (CM). For example, the

CM Acuity Tool (Craig & Huber, 2007; Huber & Craig, 2007a, b) system contains a patient need-severity stratification, which is juxtaposed onto an array of intervention-intensity responses pertinent to CM roles, functions, and competencies. Acuity PCS couple patient adjustment characteristics with specific provider supports, which are provided as interventions that are required for stability and safety. Patient adjustment strata encompass severity in at least two aspects—traditional symptomatology or severity of illness and levels of demand or dependence. These items constitute the patient's need-severity (Craig & Huber, 2007). The interventions that are required to support the patient's needs should be in proportion to the levels of severity in corresponding degrees of intensity (Figure 23.1). Interventions can be represented at various levels of detail and need to be specific to the provider. However, the ability to quantify interventions by dosage-specific amounts, intensities, frequencies, and duration (Huber et al., 2003) represents the next leap in nursing leadership. This leap will use acuity PCS to advance the refinement of nursing practice by attributing and communicating

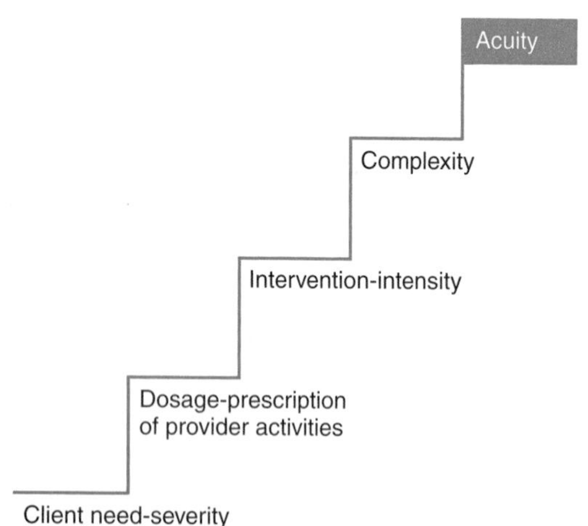

Figure 23.1
Craig-Huber Acuity Building Blocks. Acuity is derived from its foundation in client need-severity with the critical intermediate steps to account for provider activity dosage-prescription, CM intervention-intensity, and degrees of complexity.

the specific actions of nursing professionals on behalf of their patients and clients.

Nursing or profession-centric acuity PCS are the data infrastructure workhorses that have been harnessed to determine staffing mixes and minimums, as well as staffing competencies and performance outcomes. The overarching message in this chapter is that nurses need to learn how to think critically about or judge the construction of classification systems that produce acuity ratings and how to use or analyze acuity as a forward technology of nursing and practice leadership.

DEFINITIONS

Patient acuity is a key concept related to patients' needs for nursing care. To manage human resources in a service delivery system, both patients' needs for nursing care (patient acuity) and the amount of nurse time that is required to meet patients' needs for care (nursing intensity) need to be specifically and more accurately measured. By thus describing patients' care requirements, better projection of adequate nurse care resources can be made. PCS have been used to measure patient acuity to validate care requirements and then attach nursing resources to those requirements. Nurse classifications of patient acuity are called *acuity PCS.*

Nursing **workload** is a measurement of the nursing work activities and the dependence of the clients on nursing care. Thus both direct and indirect nursing care activities are a part of nursing workload (O'Brien-Pallas et al., 1997). Traditionally, nursing workload in a hospital is a function of two variables: the number of patient days and the hours of nursing care required per patient day. Workload is the use of time, and time is the basis of nursing workload measurement. **Acuity** is defined as the severity of illness or client condition. Acuity can translate into volume (census, visits, or encounters) or severity or intensity. Patient classification systems have been used since the 1960s to measure in some fashion clients' needs for care and care activities and assign acuity scores. They have become the basis for workload systems that determine staffing (Prescott & Soeken, 1996a, b).

LEADING & MANAGING DEFINED

Patient Classification System (PCS)

- Organized strategy for the timely matching of patient needs to caregiver skills (Malloch & Conovaloff, 1999).

Workload

- Degree of difficulty and time requirements associated with (e.g., CM, nurse) interventions (Balstad & Springer, 2006).
- Required number of hours of staff time per workload interval and the amount of time necessary to perform all activity surrounding patient care (Cusack et al., 2004).
- Nursing-care intensity points per nurse (Fagerstrom & Rauhala, 2007).
- Quantity determined by contact frequency (King et al., 2004).
- The quantity that lacks an accepted definition and measurement standard involving the measurement of the volume and level of nursing work. Work is frequently gauged by patient acuity and/or amount of task-oriented activity performed. An index of workload may be a stronger predictor of adverse patient events than the patient/nurse ratio (Ream et al., 2007).

Acuity

- The rating of complexity in patients' conditions or clients' cases (Craig & Huber, 2007).
- Patient need-severity in two prominent domains (clinical and psychosocial) coupled with practitioner (e.g., nurse, case manager) intervention-intensity that drives patient, client, or case complexity from lower to higher (Craig & Huber, 2007).
- Single patient's workload value or average workload of all unit's patients (Claudio, 2004).
- Numeric patient profile method to estimate and measure patient care (Malloch & Conovaloff, 1999).
- Mental health care measured by response difficulty through the caseload index approach (CLI) (King et al., 2004).
- Reflection of the "early hopes of creating systems for quantifying pt severity… [it is a] form completed tallying tasks, procedures, and characteristics associated with each patient" (Shaha & Bush, 1996).
- Amount of task-oriented activity performed (Ream et al., 2007).

Nursing Intensity

- A degree of work represented by four areas—severity of illness, patient dependency, complexity of care, and time (Prescott, 1991; Patient Intensity for Nursing Index [PINI]).

Acuity System

- Strategy of assignment of adequate number of staff based on patient-care needs (Claudio, 2004).
- Labor standards (or staffing allowances) lead to mathematical prediction of the amount of nursing care ("allowed"), generally per patient and then per shift, as a cumulative whole (Shaha & Bush, 1996).
- Operationalized assessment of patient need-severity coupled with nursing personnel or case manager intervention-intensity to enable the calculation of distinct classes of complexity (acuity) for process, performance, and outcomes endeavors (Craig & Huber, 2007).

Dosage

- Provider activity prescription by four dimensions—amount, breadth, duration, and frequency (Huber et al., 2001).

Acuity Creep

- Undesired phenomenon in which patient classification ratings are increased or changed over time as users become adept at system (Cusack et al., 2004).

Census

- Patient count per time per area (Cusack et al., 2004).

Caseload

- Volume of patients assigned to an individual (e.g., case manager, nurse) (Balstad & Springer, 2006).

Effective Communication

- Communication that is timely, accurate, complete, unambiguous, and understood by recipient for error reduction and resulting in improved patient safety (TJC, 2008).

Staffing Effectiveness

- Number, competency, and skill mix of staff in relation to the provision of needed services (O'Leary, 2002).

Nursing intensity is defined as both the amount of care and the complexity of care needed by patients in hospitals. Werley and colleagues (1991) operationalized intensity as nursing care hours and staff mix. Prescott (1991) identified four major dimensions to nursing intensity. The four components—severity of illness, client dependency on nursing, complexity, and time—are related to each other and have been combined into a 10-item nursing intensity scale, called the *Patient Intensity for Nursing Index (PINI).* Prescott and Soeken (1996a, b) have developed a companion measure for ambulatory care called the *Patient Intensity for Nursing Ambulatory Care (PINAC).* Three PINI conceptual components of complexity, dependency, and severity were modified for PINAC to severity of illness, patients' psychosocial needs, and complexity of care. Type of visit also was included as a descriptor. Intensity is usually a composite measure of the amount of work or time involved with a level of complexity of the care required (Detwiler & Clark, 1995). Nurse staffing intensity, which is expressed as the ratio of RNs to patient census in hospitals, has been associated with lower mortality in hospitals (Aiken et al., 2002).

PATIENT ACUITY SYSTEMS

Patient **acuity systems** assign acuity levels to patient risk stratification for sources of potential harm or illness worsening. Acuity systems in nursing are defined as a strategy of assigning an adequate number of staff based on patient-care needs (Claudio, 2004). Labor standards (or staffing allowances) lead to a mathematical prediction of the amount of nursing care ("allowed"), generally per patient and then per shift, as a cumulative whole (Shaha & Bush, 1996).

In traditional PCS that truly represent the client's acuity, the majority of the PCS' components focus on the client and the immediate personal caregiver constellation, especially the person's primary care provider. For example, the most experienced case managers know that the best and most versatile plans of care have several levels or strata of back-up plans to facilitate optimal independence and to support the solitary patient or the client-care provider dyad. In acute care settings, nurses know that the best PCS have sufficient detail to reflect each patient's severity of symptoms, risks for deterioration, and levels of needs. In both settings, practitioners know that good PCS are able to show changes, especially deterioration, by increments of magnitude that are appropriately graded and in time frames that are meaningful.

In the traditional patient-centered PCS, studies that illustrate the types of investigations useful for discovering information about the patient's need-severity include Armola and Topp (2001), Bolin and colleagues (2006), Butler and colleagues (2007), Clark and colleagues (2001), Craig and Huber (2007), and Cusack and colleagues (2004).

In 2001, a study by Armola and Topp (2001) looked at 12 different variables in patients with acute heart failure to determine which may best discriminate short versus long length of stay (LOS) for individual patients and which may herald likelihood for readmission within 30 days. The findings reveal that, in this examination, two variables could be used to discriminate between patients who were more likely to have longer LOS—those who had a revolving parade of different medical students, interns, and residents caring for them and patients with high serum sodium levels.

Bolin and colleagues (2006) looked at differences in patient acuity in a 10% sample (n = 197,589) of the national nursing home resident assessments using the 2000 Minimum Data Set to explore differences in acuity at admission to rural versus nonrural nursing home facilities. The client-based information that was discovered is that lower acuity levels correlated with patients' admissions to rural nursing homes for long-term or chronic care.

Butler and colleagues (2007) used a numeric rating scale to show functional limitations in an ambulatory case management setting, specifically in a corporate for-profit workers' compensation setting. They investigated the dosage and timing of nurse case managers' contacts with workers who experienced work-incurred back injuries. Focusing on the workers, the assessment scales collected acuity-defining data from pain scores, workers' satisfaction ratings, and health care use behaviors, as well as the employing firm's responses to their back injuries. An interesting finding was identified. Although work supervisor contacts proved effective only during the first 24 hours after on-job injury, "early nurse case manager contacts (markedly) improve workers' satisfaction with the way the firm is treating them" (Butler et al., 2007, p. 319). The most important discovery was that "early nurse case manager contacts have a very large effect on employment outcomes, roughly doubling the likelihood that an injured worker will remain on the job without taking time off" (Butler et al., 2007, p. 319).

Clark and colleagues (2001) used a risk stratification that paralleled acuity levels in a traditional patient classification system concerning outpatient diabetes management. This risk stratification monitors changes in PCS for diabetic therapy regimen focused on improving glycemic control, increasing monitoring and management of diabetes complications, and increasing patient and provider satisfaction. Several specific measurements are followed with evaluation at a 12-month end stage. The intervention-specific findings were that (1) patients in a low-risk group (defined by an HbA_{1c} value less than 7%) increased by 51%; (2) 97% of patients in a moderate-risk group (defined by an HbA_{1c} value more than 8%) had changes in their treatment regimens; (3) patients in the group at high risk for CHD (defined by an LDL value greater than 130 mg/dL) decreased from 25% to 20%; and (4) patients in a lower risk group (defined by blood pressure readings less than 130/85 mm Hg) increased from 24% to 47%, with 63% of these changes associated with changes in medication prescriptions. Not surprising, both patients and providers expressed significant increases in satisfaction with the outpatient diabetes management program.

Acuity and Dosage: Theory and Practice

Craig and Huber (Craig & Huber, 2007; Huber & Craig, 2007a, b) discussed the highly patient-centered acuity system called the *Case Management Acuity Tool Kit* developed in 2000. At the Tool Kit's heart is the Acuity Tool, which has a primary focus on delineating the CM client's need-severity level in two large domains—clinical and psychosocial.

This structure permits users to drill down within these domains to define driver/sub-driver combinations of specific illness or challenge areas for the client and care provider. Drivers in the clinical management domain include three indicator categories: physical status, primary disease-related symptoms, and secondary co-morbidity-related symptoms. Drivers in the psychosocial caregiver domain also include three indicator categories: patient status; family-caregiver; and satisfaction. Since their inception in 2000, these categories have undergone refinement and improvement for specific CM delivery models, settings, and patient populations. For example, the CM Acuity Tool's original development had a focus on insurance-plan clients who receive CM via telephonic contacts and nationwide care management. In 2005, the Tool's modifications generated an acuity patient classification system for clients who receive care in a single-payer (government) system who receive telephonic and home visitation contacts in a regional program of small city, suburban, and rural settings. A subsequent application of the Acuity Tool Kit is for rare disease CM also delivered in a national telephonic format model.

In the original acuity classification system, the driver/sub-driver combinations allow a well-differentiated description of the main problems that are driving up the acuity score in the case and thus the CM case's level of complexity. The problems are specific to two domains that directly reflect the client and a third domain that spans quality and cost indicator categories, which is a more case manager–focused perspective. Subsequent improvements to the client acuity classification allowed more in-depth problem description and pinpoint data capture for process, performance, and outcomes reporting that increased the ability to redirect focus onto client-specific areas of demand and need. In this regard, the driver/sub-driver combinations are increased from three domain-level ratings to nine domain-level ratings and populate an acuity scale from 5 to 1, heaviest or most complex to lightest or least complex, respectively.

Dosage-Prescription in Nursing and Case Management

The work of Craig's (Craig & Huber, 2007; Huber & Craig, 2007a, b) CM Acuity Tool also fits into this nursing classification of patient-acuity PCS. Craig's Acuity Tools Suite represents work that is based largely on the severity of illness of clients in two spheres called *domains:* (1) the clinical domain, which includes primary and co-morbid disease indicators; and (2) the psychosocial domain, which includes the presence and capabilities of the client's personal caregiver constellation, psychosocial behavior, satisfaction, and adherence to plan by clients and personal caregivers. These items are heavily represented in the CM Acuity Tool and funnel into the intervention-intensity drivers that indicate the overall type, amount, frequency, and duration of CM activity that nurse case managers use expert judgment to quantify. Activity parameters coordinate with the Huber-Hall dosage-prescription model (Huber et al., 2001, 2003) and offer opportunities for research exploration of dosage and acuity applications. The two need-severity degree levels identified through the Tool's format are combined with the degree of intervention-intensity to produce a three-item sum in the original Tool developed in 2000. The sum of these three factors is translated by an algorithm into a Likert scale that in the initial Tool ranged from 1 to 4 in acuity (1 lightest, 4 heaviest). Subsequent Acuity Tool applications use an improved acuity range of from 1 to 5.

Two separate instruments in the Acuity Tool Kit are the Caseload Matrix and AccuDiff© or acuity differentials. The Caseload Matrix is a stratification of case acuities calculated into caseload weights. The caseload weights are juxtaposed by the numbers of cases that case managers carry at any given time and provide a measure of caseload acuity, quantified as light, light$^+$, average, average$^+$, heavy, and heavy$^+$ caseloads. Caseload acuity weights offer robust data-derived parameters that go beyond case counts. The caseload acuities can be used for making rational decisions regarding new case assignment, case redistribution for illness or holiday coverage, and performance recognition and reward. Patient acuity scoring generates the ability to calculate acuity differentials, which compare changes in case acuity at different points in time. The AccuDiff© measurement compares the acuity scores at the beginning and ending of cases and whenever precipitous changes in acuity occur such as at and after crises. Updates to Acuity Tool realize the ability to capture multiple driver/sub-driver combinations due to the migration from a paper-based tool to an electronic informatics format.

The Huber-Hall model of dosage (Huber et al., 2001, 2003) presents a unique way that client-centric activities are extrapolated by using the four cornerstone concepts of nursing and care management **dosage**—amount, breadth, duration, and frequency. In this clinical trial study of clients with substance abuse disorders, the severity of the needs of the clients as individuals and as constituents within different patient populations dictated the dosage-prescriptions they received, the differences by dosage dimensions, and the various outcomes. The dosage model constructs the scaffolding upon which to frame patient-centered care delivery activities. Although they would plan to deliver specific amounts and spacing of medications and treatments by prescription, certain activities of nursing and CM care would be structured for delivery in certain quantities and concentrations at certain prescribed interval frequencies and for certain persisting spans of time.

OVERVIEW OF PATIENT ACUITY SYSTEMS

Acuity and the PCS have changed and matured since their inceptions in the 1960s. Many variations exist, and there is room for improvement. However, these simple devices constitute one of the fundamental tools needed to convey essential clinical, psychosocial, and functional details about every patient and client under the watchful protection of a nursing professional. Nurses and care managers have the opportunity, knowledge, and ability to provide resourceful leadership

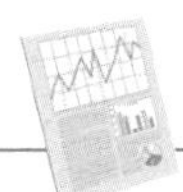

Research Note

Source: Craig, K., & Huber, D.L. (2007). Acuity and case management: A healthy dose of outcomes, Part II. *Professional Case Management, 12*(4), 199-210.

Purpose

The purpose of this series of three articles was to present dosage and acuity as two aspects of making a business case for case management by using more precise and valid measurement tools to get the right data. This research focused on the Acuity Tools Project, which resulted in a suite of instruments and measurements of case acuity in case management practice.

Discussion

Part II features an in-depth discussion of three parts of the Acuity Tools Project: the Acuity Tool, Caseload Matrix, and AccuDiff© instruments and how they can be used to calculate valid caseload acuities. Once weighted acuity scores are generated for each case assigned to a case manager, then caseload acuity can be analyzed. Subsequently, caseload differences across case managers can be analyzed and better managed. The Acuity Tools Suite was used to calculate four aspects of case manager case acuity: individual case acuity, overall caseload acuity profiles, case length, and acuity differentials.

Application to Practice

The evidence base for practice needs a foundation of rigorous measurement and valid data capture that is specific and sensitive. The Acuity Tools Suite provides case managers with a valid and reliable way to analyze and present data-driven evidence to describe their actual practice, complexity and all. This then forms the infrastructure for demonstrating the business and professional worth of case management.

using the wealth of data from well-designed acuity systems that keep the patient's best welfare at the center of the equation.

The PCS acuity factors arise as organic or natural components of each individual's health status and life situation. In contrast, disease and medical staging classifications extrapolate from a population to a disease stage rather than to a person.

Disease classification systems are the precursors of traditional PCS. Modern PCS represent the nursing adaptation of the prominent disease staging or medical risk classification systems that physicians, oncologists, and epidemiologists have employed in great number. The disease staging classifications abound in medical-surgical textbooks and are developed by organizations specializing in particular diseases and medical conditions. If a medical quality website like the National Quality Measures Clearinghouse™ (sponsored by the Agency for Healthcare Research and Quality [AHRQ; *www.qualitytools@ahrq.gov*], U.S. Department of Health and Human Services) is searched, countless disease staging classifications can be found. Although the content in medical texts is accessible and informative to nurses, nurses are encouraged to develop and use nursing-developed PCS. Because nurses do not diagnose medical conditions, few disease staging classifications have been developed by nurses as primary researchers.

In disease staging, an individual's severity of disease is judged based on a risk stratification by medical diagnosis and is implied in the general grouping of patients. Medical diagnoses of degrees of patient sickness are based on measurements and calibrations of cellular changes, organ abnormalities, and physiological system anomalies as signs of illness. These criteria, collected and collated over thousands of individuals, are used as comparisons against which the individual's condition is contrasted for classification of degree and extent of disease presence, or staging, and for prognosis estimation. The direction of the medical disease assessment is from the general to the specific; the basis of classification is the patient population; and the most likely unit of examination is the grouping by biophysiologic components. For example, in the disease staging of a patient with lung cancer, the level of a patient's disease is classified into large divisional stages I through IV. The individual's specific condition is implied from the status within the large stratification grouping. If the group within which the patient falls does not fare well, this person is likely to not fare well. This person's characterization of functioning is subsumed to the illness or wellness of the stage to which the patient's functioning is assigned. If the cells are sick, the patient is sick.

However, in nursing the emphasis of the severity classification in PCS arises from the individual's specific adaptation to the consequences of illness, at whatever particular stage the patient's disease might be, such as inherited, newly diagnosed, chronic long-standing progression, or palliative end-of-life stage. Beyond symptomatology from the primary disease, modern acuity PCS incorporate symptoms from every cause such as secondary and co-morbid conditions with facets of self-care, mobility, psychosocial coping, and adherence. As fundamental elements of overall or holistic acuity, indicators of the individual's personal support system and its richness or sparseness are included. The personal support system spans from primary carer (caregiver) through secondary familial back-up to general community support. Such presence or absence and sound or compromised functioning can be loaded into acuity classifications systems as the data that the PCS capture. This level of data represents the individual's holistic circumstance with respect to wellness and safety, illness and dependence, and need for support and augmentation in the form of health care utilization and service provision.

Practical Tips

Tip # 1: Use Nurses' Data to Manage Better

Realize and use the power of acuity and PCS in practice. These form internal-to-nursing essential data systems that measure and capture nursing's value ("business case") and are powerful internal management-of-services data. This is not just added documentation burden; this is nursing's data.

Tip # 2: Use Acuity as a Platform for Reflective Practice

Promote reflective practice behaviors. Patient acuity matched to nurse acuity raises powerful questions such as, Should we staff to fully meet all patients' needs? If not, who decides what needs will not be met?

Tip # 3: Use Acuity Outcomes to Achieve New Goals

To optimize appropriate length of stay (LOS), employ triggers from acuity-based PCS. As outcomes parameters for reducing LOS, poorly kept I&O records and tired care plans are given new life and importance. Directives, such as (1) monitor care coordination for patients with multiple physicians and (2) assess and improve hydration status, can empower nursing staff to use familiar nursing care activities to achieve new goals to improve acuity scores and patient outcomes.

Indicators of acuity are synthesized as data elements through differing methods. Nurse researchers and frontline nursing practice professionals construct acuity factors, scales, and scores from these indicators of severity of needs and robustness of support. The holistic acuity of nursing reaches beyond patient acuity to indicate the complexity of the health care system's resources and responses. In particular, the acuity PCS of nursing practice reach into the intensity of the nursing professional's care and the larger health care system's support that is required for maximal self-sufficiency, stability, and safety relative to the specific person rather than the patient as a unit of population or the repository of a disease stage.

First-Generation PCS: Patient Classification Systems Emerge

Traditional PCS have existed since the 1960s and matured during the 1970s. Considering the 1960s and 1970s as the first generation of PCS, Malloch and Conovaloff (1999, p. 49) identified PCS as a major cause not only of distress but also of "misuse and manipulation." The acuity PCS instrument is a numeric method to profile patients that is used to estimate, measure, and predict patient care. Malloch and Conovaloff reported that, although caregivers (carers) may have recognized the value of acuity PCS, they did not "embrace PCS as a valid & reliable method to estimate and measure patient care" (Malloch & Conovaloff, 1999, p. 49). The distress and distrust, in part, stem from the phenomenon called **"acuity creep,"** in which staff become adept at misrepresenting patient care needs via acuity falsification "padding" in efforts to inflate staffing needs. Malloch and Conovaloff identified gaming behavior as "not uncommon" but fail to confirm how commonly the behavior occurs. Assigning acuity this way is prone to manipulation by nurses because they fall prey to human phenomenon when the system seems unfair or invalid. Malloch and Conovaloff offered three explanations for this misuse of acuity PCS: (1) lack of credibility resulting from an industrial theory being applied to nonindustrial phenomenon; (2) fluctuating "economies of scale" with inaccuracies in resource estimation; and (3) variabilities across care providers.

As an added consideration, the acute care bias of most PCS is an obstacle to adoption. Cusack and colleagues (2004) discussed patient intensity in the ambulatory outpatient research clinic as being based in nursing classification systems used to forecast staffing needs for inpatient settings. Most first-generation systems for classifying patients' severity of needs and soundness of psychosocial supports are coupled intimately with care-related interventions performed by nurses compared with the numerous nursing practitioners who require appropriately adapted PCS. This hand-in-glove development of PCS means that, since PCS began, indications about carer delivery levels required to meet and match the severity of needs have been woven together. These usually reflected the traditional acute care hospital settings and have remained a challenge for nursing researchers, leaders, and frontline practitioners to design and develop functional PCS for alternative settings.

The real-time acuity systems capable of matching need-severity to intervention-intensity did not exist during the first PCS generation. Census-at-midnight was the general operating principle for tracking bed occupancy and patient flow, and this volume measurement, although misleading and unserviceable, would remain the primary tracking measurement of patients for decades to come and is still in use. Estimates of acuity were intuitive and seldom grounded in clearly designed PCS rating scales. Nurses were considered equal and interchangeable except for the most critical of critical care areas. Data were calculated manually, annually, and historically on retrospective files of patients and mistake-filled or gross-level reports of dated material that poorly represented the daily fluctuations of patient care settings. The fluctuations in volumes and needs were addressed by simple overstaffing.

Shaha and Bush (1996) wrote that the traditional PCS approach of the 1970s was "not effective for determining staffing needs or for controlling costs of patient care staffing" (p. 346). Their explanation was that "acuity reflects the early hopes of creating systems for quantifying patient severity" formed from the completion of "tallying tasks, procedures, and characteristics associated with each patient" (p. 346). Although the purpose of acuity has become "clearly," according to Shaha and Bush, "to determine caregiver staffing by categorizing patients into classes...reflect(ing) needs for care," this labor-standard use of acuity-based PCS for which they had been high-jacked was "rigid and dictatorial, disruptive, cumbersome to update" (Shaha & Bush, 1996, p. 347). Using acuity and PCS to determine staffing levels on a hospital-wide or macro level was open to manipulation by "classifiers (who became) more skilled at manipulating acuities to get more staffing" (Shaha & Bush, 1996, p. 347). As "acuity creep" evolved and costs continued to rise, suspicions about the accuracy and reliability of acuity levels per classes of patients increased and acuity PCS fell to disfavor or disregard awaiting the development of systems "less susceptible to nurse manipulation" (Shaha & Bush, 1996, p. 347).

At different times, other nurse researchers and leaders discussed the reliability vulnerability in acuity classification systems. Cusack and colleagues (2004) warned developers and users of acuity-based classifications systems that they must beware of "acuity creep"—the tendency over time for acuity levels to change as users become more adept at using, and gaming, the system. Malloch and Conovaloff (1999) also discussed the demon "acuity creep," identifying it as a more sinister and intentional inflation or falsification of acuity classes to meet the needs of staffing upgrades for anticipation of needing to staff-up for the worst of patients and shifts. The disparity between acuity as a pure patient classification system and its being high-jacked to determine staffing levels reflects the practitioner as a human being versus a robot (Malloch & Conovaloff, 1999).

Second-Generation PCS: Grand-Scale Changes; Inconsistent Measurement

Other descriptions of the disease and patient classification efforts in the late 1970s stemmed from the overarching change in disease staging ushered in by the U.S. federal government in the form of diagnosis-related groups (DRGs) initially in 1979 and updated in 1983 (Malloch & Conovaloff, 1999; Swan, 2005). The DRG and managed care delivery models dwarfed other methods of PCS in the 1980s. In the DRG-managed care delivery model, payment still was conducted retrospectively but according to predetermined and proscribed, or managed, categories of related diagnoses. Malloch and Conovaloff (1999) described the impact of the change: "Introduction of managed care...transform(ed) healthcare into a business" (p. 50). The gargantuan shift in classification systems from individualized to grouped diagnoses and the restrictions on reimbursement that came with DRG payment systems caused the migration of inpatient care delivery to outpatient service provision.

During this interval, PCS were mandated by accrediting organizations such as The Joint Commission (TJC; formerly Joint Commission on Accreditation of Healthcare Organizations [JCAHO]). Technology was undergoing advances associated with the introduction of computers into health care workplaces and software development for hospital use. Although visions of seamless integrated health care delivery abounded, this did not materialize. Zhang and colleagues (2006) described the minimum staff ratios that accompanied federal legislation for nursing homes in the 1987 Nursing Home Reform Act (NHRA) as a part of the Omnibus Budget Reconciliation Act (OBRA). The NHRA under OBRA required minimum staff levels for registered nurses (RN) and licensed practical nurses/licensed vocational nurses (LPNs/LVNs) based on hours per resident-day (HPRD). Although laws were on the books and accrediting agencies were setting minimum requirements, it remained difficult to assess if hospitals were complying because of lack of consistent record retention and report generation.

Examples of PCS developed during the second PCS generation include the 76-variable Therapeutic Intervention Scoring System (TISS) (Keene & Cullen, 1983; Yeh et al., 1984) and the patient acuity level (PAL) developed by Saake

(1986) and used in research (Ream et al., 2007; Zhang et al., 2006). Swan (2005) explained the differences in tools for acute to ambulatory care by citing the tool developed by Hastings in 1987 that included more patient independence but "episodes of care" as treatment periods and levels of intensity that might range from minutes to hours depending on the outpatient care being received and delivered. Although briefer treatment periods were more common and better known during the 1980s, examples of longer treatments included outpatient dialysis and chemotherapy administration. These more sustained contacts were evolving as recurring but discrete episodes of care and required the rethinking of traditional in-hospital acuity systems.

Other PCS, often called *taxonomies,* were introduced in the 1980s, such as ones from De Groot (Malloch & Conovaloff, 1999). These new quantification schemes wedded patient classifications to nurse time expended or activity categories in numerous specialty areas within acute care facilities and in alternative settings such as outpatient ambulatory care (Swan, 2005).

Second-Generation Solution: Managed Care/Managed Staff

Managed care delivery systems and efforts to better manage RN staff were the hallmarks of the second generation of PCS. The tension between reducing nursing staff and keeping minimally adequate numbers of nurses to satisfy the accrediting organizations' mandated PCS requirements placed nursing staff in the continual crosshairs of cutbacks—fiscal constraints as horizontal crosshair and staffing-up to meet possible maximal patient acuity needs as the vertical crosshair. Attempts to satisfy the ever-present need for bedside nurses and nurse managers came in the form of labor management solutions. Nurse extenders, float pools, subcontracting, travel and registry nurses, and cross-training were commonplace (Malloch & Conovaloff, 1999). Computerized options for directing workflow began to move from other scientific application areas into hospital settings, but these seldom were used for data collection on nursing practice. Finance and hospital administrators, at the same time, saw nurses as the major expenditure of hospitals and often settled for faster but less economically sound expenditure management solutions. Decisions of finance and hospital administrators led to budgetary overshoots according to Malloch and Conovaloff (1999).

Cusack and colleagues (2004) identified three main sources of information regarding PCS for the 1990s, as follows: Prescott (1991); Haas and Hackbarth (1995); and the American Nurses Association's (ANA) staffing advisory panel (Gallagher et al., 1999). Prescott categorized necessary nursing interventions according to two components—budgeting determinants by nursing hours of care per patient-day and staffing needs by shift. Haas and Hackbarth contributed the prototype method for inpatient encounters. The work of the ANA panel regarding safe and appropriate staffing began to shift the focus from hours per patient-day to interventions and complexity of care. Cusack and colleagues reported that the seven critical factors that ANA encouraged leaders to consider are (1) patient numbers; (2) patient intensity; (3) environment architecture; (4) environment geography; (5) technology availability; (6) levels of staff experience and preparation; and (7) unit functions necessary to support delivery of high-quality patient care.

Standard practice guidelines for inpatient care, such as those developed by Milliman and Robertson and InterQual (Milliman, 2007), are the mainstay of managed care reimbursement systems. These commercial guidelines, based on patients' primary presenting diagnosis and major treatment codes, operate against idealized national standards of necessity of care, level of care, and goal length-of-stay criteria. According to Milliman literature, these "utilization management decision criteria…[are] based on medical literature and actual practice of physicians across the US…" (Milliman, 2007, p. 1). Milliman materials report the following (Milliman, 2007):

> Since early 1980s, our industry has been caught between rising demand on one side of the healthcare equation, and rising costs on the other. Medical research has shown that one way to cut spiraling costs is to reduce wasteful and unnecessary practices." (p. 2)

This quote highlights a problem that persisted during the 1980s—even the best acuity-based PCS containing severity and intensity indicators drew from physician instead of nursing literature, foundation, and practice. The PCS were less patient-centered and remained poorly aligned to pertinent nursing and case management assessments and interventions until more nursing studies began to emerge in the late 1980s, 1990s, and into the twenty-first century.

Third-Generation PCS: Multiplicity in the Marketplace

The 1990s saw the blossoming of classifications systems, instruments, and measurements that such giants of the health care industry as Aiken, Giovanetti, Prescott, and Verran germinated and grew (Malloch & Conovaloff, 1999). They explained that "enormous inefficiencies in daily caregiver and patient interaction" (p. 53) remained unresolved. New technology and new research become available, and new regulations were imposed. Administrators continued to employ macro-management principles while hospital stays were getting shorter and staff were becoming more transitory. The Health Care Financing Administration (HCFA) revised its staffing standards, and The Joint Commission began requiring clinical outcomes measures for accreditation. However, not only did "caregiver rating by skill level…remain taboo" (Malloch & Conovaloff, 1999, p. 53), but "nurse staffing is a battle" that pitted mandatory minimum staffing laws against downsizing the nursing workforce to save money.

By the second-generation stage of development, expectations about the capabilities of PCS systems became more realistic. Malloch and Conovaloff noted that traditional time-study models were becoming "a dimension of PCS rather than the essence of PCS" (Malloch & Conovaloff, 1999, p. 53). More fact-derived data were available from which improved time estimations could be developed. It became clear that the identification of standard patient classification nomenclature was essential, such as the efforts of Iowa's Nursing Interventions Classification (NIC), to evaluate patients on admission, at every shift, and at hospital discharge for seven care aspects, including the patient's clinical condition, self-care management ability, knowledge, and health behaviors. As more specificity in patient description and categorization of needs solidified, PCS become more amenable to standardization, research, and outcomes linkage. Components of patients' care profiles were supplemented by medical record documentation from insurance claims, pharmacy use, and closer-to-real-time nursing records. Care provider competency remained the most difficult component for organizations to develop and the most distressing for nurses who are reluctant to "brand" one another such that "nurses' skill levels are seldom noted or managed during patient assignment decisions" (Malloch & Conovaloff, 1999, p. 54).

Third-Generation Solution: Standards Staffing

In the 1990s, using technology, PCS became more fully automated and incorporated into hospital computer tracking and reporting systems. Although thousands of health care customers are using computers from companies such as 3M and Microsoft in numerous countries, HOROPLAN in France, Park in Korea, and Fischer in Switzerland, care provider skill levels were not advanced and PCS remained difficult to use (Malloch & Conovaloff, 1999). However, these PCS were only poorly capable of achieving shift workload allocation based on patient acuity criteria.

Fourth-Generation PCS: Nursing Informatics

Although "development…of PCS parallel the adoption of technology," Malloch and Conovaloff (1999, p. 55) explained the future of PCS in the Fourth Generation: "patient always receive exactly the care they need at the appropriate time…in the holistic, humanistic, and seamless integrated healthcare delivery system." Software and hardware devices will be low-cost, remote, and flexible. In these authors' vision, bedside monitoring technology with automatic software tracking and monitoring of caregiver-patient interactions, times, and totals will be available through "transponder signal-embedded workstation devices" (Malloch & Conovaloff, 1999, p. 55). Real-time activity charts will be produced at the toggle of a switch or the click of a character.

"(A)xiomatic to the success of PCS," Malloch and Conovaloff believed, is "overcoming obstacles to [recognize and manage] varying levels of caregiver competence" (Malloch & Conovaloff, 1999, p. 55). The primary purpose of the recognition and management of caregiver competency is to better match caregiver competencies with specific patient needs. The secondary purpose is to enhance quality outcomes for patients, clients, personal caregivers, and families, as well as to improve outcomes for nurses and for nursing, resource, and finance managers. In the fourth-generation PCS, capturing and reporting true direct patient-hours will be accomplished for use in projecting or forecasting severity of needs and requisite caregiver time, effort, and intensity for patients in similar strata, risk groups, or clinical constellations. Also, indirect work efforts (Clarke & Aiken, 2006; Cusack et al., 2004; Kane & Issel, 2005), latent variables (Bradley, 2005; Clarke & Aiken, 2006; Peters et al., 2007; Ream et al., 2007), and care provider "slack-time" (Malloch & Conovaloff, 1999, p. 55) will be incorporated in future generations of PCS.

Fourth-Generation PCS Solution: Reasoning on the Data

Computer informatics (CI) that use neural networks, algorithms, and computational intelligence in the pursuit of illness detection, disease minimization, and care interventions will be the "single biggest change in how societies grow, work, and live" (Johnson, 2006, p. 87). Confidence in CI applications will promote enhanced "reasoning on the data" that can result in improved quality of life through the emerging field of nursing informatics. By discovering patterns that enable predictions for more effective therapeutic care, nursing-informatics informed acuity systems will become more accurate and beneficial to health care delivery.

The evolution of the traditional PCS has lead to the acuity PCS in five core perspectives. The most familiar core perspective is the patient-centered classification system, as a patient acuity. The four other core perspectives are nurse acuity (nursing practitioner acuity), nursing classification of patient acuity, unit acuity, and organization acuity.

NURSE ACUITY

Nurse acuity is the next level of acuity perspective for consideration. In a classification system that focuses on nurse or provider acuity, the content of the system is framed to define and describe the components that make up the levels of time, difficulty, complexity, and skill demand that the nurses must offer to meet the need-severity levels of their patients and clients. Many studies attack the problem of matching intensities of care activities and interventions to patients' severities of need. In fact, what most clinicians and researchers consider traditional PCS actually are nurse acuity classification systems that carry the PCS name.

Cusack and colleagues (2004) monitored five direct and indirect care measures of nursing task difficulty and "activity visibility," a parameter that correlates with time-for-task. In an ambulatory outpatient research clinic, a classification system called *Ambulatory Intensity System (AIS)* was used. This is based on the 1989 work of Hastings in which three major factors are identified for outpatient workloads: patient census volumes, patient care demands, and nurse roles. *Workload* is defined as the gross number of hours of staff time required per workload interval and the specific amount of time necessary to perform all the activities surrounding an aspect of patient care. **Census** equals the patient count per time per area defined. Nurse demand identifies the skill level necessary, diagnosis, clinical symptoms, and patient-intensity acuity upon which the plan of care is established. *Nurse role* involves patient care in its direct and indirect manifestations as well as the clinical duties and administrative overlay.

The nursing AIS is designed to determine outpatient practitioner workload through the collation of encounters by acuity and by intensity as time spent per activity. Cusack and colleagues (2004) described the direct patient contacts in the ambulatory practice setting as patients' visits, interactions, and encounters that can range from a 1-minute phone call for an initial triage to an 8-hour chemotherapy treatment. Indirect patient-care contacts include items done on behalf of a specific patient and ones necessary for the coordination and delivery of care to a specific individual versus contacts done for a generic group of patients. A detailed chart of the levels of indirect and direct nursing activities required to do patient care is presented. Time ranges per skill distinctions are identified for numerous encounters.

Cusack's outpatient AIS uses methods similar to the two methods to sort encounters used in inpatient settings—prototype and factor. In the prototype method, a best-fit match is sought from four or five priority levels indicating different intensities of care and amounts of time. The disadvantage of the prototype method, according to Cusack and colleagues (2004), is its subjectivity. The factor method employs a concept of "activity visibility" that correlates with sums of activities and time spent per activity sums. The sum or category of activities means that the greater the sum is, the more "visible" the task is and the higher the acuity factor is. The disadvantage of the factor method, these authors stated, is that it does not include nursing judgment, complexity of care, simultaneous combinations of multi-tasked activities, and technical changes.

Nursing Classification of Patient Acuity

Earlier efforts at developing classification systems that incorporate both patient acuity and nursing intervention were described by Phillips and colleagues (1992) and numerous articles by Prescott (Prescott, 1991; Prescott & Soeken, 1996a, b; Prescott et al., 1991; Prescott et al., 1989). Whereas the Patient Intensity for Nursing Index (PINI) system was designed to meet both the administrative and clinical needs that exist in the acute care setting, the Patient Intensity for Nursing: Ambulatory Care (PINAC) summarized medical and nursing approaches to patient classification in ambulatory care. Phillips and colleagues (1992) compared the PINI system with two other existing and widely used classification systems: Medicus and GRASP. Phillips and colleagues concluded that Medicus and GRASP, both commercial products available for purchase, did not measure nursing resources in the same way as did the PINI system. Because of this, Phillips and colleagues advised nurse administrators to exercise caution in using estimates of nursing care costs based on different methods PCS use to measure nursing intensity. Lack of standardization jeopardizes apples-to-apples comparisons. This is a judicious warning that still stands today for any nursing classification systems based on patient acuity.

Prescott determined that the PINI system constituted a "valid measure of volume or amount of care and complexity of nursing care delivered to patients" (Prescott et al., 1991, p. 213). Constructed of four dimensions, their nursing intensity model includes (1) severity of patient illness; (2) patient dependency; (3) complexity of care; and (4) time needed for care delivery. Each dimension contains 10 items for scoring nursing care using a four-point ordinal scale. Time loading is attached to each of three factors—severity, dependency, and complexity.

The 1991 study involved daily ratings of over 6000 patients from 487 RNs in 29 ICUs and medical-surgical units in five Pennsylvania hospitals. Each nurse estimated the amount of time spent delivering nursing care to specific patients. Estimated times were contrasted with observed times and shown to correlate significantly. In addition, PINI scores were related significantly to medical severity of illness, length of stay, and disposition at discharge. PINI scores also showed significant correspondence to the number of secondary medical diagnoses present and the number of specialty consults conducted. Comparing PINI with three hospital-based PCS used in 1991 for staffing purposes, the authors indicated that PINI scores correlated significantly to these three systems. Furthermore, the PINI system showed a strong ability to sort patients into high-intensity DRGs and low-intensity DRGs.

These findings indicated that the PINI and the PINAC strategies offered value and usefulness for the systematic collection and analysis of data that successfully blend the fundamentals of patient acuity, specifically severity of illness and levels of dependency, with the nursing factors concerning intervention-intensity, time, and complexity. The scoring capabilities are exactly what are needed to systematically compare data among patients, nurses, caseloads, units, DRGs, and hospital facilities. Caution is warranted, however, about drawing conclusions regarding estimates of nursing costs across systems that employ different methods to measure nursing intensity.

An array of materials, articles, and analyses exists in nursing and CM literature that looks at the classification systems that combine nursing and patient acuity. From this unified perspective, there is a hand-in-glove fit between the patient's acuity and the nursing response acuity, which Craig and Huber (Craig & Huber, 2007; Huber & Craig, 2007a, b) called *intervention-intensity.* This combination is one that is very likely to be commandeered to solve nursing staffing dilemmas, often with poor satisfaction. One reason for this dissatisfaction revolves around the differences in workloads compared with caseloads that nurses and case managers carry.

A real and important distinction exists between caseload and workload. **Caseloads** are aligned with the patient and patient-related case acuities. Caseloads are readily transitioned to caseload weights to reflect the overall complexity of the cases or patients for whom the nursing professional has responsibility. However, nurses' workloads extend beyond the nurses' actual patients, clients, and caseloads and into the architecture of the unit and organization in which they are working. The efficiencies and inefficiencies of nursing professionals' surroundings and work processes and the added responsibilities assigned to them in their jobs as performance and ancillary duties greatly affect the workload but may have limited effect on the caseload. Workloads incorporate the general management of the organization duties assigned to nurses.

LEADERSHIP AND MANAGEMENT IMPLICATIONS

Nurses provide "around-the-clock surveillance" (Aiken et al., 2002, p. 1991) for patient safety and early detection of patient deterioration. However, according to O'Leary of The Joint Commission, modern society has left the "resource-flush world" of hospitals in the 1960s and finds itself in a troubled system of "severe staffing shortages, particularly of nurses" (O'Leary, 2002, p. 2). He explained that data about sentinel events link "serious adverse events with insufficient staffing" (O'Leary, 2002, p. 2). In 2002, O'Leary proclaimed that the linkage between patients' adverse events and nursing shortages has driven the "nurse staffing issue to the top of our public policy agenda" (O'Leary, 2002, p. 4).

According to The Joint Commission, sentinel warning signs can precede an adverse event by an "average of 6 to 8 hours" (TJC, 2008). Thus The Joint Commission standards advised that for adequately staffed inpatient settings with specifically trained personnel, **effective communication** regarding sentinel warning signs is the early recognition and response method to reduce cardiopulmonary arrests and patient mortality.

Within acute care hospitals, subacute and long-term care organizations, and outpatient treatment facilities, well-designed acuity PCS with nursing-sensitive indicators can serve as highly responsive sentinel signaling instruments. In community-based nursing practice, acuity PCS have the ability to function in both short-view and long-view contexts to identify individual clients' baseline characteristics against which changes in acuity can be visualized and acted upon.

The technology of PCS and acuity started with paper-and-pencil, time-and-motion, annual budgets, and midnight census. It marched through legislative and business pressures with monthly budgets, daily staff allocation via computerized processes, and volume census. Now, PCS technologies are poised at the threshold of achieving the perceived goal of PCS—timely matching of patient needs to care provider interventions—and a discovery is dawning. The most useful patient-centric PCS will score severity of needs in the clinical, behavioral, psychosocial, and care provider spheres and remain focused on the client. Effective PCS do not solve staffing dilemmas; they describe the need-severity and intervention-intensity of nursing or care management interventions, and they relay the overall complexity of the client's circumstances in the dynamic language of acuity capable of capturing the changes in severity, intensity, and complexity parameters over time by keeping the correct core perspective—the patient and his or her needs for care.

CURRENT ISSUES AND TRENDS

Leadership initiatives are needed to discover and quantify the correct patient need and intervention elements, develop them into instruments with comprehensive acuity scales and scores, and test the elements and instruments for reliability and validity. The elements and instruments of acuity PCS must promote optimal reflective practice that distinguishes nursing professionals in the outcomes arenas of both quality patient care and business accountability.

The momentum of the future wave of acuity PCS will propagate through a dynamic combination of factors: nursing-sensitive acuity systems capable of capturing client-specific indicators and nursing professionals' interventions operationalized into predictive dosage-prescriptions. The acuity data and dosage delineations constitute a robust way to connect nursing professionals' actions by amount, intensity, frequency, and duration directly to outcomes not only for patients but also for all health care participants—practitioners, teams, units, departments, and facilities. From the direct connections between actions and outcomes comes the ability to predict. Prediction and outcomes lead to the ability to ascribe accountability; and accountability represents, among other things, the ability to invoice. Therefore acuity and the changes in acuity created through the differential applications of predictably reliable dosages of nurses' work constitute leadership and nursing care management strategies that nurse, finance, and quality mangers and researchers

LEADERSHIP & MANAGEMENT BEHAVIORS

Leadership Behaviors

- Envisions patient classification, acuity, and dosage systems that yield valid data
- Integrates acuity systems with the whole organization's data capture systems
- Advocates for software and acuity analyses
- Inspires team members to use acuity data to demonstrate positive outcomes
- Creates a culture of data-driven change

Management Behaviors

- Develops knowledge and expertise in acuity management
- Forecasts workloads and caseloads and matches staffing
- Uses data to balance workloads and caseloads
- Manages conflicts
- Evaluates acuity and resource use
- Demonstrates value to administration

Overlap Areas

- Creates data systems for acuity
- Creates an environment rich in data use for nursing care management

should adopt, develop, and test. At this cutting-edge, advances by nursing leadership reach beyond patient acuity into the future of professional accountability.

Blending historical PCS concepts with rapidly advancing informatics applications, current trends are to put in place innovative programs that are based on a solid foundation of patient and nurse acuity. One example is the work of Griffin and Swan (2006).

Using the Virginia Nursing Outcome Database (VANOD), Griffin and Swan (2006) presented a formidable example of the way to employ nurse-sensitive indicators to discover nurse-sensitive outcomes. Griffin and Swan were able to explain the quality and effectiveness of nursing care related to patient acuity factors. The authors' explanations included how to visualize nursing contributions to quality of care, how to incorporate nurse-sensitive specifics into classifications that can be operationalized for quality of highly pertinent data, and how to use this data-derived content in annual business plans to signify the excellent work and contributions made within to the health care system by nurses and nursing discipline practitioners. To pull all of the threads together, information must contain multiple lists of components from several instrumental sources.

Griffin and Swan (2006) identified three main repositories of source content. From the American Nurses Association (ANA), the foundational work of Nursing Quality Indicators in 1994 defined indicators to illuminate RNs' contributions to improved patient outcomes. The ANA released 10 acute care nurse–sensitive indicators in 1996 and 10 community nurse–sensitive indicators in 2000. The second milestone work is the 2001 (The Joint Commission) **staffing effectiveness** indicators appearing in groups called *human resource, untoward events, workload,* and *community practice.* Eight indicators are related to staff, one indicator addresses complaints from patient caregivers, and nine indicators are in the untoward-events group. The third major source is the National Quality Forum's (NQF's) three phases of directives:

- Voluntary performance standards as quality-of-care measures for ambulatory care in 2004
- Standards for ambulatory care that identify 43 measures of individual and paired nurse-sensitive indicators grouped into eight "body" topics in Phase II
- NQF's call for identification and submission of measures from each primary area within acute care and from mental health, long-term care, and spinal cord injury treatment settings in Phase III

Griffin and Swan's (2006) work collated the source content into seven nurse-sensitive indicators for acute inpatient care that rely on eight nurse-sensitive performance indicators (PIs) that closely ally with the capture of patient acuity information. In addition, the authors identified seven workload indicators, or nursing tasks, that populate the unit acuity portion of their nursing classification system. Griffin and Swan incorporated these data into a staffing and outcomes overview strategy of classification systems and reporting capabilities that focus on activities and nurse-sensitive indicators corresponding to nursing in specific unit areas. They compress mountains of data into a one-page weighted data stratification that generates three nursing staff workload indicator categories of sub-optimal, acceptable, and delighted. The weighted data are produced quarterly and projected onto a "radar" grid representing the three staff workload categories. This work is done primarily to justify four expense categories: staff level changes, equipment needs, process improvements, and workflow needs based on nine synthesized measures: (1) staff number; (2) staff mix; (3) education and training; (4) workflow; (5) retention and recruitment; (6) equipment enhancements; (7) workflow reorganization; and (8) ancillary support staff use. In addition, nursing report cards are issued to evaluate quality and effectiveness of nursing care. Nursing report cards serve to justify nursing staffing levels by linking administrative elements of staffing with the nurse-sensitive indicators via the workload and performance indicators. The Griffin and Swan (2006) model's components offer designers all the elements needed to design a data-informed nursing classification system based on the three dimensions of patient acuity, nursing caseload and workload acuity, and multiple levels of nursing-sensitive indicators and outcomes for unit and organizational depth-of-field acuity perspectives.

Summary

- Patient acuity is the patient's need for nursing care based on severity of illness and the patient's condition.
- Patients differ as to how much they need nursing services.
- Acuity matters but is difficult to measure.
- Nursing intensity is the amount of nurse time needed to meet patients' needs for care.
- Patient classification systems (PCS) quantify patients' needs for care and attempt to match them with nursing services.
- The two core PCS elements are time and activities.
- The four dimensions of nursing intensity are severity of illness, dependency on nursing, complexity, and time.
- Patient acuity systems stratify patients by risk.
- The Case Management Acuity Tool Kit measures client need-severity in the two domains of clinical and psychosocial.
- PCS have evolved through four generations of thought and application.
- Nurse acuity forms the basis for nurse workload allocations.
- Acuity PCS can serve as sentinel signaling devices.
- The future waves of acuity PCS will connect nurse intervention activities to patient outcomes.

CASE STUDY

Highest Integrity CM Inc. is a company that provides full-service case management (CM) to insurance-program clients in their homes. Case managers contact clients through home visits, telephone calls, e-mail exchanges, and traditional postal mailings. A client's case arrives on the assigned case manager's desk with details collected by the intake nurse. Beau Wellington, a 74-year-old man, has a primary diagnosis of multiple myeloma that was diagnosed 1 month ago. He lives alone in an upstairs apartment in a rural setting about 40 minutes from the town where he will receive chemotherapy and radiation treatments. He has poor eyesight caused by retinal deterioration associated with type 2 diabetes for which he takes oral medications. His internist has attempted to switch Mr. Wellington to insulin injections and considers the client to be nonadherent and resistant. During the initial home visit, the case manager notes that Mr. Wellington has become more disinterested in his personal hygiene, his apartment is cluttered, and safety issues are present such as a detached hand rail, scatter rugs, and lack of bathtub grip bars. The client states he is reluctant to give himself insulin shots because of his poor eyesight. Also, he appears to have cognitive difficulties in learning, remembering, and sequencing new information although he is reluctant to admit this. Mr. Wellington brings out a tray of medications with about 20 bottles of pills that look like a mixture of expired and recent prescriptions. He needs to attend daily outpatient oncology treatment sessions starting within 7 days and has only one adult child who is willing to drive him in the mornings but cannot remain to bring him home. The case manager knows that a patient transport bus can be secured to bring Mr. Wellington home each afternoon for the 6 weeks of his treatment. Mr. Wellington reports having pain under his arms and side that is not well controlled and that often keeps him awake at night. He is moderately overweight and often eats food not on his diabetic diet.

The case manager needs to determine Mr. Wellington's acuity scored through the CM Acuity Tool. Three domains need to be scored from 5 (most complex) to 1 (least complex). The first domain is Clinical; the second, Psychosocial; and the third, Cost-Utility. In each domain, three driver/sub-driver combinations have components that change by the degrees from 5 to 1. For the Clinical domain, the case manager chooses the secondary or co-morbid symptoms related to diabetes as the main driver/sub-driver at the baseline assessment because more problems for the client are occurring currently from diabetes than from multiple myeloma. The degree of severity is rated as a moderate problem, or 3. The Psychosocial domain includes elements such as adherence, cognitive issues, and caregiver support, all of which present different levels of problems for Mr. Wellington. The case manager chooses the cognitive issues as the main driver of complexity and rates this as above average, or a 4, since the cause and extent are unknown and require attention. The Cost-Utility domain includes the intervention-intensity in terms of the amount of time and difficulty of outreaches the CM will need to perform to acquire the services Mr. Wellington will need within the next several weeks. This is rated as a 4 also. The sum of the domains, $3 + 4 + 4 = 11$, is converted to the acuity score of 4. Therefore Mr. Wellington's case is of above-average weight or complexity with acuity of 4. The case manager records these specific indicators in Mr. Wellington's case, which is tallied in the case manager's caseload and seen by the unit supervisor.

CRITICAL THINKING EXERCISE

Nurse Diana Witte is the program manager for a group of case managers (CMs) employed by a large national telephonic case management company. The CMs are complaining about their workload, often citing stress and lack of time to complete their work. Most try to avoid accepting new cases, if possible. Nurse Witte has met with each CM and feels the need to gather data about the scope of case assignment and workload factors for each CM. At the annual conference of the Case Management Society of America (CMSA), Nurse Witte has heard about new ways to determine case acuity but does not fully understand this concept. A quick, easy, and inexpensive system is desired.

1. How would Nurse Witte locate the needed information for understanding the acuity concept?
2. What do case-acceptance avoidance behaviors mean? How can this be resolved or restored to a positive state?
3. What criteria for selection of an acuity system would lead to Nurse Witte selecting the most rigorous acuity system to implement?
4. What organizational stakeholders need to be included?

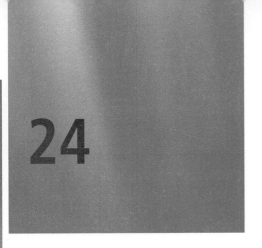

Quality Improvement and Health Care Safety

Luc R. Pelletier Lecia A. Albright

CHAPTER OBJECTIVES

- Define health care quality
- Identify your role in health care quality
- Identify two industrial models of quality
- Define PDCA
- Propose enhancements to a quality and performance improvement program based on recommendations of recent Institute of Medicine reports
- List and describe two performance measurement selection criteria
- Describe one emerging health care quality model
- Describe the costs of poor quality care
- Define mission and vision
- Propose two core value statements for an organization
- Describe two tools that a nurse can use in a quality improvement activity
- Demonstrate the use of two quality tools/techniques
- Describe the role of quality in accreditation programs
- List two examples of public data reporting systems
- Describe health care safety program components
- Define sentinel events, and describe a manager's role in risk management reporting
- Define health care risk management
- Describe the risk management interface with health care safety and performance improvement
- Exercise critical thinking to conceptualize and analyze possible solutions to a practice exercise

Health care quality is an art and science that continues to evolve. Its relevance has been heightened with ongoing reports from the Institute of Medicine (IOM) and other national organizations related to health care and health care quality. Well before these reports were published, however, professional nurses have assumed key roles in the business of measuring, monitoring, and improving health care quality. The news of health care errors is not a new phenomenon. Nurses have typically taken a leadership role in quality and performance improvement and continue to do so in their roles as board members, executives, quality directors, risk managers, and safety officers. It is important to note that identifying opportunities for improvement and continuously improving services is everyone's job. Where once there was a dedicated quality department in an organization, now best-in-class health care organizations train everyone in performance improvement techniques. It would be difficult to describe the entire field of health care quality in one chapter. The authors have distilled a large amount of information and emerging trends and have targeted specific content toward nurse managers. This system overview includes industrial, health care, and emerging models of quality, the costs of poor quality, health care quality leadership and planning strategies, resources available to the nurse manager, health care safety, and health care risk management.

DEFINITIONS

Benchmarking is a tool to assist in quality-of-care decision making. Most recently, it has been defined as "an improvement process in which an organization measures its strategies, operations, or internal process performance against that of best-in-class organizations within or outside its industry, determines how those organizations achieved their performance levels, and uses that information to improve its own performance" (Sower et al., 2008, p. 4). **Best-in-class** is defined as "a standard that [an organization] should aspire to attain" (p. 5). A **patient safety practice** is "a type of process or structure whose application reduces the probability of adverse events resulting from exposure to the health care system across a range of conditions or procedures" (Shojania et al., 2001, p. 29).

Continuous quality improvement (CQI) is defined by the American Society for Quality (ASQ) as "a philosophy and attitude for analyzing capabilities and processes and improving them repeatedly to achieve customer satisfaction" (ASQ, 2007). Further, the Agency for Healthcare Research and Quality defined CQI as "techniques for measuring quality problems, designing interventions and their implementation, along with process re-measurements" (Shojania et al., 2004, p. 16).

Evidence-based practice is defined by Sackett and colleagues (1996) as "the conscientious, explicit, and judicious use of current best evidence in making decisions about the care of individual patients" (p. 71). More recently, evidence-based practices have been defined as "those clinical and administrative practices that have been proven to consistently produce specific, intended results" (Hyde et al., 2003, p. 15).

Health care quality indicators "provide an important tool for measuring the quality of care. Indicators are based on evidence of 'best practices' in health care that have been proven to lead to improvements in health status and thus can be used to assess, track, and monitor provider performance" (Hussey et al., 2007, p. i).

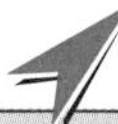

LEADING & MANAGING DEFINED

Benchmarking

An improvement process in which an organization measures its strategies, operations, and internal process performance against that of best-in-class organizations.

Best-in-Class

A standard that an organization should aspire to attain.

Patient Safety Practice

"A type of process or structure whose application reduces the probability of adverse events resulting from exposure to the health care system across a range of conditions or procedures" (Shojania et al., 2001, p. 29).

Continuous Quality Improvement (CQI)

"A philosophy and attitude for analyzing capabilities and processes and improving them repeatedly to achieve customer satisfaction" (ASQ, 2007). Further, CQI is a set of techniques for measuring quality problems, designing interventions and their implementation, along with process re-measurements.

Evidence-Based Practice

"The conscientious, explicit, and judicious use of current best evidence in making decisions about the care of individual patients" (Sackett et al., 1996, p. 71). More recently, evidence-based practices are defined as those clinical and administrative practices that have been proven to consistently produce specific, intended results.

LEADING & MANAGING DEFINED—cont'd

Health Care Quality Indicators

"Provide an important tool for measuring the quality of care. Indicators are based on evidence of 'best practices' in health care that have been proven to lead to improvements in health status and thus can be used to assess, track, and monitor provider performance" (Hussey et al., 2007, p. i).

Performance Measure

"A quantitative tool (e.g., rate, ratio, index, percentage) that provides an indication of an organization's performance in relation to a specified process or outcome." (The Joint Commission [TJC], 2008b, ¶ 13).

Performance Measurement System

"A vendor that provides an automated database to facilitate performance improvement in health care organizations by collecting and disseminating data pertaining to process/outcome measures of performance. Beginning with first-quarter 2001 data, measurement systems are required to provide feedback reports that include both control charts and comparison analysis to their client organizations" (TJC, 2007, ¶ 20).

Quality

Term referring to the characteristics of and the pursuit of excellence.

Health Care Quality

The extent to which health services provided to individuals and populations improve desired health outcomes. The care should be based on the strongest clinical evidence and provided in a technically and culturally competent manner with good communication and shared decision making.

Quality Improvement Program

An overarching organizational strategy to ensure accountability of all employees, incorporating evidence-based health care quality indicators, to continuously improve care delivered to various populations. It is the organization's blueprint for achieving and maintaining performance excellence.

Risk Adjustment

A process in which differences among clients or variables such as age or disease severity are weighted or adjusted for in outcomes analyses.

Risk Management

A "process designed to protect the financial assets of the organization and to maintain high-quality medical care" (Velianoff & Hobbs, 1998, p. 91).

Risk Management Program

An organization-wide program to identify risks, control occurrences, prevent damage, and control legal liability.

Sentinel Event

An unexpected occurrence involving death or serious physical or psychological injury.

Standards

Written value statements.

Total Quality Management (TQM)

"A term coined by the Naval Air Systems Command to describe its Japanese style management approach to quality improvement. Since then, TQM has taken on many meanings. Simply put, it is a management approach to long-term success through customer satisfaction. TQM is based on all members of an organization participating in improving processes, products, services and the culture in which they work. The methods for implementing this approach are found in the teachings of such quality leaders as Philip B. Crosby, W. Edwards Deming, Armand V. Feigenbaum, Kaoru Ishikawa and Joseph M. Juran" (ASQ, 2007).

A **performance measure** is "a quantitative tool (e.g., rate, ratio, index, percentage) that provides an indication of an organization's performance in relation to a specified process or outcome" (The Joint Commission [TJC], 2008b, ¶ 13).

A **performance measurement system** is "[a] vendor that provides an automated database to facilitate performance improvement in health care organizations by collecting and disseminating data pertaining to process/outcome measures of performance. Beginning with first-quarter 2001 data, measurement systems are required to provide feedback reports that include both control charts and comparison analysis to their client organizations" (TJC, 2007, ¶ 20).

Quality refers to characteristics of and the pursuit of excellence. **Health care quality** is defined as "the degree to which health services for individuals and populations increase the likelihood of desired health outcomes and are consistent with current professional knowledge" (Lohr, 1990, pp. 128-129).

A **quality improvement program** is an overarching organizational strategy to ensure accountability of all employees, incorporating evidence-based health care quality indicators, to continuously improve care delivered to various populations. It is the organization's blueprint for achieving and maintaining performance excellence.

Risk adjustment is a process in which differences among clients or variables such as age or disease severity are weighted or adjusted for in outcomes analyses or benchmarking efforts (Maas & Kerr, 1999).

Risk management is defined as "an interdisciplinary process designed to protect the financial assets of the organization and to maintain high-quality medical care" (Velianoff & Hobbs, 1998, p. 91).

A **risk management program** is defined as an organization-wide program to identify risks, control occurrences, prevent damage, and control legal liability; it is a process whereby risks to the institution are evaluated and controlled.

A **sentinel event** is an unexpected occurrence involving death or serious physical or psychological injury, or the risk thereof. Serious injury specifically includes loss of limb or function. The phrase "or the risk thereof" includes any process variation for which a recurrence would carry a significant chance of a serious adverse outcome. Such events are called "sentinel" because they signal the need for immediate investigation and response (The Joint Commission, 2009, p. 1).

Standards are defined as written value statements. These statements form the rules that apply to key processes and the results that can be expected when the processes are performed according to specifications. The three basic types of standards for health care quality are (1) structure, (2) process, and (3) outcome standards (Katz & Green, 1997).

Total quality management (TQM) is described as follows (ASQ, 2007):

> ...a term coined by the Naval Air Systems Command to describe its Japanese style management approach to quality improvement. Since then, TQM has taken on many meanings. Simply put, it is a management approach to long-term success through customer satisfaction. TQM is based on all members of an organization participating in improving processes, products, services and the culture in which they work. The methods for implementing this approach are found in the teachings of such quality leaders as Philip B. Crosby, W. Edwards Deming, Armand V. Feigenbaum, Kaoru Ishikawa and Joseph M. Juran.

HEALTH CARE QUALITY IN THE TWENTY-FIRST CENTURY

Professional nurses have an obligation to reasonably ensure that the care they provide is evidence-based and that work processes are consumer-centric. Providing "quality" health care is "the degree to which health services for individuals and populations increase the likelihood of desired health outcomes and are consistent with current professional knowledge" (Lohr, 1990, pp. 128-129). Nurses, as leaders and managers, have served as health care quality professionals in varied health care settings and have promoted standardization, measurement, and continuous quality improvement in a myriad of delivery settings. Professional nurses have consistently held the practice of quality management in high regard and have the effective care of clients as their primary focus. Nurses are bound by their professional association's *Code of Ethics* (American Nurses Association [ANA], 2005) and scope of professional standards to participate in the continuous improvement of the services they provide.

Although the manufacturing industry has dutifully explored ways to enhance its business practices, health care has lagged behind, and only within the past 20 years or so has it embraced improvement concepts. Health care has borrowed and applied models of continuous quality improvement and total quality management with principles and practices originally developed for the manufacturing industry. As industry has had its quality gurus, so too has the health care quality movement been fostered by professionals who have focused on continuous improvement.

Donald M. Berwick, MD, co-author of the book *Curing Health Care: New Strategies for Quality Improvement* (Berwick et al., 1990), was an early pioneer in identifying how the concepts of TQM programs could apply to health care. In 1991, the National Demonstration Project on Quality Improvement in Health Care was conducted as a collaboration between members of the John A. Hartford Foundation, the Harvard Community Health Plan, the Juran Institute, the Hospital Corporation of America, and other health care organizations (Institute for Healthcare Improvement [IHI], 2004). The goal was to apply the methods and tools of industrial quality improvement in a variety of organizations to determine whether they could apply to a service industry. Berwick was a principal investigator for this project. As a result of this endeavor, the Institute for Healthcare Improvement (IHI) was founded and became an early advocate for the concepts of process improvement and team problem solving in health care organizations.

In the mid-1990s, the Joint Commission on Accreditation of Healthcare Organizations (JCAHO) (now The Joint Commission [TJC]) began incorporating the principles of continuous quality improvement into its revised standards. Starting in 1996, the Institute of Medicine (IOM), through its Committee on Quality of Health Care in America (CQHCA), has convened the nation's quality leaders and other public and private stakeholders to assess and improve health care for all. These leaders have promoted continuous quality improvement in health care through education, research, and evaluation. Through their dedication and insights, they have defined health care quality for this generation and those ahead. Tenets promoted by these health care leaders and organizations, and embraced by health care quality professionals, include the following:

- Processes and systems are the problems, not people.
- Standardization of processes is key to managing work and people.
- Quality can be enhanced only in safe, nonpunitive work cultures.
- Quality measurement and monitoring is everyone's job.
- The impetus for quality monitoring is not primarily for accreditation or regulatory compliance, but a planned part of an organization's culture to continuously enhance and improve its services, based on continuous feedback from employees and customers.
- Consumers and stakeholders must be included in all phases of quality improvement planning.
- Consensus among all stakeholders must be gained to have an impact on quality.
- Health policy should include a focus on continuous enhancement of quality.

A framework for understanding health care improvement has been proposed by the IOM Committee on Quality of Health Care in America (Box 24.1). These six aims for health care quality improvement propose that health care systems ensure that care is safe, effective, patient-centered, timely, efficient, and equitable.

Box 24.1

Institute of Medicine's Specific Aims for Health Care Quality Improvement

- *Safe:* "Patients should not be harmed by the care that is intended to help them, nor should harm come to those who work in health care" (IOM, Committee on the National Quality Report on Health Care Delivery, 2001, p. 47).
- *Effective:* "Refers to care that is based on the use of systematically acquired evidence to determine whether an intervention, such as a preventive service, diagnostic test, or therapy, produces better outcomes than do alternatives—including the alternative to do nothing" (IOM, Committee on the National Quality Report on Health Care Delivery, 2001, p. 49). Evidence-based practice requires that those who give care consistently avoid both underuse of effective care and overuse of ineffective care that is more likely to harm than help the patient (Chassin, 1997).
- *Patient-centered:* "Refers to health care that establishes a partnership among practitioners, patients, and their families (when appropriate) to ensure that decisions respect patients' wants, needs, and preferences; and that patients have the education and support they need to make decisions and participate in their own care" (IOM, Committee on the National Quality Report on Health Care Delivery, 2001, p. 50).
- *Timeliness:* "Refers to obtaining needed care and minimizing unnecessary delays in getting that care" (IOM, Committee on the National Quality Report on Health Care Delivery, 2001, p. 53).
- *Efficient:* "Refers to a health care system where resources are used to get the best value for the money spent" (Palmer & Torgerson, 1999, p. 1136). "The opposite of efficiency is waste; the use of resources without benefit to the patients a system is intended to help. There are at least two ways to improve efficiency: (a) reduce quality waste and (b) reduce administrative or production costs" (IOM, CQHCA, 2001, p. 54).
- *Equitable:* "Providing care that does not vary in quality because of personal characteristics such as gender, ethnicity, geographic location, and socioeconomic status" (IOM, CQHCA, 2001, p. 6).

From Pelletier, L.R., & Hoffman, J.A. (2002). A framework for selecting performance measures for opioid treatment programs. *Journal for Healthcare Quality, 24*(3), 25. Reprinted with permission from the National Association for Healthcare Quality.

COLLABORATION AND HEALTH CARE QUALITY AS NURSING IMPERATIVES

Collaboration should be a goal of any interaction, regardless of the workplace or situation. Collaboration is an imperative set by the American Nurses Association (ANA). The ANA, in its release of a revised *Code of Ethics for Nurses with Interpretive Statements* (2005), proposed that "The nurse collaborates with other health professionals and the public in promoting community, national, and international efforts to meet health needs" (Provision 8). Collaborative partnerships are part of this imperative and shape the way professional nurses act clinically and how they participate in quality improvement efforts.

Collaboration is about relationships. Conflict is typically the result of a poor interpersonal relationship with a colleague. To overcome conflicts, it is necessary to strengthen, not shy away from, the relationship of the two opposing parties. The Pew Health Professions Commission (PHPC) talked about practicing relationship-centered care as one of 21 health profession competencies for the twenty-first century (O'Neil & PHPC, 1998, p. 23). Relationship-centered care in this context surely involves nurse and client/family interactions, but it also stresses the importance of collaborative interdisciplinary relationships. These 21 competencies are necessary ingredients for professional relationships and can become guideposts for successful professional working relationships within a continuous improvement framework.

The 21 competencies also include a professional nurse's responsibility and accountability to health care quality. The specific statements related

Box 24.2

Twenty-One Competencies for the Twenty-First Century

1. Embrace a personal ethic of social responsibility and service.
2. Exhibit ethical behavior in all professional activities.
3. Provide evidence-based, clinically competent care.
4. Incorporate the multiple determinants of health in clinical care.
5. Apply knowledge of the new sciences.
6. Demonstrate critical thinking, reflection, and problem-solving skills.
7. Understand the role of primary care.
8. Rigorously practice preventive health care.
9. Integrate population-based care and services into practice.
10. Improve access to health care for those with unmet health needs.
11. Practice relationship-centered care with individuals and families.
12. Provide culturally sensitive care to a diverse society.
13. Partner with communities in health care decisions.
14. Use communication and information technology effectively and appropriately.
15. Work in interdisciplinary teams.
16. Ensure care that balances individual, professional, system, and societal needs.
17. Practice leadership.
18. Take responsibility for quality of care and health outcomes at all levels.
19. Contribute to continuous improvement of the health care system.
20. Advocate for public policy that promotes and protects the health of the public.
21. Continue to learn and help others learn.

From O'Neil, E.H., & the Pew Health Professions Commission (PHPC). (1998). *Recreating health professional practice for a new century: The fourth report of the Pew Health Professions Commission.* San Francisco: PHPC.

to health care quality include "Take responsibility for quality of care and health outcomes at all levels," and "Contribute to continuous improvement of the health care system" (O'Neill & PHPC, 1998, pp. 29-43) (Box 24.2).

INDUSTRIAL MODELS OF QUALITY

Industrial models have heavily influenced the way quality is currently understood and measured in health care settings across the continuum. Industry leaders who have influenced nursing's understanding of health care quality include Walter Shewhart, Joseph Juran, Philip Crosby, and W. Edwards Deming. These leaders provided blueprints from which nursing quality management programs have been derived.

Shewhart (Deming, 2000b) explored causes of variation in work processes. He quantified these variations, categorizing variables as common or special cause. His *Plan, Do, Check, Act (PDCA)* model is probably the most frequently used in health care quality settings today, as follows (Figure 24.1):

- *Plan* (identify an issue and plan a process improvement)
- *Do* (map the current and proposed process, collect data, and analyze the results)
- *Check* (propose a solution and check the results of the new process)
- *Act* (adopt, adapt, or abandon the solution)

Shewhart also provided the industrial community with statistical process control techniques that are used widely today. Deming (2000a, b) adopted his work and refined it.

Juran (1989) defined quality as "fitness for use." Quality, in his work, was defined as freedom from defects plus value and continuously meeting

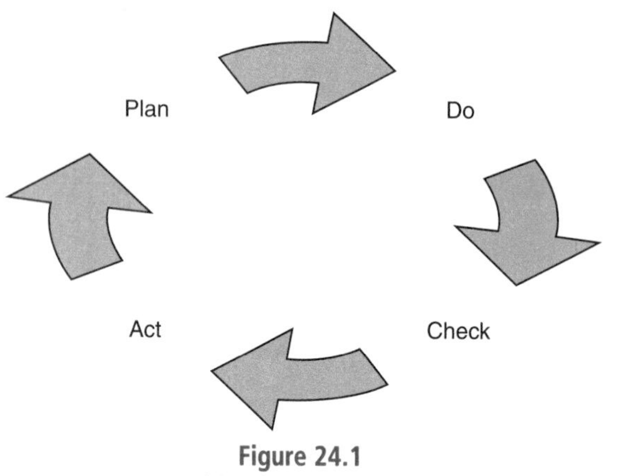

Figure 24.1
PDCA (Plan, Do, Check, Act) cycle.

customer expectations. His approach to quality centered around the use of interdisciplinary teams that used diagnostic tools to understand why industrial processes produce a product not fit for use. His framework included a three-pronged approach: quality planning, quality control, and quality improvement. Quality planning:

> ...establishes the design of a product, service, or process that will meet customer, business, and operational needs to produce the product before it is produced. Quality planning follows a universal sequence of steps, as follows:
>
> - Identify customers and target markets
> - Discover hidden and unmet customer needs
> - Translate these needs into product or service requirements: a means to meet their needs (new standards, specifications, etc.)
> - Develop a service or product that exceeds customers' needs
> - Develop the processes that will provide the service, or create the product, in the most efficient way
> - Transfer these designs to the organization and the operating forces to be carried out (Juran Institute, 2007, ¶ 1-2).

Crosby viewed quality in production terms of zero defects and measured quality in relation to conformance to requirements. He believed that the results or products of a company are made by people. He focused on systems and the consequences of poor quality. He emphasized doing the right thing the first time to prevent waste. Waste and rework were seen as costly, and good managers were those who prevented costly mistakes.

In addition to PDCA, Deming focused on statistical process control techniques and on continuous quality improvement through a culture of quality. He is credited as being influential in the success of Japanese industries. He proposed 14 points to help management staff understand and commit to quality. These points are listed in Box 24.3

Box **24.3**

Deming's 14 Points for Quality

1. Create constancy of purpose toward improving products and services.
2. Adopt the new philosophy.
3. Cease dependence on inspection to achieve quality.
4. End the practice of awarding business on the basis of cost alone.
5. Improve constantly and forever every process for planning, production, and service.
6. Institute training on the job.
7. Adopt and institute leadership aimed at helping people do their jobs better.
8. Drive out fear by promoting two-way communication.
9. Break down barriers between departments.
10. Eliminate exhortations for the workforce in such forms as posters and slogans; these methods tend to create adversarial relationships.
11. Eliminate numerical quotas for productivity; instead have leaders promote continuous quality improvement (CQI).
12. Permit pride of workmanship by removing the barriers that prevent this.
13. Encourage education and self-improvement for all workers.
14. Define management's commitment to CQI and their obligation to implement these points.

From Deming, W.E. (2000). *The new economics for industry, government, education.* Cambridge, MA: MIT Center for Advanced Engineering Studies; and Deming, W.E. (2000). *Out of the crisis.* Cambridge, MA: MIT Center for Advanced Engineering Studies.

(Deming, 2000a,b). These 14 points, although created just after World War II, have heavily influenced health care's adoption of quality principles.

STANDARDS OF QUALITY

Health care quality standards and measures can be grouped in three categories: structure, process, and outcome. Donabedian (1980) developed the initial theoretical model that identified that quality can be measured using these three aspects of a process. Donabedian's (1980) framework of structure, process, and outcomes is the most widely referenced model of quality; professional nurses have used this model to develop quality management programs and conduct improvement studies and research. Standards essentially define quality, against which performance and outcomes are measured. Standards and measures are typically developed from benchmarking activities and reviews of best practices. Therefore the selection of standards and measures is a critical activity in the quality and performance improvement process. Actually, standards establish the baseline against which measurement and evaluation are conducted. Therefore it is critical to decide who determines standards and which standards are selected to define quality. Over the past 10 years, national groups have been formed to gain consensus on performance standards and measures. The National Quality Forum is a not-for-profit, public-private membership organization created to develop and implement a national strategy for health care quality measurement and reporting.

Structure Standards and Measures

Structure standards, or structural measures, focus on the internal characteristics of the organization and its personnel. They answer the questions, Is an infrastructure in place and tools accessible to allow quality to exist? and Is the structure of the organization set up to allow for the effective, efficient delivery of services? For example, a structural standard for a long-term care facility might be to have an adequate mix of registered nurses and nursing assistants on site to ensure that comprehensive care is delivered. For specialized areas, structure standards may address whether there are enough specialists or "intensivists" to ensure quality care. Certain committees, policy statements, rules and regulations, or manuals, forms, or contracts may be needed. Structure standards regulate the environment to ensure quality. Human, organizational, and physical resources, as well as environmental characteristics, are examples of structure standards.

Process Standards and Measures

Process standards and measures focus on whether the activities within an organization are being conducted appropriately, effectively, and efficiently. Process measures focus on the behaviors of the professional nurse as a provider of care. The interventions recommended in a clinical practice guideline or best practice are examples of process standards. They relate to what the nurse will be doing and the process the nurse should follow to ensure effective, evidence-based care. Process standards look at activities, interventions, and the sequence of caregiving events, sometimes referred to as *work flow*. Typically, processes are assessed by audits, observational studies, or work flow analyses. Examples of process standards include the following: a nursing assessment is completed within 24 hours of admission; client calls are returned within 1 hour of the initial call.

Outcome Standards and Measures

Outcome standards and measures refer to whether the services provided by the organization make any difference: Were they effective? They answer the questions about the services that nurses provide and whether those services make a difference to the clients or to the health status of the population. Outcome standards address physical health status, mental health status, social and physical function, health attitudes/knowledge/behavior, utilization of services, and the client's perception and satisfaction with the care received. *Outcome* refers to a change in the current or future health status attributed to antecedent health care and client attributes of health care. Outcome standards present the possibility of measuring the effectiveness, quality, and time and resources allocated for care. Examples of outcome measures include the following: percentage of patients whose activities of daily living have improved by 80%; percentage of clients who have stopped smoking after 12 weeks of intensive psychoeducational therapy.

In measuring quality, both structure and process parameters are important but they are not sufficient in determining whether the care led to an effective outcome or whether the client learned, recovered, or improved his or her health status. Over the years, the emphasis on structure, process, and outcome aspects of health care has varied. Ultimately, various stakeholders are interested in knowing whether care resulted in a positive, expected clinical outcome, based on objective, measurable criteria.

When developing a quality and performance improvement program, nurse managers are cautioned to not first create new standards and measures. Rather, a literature review will undoubtedly yield hundreds of measures from which to choose. These measures have typically been tested for reliability and validity and have been piloted in the field. Selection criteria can then be adopted and measures chosen for a specific intervention or program. A number of selection criteria guideline statements have been developed, including statements from the following organizations (Smith et al., 1997):

- President's Advisory Commission on Consumer Protection and Quality in the Health Care Industry (1998)
- U.K. Department of Health (2002)
- Foundation for Accountability (FACCT) (2002)
- Committee on Using Performance Monitoring to Improve Community Health (Durch et al., 1997)
- The Joint Commission
- National Committee for Quality Assurance (NCQA) (2000)
- Committee on Leading Health Indicators for *Healthy People 2010*, Institute of Medicine (Chrvala & Bulger, 1999)
- National Alliance for the Mentally Ill

The performance measurement attributes common to these entities' guideline statements have been reported in the set of criteria proposed to be used for a national health care quality report (Institute of Medicine [IOM], Committee on the National Quality Report on Health Care Delivery, 2001). Common performance measurement selection criteria are listed in Box 24.4 (Pelletier & Hoffman, 2002). The adoption of these performance measurement selection criteria is the first step in developing a comprehensive performance measurement system.

More recently, an international working group on health care quality indicators defined the following as selection criteria (The Commonwealth Fund, 2004), which are similar to those previously cited:

- *Feasibility:* indicators already being collected by one or more countries
- *Scientific soundness:* indicators that are valid and reliable; existing reviews of the scientific evidence and approval by a consensus process in one or more countries
- *Interpretability:* indicators that allowed a clear conclusion (a clear direction) for policy makers
- *Actionability:* measures of processes or outcomes that could be directly affected by the health care entity
- *Importance:* indicators reflective of important health conditions representing a major share of the burden of disease, health care costs, or policy-maker priorities.

EMERGING MODELS OF HEALTH CARE QUALITY ASSESSMENT AND MANAGEMENT

A number of industry-based models for quality management and measurement have been adopted by the health care industry over the past two decades. These include Six Sigma, Lean Enterprise, the Baldrige National Quality Award, ISO 9000, and the concept of high-performance organizations. These models are briefly described in the following sections.

Box 24.4

Common Performance Measurement Selection Criteria*

- *Relevance:* The measure should address features of the health care system applicable to health professionals, policy makers, and consumers.
- *Meaningfulness and interpretability:* The measure should be understandable to at least one of the audiences. It should help inform them about the important issues or concerns.
- *Scientific or clinical evidence:* The measure should be based on evidence documenting the links between the interventions, clinical processes, and/or outcomes it addresses.
- *Reliability or reproducibility:* The measure should produce the same results when repeated in the same population and setting.
- *Feasibility:* The measure should be specified precisely. Collection of data for the measure should be inexpensive and logistically feasible.
- *Validity:* The measure should make sense (face validity), correlate well with other measures of the same aspects of care (construct validity), and capture meaningful aspects of care (content validity).
- *Health importance:* The measure should include the prevalence of the health condition to which it applies and the seriousness of the health outcomes affected.

From Pelletier, L.R., & Hoffman, J.A. (2002). A framework for selecting performance measures for opioid treatment programs. *Journal for Healthcare Quality, 24*(3), 26. Reprinted with permission from the National Association for Healthcare Quality.

*NOTE: Criteria are listed in order of their frequency, with the one mentioned most often listed first. The same label for a criterion can have different meanings depending on the framework, because the criteria are not standardized. The definitions, rather than the labels, were used to construct the figure. Feasibility was used as a category covering several criteria in some of the frameworks and as a single criterion in others. Parts of this figure were adapted from NCQA's list of desirable attributes for HEDIS measures (IOM, Committee on the National Quality Report on Health Care Delivery, 2001, p. 81).

Six Sigma

A strategy developed by Motorola and implemented successfully at General Electric (GE) and AlliedSignal Companies provided an innovative approach to reduce variation and error rates. Not surprisingly, the Six Sigma approach that these companies use is similar to tried-and-true approaches historically deployed by health care quality professionals, as previously described. In the Six Sigma breakthrough strategy, errors are measured in defects per million opportunities (dpmo). Six Sigma is achieved when the organization reaches an error or defect rate of 3.4 or less per one million. As a result of its implementation and investment of $6 million since 1995, GE boasted financial benefits of over $600 million in 1998 (Harry & Schroeder, 2000). AlliedSignal reported a 1.9% growth in operating margin in the first quarter 1999, and "cumulative impact of Six Sigma has been a savings in excess of $2 billion in direct costs" (Harry & Schroeder, 2000, p. ix). The Six Sigma strategy (Harry & Schroeder, 2000) is remarkably similar to Juran's problem-solving strategy (Plsek & Omnias, 1989), which has been applied to health care. Table 24.1 illustrates these similarities (Pelletier, 2000).

Lean Enterprise

Lean Enterprise is a model of quality measurement that was originally associated with Deming but reintroduced to the United States by Womack in the mid-1990s (Jones & Womack, 2003). The premise of this model is that operational waste needs to be eliminated in the areas of unnecessary processing, errors/defects, waiting, overproduction, inventory, excess motion by people, transportation of product, and underutilized people (Martin, 2003).

Table 24.1

Comparison of Six Sigma Breakthrough Strategy and Juran's Problem-Solving Strategy

Six Sigma Breakthrough Strategy		Juran's Problem-Solving Strategy	
Stage	Step (Objective)	Phase	Step
Identification	1. Recognize 2. Define (Identify key business issues)	Project definition and organization	1. List and prioritize problems 2. Define project and team
Characterization	1. Measure 2. Analyze (Understand current performance levels)	Diagnostic journey	1. Analyze symptoms 2. Formulate theory of causes 3. Test theories 4. Identify root causes
Optimization	1. Improve 2. Control (Achieve breakthrough improvement)	Remedial journey	1. Consider alternative solutions 2. Design solutions and controls 3. Address resistance to change 4. Implement solutions and controls
Institutionalization	1. Standardize 2. Integrate (Transform how day-to-day business is conducted)	Holding the gains	1. Check performance 2. Monitor control system

From Pelletier, L.R. (2000). On error-free health care: Mission possible! (Editorial). *Journal for Healthcare Quality, 22*(3), 9. Reprinted with permission from the National Association for Healthcare Quality.

Baldrige National Quality Award

The Baldrige National Quality Award (BNQA) establishes a set of performance standards that define a total quality organization. Named after the Secretary of Commerce, the BNQA "was established by Congress in 1987 to enhance the competitiveness and performance of U.S. businesses" (National Institute of Standards and Technology, 2007, p. 1). The standards in seven areas of excellence are (1) leadership, (2) strategic planning, (3) customer and market focus (focus on patients, other customers, and markets), (4) information and analysis, (5) human resource focus, (6) process management, and (7) business results (organizational performance results). Organizations committed to quality improvement choose to adopt the BNQA approach as another means of defining and improving their organizational processes to achieve quality outcomes. Manufacturing, service, and small business were the original award categories, but in 1999, education and health care were added. With the trend in health care to adopt industry applications and measure sets for quality improvement, it was fitting that the health care industry was recognized as one that could benefit from participating in this program. It is appropriate for health care entities to strive to achieve internationally recognized standards for performance excellence, which enable them to benchmark their "best practices" with others in the field. The first health care organization to apply and be awarded the BNQA in health care was the SSM system in St. Louis in 2002 (White, 2003). In succeeding years, the following health systems were awarded this recognition: St. Luke's Hospital of Kansas City and Baptist Hospital, Inc. (Pensacola, FL) (2003); Robert Wood Johnson University Hospital (Hamilton, NJ) (2004); Broson Methodist Hospital (Kalamazoo, MI) (2005); North Mississippi Medical Center (2006); and Sharp HealthCare (San Diego, CA) and Mercy Health System (Janesville, WI) (2007). The Alliance for Performance Excellence is a network of national, state, and local Baldrige-based organizations helping organizations achieve performance excellence using the Baldrige criteria (www.networkforexcellence.org). Various states have also developed quality awards based on the BNQA criteria (2007 State Quality Awards Directory, 2007).

ISO 9000

The International Organization for Standardization (ISO) is a network of 148 countries that have agreed on an international reference for quality requirements in business and service industries. The ISO 9000 series of standards are those that address quality management—that is, what the organization does to manage its systems and processes. Health care sector standards, originally developed in 2001, were updated in 2005 (Frost, 2006).

The achievement of an ISO 9000 registration results when a company complies with its own quality system. Again, as many health care organizations are committed to the ongoing pursuit of quality, the ISO 9000 registration process provides another type of assessment and evaluation of an organization's quality systems and sets a benchmark for achievement that is internationally recognized.

High-Performance Organizations

As organizations continue to evolve their quality models, those that are in pursuit of continuous and ongoing improvement are embracing a concept referred to as *high-performance organizations (HPOs)*. These are organizations that may already be practicing Six Sigma or Lean Enterprise or have achieved recognition through ISO 9000 registration or Malcolm Baldrige compliance. HPOs are those that have a culture of "building and sustaining a customer focused, team based organization that pays as much attention to results as it does to process" (Ward, 2004, ¶ 3).

Following are some of the attributes of an HPO:

- Leaders who communicate a strong and clear mission and vision to employees
- Strategic thinking that anticipates customer needs and market changes
- A commitment to ongoing identification of problems and a preoccupation for potential failures
- Resiliency
- Flexibility
- Creative and improvisational problem solving to address failures or "near misses"

HPOs apply the principles learned through study of high-reliability organizations (HROs). These are organizations that require reliability to ensure stable outcomes in the face of variable working conditions.

COSTS ASSOCIATED WITH POOR HEALTH CARE QUALITY

The cost associated with medical errors "in lost income, disability, and health care costs is as much as $29 billion annually" (Quality Interagency Coordination [QuIC] Task Force, 2000, p. 1) and plagues every sector in the health care industry. The number of medical errors has been described as unacceptable by an IOM report *To Err Is Human: Building a Safer Health Care System* (Kohn et al., 2000), which has been referenced widely in the professional and consumer press since its release. The IOM report has reached the highest levels in the federal government, but response to its findings and recommendations has been lackluster. The research associated with this report was preceded by other federal initiatives.

The Quality Interagency Coordination (QuIC) Task Force was established in 1998 in response to the President's Advisory Commission on Consumer Quality in the Health Care Industry to ensure that major federal agencies involved in purchasing, providing, studying, or regulating health care services are working in a coordinated manner with the common goal of health care quality improvement. The Agency for Healthcare Research and Quality (AHRQ) was given oversight of day-to-day operations (QuIC, 2001). QuIC presented its response to the IOM report to President Clinton in February 2000. President Clinton outlined a commitment of $53 million in funding for the development of a Center for Quality Improvement and Patient Safety, as well as additional funding for medical error and adverse event reporting systems at the Food and Drug Administration. The goal was to implement recommendations from the IOM report and to cut preventable medical errors by 50% over 5 years (The White House, 2000). A four-tiered approach was defined by QuIC to include the following (QuIC, 2000):

- Establish a national focus to create leadership, tools, and protocols to enhance the knowledge base about safety
- Identify and learn from medical errors through both mandatory and voluntary reporting systems
- Raise standards and expectations for improvements in safety through the actions of oversight organizations, group purchasers, and professional groups
- Implement safe practices at the delivery level (p. 12)

Tactics and strategies described in the QuIC report to reduce medical errors were targeted toward 500 federal U.S. Department of Defense military hospitals and 6000 hospitals participating in Medicare. The work of the QuIC is archived now, but it was an important early initiative regarding patient safety and the prevention of medical errors.

Both the IOM and QuIC reports defined specific strategies that could inform the development and refinement of health care safety systems nationwide. An important component of these reports is the mention of the error-reduction techniques of other industries. The federal reports provided another opportunity to advocate for patients, families, and populations. They gave health care quality professionals the evidence and research with which to defend a quality management budget, enhance information systems and technologies to track errors, and further develop quality activities and studies using proven tools and techniques. The reports are also models in defining and describing cost/benefit analyses and return-on-investment scenarios for quality and performance improvement programs. In essence, they provided a business case for quality.

A technical report published by the IOM identified key characteristics that health care microsystems use to continuously enhance the services that they provide to individuals and communities (Donaldson & Mohr, 2000). After interviewing 43 microsystems, the researchers identified eight common themes: "integration of information, measurement, interdependence of care team, supportiveness of the larger system, constancy of purpose, connection to community, investment in improvement, and alignment of role and training" (Donaldson & Mohr, 2000, p. 21).

The IOM report *Crossing the Quality Chasm: A New Health System for the 21st Century* (IOM, Committee on Quality of Health Care in America [CQHCA], 2001) recommended that Congress establish a Health Care Quality Innovation Fund "to support projects targeted at (1) achieving the six aims of safety, effectiveness, patient-centeredness, timeliness, efficiency, and equity; and/or (2) producing substantial improvements in quality for the [15] priority conditions" (p. 11). The overall goal of the funding would be to produce a "public-domain portfolio of programs, tools, and technologies of widespread applicability" (p. 11). The report recommended an initial investment of $1 billion over 3 to 5 years to support this goal. Health care organizations could take the lead either by enhancing the current resources

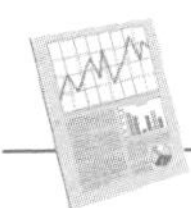

Research Note

Source: Hensing, J.A. (2008). The quest for upper-quartile performance at Banner Health. *Journal for Healthcare Quality, 30*(1), 18-24.

Purpose

In 2004, Banner Health, a large hospital system with corporate offices in Phoenix, AZ, proactively responded to external forces, emphasizing improvement in the quality and safety of patient care in hospitals. They began their 3-year plan to reach upper-quartile performance in four clinical focus areas: coronary artery bypass graft, heart failure, cerebral vascular accident, and intensive care unit measures on a system-wide basis.

Discussion

Clinical process improvement can raise the bar on clinical performance system-wide in a multi-institutional health system. Several factors contribute to successful deployment of best practices: clinical relevance, clinical leadership, focus, definition of metrics and success, prescriptiveness, and consistency of approach. The most important factor for success involved clearly defined objectives and targets. Clinician buy-in and leadership buy-in were essential. Specific and thoughtful data definitions and risk adjustment added relevance to the work.

Application to Practice

Health care enterprises need to monitor clinically relevant measures based upon nationally agreed upon metrics. Leadership must provide the strategic plan through its mission and vision statements. Clinicians and physicians need to be part of the planning and must "buy into" the process. Engaging them early on and choosing measures that are relevant to specific populations are critical. Large systems should leverage their resources and come to consensus on system-wide measures, to reduce duplication of effort. Broad-based organizational accountability for clinical performance and a supportive culture for clinicians are vital success factors.

dedicated to quality and performance improvement in their organizations or by using the funds to finance regional collaborative health care quality projects. These successes could then be described in the literature for wider application.

The third in a series of IOM quality chasm reports, entitled *Leadership by Example: Co-coordinating Government Roles in Improving Health Care Quality,* was released in 2002 (Corrigan et al., 2002). The original charge of the IOM Committee on Enhancing Federal Healthcare Quality Programs (CEFHQP) was to acknowledge that "The current federal quality oversight programs represent a patchwork of requirements and processes that have evolved over the last 30 to 35 years" (IOM, CEFHQP, 2002, ¶ 1). The committee was convened "to reexamine the various federal quality improvement and oversight programs to assess whether changes are needed to (1) provide adequate protection to beneficiaries, (2) provide strong incentives to providers to improve quality, and (3) improve the efficiency of the oversight processes by reducing redundancy" (IOM, CEFHQP, 2002, ¶ 1). This study was requested by Congress and sponsored by the U.S. Department of Health and Human Services, the California Health Care Foundation, and The Commonwealth Fund. In doing their work, the committee held workshops to obtain perspectives and information from various stakeholders with expertise in the fields of quality measurement, improvement, oversight, and research on ways to improve current federal programs (Medicare, Medicaid, Children's Health Insurance Program, Tricare, and Veterans Affairs).

From his introductory remarks at the press briefing, the committee chair outlined the major findings of the study as follows (Omenn, 2002):

- There is a lack of consistency in performance measurement requirements both across and within these government programs.
- The programs are not using standardized measures.
- There is no well-thought-out conceptual framework to guide the selection of performance measures.
- Medicare, Medicaid, and the State Children's Health Insurance Program lack computer-based clinical data, which is seen as a major impediment.
- There is also a lack of commitment to transparency and openly sharing information on safety and quality. (p. 2)

These findings were not a surprise to many nurses and health care quality professionals, who have been burdened with duplicative reporting for years. The positive message was that strong recommendations from this committee were sent to the federal government's leadership, asking them to attack these problems with a good deal of muscle to shape the measurement of performance for the whole health care sector. The charge was clear to the Secretaries of the U.S. Department of Health and Human Services, Department of Defense, and Department of Veterans Affairs (Omenn, 2002):

> Work together to establish standardized performance measures, as well as public reporting requirements for clinicians, institutional providers, and health plans in each program. The standardized measurement and reporting requirements should replace the many performance assessment activities currently under way in various programs. (p. 3)

Standardization of protocols and measures is not a new idea (Pelletier, 1998). Reducing administrative burden and duplicative reporting could easily put time back in the hands of clinicians to do what they do best: provide health care services to individuals, families, and communities.

LEADERSHIP AND MANAGEMENT IMPLICATIONS

Planning for Health Care Quality

An organization that adopts and nurtures a continuous quality improvement culture (and rewards those who identify opportunities for improvement) recognizes that change is an everyday event. One of the ways that change can be managed is to acknowledge it and make it a part of the organization's strategic planning process. Just as an organization defines its mission, vision, and core values, so too must change agents and teams define the purpose of the change (expected outcomes), the mission and vision of the change process, and the core values of the group that will be responsible for managing the change.

An organization's mission is a concise statement that answers the question: What business are we in today? (Pelletier, 1999a). Some companies refer to their mission as a *purpose.* Sharp HealthCare, a not-for-profit integrated regional health care delivery system based in San Diego, CA, (Sharp HealthCare, 2008) stated that its mission is

> ...to improve the health of those we serve with a commitment to excellence in all that we do. Our goal is to offer quality care and programs that set community standards, exceed patients' expectations and are provided in a caring, convenient, cost-effective and accessible manner.

The Visiting Nursing Service of New York's (VNSNY) (2008) mission is

> ...to promote the health and well-being of patients and families by providing high-quality, cost-effective health care in the home and community; to be a leader in the development of innovative services that enable people to function as independently as possible in their community; to help shape health care policies that support beneficial home- and community-based services; [and] to continue its tradition of charitable and compassionate care, within the resources available.

An organization's vision should accurately depict what the company is striving to become. The vision statement should be able to stand on its own and be understandable to people new to the enterprise. Sharp HealthCare's vision is "to be the best health system in the universe" (Sharp HealthCare, 2008).

It is critical for mission and vision statements to be communicated effectively and widely to internal stakeholders (employees and management personnel) and to external stakeholders (investors, clients, patients, vendors, and accreditation agencies). In this way, the statements keep employees on a path to an attainable goal. Nurse managers need to be familiar with the company's or organization's mission and vision statements. Representatives from various stakeholder groups, including patients and consumers, need be included in the development of these statements. Mission and vision statements need to be reviewed and updated periodically to accurately reflect what leadership, staff, and stakeholders believe is the purpose and future direction of the organization. This is important because mission, vision, and values form the foundation for quality and its management and improvement.

Just as a nurse's professional behavior is based on personal values, so too must an organization describe the core values that are the foundation of the enterprise or endeavor. Strategic planning often includes the development of core value statements that are in alignment with the mission and vision statements of the organization. "Value statements become part of an organization's culture; they act as a quick reference or navigation device—just as mission and vision statements do" (Pelletier, 1999b, p. 2). Marcus and colleagues (1995) defined values as "interests that reflect fundamental purpose and integrity: issues to which you hold fast as a matter of principle, with little room for compromise" (p. 430). Furthermore, "Values are operational qualities used by organizations to maintain or enhance performance" (Harmon, 1997, p. 246).

Values consciously and unconsciously guide a professional nurse's personal and professional behavior. His Holiness the Dalai Lama and Cutler (1998) said the following about values:

> Higher stages of growth and development depend on an underlying set of values that can guide us. A value system that can provide continuity and coherence to our lives, by which we can measure our experiences. A value system that can help us decide which goals are truly worthwhile and which pursuits are meaningless. Values help us with the challenges of everyday life. (pp. 192-193)

Nurses' personal and professional values come from the experiences they have shared with others in interpersonal exchanges at work and at home. To identify a group's core values, ask and record the responses

LEADERSHIP & MANAGEMENT **BEHAVIORS**

Leadership Behaviors

- Builds a culture of quality and safety
- Models evidence-based care
- Encourages use of information technology for quality improvement activities and reporting
- Participates in the spread of best practices throughout the enterprise
- Collaborates across disciplines and various stakeholders to enhance quality
- Is visible in continuous quality improvement activities
- Enables interdisciplinary quality improvement
- Evaluates quality of care and continuously identifies opportunities for improvement

Management Behaviors

- Plans for quality in care delivery
- Organizes a quality-driven service
- Directs others to achieve quality
- Monitors quality of care
- Evaluates quality of care
- Participates in ongoing quality management

Overlap Areas

- Evaluates quality of care
- Injects quality into care delivery and management of care

Table 24.2

Mayo Clinic Core Value Statements

Primary value: The needs of the patient come first.

Core Value	Description
Practice	Practice medicine as an integrated team of compassionate, multi-disciplinary physicians, scientists and allied health professionals who are focused on the needs of patients from our communities, regions, the nation and the world.
Education	Educate physicians, scientists and allied health professionals and be a dependable source of health information for our patients and the public.
Research	Conduct basic and clinical research programs to improve patient care and to benefit society.
Mutual respect	Treat everyone in our diverse community with respect and dignity.
Commitment to quality	Continuously improve all processes that support patient care, education and research.
Work atmosphere	Foster teamwork, personal responsibility, integrity, innovation, trust and communication within the context of a physician-led institution.
Societal commitment	Benefit humanity through patient care, education and research. Support the communities in which we live and work. Serve appropriately patients in difficult financial circumstances.
Finances	Allocate resources within the context of a system rather than its individual entities. Operate in a manner intended not to create wealth but to provide a financial return sufficient for present and future needs.

Courtesy Mayo Clinic. (2008). *Mayo's mission, primary value, core principles*. Rochester, MN: Author. Retrieved January 22, 2008, from www.mayoclinic.org/about/missionvalues.html

to these questions: Which three people have had the greatest influence in your personal and professional life? What are the three most important values these influential people taught you? The answers to these questions can help inform the development of mission, vision, and core value statements. An example is a set of core values or "core principles" from the Mayo Clinic, as outlined in Table 24.2.

CURRENT ISSUES AND TRENDS

A Nurse Manager's Health Care Quality Toolbox

With the paradigm shift from quality assurance to organizational performance improvement came the expectation that accredited organizations become skilled at the art and science of continuous quality improvement. This included the concepts of leadership involvement, a commitment to customers' needs (i.e., patients and families), an understanding of the principle of process versus people, a devotion to data collection and analysis as the foundation for problem solving, and the view that multidisciplinary teams working within the processes under study were the experts and therefore best equipped to drive change and improvement.

Nurse managers in accredited organizations were expected to learn these principles and tools for quality improvement, to educate staff in these tools and techniques, to identify improvement opportunities on their units, and to be able to speak to process changes that occurred as a result of data analysis. They were also tapped to

Table **24.3**

A Nurse Manager's Health Care Quality Toolbox

Tool	Description of the Tool
Data-collection tools	Checksheets and checklists facilitate the gathering of data for eventual analysis and reporting. Good data collection tools can help you count and categorize data (see Figure 24.2).
Control chart	This tool includes data points and their placement on a graph to depict variation. Its purpose is to illustrate whether the process variation is expected ("common cause") or an unexpected or unusual variation ("special cause"). Included are three lines—the mean, an upper control limit (UCL), and a lower control limit (LCL). Generally, a process is considered "out of control" when the data points stray outside of the control limits or a series of data points follow a defined pattern that illustrate lack of control in the process (see Figure 24.3).
Cause-and-effect (or fishbone) diagram	This tool resembles diagramming sentences. The "effect" is illustrated in a box at the end of a midline (or "head" of the fish). The "causes" are generally four or five categories of elements that might contribute to the effect (e.g., machines, methods, people, materials, measurements) and the specific activities. Under each of these category headings, individual items that might lead to the effect are listed. By diagramming all of the possible contributors, the predominant or root causes may be found more readily (see Figure 24.4).
Detailed flowchart	Using various shapes, this tool is used to depict a work process, from start to finish, illustrating all of the processes' action steps, decision points, hand-offs, or waiting stages. Flowcharts form the cornerstone of process improvement planning and analysis. The entire process must first be accurately defined to identify problems or process improvement opportunities (see Figure 24.5).

Continued

participate in organization-wide improvement teams designed to address overarching problem resolution or process redesign projects. Many of the early quality leaders received training in facilitation and group meeting techniques, in addition to the quality improvement (QI) tools. This enabled them to promote the team-based model of cross-functional problem solving that became the standard for most organizations. Skills and expertise in the concepts of team building, conflict resolution, statistical process control, customer service, and process improvement continue to be needed by nurse leaders in the new millennium.

Health care quality professionals and those nurses involved in quality and performance improvement activities have an enormous set of resources available to them as they plan for an enterprise-wide quality program. Tools and techniques that nurses can readily use are illustrated in Table 24.3. Figures 24.2 through 24.7 illustrate examples of templates and forms to be included in a nurse manager's quality "toolbox."

Table 24.3

A Nurse Manager's Health Care Quality Toolbox—cont'd

Tool	Description of the Tool
Pareto chart	This bar graph can help depict the "80/20" rule. In the nineteenth century, it was used to show that 80% of the wealth was held by 20% of the people. In health care, typically 20% of the issues cause 80% of the problems. The use of this tool allows a performance improvement team to focus on the "vital few" causes of the problems in a process under study (see Figure 24.6).
Scatter diagram	This graph describes the relationship between two variables that are continuous. It is used when the potential causes of effects under study cannot be easily categorized, such as in a Pareto chart or cause-and-effect diagram. Data points are plotted along the vertical and horizontal axes of the graph, and a correlation between the two variables can either be weak or strong, based on the pattern of the data points (see Figure 24.7).

Data Collection Sheet

Organization/Unit: ____________________ Date: __________

Process: ____

MEASURE	DATE	TIME	WHERE	WHEN

Figure 24.2
Sample data collection sheet for a nurse manager's quality toolbox.

Control Chart
Upper Control Limit
+2 standard deviation
+1 standard deviation
Median
−1 standard deviation
−2 standard deviation
Lower Control Limit

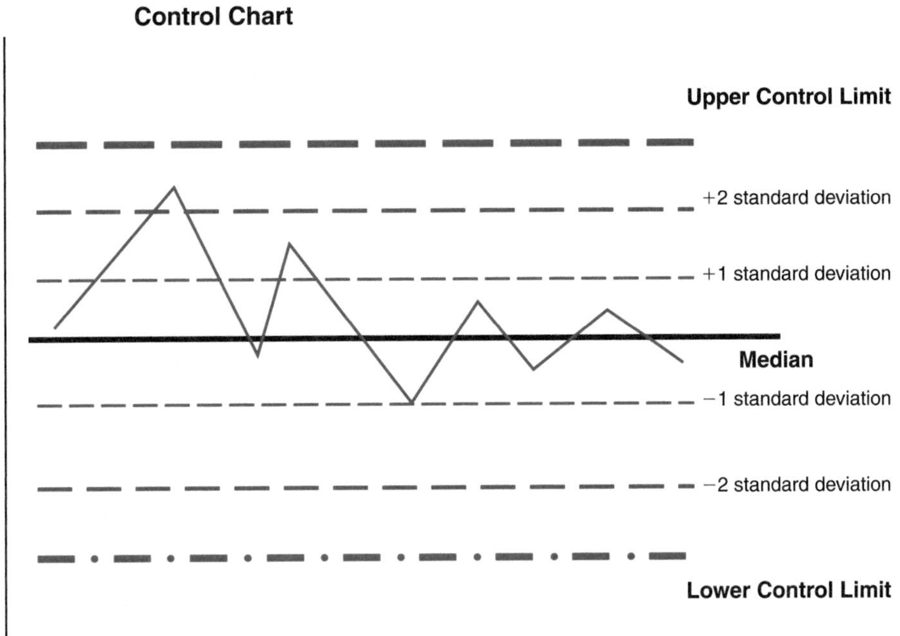

Figure 24.3
Sample control chart for a nurse manager's quality toolbox.

Cause-and-Effect Diagram
Organization/Unit:
Date:
Process:
Environment
Personnel/
people
Cause
Subcause
Clear description of problem, undesired outcome, result, or effect
Equipment/
machinery/
hardware
Policies/
procedures/
protocols
Time

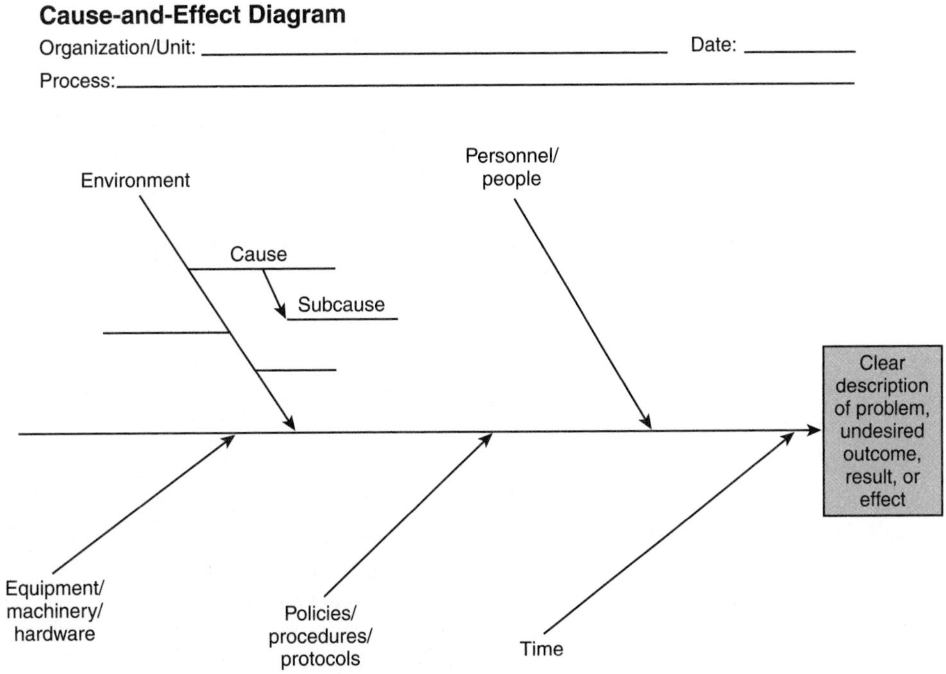

Figure 24.4
Sample cause-and-effect diagram for a nurse manager's quality toolbox.

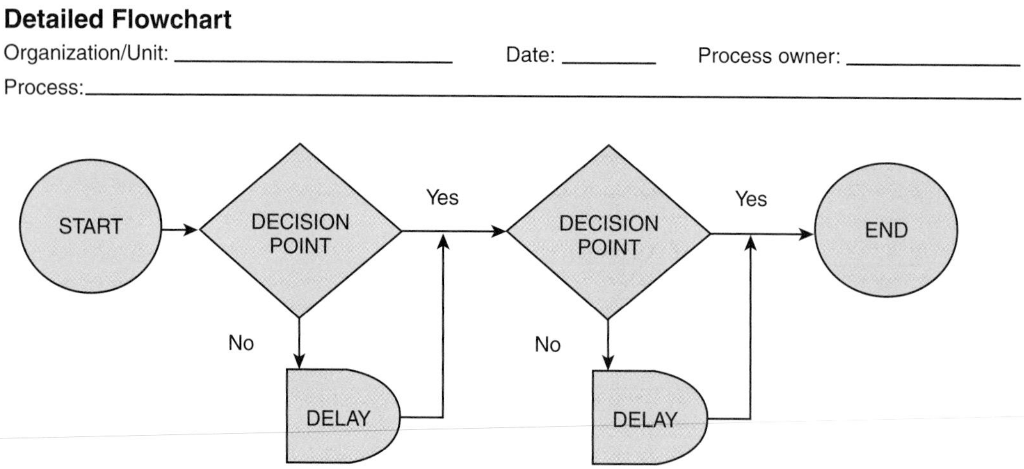

Detailed Flowchart
Organization/Unit:
Date:
Process owner:
Process:
START
DECISION POINT
Yes
DECISION POINT
Yes
END
No
No
DELAY
DELAY

Figure 24.5
Sample detailed flowchart for a nurse manager's quality toolbox.

Pareto Chart
100
75
60
45
30
15
0
Frequency
1
Causal Factors

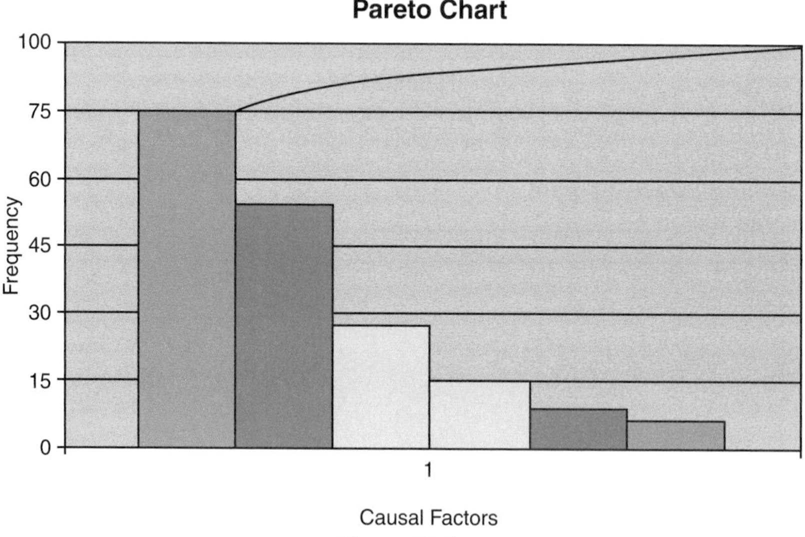

Figure 24.6
Example of a Pareto chart for a nurse manager's quality toolbox.

One excellent resource for hospital-based quality programs is the American Nurses Association's National Database of Nursing Quality Indicators (NDNQI) (ANA, 2009). This database comprises nurse-sensitive indicators collected at the nursing unit level and provides the ability of participants to benchmark performance with national averages.

In addition, the Internet can provide professional nurses with administrative and clinical tools to support a quality and performance improvement program, regardless of the delivery setting.

A health care quality glossary can also assist professional nurse managers in navigating the health care quality field. A glossary of frequently used terms is discussed in the Definitions section

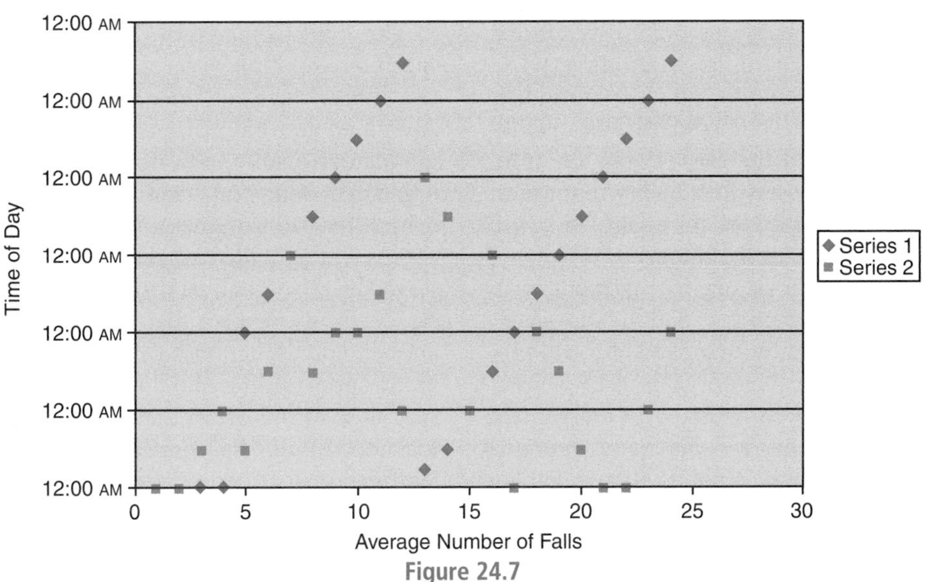

Figure 24.7
Example of a scatter diagram for a nurse manager's quality toolbox.

and synopsized in the Leading & Managing Defined box.

HEALTH CARE SAFETY AND HEALTH CARE RISK MANAGEMENT

Accreditation and Regulatory Influences on Quality

Health care organizations have always been required to meet standards for federal and state reimbursement regulations (Medicare and Medicaid) and state licensure rules and regulations in order to operate. These regulations have traditionally defined requirements for quality. However, the private accreditation process has probably had the most significant impact on the development of quality improvement systems in health care. It has been through organizations such as The Joint Commission (TJC; formerly the Joint Commission on Accreditation of Healthcare Organizations [JCAHO]), The American Osteopathic Association's Healthcare Facilities Accreditation Program (HFAP), the Commission on Accreditation of Rehabilitation Facilities (CARF), the National Committee for Quality Assurance (NCQA), and others that performance standards have been promulgated and universally adopted. In each of these accreditation processes, the concept of system-wide quality improvement provides the framework for the standards. Although accreditation is not mandatory, eligibility to participate in and receive reimbursement from managed care organizations or federal and state program funding sources is often tied to the achievement of accreditation by one or more of the voluntary accreditation organizations.

Of all of these voluntary accreditation programs, TJC has had the greatest degree of impact on the health care industry. Founded in 1951, it led the way in establishing a set of performance standards for hospitals to follow to become accredited. Over the years, its accreditation standards and programs have evolved to reflect the myriad of types of providers that now constitute the health care system, thus expanding its role beyond hospital accreditation. Currently, TJC sponsors accreditation programs for organizations that provide services in the areas of ambulatory care, assisted living, behavioral health, critical access hospitals, health care networks, hospitals, home care, laboratory, long-term care, and office-based surgery.

Throughout its evolution, TJC has continually adjusted its performance standards for quality. During the 1980s and the early 1990s, TJC promoted a "10-Step Process for Quality Assurance" that provided the framework for quality in hospitals. In 1994, TJC identified the need to enhance overall quality of care via an improvement in its own accreditation processes, and it completely revised the accreditation standards for all programs. Instead of chapters organized by department, the new approach revised and reorganized the requirements into *cross-functional processes of care and services* (e.g., Patients Rights, Patient Assessment, Patient Family Education), to more appropriately reflect the manner in which care is delivered. A new chapter entitled "Improving Organizational Performance" was introduced that created specific standards focused on quality that were based on the principle of continuous improvement rather than on pre-established thresholds for performance of individual health care quality indicators. This change reflected the influence of the industrial quality movement on health care in the early 1990s.

With this major restructuring of TJC standards, the new era of thinking in terms of *process improvement* rather than *quality assurance* began, not only for TJC-accredited organizations but also for other accrediting bodies. The description for this organization-wide programmatic approach, or *performance improvement (PI)*, established the expectation that quality initiatives in the organization were no longer the responsibility of a single quality assurance nurse or department but, rather, the responsibility of the enterprise's leaders. Standards in the newly developed "Leadership" chapter established the expectation that the outcomes of performance improvement measures be elevated to review by the administrative and clinical leaders of the organization. This review of performance measurement at senior levels of the organization provides the information that leaders require to provide oversight to the quality of care being provided to all patients and families (customers).

The Joint Commission PI standards delineate specific requirements for data collection in high-risk areas such as medication management, restraints, and blood transfusions. Beyond these mandatory quality indicators, the leaders of each organization are expected to set their own priorities for measurement that reflect the types of services provided to the various populations served by the organization. The PI and Leadership standards also expect that the outcomes of data analysis and the actions taken to address improvement opportunities should be communicated to staff. It is in this arena that a nurse manager can make the PI process "come alive" for nursing staff. Staff can relate to and understand data outcomes that are based on measurement of the everyday processes in which they work. The nurse manager should involve staff in identifying relevant and significant data collection measures for their unit/department that will have a direct impact on changing and continuously improving care processes. A sample data collection sheet is displayed in Figure 24.2.

Nurse managers need to stay abreast of changes in the standards of their organization's primary accrediting and regulatory agencies to ensure that quality outcome measures for their units/departments remain current and viable. In addition to keeping up with these requirements, many hospitals are pursuing or have plans to pursue Magnet™ recognition of their hospital's nursing practice as awarded by the American Nurses Credentialing Center through its Magnet Recognition Program® (American Nurses Credentialing Center, 2009). To be positioned to score well on an application for the Magnet Recognition Program®, nurse leaders must take an active role in the development of robust and effective quality measures. A step further might be to participate in local, regional, and national committees that set performance standards. This can be done through professional associations such as the American Nurses Association and the National Association for Healthcare Quality.

As new standards are introduced, either through participation in voluntary accreditation programs or because of regulatory requirements, policies and procedures at the unit/department level must be updated and/or revised. Staff must be educated about the impact and meaning of the standards that are applicable to the care they provide. Documentation requirements may change, and this may affect the outcome of clinical data measures and/or reimbursement. Nurse managers need to provide leadership in adopting and adapting to ongoing changes in these arenas. Many organizations do not have the luxury of devoting one individual or department solely to managing accreditation or regulatory compliance processes. At best, in those organizations that have dedicated individuals or departments for this purpose, they serve as facilitators for the accreditation and licensing processes. Since 2006, TJC surveys have been conducted on an unannounced basis. This requires that managers throughout the organization be in a continual state of readiness (i.e., to have their departments and staff in compliance with all applicable standards at all times). Thus the onus of responsibility and accountability for continuous readiness has moved from a single regulatory or quality department to all leaders and managers in the organization.

Data Collection and Public Reporting of Quality Outcomes

By 1998, The Joint Commission had developed a requirement for accredited organizations to participate in their ORYX® initiative. This program required accredited health care organizations to select six outcome measures that reflected the operations of their organizations and to choose a performance measurement vendor to aggregate and analyze the data and submit them on a quarterly basis to The Joint Commission. Similarly, since 1991, the Health Plan Employer and Data Information Set (HEDIS®) outcomes have been an integral part of the NCQA accreditation process for managed care plans. Of note, CARF has required both program evaluation and quality outcomes measurement as components of its accreditation process since the 1980s, about a decade before the other accreditors.

One drawback to The Joint Commission's initial ORYX® process, and that of the quality reporting required by other accreditors, was an inability to compare performance outcomes across and among health care organizations. This was due primarily to the variability allowed in selection of measures and reporting systems. Also, as most organizations that analyzed their ORYX® data discovered, there was a limitation in identifying improvement opportunities with data that were purely outcomes-based. In further refinement of its ORYX® process, The Joint Commission devised its Core Measures program (The Joint Commission, 2007). Three measures, initially derived from the Centers for Medicare & Medicaid Services' (CMS; formerly the Health Care Financing Administration [HCFA]) 6th Scope of Work, required both outcome and process measures. The initial measures were acute myocardial infarction (AMI), community-acquired pneumonia (PN), and heart failure (HF) and comprised 10 process measures, often referred to as the "starter set." Beginning in July 2002, accredited hospitals were required to begin collecting data on the Core Measures (with some exceptions, such as pediatric and psychiatric hospitals) and submit the data to The Joint Commission. Although participation in the ORYX® program was mandatory for each organization to be accredited, the results of Core Measures were not initially made public. Currently, the Core Measure sets include, in addition to the three just mentioned, the Surgical Care Improvement Project (SCIP) and the Pregnancy (PR) Core Measure set. Additional Core Measure sets, designed to measure care outcomes in those programs not previously covered under the original Core Measures initiative include Children's Asthma Care, Hospital Based Outpatient Department Quality Measures and Hospital Based Inpatient Psychiatric Services, with collection beginning during the 2008 calendar year.

Since the 1980s, CMS has mandated that the cost and quality of services provided to its Medicare recipients be evaluated through its peer review organizations (PROs). These PROs evolved into state and regional quality improvement organizations (QIOs) that have continued their statutory mandate through the "Statement of Work" projects. At the time of this publication, hospitals are working under the "8th Scope of Work." The statutory mission is "…to improve the efficiency, effectiveness, economy, and quality of services delivered to Medicare beneficiaries" (U.S. Department of Health and Human Services [USDHHS], 2004b, p. 1). The previous 6th and 7th Scopes of Work projects focused on clinical quality measures in specific diagnostic categories such as heart failure and pneumonia. The 8th Scope of Work integrates the process and outcome measures with other measures to comply with the national "Quality Initiative" for health care described below. The *Current Specification Manual for National Quality Measures* is a guide that combines both the CMS measures and The Joint Commission Core Measure sets "…to achieve identity among common national hospital performance measures and to share a single set of common documentation" (TJC, 2008a).

CMS has historically mandated data submission programs for non-hospital health care organizations to qualify for participation in their Medicare programs. For long-term care facilities, CMS has required the submission of data through its Minimum Data Set (MDS) program. For home health care, CMS requires submission of data to the Outcome and Assessment Information Set (OASIS) that includes clinical quality, cost, and administrative measures. In both these initiatives, the results for individual health care organizations were not also originally made public.

In fall 2001, the U.S. Secretary of Health and Human Services announced the Bush Administration's commitment to quality health care through the publication of consumer information, along with quality improvement data, through CMS's QIOs. Their program, "The Quality Initiative" began in 2002 with the Nursing Home Quality Initiative (NHQI) and continued in 2003 with the Home Health Quality Initiative (HHQI). Its purpose was to allow consumers to make informed choices about their health care providers and to encourage providers to improve their care. In 2004, The Quality Initiative was broadened to include renal dialysis or end-stage kidney disease (ESRD) and has now expanded to a Physician's Quality Reporting Initiative (PQRI).

The hospital project, the Hospital Quality Initiative (HQI), began in 2003 and differed from the Nursing Home and Home Healthcare Initiatives in that they had existing data measure sets and methods for data transmission before the start of their initiatives. At the time the HQI began, hospitals had no comprehensive data from which to draw and they had never been mandated to report data to CMS. With the advent of the HQI, that situation changed. In 2005, the first publication of the website "Hospital Compare" *(http://www.hospitalcompare.hhs.gov/Hospital/Search/Welcome.asp?version=default&browser=IE%7C7%7CWindows+Vista&language=English&defaultstatus=0&pagelist=Home)* debuted, giving consumers their first ability to view hospital data in a publicly reported forum. Data outcomes from participating hospitals are published and updated quarterly.

Since its inception, additional measures have been added to the HQI. In addition to the process measures for the three conditions on the starter set, the Hospital Compare website also documents outcome measures of 30-day risk-adjusted mortality for some of the conditions like heart failure and acute myocardial infarction. The components of the HQI reported via the Hospital Compare website are as follows:

- The National Voluntary Hospital Reporting Initiative (NVHRI), consisting of the starter set of 10. (The standardized starter set of measures [Table 24.4])
- An additional 16 quality measures that expand on the "starter set" measures and include the SCIP measures and the 30-day mortality outcomes (Table 24.5); these measures are combined and grouped into four broad outcome measure categories and are continuously refined.
- The Hospital Consumer Assessment of Healthcare Providers and Systems (HCAHPS); a patient survey that collates information on patient perspectives on hospital care.

Table 24.4

The National Voluntary Hospital Reporting Initiative: Ten-Measure Starter Set*

Performance Measures	Measure Description
AMI—Aspirin at Arrival	Acute myocardial infarction (AMI) patients without aspirin contraindications who received aspirin within 24 hours before or after hospital arrival
AMI—Aspirin Prescribed at Discharge	Acute myocardial infarction (AMI) patients without aspirin contraindications who are prescribed aspirin at hospital discharge
AMI—ACEI for LVSD	Acute myocardial infarction (AMI) patients with left ventricular systolic dysfunction (LVSD) and without angiotensin-converting enzyme inhibitor (ACEI) contraindications who are prescribed an ACEI at hospital discharge
AMI—Beta Blocker at Arrival	Acute myocardial infarction (AMI) patients without beta blocker contraindications who received a beta blocker within 24 hours after hospital arrival
AMI—Beta Blocker at Discharge	Acute myocardial infarction (AMI) patients without beta blocker contraindications who are prescribed a beta blocker at hospital discharge
HF—LVF Assessment	Heart failure (HF) patients with documentation in the hospital record that left ventricular function (LVF) was assessed before arrival or during hospitalization or is planned for after discharge
HF—ACEI for LVSD	Heart failure patients with left ventricular systolic dysfunction (LVSD) and without angiotensin-converting enzyme inhibitor (ACEI) contraindications who are prescribed an ACEI at hospital discharge
PNE—Initial Antibiotic Timing	Pneumonia patients who receive their first dose of antibiotics within 4 hours after arrival at the hospital
PNE—Pneumococcal Vaccination	Pneumonia patients age 65 and older who were screened for pneumococcal vaccine status and were administered the vaccine prior to discharge, if indicated
PNE—Oxygenation Assessment	Pneumonia patients who had an assessment of arterial oxygenation by arterial blood gas measurement or pulse oximetry within 24 hours prior to or after arrival at the hospital

From Centers for Medicare and Medicaid Services (CMS). (2004). *Hospital Quality Alliance (HQA) ten measure "starter set."* Baltimore: Author.

*Online references: *www.cms.hhs.gov/quality/hospital/HeartAttack.pdf* and *www.cms.hhs.gov/quality/hospital/Pneumonia.pdf*

Table 24.5

Hospital Measures Reported on the Hospital Compare Website

Outcome Measure	Process Measure
Acute Myocardial Infarction (AMI) Heart Attack	Aspirin at Arrival Aspirin Prescribed at Discharge ACE Inhibitor or Angiotensin Receptor Blocker (ARB) for Left Ventricular Systolic Dysfunction Adult Smoking Cessation Advice/Counseling Beta-Blocker Prescribed at Discharge Beta-Blocker at Arrival Fibrinolytic Therapy Received within 30 Minutes of Hospital Arrival Primary Percutaneous Coronary Intervention (PCI) within 90 minutes of Hospital Arrival AMI 30-Day Mortality
Heart Failure (HF)	Discharge Instructions Evaluation of Left Ventricular Systolic Function ACE Inhibitor or Angiotensin Receptor Blocker (ARB) for Left Ventricular Systolic Dysfunction Adult Smoking Cessation Advice/Counseling HF 30-day Mortality
Pneumonia	Oxygenation Assessment Pneumococcal Vaccination Blood Culture Performed in the Emergency Department Prior to Initial Antibiotic Received in the Hospital Adult Smoking Cessation Advice/Counseling Initial Antibiotic Received within 6 Hours of Hospital Arrival Appropriate Initial Antibiotic Selection Influenza Vaccination
Surgical Care Improvement Project (SCIP)	Prophylactic Antibiotic Received One Hour Prior to Surgical Incision Prophylactic Antibiotic Selection for Surgical Patients Prophylactic Antibiotics Discontinued within 24 Hours After Surgery End Time Surgery Patients with Recommended Venous Thromboembolism Prophylaxis Ordered Surgery Patients with Recommended Venous Thromboembolism (VTE) Prophylaxis Within 24 Hours Prior to Surgery to 24 Hours After Surgery
Hospital Consumer Assessment of Healthcare Providers and Systems (HCAHPS)	Communication with Nurses Communication with Doctors Responsiveness of Hospital Staff Pain Management Communication about Medicines Discharge Information Cleanliness of Hospital Environment Quietness of Hospital Environment Overall Rating of Hospital Willingness to Recommend Hospital

Source: Retrieved May 14, 2008, from *www.hospitalcompare.hhs.gov* and *www.medicare.gov.*

HCAHPS data were published on the Compare website for the first time in Spring 2008.
- Inpatient payment and volume information for selected diagnosis-related groups (DRGs).

Another component of the Hospital Quality Initiative is related to payment for good outcomes. Although submission of data is voluntary, Section 501 of the Medicare Prescription Drug Improvement and Modernization Act (Medicare Modernization Act [MMA]) provided that organizations that do not submit these data would receive 0.4% smaller amount in Medicare's annual payment updates for fiscal years 2005, 2006, and 2007. CMS is evaluating the efficacy of a "pay-for-performance" system via its Premier Hospital Quality Incentive Demonstration (HQID). Performance measures included in the HQID demonstration project are heart attack, heart failure, pneumonia, coronary artery bypass graft, and hip and knee replacements. Composite scores for these measures will be publicly reported, and those hospitals in the top 50% will be recognized as "top performers." Those participating in HQID and performing in the top 20% will be recognized and given a financial bonus.

Over the past 10 to 15 years, many states also began to require health care organizations to submit data for the purpose of public reporting. Pennsylvania was one of the first states to enact legislation, creating the Health Care Cost Containment Council (HCCCC), whose responsibilities include giving "…comparative information about the most efficient and effective health care providers to the public" (Commonwealth of Pennsylvania, 2004, ¶ 2) and "to collect, analyze and make available to the public data about the cost and quality of health care in Pennsylvania" (Commonwealth of Pennsylvania, 2004, ¶ 5).

Initially, health care providers were resistant and concerned about issues such as data integrity and the lack of risk adjustments that would ensure that the results were comparable. They were convinced that, without safeguards built into state reporting systems, their organizations might look "bad" to the public. Data-analysis systems have certainly evolved and improved over the years to address these concerns. A majority of states have now enacted legislation requiring public reporting, and with federal reporting requirements increasingly linked to reimbursement, providers must participate in data submission for public reporting or risk losing accreditation, income, and community status. As an example, organizations must be diligent in documentation of initial assessments, because care for patients with poor outcomes (e.g., skin breakdown) that are not recorded as being "present on admission," (POA) will no longer be reimbursed. Terms like "never events" represent a category of adverse outcomes that, in the view of insurers, should never happen and for which they are no longer willing to pay. Nurse managers need to be cognizant of the variety of measures being collected for state, federal, and accreditation purposes that apply to their units and patients. These managers and their staffs often have to participate in the data-collection effort and discuss outcomes at quality improvement committees. Managers are held accountable to implement corrective action plans focused on their unit/department to address issues of noncompliance with quality indicators such as Core Measures (e.g., not documenting education about smoking cessation for AMI patients). In the future, patients and families may inquire about the organization's publicly reported outcomes, so it is imperative that managers are conversant with this topic.

Health Care Safety and Quality Improvement

A landmark report from the IOM in 1999 (Chrvala & Bulger, 1999) launched a major national focus on the safety of health care systems and processes. In fact, the conclusion that 98,000 deaths in health care organizations were preventable was considered a call to action, not only by health care providers but also by business and government. Not surprisingly, health care safety became the focus as a key component of the accreditation process. Soon after the millennium, new standards were established by The Joint Commission and other accrediting, regulatory, private, and public organizations to address the issue of health care safety within health care organizations.

Box 24.5

Components of a Health Care Safety Program

- Leadership commitment as evidenced through the allocation of resources for health care safety
- Assignment of individual(s) to manage the program
- Interdisciplinary (cross-organizational) participation, coordination, and communication about safety activities
- Education of patients and families about health care safety issues
- Disclosure of unanticipated outcomes of care to patients and families
- Education of staff on safety-related topics and training in team techniques
- Data collection and analysis in safety-related areas, including the following:
  - Incident reporting
  - Medication errors
  - Infection surveillance
  - Facility/environmental surveillance
  - Staff willingness to report errors
  - Staff perceptions of and suggestions for improving safety
  - Patient and family perceptions and/or suggestions for improvement regarding safety
- Definition of terms related to safety, including sentinel events, "near misses" and what is reportable, and the development of policies and procedures to address each category of event
- Management of sentinel events
- Adherence to The Joint Commission National Patient Safety Goals
- Establishment of a risk reduction process to include Failure Modes Effects and Criticality Analysis (FMECA)

In July 2001, new standards were introduced that required all hospitals accredited by The Joint Commission to establish and implement a formal patient safety program. Additional standards to integrate health care safety programs into organization-wide processes have been added over time. The components of a health care safety program are listed in Box 24.5.

Those individuals and organizations committed to health care safety initiatives believe that a rigorous, ongoing, and proactive approach to the identification of risks will result in the prevention of errors as well as provide the framework to respond most effectively when errors do occur.

Just as a paradigm shift was required to move from a quality assurance mindset to performance improvement, the new paradigm for health care safety requires that organizations create a non-punitive culture for error reporting. This is application of the "process or system, not people" philosophy in its truest form. Systems that single out caregivers who commit errors must be eliminated. More important, nurse managers must learn the principles of the non-punitive approach (i.e., they applaud and commend staff for reporting errors or "near misses"). In fact, in some industrial models, those managers or staff who detect and report errors or system failures in their areas are rewarded. An example of the effectiveness of this approach is reported in a study conducted by Harvard Business School professor Amy Edmondson. She found that the nursing units in one hospital that were considered to be the best performing were those that had higher detected rates for adverse drug events (Hesselbein & Johnston, 2002). Certainly, the conclusion was not that more errors were committed on this unit but that the staff's willingness to report errors contributed to the improvement of the unit's overall processes, resulting in a positive reputation within the hospital.

Examples of organizations that have created health care safety programs and initiatives since the IOM reports were released are the Veterans Affairs (VA) National Center for Patient Safety, the Leapfrog Group for Patient Safety, and the National Quality Forum (NQF). The VA National Center for Patient Safety (NCPS) is committed to the reduction of error and improvement of quality through proactive approaches to risk reduction (U.S. Department of Veterans Affairs, 2004). This is accomplished through focusing on prevention, creating non-punitive environments, and conducting safety research through such concepts as human factors analysis and studying high reliability organizations (HROs) in other industries such as aviation and nuclear energy. The VA has created numerous educational programs through the NCPS and freely shares them with all health care providers who want to learn about health care safety tools and techniques. They have taken the lead in adopting the methodology and tools of health care Failure Modes Effects Analysis (FMEA).

The Leapfrog Group for Patient Safety was founded by the Business Roundtable (an association of Fortune 500 CEOs) and consists of more than 150 public and private organizations that provide health care benefits to their employees (The Leapfrog Group for Patient Safety, 2004). This coalition is committed to the identification of health care risks and the adoption of proven strategies, such as computer physician order entry (CPOE) and appropriate ICU staffing, to reduce these risks and improve care. Their purpose is to create an incentive for providers to make "leaps" in improving quality and reducing errors by adopting these proven strategies. Their plan is to reward those that make "leaps" with monetary incentives. The Leapfrog Group has influenced regulators and accrediting bodies by sharpening their focus on health care safety. The Leapfrog Group publishes on their website the results of their annual survey that is completed by participating hospitals. Consumers can review and compare numerous hospitals in a region and determine where they want to receive care based on this "report card" posted on the Leapfrog website.

The National Quality Forum (NQF) is another group that consists of a consortium of organizations that work collaboratively to address health care quality and safety (The National Quality Forum, 2009). In 2003, The NQF published a list of 30 consensus standards to address safe practices that, if implemented, would yield improvements in the safety of care. Examples of this initial list included establishment of a culture for safety, adoption of protocols to prevent wrong-side surgery, and implementation of effective admission assessments to identify and treat underlying conditions early in the care process. The NQF Safety Practices were updated in 2006, and a total of 34 practices were included in 2009 Safe Practices. New Safe Practices in the 2009 set were added in areas such as pediatric imaging, glycemic control, organ donation, catheter-associated urinary tract infection, and multi-drug resistant organisms. A number of previously endorsed practices were updated based on new evidence, including the pharmacist's role in medication management and pressure ulcers and an entire chapter on health care–associated infections (NQF, 2009). Current safety topics that the NQF has endorsed and recommend include implementation of effective "hand-off" communication, initiation of rapid response teams, and management of methicillin-resistant *Staphylococcus aureus* (MRSA) infection.

Nurse managers can personally create an environment that is devoted to health care safety by doing the following:

- Learning the concepts and tools related to risk identification, analysis, and error reduction
- Adopting and embracing the concept of non-punitive error reporting
- Advocating for the establishment of a non-punitive culture if it is not currently a strong ideal within the organization
- Encouraging staff to be constantly vigilant in identifying potential risks in the care environment
- Creating a sense of partnership with patients and families to promote communication about safety concerns and soliciting their suggestions to correct and prevent potential risks
- Becoming a role model for staff and peers in practicing health care safety concepts

Practical Tips

Tip # 1: Quality is the Centerpiece

Make quality a centerpiece of your practice. The theory is well accepted, and vast resources are available. Pick one issue, search out resources, and share these with your work group to start a dialogue.

Tip # 2: Use a Checklist

Use the components listed in Box 24.5 and make a checklist. Assess your organization using this checklist.

Tip # 3: Get Involved in Quality

Become active on your area's quality councils, and expand your knowledge and experience related to quality.

Sentinel Events

One element included in The Joint Commission standards for both the Leadership and Performance Improvement chapters addresses a key component in health care safety—that of the organizational response to sentinel events. A sentinel event is defined by The Joint Commission as follows (TJC, 2009):

> A sentinel event is an unexpected occurrence involving death or serious physical or psychological injury, or the risk thereof. Serious injury specifically includes loss of limb or function. The phrase "or the risk thereof" includes any process variation for which a recurrence would carry a significant chance of a serious adverse outcome. Such events are called "sentinel" because they signal the need for immediate investigation and response.
>
> The terms "sentinel event" and "medical error" are not synonymous; not all sentinel events occur because of an error and not all errors result in sentinel events.

In 1999, the JCAHO (now The Joint Commission) began requiring health care organizations to respond to sentinel events in a systematic and formal way (i.e., expecting that a Root Cause Analysis [RCA] be conducted by the staff involved with the event). Time frames for concluding this analysis and guidelines for conducting a "credible" process were outlined in the standards. Organizations not familiar with the quality tools for conducting RCAs (primarily flowcharting and cause-and-effect diagramming) had to quickly learn them. The purpose of the RCA is to "drill down" to the most common cause(s) for the event and determine what process improvements can be made to prevent the sentinel event from occurring in the future. Controversy over whether a sentinel event was reportable to The Joint Commission and what information could be shared with the accreditor from a risk management and legal perspective resulted in the creation of a number of alternatives for submission of the required RCAs. The detailed requirements for reporting and submitting RCAs are contained in the Sentinel Event policy and can be found on The Joint Commission website *(www.jointcommission.org/SentinelEvents/PolicyandProcedures/)*. Specific sentinel event outcomes are considered "reviewable" by The Joint Commission. Reviewable sentinel events are events that have resulted in an unanticipated death or major permanent loss of function, not related to the natural course of the patient's illness or underlying condition, or one of the following events (even if the outcome was not death or major permanent loss of function) (TJC, 2008e):

- Any patient death, paralysis, coma, or other major permanent loss of function associated with a medication error.

- A patient commits suicide within 72 hours of being discharged from a hospital setting that provides staffed around-the-clock care.
- Any elopement, that is unauthorized departure, of a patient from an around-the-clock care setting resulting in a temporally related death (suicide, accidental death, or homicide) or major permanent loss of function.
- A hospital operates on the wrong side of the patient's body.
- Any intrapartum (related to the birth process) maternal death.
- Any perinatal death unrelated to a congenital condition in an infant having a birth weight greater than 2,500 grams.
- A patient is abducted from the hospital where he or she receives care, treatment, or services.
- Assault, homicide, or other crime resulting in patient death or major permanent loss of function.
- A patient fall that results in death or major permanent loss of function as a direct result of the injuries sustained in the fall.
- Hemolytic transfusion reaction involving major blood group incompatibilities.
- A foreign body, such as a sponge or forceps that was left in a patient after surgery. (p. SE-2)

Organizations that have initiated comprehensive and robust health care safety programs are committed to the process of ongoing risk identification and prevention. These organizations encourage the staff to identify potential errors and report any "near misses" that occur. Even if an adverse event is not considered "reviewable," such organizations conduct RCAs on these identified risks to prevent similar errors from occurring in the future.

The Joint Commission accreditation standards also now require that organizations go a step beyond the RCA process in their health care risk reduction and management programs. A set of standards in the Leadership chapter requires the leaders to ensure that an integrated patient safety program is implemented. This includes the establishment of an interdisciplinary group to manage the program, definition of the program's scope, integration of the program into all components of the organization, systems to immediately respond to system or process failures, systems for reporting these failures both internally and externally, defined processes for response to unanticipated adverse events, proactive risk assessment programs, systems to support and care for staff who have been involved in an adverse event, and at least annually, a formal process for reporting to the organization's governing body on the program's components (TJC, 2008d, pp. LD-18-19). One of the methods for proactive risk assessment that accredited hospitals are expected to implement is the process of Failure Modes and Effects Analysis (FMEA). The expectation is that an FMEA will be performed on at least one identified high-risk process annually. The FMEA is conducted by an interdisciplinary team of professionals who own the process being studied and is facilitated by someone with knowledge and skills in quality improvement tools. The FMEA begins with flowcharting the steps of the process being studied. The team assesses risk points within the process steps, and these key risk points are ranked in terms of their impact on the potential failure of the system. Scores for severity and probability are calculated to give a "hazard" score to the identified breakdown, and detectability of the failure mode is factored into the analysis of its impact on the overall process. The team then "designs out" the most critical of the potential failures and recommends process improvements for prevention of the failures. Once these prevention strategies are identified, action plans for implementing them are reported to the enterprise leaders and endorsed for implementation (see the VA National Center for Patient Safety website for a detailed description of the Healthcare Failure Mode and Effects Analysis [HFMEA™] at *www.patientsafety.gov/HFMEA.html*).

PART IV

National Patient Safety Goals

Since the late 1990s, The Joint Commission has been collecting data on sentinel events and the outcomes of their RCAs for the purpose of sharing those data with health care organizations to prevent similar sentinel events from occurring. The results of the aggregation of this data collection are published by

The Joint Commission in a series of newsletters entitled *Sentinel Event Alerts.* These *Sentinel Event Alerts* address events such as wrong-sided surgery, infant abduction, infection control issues, fires, and medication error events, among others. At the time of this publication, 39 *Sentinel Event Alerts* have been published (TJC, 2008c). The original intent of these alerts was for health care organizations to review the "lessons learned" from those facilities that had experienced these sentinel events and to incorporate the recommendations for prevention described in each publication. This process was entirely voluntary and initially not tied to the accreditation process. However, certain sentinel events continued to plague the health care industry (e.g., wrong-sided surgery, suicide risk, patient falls, and the frequency of certain deadly medication errors). With the emphasis on health care patient safety (including the adoption of their own set of patient safety standards), the impact of the IOM report, and the industry-wide emphasis on error prevention as a backdrop, The Joint Commission formalized the information contained in their sentinel event database into a new accreditation requirement called the *National Patient Safety Goals.*

In 2002, The Joint Commission's Board of Commissioners approved an initial list of six National Patient Safety Goals (NPSGs) that represented the most commonly occurring and/or serious events from its sentinel event database, combined with the recommendations of an interdisciplinary task force. Each goal had evidence-based or expert-based recommendations to define how to successfully implement the goal. These new NPSGs went into effect in January 2003 and were included as a component of the accreditation process. The Joint Commission Board reevaluates the goals annually. New goals are added to the list if necessary, and/or existing goals may be replaced with new goals that reflect processes in which there are safety concerns (e.g., the list of NPSGs for hospitals added a goal for hand hygiene in 2004, goals for medication reconciliation and hand-off communications in 2006, and a goal for anticoagulation therapy in 2008). Annually, the updated lists are published in the summer, with an implementation date of January 1 of the following year, providing a 6-month time period in which accredited organizations must design and implement the processes necessary to become compliant with the new standards. Each organization must demonstrate compliance with all applicable NPSG recommendations during the time of their accreditation survey. These goals have become the underpinning of the survey process. Those organizations that effectively implement the NPSGs find that they are more apt to have a successful survey outcome in this era of unannounced surveys. Nurse managers can serve as role models by fully embracing the NPSGs on their units/departments and communicating their belief that implementation of these standards leads to safer patient care.

Health Care Risk Management

Risk management is defined as "an interdisciplinary process designed to protect the financial assets of the organization and to maintain high-quality medical care" (Velianoff & Hobbs, 1998, p. 91). Risk management as a leadership and care management concept is different from the client outcomes concept of risk adjustment, in which differences among clients or variables such as age or disease severity are weighted or adjusted for in outcomes analyses or benchmarking efforts (Maas & Kerr, 1999).

Risk management is an integral component of an organization's quality improvement and health care safety programs. A *risk management program* is defined as an organization-wide program to identify risks, control occurrences, prevent damage, and control legal liability; it is a process whereby risks to the institution are evaluated and controlled. The term has been used in health care since the 1970s, triggered by the quality assurance movement and malpractice claims.

Risk management is a process whereby risks to the institution are evaluated and controlled to *reduce* or *prevent future loss.* Before the advent of comprehensive performance improvement and health care safety programs, one of the primary purposes of risk management was to prevent financial loss resulting from malpractice claims. The Joint Commission has traditionally required a risk management program for the entire organization as a part of its quality improvement efforts. Because a risk management program is structured to identify, analyze, and evaluate risks, these programs have now been incorporated as key components in organization-wide health care safety and PI programs. A risk manager is one of the "first responders" in a serious or sentinel event situation. Risk managers should facilitate the process by which the organization's definition of risk categories is established (i.e., what constitutes a "near miss," what is reportable on an incident report, what is included in the organizational definition of sentinel event). A new concept called "enterprise risk management" addresses the evaluation of all risks confronting an organization in order to maximize safety and risk reduction. The idea is to prevent undesirable events from happening and to minimize the impact of unpreventable risks. The concept of enterprise risk management dovetails with the overall requirements of a comprehensive organization-wide approach to health care safety.

Risk management focuses on overall processes to reduce the causes and frequency of untoward or lawsuit-potential events. If an adverse event occurs, risk management personnel work to reduce the severity and impact of a financial loss (Velianoff & Hobbs, 1998). Risk managers are called on to respond to adverse events and perform the following functions:

- Assess the situation for ongoing risk potential and take measures to prevent further risk or damage from occurring
- Ensure that patients and staff are removed from immediate threat
- Secure/sequester any equipment, supplies, documents, or other elements involved with the event and take them out of service as applicable/appropriate
- Investigate the facts and circumstance of the event
- Determine whether the event meets the definition of "sentinel event" or whether it meets another risk category definition
- Make reports as needed/required to appropriate outside agencies or regulators
- Communicate with the patient, family, and staff involved in the event
- Communicate with administrative and clinical leaders and legal counsel as appropriate
- If necessary, organize the first meeting of the clinical team to conduct the RCA of the sentinel event
- Ensure that follow-up actions related to recommendations for improvement/prevention are implemented
- Collect data on the event and incorporate it into the organization's risk management database

Risk managers coordinate activities such as administering insurance coverage and risk financing, managing claims, collaborating with legal counsel, administering the risk management operations, analyzing the risk management database, conducting in-service training and education, communicating risk management information, and monitoring ongoing compliance to state, federal, and local regulations and laws (e.g., the Emergency Medical Treatment and Active Labor Act of 1986 [EMTALA] and the Health Insurance Portability and Accountability Act [HIPAA]).

As a tool for ongoing risk identification and reporting, *incident reports* form the core of organizational reporting from a risk management perspective. The purpose of an incident report is to provide a factual accounting of an incident or adverse event to ensure that all facts surrounding the incident are recorded. A successful incident-reporting process is one in which 100% of all appropriate incidents/adverse outcomes are reported to the risk manager. This goal is more apt to be achieved in those organizations that have adopted a non-punitive culture for reporting errors. The data contained in an incident report also alert the risk manager about facts and circumstances that may contribute to a potential malpractice or lawsuit claim. The incident-reporting system provides the risk manager with the opportunity to investigate all serious situations immediately. Data from incident reports are collated, analyzed, and used by leaders to identify risk areas that have ongoing trends or to point to areas that have emerging risk potential.

These data can inform the choices that the organization's leaders make in selection of processes to target for FMEA projects or to "drill down" further via an RCA to study an adverse outcome or "near miss" more fully. Aggregated data from the organization's health care risk management program are reported through the performance improvement and health care safety reporting systems to coordinate information about overall organizational risks. Performance measures of action plan elements resulting from an RCA or FMEA can be incorporated into a unit's/department's set of quality measures. Nurse managers can set the expectation for 100% reporting of risk events and "near misses" on their units/departments. Through diligent follow-up and the adoption of a non-punitive culture, managers can set the tone for a truly proactive risk reduction program.

In addition to internal reporting, many states (most via their health care licensure agencies, such as a department of health) have implemented mandatory adverse event reporting requirements, resulting in a new role for many health care risk managers. In organizations in these states, often the risk manager is accountable for the reporting of incidents that are on the mandated list. Most of these mandatory reporting programs also require the submission of formal RCAs as a follow-up to the initial report, including actions taken and assessment of the effectiveness of those actions. If the regulatory agency determines that the organization has not appropriately responded to the identified risks, it may result in further requirements for reporting and follow-up. This expanded role of the health care risk manager in external reporting creates a need for collaboration with the quality professionals in the organization. Working together as a team, the risk manager and quality manager will often share responsibilities for facilitation of RCA and FMEA teams to meet all of the internal and external accreditation and regulatory reporting requirements.

Clearly, health care quality has been an accountability of nurses since the profession's inception. Over the years, nurses have assumed roles in various health care settings for oversight of quality and performance improvement, as well as health care risk management. The IOM reports, the CMS requirements for public data reporting, and the Leapfrog initiative have raised public awareness about quality and safety outcomes in health care organizations. These quality and safety issues have challenged health care quality professionals and nurse managers for decades. A heightened public awareness combined with increasingly stringent standards for reporting quality outcomes is driving the need for health care organizations to address these issues. Professional nurses, in direct care, managerial, and executive roles, need to continue to be at the forefront, leading the charge in adoption of quality and safety initiatives that continuously enhance the quality of care and services provided to patients/clients, families, and communities.

Summary

- Quality and safety are key dimensions of health care.
- Nurses are key players in ensuring the delivery of evidence-based quality health care.
- Health care quality is an art and science that continues to evolve.
- Quality management and performance improvement are an organization's efforts to provide services according to accepted professional standards and in a manner acceptable to various organizational stakeholders.
- Nurses have a professional responsibility to be accountable for quality of care and health outcomes at all levels and to contribute to continuous improvement of the health care system.
- Health care professionals can use an identifiable model of *Plan, Do, Check, Act (PDCA)* to explore causes of variation in work processes.
- Nurse managers are cautioned to not first create new standards and measures; rather, a literature review often will reveal valid and reliable measures.
- Six Sigma and Lean Enterprise are emerging quality measurement models being applied to health care.

- A quality improvement program should pervade the entire organization, and continuous improvement should be a part of everyone's job.
- Performance standards are critically important and are the first step of a quality improvement program.
- Evaluation is based on mutually agreed-on performance standards and goal setting.
- Structure, process, and outcomes are types of performance standards.
- Mission, vision, and core value statements are the foundation on which an organization builds a quality infrastructure.
- Accreditation standards formed the basis for some of the first mandatory requirements for outcome measurement reporting (e.g., ORYX® and HEDIS® measures).
- Public reporting of process and outcome measures is now a reality, and at some point in the future, all health care organizations will be required to participate in these public reporting arenas.
- Patient safety programs are now a key component and focus of quality initiatives in health care organizations.
- The organization's leaders should establish the expectation that the entire organization, as well as patients and their families, should be involved in the identification of potential or actual errors.
- Risk management is an extension of quality improvement.
- A risk management program is an organization-wide program to identify risks, control occurrences, prevent damage, and control legal liability.
- There are certain known risk-prone areas in health care and known ways of preventing errors.
- High-performance organizations (HPOs) employ creative and improvisational problem solving.
- A non-punitive culture promotes error reporting.

CASE STUDY

Nurse Katharine Lauren has been asked by senior leadership to spearhead a group to evaluate patient falls to decrease their frequency and ideally prevent them from occurring. Based on the risk management data available, she selects nurses and nurses' aides for her team from the four patient care units in which patient falls are most prevalent. She adds a pharmacist and physician to her team to represent the interdisciplinary aspects of the fall issue. Nurse Lauren then applies the Plan, Do, Check, and Act (PDCA) process to her project on patient falls.

In the "Plan" phase, she and the team use flowcharting to visually illustrate the steps that occur when a patient falls. Next, the team brainstorms a list of all of the problems that are associated with a patient fall. From this list, Nurse Lauren directs the team to categorize these factors into five or six groups, using an affinity diagram. Once the categories are defined, the team uses a cause-and-effect (fishbone) diagram to identify all of the potential causes that lead to the eventual effect of a patient fall. From this fishbone diagram, specific factors are considered as potential root causes (e.g., no fall assessment, bed too high, patient confusion, slippery floors, poor lighting, medications that can cause dizziness, no assistance with ambulation, call bells not answered promptly).

Nurse Lauren suggests collecting more data on each of these potential root causes. She further suggests that the data be stratified by patient age and gender, time of day, patient diagnoses, patient location, and staffing. She and the team design a data collection tool that will allow all of the data to be collected on one form.

After the data are collected, the team uses a Pareto chart to visually illustrate the most frequently occurring problems in descending order. By using this technique, they find that inadequate patient assessment and reassessment, call bells not answered promptly, and beds too high are the most common factors in patient falls. They also use Pareto charts to further define the stratification categories. When using this tool, they find that women older than 75 years with postoperative hip surgery seem most likely to fall on the evening shift. Most of the occurrences are on 4 South (the postsurgical unit).

During the "Do" phase, Nurse Lauren and the team design an assessment tool for the 4 South staff to collect data on all of the key factors identified earlier. For the trial, however, only the rooms of those female post–hip surgery patients older than 65 years are designated with a special symbol created by the team to represent a Fall Risk. Stickers with this symbol are also put on the call bell system lights for these rooms. Staff members are educated to the issue regarding quick call bell response and are requested to be especially vigilant in responding to the rooms with the special stickers. The data are collected for a 4-week trial period.

In the "Check" phase, the team reconvenes to evaluate the data collected in the trial. The data demonstrate a 37% reduction in patient falls from the same month in the previous year—just from addressing call bell response and none of the other factors.

Because the data on a sole factor demonstrated such a clear improvement, the team proceeds with development of a fall protocol, incorporating action plans to implement interventions for the other key factors identified earlier. The trial is expanded to another unit. When the data are analyzed for these two units and compared with the two other units with high fall occurrences, it is clear to the team that the protocol is having a positive impact on patient fall reduction. Throughout the process, nursing staff on the two trial units are solicited for feedback on the project, and their recommendations are incorporated into the protocol.

In the "Act" phase, the new Fall Prevention Protocol is adopted. Before its official "launch" in the organization, physicians, pharmacists, and nursing personnel are educated on the protocol. Data are collected not only on the outcomes but also on compliance with the interventions included in the protocol. After 3 months, the data demonstrate that those units with the lowest frequency of falls were those that had adopted the new protocol with enthusiasm and commitment. Nurse Lauren shares the data with the Nursing Leadership group, using control charts to demonstrate the outcomes. Based on the results, and in consultation with the risk manager and the Performance Improvement Council, the group expands the definition of Fall Risk to include those patients who experienced a "near miss" (i.e., a fall in which the patient was assisted when falling and did not reach the floor). Data will now be collected on these patient occurrences and on their contributing factors. In so doing, leaders believes that overall patient safety can be further enhanced. Nurse Lauren and her team receive an award at the hospital's annual Quality Day for contributing to significant improvements in patient safety and quality of care.

CRITICAL THINKING EXERCISE

Nurse Manager Todd Jonathan has just completed an online course on change and negotiation in health care. He has also served as the nursing department's quality improvement coordinator for 6 months, and he has been given accountability for program development. Nurse Jonathan thinks that some of the health care quality indicators that nursing is using are out of date and may not be evidence-based. Furthermore, he does not see that the indicators address critical issues that the American Nurses Association (National Database of Nursing Quality Indicators), the Centers for Disease Control and Prevention (CDC; Handwashing Guidelines), and The Joint Commission have been emphasizing, especially in the areas of infection control and safety. He wants to ensure that the program is current, evidence-based, and responsive to accreditation and other regulatory standards.

1. What should Nurse Jonathan do first to address this issue?
2. Describe the written materials he must prepare.
3. What sources can Nurse Jonathan investigate to find national standardized performance measures related to nursing?
4. Because the nursing quality management program does not currently have mission and vision statements, what is the process he should employ to develop them?
5. How should Nurse Jonathan address resistance to change in this situation?

25 Measuring and Managing Outcomes

Sean P. Clarke Matthew D. McHugh

CHAPTER OBJECTIVES

- Define key terms related to outcomes research and outcomes management
- List and discuss fundamental issues in analyzing data on patient outcomes
- Explain the steps involved in outcomes management in clinical practice
- Describe key challenges in patient outcomes research
- Discuss the relevance of research findings for outcomes management
- Illustrate current and future trends in the health care system relevant to nurse leaders' responsibilities regarding health outcomes
- Identify practical tips for leadership in outcomes management
- Exercise critical thinking to conceptualize and analyze possible solutions to a practice exercise

Outcomes research aims to understand the end results of health care practices and interventions. These end results include the effects that people experience and care about, such as health status, ability to function, quality of life, and mortality. Outcomes research that links the process of care to the outcomes that people experience has become a vital component to improving quality of care and increasing patient safety (Agency for Healthcare Research and Quality, 2004).

Nurses have always been focused on patient outcomes. Popular images of Florence Nightingale's enduring impact on health care and nursing tend to center more on her caregiving activities and her creation of roles and structures for trained nurses in hospitals. However, perhaps even more important, Nightingale pioneered the systematic use of client outcomes in the form of mortality data that demonstrated the use of interventions to improve health care. Collecting and analyzing data specific to nursing care and using it to guide process improvement technique, she reduced the mortality rate in a military hospital in the Crimea from 60% to 1% (Kalisch & Kalisch, 1978). By accomplishing this, Nightingale can be considered the founder of nursing outcomes measurement and management.

In this chapter, some basic ideas about outcomes and outcomes management will be reviewed, along with what outcomes research is, how it is conducted, and how it can be used by managers. Particularly important for managers are lessons that can be gleaned from outcomes research about measurement, design, and analysis of indicator data and an ability to read and apply the findings of outcomes research.

DEFINITIONS

Key terms related to outcomes and their measurement and management include *outcomes*, *indicators*, *outcomes management*, *outcomes research*, *nursing outcomes research*, and *risk adjustment.* There are a variety of definitions for these terms from researchers, theorists, and writers from a variety of disciplines, as well as government regulators and accreditation bodies. Simply put, an **outcome** is the result or results obtained from the efforts to accomplish a goal (Huber & Oermann, 1998). When most nurses consider outcomes, they think of the consequences of a health care intervention or treatment. The term *outcomes* has also been defined as "end results, or that which results from something" (Lang & Marek, 1990, p. 158) and as the conditions in patients and others that health care delivery aims to achieve (Peters, 1995). Donabedian (1985) described outcomes as changes in the actual or potential health status of individuals, groups, or communities.

Indicators are "valid and reliable measures related to performance" (Oermann & Huber, 1999, p. 41). They are the specific tools used to make quality visible to stakeholders in health care. Outcomes are measured or quantified by observing or describing indicators. Because quality is so important yet so elusive to define, a variety of accrediting and regulating bodies and a number of trade and professional associations (some that have formed coalitions or alliances), as well as health care quality assessment organizations, have developed standardized health care performance indicator data sets. For example, the American Nurses Association (ANA) developed the National Database of Nursing Quality Indicators (NDNQI) based on their Nursing Quality Indicators initiative (American Nurses Association [ANA], 1996, 2004). According to the ANA, outcome measures or indicators measure how nursing care is affecting clients. For example, the ANA includes the measurement of urinary tract infection incidents after 72 hours of hospitalization as an indicator of nosocomial infection rate.

Indicators are used as measures of all three of Donabedian's (1985) aspects of quality: structure, process, and outcomes. Donabedian's framework is useful to understand the relationship between outcomes and the structure and processes that have produced them. This suggests that nurse managers and leaders should focus on structure and process factors because these can be modified to influence patient outcomes (Donabedian, 2005). Understanding and developing both the nurse-level and organizational-level characteristics has the potential then to improve quality and outcomes. For example, structural indicators such as the mix of registered nurses (RNs), licensed practical nurses/licensed vocational nurses (LPNs/LVNs), and unlicensed assistive personnel caring for clients can be important for assessing organizational impacts on the delivery of nursing care. These can be measured by the full-time equivalent

LEADING & MANAGING DEFINED

Outcomes

The result(s) obtained from the efforts to accomplish a goal.

Indicators

"Valid and reliable measures related to performance" (Oermann & Huber, 1999, p. 41).

Outcomes Management

"A multidisciplinary process designed to provide quality health care, decrease fragmentation, enhance outcomes, and constrain costs" (Huber & Oermann, 1998, p. 4).

Outcomes Research

A field (or subfield) in health services research that examines improvements in functional status and quality of life.

Nursing Outcomes Research

Nursing outcomes research focuses on determining the effect of different contexts and conditions, related specifically to nurses and nursing care, on the health status of patients.

Risk Adjustment

Involves accounting for patient factors, the intrinsic risks that a patient brings to the health care encounter in the form of clinical and/or demographic factors.

(FTE) ratio of RNs with direct care responsibilities to LPNs/LVNs and unlicensed assistive staff.

Outcomes management, as originally described by Ellwood (1988), is a process used to assist managers and others make rational patient care–oriented decisions based on what is known about the effect of those choices on patient outcomes. The care process in outcomes management is what is being managed to achieve outcomes. To understand outcomes, the entire care process needs to be carefully examined and variation in outcomes must be analyzed. **Outcomes management** is defined as "a multidisciplinary process designed to provide quality health care, decrease fragmentation, enhance outcomes, and constrain costs. The core idea of outcomes management is the use of process activities to improve outcomes" (Huber & Oermann, 1998, p. 4).

Outcomes research is a field (or subfield) in health services research that examines what many ultimately believe are the actual goals of health care—improvements in functional status and quality of life. What makes outcomes research distinct from the vast bodies of research that examine endpoints in patients (i.e., much clinically oriented research) is that outcomes researchers seek to tease out the effects of patient-level care and systems-level environments from the background demographic, psychosocial, and clinical characteristics of patients as influences on endpoints. The purpose is to understand which patients or clients fare well and which do not in relation to treatments selected and/or the organizational context of care delivery (Kane, 2006a; Mitchell et al., 1998). An example of a provider characteristic that might be investigated as a predictor of patient outcomes might be professional background (e.g., physicians versus advanced practice nurses; RNs versus LPNs/LVNs).

Nursing outcomes research is a subspecialty within the larger field of health outcomes research. Nursing outcomes research focuses on determining the effect of different contexts and conditions, related specifically to nurses and nursing care, on the health status of patients. Nursing outcomes researchers are interested in the structures or management strategies for nursing care delivery that can achieve optimal outcomes for various clinical populations, as well as the mix of health care workers best equipped to care for them. Studies may aim to inform managers' decisions to recruit specific types of workers, such as RNs (as opposed to other types of nursing workers) or nurses with specialized experience or training. Other types of outcomes research are intended to assist managers and clinicians in determining the types of patients who benefit most from certain nursing interventions.

OUTCOMES MANAGEMENT

The process of managing outcomes includes the following five steps:

1. Data are collected about outcomes.
2. Trends are identified from data analysis.
3. Variances are investigated.
4. Appropriate service delivery changes are determined.
5. Changes are implemented and reevaluated.

In managing outcomes, the information derived from measuring client outcomes is collected, trends are identified, variances are examined, and appropriate care needs are determined to improve care to an individual, group, or population. Goals of this process include quality improvement and risk reduction. Variance analysis is one outcomes management tool. A variance is a deviation from what is expected. For nurses, this may mean a departure from the anticipated clinical trajectory. Variances may be positive or negative but are most useful for trends analysis.

Outcomes research and measurement examines the effectiveness of nursing care in improving client outcomes. Outcomes data and information about factors or approaches that promote favorable outcomes can help nurses assist clients and their families in meeting health needs and care needs across the continuum of care. Reading outcomes research can also help nurses select interventions that are the most useful in accomplishing the desired improvement in the client's health status. Identifying the most effective interventions can provide invaluable information to empower clients to self-manage their symptoms and care for themselves (Oermann & Huber, 1997, 1999).

As in any area of clinical care or the management of health services, ideally, practice is at least partially guided by research evidence. Although outcomes research has a great deal in common with other forms of research, it involves some special elements. In particular, outcomes researchers are especially concerned about understanding "real" differences between expected and observed outcomes and between outcomes on different units, in different institutions, or at different points in time. There are at least two reasons why managers need to understand how outcomes research is conducted: first, the broad concepts can help them analyze and interpret their own data; and second, when correctly interpreted and extrapolated, the findings of outcomes research can assist managers and clinicians to make better decisions for the populations they care for and establish environments for delivering care that favor high quality outcomes.

Increasingly, managers are accountable for outcomes in clinical care—to the point that annual performance reviews and salary increases are contingent upon achieving targeted outcomes. Outcomes research can provide key data for managerial decision making to improve quality of care. Data derived from outcomes research can be used to answer the following types of questions:

- What mix of staffing skill level and education is appropriate to achieve optimal outcomes for a clinical population with a particular level of patient acuity?
- What level of technology and ratio of technology and staff achieve the best outcomes for high-risk patients?
- What is the optimal organizational structure to maintain efficiency, safety, and patient satisfaction at institutions that provide high volumes of services?

Although the answer to each of these questions depends on the specific individual and institutional contexts and economic considerations at the time, data from outcomes research can be used to inform decision making.

INFLUENCES ON OUTCOMES

It is critical that all consumers of outcomes data, including managers, understand how to interpret outcomes data. Providers' interventions are aimed at achieving positive outcomes and avoiding negative ones. Outcomes are influenced by a number of factors—the specific treatment delivered is only one. A model of factors influencing outcomes is useful as a guide for managers. Iezzoni (2003a) and Kane (2006b) summarized the factors influencing outcomes and expressed this in the form of a mathematical "function" as follows:

Outcomes = f (patient clinical charateristics and risk factors, patient demographics, organizational characteristics of the setting, treatment, random chance)

Beginning efforts at outcomes measurement tend to focus almost exclusively on the effects of treatment (for nurses, usually the process of nursing care on outcomes—but that often encompasses the actions of the entire multidisciplinary health team). Correctly interpreting health outcomes data across settings or providers (whether in practice or in research) and attributing differences and outcomes to the right causes or sources require attention to two major challenges. The first lies in ensuring that consistent definitions and data collection processes have been identified and accurate measures of the phenomena of interest are used. This includes the outcomes, treatment, and any other risk factors thought to influence outcomes. The second, shared with all research dealing with dependent variables influenced by many factors, is that of risk adjustment (Iezzoni, 2003a). **Risk adjustment** involves accounting for patient factors, the intrinsic risks that a patient brings to the health care encounter in the form of clinical and/or demographic factors, before drawing conclusions about the meaning of different values for indicators. Analyses of outcomes across groups are meaningful only if these analyses account for relevant individual characteristics.

MEASUREMENT OF OUTCOMES

Jennings and colleagues (1999) have presented a framework for classifying outcome indicators into three categories: patient-focused, provider-focused, and organization-focused.

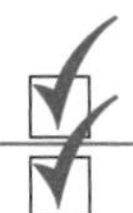

Practical Tips

Tip # 1: Verify Data First

The first steps in interpreting outcomes data are best carried out without being dismissive or panicked. Consistency and accuracy in data collection and entry are obvious areas that should be verified before taking action.

Tip # 2: Focus on Nursing's Data

Outcomes data and outcomes research findings are both essential tools for managers seeking leverage for resource allocation decisions. Collect, analyze, and use your nursing data.

Tip # 3: Present Accurate Data

High quality outcomes data can be costly, and there are limits to the quantity of information that can be effectively incorporated into managerial decisions. Clearly presented accurate data that tell a compelling story should be the goal of those who work with outcomes data in clinical settings.

Tip # 4: Use Data for Performance Appraisal

Outcomes data are increasingly forming one of the main bases for managers' performance appraisals—managers' understandings of outcomes data collection and interpretation need to keep pace.

Tip # 5: Use Data for Strategic Planning

The policy contexts of outcomes and outcomes research are rapidly heating up and need to be among the areas that managers and leaders include in their environmental scans for strategic planning.

Patient-focused outcomes can include such indicators as disease status, symptom experience, or pain. Other outcomes indicators incorporate a broader impact of disease and its management on clients' lives. These include quality of life, functional status, health status, and patient satisfaction. There are also provider and organizational outcomes. Provider-focused outcomes include such phenomena as nurse burnout, turnover, and job satisfaction. Organizational-focused outcomes may include patient or provider outcomes that are aggregated to the organizational level such as organizational mortality rates, error rates, or other rate-based outcomes. Cost indicators are often at the organizational level.

ELEMENTS OF OUTCOMES RESEARCH

Various types of indicators can be used for managerial decision making, highlighting the improvements in organizational-level factors or nursing care processes and assisting managers to make various investments in human and material resources in their settings. Indicators can also be used in controlled research examining the factors associated with the quality of care.

Variable Selection

When reading outcomes research, managers should be aware that researchers are often faced with considerable challenges when selecting outcome measures. The specific measures used should influence how managers interpret and apply study findings. For instance, outcomes can be generic or condition-specific, but they must be described adequately. An outcome that is not clearly defined is impossible to measure, and any conclusions or decisions by managers based on the research data may be flawed. Another issue for managers to consider is the reason or question driving the research and its influence on the selection of the outcome measure. For example, a study examining the relationship between the level of nurse expertise and patient outcomes generally would be insufficient to provide specific guidance on an intervention to influence the expertise level of nurses on any one hospital or unit. Managers should also consider whether the data or measurement instruments that were available to researchers influenced the selection of outcome. For example, consider the outcome measure in a study examining the influence of excessive workload on nurse injuries. It would be important to know whether the injury data were from nurse self-reports, an injury data-base, manager reports, insurance records, or some other source and what the potential limitations or biases are of each of these sources.

Risk Adjustment

Analyses of outcomes across groups are meaningful only if those analyses account for relevant individual differences in the patient populations being served. Returning back to the outcomes research model, when the interest in determining the effect of a particular intervention or process of care such as patients-to-nurse ratio on health status of patients, all of the other factors that may contribute to variation in the patients' health status must be accounted for. Thus, for example, comparing the effect of a better patients-to-nurse ratio on acute myocardial infarction (AMI) outcomes in patients without co-morbidities with those in older individuals with multiple co-morbidities would be inappropriate because it may be the patient factors, not the patients-to-nurse ratio that cause the different outcomes. Risk adjustment can be an involved and technical pursuit; but if given inadequate attention, patterns and associations that are found in outcomes research have little credibility because differences across the units or hospitals on outcomes cannot be interpreted as necessarily reflecting variations in quality of care. One caution is important. Certain types of outcomes are so dramatic and so closely tied to failures on the parts of systems for providing care (e.g., transfusion errors, severe pressure ulcers) that risk adjustment is unlikely to alter the interpretation of the relevant indicators. The literature contains some excellent references that discuss the state of the science in risk adjustment techniques (Elixhauser et al., 1998; Iezzoni, 2003b).

MEASUREMENT OF NURSING INTERVENTION OR TREATMENT

To understand the effect of the nursing treatment, intervention, or process of care being investigated, that phenomenon must be defined and measured accurately. In instances in which the intervention is straightforward, such as the implementation of a new technology or a new program, it may be easier to isolate the effect of treatment. There are times, however, when measures of the direct process of care are impossible or too labor-intensive to measure directly because they require intensive monitoring or recording of what nurses are actually doing. In those instances, proxy measures such as structural or organizational elements may replace them. For example, nurse staffing is a structural factor indicating the number or concentration of nurses often in ratio to patients. Nurse staffing measures usually do not directly assess the process of care, that is, what nurses do in their work with patients. However, it is seen as a valuable proxy measure for the process of care and quality. Proxy measures need to be evaluated for how accurately they represent the concept that they substitute for.

OUTCOMES RESEARCH DESIGN

With all of the factors that may influence outcomes, designing studies aiming to isolate the effect of nursing interventions or processes of care (or of certain organizational conditions) on outcomes and eliminating confounding sources is a challenging proposition. A range of design approaches are possible—selection depends upon the question being studied, the environment in which the investigation is to be carried out, and the subjects, instruments, and/or data available for study. The randomized controlled trial (RCT) is often described as the gold standard, but there is bias in any study and there is some concern that RCTs do not reflect the world in which managers and other decision makers must operate. One alternative is the practical clinical trial

(PCT), which aims to (1) select clinically relevant alternative interventions to compare, (2) include a diverse population of study participants, (3) recruit participants from heterogeneous practice settings, and (4) collect data on a broad range of health outcomes (Tunis et al., 2003). A great deal of nursing outcomes research uses quasi-experimental designs with either cross-sectional or longitudinal data. There are a variety of designs, measuring the outcome in relation to the treatment at any number of points and with possible control populations, each having its own strengths and weaknesses (Campbell & Stanley, 1963). In many other cases, however, researchers must turn to the analysis of data that were collected for different purposes—a practice known as *secondary analysis.* This design may save some time and money but requires much caution to avoid drawing erroneous conclusions (the measures, their reliability and/or validity, and the contexts in which they are collected may not be ideal). Knowing the potential bias that may arise because of the design of a study and the methods that a researcher used to address those biases is an invaluable skill for managers who wish to interpret outcomes data for management decision making. Classic texts such as Campbell and Stanley (1963) provide background in this area.

LEADERSHIP AND MANAGEMENT IMPLICATIONS

Leaders in today's health care delivery system are charged with the responsibility of producing quality services that achieve desired outcomes. Consumers must perceive that the outcomes of care justify the cost of services, and the services offered need to be valued by payers and purchasers of care. Outcomes research can provide nurse managers with an evidence-based foundation for leadership decisions and for making changes in practice. The process of determining the appropriate changes that need to be made in service delivery, making those changes, and reevaluating outcomes based on the changes are hallmarks of outcomes management.

Managers and executives today have a wealth of information available to them, and they are challenged with determining which data indicate a need for action in areas or aspects of care in the settings for which they are responsible. A significant body of literature in nursing outcomes research that continues to grow is a valuable point of reference for managers. There is, for instance, a large and expanding body of literature suggesting that lower staffing levels and skill mix in acute care hospitals are associated with increased risk of negative outcomes (Clarke, 2005). Insufficient nurse staffing, particularly of RNs, has been associated with a number of unfavorable outcomes including increased surgical mortality, failure to rescue, and rates of complications due to errors in care such as urinary tract infections, intravenous line infections, decubitus ulcers, and patient falls (Aiken et al., 2002; Kane et al., 2007). However, the specific context of the care environment and the patient population of interest call for continual monitoring of outcomes against internal and external benchmarks. Several data systems support the monitoring of nursing-sensitive outcomes. For example, the ANA has developed a system of quality indicators and measurement tools called the *NDNQI,* which are aimed at measuring the quality of nursing care in acute care settings (Gallagher & Rowell, 2003). The National Quality Forum (NQF) has also endorsed a set of voluntary consensus standards for nursing-sensitive care that quantify the contribution of nursing to patient safety, health care outcomes, and the professional work environment (National Quality Forum, 2004; Naylor, 2007). Also, agencies such as the Centers for Medicare and Medicaid Services (CMS) (previously known as the *Health Care Financing Administration [HCFA]*) and The Joint Commission (previously the Joint Commission on Accreditation of Healthcare Organizations [JCAHO]) incorporate outcome-based reporting requirements into their regulatory and accreditation processes (Huber & Oermann, 1998).

Managers and executives in practice struggle with decisions around the minimum number of data elements needed to satisfy payers and regulators versus how to be sufficiently comprehensive and inclusive in measure selection and what elements are needed in the dataset. Issues of feasibility, practicality, collectability, and comprehensiveness will be part of this unfolding area of nursing administration. In terms of a guide or framework for selecting outcomes for tracking purposes, balanced scorecards and dashboard approaches are gaining popularity. Dashboard approaches seek to identify the key factors for which a nurse manager needs to frequently monitor data to manage quality and costs. The balanced scorecard uses four areas for data evaluation—internal business processes, learning and growth, customer, and financial—and directs managers to select indicators from each of these areas (Park & Huber, 2007). Some research has examined whether this is a feasible approach (Hall et al., 2003).

CURRENT ISSUES AND TRENDS

Leaders and managers in nursing need to track developments in outcomes measurement and how outcomes measures are used. By feeding observations from the field back to researchers, regulators, and consensus groups, they can direct the creation of complete sets of clinically and practically important outcomes for regular use and the design of methods for measuring and managing them. Nurse leaders also have a crucial role in determining the important outcomes sensitive to nursing care, acquiring computerized data support for nursing-sensitive outcomes, and then participating in leading and managing multidisciplinary teams toward comprehensive outcomes management.

More than ever, the consequences of decisions in health care involving nursing services need to be clarified, investigated, and better matched to outcomes management. The nursing workforce supply is aging, and nurses report less favorable work environments, low relative earnings, and more satisfying alternative job opportunities. It has become a struggle to keep up the increase in demand for health care posed by an aging population. This has resulted in an impending workforce crisis that will require managers to make intelligent decisions regarding how and where to invest resources. Outcomes research will be vital for understanding the consequences of deploying various configurations of staff in different circumstances, especially when traditional models of care are no longer viable because the certain types of nursing staff are no longer available in sufficient numbers. Nurse managers especially need these data to make empirically based decisions regarding the effective management of their workforce, the maintenance and improvement of facilities operations, and the optimization of quality of care within the systems where they work.

Outcomes research is also shaping the policy environments and constraints in which managers must operate. For example, according to the ANA, 27 states had some form of nurse staffing legislation enacted, proposed, or under study as of August 2007 (ANA, 2007). The forms of the staffing proposals vary from public reporting of staffing levels to mandated staffing ratios. In 1999, then California Governor Gray Davis signed into law Assembly Bill 394 (AB 394) requiring the State Department of Health Services to adopt regulations establishing minimum nurse-to-patient ratios. The legislative intent behind the California nurse staffing ratios was to improve quality of care, patient safety, and nurse retention (California Department of Health Services, 2003). A significant, though not entirely consistent, body of evidence from outcomes research demonstrating the link between inadequate nurse staffing and unfavorable quality-of-care outcomes informed the intent of the regulations (California Department of Health Services, 2002, 2003).

Another area receiving growing attention is the trend toward pay-for-performance reimbursement systems that tie a pre-established portion of payment of services to the achievement of specific levels of measurable, targeted outcomes or being among the highest scoring organizations on specific measures. Where specific nursing services and interventions are linked to improvements and consistency in achieving outcomes that are pay-for-performance indicators, managers and institutions will have a tangible incentive for altering practice or organizational structure to achieve better outcomes.

As consumers, regulators, and payers increase their focus on outcomes, managers must proactively engage in outcomes management and participate

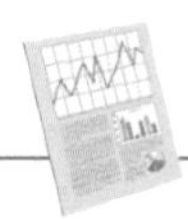

Research Note

Source: Burritt, J.E., Wallace, P., Steckel, C., & Hunter, A. (2007). Achieving quality and fiscal outcomes in patient care: The clinical mentor care delivery model. *Journal of Nursing Administration, 37*(12), 558-563.

Purpose

As the care environment becomes more complex and the characteristics of the patient population become more diverse, contemporary patient care requires sophisticated clinical judgment and reasoning in all nurses. Nurses, however, are not equivalent in their level of development regarding these abilities and their contribution to quality of care. Traditional models of care lack the structure and process to close the expertise gap, creating potential patient safety risks. As administrators struggle to compensate for a shortage of nurses, a premium will be placed on nurses with high levels of expertise because of their contribution to quality of care. The purpose of this study was to examine an innovative clinical mentor model, whereby senior, experienced nurses were relieved of direct patient care assignments in order to oversee nursing care delivery.

The clinical mentor model comprised 34 full-time equivalent positions that provided 24/7 coverage on 12 patient care units, including medical-surgical, cardiac care, intensive care, obstetrics, and emergency services. This intervention was evaluated in terms of its impact on quality and fiscal outcomes. Data on both adult patient outcomes and nurse satisfaction measures were collected as part of a 372-bed hospital's pre-existing quality program at intervals of 6 months before and after the introduction of the intervention. Patient outcomes on adults included fall rates, nosocomial pressure ulcers, failure to rescue, length of stay, and complication rates and were pre-defined to be consistent with the nurse-sensitive measures of care identified by the NQF. Lake's (2002) modification of the Nursing Work Index-Revised, the Practice Environment Scale of the Nursing Work Index (PES-NWI), was utilized for the measure of nurse satisfaction. This is also a NQF-endorsed measure.

Discussion

For clinical patient outcomes, 2-sample, 2-tailed t-tests demonstrated that the prevalence of stage 2 or greater pressure ulcers was significantly lower by 38% ($p < 0.05$) in the post-implementation phase. There was a significant reduction of 47% in the number of adverse events that made up the failure-to-rescue measure. Patient falls decreased by 20%, but this did not reach significance.

For financial outcomes, the impact of complication avoidance was estimated to save a total of 3192 excess days and charges of $2,813,418. Nurses reported improvements in all aspects of the nursing practice environment that were measured by PES-NWI. Significance testing was not performed on the difference between baseline and post-intervention scores, however.

Application to Practice

Nurse executives are consistently being challenged with ensuring safety, quality, and fiscally responsible patient outcomes in a highly competitive, regulated health care market. Capitalizing on the clinical expertise in all staff members has never been more important. While additional research is needed that uses control group designs and risk adjustment, the clinical mentor program exemplified a theoretically based strategy to maximize the expertise of the nursing staff and demonstrated improvements in cost-effective patient and nurse outcomes.

LEADERSHIP & MANAGEMENT BEHAVIORS

Leadership Behaviors

- Inspires outcomes thinking
- Enables the identification and use of evidence-based knowledge to drive outcomes
- Describes a vision for both client and systems outcomes
- Enables outcomes measurement using computerization and large nursing databases
- Removes barriers to outcomes improvement
- Articulates the value of nursing outcomes and practice

Management Behaviors

- Identifies outcomes of care and service
- Measures outcomes
- Manages the process of outcomes measurement
- Analyzes variances
- Takes corrective action when variances occur

Overlap Areas

- Determines outcomes to be measured and managed
- Leads and manages outcomes evaluation

in the ongoing development and implementation of nursing-sensitive indicators of quality. Maintaining an awareness of the advances and developments in outcomes research and the management techniques necessary to achieve improved outcomes is essential to maximizing system performance.

Summary

- Nursing outcomes research offers managers information to integrate into solutions but also challenges managers to use evidence to adapt to the evolving health care landscape.
- Nursing outcomes research is particularly suited to understanding those elements in the nursing care delivery environment that managers can modify to influence patient outcomes and quality of care.
- Specific nursing outcomes research methods and measurement databases and instruments are available to managers to effectively incorporate outcomes data-based decision making and outcomes management into the nursing practice environment.
- As health care systems continue to become more outcomes- and performance-driven, nurse managers and leaders must be influential in the development of outcomes research and management systems that are sensitive to the care that nurses provide and create work environments that support these systems.

CASE STUDY

Nurse Maria Garcia works for a managed care type of health maintenance organization (HMO). The nurses at the HMO have noticed a problem with women's health care. Little concern or counseling regarding menopause and health care is being provided. Nurse Garcia sees menopause counseling as a prime opportunity for nurses to deliver needed preventive and wellness care to adult women and their families. Furthermore, the National Committee for Quality Assurance (NCQA) that accredits managed care organizations is projected to include menopause counseling in its upcoming HEDIS® data set. It already has developed a national database of standardized performance and accreditation information for benchmarking. Nurse Garcia wants to take the lead in developing a menopause counseling program. However, several questions have arisen: How much will this cost? Which personnel should do this? What should be included in the program? What groups should be targeted?

1. What is the problem?
2. Why is it a problem?

3. What are the key issues?
4. What should Nurse Garcia do first?
5. How should Nurse Garcia handle this situation?
6. What outcomes should be used for this new program?
7. What outcomes measures might be useful?

CRITICAL THINKING EXERCISE

Pearl is the manager of a surgical unit at Great Swamp Memorial Hospital where many elderly orthopedic patients are admitted. Her clinical director and the quality improvement director for the hospital wish to speak with her this morning about high rates of pressure ulcers on her unit in the most recent institutional cross-sectional survey of patients. Patients on Pearl's unit had not only a very high number of ulcers but also a high number that were not documented on admission, suggesting that they occurred during the patients' hospital stays. Pearl and others are particularly concerned. Public reporting of pressure ulcer rates is on the horizon in her state, and in a few months, added hospital days and costs related to nosocomial pressure ulcers will no longer be billable to the Medicare program and other health insurance carriers.

1. What are the structure, process, and outcomes elements associated with pressure ulcer incidence?
2. What would Pearl want to clarify about these data and how they were collected before getting too far into a discussion about next action steps?
3. If Pearl or her colleagues wanted to compare the unit's rates of pressure ulcers with those of other units or hospitals (or even to last year's figures), what cautions should be applied? Where would they go to find benchmarks?
4. Imagine that this problematic indicator is a new development. Draw up a list of potential explanations that reflect a "real" decline in quality of care related to pressure ulcer prophylaxis on Pearl's unit or an "artifactual" one (one related to something other than quality of care).
5. Drawing on your background and a search of the Internet, outline some investments of resources that could be attempted to change this situation.
6. How would Pearl and her colleagues know if the approaches in No. 5 worked? What kinds of data would you suggest they gather?

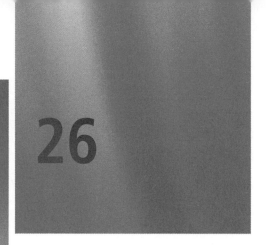

26 Confronting the Nursing Shortage

Amelia Sanchez McCutcheon

CHAPTER OBJECTIVES

- Define nursing shortage
- Describe current nursing shortage issues and trends
- Critically analyze factors that contribute to a nursing shortage, and discuss possible strategies to address the nursing shortage
- Link leadership and management concepts to strategies to confront the nursing shortage
- Use critical thinking to conceptualize and analyze possible solutions to a practice exercise

The nursing shortage is a major phenomenon affecting nurses and the provision of patient care. The Bureau of Labor Statistics' (BLS) (2007) *Employment Outlook: 2006-16* report projects a shortfall of over a million new and replacement registered nurses (RNs) to meet the demand for nursing care in 2016. The report also projects the need for a 90% increase in the number of nursing graduates. At the same time, enrollment in nursing schools and the number of nursing graduates are not keeping up with this target. The American Association of Colleges of Nursing's (AACN) (2008a) *2007-2008 Enrollment and Graduations in Baccalaureate and Graduate Programs in Nursing* report showed only a 5.4% increase in enrollments and a 7.4% increase in graduates from 2006 to 2007.

Nursing shortages have been cyclical over the past few decades; however, the current shortage may last longer because of a variety of factors, such as the large number of RNs approaching retirement age and the growth and aging of the U.S. population. For example, the report by the Bureau of Health Professions (BHPr) (2006) titled *The Registered Nurse Population: Findings from the March 2004 National Sample Survey of Registered Nurses* showed that the average age of registered nurses was 46.8 years in 2004 compared with 45.2 years in 2000. This "graying" factor makes the nursing shortage an even greater issue in light of the fact that the proportion of RNs younger than 30 years was only 8% in 2004, a decrease from 9% in 2000 and 25% in 1980.

DEFINITIONS

A nursing shortage is a condition in which the delicate balance of nurse supply and nurse demand is not at equilibrium. A **nursing shortage** is defined as a situation in which the demand for employment of nurses (how many nurses employers would *like* to employ) exceeds the available supply of nurses willing to be employed at a given salary. A nurse shortage is not just a matter of understaffing; in fact, understaffing can occur in conditions of shortage, equilibrium, or surplus, depending on local factors such as tight budgets or poor working conditions. The hallmark of a nursing shortage is the discrepancy between the supply and demand for RNs.

LEADING & MANAGING DEFINED

Nursing Shortage

Situation in which the number of nurses that employers would *like* to employ (demand) exceeds the number of nurses willing to be employed at a given salary (supply).

Span of Control

The number of staff reporting directly to a manager.

Transformational Leader

A leader who inspires and transforms followers.

Turnover

Termination of membership in an organization.

A nursing shortage can be identified by opinions of nurses, the public, or experts. Nurses or the public may believe there is a shortage based on a variety of factors. Experts generally use indicators such as employer reports, vacancy rates, turnover, recruitment difficulty, staffing levels, RN supply per population, or forecasting models to determine a nursing shortage.

Definitions of other factors surrounding a nursing shortage are as follows:

- **Span of control:** The number of persons who report directly to a single manager; affects the functions of planning, organizing, and leading (Hattrup & Kleiner, 1993).
- **Transformational leader:** A leader who inspires and transforms followers by raising their sense of the value of the task and their sense of importance (Bass, 1998). Bass outlined four components of transformational leadership: (1) charisma or idealized influence, (2) inspirational motivation, (3) intellectual stimulation, and (4) individualized consideration.
- **Turnover:** The termination of membership in an organization. The turnover rate is derived by dividing the total number of nurses who left a unit in 1 year by the total number of nurses employed on that unit.

CURRENT ISSUES AND TRENDS

Registered nurses make up the largest health care occupation in the United States, holding about 2.5 million jobs in 2006, with about 59% of jobs in hospitals and more than 1 in 5 (21%) working part-time (BLS, 2007, HRSA, 2007). Despite large numbers, the supply of RNs has not been in balance with demand or stable over time. Since the early 1900s, U.S. nursing has undergone repeated cycles of shortage and surplus. Although the length of each phase varies, clearly the alternation between shortage and surplus has been more frequent since the mid-1960s. Shortage phases have lasted longer, with only brief periods of surplus. Figure 26.1 shows the cycles of nursing shortage and surplus from 1901 to 2009.

These cycles are interrelated with social and economic forces, shifts, and changes. For example, the nursing shortage from about 1915 to 1920 resulted from the inability to recruit qualified and suitable students, since students provided most of the service on hospital wards (King, 1989). A little more than a decade later, in the context of the Great Depression (1929-1932), a surplus prevailed (Carlson et al., 1992). The 20 years after World War II (1945-1965) saw yet another nursing shortage (Grando, 1998). The availability of financial aid via the Nurse Training Act of 1964 increased nursing enrollments, and wage increases triggered increased labor force participation, thus lowering job vacancy rates during the next cycle (1965-1970). During the 1970s, nurse job vacancy rates climbed steadily, and a chronic shortage existed from 1970 to 1980 (Carlson et al., 1992). The recession in 1981 again converted the cycle to one of surplus until about 1985, when the results of implementing diagnosis-related groups (DRGs) passed and more ill patients were housed in hospitals. A shortage

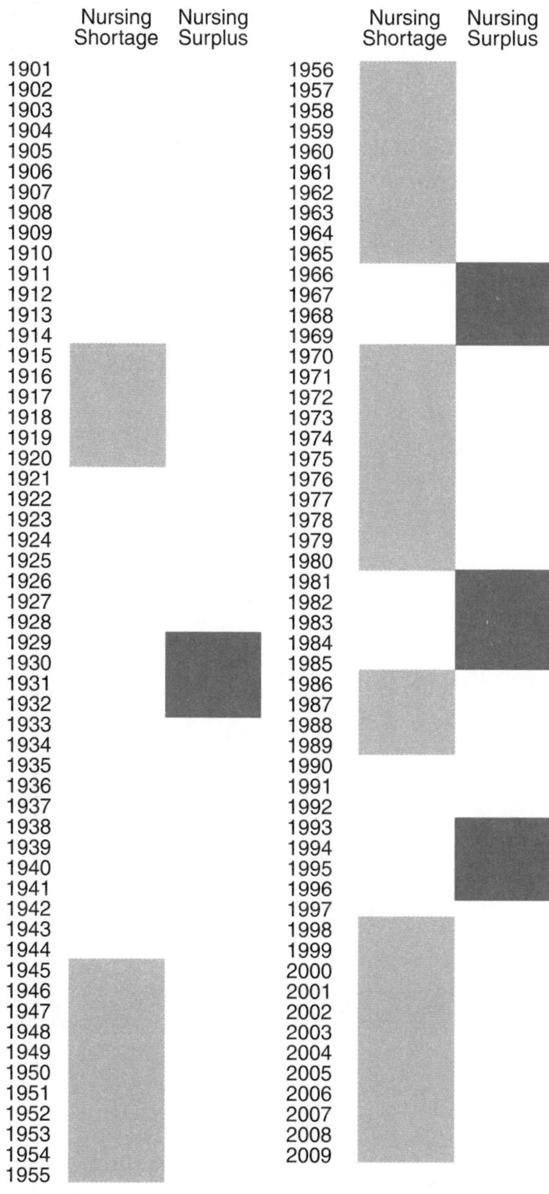

Figure 26.1

Nursing shortage and surplus cycles. (Copyright © Diane L. Huber, 2009. All rights reserved.)

again was noted from about 1986 to 1992, marked by an increase in the hospital RN vacancy rate at a national average of 11% (Buerhaus et al., 2005). By 1992, managed care, capitated reimbursement, cost containment, and downsizing hit the hospital industry, and only 5 years later nurses once again experienced a surplus environment. However, this cycle again reversed by 1998, when the beginning of a shortage was once again in evidence. By 2001, the hospital RN vacancy rate was at a national average of 13% and ranged up to 20% (Bureau of Health Professions [BHPr], 2006; Health Resources and Services Administration [HRSA], 2007). This cycle of shortage entered its eleventh year in 2008 and extended into 2009. The effects of the recession starting in 2008 and continuing into 2009 are not yet clear. In mid-2009, the Health Resources and Services Administration (HRSA) characterized the nurse shortage as moderate with areas of severe shortage (HRSA, 2009).

Clearly, the cycling through surplus and shortage increased in frequency in the last quarter of the twentieth century. Such rapidity of change disrupts individual nurses' lives and careers and makes the economic welfare of nurses precarious. Policies and practices related to recruitment into nursing as a career, recruitment and attraction to specific jobs, and retention in both job and career swing with the immediate crisis. This robs nursing of stability and long-term growth. Both historical indicators and research on nursing shortages have indicated that the basis of the problem relates to the nature of the work, low wages, poor working conditions, and hospital administrators' desire to keep nursing costs down at all costs (Carlson et al., 1992; Grando, 1998; King, 1989). Without a doubt, as the shortage/surplus cycles have increased in cycle time, planning change in the nurse labor force has become more difficult. Projecting the future demand for nurses requires careful attention to social and economic forces. The future projected demand for nurses is tied to an increase in chronic illnesses and an increasingly geriatric population.

The year 1998 marked the beginning of the current shortage. Unlike some previous shortage cycles, the current shortage is not resolving quickly (Buerhaus et al., 2008; Huston, 2003; Kimball & O'Neil, 2002). The latest projections are gloomy. According to the U.S. government (BLS, 2007; HRSA, 2007), more than one million nurses will be needed by 2016. If current trends persist, by

2020 only 64% of projected demand will be met, thus a shortage of 36%, as evident in Figure 26.2 and Table 26.1 showing the projected U.S. full-time equivalent (FTE) RN supply, demand, and shortages (BHPr, 2004). The projected RN shortage numbers are as follow:

- 405,800 in 2010
- 683,700 in 2015
- 1,016,900 in 2020

The report *What is Behind the Health Resources and Services Administration's Projected Supply, Demand, and Shortage of Registered Nurses?* (BHPr, 2004) projects that by the year 2015, all 50 states will experience a shortage of nurses. The predictions for some states are especially grim. Table 26.2 shows the following seven states, with the highest projected number of registered nurses needed who will not be available, in descending order: California, Texas, Florida, New York, Pennsylvania, New Jersey, and Tennessee. The number of nurses needed over what will be available in these seven states

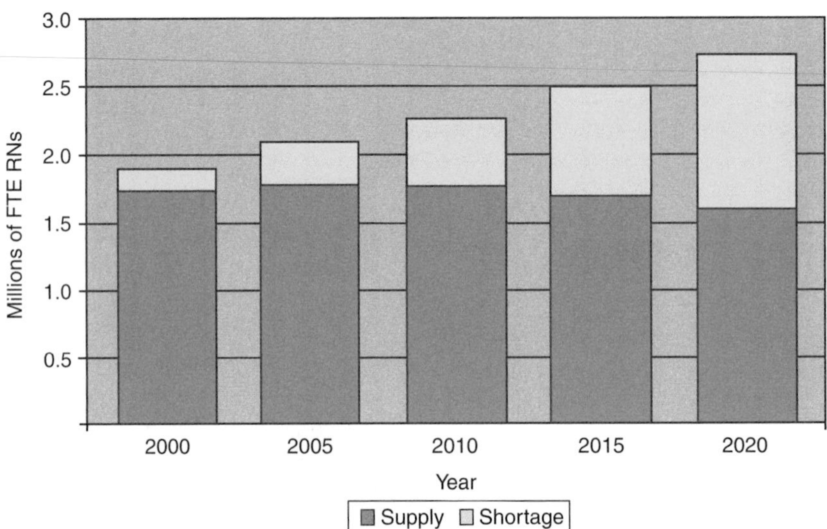

Figure 26.2
Projected U.S. FTE RN shortages, 2000 to 2020. (From Bureau of Health Professions. [2006]. *The registered nurse population: Findings from the 2004 National Sample Survey of Registered Nurses.* Rockville, MD: U.S. Department of Health and Human Services, Health Resources and Services Administration. Retrieved November 20, 2008, from http://bhpr.hrsa.gov/healthworkforce/rnsurvey04/.)

Table 26.1

Projected U.S. FTE RN Supply, Demand, and Shortages

	2000	2005	2010	2015	2020
Supply	1,890,700	1,942,500	1,941,200	1,886,100	1,808,000
Demand	2,001,500	2,161,300	3,347,000	2,569,800	2,824,900
Shortage	(110,800)	(218,800)	(405,800)	(683,700)	(1,016,900)
Supply ÷Demand	94%	90%	83%	73%	64%
Demand Shortfall	6%	10%	17%	27%	36%

From Bureau of Health Professions. (2006). *The registered nurse population: Findings from the 2004 National Sample Survey of Registered Nurses*. Rockville, MD: U.S. Department of Health and Human Services, Health Resources and Services Administration. Retrieved November 20, 2008, from http://bhpr.hrsa.gov/healthworkforce/rnsurvey04/.

Table **26.2**

Seven States with the Highest Number of Nurses Needed Who Will Not Be Available

State	2010	2015	2020	% of U.S. Population in 2010	% of U.S. Population in 2007	Population Rank	Shortage Rank
California	47,600	80,700	116,000	11.7	11.9	1	1
Texas	41,900	60,900	83,600	10.3	7.8	2	2
Florida	32,700	54,100	81,200	8.1	6.0	4	3
New York	21,500	36,600	54,200	5.3	6.3	3	4
Pennsylvania	21,100	36,600	54,800	5.2	4.1	6	5
New Jersey	19,600	29,900	42,400	4.8	2.8	11	6
Tennessee	18,500	26,000	35,300	4.6	2.0	17	7
Total of 7 States	164,800	268,900	389,800	50.0	40.9		
% of U.S. Total	50.0%	47.5%	46.0%				
U.S. Total	**405,800**	**683,700**	**1,016,900**				

From Bureau of Health Professions. (2006). *The registered nurse population: Findings from the 2004 National Sample Survey of Registered Nurses*. Rockville, MD: U.S. Department of Health and Human Services, Health Resources and Services Administration. Retrieved November 20, 2008, from http://bhpr.hrsa.gov/healthworkforce/rnsurvey04/.

constitutes 50% of the country's total need. The percentage ranking of projected shortage of five of the seven states (New Jersey and Tennessee excluded) is the same as that of the percentage population ranking.

The U.S. shortage is confounded by the fact that many other countries are experiencing similar shortages. The International Council of Nurses (2003) reported the following statistics—the projected shortfall in Canada is 78,000 RNs by 2011 and 113,000 by 2016; a similar shortage is expected in Europe when the difference in population size is considered. Projected shortfalls in European countries include the following: United Kingdom—22,000; Denmark—22,000 (by 2025); Germany—13,000; Netherlands—13,000; and Switzerland—3,000. In France, 6% of the nursing workforce left the public sector in 2001, compared with 4% in 1997; 18,000 nurses leave public hospitals every year, and the private sector reports a worse situation. Another 33 countries, most of which are in Oceania, Africa, Central America, and the Caribbean, also reported nursing shortages, worsened by the outflow of nurses to richer countries. The exceptions are Spain, Hong Kong, Korea, Taiwan, and the Philippines. The Spanish government stated 13,000 nurses are unemployed, and it was working to find jobs for them in the United Kingdom. Spain's national nursing associations are challenging this figure. They reported a reduction in demand as a result of hospital downsizing. Hong Kong, Korea, and Taiwan reported a surplus of nurses. The Philippines has a unique situation, reporting a balanced supply and demand but leaning toward a nurse surplus. Thousands of Philippine nurses continue to be recruited by the international market, particularly the United States. The recruitment eagerness is mutual; the most common reason Philippine nurses leave their country is to earn sufficient income to have a better standard of living and at the same time be able to financially help their families in the Philippines.

A nursing shortage has been shown to have adverse effects, including decreased access to care, decreased job satisfaction, and increased turnover. For example, an inadequate number of nurses to staff the operating room results in decreased OR capacity, which in turn increases wait time for surgical procedures. The concern about the effect of RN shortages on the quality of patient care is growing. Needleman and colleagues (2002), Kovner and colleagues (2002), and Kovner and Gergen (1998) discussed the evidence demonstrating that hospitals with lower staffing of RNs to patients experienced more adverse patient outcomes than did hospitals with higher RN staffing. The meta-analysis conducted by Kane and colleagues (2007) found that the shortage of RNs and the increased workload can negatively impact the quality of patient care. Duffield and colleagues (2007) found that stabilizing the work environment, whether by having a low nurse turnover, having a stable nurse leadership, or providing adequate competent staff, enhances patient outcomes.

Cycles of nurse shortage and surplus have been the focus of study and discussion over the years. Many factors contribute to these phenomena. Just as numerous factors contribute to the nursing shortage, multiple possible solutions are needed to resolve it. An analysis of these factors will highlight the nurse shortage as a current and future issue. Then leadership and management implications will be discussed.

FACTORS THAT CONTRIBUTE TO THE NURSING SHORTAGE

The nursing shortage is a national and international phenomenon. The causes are complex and interactive. There is no one simple, quick fix. In this analysis of the causes of the nursing shortage, the U.S. Health Resources and Services Administration's (HRSA) (BHPr, 2004) Nursing Supply Model (Figure 26.3) and Nursing Demand Model (Figure 26.4) will be used as guides. HRSA used these two models to project the nursing shortage. The assumption of this analysis is that to best understand the factors that contribute to the nursing shortage, the factors impacting nursing supply and factors influencing demand for nursing services must be examined.

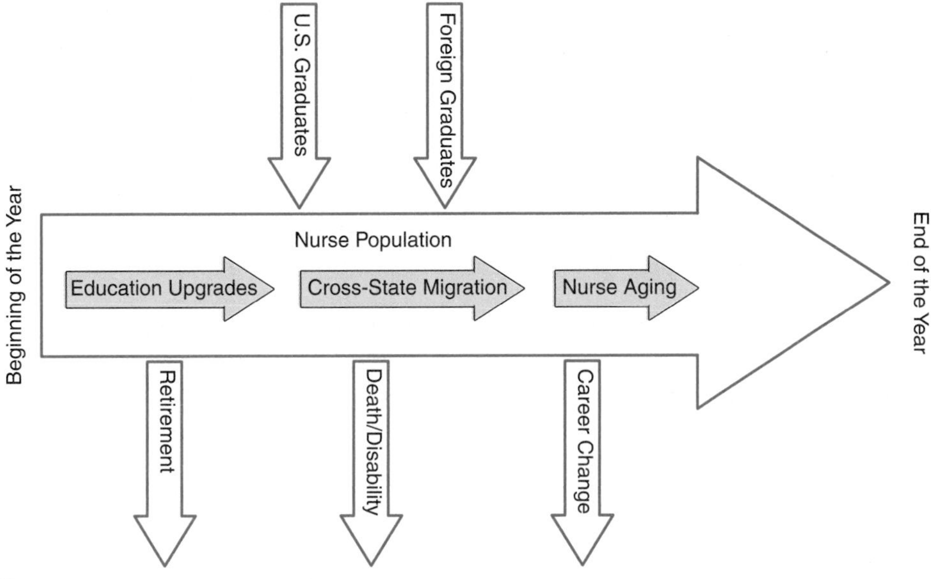

Figure 26.3
Nursing Supply Model. (From Bureau of Health Professions. [2004]. *What is behind the Health Resources and Services Administration's projected supply, demand, and shortage of registered nurses*? Rockville, MD: U.S. Department of Health and Human Services, Health Resources and Services Administration. Retrieved November 20, 2008, from http://bhpr.hrsa.gov/healthworkforce/reports/nursing/rnbehindprojections/index.htm.)

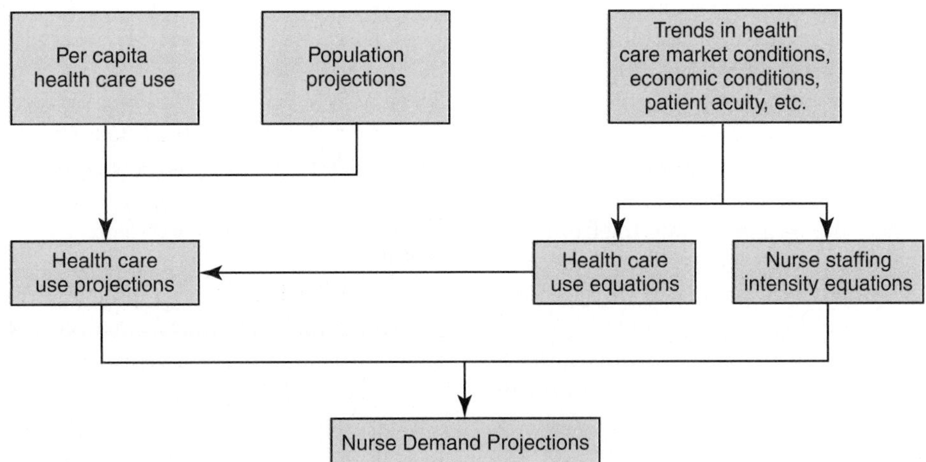

Figure 26.4
Nursing Demand Model. (From Bureau of Health Professions. [2004]. *What is behind the Health Resources and Services Administration's projected supply, demand, and shortage of registered nurses*? Rockville, MD: U.S. Department of Health and Human Services, Health Resources and Services Administration. Retrieved November 20, 2008, from http://bhpr.hrsa.gov/healthworkforce/reports/nursing/rnbehindprojections/index.htm.)

Supply

The Bureau of Health Professions (2004) projects the number of licensed RNs to remain relatively constant (2.7 million) between 2000 and 2020. The number of licensed RNs is projected to increase slightly through 2012 but will start decreasing because of the number of retiring RNs exceeding the number of new graduates.

Factors that affect nursing supply include the following:

- Nursing education factors: Those impacting the number of new nursing graduates
- Demographic factors: Those affecting the nature of the current RN workforce, thus the number of practitioners who can continue to work
- Work environment factors: Those influencing the ability of the workplace to recruit and retain nurses

Nursing Education

The ability of the education system to produce new graduates is affected by low enrollment, a shift from associate degree to baccalaureate-prepared RNs, and a shortage of nursing school faculty.

First, enrollments in nursing schools and the number of graduates are not growing quickly enough to meet the projected demand for nurses. There was a 5.4% increase in enrollment and a 7.4% increase in graduates from 2006 to 2007 (AACN, 2008a). At the same time, enrollment must increase by 40% and new graduates must increase by 90% to meet the projected demand for nurses in 2020 (BHPr, 2006). Buerhaus and colleagues (2000) reported that women graduating from high school in the 1990s were 35% less likely to become nurses than women who graduated in the 1970s. Reasons for this trend include (1) increasing career opportunities for women such as medicine, business, engineering, and other careers traditionally chosen by men; (2) difficult working conditions; and (3) a decrease in the attractiveness of the nursing profession (Buerhaus et al., 2000).

Second, the shift from associate degree to baccalaureate-prepared RNs has also affected the growth in supply. Baccalaureate-prepared RNs need twice as long to complete their education and enter the workforce than those graduating from associate degree programs. The number of new licenses in nursing is projected to be 17% lower in 2020 than in 2002 (National Center for Health Workforce Analysis, 2002).

Third, a shortage of nursing school faculty is limiting enrollments. The AACN's (2008a) *2007-2008 Enrollment and Graduations in Baccalaureate and Graduate Programs in Nursing* report points to a faculty shortage as the main reason (71.4%) for U.S. nursing schools turning away 40,285 qualified applicants to baccalaureate and graduate nursing programs in 2007. The other reasons were insufficient number of clinical sites, classroom space, and clinical preceptors, as well as budget constraints. To further confound the shortage, the average ages of nurse faculty pose a probable large surge of retirements in the near future. AACN's report (2008b) on *2007-2008 Salaries of Instructional and Administrative Nursing Faculty in Baccalaureate and Graduate Programs in Nursing* shows the following average ages of doctoral-prepared and master's-prepared nurse faculty:

- Professors: 59.1 years (PhD); 58.9 years (master's)
- Associate professors: 56.1 years (PhD); 55.2 years (master's)
- Assistant professors: 51.7 years (PhD); 50.1 years (master's)

The AACN's (2007) *2007 Survey on Faculty Vacancies* report shows a national nurse faculty vacancy rate of 8.8%, which equates to approximately 2.2 faculty vacancies per school.

Demographic Factors

Understanding the demographic nature of the RN workforce requires an examination of the factors affecting the number of practitioners who may continue to work, that is, the aging of and the changing composition of the RN workforce. These factors have implications for human resource initiatives.

Aging of the RN Workforce

The aging of the RN workforce is affected by the following two factors: the higher average age of recent graduating classes; and the aging of the existing pool of licensed nurses.

The data from the Bureau of Health Professions (BHPr, 2006) were used in this section unless otherwise indicated. There were 2.9 million RNs in the United States in 2004 (about 83% are employed in nursing), an increase of 7.9% between 2000 and 2004. This increase is comparatively low compared with the 14.2% increase between 1992 and 1996.

There has been a significant decline in the proportion of RNs younger than 30 years. Between 1980 and 2004, the proportion of RNs in the licensed pool who were younger than 30 years declined from 25% to 8%. Graduates of associate degree programs, the largest source of new RNs, are on average 33 years old—considerably older than in 1980, when the average age was 28.

The "graying" factor makes the nursing shortage an even greater issue, as the RN loss is projected to be 128% higher in 2020 than in 2002. The "graying" of the existing licensed pool who were nurses is evident in the following data. The average age of the RN population in March 2004 was 46.8 years, compared with 45.2 years in 2000. About half of RNs are projected to be older than 50 years by 2010 (Buerhaus et al., 2003). Nurses appear to be leaving the RN licensed pool, through death or retirement, at a faster rate than ever, with an average retirement age of 49 years. Between 1988 and 1992, 30,000 RNs left the license pool; 23,000 left between 1992 and 1996. The loss of RNs between the 1996 and 2000 surveys increased sixfold to sevenfold, to nearly 175,000, which points to a critical situation.

Changing Composition of the RN Workforce

The reliance on older RNs and on internationally educated RNs has increased significantly in the past 10 years. Of the 2.9 million RNs in the United States, more than 41% were 50 years of age or older, compared with 33% in 2000 and 25% in 1980. Buerhaus and colleagues (2007) reported foreign-born RNs accounted for 36.8% (93,000) of the estimated 252,479 RN employment growth between 2002 and 2006, and more than 50% in 2004 to 2006.

Work Environment Factors

Nurse vacancy rate and turnover rate are measures of nursing shortage. The average nursing vacancy rate is increasing: 13% in 2001 (First Consulting Group, 2001); 13.9% in 2003; and 16.1% in 2005. The turnover rate is slowly decreasing: 15.5% in 2003; and 13.9% in 2005 (AACN, 2008c). However, the turnover rate for first-year nurses remains high: one survey reported 27.1% in 2007 (PricewaterhouseCoopers, 2007); and another found 13% (Kovner et al., 2007). Kovner and colleagues also found 37% of first-year nurses reported that they felt ready to change jobs.

Several work environment factors have been cited as reasons for increased turnover (Buerhaus et al., 2000; Tri-Council for Nursing, 2004), including workload, autonomy, relations with managers, and compensation. Such factors influence job stress, in turn leading to job satisfaction or dissatisfaction (Moos, 1994). Job satisfaction is a strong predictor of turnover and intent to stay (Blegen, 1993; Davidson et al., 1997; Irvine & Evans, 1995; Larabee et al., 2003; Shader et al., 2001). For example, in a meta-analysis of 18 studies (16 were nursing), Irvine and Evans found a strong negative relationship between job satisfaction and intent to stay, suggesting that the more unhappy staff members are, the more likely they are to leave the organization. In 2004, RNs (76%) working in hospitals reported being satisfied in their work. This is significantly lower than for U.S. workers in general (85%) and for professionals (90%) (BHPr, 2004). RNs in nursing homes (75%) and hospitals (76%) were least satisfied; whereas RNs in nursing education (82%) were most satisfied.

Workload

One of the findings of a study by Aiken and colleagues (2002) was that nurses with the highest nurse-to-patient ratios (fewer nurses for the number of patients) were more likely to describe feelings of burnout, emotional exhaustion, and job dissatisfaction than nurses with lower ratios (more RNs for the number of patients). In addition, 43% of nurses who reported high levels of burnout and dissatisfaction intended to leave their jobs within a year. In contrast, only 11% of nurses who did not complain of burnout or dissatisfaction expressed intent to leave their current jobs. Buerhaus and colleagues (2005) found that insufficient staffing is raising the stress level of nurses, impacting job satisfaction, and causing nurses to leave the nursing profession.

Autonomy

Professional autonomy, or control over the practice environment, was identified as the strongest predictor of nurses' identification with the organization (Apker et al., 2003). Nurses who did not believe their jobs provided sufficient freedom were less likely to experience feelings of affiliation and loyalty toward their employers.

Relations with Managers

The manager's leadership style was found to be a significant predictor of nurses' job satisfaction (Bakker et al., 2000; Duffield et al., 2007; Loke, 2001; McCutcheon et al., 2004) and retention of nurses (Irvine & Evans, 1995; Leveck & Jones, 1996; Medley & Larochelle, 1995; Shader et al., 2001). Duffield and colleagues (2007) found that nursing leadership at the unit level is important for job satisfaction and intention to leave, which in turn impact on safety and patient outcomes.

Compensation

The National Center for Health Workforce Analysis (2002) reported that, on average, RNs have seen no increase in purchasing power over the past 9 years. Conversely, the average salary for elementary school teachers has always been greater than that for RNs and is growing at a faster pace. For example, in 1983, the average elementary school teacher earned $4,400 more than the average RN; and in 2000, elementary school teachers earned about $13,600 more (Figure 26.5).

An increase in salary for nurses relative to the salary in other occupations will increase the

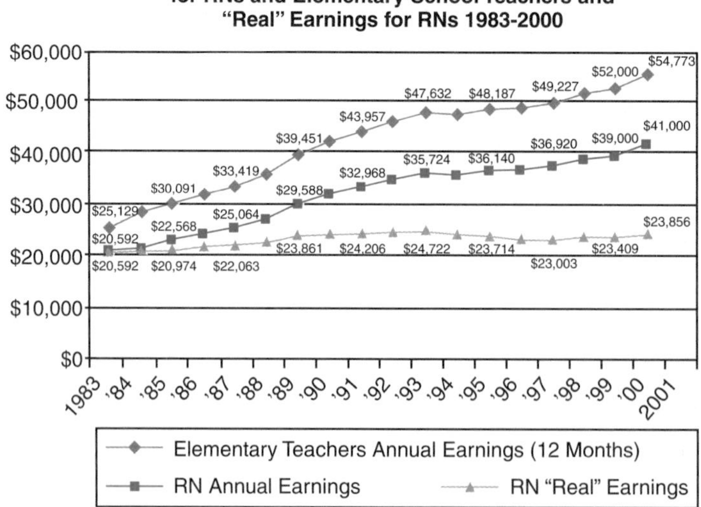

Figure 26.5
Comparison of actual earnings for RNs and elementary school teachers and "real" earnings for RNs for the years between 1983 and 2000. (From National Center for Health Workforce Analysis. [2002]. *Projected supply, demand, and shortages of registered nurses: 2000-2020.* Rockville, MD: U.S. Department of Health and Human Services, Health Resources and Services Administration. Retrieved May 21, 2004, from www.bhpr.hrsa.gov/healthworkforce/reports/rnproject/report.htm.)

attractiveness of nursing as a profession. An increase in salary would increase the supply of nurses by motivating part-time RNs to work full-time or work more hours; RNs to delay retirement or return to work from retirement; licensed RNs working in non-nursing jobs to return to nursing; and young people to enroll in nursing programs.

Demand

Demand for RNs is projected to increase 40% over the next two decades, with the majority of employment growth occurring in hospitals (BHPr, 2004). In this analysis, the following factors that affect the demand for nursing services are discussed: (1) demand for health care services; and (2) health delivery system–related issues.

Demand for Health Care Services

The recent increase in demand for RNs is projected to continue as a result of accelerating demand for health care services, which is affected by population growth, a rising proportion of people older than 65 years, economic growth, and advances in technology.

Changing Demographic Nature of the Population

Population growth and aging Baby Boomers are the major factors changing the demographic nature of the population, which in turn are affecting the demand for RNs. The Bureau of Health Professions (2004) reported the following statistics. The U.S. population will grow 18% between 2000 and 2020, which equates to an additional 50 million people requiring health care. Increased life expectancy resulting from advances in science and medicine accounts for most of this population growth, as well as the increase in the proportion of the population older than 65 years. A rapid increase in the elderly population is projected to start around 2010, when those at the top end of the Baby Boom generation reach age 65 (Figure 26.6). The subgroup of people 65 years old and older will grow 54% between 2000 and 2020, which equates to an additional 19 million people in this age-group. This is equivalent to a tsunami wave that cannot be stopped yet has huge implications for health care delivery financing.

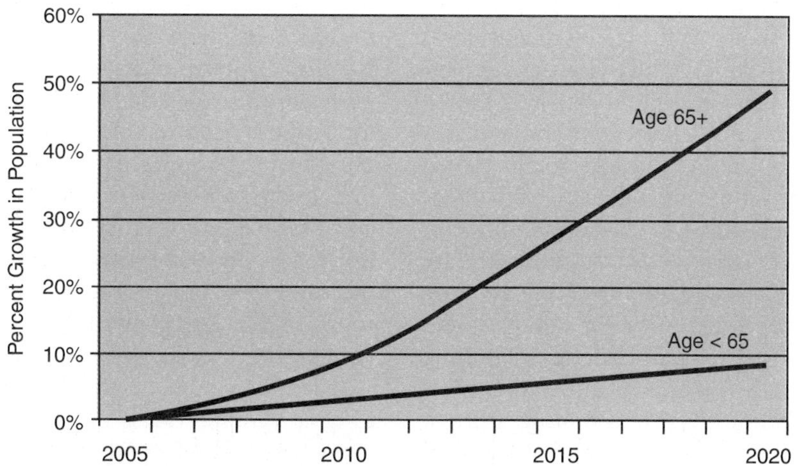

Figure 26.6

Population growth, 2000 to 2020. (From Bureau of Health Professions. [2006]. *The registered nurse population: Findings from the 2004 National Sample Survey of Registered Nurses.* Rockville, MD: U.S. Department of Health and Human Services, Health Resources and Services Administration. Retrieved November 20, 2008, from http://bhpr.hrsa.gov/healthworkforce/rnsurvey04/.)

PART V

Individuals older than 65 years, particularly those ages 85 years and older, have the greatest per capita demand for health care and thus the greatest need for the services of RNs. These individuals tend to have (1) a higher incidence of chronic conditions such as arthritis (50%), hypertension (36%), and heart disease (32%); and (2) a higher occurrence of multiple conditions requiring more regular care. Thus with living longer comes the increased prevalence of chronic medical conditions (Administration on Aging, 2002; Alliance for Aging Research, 2002; Wolff et al., 2002). As a result, this population uses a larger portion of the available health care services and resources. They visit physicians twice as often as those younger than 65 years, account for 38% of hospital discharges (they represent 13% of the population), and have annual per capita health care expenditures of $5400 compared with $1500 for those younger than 65 years. Individuals with one chronic condition had 7.5 times more inpatient admissions compared with those without chronic conditions (Wolff et al., 2002).

Health Delivery System

Health delivery systems form the structure around how care is delivered, where it is delivered, and how it is paid. For example, Medicare and Medicaid reimbursement, along with regional and local customs and culture, influence the demand for nursing services (Tri-Council for Nursing, 2004). It is commonly known that socioeconomic determinants such as culture, income, educational level, and age affect an individual's health practices, which in turn affect the person's health status and subsequent use of and access to health care services. Thus the demand for nurses may be more or less intense depending on local health system characteristics. For example, a General Accounting Office report (GAO-03–460) (2003) on emergency department overcrowding found waiting times to be longer in communities with more uninsured people. In rural areas, services or specialists may not be available without long-distance travel, which could result in delays in diagnosis, treatment, and care. Such delays could adversely affect outcomes, resulting in patients becoming more ill. Increased acuity of patients puts more demand on critical care services such as emergency and intensive care areas, thereby increasing the need for nurses. A combination of decreased supply and increasing demand creates a serious nursing shortage situation.

LEADERSHIP AND MANAGEMENT IMPLICATIONS

Health workforce dynamics are a current issue for leadership and management in nursing. Nurse leaders and managers have the responsibility for managing scarce resources, including the human capital resources within nursing service delivery. Chief among these resources is the adequate and appropriate mix of RNs and assistive personnel. Because the RN workforce has not been stable, workforce dynamics are an ongoing issue in clinical practice. Therefore the current nurse shortage (one that is projected to continue) becomes one of the preeminent current issues in nursing leadership and care management.

Just as multiple factors contribute to the nursing shortage, multiple possible solutions may exist to resolve it. Leadership is needed at all levels, both in the profession and in associated organizations. Several initiatives have been developed by hospitals, other health organizations, and health professional associations in response to the factors contributing to the nursing shortage. These initiatives include formal recruitment and retention programs, collaboration between education and practice settings to recruit more people into nursing, sign-on bonuses and other types of hiring incentives, and actions to improve the work environment of nurses (American Hospital Association [AHA], 2002).

The strategies that are most likely to provide for a stable nursing workforce now and in the future cluster into the following areas:

- Strategies aimed at increasing supply: (1) education-related strategies; (2) regulatory and policy issues; and (3) work environment–related strategies to increase the number of

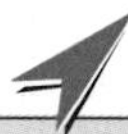

LEADERSHIP & MANAGEMENT **BEHAVIORS**

Leadership Behaviors

- Creates and communicates a sense of purpose
- Discovers and creates possibilities to recruit and retain nurses
- Motivates nursing staff's sense of value and importance
- Builds and sustains trust and commitment
- Develops leaders
- Transforms followers
- Makes decisions

Management Behaviors

- Communicates objectives
- Administers, maintains, focuses on work environment systems, and controls
- Sets staffing budgets, monitors progress
- Develops schedules
- Organizes the group
- Implements the plans
- Thinks critically
- Takes appropriate risks
- Measures performance
- Delegates tasks
- Makes decisions

Overlap Areas

- Communicates purpose and objectives
- Makes decisions

nurses staying in the profession. The first two strategies are aimed at increasing the number of nurses entering the profession. The third strategy is designed to increase the number of nurses staying in the profession.

- Strategies affecting demand, specifically health delivery system–related strategies aimed at reducing the demand for nursing services.

Most of the proposed solutions are derived primarily from the following sources:

- Bureau of Health Professions (2002), which outlined the Nursing Reinvestment Act
- Joint Commission on Accreditation of Healthcare Organizations (JCAHO, 2002)
- Tri-Council for Nursing (2004)
- American Nurses Association (2008)

The Tri-Council consists of the AACN, the American Nurses Association (ANA), the American Organization of Nurse Executives (AONE), and the National League for Nursing (NLN). An overarching strategy is collaboration. Nursing needs to partner and network with the public colleges and universities, the professional associations, and the various stakeholders of health care services.

Strategies to Increase Supply of Nurses

The following strategies designed to increase supply will be discussed: (1) education-related strategies aimed at increasing the number of nurses entering the profession; (2) regulatory and policy issues; and (3) work environment–related strategies to increase the number of nurses staying in the profession.

Education-Related Strategies

The following education-related strategies are grouped into three basic types based on the desired outcome, keeping in mind that the main goal is to increase the supply of nurses:

- Strategies to increase program capacity: advocate for increased nursing education funding under publicly funded initiatives.
- Strategies to increase nursing school enrollment: encourage young, more diverse population of nursing students; enhance image of nursing; articulate a clear vision of nursing; and provide financial incentives to students.
- Strategies to increase nursing program efficiency: offer accelerated nursing programs; promote distance and online learning; and enhance the use of high-fidelity clinical simulation.

Strategies to Increase Program Capacity

May and colleagues (2006) recommended more public financing to enable nursing schools to increase student capacity. These initiatives included faculty loans and subsidies for nursing faculty salaries. Whereas Cooper and Aiken (2006) recommended a priority on building adequate educational infrastructure to meet nursing workforce needs, JCAHO (2002) recommended the establishment of the federal funding of a graduate nursing residency program.

Several public funding initiatives have been put in place to improve the resources for nursing education:

- On August 1, 2002, The Nurse Reinvestment Act was signed into law. Two of the initiatives funded by The Act to help the nursing faculty shortage are (1) the fast-track faculty loan cancellation program for nursing students who agree to teach at a school of nursing and (2) the career ladder grant program that creates partnership between health care providers and nursing schools for advanced nursing education.
- In June 2005, the U.S. Department of Labor (2005), through the President's High Growth Job Training Initiative, provided grants to address the nurse faculty shortage.
- In 2006, nursing was designated by the U.S. Secretary of Education as an "area of national need" under the Higher Education Act's Graduate Assistance in Areas of National Need (GAANN) program. This program provides capitation grants for nursing schools offering PhD programs to increase the number of faculty and students.
- In January 2007, the Nurse Education, Expansion and Development Act (NEED Act) was introduced in the House. The NEED Act allows grants for nursing schools to increase the number of faculty and students.
- In October 2007, the Labor, Health and Human Services and Education Act was passed allocating funding for the Title VIII nursing workforce development programs. These programs are the primary source of federal funding for nursing education. Title VIII was expanded and improved by the Nurse Reinvestment Act. The major grant program areas are Advanced Education Nursing; Workforce Diversity; Nurse Education, Practice and Retention; Nurse Loan Repayments and Scholarships; Nurse Faculty Loans; and Comprehensive Geriatric Education.
- In December 2007, the Robert Wood Johnson Foundation (RWJF) and the AARP Foundation launched the Center to Champion Nursing in America funded by a $10 million grant from RWJF. One of the main objectives of the Center is to advocate for increased funding (federal and state) for nursing education for new nurses and nursing faculty.
- The Troops to Nurse Teachers (TNT) Act of 2008 is a partnership between military and civilian nursing schools to address the nurse faculty shortage. Modeled after the Department of Defense's Troops to Teachers program, the TNT program offers fellowship, scholarship, and transitional assistance programs for eligible commissioned officers of the Nurse Corps who can serve as faculty in nursing schools.

Schools are collaborating with clinical partners in developing initiatives to build program capacity. These initiatives include using clinical expert practitioners to increase the nursing faculty supply; increasing clinical student placement (practicums); and sharing physical resources to overcome clinical, classroom, and research space limitations.

Strategies to Increase Student Enrollment

Encourage a Young, More Diverse Population of Nursing Students. To attract young people into nursing, a national media "Nurses for a Healthier Tomorrow" campaign was launched by a coalition of 43 nursing and health care organizations working together to raise interest in the nursing profession among middle and high school students (Nurses for a Healthier Tomorrow, 2005). The campaign included conducting nationwide focus

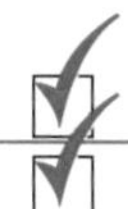

Practical Tips

Tip # 1: Monitor Career Options

Nurse shortages have occurred in cycles, but the present one seems to be stuck in shortage for a long time. Monitor your personal career options and plans with regard to nurse workforce realities. What would help your career?

Tip # 2: Be Proactive With Retention

If you are in a leadership or management role, evaluate how you can be proactive in nurse retention. Make your unit a Magnet™ one.

Tip # 3: Activate an Action Plan

This chapter presents many strategy options. Choose one that is within your power (e.g., reach out to a nurse faculty colleague to network and create synergy), and activate an action plan to make a difference in one discrete issue affecting nurses or nursing practice.

groups with students 6 to 15 years of age; raising funds in sponsorship; launching a website; and creating a televised public service announcement.

A related strategy is to encourage gender, racial, and ethnic diversity. The AACN (2001) promotes increasing diversity in nursing programs as one of the solutions to the nursing shortage. The AACN reported that the overwhelming majority of baccalaureate nursing students are female (91%) from non-minority backgrounds (73.5%). These numbers do not reflect the nation's population of 51% female and 33% minority group. Several reasons provided why men and minority group members do not pursue nursing include role stereotypes, economic barriers, few mentors, gender biases, and increased opportunities in other careers.

A report by the National Advisory Council on Nurse Education and Practice (2003) stated that it is essential to have a culturally diverse nursing workforce to meet the health care needs of the population. Minority nurses have contributed significantly to providing health care services in the United States and to leadership in developing models of care addressing the unique needs of minority populations.

Enhance the Image of Nursing. To attract people into nursing, the profession must be communicated as a positive, satisfying, and inspiring career. Nursing must provide for a balanced work life, offer leadership opportunities in which nurses may hone their management skills, and create an environment in which young nurses may plan to move toward higher pay and better hours. Wieck (2003) recommended expanding the image of nursing from caring and caregiver to opportunities and outcomes. Young people want opportunities to succeed and outcomes against which they can measure their success. Nursing must be advertised by focusing on such specialties as operating room nursing and emergency nursing, which are outcome-driven and meet many young people's desires for a fast-paced, high-intensity work environment. Nursing must learn from Drucker's (1999) model of productivity—that is, young people value productivity and want to be rewarded for it. If the nursing profession cannot adapt to this model, the emerging workforce will pursue other careers that can.

A survey (Seago et al., 2006) of 3000 college students in science and mathematics courses in California found that students generally had favorable perceptions of nursing. Two thirds of the students believed nursing provides good income potential, job security, and interesting work. However, compared with other professions, nursing had a lower perceived independence at work and was more typically perceived as a "woman's occupation." Work is needed to alter the image of nursing as primarily a woman's occupation and to transform the work environment of nurses to make a career in nursing more attractive (Seago et al., 2006).

Communicating the significant contributions of nursing and important nursing practice innovations and discoveries enhances the image of nursing. Nurses need to reach out to the media and seek their help in increasing the public's awareness of the relationship between nursing and patient outcomes, that is, the relationship between nursing variables and quality of care. For example, lower hospital mortality rates have been associated with higher RN skill mix (Hartz et al., 1989). This important research is an example of rigorous evidence of the significant contribution of nurses to health care that can elevate the prestige and image of nursing, thus attracting people to careers in nursing.

National and regional campaigns help show the nursing profession in a positive light. An example at a national level is the "Campaign for Nursing's Future" launched by Johnson & Johnson (2002). The campaign provided television advertising to celebrate nurses, a website, recruitment video, and brochures mailed to middle and high schools across the country. An example at a local level is a half-hour television special, "Medical Miracles. Nurses: Celebrating Our Heroes," showcasing nursing at the Cleveland Clinic Foundation.

Create a Clear Vision of Nursing. For a long-term solution, there is a need to formulate and articulate where the nursing profession is going. Wieck (2003) discussed having a nursing vision so that young people may see opportunities for great rewards and experiences. A lifelong nursing career path, which includes a series of value-added aspects (e.g., the nurse as a doer, a thinker, a practitioner, and a researcher), is recommended. Nursing needs to recruit outstanding students and appropriately educate the nursing workforce.

Provide Support to Students. Tuition and scholarships are strategies to be considered. The Nurse Reinvestment Act (2002) offers educational scholarships in exchange for commitment to work in organizations with critical nursing shortage. Other programs providing financial support to students are the President's High Growth Job Training Initiative; the Higher Education Act's GAANN program; and the NEED Act.

Strategies to Increase Nursing Program Efficiency

Accelerated nursing programs could quickly produce competent nurses if the integrity and quality of the nursing education provided are maintained. One approach is a 3-year (30 months) baccalaureate nursing degree instead of the current 4-year (32 months). Another approach is the accelerated degree (baccalaureate and master's degree) program for students holding a non-nursing degree (e.g., "second-degree nursing students") AACN, 2009). Accelerated baccalaureate nursing programs (12 to 18 months long) offer a quick route to becoming a registered nurse. Accelerated generic master's degrees take 3 years (1 year to complete baccalaureate-level nursing courses and 2 years of graduate study). Other strategies to increase nursing program efficiency include offering distance and online learning and using high-fidelity clinical simulation.

Distance and Internet-based training tools are being used increasingly in education and the workplace from virtual training and curriculum management to delivering professional development. Software is now available to make it easier for faculty and training personnel to teach and learn with virtually anyone, anywhere, and anytime. For example, the University of Virginia Darden School of Business uses software to offer a distance and strong collaborative learning tool in its MBA program (University of Virginia, 2006). The software enables the school to deliver innovative content in graduate-level distance learning programs, to enhance collaborative learning, and to conduct web conferencing. Benefits cited include engaged students in collaborative learning; archived key sessions for immediate retrieval; provided individuals contemplating enrollment with prompt communications from faculty and staff; and enabled real-time interactive experiences and a collaborative environment for students and faculty to more easily critique presentations, homework, and other projects. Their MBA students are often working full-time; thus the Internet-based learning tool saves time and expenses since the need to travel is minimized when students can view presentations at home or at work any time.

Another strategy to increase nursing program efficiency is high-fidelity medical simulations, which are now in widespread use in medical education and medical personnel evaluation (Issenberg et al., 2005; Scalese et al., 2008). Simulation is an educational tool that allows interactive activity by recreating all or part of a clinical experience without exposing patients to the associated risks. The available technologies used in simulation for education of health care professionals range from task training models to highly sophisticated computer-driven models (Maran & Glavin, 2003).

Simulation-based education allows students to carry out the practice required to master various techniques in a risk-free environment. Simulators can be available at any time and can reproduce a wide variety of clinical conditions on demand. Simulators are used to teach basic skills (e.g., respiratory physiology, cardiovascular hemodynamics) and advanced clinical skills (e.g., management of difficult airways, tension pneumothorax, pulmonary embolism, shock) (Good, 2003). Simulators allow faculty to obtain reliable evaluation of competence in multiple areas. Quality, high-fidelity medical simulations are educationally effective, and simulation-based education complements medical education in patient care settings. Nurses need to adopt simulations in nursing education in schools and the workplace.

Regulatory and Policy Issues

Regulatory and policy issues, such as licensure and nursing practice acts, can be barriers for recruitment of nurses, particularly internationally educated nurses. Registration application, review, and approval could take 1 to 2 years. This has resulted in some nurses doing non-nursing jobs while waiting for eligibility to write the RN examinations and work. Requirements before writing board examinations have also been restrictive. For example, RNs from the United Kingdom who are working in medical units and have no desire or plan to work in obstetrics are being required to take an obstetrical course to be eligible to write their RN examinations in North America. Regulatory bodies need to review their policies and procedures to ensure these policies and procedures are up-to-date and not contributing to the nursing shortage.

If enrollment does not increase dramatically, internationally educated RNs are likely to play an increasingly important role in providing nursing care in the United States. The use of internationally educated RNs in the United States may not be favored by (1) unions, because of a possible negative impact on wages; (2) patient advocates, because of possible effects on quality of care; and (3) other associations and foreign governments, because of possible worsening of shortages in their own countries. Conversely, the use of internationally educated RNs may be supported (1) by provider and payer groups, because of possible reductions in labor costs and (2) by foreign governments, because of possible benefits for foreign-born RNs, namely, the opportunity to work in the United States and send money home. Policy makers must encourage debate and the formulation of policies in the use of internationally educated RNs.

Work Environment–Related Strategies

One of the strategies proposed by a special JCAHO Expert Roundtable (JCAHO, 2002) is transforming the nursing workplace. Flynn (2005) recommended the creation of a safe and supportive workplace environment. The assertion is that a work environment that supports nursing practice increases nurses' job satisfaction and retention. Thus one way to address the current nursing shortage and prevent future crises would be to create and maintain Centers of Excellence in leadership and management aimed at advancing the profession and practice of nursing through the following strategies:

- Establishing appropriate leadership and management structures that provide consistent support to nurses
- Providing nurses with sufficient autonomy
- Ensuring adequate nurse staffing
- Implementing flexible schedules and appropriate compensation and benefit programs

Establish Appropriate Leadership and Management Structures

Nurse leaders have the ability to control or influence most variables that affect nurse retention. For example, the leadership style of the nurse managers on individual nursing units influences the retention of nurses (Irvine & Evans, 1995; Leveck & Jones, 1996; Medley & Larochelle, 1995) and nurses' job satisfaction, which subsequently affects turnover (Bakker et al., 2000; Loke, 2001; McCutcheon et al., 2004; Stordeur et al., 2000; Stordeur et al., 2001). McCutcheon and colleagues (2004) found that the higher the nurses rated their manager as having a transformational leadership style, the higher the nurses' job satisfaction and the lower the unit turnover rate. Similar findings were reported by Medley and Larochelle (1995) and Stordeur and colleagues (2000). When managers with high transformational leadership scores were compared with managers who had high transactional leadership scores, transformational managers were more likely to have staff nurse followers with higher job satisfaction scores. Transformational leaders exert a significant positive impact on staff satisfaction by providing support, encouragement, positive feedback, and individual consideration and promotion of open communication. These leadership behaviors tended to generate a favorable climate on the unit, characterized by increased cooperation and teamwork and fewer interpersonal conflicts.

Frontline nurse managers are in the best position to impact retention because they have direct knowledge of the issues impacting nurses and patient care delivery on their units. Nurse managers are also best situated to promote change in creating more positive work environments for nurses, but they need adequate supports and resources (Anthony et al., 2005). The nurse manager should be able to predict which nurses are most in need of retention attention and be able to identify factors in the work environment that are impacting nurse satisfaction levels. The nurse manager then has the ability to moderate nurses' job satisfaction levels and can thereby influence nurse retention (Andrews & Dziegielewski, 2005).

It is important for nursing to recruit and train managers who exhibit supportive and participative leadership styles, such as the transformational leadership style (Bass, 1998). It is critical that nurse leaders have the knowledge and skills necessary to influence nurse retention. Some organizations are implementing comprehensive leadership development programs (Herrin & Spears, 2007). These programs include individual development plans, provision of leadership training, and one-to-one assessment and coaching in a clinical setting. The focus is on training to develop the skills required to retain nursing staff. For example, because involving staff in collaborative practice and decision making increases nurse retention, these leadership skills are emphasized.

Another factor that affects turnover is span of control (McCutcheon et al., 2004), which is defined as the number of staff reporting directly to the manager (Hattrup & Kleiner, 1993). McCutcheon and colleagues found that the turnover rate increases by 1.6% for any increase of 10 in the size of the manager's span of control. For example, a manager with a span of control of 50 is predicted to have a unit turnover rate of 8%. The wider the manager's span of control, the higher is the unit turnover. Possible explanations for this effect may be found in the findings of Green and colleagues (1996) and Gittell (2001). Green and colleagues found that when the work unit increases in size, relationships between managers and staff become less positive. Managers cannot develop close relationships with staff and provide support and individual consideration while seeing to the daily operations of their unit. Similarly, Gittell (2001) found that small supervisory spans have positive effects on group process; that is, managers with smaller

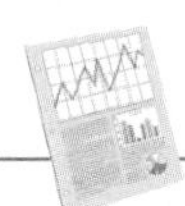

Research Note

Source: McCutcheon, A., Doran, D., Evans, M., McGillis-Hall, L., & Pringle, D. (2004). *The impact of the manager's span of control on leadership and performance.* Ottawa, Canada: Canadian Health Services Research Foundation. Retrieved May 15, 2009, from www.chsrf.ca/final_research/ogc/pdf/doran2_e.pdf

Purpose

The purpose of this study is to examine the relationships between leadership style, span of control, and outcomes using a conceptual model linking concepts from three theories: Transformational Leadership Theory, Span of Control Theory, and Contingency Theory. The sample consisted of 717 nurses, 41 nurse managers, and 51 patient care units drawn from four types of units (medical, surgical, obstetrics, and day surgery) and seven hospitals. Hierarchical linear modeling and multiple regressions were used to test the study hypotheses.

Discussion

The study findings support the theoretical relationships between leadership style, span of control, and outcomes. Results of the study supported the argument that transformational leadership matters—the higher the nurses rated their manager as having a transformational leadership style, the higher the nurses' job satisfaction and the lower the unit turnover rate. Transactional leadership style had a similar effect on nurses' job satisfaction, although to a lesser extent. Management-by-exception leadership style, on the other hand, decreased nurses' job satisfaction.

The study findings also supported the argument that span of control matters—the wider the span of control, the higher the unit turnover rate. A very important and interesting finding is the significant moderating influence of span of control on the effects of leadership on nurses' job satisfaction. Increased span of control decreased the positive effects of transformational and transactional leadership styles on nurses' job satisfaction while increasing the negative effects of management-by-exception and laissez-faire leadership styles on nurses' job satisfaction. These findings demonstrated that no leadership style can overcome a wide span of control.

Application to Practice

Recommendations for practice include designing and implementing management education programs that focus on effective leadership, such as a transformational style of leadership and the development of guidelines regarding the number of staff a nurse manager may effectively supervise and lead. Recommendations for theory and research include further testing of the proposed relationships in the study's theoretical model and continued examination of how various organizational factors affect leaders, staff, work groups, and organizations.

spans tend to relate better with the staff. Managers with smaller spans work with and provide intensive coaching and feedback to their staff.

In addition to the effect of the manager's span of control on turnover, McCutcheon and colleagues (2004) found span of control influenced the relationship between the manager's leadership style and nurses' job satisfaction. The positive effect of transformational leadership style on nurses' job satisfaction is significantly reduced in units in which managers have wider spans of control.

The results of a review of literature on span of control support the importance of the manager's span of control in creating a positive work environment (McCutcheon, 2005; McCutcheon et al., 2004).

Increase Autonomy

Apker and colleagues (2003) stressed the importance of developing nursing jobs and management practices that increase nurses' professional autonomy in their practice. For example, nurse leaders may establish organizational structures such as shared governance, continuous learning, and nursing research. These structures encourage nurses to take part in making decisions that influence patient care and nursing practice, and they encourage greater participation in clinical decision making with physicians and the interdisciplinary team. Nurse leaders also need to extend professional autonomy into quality-of-work-life issues such as promotion and advancement, flexible scheduling, and organizational culture that promotes respect and collaboration.

The Nurse Investment Act (BHPr, 2002) offered grants to help health care facilities retain nurses and improve patient care through increased interprofessional collaboration and more involvement by nurses in the decision-making process. One of the objectives of the newly created Center to Champion Nursing in America (Robert Wood Johnson Foundation & AARP Foundation, 2007) is to advocate for hospitals and other health care organizations to include nurse leaders on their governing boards. Nurse leaders can provide "critically needed practical perspective" on improving quality and safety of patient care.

Ensure Adequate Competent Staff

The following strategies help ensure adequate competent staff: (1) comprehensive orientation programs for new nurses; (2) sufficient staff development programs; (3) retention of experienced nurses; and (4) nurse leaders participating in decision making.

A comprehensive orientation program is necessary to help ensure adequate competent staff and retain new nurses. An estimated 33% of newly graduated nurses younger than 30 years intend to leave their positions within 1 year of hiring (Nelson et al., 2004, as cited in Hayes & Scott, 2007). Over a third of the hospitals (n = 32) studied by May and colleagues (2006) reported use of orientation programs as a retention strategy. Many hospitals had lengthened or redesigned their orientation programs to address the increasing complexity of patient care. Residency and mentorship programs also are being expanded to help new RNs settle into beginning practice. Another strategy to ensure adequate competent staff is to establish and sustain sufficient staff development programs and continuing education.

The high rates of RN departure from the workforce include the large nurse cohort between 62 and 65 years of age as nurses qualify for Social Security and Medicare benefits (BHPr, 2004). Although the impact on alleviating the nursing shortage is modest, delaying retirement by an average of 4 years would increase the FTE RN supply by nearly 158,000 (9%) in 2020 (BPHr, 2004). A strategy to ensure adequate competent staff is the retention of experienced nurses. Experienced RNs have a wealth of clinical expertise, nursing knowledge, skills, and judgment. Initiatives that may help retain older RNs include clinical ergonomic adaptations to minimize the physical strain in the work environment, flexible scheduling and part-time work, new roles (e.g., mentorship, internship), and economic incentives.

Another strategy to ensure adequate competent staff is for nurse leaders to be part of the senior management team. Nurse leaders must have a strong voice in executive decisions that affect the ability of managers to ensure the provision of adequate competent staff. Reid Ponte (2004) pointed out that the AONE recommends (1) a conscious valuing of the nursing's contributions to the quality of patient care, and (2) designing the nursing infrastructure within an institution wherein nurse leaders, at the senior level and at the unit level, have a manageable span of control and are positioned within the organizational key decision-making hierarchy. Two of the main objectives of the Center to Champion Nursing in America (Robert Wood Johnson Foundation & AARP Foundation, 2007) corresponded to the AONE recommendations to (1) educate policy makers and the public about issues facing nursing and evidence showing the relationship between higher nurse staffing levels and improved care quality, and (2) include nurse leaders on the governing boards of hospitals and health care organizations to provide "critically needed practical perspective" on improving patient care quality and safety.

Other strategies to retain staff, thus ensuring adequate competent staff, include the implementation of flexible schedules and appropriate compensation and benefit programs. In a survey of 428 inactive nurses in Mississippi younger than 60 years, 48% reported that they would be willing to work if they could work part-time, whereas only 9% were willing to work full-time. Thirty-six percent responded that they would be willing to return to work if the patient load decreased. Out of the disabled RNs, 26% were willing to work light duty, whereas 41% were willing to perform non–patient care activities. Primary reasons for leaving nursing were parenting (28%), shift length (14%), and salary (13%). Refresher courses and a flexible work environment were reported as important factors in the decision whether or not to return to work (Williams et al., 2006). Similarly, a small survey (n = 33) of factors that would influence inactive RNs in Missouri to return to practice found that money, improved working conditions, refresher courses, and health insurance were positive incentives that could motivate RNs to return to practice. After years of almost zero salary growth for nurses, nursing needs to implement appropriate compensation and benefits commensurate with nurses' contributions to health care. Although pay often is not listed as a major factor motivating nurses, clearly, society judges value, esteem, and image through compensation.

Strategies to Decrease Demand for Nursing Services

The following strategies focus on health delivery system–related aspects and are aimed at reducing the demand for nursing services: strengthening primary prevention; improving chronic disease management; adopting different delivery-of-care models; and increasing use of technology, research, and innovation.

Strengthening Primary Prevention

Primary prevention will reduce the demand for health care, thus nursing services. Examples of primary prevention efforts that have been effective are campaigns such as mandatory seatbelt use, legislation on driving under the influence of alcohol, and prohibiting smoking in the workplace and indoor public places. Colin-Thomé & Belfield (2004) recommended the following programs to strengthen primary care: health promotion programs on nutrition, obesity, exercise, and smoking cessation; and targeted screening programs.

Programmatic changes for reimbursement are needed to strengthen primary health care and increase access to health care services for specific populations. One of the strategies recommended by PricewaterhouseCoopers' Health Research Institute (2007) to address the nursing shortage was designing more flexible roles for advanced practice nurses to increase their use as primary care providers.

Improving Chronic Disease Management

The care of individuals with chronic diseases takes a large proportion of health care resources. For example, individuals with chronic conditions are more likely to see their family physician, to be admitted as inpatients, and to stay in hospitals longer (Colin-Thomé & Belfield, 2004). Chronic diseases include asthma, arthritis, diabetes, chronic obstructive lung disease, dementia, and heart failure. With the right care and support, individuals with chronic conditions can learn to manage their own care, which in turn can lead to slowing down of deterioration, preventing complications, preventing unnecessary hospital admissions, and when admitted, earlier discharge. Improving their care will improve the quality of life of these individuals and free up resources to address other needs for health care, such as reducing surgical wait lists and decreasing demand for nursing services.

Some of the recommended strategies by Colin-Thomé and Belfield (2004) to improve the management of chronic diseases included conducting health promotion programs such as reducing falls in older people; weight control, exercise, and smoking cessation; and early detection of dementia and support to residential and nursing homes. The Nurse Reinvestment Act provides training grants for programs to train and educate nurses in providing geriatric care for the elderly (BHPr, 2002).

Adopting Different Delivery-of-Care Models

One strategy to reduce the demand for RNs is to develop new roles and new ways of working (e.g., changing the way nurses are utilized, which in turn creates a demand for nurses with varying levels of education). Also, having non-licensed personnel perform non-nursing functions, such as supply and equipment restocking, increases nurses' ability to deliver care.

Other examples are some of the recommendations discussed by Colin-Thomé and Belfield (2004) to improve health care delivery in the United Kingdom. One recommendation was to improve access to primary care by developing the role of nurses in assessing and managing certain conditions previously seen to be mainly the family physician's responsibility. Another recommendation was to help people make the right choices by providing advice and information, either by telephone or with written materials. A third recommendation was to provide more secondary care in the community so that patients who are normally seen in hospitals can be cared for in the community. Some examples of this are chemotherapy programs, secondary prevention clinics, and cardiac rehabilitation delivered in the community setting to manage minor illnesses and treatment of injuries.

Increasing Use of Technology, Research, and Innovation

Technology, research, and innovation can reduce the demand on services and enhance the capacity of a reduced nursing workforce. For example, technological advances in surgery, such as laparoscopic and minimally invasive surgeries, have made it possible to do major surgical procedures as outpatient day surgery or as inpatient surgery with significantly shorter lengths of stay, thereby decreasing the demand for nursing services.

The amount and complexity of paperwork and documentation, both clinical and administrative, takes much of nurses' time. Electronic charting is being seen as a solution. However, standardization and streamlining of processes must first occur for electronic charting to reduce the time nurses spend on documentation.

Other Strategies

Two overarching strategies are (1) accurate and comprehensive workforce data and (2) stronger partnerships and alliances.

Accurate and Comprehensive Workforce Data

In planning and implementing solutions to the nursing shortage, the need for comprehensive, valid, and reliable workforce data has been recognized (Richardson, 2002). Such data are necessary to allow long-range forecasting in nursing human resources planning and system reforms (Little, 2007). Ryten (as cited in Richardson, 2002) emphasized that the lack of current and complete workforce data for nurses limits the ability to respond to nursing workforce issues and support successful nursing human resource planning.

Nooney and Lacey (2007) recommended devising nursing workforce solutions at both the state and national levels. The authors described the process used to project nurse supply and demand in North Carolina using the 2005 Health Resources and Services Administration's Nurse Supply Model and Nurse Demand Model. The models were found to work well for state-level forecasting providing that the default data accompanying the models are appropriately assessed against independent data sources specific to the individual state.

Stronger Partnerships and Alliances

Another overarching strategy is the need to build stronger partnerships and alliances with colleges and universities, professional associations, health care employers, government, community organizations, corporations, foundations, and the public. Improving the current nursing shortage will require stakeholders to work together. To address the systemic issues underlying the nursing shortage and develop sustainable solutions, active and collaborative participation of all groups that share concern about the nursing shortage will be required (Kimball, 2004). A study by Cooksey and colleagues (2004) of the 5 years of state-level efforts to address the nursing shortage in five midwestern states (Illinois, Iowa, Kansas, Missouri, and Nebraska) highlighted the role of collaboration, creativity, and flexibility. In each of these five states, taskforce groups were formed and later became influential nursing coalitions advocating for permanent state nursing centers with the main objectives of collecting and analyzing nurse workforce data, improving recruitment and retention, and enhancing the nurse practice environment.

CONCLUSION

In conclusion, factors related to the nursing shortage influence multiple aspects of society. Nurses serve the public good by taking care of the health of people who cannot take care of themselves. Thus, although one could argue that the nursing shortage is a leadership and management issue, individuals and various organizations (e.g., public and private, health care organizations, government, foundations) at all levels need to be a part of the solution. As well, for us to effectively confront the nursing shortage, various targeted strategies need to be implemented across the country.

Summary

- The nursing shortage is a major national and international phenomenon.
- Nursing shortages have been cyclical over time.
- The current shortage is predicted to continue into the future, partly because of the "graying" of America.
- A nurse shortage is a condition in which demand and supply are not in equilibrium.
- The nursing shortage is complex and the result of multiple factors.
- Demographic factors highlight trends and suggest strategies.
- Supply and demand are major parameters.
- Strategies to confront the nursing shortage include those aimed at education, regulatory and policy issues, work environment, and health delivery systems.
- At all levels, nurses need to develop innovative responses to a nurse shortage.

CASE STUDY

Nurse Manager Rebecca Pena's 80-bed surgical unit has been suffering from a severe nurse shortage. She recognizes the following problems: lack of staff involvement, high turnover rate, high use of sick time and low patient satisfaction. Rebecca wants the opportunity to work with the staff in developing a vision that will empower the staff and improve staff satisfaction, recruitment, and retention, thereby improving patient care and outcomes. She knows she must use both leadership and management skills to accomplish this important goal. First, she begins with a clear articulation of her vision.

Nurse Manager Pena knows she needs to develop strategies that will help her team achieve this vision. The strategies need to be consistent with organizational priorities, which include patient satisfaction, staff satisfaction and empowerment, and improved performance outcomes. These targeted strategies might include action plans developed to address recruitment and retention, improvement in patients, and organizational outcomes. Her first strategy is to create a small interdisciplinary team to lead the development and implementation of several specific strategies. The initial step is the identification of program, unit, and staff needs; key issues; and challenges. This is achieved by conducting a survey and seeking input from focus groups. Second, she organizes a retreat for teambuilding, discusses the results of the survey and focus groups, and crafts a consensus-based vision and a plan to achieve the vision. Third, she determines a strategy to implement the plan, which includes the development of a shared governance structure that promotes staff participation in decision making.

The governance structure includes three subcommittees reporting to the main unit committee. The three subcommittees are the Excellence, Safety, and Accountability Subcommittee; the Respect and Collaboration Subcommittee; and the Mastery, Discovery, and Innovation Subcommittee. The Excellence, Safety, and Accountability Subcommittee's responsibility includes the development, implementation, and evaluation of standards of care, clinical practice guidelines and pathways, and quality and safety indicators. The Respect and Collaboration Subcommittee is responsible for the following items: respectful workplace, positive team working relationships, clarification of roles, and staff satisfaction. The Mastery, Discovery (Research), and Innovation Subcommittee leads the planning, implementation, and evaluation of staff education, research, and innovation. After implementing her grassroots-based interprofessional team-building strategies, a self-sustaining and effective interprofessional team is created. Positive performance outcomes at the patient, staff, unit, and organizational level are being achieved through the governance structure and process.

CRITICAL THINKING EXERCISE

Rebecca Pena is the manager of an 80-bed surgical unit, which is split into two units—one located on the 6th floor of Building A and the other located on the 3rd floor of Building B. Nurse Pena started 2 weeks ago. She has noticed that most of the staff are pleasant but quiet. The staff tend to come to her for small things on a regular basis. Although there are numerous hospital committees, there are no committee representatives from this unit. In addition, there are no existing unit-based committees. Nurse Pena is the third manager on this unit in the past 2 years. Her colleagues mentioned that her unit has had difficulty recruiting and retaining not only managers but also staff. The unit has a high absenteeism rate and a very high agency nursing usage. These rates suggest that an underlying nurse shortage is occurring. The unit's patient satisfaction scores are the lowest in the hospital.

1. What are the problems that need to be addressed?
2. How will the unit's functioning be improved once the problems are addressed?
3. What strategies need to be implemented to address the problems?
4. To what extent are these strategies consistent with solutions to a nurse shortage?
5. What outcomes should Nurse Pena aim to achieve?

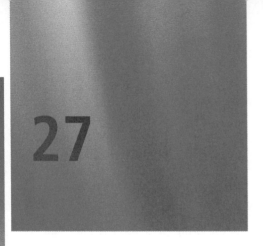

Staff Recruitment and Retention

Linda L. Workman

CHAPTER OBJECTIVES

- Discuss why organizations need to perceive and treat the human resources (health care employees, including nurses) within the organization as their primary business asset
- Examine internal and external health care processes that have affected the nursing shortage
- Differentiate factors that contribute to staff nurse shortage versus managerial nurse shortage
- Evaluate turnover rates, impact, and related costs
- Analyze the impact of generational differences on worker expectations and practices
- Address the role of the registered nurse in the delivery of quality health care services
- Describe major factors that affect registered staff nurses' and managerial nurses' recruitment and retention
- Analyze recruitment and retention strategies used by managers and/or organizations that have had a positive impact on nurse recruitment and retention
- Examine the positions professional organizations have taken relative to the nursing shortage, recruitment, retention, and strategies for management
- Apply critical thinking to conceptualize and analyze possible solutions to a practice exercise

Recruitment and retention of registered nurses in health care services has never been such an imperative as it is today. The nation is facing a critical nursing shortage. This nursing shortage is unlike either of the immediately prior two shortages (Buerhaus et al., 2000; Prescott, 2000). According to Prescott, this shortage is driven by supply-side economics (the amount of labor available to work), not just misdistribution of nurses or demand-side economics (employers' willingness to hire nurses). The following are some of the numerous causes related to this shortage (Buerhaus et al., 2000):

- Decrease in the U.S. birthrate since the 1950s
- Increase in the number of nurses approaching retirement
- Decrease in the number of students entering into nursing in the 1980s
- Increase in the number of students in their 30s who enrolled in associate degree programs during the 1980s
- Inability of schools of nursing to accommodate the number of students applying
- Decrease in the number of qualified faculty available to teach the students
- Increase in the number of positions available to nurses in the workplace
- Increase in the need for nurses in hospitals to manage the high-acuity patient populations
- Increase in patient volume in acute, specialty, and long-term care facilities related to the increased aging population

The number and percentage of nurses preparing for retirement in the next 15 years is of significant concern, since this group accounts for approximately 40% to 50% of the current workforce (Buerhaus et al., 2000;

The HMS Group, 2002). If the projections of Buerhaus and colleagues and The HMS Group are true, by the year 2020, the nursing workforce will remain at about its current size, which will be nearly 20% below the required need. This means that the nursing workforce, even at more than 2 million strong, will be short approximately 400,000 nurses. This shortage is of particular concern because of the 78 million Baby Boomers who will be retiring by the year 2015, a factor expected to cause health care demands to soar.

In September of 2004, Health Resources and Services Administration (HRSA) (2004) published a report entitled *What is behind HRSA's Projected Supply, Demand, and Shortage of Registered Nurses?* Included in this report was a table (Exhibit 24, p. 27) in which they noted the projected shortage from 2000 through 2020 (see Table 26.2 in Chapter 26). The report further indicated that RN supply shortage would occur in 31 of the 50 states and that 15 of those states would experience a supply reduction of 15% to 52%.

Although these figures are daunting, Auerbach and colleagues (2007) revised their forecast, noting a smaller shortage than originally projected based on trend analysis through 2005. The results of this analysis indicated that there was a larger-than-expected increase in overall interest in nursing as a second career choice, especially among people in their late 20s and early 30s. Based on the influx of nurses, their projection was that the shortage would be approximately 800,000 by the year 2020. Clearly, recruitment and retention will be major factors in the future. Multiple approaches will be needed, coming from both political arenas and the marketplace if the shortage is to be averted or minimized in the future. Actions noted by Auerbach and colleagues (2007) for addressing the shortage were directed toward workforce planning by policy makers. They recommended that initiatives include strategies for engaging high school and college graduates to select nursing as a career, finding ways to increase nursing education program capacities, providing incentives for hospitals to continue efforts to retain the older RNs, and clarifying how the use of foreign nurses will be addressed. They further noted that, in order to increase educational program capacity, faculty would have to be recruited and developed. This issue needs to be dealt with now, given that the average age of nurse educators in 2005 was 55 years (Davidhizar, 2005).

DEFINITIONS

Issues surrounding the nursing shortage have highlighted the important leadership and management interventions related to recruitment and retention of nursing personnel. **Recruitment,** defined as replenishment, is the process used by organizations to seek out or identify applicants for potential employment (Dictionary.com, 2004a). The impact is to ensure that an adequate number and quality of workers are available for selection and employment. **Retention** is the act of retaining. It is defined as the ability to continue the employment of qualified individuals, that is, nurses and/or other health care providers/associates who might otherwise leave the organization (Dictionary.com, 2004b). The impact of this action is to maintain stability and enhance quality of care while reducing cost to the organization. **Selection** is defined as the job of determining the most qualified candidate for a job. This process includes reviewing, sorting, ranking, and offering of candidates recruited for a job. **Staff vacancy** is defined as an employee position—full-time or part-time equivalent—that is budgeted but not filled. **Turnover** is defined as the loss of an employee because of transfer, termination, or resignation. **Transfer** is the movement of an employee whose performance is satisfactory from one area to another within the same institution or corporation. **Termination** is the discharge of an employee who is performing at a less-than-satisfactory level or is not a good match for the organization. **Resignation/voluntary turnover** is the failure to retain an employee who is performing at or above satisfactory level. Although all turnovers have an associated cost to the organization, the most costly are those dealing with termination and resignations.

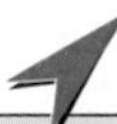

LEADING & MANAGING DEFINED

Recruitment

The process used by organizations to replenish employees.

Retention

The ability to continue the employment of qualified individuals.

Selection

Determination of the most qualified candidate for a job.

Staff Vacancy

A budgeted but not filled employee position.

Turnover

Loss of an employee because of transfer, termination, or resignation.

Transfer

Movement of an employee whose performance is satisfactory from one area to another within the same institution.

Termination

Discharge of an employee who is performing at a less-than-satisfactory level or is not a good match for the organization.

Resignation/Voluntary Turnover

Failure to retain an employee who is performing at or above satisfactory level.

THE NURSING SHORTAGE

According to Atencio and colleagues (2003), the changes in the nursing workforce were being felt in acute care institutions. The national vacancy rate in 2000 was 21.3%, while acute care hospital vacancy rates nationally were at 10.2%. The vacancy rate by services within acute care hospitals ranged from 9% to 15%: 14.6% for critical care, 14.1% for medical/surgical, and 11.7% for emergency department, with the lowest rates in the OR/perioperative (9.4%) and obstetric (9.65%) areas. Vacancies and turnover varied by region across the United States. Overall, the vacancy range was 9.3% to 12.2%, and the turnover range was 17.4% to 24%. The western and southern regions had both the highest vacancy and turnover rates, with vacancy rates at 12.2% and 11.0% and turnover rates at 22.2% and 24%, respectively. The region with the lowest vacancy rate was the Midwest (8.95%), and the lowest turnover rate was in the Northeast (17.4%). The western region, however, reported having the largest proportion of RNs in the age range of 50 to 59 years, whereas the southern region reported having the largest proportion of RNs in the age ranges of 20 to 29 years and 30 to 39 years. During this same period, the national vacancy rate for RN managers was 6.5%, with the western and southern regions having the largest rate at 8.5% and 8.2%, respectively. Urban and suburban hospitals reported higher vacancy rates than did rural hospitals, and individual and multihospital systems reported higher average RN vacancy rates than did integrated delivery systems. The percentage of facilities that used temporary staff such as agency staff or travelers to compensate for vacancies was approximately 54%. Range of usage (53% to 24%) varied by specialty service—critical care, medical/surgical, and emergency departments required the most, and obstetrics and OR/perioperative areas required the least. The impact of the shortage and use of higher-paid agency or traveler workers was a significant financial expense for 69% of the organizations. In addition to the cost, 51% of the organizations reported overcrowding in the emergency area, and 26% reported going on diversion for an average of 4 hours per week. Other impacts included restriction in admissions, increased waiting time for surgery, and reduced or eliminated services. Approximately 17% of the organizations reported that the shortage had a serious impact on nurse staffing and staff, including increased overtime usage, higher stress, restricted expansion, changes in recruiting and hiring practices, decreased quality of care, and increased difficulty in scheduling coordination. Chapter 26 further details the statistics related to the nurse shortage. Recent data are difficult to locate due to the lag time in data collection and reporting to the public.

This shortage is further being fueled by the international demand for nurses. According to Daniel and colleagues (2000) and Gamble (2002), international recruitment of nurses has once again surfaced as a way of addressing the nursing shortage, specifically in the United States, United Kingdom, Canada, and Western Europe. The International Council of Nurses (ICN) (2006) reported worldwide population aging projections in the first quarter of the twenty-first century. The results clearly indicated that aging population is an issue around the world, with greater than 1 billion people older than 60 years. The distribution of this population includes approximately 700 million in developing countries (which will increase nearly 240% from the 1980 levels). Included in this latter group are five of the ten largest populations in the world—China, India, Indonesia, Brazil, and Pakistan. This projection also indicated that the four countries with the oldest populations (with 31% older than 60 years) in the world—Japan, Italy, Greece, and Switzerland—would also be severely affected. Given the global magnitude of this shortage, few countries have nurses in excess; as a result, recruiting nurses internationally often creates an even more severe shortage in their home country.

INTERNATIONAL RECRUITMENT

International recruitment has been of major concern to the ICN. The ICN (1999) released a position statement, *Nurse Retention, Transfer and Migration*. In this document, the ICN linked the nursing shortage (inadequate supply of nurses) to lack of quality in health care. The statement addressed the individual nurse's rights, as well as positive and negative issues related to migration. It also delineated roles that national nurses associations should take to raise nurse awareness of potential constraints and ensure that countries seeking to recruit nurses had policies and practices relative to fair and humane treatment of nurses. The ICN supports the migration of nurses as a short-term strategy for addressing the nursing shortage, viewing nurse migration as a way of increasing the nurse's career opportunities and personal self-interests. Nurse migration is further viewed by the ICN as a way of increasing multicultural practice and learning opportunities within the nursing profession. This is especially so because nurses have identified two major reasons for leaving their home country—economic security and professional opportunity—although personal safety/security in the workplace and/or country has also been noted. However, concerns related to recruitment practices led the ICN in 2001 to issue a position statement on ethical nurse recruitment. In this document, 13 key principles specific to the recruitment of international nurses were identified as needing to be addressed (Box 27.1).

Box 27.1

ICN Ethical Nurse Recruitment Principles

1. Effective human resources planning and development
2. Credible nursing regulation
3. Access to full employment
4. Freedom of movement
5. Freedom from discrimination
6. Good faith contracting
7. Equal pay for work of equal value
8. Access to grievance procedures
9. Safe work environment
10. Effective orientation/mentoring/supervision
11. Employment trial periods
12. Freedom of association
13. Regulation of recruitment

Adapted from International Council of Nurses (ICN). (2001). Ethical nurse recruitment: Position statement. Geneva: Author.

These principles are relevant because they address changes that need to take place to ensure that nurses are treated fairly and equably in the international market place. Unethical recruitment of nurses in the past has led to nurses being exploited and misled into accepting job responsibilities and work conditions incompatible with their qualifications, skills, and experiences. The ICN further condemns the recruitment of nurses into countries where authorities support human rights violations. Sparacio (2005) addressed the complexity of international recruitment and the ethical impact of "brain drain" on the country from which nurses are being recruited. The California Nurses Association (CNA) and National Nurses Organizing Committee put forward a resolution, which was adopted by the CNA's 2005 House of Delegates, outlining a code of practice for international nurse recruitment (Dumpel, 2005). This code was directed at the concerns and unlawfulness of international recruitment relative to the health care impact. The code specifically targeted human rights issues relative to accessibility and quality of care within the home country. It also addressed concerns related to the potential health and patient safety issues secondary to recruitment of international nurses into the United States. According to Dumpel (2005), the California Board of Registered Nurses (BRN) in 2002 also opposed expansion of the international sites for NCLEX licensure testing approved by the National Council of State Boards of Nursing (NCSBN). The NCSBN expanded the testing to three new sites—Hong Kong, People's Republic of China; London, England; and Seoul, Korea. Their opposition was directed at the global nurse shortage, patient harm from fraudulent licensure, high financial stakes, and risk related to examination security.

AMERICAN NURSES ASSOCIATION'S CALL TO ACTION

In September 2001, the American Nurses Association (ANA) (2001)—in conjunction with the American Organization of Nurse Executives (AONE), Sigma Theta Tau International (STTI), and 60 other professional nursing organization and 19 steering committee organizations—held a summit meeting to begin to analyze the nursing shortage problem and to develop a strategic plan entitled *Nursing's Agenda for the Future: A Call to the Nation* (ANA, 2002). The outcome of this meeting was a vision statement and 10 domains for action. The vision statement was as follows (ANA, 2002):

> Nursing is **the** pivotal health care profession, highly valued for its specialized knowledge, skill and caring in improving the health status of the public and ensuring safe, effective, quality care. The profession mirrors the diverse population it serves and provides leadership to create positive changes in health policy and delivery systems. Individuals choose nursing as a career and remain in the profession because of the opportunity for personal and professional growth, supportive work environments and compensation with roles and responsibilities. (p. 7)

The 10 domains that emerged from this summit were derived from the research literature and the Institute of Medicine's study *Crossing the Quality Chasm: A New Health System for the 21st Century*, published in 2001. The domains are as follows (Institute of Medicine, 2001, p. 7):

1. Leadership and planning
2. Delivery systems
3. Legislative/regulatory/policy
4. Professional/nursing culture
5. Recruitment/retention
6. Economic value
7. Work environment
8. Public relations/communication
9. Education
10. Diversity

In addition to the vision and domains, a short-term plan was developed that outlined the desired future state, strategies for achieving the desired state, objectives to support the primary strategy, and the co-champions for each. The project was extremely comprehensive given that the nursing shortage and its impact on health care are not linear. On the contrary, the problem is extremely complex. The group recognized that in order to actualize the *Nursing's Agenda for the Future: A Call to the Nation* by 2010, extensive partnerships would be required to bring about strategic change, and change would have to occur, for example, in health care leadership, health care organizations, academic programs, health care policy, governmental agencies, health care and professional regulatory agencies, governmental and private funding, professional practice groups, and consumer groups.

The ANA (2002) as part of the *Nursing's Agenda for the Future: A Call to the Nation* developed a "Desired Future Statement (Vision)" for each of the 10 domains. The statement for the domain of "Recruitment and Retention" clearly delineated the comprehensiveness of the undertaking, as follows (ANA, 2002):

> Nursing is comprised of a diverse body of individuals committed to promoting and sustaining the profession through addressing diversity, image, education, funding, practice models and environments, and professional development. (p. 17)

The vision was derived from the nursing research literature and incorporated the recurring themes related to recruitment and retention. Five strategies were formulated to achieve this vision. The strategies also addressed the two-pronged recruitment issue of the shortage (supply-side economics) and recruitment of (1) students for nursing education programs and (2) qualified nurses for health care agencies. The strategies also targeted retention issues to be addressed within health care agencies and academic programs focusing on the development of career-based opportunities within health care, development and funding of creative educational initiatives, creation of a desirable and appealing image for nursing as a career choice, formulation and implementation of professional practice models, work environments that ensure career satisfaction, and development of comprehensive recruitment and retention strategies that will appeal to a diverse customer group/population (ANA, 2002). These global strategies were then broken down for the primary strategy in each of the domains, with work on the remaining strategies to be developed. The ANA also identified strategies that could be used to enhance student and faculty recruitment and/or retention (Table 27.1).

Table 27.1

Student-Related and Faculty-Related Strategies for Recruitment and Retention

Recruitment and Retention Strategies	Students	Faculty
Develop professional mentoring models	X	
Create a specific curriculum to address diversity	X	X
Obtain funding to support minority enrollment	X	
Develop and distribute promotional and recruitment materials to attract individuals from diverse backgrounds into nursing	X	
Recruit retired nurses to form professional mentoring corps		X
Provide joint educational and service standardized internships and residencies	X	X
Co-op program/student clinical assistant (SCA) program	X	
Negotiate professional paid development opportunities with employers		X
Create a website for leadership development that can be used by education, service, and professional organization members	X	X

The multifaceted approach undertaken by the organizations that participated in the Nursing Professional Summit called by the ANA in 2001 addressed issues that were consistent with the findings identified by Goodin (2003). Goodin's findings were based on a comprehensive, integrative review of the nursing shortage literature in the United States from 1999 to 2001. The findings of this analysis revealed that the major contributors to the nursing shortage and factors affecting recruitment and retention were directed at four major themes. The themes and examples of the related intervention approaches are listed in Box 27.2.

To meet the demand for nurses now and in the future, actions need to be taken that are directed at what drives young people and career switchers to choose nursing as a career. Erickson and colleagues (2004) reported on an initiative undertaken by Partners Healthcare in Boston. The goal was to gain insights into the dynamics of career selection by young people and career switchers. To determine this information, a consulting firm was hired to conduct focus groups and telephone interviews. Specific questions used in this qualitative approach focused on the following: How were decisions made relative to choosing a career? How did significant

Box 27.2

Themes and Related Intervention Strategies

Aging Workforce

- Strive to minimize work demands on older nurses
- Find ways to increase reimbursement or salary equity for experienced nurses
- Develop care management approaches that increase health and decrease physical injury of nurses
- Find ways to increase use of nurse expertise as workload burdens increase
- Develop strategies for retaining older nurses

Declining Enrollment

- Target younger students in elementary and junior high school
- Target nontraditional students (e.g., males, minorities)
- Continue to develop diverse tracks for varied entry levels into nursing
- Continue to develop methods for bringing nonpracticing nurses back into the workforce and foreign nurses into the workforce
- Work to ensure that there are adequate faculty to teach students
- Provide career opportunities and lifelong learning opportunities for nurses

Changing Work Climate

- Work to ensure that nurses have the opportunity to practice care delivery versus managing the system
- Provide opportunity for ongoing education that will allow nurses to move within specialty areas of care
- Organizationally support ongoing education
- Develop new approaches for relieving nurses in times of high patient care demands
- Increase flexibility
- Promote assignments/workload that is reasonable and achievable
- Avoid use of mandatory overtime
- Develop strategies for accommodating lifestyle needs of new graduates

Continued

Box 27.2

Themes and Related Intervention Strategies—cont'd

Poor Image of Nursing

- Work to change the image of nursing among young potential nurses through Career Days for middle school students and Shadow Days for junior and senior high school students
- Develop web-based career information
- Involve practicing nurses in recruitment initiatives and school activities
- Provide community programs and individual activities that address the rewarding challenges of nursing
- Continue to work with the TriCouncil and external organizations such as Johnson & Johnson to develop targeted campaigns
- Reform educational and credentialing mechanisms to empower nurses in the workplace
- Lobby Congress to pass legislation that promotes nursing as a career and provides funding of students—scholarship, loan forgiveness, retention grants, elder care

influences in one's life affect career choice? What was the individual's perception and image of nursing? As a result of this study, vital information was identified reflecting differences in the two groups. Outcomes of the study included two major marketing strategies that would promote the image of nursing as a career choice: "Be Somebody" and "Valuable Partner." In addition, the following nine strategies for promoting nursing as a career were identified (Erickson et al., 2004, p. 86):

1. Classroom ambassadors program
2. Job-shadowing experiences
3. Bring-your-child-to-work day
4. Volunteer health care settings opportunities for students and adults
5. Part-time employment opportunities for students and adults need to be developed
6. Presentation to clubs/organizations regarding nursing
7. Participation at community health fairs
8. Advertising campaigns directed at job satisfaction, making a difference in people's lives, flexible scheduling, and competitive salary and benefits
9. Advertising that directs people to dynamic, comprehensive web sites that offer positive, motivating information about nursing and its reward

RECRUITMENT

As identified by the studies and actions just mentioned, recruitment has taken on a completely new perspective. It has always been about the replacement of non-retained staff and the hiring of staff to fill newly created and/or expanded positions. With the changes that have occurred in health care over the past two decades, the concept of recruitment has begun to focus more and more on the identification and development of pre-employment hires. This means marketing the agency to potential pre-nursing students and active nursing students. Recruitment, therefore, has become more complex and more linked to partnerships than ever before. These partnerships are not only with schools of nursing but also with elementary and secondary schools and other community agencies. Co-op programs and/or student clinical assistant (SCA) programs (Henriksen et al., 2003) and other related preceptor programs create a model for attracting and retaining new graduates. These and other student-related activities blend the student-employee role, thus changing recruitment to a retention strategy once the student gets linked in a nursing capacity to the health care facility. These linkages in the form of precepting and mentoring activities have also been shown to have a positive impact on job satisfaction among experienced RNs (McClure et al., 1983).

Following work with the AONE and American Association of Colleges of Nursing, Johnson & Johnson (J&J) (2008) launched a multi-year nursing initiative, *The Campaign for Nursing's Future,* in February 2002. This campaign grew out of J&J's concern over the nursing shortage—current and future. According to J&J, the "public awareness campaign is designed to enhance the image of the nursing profession, recruit new nurses and nurse faculty, and help retain nurses currently in the profession" (p. 1). The campaign was international in nature and covered a broad spectrum of activities that were directed at enhancing the image of nursing as a profession (e.g., fundraising for scholarships [student and faculty]; research, awards, and support to nursing schools program expansion; national television, print, and interactive advertising; development and maintenance of a website; and production and distribution of recruitment and retention materials). These activities clearly put nursing forward in the public arenas and raised the status of nursing as a profession. According to Donelan and colleagues (2005), this campaign has had a positive effect on nursing recruitment and enrollment in schools of nursing. The campaign was a major private corporate sector initiative and has provided valuable insights into ways to examine challenges confronting the nursing workforce.

Clearly, recruitment needs both long-term and short-term strategies. Although the long-term plan is extremely important, most of the organization's resources tend to go to short-term initiatives—filling vacant and/or newly created positions. The recruitment focus of this chapter is directed at short-term strategies.

Recruitment of Professional Nurses

In 1983, a study was conducted (1) to identify variables in hospital organizations and their nursing services that create a magnetism that attracts and retains professional nurse staff and (2) to identify particular combinations of variables that produce nursing practice models within hospitals in which nurses receive professional and personal satisfaction to the degree that recruitment and retention of qualified staff are achieved (McClure et al., 1983). The study included 41 of 165 hospitals from 10 geographic regions (designated by the Bureau of Labor Statistics). The hospitals were nominated by Fellows in the American Academy of Nursing (AAN). Each AAN Fellow was asked to nominate 6 to 10 hospitals of varying sizes in their region of the country that demonstrated success in recruiting and retaining staff. The final selection of the institutions for inclusion in the study was done after a review and ranking of the top 10 choices in each region based on established criteria and recruitment and retention data provided by each institution. Originally, 46 hospitals were chosen, but 5 were unable to participate. The results of the study clearly showed that the three major variables of administration, professional practice, and professional development, with related attributes, positively affect hospitals' ability to recruit and retain registered nurse staff. These variables and related attributes are listed in Box 27.3.

This study was one of the first to describe organizational and leadership factors that are important to the recruitment and retention of nurses in the workplace. As noted by the variables just mentioned, the nurses specifically wanted a leadership and organizational structure that supported participatory involvement, as well as flexibility for work scheduling and personal/professional development. In addition, nurses wanted to work in an institution that had a clearly defined professional practice model that used the skills and knowledge of the professional nurse. Nurses were also interested in working in an organization that allowed them to be "able to practice nursing." Managerial visibility and support were viewed as strengths in promoting autonomy. Nurses also wanted to have control over their practice (autonomy) and collaborative relationships with physicians relative to care management. This study and the follow-up study conducted by Kramer and Hafner (1989) 5 years later were the basis for the ANA's Magnet Recognition Program®.

The America Nurses Credentialing Center (ANCC) implemented the Magnet Recognition Program® in the 1990s, with the first award going to the University of Washington Medical Center

Box 27.3

Organizational and Nursing Service Variables of Magnetism That Attract and Retain Professional Nurses

Administration	Professional Practice	Professional Development
Management style	Quality of patient care	Orientation
Quality of leadership	Professional practice models	In-service/continuing education
Nursing managers	Autonomy	Formal education
Nursing directors	Consultation and resources	Career development
Organizational structure	Teaching	
Decentralization	Image of nursing	
Committees		
Staffing		
Personnel policies		
Work schedules		
Promotion opportunities		

in 1994. According to the ANCC (February 27, 2008), Magnet™ recognition has since been awarded to 286 health care organizations in 45 states, as well as one in Australia and one in New Zealand, for their excellence in nursing service. This clearly indicates the importance placed on this program nationally relative to recruitment and retention by hospitals and other health care organizations.

Recruitment initiatives in the past several years have used strategies targeted at nurse satisfiers as reported in the nursing and health care literature. Satisfiers have included strategies such as professional practice model usage, preceptor/mentorship opportunities, increased flexibility in work scheduling, low patient-to-RN ratios, a collaborative practice environment, Magnet™ recognition status, environment of respect and value, and a competitive compensation model. Strategies commonly used that are related to nurse recruitment of new and experienced nurses are identified in Box 27.4.

Human Resources, Managerial, and Staff Roles Associated with Recruitment

In the context of a nurse shortage, recruitment is a major human resources (HR) strategy. Because the organization needs to find and hire the best qualified nurses who also "fit" with the culture and are willing to work for a specific salary and work conditions, both recruitment and retention are important. Both managers and staff contribute to successful recruitment and retention. A complex and detailed process is followed for effective recruitment and retention. The nine major processes or phases of recruitment are as follows:

1. Position posting
2. Advertising
3. Screening
4. Interviewing
5. Selecting
6. Orienting
7. Counseling/coaching
8. Performance evaluation
9. Staff development

Position Posting

Position posting for recruitment begins after determination of vacancies based on position controls developed for each of the clinical/service areas. The vacancies are identified based on the full-time equivalent (FTE) status for each of the positions. Once the positions have been identified and the shift/holiday schedules are determined, the first step is to post them internally for staff

Box 27.4

Recruitment Strategies

- Flexible hours
- Competitive salaries
- Bonus pay
- Relocation pay
- Fixed shifts
- Weekend option program
- Part-time pay with bonus hours
- Flexible benefits packages
- Scholarships for BSN or graduate studies
- Tuition benefit plan
- Educational loan repayment
- Residency programs and RN specialty internships
- Onboarding
- Refresher courses—return to work
- Professional development opportunities
- Career opportunities
- Specialty certification reimbursement
- Low nurse-to-patient ratios; higher numbers of RNs for the patient load (workload staffing)
- Shared governance/leadership models
- Care delivery model that promotes professional care at the bedside
- Clinical ladder/career ladder
- Free parking
- Magnet™ recognition
- Culture of safety: zero tolerance for incivility
- Research/evidence-based practice
- NCLEX review course
- Qualified managerial support
- Clinical support: staff educators, clinical nurse specialists
- Workforce diversity
- Interdisciplinary collaboration opportunities

review and selection. The length of this posting time is determined by each organization and/or respective collective bargaining contracts. Positions not filled within a defined period are then posted externally to the organization. Based on the need and/or limited number of nurses in a given specialty, recruitment agencies may be contacted at this time to conduct a regional, statewide, or national search for the position.

Advertising

Advertising includes the development of an institutional advertisement outlining the positions or job opportunities within an organization. The advertisement addresses the area of need and specific information that would be likely to attract an employee (RN) to the position. The HR department determines distribution sites, with input from the specific departments. Sites may include professional journals or newspapers, local or regional newspapers, radio, or the organization's website. An advantage of online advertisement is that the application process can be made available at the same time, making it a one-stop process for the person seeking employment.

If the recruiter is planning to attend special events, information about the position will be taken for posting along with the application forms. In addition, information about the organization and related benefits and specialty strengths will be highlighted. A shortcoming that needs to be addressed related to advertising is that organizations often spend an enormous amount of money on advertising only to miss the most important aspect, that of a quick, effective, courteous follow-up with potential candidates (Curran, 2003). All of the positive results that the expensive advertising and recruiting efforts have produced with regard to candidates for a position can be lost depending on how the institution follows up with candidates. For example, if potential candidates for a position have been encouraged to apply through advertising and recruitment efforts and then log on to an institution's website and find that they cannot complete an application for the job, in frustration they may decide not to pursue the job (Curran, 2003). In addition, if candidates cannot obtain a response about the status of their application after submitting it, they may decide that they do not want to work for this type of institution. If recruitment and advertising efforts are to be productive, these kinds of flaws in the system must be avoided.

Screening

Screening is the process in which the application is reviewed before determining whether the nurse meets the pre-established criteria for the position. During this activity, the reviewer selects who should be interviewed. It is important to remember that if an organization is classified as an *equal opportunity employer,* the reviewers are required to follow the guidelines established by the federal government.

Interviewing

Interviewing is the time for clarification of information presented in the application and dossier submitted by the applicant. The job description is the basis for a hiring interview. The interview can be conducted in person or over the telephone, in a group/committee or one-on-one meeting. For best results, predefined questions should be used to interview all candidates for the position. Also, questions should be directed at the work expectations outlined in the position description and/or practices. Open-ended questions and follow-ups are recommended. For example, the following questions or discussion points can be posed:

- *Tell me about your current position.*
- *What do you like least about it?*
- *What do you like best about it?*

To get more in-depth responses and to determine behavior-specific examples, questions can be framed as follows:

- *Think of a time in your experience when X was needed, and describe how you did X.*
- *How did you handle X?*

It is appropriate to ask the candidate about aspects of his or her practices related to the job, such as the following:

- *Given the varied work hour requirements, how would you handle this?*
- *What problems do you see the work hour requirements presenting?*
- *Based on the work requirements relative to lifting, how would you go about transferring a patient whose body weight is more than 350 pounds?*

The information obtained through this process will help the committee or manager assigned to the recruitment process determine the applicant's "fit" with the unit and/or organizational culture, as well as consistent data for comparison of candidates. Use of formalized questions is often referred to as a *structured interview* or *targeted selection process* (DDI, 1997, 2004; Lipsey, 2004). The targeted selection process is built on analysis of work per job, organizational values, clear identification of competencies for key positions, and development of interview skills and confidence of the interviewers. Using the targeted interview ensures that all candidates are interviewed based on the same criteria. In addition, during the targeted interview process, the interviewer asks questions that are directed at having the candidates describe typical situations that they have encountered in previous jobs. Use of the targeted interview method allows the interviewers to gain data from the candidates to more fully evaluate their values and practice patterns. It further allows for objective comparison of candidates based on their responses, and it decreases personal biases and assumptions. Questions that should be avoided during the interview relate specifically to personal information about the candidate, such as the following: age, marital status, living arrangements, children, limitations or disabilities, religion, substance abuse, and membership in professional organizations.

Selecting

Selecting is the determination of who will be offered an opportunity for employment (termination of the recruitment process). A committee or manager may complete the selection process. For best results, data used in the screening and interviewing phases should be used when comparing candidate responses and other related data. The selection process also involves the formal activity of making an offer to the candidate. Who does this activity varies according to institutional policy, but it usually involves either the manager or HR personnel. At the time the job offer is made, the employee is informed of the position/job being offered, the FTE allocation (full-time [FT] or part-time [PT]) for the position, and the salary offer and benefits. Regardless of who makes the final offer, HR plays a role in determining the salary range.

Selection of an employee who is a match with the core values of an organization has been shown to have important implications. It facilitates ease of employee transition into the new role and fit with staff within the unit and organization. Employee fit and related retention have also been shown to have an impact on cost savings within the organization. According to Lipsey (2004), return on investment of hiring the right versus the wrong person (poor performer) is more significant than just the costs of simple replacement of an employee. The costs of hiring the wrong person are associated with not only the recruitment, replacement, and hiring expenses but also the secondary costs. Secondary costs of hiring a poor performer include increased dollars wasted on training and development, decreased productivity and increased errors, lost opportunities to improve processes and/or outcomes, decreased or poor staff morale that results from staff struggling to pick up slack of the poor performer, and dissatisfied customers. The secondary costs have a significant impact on the organization and workers and are often much greater than those associated with the initial recruitment process.

Orienting

Orienting is an important activity for bringing new employees into the organization, department, and unit. It is the employee's introduction to the culture and values of the organization and discipline. Changes in orientation format and content have occurred as a result of study outcomes that have shown the relationship between job satisfaction and staff retention. The newest approach to orienting is referred to as "onboarding" (HR Solutions, 2007; Lee, 2008; Platz, 2008). The approach is directed at fully engaging and integrating the employee into the organization by focusing on how to assist him or her in successfully preparing for the job. Onboarding expands the orientation beyond the employee's initial introduction to the organization and role expectations by providing ongoing coaching and mentorship through a defined program (Lee, 2008; Northwestern University, 2008). These programs usually last from 3 months to 1 year. This approach is consistent with expectations expressed by the new nurse graduate (Casey et al., 2004; Halfer, & Graf, 2006; Manion & Bartholomew, 2004; Orsini, 2005), especially those in the Generation Y group (Hart, 2006). Onboarding is also consistent with a Magnet™ culture (Upenieks, 2003). Onboarding has also brought about a change in learning in that, whereas once it was a fairly passive didactic experience, it has moved to an interactive process built around self-learning and renewal.

Many hospitals have adopted residency and/or internship programs with RN preceptors working one-on-one with the new graduate. According to Casey and colleagues (2004), residency/internship programs have an important role in transitioning graduate nurses into the RN role. The success of these programs has been closely tied to the new graduates' "intent-to-stay" and retention.

Counseling and Coaching

Counseling and coaching are strategies used to promote a sense of community for new and ongoing employees. These strategies create a professional and social network for new employees, an attribute identified in Magnet™-recognized institutions. Use of these strategies also creates a sense of a non-punitive culture in which staff can learn and grow. Graduate nurses have indicated the need for positive support and timely verbal feedback from preceptors to gain the confidence and competence needed during their transition into the RN role (Casey et al., 2004). According to Manion and Bartholomew (2004), healthy working relationships and group cohesion enhance retention for both new and experienced employees. For this to happen, the leaders at all levels need to work with employees to ensure group cohesiveness in a family-like environment.

Performance Evaluation

Performance evaluation is a mechanism for giving feedback to employees—new and experienced. In addition to new employees receiving ongoing

Practical Tips

Tip # 1: Use the Evidence Base

There is a long history of nursing research about recruitment and retention. Translate this knowledge into a persuasive argument (with rationale) for organizational resources that are sufficient and targeted toward a steady, stable program that builds a stable workforce for your workplace. List three ongoing initiatives (e.g., new hire onboarding) that will receive sustained and intensive program support going forward.

Tip # 2: Do Career Planning

Use self-awareness and reflection to identify your own personal recruitment and retention needs. Use this going forward to integrate into your career planning. This could perhaps be based on a standardized tool such as the Meaningful Retention Strategy Inventory (MRSI).

Tip # 3: Recruit Based on "Fit"

Hiring new RN employees is a major opportunity for any work group. The concept of "fit" is very important. Work to form and be a cohesive work group that emphasizes the crucial aspect of hiring in knowledge workers who complement the group's work styles and culture. This can greatly affect staff satisfaction and investment in the work group's productivity.

evaluation during their onboarding by an assigned preceptor/coach, they are expected to receive an initial performance evaluation within the first 60 to 120 days, depending on the policies of the organization. This feedback is directed at the individual employees' progress relative to their onboarding program (formative evaluation). During this evaluation, the employee and managerial staff also should take the time to evaluate the employee's "fit" with the organizational and departmental culture (summative evaluation). Strategies to address further needs and/or employment status should be decided at this time. A full performance evaluation then occurs at the end of the orientation period and annually thereafter. Feedback regarding ongoing performance needs to be provided to employees on a regular basis. Performance evaluation needs to focus on the employee's achievement toward defined goals, with feedback directed at the individual's contribution to the development of peers and clinical and/or leadership practices. The meeting can be conducted using a formal or informal process, one-on-one or in a group.

Staff Development

Staff development has been identified in the literature as an important factor in job satisfaction. It provides employees with an opportunity to improve their practice, level of competency, or other areas of self-interest. Programs for staff development are usually determined based on staff surveys conducted annually. Programs developed are usually posted for staff selection, and the institution provides scheduling flexibility and funding for employees to participate.

Staff development, as defined in the Magnet™ study (Kramer & Hafner, 1989; McClure et al., 1983), identified four areas of professional development beyond orientation. The four areas included in-service education, continuing education, formal education, and career development. Professional development was valued for its economic potential. However, other attributes identified were personal and professional growth opportunities, career advancement opportunities, and preceptor skill development. Nurses also reported that the variety of programs available provided increased flexibility, as did the instructional methods used. Nurses in these institutions viewed education as being valued. Administrative support was provided and available, as were clinical and managerial resources. Professional development opportunities overall were shown to have a positive influence on nurse satisfaction.

RETENTION: NEW GRADUATES AND QUALIFIED EXPERIENCED REGISTERED NURSES

Renewed attention has been directed at retention of nurses over the past 10 to 15 years (Upenieks, 2003). The turnover rate of a new graduate ranges from 21% to 60% in the first year (Halfer & Graf, 2006; Shermont & Krepcio, 2006), the average age of the nurse is 45 years, and nurses begin to phase into retirement beginning at age 55 years (Mion et al., 2006). In light of these facts, it is little wonder that nursing has begun to focus attention on expanding retention programs beyond the promotion of job satisfaction, safety, respect, and financial security (401 [k] plans, gain sharing, IRAs) (Kramer & Hafner, 1989; McClure et al., 1983) to the development of infrastructure services that meet the diverse needs of current employees. The primary focus of these changes is to promote nurse autonomy and the nurse role on the interdisciplinary team while providing services that will enhance the work and life of the nurse both inside and outside of the organization. Today more than ever it is imperative that nurses and other health care workers experience a sense of community in the workplace (Manion & Bartholomew, 2004). After all, many spend more time at work than at any other single place.

In 2001, the Nursing Executive Center identified three categories and nine subcategories of reasons that nurses had given for remaining at a Destination Hospital. These categories and their related subcategories are listed below in the order of greatest importance (Nursing Executive Center, 2001, p. 23):

1. High-Quality Care
   1.1 Hospital's commitment to providing high-quality patient care
   1.2 Hospital's reputation as outstanding setting for clinical care
2. Strong Nurse Leadership
   2.1 Quality of direct manager
   2.2 Quality of overall nursing leadership
3. Meeting the Baseline
   3.1 Salary
   3.2 Scheduling options
   3.3 Benefits package
   3.4 Hospital's reputation for assigning nurses lower numbers of patients
   3.5 Location/convenience (p. 23)

Although the categories and subcategories are still relevant today, the strategies for meeting each of these have expanded. Diversity within the nurse pool has varying needs, and it is important that these needs be addressed in creative and innovative ways if nurses are to be retained in the health care industry.

One of the primary issues of diversity that affects both recruitment and retention is the generational differences among workers. Age-related cohorts appear to hold divergent perceptions, needs, and attitudes toward work that may be challenging to fulfill or manage. Both retention and recruitment can be affected if clashes or conflict ensues.

Generational workforce diversity refers to the differences in employees' perspectives of the job security, work behaviors and related skills, work expectations associated with the job, and value placed on employer versus personal/family needs, as associated with the generation/period of the employees' birth. Generational workforce group and related periods usually include the following categories:

- Mature/Silent Generation: born between 1909 and 1945
- Baby Boomers: born between 1946 and 1964
- Generation X: born between 1965 and 1981
- Generation Y/Next Generation/Millennium Generation: born between 1982 and present

With four generational groups now in the workplace, it is important that managers and staff consider differences when developing strategies for change or rewards. Each generation has its own perspective, and diversity exists even among each generation. It is imperative, therefore, that generational groups have representation or opportunity for input in planning and decision making. In addition, it is important to develop a variety of alternatives from which employees can select rather than targeting a single approach. Strategies commonly used for nurse retention of new and experienced nurses are identified in Box 27.5.

Box 27.5

Retention Strategies Used to Retain New Graduates and Experienced Nurses

- Onboarding
- Mentoring/precepting program opportunities
- Professional development opportunities
- Financial support associated with credentialing
- Realignment of salary structure/compression management
- Part-time pay with bonus hours
- Flexible hours/schedules
- Bonus pay
- Bonus pay for recruitment of employees
- Profit/gains sharing program
- Scholarships for BSN or graduate studies
- Free parking
- Fixed shifts
- Shift bidding
- Creation of autonomous self-managed units
- Initializing of new technology into practice
- Shared governance/leadership models
- Career advancement program
- Clinical ladder/career ladder
- Support services—discussion groups and social networking activities
- Volunteer roles—inside and outside the organization
- Specialty equipment for use in care delivery
- Technology to support the work
- Streamlined processes
- Culture of safety
- Physician-nurse collaborative partnership
- Carved out roles for specialty functions
- Creation of a community culture
- Magnet™ recognition
- Concierge services
- Child/elder care
- Provision for sabbatical
- Phased retirement

As noted earlier in the chapter, significant efforts have been directed at the recruitment and retention of new graduates. However, in the past few years, equal effort has been directed at the retention of experienced older nurses because of their depth of knowledge relative to the organization and their clinical expertise. Retention factors related to the older nurse have been shown to vary significantly from that of the new graduate, as older nurses find it harder to manage the physical demands of hospital work and are focusing on establishing financial security for retirement. To meet the needs of the older nurse, organizations have had to rethink the rules and roles that have been in place. According to Mion and colleagues (2006), a number of changes to be made in the area of retention are (Hare, 2007; Mion et al., 2006):

- Scheduling—decreasing frequency of rotations, reducing length of shifts, using sabbaticals
- Assignment requirements—geographic location, assignment consistency, work with preceptor
- Practice models—using specialty roles (e.g., wound nurse, audit nurse, admission and/or discharge nurse, telephone triage)
- Technology usage—lifting equipment, ergonomic computers and electrical devices, soften hard floor surfaces, cell phones, tracking systems, improved lighting
- Streamline processes—revised documentation systems, bed utilization programs, online continuing education, computer training, and multi-site computer access
- Communication and recognition opportunities—membership on unit-based and organizational committees, participation in shared governance activities, volunteer roles as institutional representatives, ambassador programs

These and other changes are important if experienced nurses are to be retained at the bedside (Ward-Smith et al., 2007).

Probably the single most important factor in retention of nurses, however, is managerial leadership (Acree, 2006; Anthony et al., 2005; Cunningham, 2005; Force, 2005; Kleinman, 2004).

Leadership has been defined in a number of ways, but the outcome is consistent—it is working through others to achieve intended goals. The two leadership styles that predominate in the literature today are *transformational* and *transactional.* Acree (2006) presented Bass's definition of transformational and transactional leadership and noted that transformational leadership consists of four major components: "idealized influence (charisma), inspiration (engagement and confidence building), intellectual stimulation (problem awareness/solving) and individualized consideration (supportive, encouraging, and provision of developmental experiences" (p. 35). "Transactional leadership has two major components: contingent reward (reward for an agreed-upon effort) and management by exception (leader intervention only if something goes wrong or standards are not met)" (p. 35). Managerial use of transformational leadership has been shown to have the greatest impact on nurse job satisfaction. This is no surprise given the need for ongoing support, recognition, and life-balance expressed by both new graduates and experienced nurses. To provide this level of leadership, organizations will need to commit to ongoing development of nurse managers and promote the cultural changes needed by nurse managers to actualize this level of leadership.

Organizations that have been successful in their communication and work with managers and staff have been shown to have increased stability and retention in the workforce, higher job satisfaction, higher quality patient outcomes, and fewer nurse injuries (Aiken et al., 1997; Laschinger & Wong, 1999, Mion et al., 2006). Decreased cost has also been associated with effective recruitment strategies, consistent with the Magnet Recognition Program® (Upenieks, 2003).

TURNOVER: COST AND MANAGEMENT STRATEGIES

Turnover of qualified staff not only is disruptive to the care community in which the nurse works (Manion & Bartholomew, 2004) but also is extremely costly to the organization (Jones, 2004a, b). Kuhar and colleagues (2004) suggested that a single nurse replacement cost could be as low as $44,000, but its impact on customer satisfaction is not included in calculation cost. According to Atencio and colleagues (2003), the cost of replacement is approximately two times the nurse's annual salary. Thus the average replacement cost for a medical-surgical nurse is approximately $92,442 (based on a national average salary of $46,832), whereas replacement of a critical care nurse is almost $145,000. Expenditures include a variety of costs—advertising and marketing, human resource salary costs, travel expenses for nurses interviewing, temporary replacement costs for per diem nurses, overtime usage, terminal payout, orientation costs, as well as employee and managerial costs associated with the review, interview, and selection process. Based on the projected medical-surgical nurse replacement costs identified by Atencio and colleagues, the loss of 21.3% (which represents the national average) from a staff of 100 could cost an organization as much as $1,969,014. Jones (2004a, b) indicated that turnover costs are calculated based on three pre-hire categories—advertising/recruiting, vacancy, and hiring—and four post-hire categories—orientation/training, newly hired RN productivity, pre-turnover productivity, and termination. The greatest costs listed in order of priority were associated with vacancy, orientation/training and newly hired RN productivity, advertising and recruiting, as well as hiring. Termination and hiring had the least impact on cost, and the impact of pre-turnover productivity is not yet fully understood because it is difficult to capture. Jones (2004b) reported that the cost per RN turnover was $62,100–$67,100 for a total cost of RN turnover to the division of $5,964,200–$6,436,400. Based on these and other findings, it is clear that the human capital costs associated with turnover are a tremendous burden on the organization. Money spent for replacement could have been used by the organization to improve their competitive advantage, nurse satisfaction, and consumer perception of workforce quality and expansion of services.

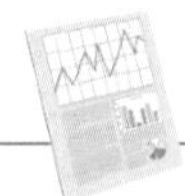

Research Note

Source: Kuhar, P.A., Miller, D., Spear, B.T., Ulreich, S.M., & Mion, L.C. (2004). The meaningful retention strategy inventory: A targeted approach to implementing retention strategies. *Journal of Nursing Administration, 34*(1), 10-18.

Purpose

The nursing shortage has driven administrators to begin to evaluate new and creative strategies for retaining qualified experienced nursing staff. With this need in mind, the authors sought to develop an inventory to be used with staff nurses and managers to identify issues that could be addressed. The purpose of this study was to determine retention strategies perceived as meaningful to nurses and to design and implement interventions directed at resolving issues that were of greatest importance.

Discussion

As part of this study, the authors developed a valid and reliable instrument, the Meaningful Retention Strategy Inventory (MRSI). This inventory was used to measure staff nurse and nurse manager perceptions of retention strategies and overall level of importance. Data were collected on nursing and managerial staff at eight of the Cleveland Clinic Health System hospitals. The results of the study indicated that staff nurses from three different age-groups were able to agree on 9 of the top 10 ranked retention strategies selected. One difference among the staff nurse groups was related to "pay increase" and "differential pay," with nurses younger than 36 years selecting pay increase and those older than 36 years and younger than 56 years selecting differential pay among their preferred choices. Another difference was associated with nurses older than 56 years, who included "respect from physicians," "respect from administration," and "educational opportunities" among their preferred choices. The results of the staff nurse and nurse manager groups also indicated consistency relative to 9 of the top 10 preferred choices. The only difference noted was that staff nurses included "shift of choice" as a preferred choice, whereas managers ranked this strategy as twenty-fifth.

Major concerns identified relative to job satisfaction and retention were in the areas of teamwork, compensation/benefits, staffing flexibility, and equipment. The retention items with the highest mean scores were categorized into three groups—people, process, and technology—for the purpose of strategy development. Activities related to each of these three categories were described, along with the impact observed and related outcomes. Each of the hospitals used institution-specific nurse/manager data to devise and implement retention strategies. Some examples of the retention strategies used per category were the following:

- *People:* flexible staffing options, development of a new compensation structure, and addition of new role to support the nurse at the bedside
- *Process:* redesigned transportation processes, changes in dietary services support, forms revision
- *Technology:* increase in use of wireless technology on pilot units, electronic medical record, new tracking systems in the emergency department (ED) and operating room (OR), ergonomic care devices

Implementation of these retention strategies was reported to have had a positive impact on nurse satisfaction and nurse retention, as well as achievement of the Magnet Recognition Program® award.

Application to Practice

Because nothing can be done to alter the aging of nurses, it is important to identify ways of positively affecting nurse retention. The availability of an instrument that is institutionally sensitive and can be used by nurse administration to objectively determine the retention strategies nurses prefer will greatly add to the development of a retention plan that is likely to bring about the positive results in a more cost-effective manner. Use of the MRSI and the structural design

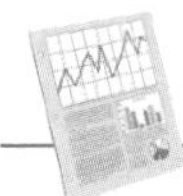

Research Note—cont'd

of this study provide an objective method for positively affecting retention within a given organization. In addition, the methods can be evaluated over time and/or replicated by other institutions to determine strategies that are most effective in influencing nurse satisfaction and retention. The inventory developed in this study also provided a valid and reliable measure for future research in nursing administration. The strategies designed and their effectiveness over time will provide useful data for future planning within nursing and health care agencies. Certainly, the use of this approach to planning is grounded in performance improvement.

The replacement cost of turnover can be determined using the formula for cost per RN hire (Figure 27.1) presented by Hoffman (1984). Other related costs associated with turnover and a nurse shortage are decreased patient outcomes. These include longer lengths of stay, increased risk for falls, medication errors, infections, gastrointestinal bleeding, and failure to rescue (Aiken et al., 2002; Needleman et al., 2002). Intrinsic costs associated with the remaining nurses include increased dissatisfaction and burnout when staffing ratios deteriorate for sustained periods (Aiken et al., 2002). Increased dissatisfaction in nurses has also been directly linked with nurses' intent to leave, which has been shown to be the greatest predictor of whether a nurse will leave the job (Atencio et al., 2003). Loss of experienced, qualified nurses has had a major impact on the care delivery within a unit of service and is a hard-to-quantify indirect cost. Changes in the community of care have negative implications and need to be avoided if possible. Factors shown to have a negative impact on retention include overload caused by increased patient assignments related to too few staff or too many patients, as well as exhaustion and nurses' associated fears of making mistakes under those conditions.

Analysis of turnover is an important continuous quality improvement process because it provides the data needed to identify and address trends and patterns related to staff retention. The human resources (HR) department usually provides turnover data because it is the repository for employee records. Turnover data are primarily reported quarterly, but that depends on organizational and/or managerial needs. Managerial staff can calculate their own unit-based turnover using the formula in Figure 27.2, presented by Hoffman (1984).

When calculating turnover data, the manager should confer with HR to verify employee numbers (resignations and terminations) that have occurred during the specified time frame. Failure to do so may result in discrepancies between HR and managerial data sets. These discrepancies may call the data into question and decrease their value at the organizational level. It should also be pointed out that transfer data are not included in turnover because the employee is not "lost" to the organization. Tracking and trending transfer data are important, however, because these steps may alert the manager to unit-based issues that need to be addressed. Tracking and trending these data can also alert the administrative team to managerial leadership issues that need to be evaluated.

$$\frac{\text{Total cost (e.g., recruitment, training, coverage)}}{\text{Total RNs hired}} = \text{Cost per RN hired}$$

Figure 27.1

Cost-per-RN hire. (Derived from Hoffman, P.M. [1984]. *Financial management for nurse managers.* Norwalk, CT: Appleton-Century-Crofts.)

$$\frac{\text{Number of terminations per year}}{\text{Average workforce per year}} \times 100 = \text{\% Turnover}$$

Figure 27.2

Turnover formula. (Derived from Hoffman, P.M. [1984]. *Financial management for nurse managers.* Norwalk, CT: Appleton-Century-Crofts.)

LEADERSHIP AND MANAGEMENT IMPLICATIONS

Whether more registered nurses are needed is an issue that needs to be further addressed. Using an economic model (supply and demand), history would suggest that with increased labor available in the workforce (supply), opportunities and pay would diminish (Prescott, 2000). If this happens, nurses will once again begin to withdraw from the marketplace, re-creating a nursing shortage. It is indisputable that a correlation exists between the number of registered nurses available on nursing units and quality patient outcomes. However, although nursing and health care organizations are moving forward to address the current shortage, efforts also need to be directed at the development of new practice models and changes in organizational systems, processes, and practices that enhance nurses' ability to successfully perform their work. Changes in health care and nurse reimbursement systems will also need to be addressed. According to Parsons and Stonestreet (2004), factors that have been closely linked with nurse retention "coalesce into two categories: the quality of administrative management systems and quality of relationships with physicians, managers, peers, and administrators" (p. 111). Bower and McCullough (2004) suggested that the development and use of technology would have to be expanded if nurses are to be deployed to their fullest potential.

According to the literature, to truly address and effectively manage the changes needed relative to this current nurse shortage, partnerships will have to be formed among health care organizations, educational programs, professional organizations, and collective bargaining groups (American Hospital Association [AHA], 2001; ANA, 2002; Nevidjon & Erickson, 2001; Prescott, 2000). To achieve the desired outcomes, extensive data analysis, strategy design, and policy changes will be required.

In addition, administration will need to evaluate its organizational structure and scope of assignment for managerial staff, because nurses repeatedly report that lack of managerial presence and support is a significant dissatisfier (Peterson, 2001). Managerial staff, specifically, need to be aware of the ongoing support and development requirements of new nurse graduates. Managers need to work with experienced staff to develop mentorship and/or preceptor models that promote the development of new graduates. Managers further need to work with support staff (staff

LEADERSHIP & MANAGEMENT IMPLICATIONS

Leadership Behaviors

- Motivates followers to lifelong learning
- Inspires staff education efforts
- Ensures access to education and training opportunities
- Enables higher-quality staff recruitment and selection
- Models lifelong learning and professional development
- Selects highly qualified candidates
- Mentors employees

Management Behaviors

- Plans for lifelong learning when formulating employee benefits
- Manages human resource processes
- Establishes a staff development department
- Monitors orientation, in-service, and continuing education
- Evaluates staff development needs
- Conducts educational and orientation sessions
- Coaches employees
- Determines employees' competence

Overlap Areas

- Provides leadership and management in human resource development
- Makes recruitment and selection decisions
- Establishes and manages a comprehensive human resource system

educators and clinical specialists) to develop unit-based registered nurse staff with skills and knowledge about how to manage workload and be accountable for outcomes while promoting growth of non-nurse caregivers and other support staff (Nevidjon & Erickson, 2001).

To meet the current and future demand for nurses and to create stability in the workplace, greater efforts will have to be directed at recruiting minorities, including males, into the profession. Nurse managers need to explore all opportunities to fill vacant positions. Special attention will need to be directed at retention of qualified, experienced staff. This can be accomplished in a number of ways. One approach that is strongly supported in the literature is to survey staff and to plan institutionally based recruitment and retention strategies jointly with staff (Kuhar et al., 2004).

Numerous strategies shown to be effective in both recruitment and retention have been outlined in the literature. It is therefore imperative that the nurse manager has a working knowledge of these strategies and uses them in the work setting. It is also important that the culture within an organization is one that supports and promotes professional nursing practice, nursing autonomy, quality patient care, and interdisciplinary collaboration as a means of achieving organizational outcomes. Another strategy is the recruitment of foreign nurses. Although recruitment of foreign nurses provides a nurse to fill a permanent position, care must be taken in this endeavor, since it is not without its drawbacks (Daniel et al., 2000). Recruiting a foreign nurse takes time (approximately 2 years), and it is an expensive process (Gamble, 2002). Several countries produce an abundance of nurses—for example, the Philippines. Although many of the Filipino nurses speak English, their understanding of the language and of U.S. culture is often limited (Daniel et al., 2000; Sparacio, 2005). Clearly, the addition of any new employee brings about a change in the culture or sense of community; adding a nurse from a different culture increases the stresses in the work environment while enhancing cultural diversity (Flynn & Aiken, 2002; ICN, 2001). Bringing a foreign nurse into an organization can be successful, but adequate planning and development of staff are required. According to Flynn and Aiken (2002), "increased recruitment of international nurses, without fundamental changes in the practice environment, will not help to solve the nursing shortage" (p. 68) or necessarily decrease nurse burnout.

Job dissatisfaction has been linked with nurse turnover or intent to leave (Aiken et al., 2001). Upenieks (2003) and Flynn and Aiken (2002) recommended that, in light of the nursing shortage, nurse administrators and managerial staff work to ensure that organizational attributes and professional nursing practice environments are as consistent as possible with practices identified by the Magnet™ studies and Magnet™ hospitals. According to the American Hospital Association (AHA) (2001), to maintain an adequate workforce, hospitals will have to actively address issues related to work design and the work environment.

Finally, nurse managers must work closely with their HR department to ensure effective and timely recruitment of nurses and to develop incentive programs that will assist in retaining and recruiting nursing staff. Managers can expect support from the HR department relative to turnover data, demographic information of nursing staff per unit/division, compensation information, job classification, work analysis, personnel management, and leadership and management education. Working with physician groups is another important partnership because nurses have consistently identified concerns over lack of perceived value by physicians as a major dissatisfier (Kuhar et al., 2004; Rosenstein, 2002). As McClure and colleagues (1983) reported in the Magnet™ study, nurses value a collaborative relationship with physicians and expect to be recognized and consulted by physicians for the contributions they bring to the management of patients.

CURRENT ISSUES AND TRENDS

The current nursing shortage is driven by a number of factors such as lack of an adequate supply of students, increased aging of the registered nurse workforce, increased demand for nurses within and outside of health care, and generational differences in nurses related to their intention to stay in nursing (AHA, 2001; Buerhaus et al., 2000). In addition to the shortage of nurses, health care is facing a reduction in all health care workers, both professional and non-professional (AHA, 2001). The overall shortages of health care workers are driving organizations to use higher-cost contractual labor. The costs associated with contractual labor, as well as changing reimbursement, increased higher consumer demand for and use of technology, increased numbers of chronically ill aging patients, and the high intensity of care services required, are significantly affecting the cost, quality, and demand for health care service. Nursing care has been strongly linked to both quality and cost; yet organizations are struggling to establish an environment and culture that promote job satisfaction and retention of nurses (Parsons & Stonestreet, 2004). Many of the recruitment practices within hospitals have proven to be counterproductive to nurse satisfaction, such as sign-on bonuses (Gamble, 2002); therefore greater attention will need to be given to nurse preferences if organizations plan to stabilize the workforce in the future. As noted earlier, onboarding of new graduates and experienced staff is a major factor in enhancing staff satisfaction and intent to stay (Mion et al., 2006; Shermont & Krepcio, 2006). In addition, strategies that improve the work life of older experienced nurses will facilitate them staying in the workforce longer (Mion et al., 2006; Ward-Smith et al., 2007).

As identified in the literature, nurse managers play a key role in both retention and recruitment of staff. The nurse manager's leadership style plays a major role in setting the tone for the unit and/or establishing a culture of retention. Manion (2004) defined a culture of retention as "an environment where people want to stay…or that meets peoples' needs" (p. 30). Manion, based on her research with nurse managers, described five themes and associated activities relative to the manager's role that contribute to the establishment of a culture of retention. These themes and related activities are as follows (Manion, 2004, pp. 30-39):

1. Put the staff first
   - 1.1 Listen and respond
   - 1.2 Appreciate and recognize
   - 1.3 Support
2. Forge authentic connections
   - 2.1 Get to know them
   - 2.2 Create a sense of community
   - 2.3 Hire the right people
   - 2.4 Have fun together
3. Coach for—and expect—competence
   - 3.1 Set high standards
   - 3.2 Support development
   - 3.3 Model behavior
   - 3.4 Manage performance
4. Focus on results
   - 4.1 Solve problems
   - 4.2 Empower and involve staff
   - 4.3 Provide adequate resources and a pleasing physical environment
5. Partner with staff
   - 5.1 Visibility
   - 5.2 Accessibility
   - 5.3 Set clear boundaries
   - 5.4 Communicate openly

These themes were also supported in research related to retention conducted by Parsons and Stonestreet (2004) with staff nurses. It is clear from the literature that considerable work needs to be done within nursing services and health care administration to establish a community/culture of caring and safety/security for nurses and other health care providers. People, for the most part, want to be able to go to work each day with a sense of pride and respect for their contributions. In return, they expect to be treated with respect and have a sense of security within the job and work environment. It is projected that this area of study and the application of related strategies will be a major thrust in the future. This approach is consistent with the Magnet Recognition Program® by the ANA (2003), the AHA report *In Our Hands* (2002), and the IOM report *Crossing the Quality Chasm* (2001).

Last, the literature clearly indicates that market and political forces have begun to create pressure in an attempt to help mitigate the nursing shortage and its impact on health care (HRSA, 2004; Runy, 2008). These actions have been directed at both the supply end through funding availability for students who choose nursing as a career, nursing program expansion, and faculty funding. In addition, more efforts are being directed at the retention of experienced bedside nurses and managerial staff.

Summary

- Nursing retention issues are strongly associated with job satisfaction and an aging workforce.
- The nursing shortage has long-term implications for quality patient care and hospitals' and health care systems' ability to provide services.
- To meet future nursing demands, changes will have to occur at the supply side, as well as policy formulation at the state, national, and international levels.
- Recruitment processes are clearly defined and amenable for use by both management and staff.
- Nurse recruitment is driven predominately by staff turnover rates.
- Nurse retention strategies based on the Magnet™ studies have proven to be successful.
- Retention rates to be effective must be multifaceted.
- Use of sign-on bonuses for the new employee as incentives for recruitment has resulted in an unstable and often non-retainable staff.
- Foreign nurse recruitment is a way of stabilizing staff turnover, but it is not without its own set of problems.
- The Philippines is one country that actively promotes, for its own economic benefit, nurses as expatriates.
- Staff turnover and related costs can be calculated by the nurse manager or reported by the HR department as a way of tracking and trending issues at the unit level.
- Nurse managers need to work closely with the HR department to ensure an adequate flow of candidates for selection and hire.
- Instruments and methods for measuring staff concerns or perceptions relative to job satisfaction and/or intent to leave are available for use by the nurse manager.
- Partnerships among health care organizations, schools of nursing, and industry/private business sector that have focused on changing the image of nursing as a career are having a positive impact on students and career switchers.
- Nurse managers and physician relationships play major roles in retention of nurses.
- Culture of retention and community in the workplace has been repeatedly reported by nurses to be of value relative to intent to leave and staff retention.
- The national multimillion-dollar marketing campaign undertaken by Johnson & Johnson addressing the caring attributes, knowledge-based practice of nurses, and nurse workforce needs within health care has clearly had a positive impact not only on recruitment of persons into nursing but also on nurses' pride.
- Nurse turnover is costly and must be managed in order to have the funding needed to maintain a competitive advantage for salaries and benefits, work-life balance, staff satisfaction, and overall nurse productivity.

CASE STUDY

Todd Samuelson, the nurse director (ND) for the intensive care unit, is reviewing the annual (FY2006) vacancy and turnover data for the four units that he manages: (1) cardiac care (CCU), (2) cardiac stepdown (CSU), (3) medicine intensive care (MICU), and (4) medical stepdown (MSU). The data reveal a vacancy rate of 30% and a turnover rate of 46% in the past two quarters for the MICU and MSU, respectively. The vacancy and turnover rates for the CCU and CSU are 8% and 10%, respectively, in both of these units. Further review of the data from the previous fiscal year (FY2005) indicated that both the MICU and MSU have been increasing volume 4% to 6% incrementally for the past 18 months. In addition, the personnel costs have increased exponentially over the past 12 months and medication error rates and staff injury are at an all-time high for the two units. Physician complaints have also increased. Before meeting with Alicia Stone, the nurse manager (NM) responsible for two of the units, Nurse Samuelson arranged a meeting with Jody George, the nurse recruiter (NR) in the human resources department.

At the meeting with Ms. George, Nurse Samuelson carefully reviewed the number and types of full-time (FT) and part-time (PT) RN positions open in the MICU and MSU, as well as the turnover data for each job classification. The information obtained showed that 7.6 positions, 4 FT and 8 PT, are open in the MICU; and 3.8 positions, 3 FT and 3 PT, are open in the MSU. During the discussion, Nurse Samuelson paid careful attention to the role of both Ms. George and Nurse Stone in the recruitment and retention processes. Ms. George reported that 35 RN applications were forwarded to Nurse Stone to review and request for interview. To date, only 12 RNs had been interviewed and only 6 (4 in MICU and 2 in MSU) have been hired in the past 6 months.

During this same period, three nurses had resigned or transferred from each of the two units. Nurse Samuelson's discussion with Ms. George also revealed that the NM responsible for these two units, Nurse Stone, had been making the decisions for interview and hire without input from the staff on either unit and that the application review process took at least 4 weeks before a decision regarding the interview was made. This delay had resulted in numerous RNs withdrawing their application and/or obtaining another job before being contacted for interview. Ms. George also reported that agency nurses and travelers have expressed frustration and dissatisfaction with the care on the unit and the way they are being treated by staff. Nurse Samuelson queried Ms. George to determine whether this information had been shared with Nurse Stone on the units. The response was "yes." Review of retention strategies implemented on the units by Ms. George and/or Nurse Stone revealed that food had been provided on occasion when staffing was extremely tight. However, no proactive actions (e.g., staff survey to identify needs and concerns, recognition activities for outstanding staff performance or contributions, staff involvement in the recruitment process, preceptor usage, or mentorship offerings) have occurred. Nurse Samuelson asked Ms. George to put together a table outlining the recruitment and retention activities that have occurred over the past 2 years for a meeting in the next week with Nurse Stone and the staff members.

Nurse Samuelson next met with the NM of MICU and MSU, Nurse Stone, to discuss the issues related to high vacancy and turnover rates. At the meeting, Nurse Samuelson inquired about the level of concern Nurse Stone had related to these statistics and asked her to discuss strategies that have been put into place to increase the hiring and decrease the turnover on both of these two units. Nurse Stone reported that she is getting poor response from Ms. George relative to the specialty requirements for critical care nurses. She also reported that the relationship between her and Ms. George is not positive, noting that interviews are not set up quickly and that a salary offer is late in coming. This makes it difficult to get back with the RN applicant in a timely manner. Nurse Stone reported that staff involvement in the recruitment and retention process has been limited because of the high staffing needs and overtime worked. Staff attitudes have not been positive lately, and from Nurse Stone's perspective, asking staff members to be involved in addition work responsibilities would further inflame them. In addition, extensive use of agency nurses and travelers has already resulted in a negative personnel budget variance. Nurse Stone further stated that she did not bring this problem to Nurse Samuelson because she was hoping to have it resolved in the near future.

After the meeting with both Ms. George and Nurse Stone, Nurse Samuelson next approached the staff to determine their concerns and responses to the nurse vacancy and turnover rates on the units. The staff revealed that, although a number of positions were open, Nurse Stone had given them time off when requested and that agency nurses and travelers were filling in for the most part. However, use of supplemental staff often cut into their ability to work overtime, something that they all did as a way of increasing their monthly salary. Several of the staff blamed the agency nurses and travelers for the increase in error rates, noting that they were too busy to monitor everything that happened on the units. The staff also indicated that many of the new RNs who had joined the staff were not a "good fit" and left within a few weeks or months of hire. When asked about their role in precepting the new RNs, only one nurse indicated that she had taken an active role as both a preceptor and mentor with three of the new RNs, only one of whom stayed. Staff attitude and lack of support were reported by this nurse preceptor as the major reasons for decreased retention of new hires. Another reason given was a lack of training support for nurses with limited medical intensive care experience and/or knowledge. Staff reported that developing staff took time away from caregiving and suggested that it needed to be provided off-unit by staff educators or clinical nurse specialists.

After the interviews, Nurse Samuelson formulated an analysis outlining the **s**trengths, **w**eaknesses, **o**pportunities, and **t**hreats (SWOT) on each of the units relative to the recruitment and retention of staff. To implement change, Nurse Samuelson established a unit-based work group on each of the units because an action and implementation plan with defined outcome goals and timeline was needed.

CRITICAL THINKING EXERCISE

As a nurse manager of a cardiac critical care unit (CCCU), Maria Gonzales is struggling to retain qualified experienced nurses who are being recruited to work at a new cardiac care hospital that has just recently opened in the community. She has been asked to present a retention plan to the chief nurse officer (CNO). In preparation for the plan, Nurse Gonzales becomes aware that more then 65% of the registered nurse staff in the CCCU have 15 or more years of experience and employment at the current institution. However, these nurses are at the top of the pay scale in their job classification. In addition, 25% of the RNs have less than 1 year of experience. The complexity of the patient population is continuing to change, requiring greater use of technology, so traditional continuing education is no longer an option for staff. Based on this and other information available, Nurse Gonzales develops a plan that she believes will maximize retention and ensure stabilization of the unit.

1. How would Nurse Gonzales go about determining staff perceptions relative to job satisfaction and preferred retention strategies?
2. With what department would Nurse Gonzales work to determine common retention practices used in the community and RN pay scales for experienced CCCU nurses in the community/region?
3. Where would Nurse Gonzales go for data relative to the CCCU patients—for example, populations served, year-to-date volume, complexity of care requirements, treatment requirements?
4. Who else in the organization could Nurse Gonzales partner with in addressing this issue?
5. What do you think might be Nurse Gonzales' final recommendations to the CNO?

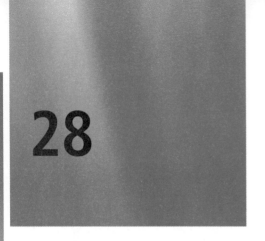

28 Staffing and Scheduling

Beth Pickard Sharon A. Eck Birmingham

CHAPTER OBJECTIVES

- Discuss the staffing management of nursing resources and its relevance to the quality, safety, and cost of health care
- Discuss the professional, legislative, regulatory, and organizational factors that influence staffing management
- Describe a framework for staffing management, including strategies, staffing plan, and outcomes
- Discuss attributes of the staffing management plan: forecasting workload, staffing patterns that meet patient care needs, position control, scheduling, demand management, staffing allocation, and caregiver assignment
- Discuss the impact of staffing on patient, fiscal, and organizational outcomes
- Explore current trends and issues as they relate to the nurse's role in revenue generation
- Critically analyze and apply chapter content in a staffing management exercise
- Exercise critical thinking to conceptualize and analyze possible solutions to a practice exercise

"Nurse staffing methodology should be an orderly, systematic process, based upon sound rationale, applied to determine the number and kind of nursing personnel required to provide nursing care of a predetermined standard to a group of patients in a particular setting. The result is prediction of the kind and number of staff required to give care to patients. This prediction of the number and kinds of personnel to give patients nursing care 24 hours a day, 7 days a week…is no small task. The aim is to provide, at a reasonable cost to the general public the agency serves, a standard of nursing care acceptable to its clientele and the nursing staff serving it." (Aydelotte, 1973, p. 3)

The nurse staffing methodology eloquently articulated by Aydelotte in the early 1970s continues as a critical human resource issue affecting the quality, safety, and cost of U.S. health care today (Aiken et al., 2002; Aiken et al., 2003; Hinshaw, 2006; Institute of Medicine [IOM], 2004; Kane et al., 2007a,b; Kovner & Gergen, 1998; Litvak et al., 2005; Needleman et al., 2002; Needleman et al., 2006; Unruh, 2008). Nursing is essential in the delivery of health care to society. Nursing's Social Policy Statement reflects the societal contract for the provision of safe and quality nursing care and services for all people (American Nurses Association [ANA], 2003). Whether in health care systems, single hospitals, ambulatory practice settings, long-term care, home care, or other health care settings, the delivery of nursing care and services is expected to meet certain standards established by organizations, state and private regulatory agencies, the profession, and in certain states, legislative mandates and public reporting of nurse staffing. The major goal of staffing management is to provide the right number of nursing staff with the right qualifications to deliver high-quality, safe, and cost-effective nursing care to a group of patients and their families (Smith, 1994; Warner, 2006).

Staffing management is cited as one of the most critical yet highly complex and time-consuming activities for nurse leaders at every level of the health care organization today (Abdoo, 2000; Sullivan et al., 2003). How well or poorly nursing leaders execute staff management impacts the safety and quality of patient care, financial results, and organizational outcomes, such as job satisfaction and retention of RNs. In the foreword to the American Organization of Nurse Executives (AONE) monograph, *Staffing Management and Methods: Tools and Techniques for Nursing Leaders,* Beyers (2000) stated, "Staffing is one of the outcomes and indicators of the effectiveness of nursing management practices" (p. xxii).

The purpose of this chapter is to assist nursing managers and students to understand the complex issues associated with staffing management in nursing. A framework for staffing management is presented and will guide the reader through the internal and external strategies that influence an organization's staffing management plan. Critical components of the staffing management plan are described and include forecasting workload, developing staffing patterns, position control, scheduling, demand management, staffing allocation, and caregiver assignment. The effects of staffing on patient, financial, and organizational outcomes are presented. Finally, current trends and issues that recognize nurses' role in revenue generation are explored.

DEFINITIONS

Staffing terminology in nursing administration is often confusing, particularly to students and novice nurse managers. The following definitions clarify and introduce staffing management terminology. **Staffing** is defined as a human resources plan to fill positions in an organization with qualified personnel. A **staffing strategy** is a set of actions undertaken to determine the organization's future human resources needs, recruit and select qualified applicants, and meet the needs of the organization (Fried & Johnson, 2002). Staffing strategies are consistent with the hospital's mission, and annual strategic goals and are executed to meet the staffing management plan of an organization. The **staffing management plan** is a structured approach to the process of identifying and allocating unit-based personnel resources in the most effective and efficient manner (Kirby & Wiczai, 1985; Nash et al., 2000). **Skill mix** is defined as the proportion of direct-care RNs to total nursing staff and is expressed as a percentage of RNs/total nursing staff (e.g., 65% RNs) (Unruh, 2003). A **staffing pattern** quantifies the total number of staff by skill level scheduled for each day and each shift (e.g., 3 RNs, 1 UAP, and 1 health unit coordinator [HUC] on Monday 7 AM to 7 PM). **Scheduling** is the process of assigning individual personnel to work specific hours, days, or shifts and in a specific unit or area over a specified period of time (Barnum & Mallard, 1989). **Staffing effectiveness** is the evaluation of the effect of staffing on patient, financial, and organizational outcomes.

Other definitions include **nurse-to-patient ratio,** which is the number of patients cared for by one nurse (e.g., 1 registered nurse [RN]: 4 patients). **Skill level** refers specifically to the licensure or certification of a staff member (e.g., RN, licensed practical nurse/licensed vocational nurse [LPN/LVN], or unlicensed assistive personnel [UAP]) (Warner, 2006). **Nursing workload** is the amount of intensity (in terms of effort required) of the work a nurse performs within a given period (Unruh, 2008). Because so many variables affect workload, there are efforts to better explicate and measure workload, such as nursing intensity (Moore & Hastings, 2006) and nurse dose (Brooten & Youngblut, 2006). **Direct-care hours** include nursing staff hours that are assigned to provide direct care to a patient or groups of patients for a specified period; the most common direct-care staff include the RN, LPN/LVN, and UAP. The **average daily census (ADC)** is calculated by dividing the number of patients cared for per day over a certain period by the number of days in a period; this may be an actual ADC or a budgeted ADC. The **average length of stay (ALOS)** is the average number of days the patient is in the hospital and is determined by dividing the total number of patient days by the total number of admissions (Finkler et al., 2007).

LEADING & MANAGING DEFINED

Staffing

A human resources plan to fill positions in an organization with qualified personnel.

Staffing Strategy

A set of actions undertaken to determine human resources needs, recruit and select qualified applicants, and meet the needs of the organization (Fried & Johnson, 2002).

Staffing Management Plan

A structured approach to the process of identifying and allocating unit-based personnel resources in the most effective and efficient manner (Kirby & Wiczai, 1985; Nash et al., 2000).

Skill Mix

The proportion of direct-care RNs to total nursing staff; expressed as a percentage of RNs/total nursing staff (Unruh, 2003).

Staffing Pattern

Quantifies the total number of staff by skill level scheduled for each day and each shift.

Scheduling

The process of assigning individual personnel to work specific hours, days, or shifts and in a specific unit or area over a specified period of time (Barnum & Mallard, 1989).

Staffing Effectiveness

Evaluation of the effect of staffing on patient, financial, and organizational outcomes.

Nurse-to-Patient Ratio

The number of patients cared for by one nurse.

Skill Level

The licensure or certification of a staff member.

Nursing Workload

The amount of intensity (in terms of effort required) of the work a nurse performs within a given period (Unruh, 2008). Because so many variables affect workload, there are efforts to better explicate and measure workload, such as nursing intensity (Moore & Hastings, 2006) and nurse dose (Brooten & Youngblut, 2006).

Direct-Care Hours

Nursing staff hours that are assigned to provide direct care to a patient or groups of patients for a specified period; the most common direct-care staff include the RN, LPN/LVN, and UAP.

Average Daily Census (ADC)

Calculated by dividing the number of patients cared for per day over a certain period by the number of days in a period; may be an actual ADC or a budgeted ADC.

Average Length of Stay

The average number of days the patient is in the hospital; determined by dividing the total number of patient days by the total number of admissions (Finkler et al., 2007).

FRAMEWORK FOR STAFFING MANAGEMENT

Staffing management is often a complex and challenging problem because of the numerous dependencies and inter-related organizational processes. A conceptual framework provides logic and order to a complex process and limits the number of staffing-related variables for administrators and scientists to consider (Edwardson, 2007). A conceptual framework for staffing management is proposed and illustrated in Figure 28.1.

This conceptual framework is organized and adapted from Donabedian's (1966) framework for the evaluation of quality of care, relating various structures (e.g., hospital characteristics) that

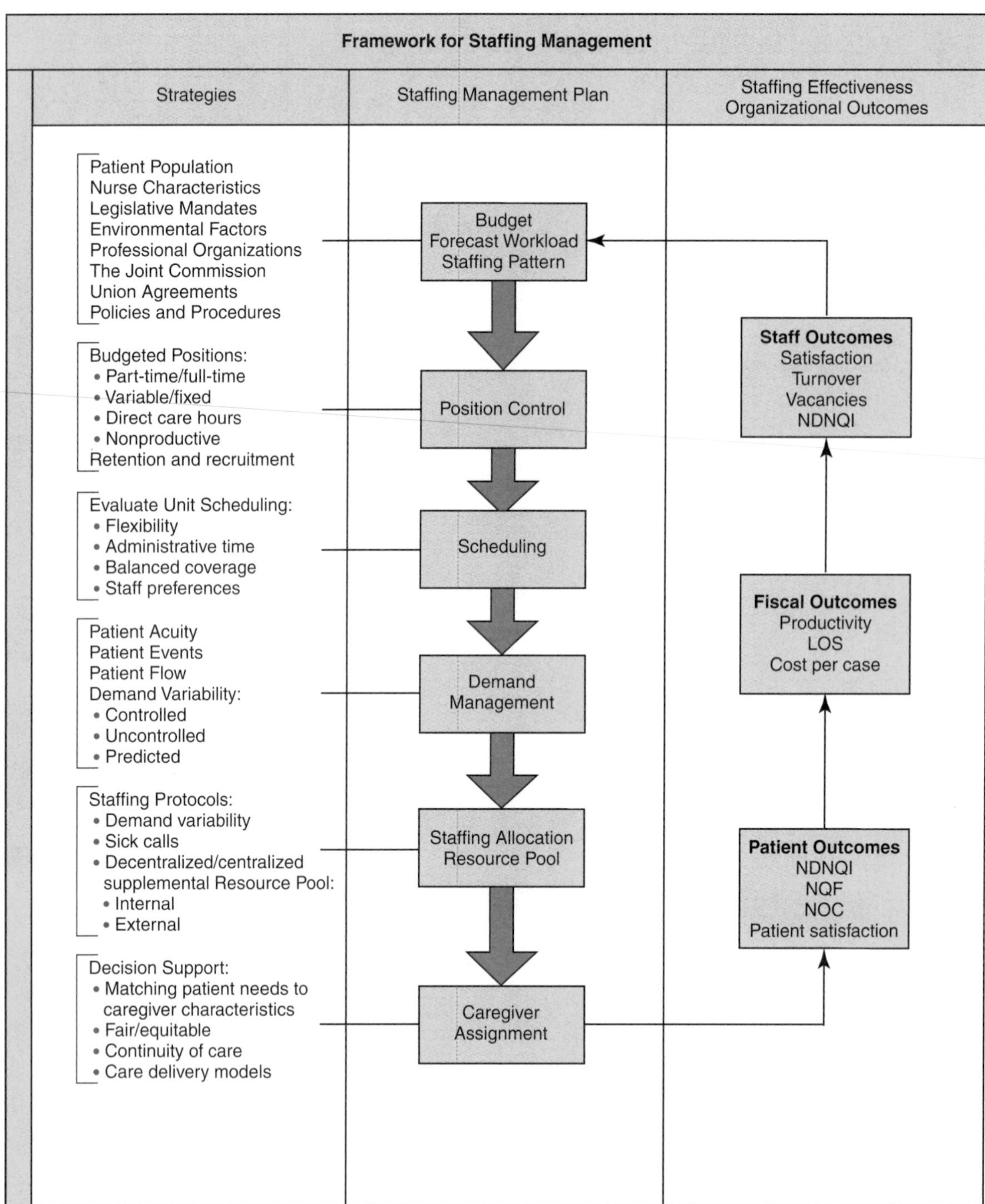

Figure 28.1
Framework for staffing management. *LOS,* Length of stay; *NDNQI,* National Database of Nursing Quality Indicators; *NOC,* nursing outcomes classification; *NQF,* National Quality Forum.

impact various processes (e.g., actual staffing) and subsequently influence various outcomes (e.g., patient quality, staff satisfaction). This framework has been adapted to guide numerous staffing studies (Cho, 2001; Eck, 1999; Edwardson, 2007; Kane, 2007a,b; Mark et al., 2007; Mark et al., 2004). In the proposed framework, structures represent the various nursing strategies, both internal and external to the organization, that directly influence an organization's ability to effectively manage the necessary processes for adequate staffing. The processes are a series of defined stages with outputs that directly affect subsequent stages of staffing. Finally, the outcomes of staffing management are multidimensional and measured in terms of organizational outcomes including patient, fiscal, and staff outcomes. The staffing management framework is not intended to address all variables, influences, stages, and outcomes but, instead, is intended to provide a guide for nursing leaders to assess staffing management in their organizations.

STRATEGIES INFLUENCING STAFFING MANAGEMENT

The following section describes the significant influences and strategies on staffing management in organizations today. It is important for nurse executives and managers to remain current on both the internal and external influences affecting staffing management. Briefly presented are (1) professional nursing resources and recommendations, (2) nursing care delivery models, (3) state legislative mandates, (4) The Joint Commission (TJC) regulation, and (5) nurse union agreements.

American Nurses Association Principles for Nurse Staffing

The American Nurses Association (ANA) has published several guiding documents that serve as resources for students, staff nurses, nursing leaders, organizations, and lawmakers to better understand the complex staffing issues associated with creating a nursing unit schedule, an organization-wide staffing plan, or a piece of staffing legislation. *Principles for Nurse Staffing* (ANA, 1999) was developed by an appointed expert panel to guide nurse staffing. The nine principles are organized into three categories pertaining to the patient care unit, the staff, and the organization. The nine principles are as follows (ANA, 1999):

I. Patient Care Unit
   A. Appropriate staffing levels for a patient care unit reflect analysis of individual and aggregate patient needs.
   B. There is a critical need to either retire or seriously question the usefulness of the concept of nursing hours per patient day (HPPD).
   C. Unit functions necessary to support delivery of quality patient care must also be considered in determining staffing levels.

II. Staff
   A. The specific needs of various patient populations should determine the appropriate clinical competencies required of the nurse practicing in that area.
   B. Registered nurses must have nursing management support and representation at both the operational level and the executive level.
   C. Clinical support from experienced RNs should be readily available to those RNs with less proficiency.

III. Organization
   A. Organizational policy should reflect an organizational climate that values registered nurses and other employees as strategic assets and exhibit a true commitment to filling budgeted positions in a timely manner.
   B. All institutions should have documented competencies for nursing staff, including agency or supplemental and traveling RNs, for those activities that they have been authorized to perform.
   C. Organizational policies should recognize the myriad needs of both patients and nursing staff. (p. 2)

These principles reflect many important values related to the analysis of patients' needs, nurses' work environments, and outcomes at the unit level.

The ANA recommended a professional model in which staffing factors taken into account include the number of patients, acuity levels of patients, contextual issues such as unit geography and technology availability, and the level of preparation, experience, and competency of caregivers. The need for these principles certainly became evident shortly after they were published when they were integrated into legislative and collective bargaining language.

As the nursing shortage has intensified, nurse staffing issues and rising concern for both the quality and cost of care have escalated. The ANA responded with an updated *Utilization Guide for the ANA Principles for Nurse Staffing* (2005). This report highlighted several policy perspectives: (1) the value of direct-care nurses' input into an organization's staffing plan; (2) the value of direct-care nurses' input into the selection and implementation of patient classification or acuity systems; and (3) the value of the clinically skilled and experienced RN who is familiar with the specific patients and nursing staff making a professional judgment regarding staffing decisions.

Nursing Care Delivery Models and Staffing Management

Nursing care delivery models significantly influence staffing management. A nursing care delivery model "is defined as a method of organizing and delivering nursing care in order to achieve desired patient outcomes" (Deutschendorf, 2006, p. 316). The model characteristics describe the nature and degrees of continuity in the assignment of nursing personnel, the type of coordination that is specific to the patient, and available nursing resources (Mark, 1992). Examples of nursing care delivery models include patient-focused care, team nursing, private duty nursing, total patient care, functional nursing, primary nursing, and various combinations. Regardless of the model type, the RN is accountable for the provision of nursing care to patients 24 hours a day, 7 days a week in the hospital setting. Specific to staffing management, the new roles of the charge nurse, clinical nurse leader, and three care delivery models are discussed.

Manthey (1990) and Person (2004) described the four fundamental elements of any nursing care delivery model as follows: (1) nurse/patient relationship and decision making; (2) work allocation and patient assignments; (3) communication among members of the health team; and (4) management of the unit or environment of care. How these fundamental elements in the care delivery model are defined has a direct impact on every aspect of staffing management.

Translating the nursing care delivery model's elements and inherent values to staffing management is a key role for nurse executives and managers (ANA, 2004). For example, many care delivery models articulate the value of the nurse and patient/family relationship. Caregiver assignment technology, or the previous 48 hours of assignments, provides charge nurses with data to implement nurse and patient continuity. The nurse-patient relationship element of the model also typically delineates the registered nurse–to–unlicensed assistive personnel (RN-to-UAP) ratios and the expected UAP role and relationship to the RN. The ratios will be executed in multiple phases of staffing management as determined by various patient unit types and, if implemented, by an acuity methodology.

The charge nurse and the clinical nurse leader have received notable attention in recent care delivery models. Many care delivery models now dedicate an RN in the charge nurse role to proactively manage the complexities of patient flow. The charge nurse, particularly on larger units and units with high patient turnover, is free of a direct patient care assignment, which is the new element in this role. This allows the charge nurse to readily assist in critical patient situations, support novice clinicians, and continuously communicate about patients with fellow charge nurses in the emergency, operating, or labor and delivery departments. In this case, the scheduling technology or schedule must incorporate an RN competent in the charge role for each shift that is not included in the caregiver assignments. Because charge nurses are critical to effectively managing patient flow and the care environment, many nurse managers involve staff nurses and physicians in the interview process to select the best charge nurses.

The American Association of Colleges of Nursing (AACN) has recommended a new professional nurse role, the clinical nurse leader (CNL) (AACN, 2003, 2007). The CNL role integrates various aspects of previous roles known in nursing, such as the case manager and clinical nurse specialist. The CNL vision statement is as follows: "The CNL champions innovations that improve patient outcomes, ensure quality care and reduce healthcare costs. The CNL integrates emerging nursing science into practice and leads this effort to enhance patient care. A recognized leader in all settings, the CNL is an advocate for reforming the healthcare delivery system and putting best practices into action" (AACN, 2003, p. 2). The new CNL role also embodies many of the key points with the AONE *Guiding Principles for the Nurse of the Future* (Haase-Herrick & Herrin, 2007).

Three of the nursing care delivery models that influence staffing management are case management, relationship-based care, and the Synergy Model. Case management is defined by the Case Management Society of America (CMSA) as "a collaborative process of assessment, planning, facilitation and advocacy for options and services to meet an individual's health needs through communication and available resources to promote quality, cost-effective outcomes" (CMSA, 2002, p. 5). In hospitals, case management is frequently associated with evidenced-based critical paths or the expected pattern of a patient's hospital stay with emphasis on variance tracking regarding the anticipated length of stay (LOS). Technologies tracking individual patients to their expected outcomes and LOS provide significant data for the direct-care RN, charge nurse, and case manager to best coordinate care and resources to achieve optimum patient outcomes and hospital reimbursement.

A second care delivery model is described in the book *Relationship-Based Care* (RBC) (Koloroutis, 2004). Person (2004) articulated continuity of care as central to the RBC model, and this value has the most significant implications for the caregiver assignments. Many RBC models integrate Jean Watson's theory of caring (Watson, 1988; Watson, 2002). Last, a Synergy Model for patient care is presented by the American Association of Critical-Care Nurses (Hardin & Kaplow, 2005). The core concepts of the model are that the needs or characteristics of the patients and families influence and drive the characteristics and competencies of the nurse. Synergy results when the needs and characteristics of the patient clinical unit, or system, are matched with a nurse's competencies to achieve the optimal patient outcomes. The patient and nurse characteristics are defined and scored and, once implemented, are reported to provide evidence for Magnet™ designation (Kaplow & Reed, 2008).

American Organization of Nurse Executives

The American Organization of Nurse Executives (AONE), a subsidiary of the American Hospital Association, is a national organization whose mission is to represent nurse leaders. They issued *Staffing Management and Methods: Tools and Techniques for Nurse Leaders* (AONE, 2000), which presents an introduction into evolving staffing measures and has a chapter dedicated to staffing management approaches in each of four hospital types: the large academic medical center, an integrated health care system, a small community hospital, and a rural hospital setting. The final chapter presents how various innovations in information systems support nurse staffing.

AONE's 2008 Legislative Agenda for public policy and advocacy includes several key points relevant to staffing management. An excerpt of the policy agenda aims to: "Develop, evaluate and support legislation that will foster the nurse executive's leadership role in the management of the care environment, especially in areas related to staffing, information technology and patient care services" (AONE, 2008). The agenda does not support mandates, such as overtime or staffing ratios, and recommends working with state and federal legislators to shape policies that promote flexibility and recognize the volatility of the patient care environment.

Practical Tips

Tip # 1: Listen to Staff Perceptions Regarding Staffing Management

Be open to staff feedback, ideas, and suggestions regarding every aspect of staffing management. Schedule a periodic open discussion at a staff meeting: What are the strengths of staffing in our area? What are the areas we would like to change? Listen carefully to the staff comments. Record the comments on a flip chart or in meeting minutes. Engage the staff in action planning toward improvements. Communicate staff ideas to your boss for additional guidance. Recommend appropriate budget changes as necessary.

Tip #2: Use Patient Acuity Data for Clinical Rounding with Staff

On a regular basis, conduct rounds with the staff based on current patient acuity information. Talk with nurses caring for high-acuity patients, and inquire: Do you have the resources to safely care for the patient today? What resources do you have? What resources are lacking in sufficiency or timeliness? If a novice nurse is caring for a moderate-acuity to high-acuity patient, inquire: Who do you consider your expert resources? Are these resources readily available? Actively listening to the responses of the staff regarding their patient in the moment will give you insights into the adequacy of staffing, teamwork, mentoring, and effective use of resources among staff directly caring for patients.

Tip # 3: Collaborate with Finance Department Colleagues

Organizations differ in their definitions of which staff and worked activities count in direct hours of patient care. Discussing and generating a working list of definitions is an excellent way to bridge fiscal language. Clearly differentiate with members of the finance department the direct, worked, paid FTEs, and hours per unit of service. Encourage finance members to participate in unit rounds, and educate them regarding patient care and nurse staffing and be open to attending fiscal seminars in return.

Staffing Recommendations by Professional Organizations

Several professional nursing specialty organizations also have published position statements and recommendations for nurse staffing in an effort to provide evidence-based guidelines for specialty areas. The National Association of Neonatal Nurses (1999a, b) has a staffing position statement and recommended staffing ratios that are also described in the "Guidelines for Perinatal Care" (American Academy of Pediatrics [AAP] & the American College of Obstetricians and Gynecologists [ACOG], 2007). The ratios delineate care provided for women and newborns in the antepartum, intrapartum, and postpartum settings, as well as the newborn nursery. The Association of Women's Health, Obstetrics and Neonatal Nurses (AWHONN) further described the specific staffing recommendations for women in the various stages of normal labor and labor with complications. The commonwealth of Virginia has used the AWHONN guidelines to legislate regulations for perinatal nurse-to-patient ratios (White, 2006).

The Association of periOperative Registered Nurses (AORN) has a position paper addressing key staffing issues in the operating rooms (OR), and the Emergency Nursing Association (ENA) also has recommendations for staffing. Finally, the American Academy of Ambulatory Care Nursing (AAACN) has published an annotated bibliography summarizing the ambulatory nurse staffing literature (2005). Haas and Hastings (2001) have outlined the methods for determining staffing requirements, skill mix, and productivity in the ambulatory care setting. Staffing recommendations by the various professional organizations are frequently adopted in clinical settings and incorporated into written staffing plans.

The Joint Commission Staffing Regulation

Private regulatory agencies, such as The Joint Commission (TJC), are widely used by hospitals today to conduct external reviews for quality and safety. The Joint Commission noted the following (TJC, 2006):

> The goal of the human resources function is to ensure that the hospital determines the qualifications and competencies for staff positions based on its mission, populations, and care, treatment and services. Hospitals must also provide the right number of competent staff members to meet the patients' needs. (p. HR-1)

The human resources standards clearly outline the complex requirements associated with staffing management today and include, but are not limited to, the adequacy of staff numbers, mix of staff levels, licensure, education, certification, experience, and continuing education.

Union Agreements on Staffing Management

The two largest nursing and health care unions are (1) the United American Nurses (UAN), a branch of the ANA; and (2) the Service Employees International Union (SEIU) District 1199. Nursing unions are organizations that represent nurses for the purpose of collective bargaining. Collective bargaining is defined as "the performance of the mutual obligations of the employer and the exclusive representative to meet at reasonable times, to consult with respect to terms and conditions of employment. This obligation does not compel either party to agree to proposals or make concessions" (Department of Veterans Affairs, 2002). In nursing, it is a process of negotiation between an employer and the union representatives of nurse employees to reach a written agreement regarding certain terms of employment. The mandatory terms of employment include subjects such as wages, hours, overtime, low census call-off procedures, recall, floating, use of UAP, seniority, sick leave, discharges, leaves of absence, and other non-mandatory topics as negotiated. These employment subjects have significant implications for staffing management; however, collective bargaining agreements vary in their specificity across organizations. Nurse executives and managers working with nursing unions must have detailed knowledge of the relevant contract implications and integrate these requirements into the staffing management plan.

Legislative Impact on Staffing Management

Nurse dissatisfaction and concern for adequate staffing to provide quality nursing care to patients and their families arose from the hospital cost-reduction initiatives throughout the 1990s. Armed with quality-of-care concerns, nurses began to organize and craft proposed staffing legislation in many states. The historical context that led to quality-of-care concerns continues to impact legislation today. Throughout the 1990s, hospital administrators relied on consultants to implement work redesign to promote patient-focused care as a method of cost reduction. The central labor reduction approach in patient-focused care was to reduce the number of RNs and increase or maintain the number of UAP. This approach for decreasing nursing RN skill mix was implemented in a "one size fits all" approach across organizations and often lacked evaluation of the skill mix change and other changes on the quality of care and nurse job satisfaction and retention (Eck, 1999; Norrish & Rundall, 2001). This was most apparent in California where a leaner RN skill mix was tried by Kaiser Permanente Northern California in the early 1990s (to 55% RNs in the total staff mix) and in 1995 (to 30%) (Robertson & Samuelson, 1996). The changes in skill mix led to widespread real and perceived increases in RN workload, patient safety concerns, and nurse and consumer complaints (Norrish & Rundall, 2001; Seago et al., 2003).

Despite patient complaints and reports of nurse dissatisfaction, little was done until 1999. Only then did the California legislature pass Assembly Bill 394 (AB 394) to mandate minimum nurse staffing ratios. The mandating of minimum nurse-to-patient ratios legislated in California ignited great debate, controversy, and study. California remains the only state with mandated ratios. Meanwhile, nurse scientists and policy experts have presented compelling arguments against mandated ratios and explicate that the local nursing leaders are in the best position to determine the actual staffing required by the particular patient population (Buerhaus, 1997; Clarke, 2005). The bold action, however, of the California's state legislative mandate stimulated focused attention on addressing nurse staffing issues.

Since the late 1990s, state legislation regarding nurse staffing issues has been commonplace. Primary trends of the enacted state legislation may limit or preclude mandatory overtime and require staffing committees and plans with direct-care nurse input. More recently, legislation provides whistleblower protection, mandates public access to staffing information, and requires implementing patient acuity methodologies to adjust for staffing workload (White, 2006).

The Illinois staffing legislation is significant because its primary elements also have been adopted in other states such as New Jersey and Washington. Illinois enacted Senate Bill 0867 (SB 0867) specifically to address the staffing plan and direct-care nurse input and provide for patient acuity measurement. Unlike the California bill, this bill does not mandate nurse-to-patient ratios. Instead, the language of SB 0867 defines that the:

> Written staffing plan for nursing care services means a written plan for guiding the assignment of patient care nursing staff, based on multiple nurse and patient considerations that yield minimum staffing levels for inpatient care units and the adopted acuity model aligning patient care needs with nursing skills required for quality patient care consistent with professional nursing standards.

SB 0867 also requires significant input among direct-care staff nurses within hospitals with regard not only to the written staffing plan but also in "the selection, implementation, and evaluation of an acuity model to provide staffing flexibility that aligns patient acuity with nursing skills required."

On the national level, U.S. Senate Bill 71, the Registered Nurse Safe Staffing Act of 2005, has been proposed as an amendment of Part D of Title XVIII (Medicare) of the Social Security Act. It would make nurse staffing systems a condition for participation in Medicare (White, 2006). The proposed federal bill requires staffing systems that determine or define appropriate staffing levels for patient care and accommodate recommendations by specialty nursing organizations and public reporting for staffing, meanwhile providing whistleblower protection and civil monetary penalties for violations.

The ANA has dedicated a new web page as part of a national campaign, entitled *Safe Staffing Saves Lives,* to help fight for safe staffing legislation (ANA, 2008). In its fight, the ANA believes staffing ratios need to be required by legislation but the number itself must be set at the unit level with RN input rather than by the terms of the legislation. In summary, state nurse staffing legislation is growing and has a significant impact on staffing management in health care today. Many states do not have established reporting or accountability processes. In light of these legislative trends, many nursing organizations are proactively establishing staffing committees with significant direct-care staff input and are exploring, selecting, and implementing new patient acuity methodologies in an effort to implement staffing plans that result in quality patient outcomes.

THE STAFFING MANAGEMENT PLAN

The staffing management plan provides the structured processes to identify patient needs and then to deliver the staff resources as efficiently and effectively as possible. An effective plan first focuses on stabilizing the unit core staffing. A staffing pattern, or core coverage, is determined through a forecasted workload and a recommended care standard. Hiring to the associated position complement and developing balanced and filled schedules, without holes, are essential building blocks for efficient and cost-effective daily resource allocation. Daily staffing allocation requires managing a variable staffing plan, measuring and predicting demand, and then providing balanced workload assignments to ensure that the correct caregivers are best matched to patient needs (Warner, 2006). A successful staffing management plan incorporates the policies inherent to the organization, patient care unit, and nurse population including union and contracting affiliations. Kane and colleagues (2007a, b) suggested nurse staffing policies that should be addressed by both patient care units and organizations, such as shift rotation, overtime, full-time/part-time mix, and weekend staffing. In addition to policies, procedures are essential for effective communication and execution of the plan.

Forecasted Workload and Staffing Pattern (Core Coverage)

Forecasting a workload for each patient care area is typically evaluated and adjusted at least annually as part of the budget process or when the patient characteristics, services, and/or volume changes. The amount of work performed by a unit is referred to as its *workload*, and workload volume is measured in terms of units of service. The unit of service is specific to the type of unit, such as the number of patients, patient days, deliveries, visits, treatments, or procedures.

Once the unit of service is determined, the number of units of service that will be provided in the coming year must be forecasted. Total patient days are commonly used in inpatient hospital areas. This is calculated by multiplying the average length of stay (ALOS) and the average daily census (ADC). The workload standard commonly used is nursing care hours per patient day, although the validity of this measure is disputed. Kane and colleagues (2007a, b) define nursing care hours per patient day (NHPPD) as the total number of productive hours by all nursing staff with direct patient care responsibilities for one patient over 24 hours.

However, not all patients require the same number of care hours, and the total number of patient days may be inadequate for planning purposes. Finkler and colleagues (2007) suggested using adjusted units of service. For example, a nursing unit can be adjusted using a system for classifying patients, such as a patient acuity system, based on the resources each classification category is expected to use. Segregating patients into acuity classifications allows the staffing pattern to be developed based on the resource requirements of the specific mix of patients forecasted for the unit. Similar calculations can be made in ambulatory and a variety of other settings. All that is required is a method to classify patients into different categories to estimate the average resource required for patients in each category (Finkler et al., 2007).

In addition to adjusting workload for a specific severity mix of patients, patient turnover on the unit is a consideration. The length of time patients stay in the hospital or, conversely, the rate of patient turnover affects resource use and workload. Reduced length of stay, or higher patient turnover, requires intensive periods of higher resources for patient admissions, transfer, discharge, and other concentrated activities that have an impact on overall workload. As patient turnover increases, the highly intensive periods of patient admission, transfer, and discharge procedures take up an increasing proportion of the hospital stay. Unruh and Fottler (2006) referred to an approach in which the nursing workload takes into account the intensity of nursing care.

Outside of state-mandated nurse staffing ratios, there is no one "gold care standard" or recommended nursing workload. Inconsistent operational definitions and methods of measuring care have been a challenge both for benchmarking resources across organizations and for research analysis related to adequate nursing care (Kane et al., 2007a, b). Therefore each organization must document and provide rationale regarding how staffing standards are determined within each patient care area.

Once the annual workload is forecasted, the skill mix required on each shift is determined. There are two general staffing methods: (1) with *fixed staffing*, staffing is built around a fixed projected maximum workload requirement and the staffing pattern is based on maximum workload conditions; (2) with *variable staffing*, units are staffed below maximum workload conditions and staff is then supplemented when needed (Bennett, 1981). An effective staffing pattern requires clear definitions for productive time, nonproductive time (i.e., benefits time, work for the organization, knowledge-related projects), worked time, paid full-time equivalents (FTEs), and hours per unit of service. In addition, staff roles must be clearly defined as to whether they are fixed or variable. The necessary number of FTEs to yield the desired care standard to the forecasted number of patients in each department must be calculated. In addition, the number of FTEs to replace staff members when they use nonproductive hours, such as benefit time, must also be included. Finkler and colleagues (2007) described the method for calculating a staffing pattern as follows:

- Determine the number of paid hours per FTE.
- Determine the percentage of productive hours to total paid hours.
- Multiply the number of paid hours per FTE by the percentage of productive hours to find the number of productive hours per FTE.
- Divide required care hours by productive hours per FTE to find the required number of FTEs.
- Divide the require care hours by the number of days per year that the unit has patients to find care hours/day. Divide that result by hours per shift to find the number of person shifts needed per working day.
- Assign staff by employee type and among required shifts per day.

Box 28.1 refers to a sample variable staff calculation. Table 28.1 provides a sample staffing pattern that includes the final step of allocating total FTEs

Box 28.1

Variable Staff Calculation

2,080 paid hours per FTE
80% productive hours to total paid hours
2080 × 0.8 = 1,664 productive hours per FTE

71,830 care hours ÷ 1,664 = 43.17 FTEs

71,830 care hours ÷ 365 days per year = 197 hours of care per day

197 hours of care per day ÷ 8-hour shifts = 24.6 person shifts

Table 28.1

Sample Staffing Pattern for a Wednesday for an Intermediate Care Nursery (40 Beds)

Staff Type	7 AM–7 PM Shift	7 PM–7 AM Shift	Skill Mix	Total
Fixed 8-Hour Day Staff				
Nurse Manager	1			1
Nurse Educator—shared	0.5			0.5
Lactation Specialist	1			1
Variable Staff				
Charge Nurse	1*			1
RN	8	7	75% RN	15
LPN	0	1	5% LPN	1
UAP	2	2	20% UAP	4
HUC	1	1		2

*Charge Nurse on days without a direct-care assignment.
HUC, Health unit coordinator; *LPN,* licensed practical nurse; *RN,* registered nurse; *UAP,* unlicensed assistive personnel.

across shifts and by skill mix. In many patient care areas, the staffing pattern may be different by day of week. For example, a post-surgical unit may have a lower patient census on weekends; thus a different staffing pattern may apply. Factors such as program guidelines and physician practice patterns must be considered (McKinley & Cavouras, 2000).

Position Control

Once the staffing pattern for each unit has been established, the next step to ensuring safe staffing coverage is to provide a structured measurement and evaluation of position control. Future schedule coverage and adequate staffing first require that unit staff are available to work the needed shifts. Therefore the hours of care requirement on a unit must be converted to the correct number of full-time positions. Position control is the process of providing and measuring the correct FTE, or complement, to adequately staff a given area. Full-time and part-time mix, shift lengths, weekend commitments, and available contingency, or flex staff, are components to be analyzed to produce the ideal complement. The correct complement of full-time and part-time employees requires an understanding of the institution's nonproductive time (e.g., sick and vacation time) and other budgeted activities (e.g., education time) that are not included in the direct patient care hours required for the staffing pattern. Brown (1999) provided an example equation to determine adequate FTEs needed to staff a sample medical-surgical unit, as shown in Box 28.2. An ideal measure of nursing staff adequacy, which considers intensity, was presented by Unruh and Fottler (2004, slide 3). They suggested that a staffing adequacy measure should indicate the volume of nurses of a certain skill level needed for a given volume of patients and the given intensity of nursing care required for those patients during their stay (Box 28.3).

Once position control is established to support the staffing patterns, vacancy and turnover rates need to be managed. A strategy for covering future vacant positions should be identified to prevent the use of more costly, last-minute staff resources. An organization reported actual cost savings by over-recruiting by 1.0 FTE in the ICU area, which resulted in lower use of more expensive contingency and external staff resources (Cipriano & Cutruzzula, 2007). With fiscal and human resources support, managers must strive to recruit and retain the FTE complement of the full-time and part-time mix needed for each staffing level. This will then increase the available resource pool

Box 28.2

Calculating Medical-Surgical Staff Coverage

Given:

Average daily census = 33.4
Nursing hours per patient day = 4
Constant representing 7 days per week with an FTE working 5 days = 1.4
Average nonproductive time = 1.14
The potentially productive hours in 1 workday for 1 staff person for 1 shift = 7.5

Then:

$$\frac{33.4 \times 4 \times 1.4 \times 1.14}{7.5}$$

= 28.4 total caregiver FTEs needed to staff the unit per shift

Adapted from Brown, B. (1999). How to develop a unit personnel budget. *Nursing Management, 30*(6), 34-35.

Box 28.3

An Ideal Measure of Nursing Staff Adequacy

$$\frac{\text{\# of RNs}}{\text{\# of Patient days} \times \text{Intensity of RN care for those patient days}}$$

Adapted from Unruh, L., & Fottler, M.D. (2004, June 6-8). Patient turnover and nursing staff adequacy. San Diego: AcademyHealth Annual Research meeting. Retrieved May 24, 2009, from www.ahsrhp.org/2004/ppt/unruh.ppt.

PART V

shifts to respond to higher-than-budgeted patient volume. Filled positions are the foundation for adequate balanced work schedules.

Scheduling

The scheduling process assigns personnel to work specific shifts, hours, and days in their clinical area. The schedule typically spans a period of 4 to 6 weeks into the future. With a growing forecasted workforce shortage, organizations that focus on retention strategies that include balanced, flexible, and predictable work schedules will have a competitive edge in recruiting top talent (PricewaterhouseCoopers, 2007). An assessment of scheduling procedures should include staff participation in the scheduling process, manager's administrative time spent creating and maintaining the schedule, and ability of the schedule procedures to provide the core coverage of the staffing plan. In recent years, scheduling applications have been created to balance the often-delicate polarity of employee requests and unit core coverage.

Whether using automated or manual scheduling processes, master schedules can provide fixed schedules for each day of the scheduling period. Although master schedules provide staff with predictable work schedules, they typically do not afford administration the flexibility needed to accommodate vacations and time-off requests. Skeleton schedules fix only a portion of the schedule, such as weekends, and then allow administration the flexibility to better accommodate staff requests. This is frequently a time-consuming process for nurse managers in order to provide equitable and fair schedules that also accommodate staff requests and preferences.

With today's workforce, an alternative method to a manager-constructed schedule is self-scheduling, whereby nurses on a unit work together to construct their schedules within budgetary parameters and unit-based guidelines (Hung, 2002). Setting limits for the target number of staff needed for each shift and day of the week greatly fosters a complete schedule that meets the needs of the unit and staff. The unit-based guidelines may include rules such as a rotation of who enters their schedule first, number of weekend or "off" shift days, and number of Fridays worked. The guidelines also aim to foster a fair schedule among nurses, such as equally sharing the distribution of the number of Fridays scheduled. The critical factors for success are staff input into the guidelines, a staff perception of fairness and equity, and a schedule that meets core coverage.

In recent years, computer technology has significantly automated the previous paper-intensive process of scheduling. In addition, technology has allowed the staff to participate or interact in the scheduling process with the advent of web-based employee self-service tools. From any location with Internet access, staff can view schedules, make requests, communicate schedule preferences, self-schedule, swap shifts, and even bid or sign up for extra shifts or opportunities.

A final schedule should be evaluated for adequacy of meeting core coverage. Schedule coverage variances, or schedule holes, should be analyzed as to whether inadequacies exist because of ineffective scheduling (e.g., unbalanced shifts) or because of accommodating too many requests (e.g., vacations). Staffing strategies should be identified for schedule variances caused by position vacancies and leaves of absence. Plans to fill the open shifts should be assessed before the schedule is posted to staff to prevent the often last-minute stress of inadequate available staff. As position control is the foundation for balanced schedules, balanced schedules are the foundation for adequate daily staffing allocation.

Demand Management

Demand management as a discipline focuses on (1) measuring, predicting, and understanding demand for an institution's products and services; and (2) deploying resources and management to ensure that demand is met in the way the consumer's wants and needs are satisfied. For health care, a key component of the "product and service" equation is high-quality, safe patient care, with the goal of having the patient leave the hospital in the shortest amount of time and at the lowest cost, given high-quality and safe care (Pickard & Warner, 2007).

An often-overlooked strategy for creating predictable and cost-effective staffing is the need to staff according to real-time patient information or to make staffing decisions that facilitate individual patients moving through their stay as quickly as possible with high-quality, safe care. Because most staffing plans staff to average forecasted care levels, periods of higher needed care levels, or peaks, may create serious stressors for both patients and nurses. Litvak and colleagues (2005) described three types of stressors intrinsic to health care organizations:

- Flow stress, representing the appearance rate of patients for hospital care
- Clinical stress, which is expressed in the variability in type and severity of disease
- Stress caused by competing responsibilities of health care providers

System stress introduced by demand for nurses to care for more or sicker patients has been shown to be a leading cause of adverse patient outcomes (Litvak et al., 2005). When variability is minimized and/or better predicted, a hospital has greater resources for the remaining patient-driven peaks in demand, over which it has no control. Effective staffing requires an assessment of demand variability or the required hourly nursing care for each day on each unit. Ways to control variability, hence decrease peaks and valleys, include better planning for scheduled events such as elective OR procedures, better control over bed assignments based on current unit workload, and improved planning for discharges—all of which increase the demand and stress for nursing resources. Computer technologies that continuously track and predict demand assist managers with variability analysis and prospective planning for predicted variability. Predictive modeling can forecast unplanned patient and staff events, such as admissions by day of week and unplanned sick calls (Warner, 2006).

Pickard and Warner (2007) outlined the essential components for effective demand management:

- The entire methodology must use a measure of demand (need for nursing care) based on *patient outcomes* (how well he or she is progressing) rather than just census or caregiver activities.
- The methodology must be focused on the *individual patient,* both for maximum accuracy and validity and for effective patient management.
- The methodology should incorporate *progress goals* for each patient throughout his or her stay with which actual progress may be compared.
- The methodology must *continuously measure progress in real time,* so that decisions can be made as the patient's need changes (rather than once a shift or once a day, thereby basing decisions on information than is typically 8 to 16 hours old).
- This measure of demand must be *projected* into the near future (several days ahead) to allow time for optimal staffing decisions to be made while there is still time for numerous choices among available caregivers and cost-effective options.
- The measure must be able to be *embedded in a decision support system* for staffing and patient management.
- The measure and the decision support system that uses it must be appreciated and *acceptable to all stakeholders,* especially administration and finance, to avoid organizational polarity.
- The measure should produce need for care in terms of not only quantity and skill but also the *caregiver attributes* necessary to provide optimal care for the patient.
- An *outcomes-driven acuity system,* based on an established taxonomy for assessing and documenting patient care on outcomes, greatly enhances the demand methodology's effectiveness.
- The measure should incorporate all presently and planned *electronically available data* to reduce nursing time in data gathering and to provide as much real-time valid data as possible.

Incorporating these elements is not a simple task, but doing so offers significant advantages and benefits. By focusing on the individual patient, with individual outcome progress goals for each patient, hospitals can achieve results not previously addressed with traditional models. These results include (1) best-practice staffing protocols based on "true (outcomes-oriented) demand" and the optimal staffing levels to move a patient through each phase of his or her stay as quickly as possible, (2) early identification of patients who are not moving through their hospital stay as planned, and (3) improved near-term projection and prediction of staffing needs.

Staffing Allocation and Resource Pool

Even with the best planning and most accurate prediction of supply and demand, uncontrolled events such as unexpected high demand and sick calls are intrinsic to the health care environment. Key to effective staffing are protocols and processes for daily staffing decision support that are aligned with a budget-sensitive variable staffing plan. In a decentralized model, individual department managers and directors are responsible for daily staffing allocation. Units with decentralized staffing are typically units whereby volume and/or acuity may be most unpredictable and the nursing competencies are unique to that area (e.g., emergency department, labor and delivery, critical care). However, a decentralized model places the responsibility of staffing on managers, which may take them away from other duties and responsibilities.

In contrast, centralized staffing is filtered through a centralized staffing office, which maintains responsibility for ensuring adequate staffing for multiple units. Centralized staffing offers the benefit of being able to view supply and demand from an enterprise perspective. With patient acuity, nursing competencies, and available staff viewed across multiple units, staff can be optimized by increasing staff in one area and reducing staff in another to accommodate variable patient demand. Staffing protocols for obtaining supplemental staff can be standardized, such as procedures for using internal staff, per diems, and external sources (e.g., travelers and agency). The staffing office can relieve the nurse managers and/or charges nurses of the time-consuming administrative task of responding to sick calls and obtaining supplemental staff. In addition, the central staffing office provides a command center with protocols and information to manage disasters in which staff must be quickly obtained and deployed.

The downside to relying solely on a centralized staffing office is that it can become too remote from the unit, thus losing some of the intelligence that may be considered when making staffing decisions (Lauw & Gares, 2005). Combinations of centralized and decentralized models are most commonly used. Policies and procedures clearly define the roles and responsibilities and communication among areas. But as with any of these staffing models, the key to eliminating chaotic, last-minute staffing decisions is to move more of the staffing decisions and protocols to the near future, or next 2 to 3 days. Assessment and analysis of staffing needs in the near future provides more available options, including more competent staff, at optimal costs.

Computerized staffing systems play a pivotal role in providing a "single version of the truth" and providing decision support such as staffing variances across units, workload indicators, employee competencies, and decision costs. Information for staffing decisions must be readily available and accurate. Staffing systems serve as a communication tool for all staffing "stakeholders" including employees, unit managers, centralized staffing office, and executives. Staffing systems also offer automated open-shift management, which posts open shifts electronically to qualified staff. Protocols are provided as to which personnel are the best qualified and at the best cost to fill needed shifts. The staffing system measures and reports the staffing management performance at both the unit and organization level, providing staffing indicators as to the staffing effectiveness of the organization.

Access to nurses outside the unit to cover transient shortages is critical to meet last-minute, unplanned nurse shortages, such as sick calls, and high patient demand. Supplemental staffing resources, frequently referred to as the *staffing pool,* are defined as a group of nurses who supplement the core unit staffing. This includes per diem nurses, float pool nurses, part-time nurses desiring additional hours, seasonal nurses, agency nurses, and traveling nurses. The scope of clinical competency, pay rates, and contractual arrangements vary among these internal and external pools of nurses as well. For example, select nurses may be competent to work on all of the medical-surgical units, whereas other specialty nurses may be competent to work in only one area, such as labor and delivery, the emergency department, the dialysis unit, or the perioperative areas.

Supplemental staffing resource guidelines have to be established as to when supplemental resources may be assigned to a unit and what type of supplemental staffing resources may be used at each stage of the staffing process. These guidelines are designed to prevent depleting supplemental resources by using them for core staff coverage and, instead, to reserve them for unexpected intervals of high need. A guideline example may be to first fill a sick call with a part-time nurse who has signed up to work extra shifts, then to use a supplemental float pool nurse, and then to use an external agency nurse if previous resources are unavailable. The costs associated with each resource progression are then inherently built into the staffing decision model. Additional strategies for covering long-term family medical leaves are also needed to meet core coverage. Still, strategies for covering these longer-term shortages are critical; otherwise, a manager is depleting the resource pools intended for last-minute and transient shortages.

Operational metrics for the supplemental resource pool not only are defined for daily staffing allocation but also may be defined during the scheduling stage. The operational total nurse vacancy rate for scheduling purposes is defined as all budgeted nurse positions that are vacant during the scheduling period, including the unfilled or vacant positions and positions for which nurses are on short-term or long-term leaves of absence (e.g., Family and Medical Leave Act [FMLA], workers' compensation) (Jones et al., 2005). For example, if a unit has an operational RN vacancy rate of 5% to 10%, it may be approved to cover the shortage with part-time nurses working additional shifts and possibly overtime but would not be approved for agency nurses. Alternatively, a unit with a 22% operational RN vacancy rate may be approved for the higher agency labor expense. Defining operational vacancy rates and budgeting for the vacancy coverage are important aspects of cost-effectively managing staff shortages. As such, protocols driven by operational vacancy rates generate consistency in how higher labor costs are aligned with the greatest need. In addition, wages, benefits, transfer, and work policies of supplemental internal float pools should be carefully designed so that the stability of unit-based core nursing staff is not compromised.

Caregiver Assignments

Nurse managers are responsible not only for forthcoming schedules and immediate staffing but also for ensuring that the "assignments reflect appropriate utilization of personnel, considering scope of practice, competencies, patient/client/resident needs and complexity of care" (ANA, 2004, p. 9). The caregiver assignment is defined as the task of assigning the scheduled staff to specific patients for the shift duration. Nurse managers typically delegate assignment making to the charge nurse on the inpatient nursing units, as well as managing the flow of patient admissions, discharges, and transfers during their shift (ANA, 2004; Sherman, 2005). The charge nurse is responsible for matching the qualified caregivers to meet the patients' needs and for providing a balanced workload across caregivers. Often the nursing care delivery model articulates the value for nurse-to-patient continuity across time; thus access to the previous 48 hours of caregiver assignments facilitates providing continuity of care. A balanced workload enables nurses to provide reasonable equity in nursing care delivery to patients and their families. In addition, the staff members expect the charge nurse to create equitable assignments as a valued measure of fairness in workload distribution. Many organizations require an annual charge nurse competency demonstrating effective assignment making.

Those making caregiver assignments must know the patient acuity, family/visitor situation, and scheduled patient events such as tests or procedures that require RN care and accompaniment off the unit. The charge nurse must know the staff experience and competencies and the patient preferences. The staff competencies may range from simple, in which all staff possess every competency, to very complex, in which only a select few possess every competency because of the cost of maintaining competencies or because of the scarcity of credentialed nurses. Foresight and access to timely information regarding planned and unplanned admission, discharges, and transfers are equally critical for the charge nurse to avoid patients having to wait for care and certain caregivers being overloaded.

Proper assignments also consider staff in orientation, nursing students needing appropriate nurse preceptors, and the number of licensed practical nurses/licensed vocational nurses (LPNs/LVNs) and UAP to appropriate RN staff. Effective staff assignments aggregate patients assigned to each nurse in physical proximity yet maintain workload balance. This proximity fosters patient observation and nurse availability and increases nurse efficiency by limiting walking distances. Also, infectious disease factors relate to staff nurses assignments (e.g., chickenpox and pregnancy). The data requirement for caregiver assignments and values related to continuity, equity, and balance are evolving in complexity and often challenge highly experienced charge nurses. Charge nurses now may benefit from caregiver assignment technology that provides key patient, staff, and environmental information and supports effective assignment decision making. A side benefit of using automated technology to make effective caregiver assignments is fast storage and retrieval that meets the 3-year archive requirement for TJC and related requirements of the state for public reporting of staffing.

In the staffing management framework, the caregiver assignment is the point at which individual patient outcomes can be measured as to whether adequate staffing and adequate knowledge and skill were provided to facilitate the patient to his or her next level of wellness or contributed to an adverse event. Furthermore, quality indicators such as those sensitive to nursing care identified in the National Database for Nursing Quality Indicators (NDNQI) and patient and staff satisfaction surveys provide feedback regarding staffing effectiveness.

LEADERSHIP & MANAGEMENT BEHAVIORS

Leadership Behaviors

- Integrates hospital mission, values, strategic goals, and care delivery model attributes into staffing management
- Integrates staffing legislation, regulations, and professional recommendations into staffing management
- Advocates for technology to support nursing staffing management
- Involves staff members in staffing management
- Develops leader knowledge and expertise related to staffing management
- Designs systematic methods to evaluate patient, financial, and organizational outcomes

Management Behaviors

- Forecasts workload, creates staffing patterns, and manages position control
- Provides staff self-scheduling within unit and organizational guidelines
- Integrates demand management and patient acuity data into daily resource planning
- Allocates staffing resources and supplemental resources effectively
- Assigns caregivers to patients for the provision of safe, competent, and quality care
- Evaluates staffing effectiveness and recommends changes as necessary

Overlap Areas

- Creates and manages a safe staffing environment
- Balances staffing needs with financial pressures

ORGANIZATIONAL OUTCOMES AND STAFFING

Staffing Effectiveness

Hospital organizations examine the relationships between staffing and nurse-sensitive outcomes to meet TJC staffing effectiveness requirements. In TJC human resources standards (TJC, 2006):

> Staffing effectiveness is defined as the number, competency and skill mix of staff in relation to the provision of needed care and treatment. Effective staffing has been linked to positive patient outcomes and improved quality and safety of care. This standard is designed to help healthcare organizations determine and continuously improve the effectiveness of their nurse staffing (including registered nurses, licensed practical nurses and nursing assistants or aides) through an objective evidenced-based approach. (HR-6)

This standard describes the required data collection of clinical quality and human resource indicators, analysis, trending over time, and subsequent improvement plans as deemed appropriate.

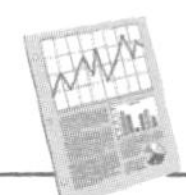

Research Note

Source: Kane, R., Shamliyan, T., Mueller, C., Duval, S., & Wilt, T. (2007b). The association of registered nurse staffing levels and patient outcomes. *Medical Care, 45*(12), 1195-1204.

Purpose

The purpose of this study was to examine the associations between RN staffing and patient outcomes in acute care hospitals among 96 eligible research studies published between 1990 and 2006. A systematic literature review and meta-analysis was conducted as part of a larger study by the Agency for Healthcare Research and Quality (AHRQ). A meta-analysis is a statistical method of analyzing the outcomes across similar studies and, in this case, serves to synthesize what is known about the association between staffing and patient outcomes.

Discussion

Of the potential 2858 studies, 96 studies were included after the inclusion criteria were applied. The independent variables of interest included RN-to-patient ratios and RN full-time equivalents (FTEs) per patient day, and the dependent variables included patient-nurse sensitive outcomes. The evidence indicated that there is a statistically and clinically significant relationship between RN staffing and hospital-related mortality, failure to rescue, and many other patient outcomes. These findings were also consistent in surgical patients and in intensive care units (ICUs). *Failure to rescue* is defined as the number of deaths in patients with adverse occurrences divided by the number who developed adverse occurrences. The patient outcomes included hospital-acquired pneumonia, pulmonary failure, unplanned extubation, increased length of stay, cardiopulmonary resuscitation, and nosocomial bloodstream infections. This analysis supported the previous findings that increased nursing staffing in hospitals is associated with improvements in patient care outcomes. The primary independent variable was a measure of the volume of nursing care, tempered by nurse training levels. Differences in the nurse work environments at both the unit and hospital levels also influenced this relationship.

Application to Practice

The findings of this AHRQ-funded study support the need for continued rigorous attention among nurse leaders at every level of the hospital organization to staffing management and adequacy, nurse education and continuing education, and creating positive work environments. Nursing leadership in these areas is critical to the quality and safety of patient care.

In the staffing effectiveness standard, a list of 34 approved nursing-sensitive outcome screening indicators is provided in the following categories: patient satisfaction/complaints; clinical (e.g., urinary tract infections); National Quality Forum (NQF) measures (e.g., falls with injury); and human resource indicators (e.g., overtime, staff vacancy, turnover) (TJC, 2006). Potter and colleagues (2003) described their application of these requirements at Barnes-Jewish Hospital in St. Louis to provide baseline data to evaluate the effect of future changes in care delivery and staffing. For example their investigation revealed that predictive modeling can forecast unplanned patient and staff events, such as admissions by day of week and unplanned sick calls (Warner, 2006); thus as the RN hours decreased, the patients' perception of pain increased.

Many nursing organizations achieve this standard through membership in the NDNQI and submit quarterly data for analysis and benchmarking services. The NDNQI is an official quality database management organization for the ANA administrated by the University of Kansas, School of Nursing. The analyses of the effect of staffing variables on nursing outcomes also provide organizations with robust evidence toward Magnet™ designation, a national honor of excellence awarded by the American Nurses Credentialing Center (ANCC), also an ANA organization for excellence in nursing care of patients and families and in the work environment.

Evaluating the nurse satisfaction and its influence on nursing turnover are two of TJC human resource and NDNQI indicators. The NDNQI offers nurse satisfaction, turnover, and other survey measurements. An additional survey relevant to staffing management is the Decisional Involvement Scale (DIS) by Havens and Vasey (2003). It is an easy-to-use survey instrument, well liked by staff nurses, that measures nurses' satisfaction with their involvement in decision making and has a specific item regarding satisfaction with input into staffing and scheduling processes. Use of this tool is an excellent method of integrating research into shared governance structures by engaging nurses in meaningful ways. An ultimately critical factor, nurse turnover measurement and associated organizational costs, is well explicated by Jones (Jones, 2004; Jones & Gates, 2007) to assist organizations in managing turnover. The link between staffing levels and retention is important to consider because turnover is costly; the cost to replace one RN is estimated to range between $62,100 and $67,100 (Jones, 2005).

Evidence of Staffing on Outcomes: Staffing Matters

The effect of adequate staffing on positive patient and organizational outcomes is well documented by scientific evidence. A crucial role for chief nursing executives, directors of nursing, and nurse managers is to articulate and execute strategies in the hospital organization to help ensure adequate staffing to promote safe, high-quality patient, staff, and organizational outcomes. Balancing these decisions with and conducting cost-effectiveness analyses is the current challenge for organizations and future research (Jones & Mark, 2005; Pappas, 2007). Comprehensive reviews of staffing evidence and sentinel works are not presented here but are available elsewhere (Aiken et al., 2001; Aiken et al., 2002; Aiken et al., 2003; Needleman et al., 2002; Needleman et al., 2006; Unruh, 2008). These studies, literature reviews, and a recent meta-analysis by Kane and colleagues (2007a, b) demonstrate the strong evidence linking inadequate staffing with adverse events and failure to rescue.

New evidence in staffing management builds upon what little is known about the effect of supplemental staffing, the California-mandated staffing ratios, and nurses' participation in unions. Aiken and colleagues (2007) examined the characteristics of supplemental nurses and the relationships of the supplemental staff to nurse outcomes and adverse events. Their findings suggest that widely held negative perceptions of temporary nurses may be unfounded. Both national and the state of Pennsylvania RN survey data in 2000 showed that an estimated 6% of hospital staff were employed by supplemental staffing agencies. The supplemental nurses were equally, if not more, educated than the permanent staff, and the supplemental nurses were not associated with a negative impact on quality-of-care indicators. In 2007, the PricewaterhouseCoopers report indicated a 5% use of supplemental staffing of the total nursing hours, and executives surveyed predict this trend will continue to sustain operations.

Donaldson and colleagues (2005) presented one of the first studies evaluating the impact of California's Assembly Bill 394 mandating staffing ratios at the unit level in 68 hospitals. The California Nursing Outcomes Coalition (CalNOC) examined 268 patient care units including medical, surgical, and observational units. The RN increase as a percentage of total hours was validated from 57% to 65% RN for an overall compliance with the new regulation. This also represents a 20.8% increase in RN hours per patient day. Data validation of ratios was not available at the shift level per unit. The increase in RN staffing was not associated with a significant reduction in patient falls or pressure ulcers. The authors suggested that further research is needed to complement the staffing measure with other multi-factorial factors known to reduce the incidence of falls and pressure ulcers.

Finally, there is little known about the impact of nurse union participation on quality of care. Seago and Ash (2002) explored the relationship between RN union status and outcomes for one cardiac patient population using the California Hospital Disclosure Report database in which 35% of California hospitals have nursing unions. The significant study finding among the sample of 343 hospitals was that hospitals with nursing unions have a 5.7% lower mortality rate for patients with acute myocardial infarction (AMI), while controlling for relevant patient and organizational factors, including staff hours. These scientists raise the question for future research regarding the explicit mechanisms within union participation that affect patient outcomes, such as possible work environmental factors (e.g., stability, autonomy, and collaboration with physicians) that may have implications for all nurse executives.

In summary, the rich body of staffing evidence continues to build upon what is known about the profound effect of RN staffing on safety, quality, and cost of patient care delivery. Nurse executives and leaders at all levels must incorporate relevant scientific findings, the evidence base for practice, into staffing administrative policy and practice and lead the evaluation of all innovations in care delivery. Health care services researchers with interest in staffing management are guided by a research agenda for future quality and safety, cost-effectiveness, and delivery of care generated by national experts (Jones & Mark, 2005).

CURRENT ISSUES AND TRENDS

Nursing care, for the most part, is reported as a hospital expense and frequently cited as representing two thirds or more of hospital labor costs. Nursing is not viewed as important to hospital revenue generation. Because nurses represent the largest personnel budget line of hospital operations, they are the target of labor reduction strategies, and this too-often occurs without an evaluation of the effect on patients or the staff morale and turnover. With the advent of pay-for-performance (P4P) and forthcoming Centers for Medicaid & Medicare Services' (CMS) provision 1533-F, this paradigm of "nurses as expense" is likely to change. CMS provides health care coverage for 80 million Americans for Medicaid, Medicare, and state children's programs and represents the largest payer in the world, administering $800 billion in benefits per year. CMS (2009, p. 1) stated, "Quality based purchasing, also known as pay-for-performance (P4P), is a quality improvement and reimbursement methodology which is aimed at moving towards payments that create much stronger financial support for patient focused, high value care."

Since CMS provision 1533-F became effective October 1, 2008, hospitals are not being reimbursed for hospital-acquired conditions (HACs)—that is, conditions such as skin pressure ulcers, urinary tract infection, ventilator-acquired pneumonia, and falls with injury that occurred within the hospital stay and were not present on admission (POA).

Among the 14 HACs in the provision, at least 9 of the conditions are sensitive to nursing care intervention. Thus hospitals will have new financial incentives to support both nursing education and appropriate staffing to prevent HACs and increase reimbursement.

The PricewaterhouseCoopers report *What Works: Healing the Healthcare Staffing Shortage* suggested the following (2007):

> Rainmaker roles may change for hospitals. Employment changes and [P4P] reimbursement may combine to flip the workforce dynamic in hospitals. Traditionally physicians were rainmakers who brought in revenue and nurses were overhead. Through new, [P4P] programs that focus on clinical quality and patient satisfaction, nurses will have a significant impact on the key metrics that will drive reimbursement updates. (p. 2)

Furthermore, there are national policy initiatives to identify and make visible nursing care in the U.S. health care reimbursement system. Historically, nursing care has been bundled within the "room-and-board" hospital charges, which do not capture the variability in nursing care costs (Thompson & Diers, 1985). Given the variability in nursing care intensity and cost of nurse staffing, this traditional costing system has resulted in cost compression and distortion in the current inpatient prospective payment system (Dalton, 2007). A proposed solution separates nursing care from the room and board charges and accounts for this care as a variable, direct cost within the billing system based on actual nursing time delivered to patients (Welton, 2007; Welton & Harris, 2007; Welton et al., 2006). This proposal has generated national dialogue among health care leaders with CMS that would make nursing care visible as part of reimbursement reform.

In the summer of 2007, the Robert Wood Johnson Foundation and the Rutgers Center for State Health Policy sponsored an Economics of Nursing Invitational Conference attended by key national health care leaders (Unruh & Hassmiller, 2007). At this conference, three questions were discussed: (1) How we can make a business case for improving nursing care? (2) Should public and private payers specifically account for the intensity of nursing care? And if so, how? and (3) What are the challenges and directions for nurses in P4P? Several significant policy recommendations emerged, and members committed to follow-action. The current issues in health care policy raise the visibility and importance of nursing care in our society and may not only illuminate nurses as rainmakers but also stimulate organizational, state, and federal incentives that support safe, high-quality nursing care for all.

Summary

- Staffing management in nursing and its complex terminology are defined and described in the broader context of health care safety, quality, and cost.
- A conceptual framework for staffing management is presented.
- The ANA and other professional nursing societies provide valuable recommendations for nurse staffing.
- The recent rapid enactment of state legislation for nursing staffing plans, direct-care staff involvement, and acuity methodologies have significant impact on staffing management.
- Numerous strategies for forecasting workload are available to generate staffing patterns, position control, and schedules with significant staff input.
- New methodologies for demand management and patient acuity will greatly assist leaders in predicting and cost-effectively managing patient care.
- The complexity and importance of caregiver assignments will continue to evolve the use of technology to ensure consistency within the care delivery model accounting for competency, continuity, fairness, and balanced workload.
- A body of evidence is growing regarding the effect of staffing on patients', financial, and organization outcomes.
- Nurses have an opportunity in new CMS regulations to become rainmakers in health care.

CASE STUDY

Susan Smith is the new nurse manager of a large surgical intensive care unit (SICU). When she began her new job, she was faced with constant last-minute staffing shortages requiring excessive overtime and agency use. Nursing staff were working multiple overlapping shift lengths to fill the continual shortages. Staff morale was low with high turnover and high absenteeism, and organizational loyalty was lacking among the nursing staff. Nurse Smith visited nearby intensive care units and collaborated with colleagues looking for best practices to stabilize the unit's staffing.

Based on her findings, Nurse Smith first analyzed her core coverage and developed a staffing pattern that met forecasted patient care needs. She determined that overlapping shifts did not provide balanced coverage during a 24-hour period and developed a staffing pattern using 12-hour shifts. She then converted her staffing pattern to full-time positions to determine whether the current and open positions provided the unit-based staff needed to cover a 4-week schedule. The position control showed that the budgeted unit position, if filled, did provide the total positions needed to schedule and staff the unit. However, based on the literature review, Nurse Smith decided to convert some of the full-time positions to part-time to provide more flexibility in scheduling. With a high vacancy, Nurse Smith consulted and worked with the human resources department to develop new strategies for recruiting ICU nurses and for obtaining ICU competency certification for a core group in the organization's supplemental resource pool. She also obtained budget authorization to obtain two full-time ICU travel nurses for a 2-month interval, which was less costly than agency use. This also helped establish full unit-based coverage for the initial schedule until the vacant positions were filled.

Nurse Smith surveyed the current nurses to determine satisfaction with current staffing and ideas for improvement. She determined two consistent findings among the staff. The first finding was that nurses described being stressed by high workload demands and left with a feeling of not providing adequate care. A unit-based committee was formed to evaluate patient care assignments and developed a standard procedure for ensuring workload assignments were manageable and safe. Improved communication with the operating room for transfers into the unit provided better planning for scheduled admissions, preventing episodes of high nursing intensity with admissions. Protocols were established for when workloads were exceeding unit-based standards for safe, quality care.

The second finding was that nurses were tired of the excessive calls to their homes to sign up for extra shifts. By using best practices from other units, staffing decisions were moved from last-minute to evaluating staffing 2 to 3 days in advance. By using new computer technology, open shifts were posted in advance for staff to sign up for extra shifts. Staff also provided their availability to fill shifts on short notice so that only those nurses who were available were called. Staff found they were willing to sign up for availability if it prevented the last-minute unexpected calls. The result of this forward-looking planning was consistent with the literature noting that nurses want control over their work schedule and the ability to balance work with their lifestyle.

Within 3 months, vacant positions were filled and the supplemental travelers were no longer required to fill core staffing. Agency usage was eliminated, and overtime decreased. Initial schedules were posted only with all shifts filled. ICU-competent nurses from the supplemental resource pool were used only to fill last-minute sick calls. A second nursing survey was conducted that showed increase in staff satisfaction, which also had a positive impact on nursing turnover.

CRITICAL THINKING EXERCISE

Nurse Manager Susan Klein is preparing annual goals for her upcoming one-on-one meeting with her pediatric director of nursing. Susan has been the nurse manager on the 30-bed neonatal intensive care unit (NICU) in an academic medical center for the past 7 years. Two years ago, her hospital was awarded Magnet™ recognition, but this past year there has been some union organizing activity among the nurses in the medical-surgical areas. She examined her past fiscal year administrative data: average patient LOS exceeded budget by 1.7 days; 16 patients were diverted to surrounding hospitals because of full capacity; family satisfaction with infant care scores remained >95%. With an 85% response rate, nurse satisfaction dropped in the areas of satisfaction with their schedule and available UAP support and the labor budget was on target after adjustment for high volume and acuity.

1. What are the opportunities for the nurse manager in the upcoming year?
2. What information does the nurse manager, case manager, and staff nurses need?
3. In what ways could the staff be involved?
4. What neonate (patient) and family issues are involved?
5. What staffing management issues are involved?
6. What clinical, financial, and organizational outcomes might demonstrate improvement?

29 Collective Bargaining

Karen W. Budd

CHAPTER OBJECTIVES

- Understand collective bargaining and its relationship to nurse leaders and managers
- Define and describe terms related to collective bargaining and nursing leadership and management
- Chronicle the history of U.S. collective bargaining legislation and its impact on nursing
- Examine the process of collective bargaining in relation to the tension that often develops between unionized nurses and their managers
- Analyze ways and means to lessen the tension between unionized nurses and their management/leadership team
- Exercise critical thinking to conceptualize and analyze possible solutions to a practice exercise

Since the late 1960s, nurse managers and staff nurses alike increasingly have found themselves either directly or indirectly involved in collective bargaining issues. Collective bargaining consists of a process of negotiations between the management of an organization and a group of employees, typically represented by a labor union. Management and employees negotiate over terms and conditions of employment, attempting to reach agreement on items employees believe to be fair and management believes it can live with in terms of the organization's operational needs and financial resources. The negotiated terms and conditions of employment are spelled out in a *collective bargaining agreement.* The collective bargaining process is governed by federal and state laws, administrative agency regulations, and judicial decisions. Where the federal law and state law overlap, federal law usually prevails (Legal Information Institute [LII]: Wex, 2007a, b).

Attention to collective bargaining and unions has intensified in nursing (DeMoro, 2007). Nursing is in the midst of a shortage that likely is a result of the work redesign, downsizing, closures, reengineering, altering staff mix, and takeovers that began to occur in the health care delivery system in the early 1990s (Porter-O'Grady, 1992). Such rapid change created untenable working conditions, threatened nurses' job security and benefits, and sparked unionizing drives (AJN Headlines, 1993). Collective bargaining was found to be an important tool by which staff nurse employees, as a collective, could balance the power of their employer and negotiate an improvement in wages, benefits, and working conditions (Clark et al., 2000).

The firm belief and position taken by most union members is that "even if an employer is in a position to pay higher wages and benefits and to improve working conditions, many employers will not do so unless forced to do so, directly or indirectly, by a strong union" (Rainsberger, (2006b, §20). Despite the fact that more nurses are being employed than ever before (Lovell, 2006), the shortage is predicted to continue at least until 2020 (Auerbach et al., 2007). Thus collective bargaining likely will continue to be used as a tool by staff nurses to gain control over their work environment. If they are to be effective, nurse managers must be well-informed about the process and their relationship to it.

DEFINITIONS

The lexicon of terms associated with collective bargaining is long and specific. Some of these terms have a precise meaning that is defined by law and is specific to the rules and regulations of collective bargaining activities. For example, the National Labor Relations Board (NLRB) provides definitions of terms in its guide to the National Labor Relations Act (NLRA) (NLRB, 1997). The following definitions are part of the collective bargaining terminology:

- *Arbitration (interest):* The use of an impartial third party(s) to arrive at a solution to a dispute between parties concerning the contents of a collective bargaining agreement. The decision of the arbitrator(s) is usually, but not always, binding on the parties at interest.
- *Arbitration (grievance):* The use of an impartial third party(s) to settle a dispute between the parties to a collective bargaining agreement as to the meaning and application of certain language in the bargaining agreement. The decision of the arbitrator(s) is usually, but not always, binding on the parties to the collective bargaining agreement.
- *Bargaining agent/representative:* The organization selected by employees in a bargaining unit, under regulations of the appropriate labor agency, to represent exclusively the employees in that unit in all negotiations with their employer. This pertains to all parts of the employment relationship mandated by the applicable state or federal statutes. Frequently the local bargaining agent/representative will be affiliated with a national or international bargaining agent/representative.
- *Bargaining unit:* The employees or jobs that are joined together as a group by the authorized agency (NLRB or a state labor agency) for purposes of bargaining collectively with the employer. The appropriate labor agency determines that certain employees or jobs have a commonality that supports the negotiation of one contract agreement to cover their employment relationships with the employer.
- *Certification:* The official designation by the appropriate labor agency of a bargaining agent/representative as the exclusive representative of employees in a bargaining unit concerning matters of employment that are required to be negotiated between management and that agent/representative.
- ***Collective bargaining:*** The process used by representatives of an employer and the certified bargaining agent/representative for a group of employees to reduce to writing and sign an agreement covering terms of employment that are either mandated or allowed by applicable state or federal law.
- *Contract:* The written agreement between the employees in a bargaining unit and the employer concerning some or all of the conditions of employment applicable to any or all of the employees in the bargaining unit.
- *Good faith bargaining:* The performance of the mutual obligation of the employer and the representative of the employees to meet at reasonable times and confer in good faith with respect to wages, hours, and other terms and conditions of employment specified under the applicable state or federal law. This obligation does not compel either party to agree to a proposal or to make a concession.
- *Grievance:* The allegation by an employee or employees or certified bargaining agent/representative that management has violated the collective bargaining agreement (contract) between the parties.
- *Grievance procedure:* A written plan outlining the actions to be taken by both the employees and their certified bargaining agent/representative and the employer to adjust a grievance. This plan usually involves progressive steps through the employer's administrative structure that end with external arbitration (if agreement is not reached internally).
- *Impasse:* A deadlock in negotiations between management and employee representatives over the terms and conditions of employment specified by the appropriate state or federal law.

- *Management rights:* Policies or practices that the applicable national or state collective bargaining law says are not subject to negotiation.
- *Mandatory bargaining items:* Policies or practices that the applicable national or state collective bargaining law says management *must* negotiate with its employees' agent/representative.
- *Mediation:* The use of a neutral third party to facilitate negotiations between management and the bargaining agent/representative.
- *Non-mandatory bargaining items:* Policies or practices that the applicable national or state collective bargaining law says management *may* negotiate with its employees' agent/representative.
- *Prohibited bargaining items:* Policies or practices that the applicable national or state collective bargaining law, or other law, says management *may not* negotiate with its employees' agent/representative.
- *Unfair labor practice:* An allegation made by an individual, an employer, or a labor organization of a violation of the applicable state or federal law concerning bargaining.

BACKGROUND

The National Labor Relations Act

The main body of law for collective bargaining in private industry, including the health care industry, is the Wagner Act or National Labor Relations Act (NLRA), which was enacted in 1935. Under the NLRA, or *labor's bill of rights,* employees have the right to organize, to engage in collective bargaining, and to strike. Employers cannot (1) interfere with employees' collective bargaining; (2) try to influence the employees' union; (3) refuse to bargain collectively in "good faith"; and (4) attempt to discriminate against the union (Wagner, 2002). To engage in any of these activities is to engage in an *unfair labor practice (ULP).*

Since enactment of the NLRA, the matter of labor's relationship with management, both as individual workers and as collectives represented by unions, has been governed by federal law and, increasingly over the years, by state law. The labor-management relationship also is governed by rules and decisions from regulatory agencies, at both the federal and the state level. In circumstances of conflict between federal and individual state requirements, typically the federal requirements supersede those of an individual state.

National Labor Relations Act Amendments

Two major amendments have been made to the NLRA. Believing the provisions of the NLRA were too heavily weighted in favor of labor, Congress first amended it in 1947 (the Taft-Hartley Act). This amendment, referred to as the *slave labor bill* by labor leaders, allowed the President to appoint a board of inquiry when a strike was judged to be a danger to national health or safety. The Taft-Hartley Act also added a list of ULPs targeted at labor that balanced the NRLA's list of ULPs directed at unfair management practices (Wagner, 2002). (See Box 29.1 for a sample of labor and management ULPs.)

LEADING AND MANAGING DEFINED

Collective Bargaining

The process used by representatives of an employer and the certified bargaining agent/representative for a group of employees to reduce to writing and sign an agreement covering terms of employment that are either mandated or allowed by applicable state or federal law.

Collective Action

Action, such as mass resignations, taken by employees or professional organization groups to bring about changes in terms of employment.

Box 29.1

Unfair Labor Practices

Committed by Employers

- **Threatening** employees with loss of jobs or benefits, or interfering with, restraining, coercing, or retaliating against employees if they join or vote for a union or engage in union activity (e.g., management cannot dominate a labor organization or threaten to close down the entire employment operation)
- **Interrogating** employees about their opinion, current activity, or future intentions pertaining to union activity if this is intended to restrain or coerce the employees
- **Promising** wage increases or benefits to employees to discourage their union support
- **Spying** on employees by having "friendly" employees attend meetings and report back

Committed by Employees/Unions

- **Force** or violence on the picket line, or in connection with a strike
- **Mass picketing** in such numbers that non-striking employees are physically barred from entering the premises
- **Threats** to employees who oppose the union that they will lose their jobs if the union wins a majority or unless they support the union's activities (even though they are non-union members of the bargaining unit)
- **Illegal representation** by entering into an agreement with an employer who recognizes the union as the exclusive bargaining representative when it has not been chosen by a majority of the employees
- **Fining or expelling** members for:
  - Filing ULP charges with the board or for participating in an investigation conducted by the board
  - Crossing a picket line that is unlawful under the NLRA or that violates a no-strike agreement
  - Crossing a picket line after they resigned from the union

Adapted from National Labor Relations Board (NLRB). (1997). Basic guide to the National Labor Relations Act: General principles of law and procedures of the National Labor Relations Board. Washington, DC: U.S. Government Printing Office, pp. 27-28, 40.

Then, 26 years later after the NRLA was enacted, an amendment of particular importance to nurses was passed. When the NLRA was enacted, not-for-profit hospitals were excluded from the law. In 1974, Congress extended the coverage of the Act to private not-for-profit hospitals and nursing homes. For the first time, these employees, including RNs, could engage in federally protected labor union activity. Nurses now were allowed to bargain collectively over wages, hours, and other terms and conditions of employment.

Private Versus Public Institutions

Although nurses work in both privately owned and publicly owned institutions, different laws and regulations apply, depending on the ownership structure. In the private sector, employees typically are under the jurisdiction of the NLRA, and the NLRB is the governing agency responsible for administering the law. The NLRB conducts representation elections, certifies the results, and serves as a deterrent to ULPs by both employers and unions. The processes of the NLRB are begun only when requested.

In the public sector, employees routinely are under the jurisdiction of a state labor agency. State laws and agencies frequently are patterned after the federal approach, but many states have adopted a narrower view of the employment relationship, which must be bargained by employers with their organized employees. Most of the state statutes permitting collective bargaining for public employees have been enacted since the late 1970s. One exception to the rules for public sector employees is the U.S. Department of Veterans Affairs (VA). These employees, along with other federal public sector employees, are governed by the Federal Service Labor-Management Relations Statute (FSLMRS), which is administered by the Federal Labor Relations Authority (FRLA).

Unionizing Activities of Nurses

The question of whether it is professional for nurses to take collective action associated with unionizing has been a source of tension within nursing throughout much of the twentieth century and continues to the present (McNeese-Smith, 2006). The use of collective bargaining by blue collar workers and the aggressive, strong-arm tactics of union organizers may be some underlying reasons for the tension. Inherent in the term "professional" are the characteristics of specialized, higher education; autonomy to practice the learned specialized skills; and compensation as determined by the professional for the performance of the specialized skills (Jacox, 1971). Indeed, the struggle to be identified as a profession rather than an occupation was the motivation in 1911 for organizing the American Nurses Association (ANA) from the Nurses' Associated Alumnae and the American Society of Superintendents of Training School for Nurses (Flanagan, 1976).

The American Nurses Association and Collective Action

As a professional association, the ANA had a dual mission to fulfill, which was to "work for the welfare of the community and for the welfare of members of the profession" (Jacox, 1971, p. 241). These dual foci involved defining safe and effective autonomous practice and then developing a code of ethics that demonstrated the boundaries of the nurse's professional practice with a client. In return for control over practice, society expected nurses "to ensure that their practice [was] safe" (Jacox, 1971, p. 243).

Nurses, however, always have been employed in hierarchical organizations in which, although they may have some degree of practice autonomy, they are constrained by the rules of the employer. As a result, the employer rather than the nurse determines "the conditions under which he practices, how he practices, and how much he is paid" (Jacox, 1971, p. 251). Thus, in the interest of fulfilling its mission, the ANA has supported **collective action** throughout its history.

Although it did not have an economic security and general welfare program before World War II, ANA did promote equitable wages and conditions of employment for nurses. In 1941, the California Nurses Association, a constituent nursing association of ANA, successfully argued for a 15% increase in salaries for its members before the War Labor Board (Shepard, 2004). Prompted by this success, in 1945 the ANA appointed a committee to study collective bargaining on a national level. The first platform with planks reflecting interest in promoting the economic and general welfare of nurses was adopted in 1946 at the ANA Convention. Also adopted was a statement reflecting the position that the state and district associations should represent their memberships for collective bargaining (Ketter, 1996).

The Sixties

The late 1960s was productive for collective bargaining, after the issuance of an executive order by President John F. Kennedy in 1962 that protected the collective bargaining rights of nurses and others employed in federal hospitals. Large numbers of nurses organized, especially those working in VA hospitals. By 1969, the number of RNs under contract jumped from 8,000 to more than 30,000. The number tripled in the next 5 years, jumping to 90,000 (Forman, 1989).

Even in non-profit hospitals in which collective bargaining rights were not yet protected by the Taft-Hartley Act, nurses were taking collective action. In 1965, in Youngstown, Ohio, 60% of the nursing staff at one hospital were employed part-time and were given a 5-cent raise in contrast to the full-time nurses' 10-cent raise. When attempts to discuss the discrepancy with management fell on deaf ears, the part-time nurses contacted the Ohio Nurses Association (ONA), a constituent nursing association of ANA, for assistance. When, after months of waiting, the hospital would not recognize ONA as the nurses' official representative, 85% of the nursing staff submitted letters of resignation that were to be effective at the end of October, 1966 (Patton, 1998).

Each of the 335 letters stated, "We reserve the right to withdraw this resignation upon satisfaction that the Youngstown Hospital Association is willing to recognize and bargain with the Ohio State Nurses Association in a bona fide effort to establish conditions under which we can practice our profession in a responsible and honorable manner" (Shepard, 2004, p. 51). At the eleventh hour, the hospital did in fact agree to recognize ONA as the nurses' representative. When no agreement was reached after 10 weeks, however, the letters of resignation were re-submitted. The mass resignation lasted for 13 weeks until, with the assistance of a federal mediator, an agreement was reached (Patton, 1998).

The Seventies and Eighties

By 1972, more than 100 contracts had been negotiated by ANA constituent state nursing associations (Ketter, 1996). Collective bargaining issues continued to be prominent among nurses in the 1970s and into the 1980s, and unionization among nurses rose steadily even though the labor union influence as a whole in the United States began to diminish (Breda, 1997; Cutcher-Gershenfeld et al., 2007). As advocates for patients, nurses looked to the experience of skilled union negotiators to help them gain control of their practice.

In 1984, the Minnesota Nurses Association (MNA), representing 6000 nurses in 17 hospitals of the Twin Cities, led a 39-day strike against the hospitals, which were represented by Health Employers, Inc. (HEI). The overt issues involved layoffs, which were partly "due to changes in the Medicare reimbursement structure (DRGs), and the application of seniority" (Minnesota Nurses Association, 2008, § 78). In the view of LaTourneau, a physician (MD), and Hybben, a chief nursing officer (CNO) (LaTourneau & Hybben, 1990), the covert issues were the nurses' search for control over their practice and their strength in collective bargaining that had been building through the 1970s.

The hospitals responded to the strike by putting contingency plans in place whereby patients were discharged, non-urgent admissions were postponed, and employees were laid off as hospital capacity decreased. Physicians performed outpatient procedures and therapies in their offices. The hospitals continued to argue at the negotiating table that cost-containment constraints were insurmountable, and after 39 days, the MNA settled at the same package offered before the strike. On the surface, the strike had accomplished very little for the nurses. Through the next years, outpatient procedures put in place during the strike increased and hospital days and RN jobs decreased. Upon reflection, however, LaTourneau and Hybben (1990) described intangible accomplishments of the strike as follows:

> The corporate cultures during the strike shifted from one based on structural authority to one that required situational competence, openness, and acceptance.... Communication became important for recognition, as well as for information sharing. A person who could identify the key questions became as important as those who could answer them. There was a strong diverse work force emerging that demanded to be heard. (§ 9)

The Nineties

In the 1990s, unionization of nurses experienced a strong up-swing in response to (1) redesign of the health care work environment by administrators and fiscal consultants and (2) lack of support by nurse leaders who implemented the work redesign programs. The major sources of conflict were and continue to be issues of nurses' economic welfare, staffing ratios, mandatory overtime, floating, and governance. Work redesign created a dramatic alteration in staff mix by drastically reducing the number of RNs caring for patients and increasing the use of non-nurse assistive personnel. Nurses argued that such externally induced rapid changes compromised patient safety (Buerhaus et al., 2007). Administrators and consultants argued that nurses wanted merely to save their jobs rather than to assist the fiscal needs of the organization.

Support for Nurses' Patient Safety Argument

Several landmark reports and studies have been released since work redesign began that support nurses' allegations that substituting RNs with unlicensed assistive personnel was dangerous to patients (e.g., Aiken et al., 2002; Institute of Medicine, 2004; Needleman et al., 2002). For instance, Aiken and colleagues (2002) clearly demonstrated the link between low RN staffing and poor patient outcomes. Based on a sample of 10,000 nurses and 230,000 patients in 168 Pennsylvania hospitals from 1998 to 1999, they found that each additional patient assigned to a nurse resulted in a 7% increase in 30-day patient mortality and a 7% increase in failure-to-rescue rate. Furthermore, when nurses had eight patients instead of four, their patients had a 31% higher chance of dying within 30 days of admission.

Despite evidence to the contrary, however, nurses continue to find lack of support from hospital administrators and other health care team members for linking poor patient outcomes to an unsafe RN-to-patient ratio and an unsafe RN work environment created by policies such as mandatory overtime. In a national survey of RNs, MDs, CNOs, and chief executive officers (CEOs), Buerhaus and colleagues (2007) asked whether the nursing shortage was of concern. Although the majority of the sample did respond that the shortage was very concerning, 32% of the CEOs, 25% of the CNOs, and 19% of the MDs perceived there was no shortage as compared with 13% of the RN respondents. Nevertheless, of those responding that the shortage was of concern, significantly fewer MDs and CEOs than RNs and CNOs thought the shortage was a problem for nurses' ability to maintain patient safety and for the quality of nurses' work life.

UNIONS REPRESENTING NURSES

Stressed, discouraged, dissatisfied nurses look to unions and collective bargaining as a means to gain control over their work environment. Unions respond by aggressively seeking out RNs to strengthen their organizations. In 2007, 19.4% of employed RNs were union members compared with 16.4% in 1983 (Hirsch & Macpherson, 2008).

The largest RN union is the United American Nurses (UAN), which was established in 1999 as a separate affiliate of ANA. In 2001, it also became an affiliate of the AFL-CIO. Its membership comprises ANA members whose local units are organized by the relevant constituent state associations and whose financial support comes from the dues of those members. Another RN union is CNA/NNOC. The California Nurses Association (CNA) split off from the ANA in 1995 and then went national in 2004 as the National Nurses Organizing Committee (NNOC). The vision of CNA/NNOC, which has energized an aggressive national organizing campaign, is "CNA/NNOC contract standards coast to coast" (DeMoro, 2007, p. 26).

The UAN and CNA/NNOC are just two of many unions that represent RNs in their work. The other major health care workers' union is the Service Employees International Union (SEIU) District 1199, which originally started as a union to represent pharmacists and then health care workers other than RNs. It now also represents RNs through its Nurse Alliance of SEIU, which is within the renamed *SEIU Healthcare*.

Non–health care unions also represent RNs. For example, some RNs are represented by traditional trade unions such as the Teamsters, the United Auto Workers, a grocery workers union, or even a meatpackers union. In 2006, seven non-RN AFL-CIO unions and the UAN created an Industrial Coordinating Committee (ICC) called "RNs Working Together." The seven unions are the American Federation of State, County and Municipal Employees; the American Federation of Teachers; the Communications Workers of America; the American Federation of Government Employees; the United Steelworkers; the Office and Professional Employees International Union; and the United Auto Workers (Genovese, 2006). The purpose of the ICC is to pool resources so that issues important to nurses such as "staffing, workplace safety, and professional practice" can be addressed with the voice of close to 200,000 nurses (Genovese, 2006, §5).

As the first decade of the new century nears an end, issues contributing to the nursing shortage that began in the mid-1990s continue on

Practical Tips

Tip #1: Engage in Self-Reflection

Think through your position of whether nurses who belong to unions are unprofessional. Then become informed about why nurses may take an opposite position. Try to understand the emotions involved. Understanding brings the ability first, to set aside your emotional response, and second, to focus your attention on determining the best leading and managing behaviors for the situation.

Tip #2: Become Knowledgeable About the Rules, and Stay Informed

If you are in a collective bargaining situation, become very familiar with the collective bargaining agreement. Make it visible to staff and other leaders that you are using it as a basis for relevant problem solving.

---

with little resolution. One such issue is that of an unsafe environment for nurses and their patients resulting from management decisions such as mandating nurses to work overtime. Although mandating work is perhaps the most easily understood violation, other poor management decisions also have left nurses out of the decisions that affect their practice and have resulted in staff nurses organizing for collective bargaining.

COLLECTIVE BARGAINING STRUCTURE, SCOPE, AND PROCESS

Collective bargaining is a legally prescribed *process* whereby management is compelled to negotiate conditions of employment with its employees. The outcome of the negotiations is a collective bargaining agreement. As is suggested by the definition of terms at the beginning of the chapter, however, there is more to collective bargaining than its definition might suggest. The collective bargaining negotiations take place within the context of a legally prescribed *structure* and *scope* in addition to *process.*

Structure

The structure for collective bargaining ultimately determines who sits at the negotiating table. At a broad level, the structure includes procedures for taking collective action to elect a bargaining agent; setting out a framework of prohibited behaviors (ULPs); and determining the specific group of employees included in the bargaining unit.

Electing a Bargaining Agent

The NLRA protects the rights of employees to organize themselves. Before bargaining can begin, either an employer must formally recognize the employee's representative or the NLRB certifies the representative elected by the majority of the employees to be covered by the agreement. When a union or a group within wants to organize a facility, a carefully constructed campaign will have been conducted during which a core group with common issues and concerns is identified. This group conducts a campaign designed to generate support for a representation election. According to the Michigan Nurses Association (2007):

> To seek voluntary recognition by the employer, a public petition must be signed by a majority of nurses....More than likely, an employer will refuse to voluntarily recognize the bargaining unit of nurses and its designated representative. When this occurs, it is necessary to establish majority status through a representation election conducted by the [NLRB].
>
> To file a petition for a representation election, the published petition must be signed by at least 30 percent of the nurses in the proposed unit. However, it is advised that a petition not be filed

> with the regional NLRB office until signatures have been obtained from a clear and substantial majority, excluding supervisors and managers.
>
> Upon receipt of a petition, the regional director of the NLRB will attempt to reach agreement between the employer and the [union] on several issues, including the definition and scope of the proposed unit. In the event that agreement is not reached, a hearing may be scheduled.
>
> After the pre-election issues have been determined, the NLRB will set the date for an election by mutual agreement of the two parties (employer and [union]). After the NLRB has set the date of the election, copies of the Board's official Notice of Election will be posted at the employer's facility in places where notices to employees are normally posted. This notice will include the date, hours, and places of the election; payroll period for voter eligibility; description of the voting unit; a sample of the ballot; and general rules as to the conduct of the election.
>
> If the majority of voting nurses (50 percent plus one) select [the union], it will be certified by the NLRB as the exclusive bargaining agent. The employer is then required to recognize this agent and to bargain in good faith for a collective bargaining agreement. If a majority of voting nurses opposes representation, the Board will certify these results; a tie is considered a loss (§ 10-16).

The Bargaining Unit

The NLRA states the unit is determined by whether a group of employees form a community of interest relative to wages, hours, and conditions of employment. The NLRB has determined that RNs make up a community of interest and should occupy their own bargaining unit rather than be included with other professionals such as social workers.

Determination of the bargaining unit status of an individual employee is based on the position of the employee in the agency, not on whether the individual pays dues to the union. Some members of the bargaining unit may not pay union dues, and only members of the bargaining unit may have automatic payroll deduction of dues. Although certain limited services offered by the union might favor members over non-union employees, when the collective bargaining agreement is negotiated by management and the union, "its terms and conditions cover all employees in the bargaining unit irrespective of their union membership" (U.S. Army CPOL, 2006, § 3).

Unfair Labor Practices

The NLRA prohibits employers from interfering with the employees' selection of the representative (labor union) for collective bargaining and requires that the employer bargain with the representative who is selected. The law also places certain restrictions on the tactics that either side may use in bargaining (e.g., strikes, lockouts). The NLRA prohibits employers and unions from engaging in ULPs (LII: Wex, 2007a). For example, the NLRA forbids management and labor to refuse to bargain in good faith. Furthermore, it forbids an employer to do any of the following (NLRB, 1997):

> ... interfere with, restrain, or coerce employees in the exercise of the rights guaranteed in section 7. Any prohibited interference by an employer with the rights of employees to organize, to form, join, or assist a labor organization, to bargain collectively, to engage in other concerted activities for mutual aid or protection, or to refrain from any or all of these activities, constitutes a violation of this section. This is a broad prohibition on employer interference, and an employer violates this section whenever it commits any of the other employer unfair labor practices. (pp. 27-28)

Box 29.1 contains ULPs prohibited by employers and those prohibited by employees/unions.

Impasses

Showing the desire to negotiate, or bargaining in good faith, does not mean having to make concessions or agree with the other side; at times, the process may be at an impasse. Should that occur, several options are possible to resolve the dispute such as mediation, fact-finding, and arbitration. The procedure to follow likely was a part of the grievance procedure of the previous contract.

Because no such procedure exists in first contract negotiations, however, for several years organized labor has sought an amendment to the NLRA. Known as the *Employee Free Choice Act (EFCA)*, it would provide for mediation if the two sides could not come to terms on a first collective bargaining contract after 90 days. After 120 days, the Act would empower an arbitration board to settle a dispute. The bill passed the U.S. House of Representatives on March 1, 2007; on June 26, 2007, the U.S. Senate voted 51 to 48 to invoke cloture on considering the bill. Because 60 votes were required, however, the bill was not considered. Labor proponents believe the amendment is essential because of the documented history of avoidance in signing contracts by some organizations (Malmgren, 2008).

Scope

The specific elements of work life that may be included in the subjects of collective bargaining remain a source of confusion. For example, nurses may believe that they can bargain collectively over nurse staffing ratios. In every case, it is imperative that the applicable laws be reviewed and understood. For nurses who are covered by the Fair Labor Standards Act (FLSA), there is a broad category of mandatory items including wages and overtime pay that the employer must bargain over once an employee organization has been certified to represent the nurses for collective bargaining. Employees covered by FLSA include all employees of an enterprise that are engaged in the operation of a hospital (Department of Labor, 2007).

The NLRB (1997) describes the scope of bargaining in terms of mandatory and non-mandatory subjects as follows:

> The duty to bargain covers all matters concerning rates of pay, wages, hours of employment, or other conditions of employment. These are called "mandatory" subjects of bargaining about which the employer, as well as the employees' representative, must bargain in good faith, although the law does not require "either party to agree to a proposal or require the making of a concession." In addition to wages and hours of work, these mandatory subjects of bargaining include but are not limited to such matters as pensions for present employees, bonuses, group insurance, grievance procedures for discharge, layoff, recall, or discipline, and union security. Certain managerial decisions such as subcontracting, relocation, and other operational changes may not be mandatory subjects of bargaining, even though they affect employees' job security and working conditions. The issue of whether these decisions are mandatory subjects of bargaining depends on the employer's reasons for taking action. Even if the employer is not required to bargain about the decision itself, it must bargain about the decision's effects on unit employees. On "non mandatory" subjects, that is, matters that are lawful but not related to "wages, hours, and other conditions of employment," the parties are free to bargain and to agree, but neither party may insist on bargaining on such subjects over the objection of the other party. (p. 36)

For nurses covered by state collective bargaining labor laws, categories of mandatory bargaining items may differ and requirements may vary from state to state. The following example from Iowa's Code demonstrates the possible breadth in scope that may be found (Iowa Public Employment Relations Act, 1999 supp.):

> The public employer and the employee organization shall meet at reasonable times, including meetings reasonably in advance of the public employer's budget-making process, to negotiate in good faith with respect to wages, hours, vacations, insurance, holidays, leaves of absence, shift differentials, overtime compensation, supplemental pay, seniority, transfer procedures, job classifications, health and safety matters, evaluation procedures, procedures for staff reduction, in-service training, and other matters mutually agreed on.

> Negotiations shall also include terms authorizing dues check-off for members of the employee organization and grievance procedures for resolving any questions arising under the agreement.... All retirement systems are excluded from the scope of negotiations. (§ 20.9)

Box 29.2 lists items typically contained within an RN collective bargaining agreement (Budd et al., 2004).

Process

The complete collective bargaining process actually occurs in three stages. The first stage occurs before negotiations begin; the second stage includes the negotiations; and the last stage is the implementation of the negotiated agreement.

First Stage

The composition and selection method of the employees' negotiating team likely will have been spelled out in the by-laws of the bargaining unit. Generally, the team comprises five to seven persons, including the certified union representative.

Before the employees' negotiating team goes to the bargaining table, it will have carefully formulated a proposal of demands based on the issues and ideas of the bargaining unit members. If this is a first-time collective bargaining situation, the proposal will be based on the issues that prompted the RNs to organize. If it is a contract renegotiation situation, the existing agreement will be used as the basis for the new proposal. In either case, the employees' certified representative and the rest of the negotiating team will have prepared themselves to defend the proposal by reviewing relevant research findings and statistical data to support its demands (Nyman, 1981). Also included in this stage is the actual scheduling of the time and place for the negotiations to begin, a potential ULP if management refuses to respond (Rainsberger, 2006a).

Box 29.2

Subjects Found in RN Labor Agreements

- Mandatory and voluntary overtime
- Acuity-based staffing systems
- Use of temporary nurses
- Protections from reassignments, work encroachment by non-nurses, and mandated non- nursing duties
- Provisions for work orientation and continuing education
- Whistleblower protection
- Health and safety provisions, such as free hepatitis B vaccine
- "Just cause" language for discipline and termination
- Provisions for nursing and multidisciplinary practice committees

Adapted from Budd, K.W., Warino, L.S., & Patton, M.E. (2004). Traditional and non-traditional collective bargaining: Strategies to improve the patient care environment. *Online Journal of Issues in Nursing, 9*(1), § 12.

Second Stage

The negotiations that take place during the second stage are the *raison d'être* of collective bargaining, and a substantial body of knowledge has been built by scholars in a wide variety of fields to guide those that are faced with the task of negotiating change. A theory found useful by many not only to understand the nature of collective bargaining but also for designing and conducting negotiations (Bacon & Blyton, 2007; McAndrew & Phillips, 2005) is Walton and McKersie's *A Behavioral Theory of Labor Negotiations* (1965). The framework of negotiating activities is based on three assumptions. The first assumption is that "the agenda in labor negotiations...usually contains a mixture of conflictful and collaborative items. The need to defend one's self-interest and at the same time engage in joint problem-solving vastly complicates the selection of bargaining strategies and tactics" (p. 3). A second assumption is that an important dimension underlying the negotiations is the attitudes, feelings, and relationships of those at the table. Because the theory deals with labor negotiations and not negotiations in general, the third assumption is that the "negotiations...involve complex social units in which the constituent members are very interested in what goes on at the bargaining table and have some influence over the negotiators" (p. 3).

The theory specifies four systems of activities that account for the behavior in negotiations. Each interrelated system has its own tactics, skills, and functions. These functions are to resolve conflicts of interests, find common interests, or influence attitudes between the groups and to achieve consensus within the groups. Walton and McKersie (1965) labeled the four systems *distributive bargaining, integrative bargaining, attitudinal structuring,* and *intraorganizational bargaining* (Box 29.3). Negotiations between labor and management occur by overt use of distributive or integrative bargaining techniques or by a mixture of the two.

Distributive Bargaining

Also called "*competitive, zero sum, win-lose* or *claiming value*" (Wertheim, n.d., p. 3), the distributive approach is traditional, position-based argumentation. One side presents its proposals and then argues, with supporting evidence, why its proposals are better than the other side's (U.S. Army CPOL, 2005). It is most commonly used for conflicts-of-interest issues in which the issue is how to distribute or divide limited resources. This bargaining approach tends to end either in compromise or in stalemate.

Tactics used in the traditional approach have been described by McKersie and colleagues (2008) as "negotiations where labor and management begin by overstating their real positions, followed by a series of offers and counter-offers en route

Box 29.3

Types of Labor Negotiation Behavior

Distributive Bargaining

- Activities are directed toward achieving goals that are in conflict with the other side's goals.
- Pay-off is a fixed sum, and each side tries to maximize its share.
- Joint decision-making process is focused on an issue and strategies for winning.
- Functions to resolve conflicts of interest.

Integrative Bargaining

- Activities are directed toward goals that are *not* in conflict and are integrated with the other side's goals.
- Each side tries to increase the size of the joint gain irrespective of the pay-off.
- Joint decision-making process is focused on problem solving.
- Functions to find common interests and solve problems.

Attitudinal Structuring

- Activities are directed toward changing attitudes and relationships.
- Socio-emotional interpersonal process is focused on structuring the attitudes toward and relationships with the other side.
- Functions to build trust and cooperation.

Intraorganizational Bargaining

- Activities are directed toward aligning the goals of the chief negotiator's organization with those of the chief negotiator.

Adapted from Walton, R.E., & McKersie, R.B. (1965). *A behavioral theory of labor negotiations: An analysis of a social interaction system.* New York: McGraw-Hill.

to an agreement" (p. 67). At the first meeting, the union's spokesperson makes an opening statement, during which the union's position is stated and the general reasons for making the demands are given. Management's representatives respond in general and usually agree to reply in writing before the next meeting. At the second meeting, generally management's spokesperson speaks first, summarizing its position, and the union responds. Likely the reply is negative at first, but then a compromise will be offered for at least one of the demands. Management then will be expected to reply to the compromise with a counter-proposal. "The cycle of proposals followed by counter-proposals continues [for several meetings] until a formula acceptable to both sides has been reached" (Nyman, 1981, p. 17).

Integrative Bargaining

"Also called collaborative, win-win or creating value" (Wertheim, n.d., p. 3), the integrative, interest-based approach emphasizes collaboration instead of compromise. Spangler (2003) illustrated the difference as follows:

> The classic example of interest-based bargaining...is that of a dispute between two little girls over an orange. Both girls take the position that they want the whole orange. Their mother serves as the moderator of the dispute and based on their positions, cuts the orange in half and gives each girl one half. This outcome represents a compromise. However, if the mother had asked each of the girls why she wanted the orange—what her interests were—there could have been a different, win-win outcome. This is because one girl wanted to eat the meat of the orange, but the other just wanted the peel to use in baking some cookies. If their mother had known their interests, they could have gotten all of what they wanted, rather than just half. (¶ 4)

Rather than the adversarial methods used in traditional positional bargaining, the process used in interest-based bargaining is for "the bargaining parties jointly [to] identify issues, pinpoint separate and mutual interests, select criteria for solutions, brainstorm options, and reach solutions through consensus agreement" (Stepp & Bergel, 2008, p. 34). The agenda item represents a problem to be solved, not an issue to be settled (Madden, 1969). The steps of the process are as follows (Spangler, 2003):

- Identify the interests of each side. (Ask "why" questions.)
  - Find out why the other side is making its demands.
  - Determine how they perceive your demands.
  - Clarify your underlying interests.
- Brainstorm a list of options.
- Create a win-win outcome with each side getting as many interests as possible.

In this type of bargaining, negotiators from both management and the union work in teams, sitting around a table rather across from each other as they would in traditional bargaining (Lavigna, 2002). Lavigna called this type of bargaining "consensus bargaining" and identified a four-step process. First, all interests and then mutual interests are identified. Second, negotiating teams develop many options for the mutual interests. Third, objective standards for evaluating the options are agreed upon. Finally, "teams then apply the standards and identify the options on which they can reach consensus. As the teams agree to options, union and management representatives jointly draft contract language" (p. 380).

Mixed Bargaining

Although Walton and McKersie's theory stated that distributive and integrative bargaining are core ingredients of all negotiations, most negotiators have been trained in the techniques of traditional, positional bargaining (Heumann & Hyman, 1997). Roberts and Lundy (2003) noted, however, that because the "key features of interest-based bargaining are mutual respect, consensus decisionmaking, and the valuation of the relationship between the parties," (§ 5) this bargaining method is the more successful approach for addressing nursing concerns. Factors affecting the success of integrative collective bargaining have been found to be "the degree of trust developed from previous negotiations, the level of expertise/style demonstrated by the negotiators, the clarity of the

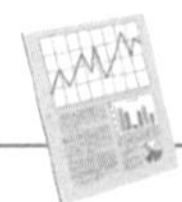

Research Note

Source: McKersie, R.B., Sharpe, T., Kochan, T.A., Eaton, A.E., Strauss, G., & Morganstern, M. (2008). Bargaining theory meets interest-based negotiations: A case study. *Industrial Relations, 47*, 66-96.

Purpose

Noting that use of interest-based negotiation (IBN) techniques were being reported by over half of union and management negotiators, these researchers sought to describe if and how IBN was related to other negotiating methods during collective bargaining. Using mixed methods composed of participant observation, surveys, and interviews, the complex 2005 national contract negotiations between Kaiser Permanente and the Coalition of Kaiser Permanente Unions were described.

Discussion

A team of six investigators participated as observers in the national contract negotiations conducted on behalf of 44 bargaining units with 86,000 employees, represented by 10 unions; and the management of Kaiser Permanente, which included the Kaiser Health Plan and Hospitals and the Permanente Medical Groups. The first of two phases of negotiations was focused on topics of common interest by eight bargaining task groups (BTGs). Interest-based negotiating (IBN) or integrative bargaining was the process used most frequently in this phase, and the teams that used it most were more satisfied with the outcome of this phase. The second phase was the final week of negotiations when the economic package was addressed. Distributive or positional bargaining predominated during this second phase, and extreme positions generated strong emotional responses. The researchers concluded, however, that the trust developed through the work of the BTGs and the trust that the chief negotiators had built through the years assisted with resolving conflict and finding compromise.

Application to Practice

The development of a culture of trust is vitally important to successful resolution of negotiations. When tensions surface during any negotiation, and regardless of the process or technique being used, they must be dealt with before the process can proceed.

bargaining issues and the ability of facilitators to use problem solving-based techniques" (Caverley & Cunningham, 2006, p. 62). Both the traditional, distributive bargaining technique and the interest-based, integrative bargaining technique have been used as predicted by Walton and McKersie's theory in contract negotiations with hospitals and unions representing nurses.

Third Stage

In principle, the third stage, which is implementing the collective bargaining agreement, should be a matter of course. Within the agreement should be procedures such as grievance and arbitration for handling any infringements of its specific content (Nyman, 1981). Building upon, nurturing, or changing the trust relationship and other attitudes that might have been fostered or that are in need of repair by both sides during the second stage also is a function of this stage.

LEADERSHIP AND MANAGEMENT IMPLICATIONS

Writing for the *Labor Studies Journal*, Clark and Clark (2006) recognized that despite nurses' "traditional reticence" to join unions, they might be a particularly "fertile target for union organizers" if unions could "help them address one of their most important concerns—the quality of patient care" (p. 52).

LEADERSHIP & MANAGEMENT BEHAVIORS

Leadership Behaviors

- Creates unit and organizational climate that values nurses
- Guides nurses in conflict resolution strategies
- Creates a vision of professionalism and collectivity
- Inspires professional autonomous behavior
- Communicates relevant work-related information
- Leads others to value and respect the work of nurses
- Advocates for nurses' values and needs
- Inspires trust and respect and pushes the envelope

Management Behaviors

- Plans career growth opportunities
- Structures the work environment for professional autonomy
- Manages work-related conflicts
- Organizes the flow of work-related communication
- Acquires specific state and federal collective bargaining rules, regulations, and information
- Administers the collective bargaining contract fairly and equitably
- Ensures that management's rights and employee's rights are respected

Overlap Areas

- Leads and manages the unit and organizational climate for nurses
- Manages the flow of communication
- Enhances organizational respect for nurses
- Serves as a role model at all times
- Applies critical thinking skills and serves as a mentor and team builder
- Keeps the patient as the central focus and uses patient-centered language as a problem-solving technique

High patient-to-nurse ratios, use of mandatory overtime, and floating are the management practices nurses believe jeopardize the quality of patient care. For nurses to provide high levels of safe care, they need to be supported by management in addressing these issues. In addition, nurses need to feel respected and to have input into matters that affect their work life. If they do not trust their management, invariably they will turn to a third party to represent them to management. Unresolved problems and conflicts between staff nurses and management likely will become union contract demands.

Leaders and managers are the key to a satisfying work environment for nurses. Leadership is demonstrated by seriously addressing the issues and making appropriate changes. If discontent leads to unionization, then nurse leaders and managers are obligated to follow applicable laws and rules. Once a contract is negotiated, personnel policies may need to be reviewed and revised as appropriate. Managers will be responsible for administering the contract from the employer's perspective, usually under the direction of the central human resources office.

Although many unions promise to mandate favorable staffing ratios and, in some states, staffing ratios have been legislated, root causes of the nursing shortage must be addressed at the worksite. An increase in the numbers of RNs in the employment pool cannot be mandated or legislated. The challenge to both staff and management RNs is as follows:

- Set up some form of governance model that empowers the staff nurse through the work of councils led by staff nurses.
- Work through the staff nurse council and eliminate mandatory overtime and other unacceptable practices identified by staff nurses. Work-life balance should be a key goal.
- Provide professional leadership and management around the clock.
- Reward positive performance, and eliminate punitive thinking and action.
- Work toward a cooperative labor-management relationship, keeping the focus on the patient.
- Develop and use patient-focused language.

CURRENT ISSUES AND TRENDS

The "Kentucky River Cases"

Because the 1947 Taft-Hartley amendment to the NLRA excluded supervisors from unions, through the years RNs' rights to organize have been challenged by employers based on the question of whether RNs should be considered supervisors or professional health care workers (Bodley et al., 2003). Whereas supervisors are excluded from collective bargaining by the Act, professionals are not. At issue is the definition of *supervisors* found in the Taft-Hartley Act:

> The term "supervisor" means any individual having authority, in the interest of the employer, to hire, transfer, suspend, lay off, recall, promote, discharge, assign, reward, or discipline other employees, or responsibly to direct them, or to adjust their grievances, or effectively to recommend such action, if in connection with the foregoing the exercise of such authority is not of merely routine or clerical nature, but requires the use of independent judgment. (§ 2[11], 61 Stat. 141)

In general, through the years, the NLRB held the view that an RN's direction of other employees while exercising professional judgment in the care of clients was distinct from the exercise of supervisory authority, or "independent judgment" in the interest of the employer (Ketter, 1994). In 1996, the NLRB made such a ruling against Kentucky River Community Care, Inc., which employed 110 professional and non-professional employees at a mental retardation and mental illness facility in Pippa Passes, KY (Bernat, 2001).

When the Kentucky State District Council of Carpenters attempted to represent the 110 employees, the employer objected to including the six registered nurses at the facility in the unit, claiming they were supervisors. Noting the nurses did not meet the criteria of the Act (e.g., they did not hire or fire), the NLRB ruled in favor of the union. "The U.S. 6th Circuit Court of Appeals reversed the decision, [however], and the NRLB took it to the U.S. Supreme Court. In a 5 to 4 decision, the high court ruled in favor of the employer and against the NLRB and the union. The nurses were supervisors." (Bernat, 2001, p. 49).

One possibility for allowing professionals to be included by the Act was offered by Supreme Court Justice Scalia, who stated that "perhaps the [NLRB] could offer a limiting interpretation of the supervisory function of responsible direction by distinguishing employees who direct the manner of others performance of discrete tasks from employees who direct other employees" (Bernat, 2001, p. 50). To clarify its definitions of "independent judgment," "assign," "direct," and "responsibly," in 2003 the Board invited the filing of amicus briefs with reference to three cases, Oakwood Healthcare, Golden Crest Healthcare, and Croft Metals Inc., known as the "Kentucky River cases." In response, the ANA and UAN (Bodley et al., 2003) jointly authored a brief in which professional nursing practice was described in terms of the regulated practice environment of state practice acts, hospital policies and procedures, and practice standards. The brief concluded the following (ANA, UAN, 2003):

> Nurses must practice within the scope of their license and, in doing so, may delegate to others certain tasks that they do not have to accomplish personally. Equating such delegation with the exercise of independent judgment or with the assignment or direction of work as defined by the Act ignores the strictly circumscribed legal and ethical environment under which all RNs, including charge RNs, must operate. (p. 29)

In 2006, the Board finally released its decision on the three cases (NLRB, 2006):

- In the case of Oakwood Healthcare, it found that the supervisory authority was exercised by permanent charge nurses since "significant overall duties" were assigned to employees by them. Such authority was not demonstrated by rotating charge nurses during "substantial" work time.
- Applying the definitions to Golden Crest Healthcare Center, for "assign" and "responsibly direct," the Board found the Golden Crest charge nurses did not meet these guidelines.

Although its employees were not health care employees, the definition for "assigning" and exercising independent judgment was applied to the lead persons of Croft Metals. "The Board found that the lead persons' exercise of judgment was either fundamentally controlled by pre-established guidelines, such as delivery schedules, or was simply routine" (NRLB, 2006, last §). Therefore the NLRB found that these employees were not supervisors.

- Excluding certain categories of nurses from collective bargaining during these years when staffing levels, mandatory overtime, floating, and other issues have become key to union organizing efforts (Clark & Clark, 2006) galvanized unions to push for federal legislation to reverse the NLRB ruling. In March 2007, the Re-Empowerment of Skilled and Professional Employees and Construction Trade Act was introduced to the House (HR 1644) and Senate (S 969). The legislation would amend the NLRA to require that, to be a supervisor, an employee would be required to spend the majority of the day performing supervisory duties (Congress May Determine Definition, 2007). On September 19, 2007, the full House Education and Labor Committee voted 26 to 20 in favor of the bill.

Summary

- Collective bargaining consists of two basic types of labor and management negotiations—distributive bargaining and integrative bargaining.
- Unionization in nursing has steadily increased over the last quarter of the twentieth century.
- Unionization is governed by federal and state legislation and administrative rules and regulations.
- Nurse managers need to be aware of the structure and scope of collective bargaining in nursing.
- Nurse managers must be willing to work collaboratively with unionized nurses to achieve healthy patient outcomes.

CASE STUDY

Monica Hendricks, a master's-prepared RN educator, has recently been hired as the director of nursing education in a unionized acute care hospital. She has had experience in unionized organizations and understands managing in a collective bargaining environment. One of the responsibilities outlined to her by her new employer is to upgrade the management team so that everyone is at least at a basic level of management expertise with knowledge and skill in collective bargaining. Eventually, she is to upgrade them further.

Ms. Hendricks thought she would have some time to get to know the staff and set up her schedule and curriculum, but shortly after her arrival, she became aware that supervisors were using the phrase "Oh, the union won't let us do that." She also noticed that staff members often extended their breaks and that the units seemed unusually disorganized. As she made her rounds, she asked the same question of all management personnel in the department: "Do you have a copy of the union contract?" No one did.

Ms. Hendricks had sufficient copies of the union contract printed for all managers and set up her classes so that every manager could attend. Then, using the clauses of the contract as a roadmap, she immediately started discussion groups to review the contract line by line. It was not long before management personnel from other departments started to wander in to her classes, where they received a warm welcome. The phrase *knowledge is power* was actualized. Ms. Hendricks was careful to alert human resources (HR) to her activities, and HR had appropriate conversations with union leadership. Over time, patients became the central focus, but not without some difficulty. After all, when you change an existing paradigm, some resistance is inevitable. However, persistence and goodwill eventually overcame resistance. Patient focus, patient-focused language, and carefully staying within the confines of the collective bargaining agreement were Ms. Hendricks' winning strategies.

CRITICAL THINKING EXERCISE

It has been 42 days since the NLRB certified a trade union as eligible to attempt to organize the nurses in Registered Nurse Janet Hargrove's hospital. At first she was in favor of the union because RNs had been laid off. Staffing ratios were very high, and staff nurses such as Ms. Hargrove had to do mandatory overtime. They were expected to orient and direct unlicensed assistive personnel, as well as newly hired, newly graduated nurses. Supplies were often short, especially on the off-shifts and weekends. In addition, although the nurses had not been given a salary raise in more than 2 years, pharmacists had received substantial pay increases because they were in such "short supply." Often, RNs were treated disrespectfully by physicians, family members, patients, and even within their own hierarchy.

What was making Ms. Hargrove question her original decision to vote for the union was that, right after the NLRA certified the campaign, a new chief nurse executive (CNE) had come on board. The new CNE immediately moved her office from the insular location it had always been to a central location with an open door. She had started around-the-clock group meetings and instituted what she called *MBWA*, or "management by walking around," on every nursing unit during all three shifts. The CNE quickly began to get to know staff members by name. She asked staff members for input in identifying three priority problems (excluding those that involved money or structural repair) that could be solved quickly. Then, by working with a volunteer staff nurse committee, the CNE solved those problems almost immediately.

Ms. Hargrove, along with other RNs, was very happy with the CNE and her new approach, but union reps warned them that goodwill by management would end unless they voted for the union. They brought in nurses from other unionized hospitals to reinforce this message and to "talk up" the union. Ms. Hargrove and her colleagues were confused. They did not know what to do.

1. What critical thinking techniques might Ms. Hargrove use to come to a decision?
2. How might Ms. Hargrove weigh the pros and cons of voting for the union or for management?
3. What is the significance of *42 days* in the first paragraph?
4. What is the significance and value of MBWA?

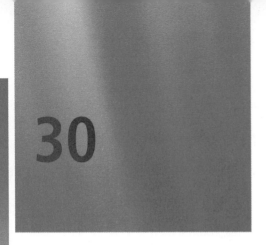

30 Financial Management

Judith Lloyd Storfjell   Therese A. Fitzpatrick

CHAPTER OBJECTIVES

- Define and describe financial management
- Describe the role nurse leaders play in managing the convergence of operations, patient care, and financial stewardship
- Identify financial management tools useful to nursing managers
- Discuss the impact staffing strategies can have on organizational costs
- Differentiate charges from costs
- Analyze cost awareness as related to nurse decision making
- Analyze ethical and legal financial management considerations
- Exercise critical thinking to conceptualize and analyze possible solutions to a practice exercise

Health care service costs continue to escalate, and the pressure to control these costs is increasing. Nurses at all levels need to become more knowledgeable and sophisticated in financial management. This is because the accuracy of resource projections and the efficiency of care provision are crucial to the viability of health care organizations. There is little operating margin to act as a buffer. At minimum, nurses need to develop and justify budgets, use computerized information systems and technology, and economize staff and supply use while ensuring that safe and appropriate care is delivered in nursing services.

Every health care management decision has both a financial and a clinical impact. It is nearly impossible to make a decision in one area without it affecting the other. This is why nurses need to be equal partners in making key strategic and operational decisions—because they understand the service being provided, and they are responsible for the quality of that service. Without nursing input, non-clinical executives and managers are left without critical knowledge about the impact of decisions on clients, services, and quality. Nurses need not only an understanding of financial issues related to clinical service delivery but also the tools to help plan and evaluate the financial impact of their many decisions and to be leaders and active participants in making effective strategic and operational decisions. Nurses in all positions need to understand their impact on both revenue and expenses and, ultimately, on the financial health of their programs and organizations.

A major organizational concern is how to allocate scarce resources efficiently and effectively. Some issues in financial management relate to who (or what level of management) decides how much of an organization's resources will go to staffing, who makes decisions about staff mix and levels, and who decides how many nursing care hours each client receives. Does shared governance mean shared control over financial resources? Can there be split responsibility, with nursing deciding client care hours but management controlling the resources to pay for those hours? According to Cleverly and Cameron (2002), the effectiveness of financial management is the product of many factors including environmental conditions, personnel capabilities, and information quality. Timely, accurate, and relevant information through the accounting process is an important ingredient of financial management. Therefore an adequate understanding of the accounting process and the data generated by it is critical to successful decision making.

DEFINITIONS

Financial management is defined as a series of activities designed to allocate resources and plan for the efficient operation of an organization. Uncertainty and risk are associated with cash flow, as well as other forces that affect the ability to meet an organization's financial needs. Thus the managerial process of planning is linked closely with financial management. **Strategic planning** is a process of assessing the organization and its departments or divisions. Strengths and weaknesses are explored and analyzed. Opportunities and external threats are identified and critiqued. External forces are considered, and their impacts are projected in relationship to the organization. Key organizational strategies are developed for financial, customer, process, and organizational learning/growth perspectives (Kaplan & Norton, 2006). A financial plan, the budget, is developed to support the implementation of this strategic plan.

Financial accounting is a core aspect of financial management. Accounting is divided into managerial accounting and financial accounting. Managerial accounting is focused on the generation and evaluation of financial information needed by managers to manage parts or all of the organization. Financial accounting is targeted toward providing information to external sources of investment, money lending, or control. Managerial accounting is designed for internal users; financial accounting is targeted toward external constituents. Managerial accounting results in a wide variety of statements and financial information that vary from organization to organization.

BACKGROUND

Health care organizations are affected by their environment—economic, political, and social—which has implications for its financial management. For example, the number, type, and location of competitors influence potential volume and subsequent revenue streams. The demographic profile of the surrounding population affects the use of services. Payer and provider types and numbers also influence financial management. Employer groups exert considerable influence when they negotiate health care for large blocks of employees. The legal and regulatory environment also influences health care service delivery. The key factors to assess in any community evaluation are the major employers, provider groups, and health care facilities in the area. In the planning of services, population

LEADING & MANAGING DEFINED

Financial Management

A series of activities designed to plan for the efficient and effective operation of an organization, allocate resources, and monitor progress.

Strategic Planning

Development of key organizational strategies for financial, customer, process, and learning/growth perspectives based on internal and external analyses.

Charge

The price asked for services or goods.

Cost

The amount of money required to deliver specific services or products, including administrative expenses.

Unit of Service (UOS)

The basic measurement of an item produced by an organization (e.g., patient days, outpatient visits, home care visits, surgeries).

characteristics are important. Other important financial management factors are the structure of the health care organization, economic principles, accounting, and finance.

FINANCIAL MANAGEMENT TOOLS

Financial Reports

Accounting is a system that keeps "account" of the financial functions of an organization and tracks its financial well-being. To do this, it follows general rules of accounting or accounting principles that guide in the systematic collection and dissemination of financial data. To understand the financial performance of an organization and to assist in decision making for the future, a variety of financial reports are generated on a routine basis (usually monthly or quarterly). To do this, accountants keep a "general ledger" (GL) into which they make "journal entries" to record financial transactions to specific "accounts." This is as important in health care organizations as in any other type of business.

The smallest functional unit that generates revenues and expenses is called a *cost center.* Some units generate direct revenue or charges, whereas others (e.g., administration) generate expenses but no direct revenue. A charge is generated for the purpose of acquiring income for the health care organization. There is a difference between the charge and the actual cost, just as there is when purchasing a piece of clothing from a department store. The **charge** is defined as the price asked for services or goods. The **cost** is the actual amount of money required as payment to cover direct production inputs used in producing the service. *Profit* is defined as the money gained as excess of charges over outlay costs in producing a service. For example, a health care facility may bill a client for $5 for the use of a vial of sterile saline when it cost the hospital $1 to purchase and process the purchase. The difference is profit.

Health care managers need accountants to keep financial records and produce financial reports. Even though financial reports are prepared for external purposes, they contain valuable management information as well. All nurse managers need to be able to understand and interpret financial information for themselves. Sometimes, the biggest stumbling block is to interpret the financial "language" or jargon. Think of these financial reports simply as management tools. The two most common financial reports or statements are (1) the balance sheet (statement of the financial position of the organization), and (2) the income statement (statement of revenues and expenses). Both are used to understand and analyze the organization's financial status. Operational decisions follow, as do reports to controlling or interested bodies such as boards of directors or trustees, banks, investors, and the federal government. Although nurses often do not see balance sheets or statements of revenue and expenses, they need to know they exist. Furthermore, nurses need to become well informed about the financial "health" of the organization. Resources and jobs may be at stake. One measure of the cultural aspect of "openness" is whether such documents are shared with staff at the operations level (bedside).

Balance Sheet

The *balance sheet* is probably the most misunderstood by clinical managers. It basically portrays the financial "health" of an organization. It has three major sections as follows:

- *Assets*—what the company "owns"
- *Liabilities*—what the company "owes"
- *Fund balance* (or *owner's equity*)—what the company is worth (subtract *liabilities* from *assets*)

Balance sheets may vary in the amount of detail they show, but they always have these three sections. The basic framework is Assets = *liabilities* + *fund balance (net assets)* (Figure 30.1). There are usually two types of *assets* and two types of *liabilities*: current and long-term. *Current assets* are those things that can be turned into cash quickly, such as bank accounts and accounts receivable (money owed to the organization by customers). *Long-term assets* (sometimes divided into *fixed* and *other assets*) are things owned by the organization that cannot be converted quickly into cash—such

HOME HEALTH AGENCY	31-Dec-08		
ASSETS		*LIABILITIES AND FUND BALANCE* (*Net Assets*)	
Current Assets:		Current Liabilities:	
Cash	$ 100,000	Accounts payable	$ 150,000
Accounts receivable (net)	$ 520,000	Accrued wages and benefits	$ 170,000
Inventory	$ 60,000	Accrued other expenses	$ 90,000
Prepaid expenses	$ 20,000	Deferred revenue	$ 30,000
Total Current Assets:	$ 700,000	Current portion of long-term debt	$ 30,000
		Total Current Liabilities	$ 470,000
Property and equipment (net of accumulated depreciation)	$ 300,000	Long-term debt (less current maturities)	$ 310,000
TOTAL ASSETS	$1,000,000	TOTAL LIABILITIES	$ 780,000
		FUND BALANCE (Net Assets)	$ 220,000
		TOTAL LIABILITIES AND FUND BALANCE	$1,000,000

Figure 30.1
Sample balance sheet.

as capital (e.g., land, buildings, equipment). The definitions are similar for liabilities. *Current liabilities* are what the company owes during the current year (e.g., wages, accounts payable to vendors, taxes), whereas *long-term liabilities* are those debts the company plans to carry beyond one year, such as mortgages for buildings and/or land. The format of the balance sheet is interesting. Notice that the "total assets" always equals the sum of total liabilities and the fund balance.

Income Statements (Revenue and Expense Statement)

The most common financial report is the *income statement*. This report has a number of different names including "profit and loss statement" (P&L), "revenue and expense statement," or "income and expense statement." Whatever title is used, its purpose is to provide a picture of operations for a specific time period—a month, quarter, or year. It reports the money coming into an organization or program *(revenue)*, and the money going out *(expense)* during this time period, and the difference between these two *(profit/loss)*. It may also compare this activity with the budget and/or a prior period for reference and trending purposes.

An *income statement* has three basic components:

- Revenue (income)
- Expenses (direct and indirect)
- Loss or gain (or profit/loss)

Revenue is generally recorded either by the source of that revenue (e.g., payers such as Medicare, Medicaid, insurance, private pay) or by the program producing the revenue (e.g., the specific clinic or inpatient unit). *Operating revenue* is that portion of total revenue generated from actual operations, exclusive of income from interest, sale of property, donations, or other "non-operating" revenue sources. *Expenses* are generally divided into *direct* and *indirect* expense. *Indirect* expenses are those expenses not directly attributable to the provision of services, such as occupancy costs or administrative salaries. Direct expenses are those costs used for the direct provision of a service, such as staff nurse wages or clinical supplies. The ratio between *indirect* and *direct expenses* can be a useful financial indicator. The *expenses* are subtracted from the *revenue* (income) to determine the *profit (gain)* or *loss* for the time period being reported. This is the famous "bottom line." Managers always want to have a positive bottom line, showing a *gain* rather than a *loss.*

Most large organization use what is called an *accrual* method of accounting. *Income* is recorded

NURSE-MANAGED PRIMARY CARE CENTER	
Revenue (Income)	12/31/2008
Net patient service revenue	$ 160,000
Grants	$ 50,000
Interest income	$ 15,000
Total Revenue	$ 225,000
Expense	
Salaries and wages	$ 140,000
Fringe benefits	$ 35,000
Professional fees	$ 10,000
Supplies and other	$ 7,100
Depreciation	$ 1,200
Miscellaneous	$ 3,700
Total Expense	$ 197,000
Gain (Loss)	$ 28,000

Figure 30.2
Sample income statement (revenue and expense statement).

when a service is provided, not when the cash is received, even though it may take weeks or months to collect the income. Similarly, *expenses* are recorded when they are due, even if they have not actually been paid. This approach gives a more accurate view of the financial operations of an organization during the specified time period. It is therefore necessary to review the *balance sheet* to determine what bills are yet to be paid *(accounts payable [A/P])* and what revenue is yet to be collected *(accounts receivable [A/R])* (Figure 30.2).

FINANCIAL INDICATORS

Certain financial ratios can be used to determine the viability of the organization—beyond just looking at the total worth of the organization. The most useful financial indicators include the following:

- Comparing current financial reports with the following:
  - Prior years or months;
  - The budget; and/or
  - Benchmarks or standards
- Calculating financial ratios including the following:
  - Liquidity ratios (current ratios)—how much cash an organization has available to pay its debts;
  - Profitability ratios; and
  - Efficiency ratios (productivity)

Some key health care financial indicators are listed in Table 30.1.

Variance Analysis

The two easiest ways to determine the financial performance of a program or service are to (1) determine whether the program is profitable and (2) compare financial performance with the projected (budgeted) performance. These comparisons are called *variances.* Actual income and expense line items in each cost center can compare with budgeted amounts for the current month and year-to-date (YTD). This can be done for both operating and cash flow budgets (Figure 30.3).

Variance analysis should start during the budgeting process by determining which indicators need to be monitored on a regular basis and which will give meaningful variance information. Although monitoring the variance of line items is a powerful management tool, it can be misleading. Too often, variances are viewed in isolation—not as a part of a suite of management tools.

If expense exceeds budget, for example, it is important to determine if this is caused by additional service volume—something that could actually be very positive if it results in increased revenue as well. Or, if volume is down, causing a corresponding decrease in revenue, then expenses will need to decrease accordingly. For this reason it is important to compare costs and revenue per unit of service—actual and budgeted. In fact, unit cost and unit revenue are probably the most important indicators to monitor.

Cost Analysis

Cost accounting, or cost analysis, focuses on cost measurement and cost reporting. An understanding of the cost of a service or product can be one of the most valuable pieces of information a manager can have. And the good news is that it is

Table 30.1

Key Health Care Financial Indicators

Indicator	Formula	Standard	Definition
Current ratio (liquidity ratio)	Current assets ÷ current liabilities	2.0 ($2 in current assets for every $1 in current liabilities)	Liquidity ratio—the higher the ratio, the better the organization's ability to meet its obligations during the current year (access to cash)
Cost per unit	Total revenue ÷ # of service units	Varies—should be lower than revenue per unit	Cost of producing one unit of service (clinic visit, home visit, patient day)
% Indirect expense	Total indirect expense ÷ total expense	25% to 45% (varies depending on the amount and type of service)	Indirect expense as a % of total expense
Gross profit %	Total revenue—direct expenses ÷ total revenue	35% to 60% (varies based on type of service)	% of revenue available for indirect expenses and profit
Profit margin	Total revenue—total expense ÷ total revenue	8% to 30% (based on budget; varies by service)	Profitability ratio—total relative profitability of an organization (considers all income and expense)
Debt-to-equity ratio	Current liabilities + long-term debt ÷ fund balance	1.0 ($1 liability for every $1 fund balance)	Solvency ratio—ability to meet obligations over a period of time (e.g., 5 years)
Days in receivables	Net accounts receivable ÷ daily operating revenue	30 to 60 days	Efficiency ratio—number of days of business in accounts receivable
Days of cash	Cash (in bank) + marketable securities ÷ daily payables (total annual payables/365)	30 days	Indicator of cash adequacy (# days company can operate with current cash)

NURSE-MANAGED PRIMARY CARE CENTER			
Revenue (Income)	YTD Actual	Budget	Variance
Net patient service revenue	$165,000	$180,000	$(15,000)
Grants	$ 55,000	$ 60,000	$ (5,000)
Interest income	$ 15,000	$ 10,000	$ 5,000
Total Revenue	$235,000	$250,000	$(15,000)
Expense			
Salaries and wages	$140,000	$150,000	$(10,000)
Fringe benefits	$ 35,000	$ 37,500	$ (2,500)
Professional fees	$ 10,000	$ 11,000	$ (1,000)
Supplies and other	$ 7,100	$ 6,800	$ 300
Depreciation	$ 1,200	$ 1,200	$ —
Miscellaneous	$ 3,700	$ 3,500	$ 200
Total Expense	$197,000	$210,000	$(13,000)
Gain (Loss)	$ 38,000	$ 40,000	$ (2,000)

Figure 30.3
Sample variance analysis. *YTD,* Year-to-date.

relatively easy to calculate. In spite of that, most nurse managers have little understanding about how much it costs to provide specific services to a patient. It is an irony that nurses are responsible for ensuring that cost-effective care is provided without any way of tracking the cost of that care.

Income statements (P&L reports) tell us how much money came in during the month (or year) and how much went out. Depending on the amount of detail provided, we can probably tell where the money came from—which payers or for which services—as well as how much of the expense was for labor, occupancy, supplies, and other cost areas. However, it typically does not tell how much it costs to serve one patient or client or to provide one unit of service.

The easiest way to determine the cost of a unit of service (e.g., an inpatient day, a clinic visit, a patient) is to divide the total expense by the total units of service. This results in the average cost per unit of service. This approach averages all patient days equally. However, to differentiate between the cost of a perinatal patient day and the cost of a day in the inpatient cardiac unit, it would be necessary to separate the direct costs of each unit and then divide the costs by the number of patient days in each unit. Spreadsheets are excellent tools for doing this.

Beware, however, that cost indicators are actionable and may be misleading. An example of a misleading cost indicator is "cost per FTE." This indicator has been used frequently by hospitals, sometimes with disastrous results. Full-time equivalents (FTEs) are not equal—either in salary or in type of skill. Different services may require different skill mixes. By indiscriminately reducing the number FTEs just to change the "average cost per FTE," both revenue production and quality of care could be seriously affected. Critical judgment is required when using any type of indicator.

Break-Even Analysis

A break-even analysis is the determination of the volume of business needed for a program or organization to cover its costs—to break even. In other words, it is the service volume at which the revenue collected will cover all fixed costs and the variable costs for that amount of business. Because fixed costs do not vary as service volume changes, revenue generated for volume over the "break-even

OUTPATIENT CLINIC	
Assumptions	
Days of operation per FTE (annual)	210
Clinic visits per day per FTE	18
Number of provider FTEs	4
Total annual visits	15,120
Average revenue per visit	$ 110
Fixed wages + benefits	$650,000
Other fixed expenses	$150,000
Variable expenses per visit	$ 40
Break-Even Analysis	
Revenue per visit	$ 110
Less variable cost per visit	$ (40)
Contribution per visit	$ 70
Fixed expense (wages and other)	$800,000
Number of visits required to break even*	11,429

*Divide total fixed expense by contribution per visit.

Figure 30.4
Sample break-even analysis. *FTE,* Full-time equivalent.

point" will no longer need to cover the fixed (overhead) expenses but will cover the variable costs and create profit (Figure 30.4). Nurse planners and managers can use a break-even analysis to determine whether to develop an additional service or to give volume discounts.

HEALTH CARE FINANCIAL STRATEGIES

There is great pressure to hold down health care costs and yet maintain high quality and availability of services. Nurses can also learn from the field of economics about how scarce resources are allocated among alternative uses. Financial resources are either short-term or long-term. Financing of the health care delivery system is important for nurse managers and leaders to understand. Political savvy can be augmented by understanding the key stakeholders, the basics of insurance and payment to providers and organizations, and methods used to control payments for care. Internally, important financial management concepts are related to both finance and accounting. Finance focuses on the next several years and what might pay off in the longer-run. Accounting has a 1-year time horizon. Thus with accounting, it is difficult to justify programs that do not return gains on investment in less than a year.

Cost management is the analysis and control of costs. In health care, revenues are important but the control and management of costs is more important to profit/surplus because increasing revenue is more difficult to accomplish.

Nurses continue to struggle with how to allocate scarce nursing resources effectively and efficiently. Financial compensation (pay and benefits) remains an issue for all nurses. Shift work and the consolidation of multiple nursing units in hospitals under one nurse manager are work stresses for nurses. Alteration of staff mix affects the financial bottom line and also morale, recruitment, and quality of reliability of service delivery. These and other issues in the dynamic health care environment press nurses to augment and enhance their skills and abilities in financial management. Because labor is the largest portion of most health care expense budgets and nursing generally consumes the majority of the labor budget, an understanding of nurse staffing strategies is critical.

Nurse Staffing Strategies

The economic principle of supply and demand is manifested on a daily basis as leaders attempt to allocate scarce clinical resources among their possible uses. A number of demographic trends have converged to create a mismatch between available nursing staff and the need for health care services. The health care system in this nation is composed of 875,785 beds, having an average length of stay of 5.6 days. Visits to the emergency department (ED) are rising and the Centers for Medicare and Medicaid Services is reporting a need for 18% more beds by the year 2012, due in large part to the aging population. Baby Boomers began turning 50 years of age every 7.6 seconds in 1996 and likewise will begin to turn 65 in 2011. During this same period, the nursing shortage will reach 29%, or 1,200,000 nurses, while the demand will increase to 43% (Colosi, 2007).

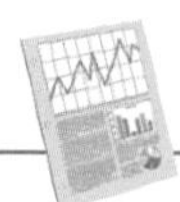

Research Note

Source: Murray, M.E., Brennan, P.F., & Moore, S.M. (2003). A model for economic analysis. *Nursing Economic$, 21*(6), 280-287.

Purpose

Technology and other health care innovations are costly. Responsible allocation of resources decisions need to be based on economic assessments. The purpose of this article was to display and discuss a model for the economic assessment of patient care innovations. A production process model was used to define the costs of resources used to produce a specific amount of output. This allowed the derivation of the average cost per unit for the innovation.

Discussion

A production process is a relationship between inputs used and outputs that result. Outputs in health care can be a patient education program, a critical pathway, or a treatment procedure. Characteristics of the production process include economic efficiency, economics of scale, marginal productivity, and the influence of time on short-term and long-term production costs. A cost analysis strategy was used to specify the inputs to the production process and determine total costs and average cost per case. The first step was specifying and defining costs. Less obvious costs, such as fringe benefits, consultation fees, printing costs, out-of-pocket expenses incurred by patients, and training time for staff, needed to be considered. The second step was developing a detailed listing of the costs involved. Using the model, the cost per unit of innovation metric was displayed and discussed using an example from a clinical trial involving the use of a computer-based home care program for postsurgical cardiac patients. The example used was an economic analysis of HeartCare, a home-based self-care technology research project. Four production processes were presented: design, pilot implementation, maintenance, and completion.

Application to Practice

Economic assessments of innovations clearly are crucial steps for nursing administrators. However, methods and measurements are difficult and complex. Selecting the best methodology is a challenge. The production process model, as a way to guide the economic analysis of health care programs, is a good strategy for answering important economic questions.

The nursing shortage is the result of a number of converging phenomena, including the aging of the nursing workforce, capacity problems in colleges of nursing, inability to retain nurses in clinical practice, and recruitment into the profession (Buerhaus et al., 2007). A supply shortage in the face of increasing demand leads to increased costs for the organization as nursing departments are required to use more expensive types of labor to fill available shifts, including overtime and bonuses for current staff and travel and per diem registry staff. Some organizations are obliged to turn away patients, thereby sacrificing revenue and severely affecting access to care within the community. Nursing leaders must also be mindful of the impact that staffing has on the quality of care, patient satisfaction, attempts to improve clinical outcomes, and the mandate to reduces errors and improve safety. Although providing supplemental staffing may be an effective short-term solution, it will not be effective in addressing the fundamental issues resulting from demographic shifts in the U.S. population.

When staffing levels or supply is inadequate to accommodate the workload or demand, the impact is significant. Aiken and colleagues (2002) determined that each additional patient assigned to a nurse resulted in the following:

- 30-Day patient mortality increased by 7%
- 7% Failure-to-rescue rate increased
- The odds of nursing job dissatisfaction increased by 15%
- The odds of nurse burnout increased by 23%

Minimum staffing standards for hospitals have become the topic of vigorous debate in state legislatures across the country. In 1999, the state of California passed Assembly Bill 394 (AB 394), which requires that hospitals provide minimum nurse-to-patient ratios. Hospitals have also been required to develop and implement patient classification systems, which may indicate that more nurses than the minimum are needed for a shift based on the acuity of the patients at that point in time (Spetz, 2004; Welton et al., 2006). The California ratios were phased in over the course of several years, but in their final form, they are as follows:

Specialty Unit	Nurse-to-Patient Ratio
Critical Care	1:2
Medical-Surgical	1:5
Telemetry	1:4
Behavioral Health	1:6
Step-down	1:3
Pediatrics	1:4
Emergency Department	1:4
Nursery	1:8
Labor & Delivery	1:2
Postpartum	1:4 to 1:6
Operating Room	1:1
Recovery Room	1:2

As of this writing, one half of all states in the nation are considering similar legislation or have recently implemented regulations requiring minimum staffing levels. For example, effective in January of 2008, the state of Illinois enacted Senate Bill 0867 (SB 0867), which amends the Illinois Hospital Licensing Act by requiring that hospitals (1) implement a written staffing plan that reflects the complexity of care, (2) develop a committee made up of 50% staff nurses to provide advice to the staffing plan, and (3) implement an acuity model that will provide direction in re-aligning staffing based on changing patients' needs (Amendment to the Illinois Hospital Licensing Act, 2008). A number of bills have been introduced in Congress, fueled by the growing body of research linking patient outcomes to staffing levels.

The costs and quality implications of these regulations are being studied. Lang and colleagues (2004) performed a systematic review of the literature related to the employee, patient, and hospital effects of nurse-to-patient ratios. They found that the literature offers minimal support for specific minimum nurse-patient ratios but that patient acuity, skill mix, nurse competence, nursing process variables, availability of technology, and institutional support for nursing also play an important role in determining the numbers of nurses required. The evidence does support a probable relationship between richer nurse staffing and a number of improved outcome measures such as failure to rescue and shorter lengths of stay.

Developing staffing strategies that not only meet the clinical needs of patients but also address the personal and professional needs of the nurse will help stem the tide of staff turnover. The cost of replacing a nurse has been estimated between \$22,000 and \$64,000, or 0.75 to 2 times an annual salary (Jones, 2005; O'Brien-Pallas, 2006). Jones (2008) adjusted these costs for inflation. Expressed in July 2007 inflation-adjusted dollars, the range is \$82,000 if the position is filled by an experienced nurse requiring a shorter orientation to \$88,000 if filled by a nurse with a longer learning curve. These direct costs include replacing the nurse during the recruitment process (often at premium rates), orientation costs of a new employee, and the indirect or administrative costs including advertising, interviewing, and background checks. The cost that is most difficult to quantify is the loss of intellectual capital or the years of experience and clinical judgment lost every time a nurse leaves the organization.

Based on the significant cost and quality impact of nurse turnover, it is imperative that organizations retain their qualified staff. A number of retention strategies suggested by nurses themselves (e.g., improvements in the work environment, establishing a culture of safety, supportive supervision, involvement in organizational decision making) have been addressed in other sections of this text.

Often cited as key drivers of retention are flexible and creative staffing and scheduling practices. Staffing and scheduling strategies are also instrumental in supporting a diverse workforce and in creating an environment that supports nurses throughout their professional life. Nurses balancing family commitments, caring for aging family members, or looking for part-time or limited hours as they approach the end of their careers would benefit from flexible scheduling (Cyr, 2005; Mion et al., 2006; Ward-Smith et al., 2007; Young et al., 2007).

Flexible scheduling includes partial or non-traditional shift lengths (e.g., 4- or 6-hour shifts), as well as non-traditional start times. These types of schedules may also include various configurations of part-time employment as well (e.g., job-sharing, combinations of shifts, seasonal employment). Organizations are also developing roles that leverage the collective wisdom and experience of the mature nurse, including recruiting retired nurses. These include carved-out roles such as admitting-discharge teams and patient educator or preceptor-mentor for new staff. Although these new creative and flexible strategies can be highly desirable for both the nurse and the hospital, managers are responsible for understanding and quantifying the operational and financial impact to the organization.

To determine how these flexible schedules can best facilitate the care process, the leader must understand and measure the department's workload. Workload is typically defined as the census, the number of patient visits, or the number of treatments administered within the department. This **unit of service (UOS)** measures the work performed within a cost center or department. Often this unit of service is adjusted for acuity or a particular mix of patients. This UOS is used in the calculation of the annual budget.

Scheduling and staffing of clinical staff in a dynamic demand environment presents many challenges. The workload on a nursing unit does not remain constant across the day or even across the days of the week. For example, a surgical unit may receive most of its admissions in the late afternoon after the patients have been discharged from the recovery room. Some nursing units may experience a high number of discharges before the weekend; therefore their workload or census may be lower on Saturday and Sunday than during the middle of the week. Although it is difficult to predict all of the elements that affect a department's workload, the data will typically point to trends. It is important to use this trend data in planning; this is often referred to as *common cause variation.* In contrast, the *special cause variation* that occurs in workload should not be used for planning. Special cause variation would include atypical spikes in volume or a day with an unusually high number of nurse sick calls. Although these events require a contingency plan, they should not drive a permanent change in the process or the budget (Figure 30.5).

The workload of a typical emergency department may fluctuate significantly over the course of the day. Figure 30.6 illustrates the shifts in volume beginning at midnight by hour of the day. It is obvious that staffing at 1700 needs to be substantially higher for a volume of 35 patients than at 0200 when 15 patients are in the department. Important to note is the regularity of the patterns across days of the week, data that will be useful in planning staffing.

The volume of patients may also fluctuate over the course of a year. For example, some organizations may see more patients during the winter season (Figure 30.7).

The fact that a typical workload does not remain constant over 24 hours a day and 7 days a week makes it easier to design flexible work shifts. Using the surgical unit as an example, it may be helpful to have an extra nurse available to help admit patients during the afternoon when the patients return from surgery. To deploy a nurse for an entire 12- or 8-hour shift would provide too much staff at some times throughout the day. Staffing is *optimized* when the *right number* of the *right type* of staff are deployed at the *right time* to meet the workload demands of the unit.

The traditional method of budgeting staff based on an average daily census (ADC) does not

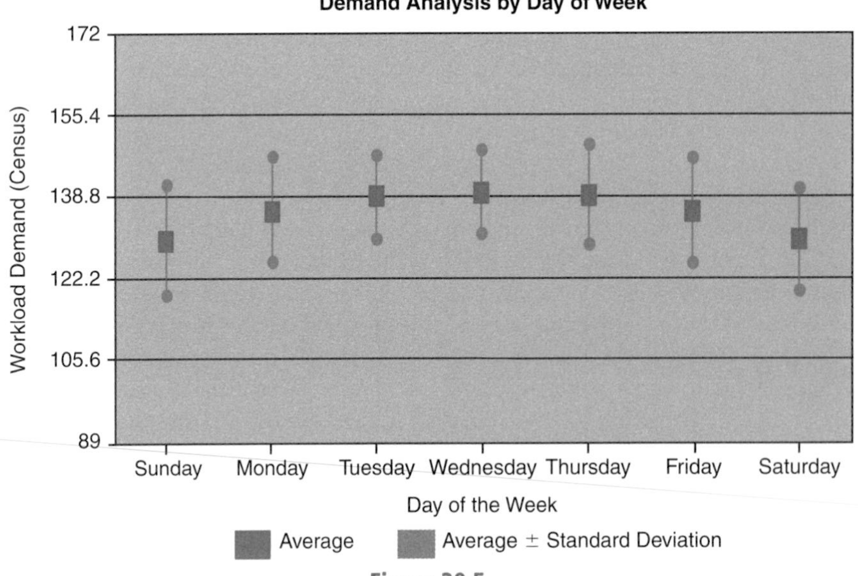

Figure 30.5
Demand analysis by day of week.

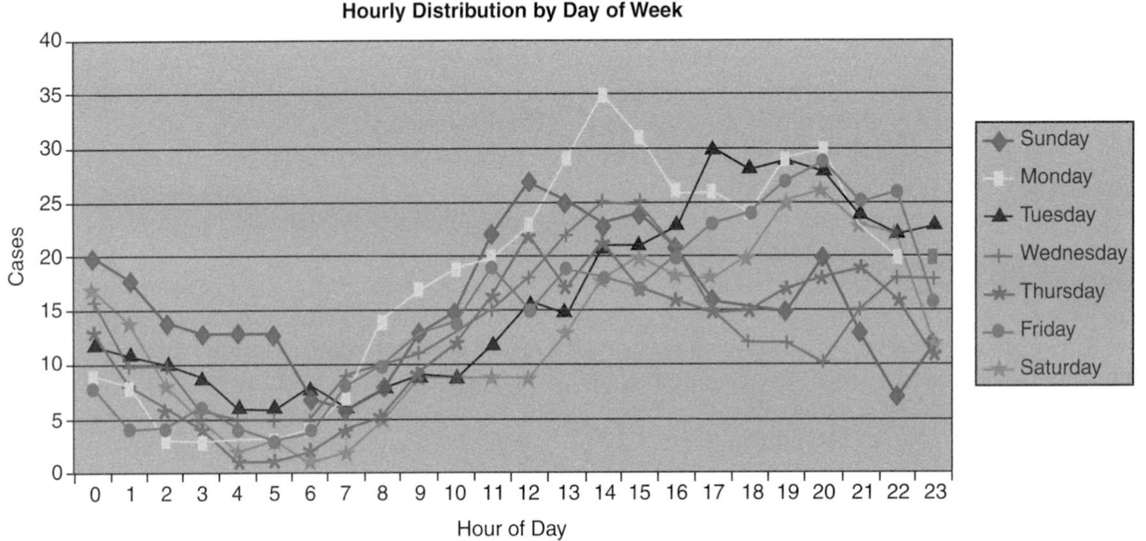

Figure 30.6
Emergency department hourly census fluctuation.

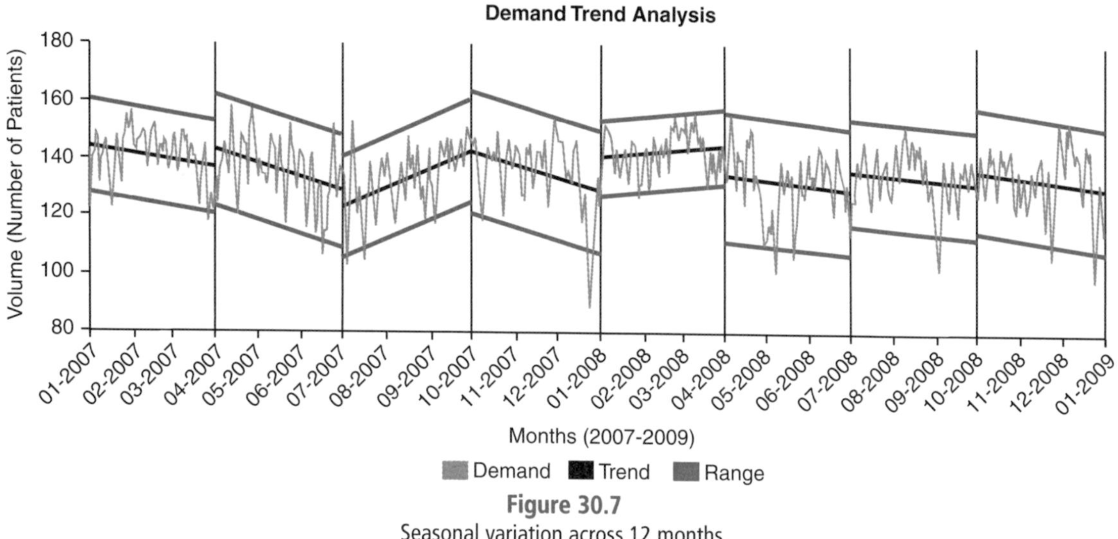

Figure 30.7
Seasonal variation across 12 months.

provide sufficient detail about the workload at points throughout the day or by day of the week to create the flexible shifts desired by many nurses. Figure 30.8 illustrates the budget for the surgical unit based on an ADC of 26.

In reality, the workload on this unit fluctuated significantly; one third of the time the census was greater than 1 standard deviation above or below the target (Figure 30.9). That means that one third of the time, or 122 days of the year, the unit had either too much staff or insufficient staff to meet the workload needs. By looking at this misalignment, it is easy to understand how nurses have become dissatisfied with staffing; they may be floated outside of their home unit on some days and be required to "work short" on others (see Figure 30.9).

However, nurse staffing is a complex endeavor because of the large number of variables that must be considered. The patient volume may be highly variable, nurses have differing sets of competencies, and human resource policies or collective bargaining agreements may define the work rules that guide staffing practices. Managers must also be mindful of the importance of considering staff preferences in their staffing and scheduling protocols. To effectively manage these often-conflicting requirements, technology or advanced mathematical tools are helpful and commercially available. By reconceptualizing these challenges as complex logistics problems, a variety of mathematical and process solutions heretofore available only to industries and organizations outside of health care can be applied in the solution of these business problems. Linear programming or mathematical optimization modeling is an effective way to find the lowest cost solution to staffing problems while meeting the myriad of system constraints such as work rules or staff availability.

How is Nurse Staffing Optimized?

Optimization models are a mathematical representation of a hospital's business situation. Key elements include the identification of the following:

- Business objectives such as:
  - Minimizing costs
  - Maximizing staff preference
  - Maximizing coverage to meet quality standards
- Decision variables such as:
  - Patient census and availability of staff

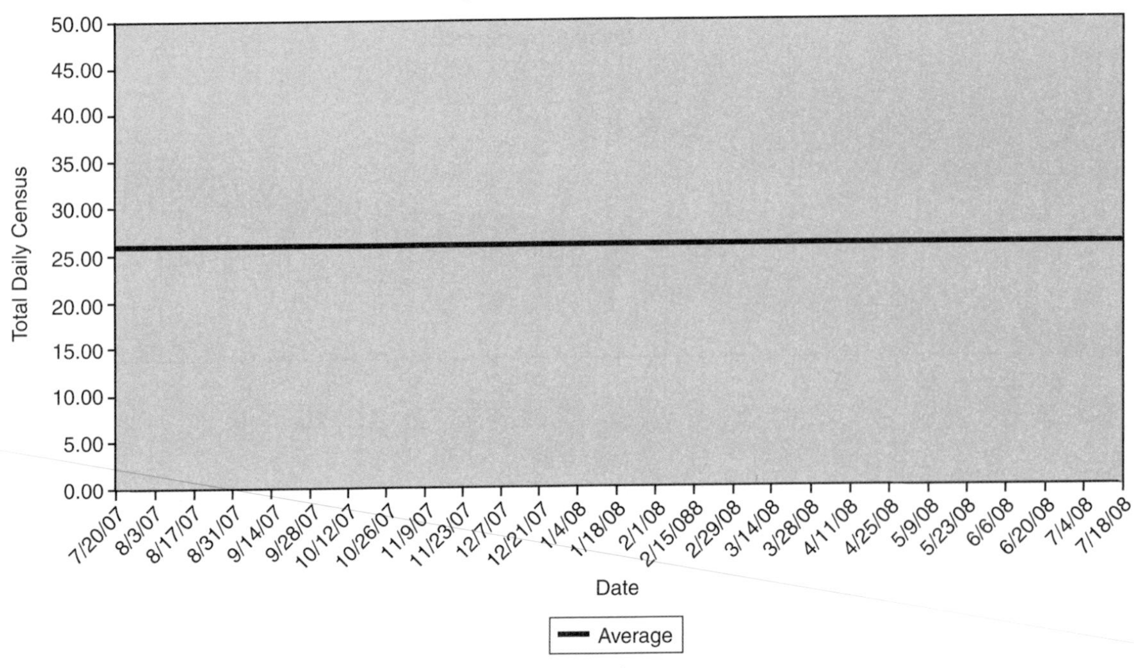

Figure 30.8
Budget based on average daily census.

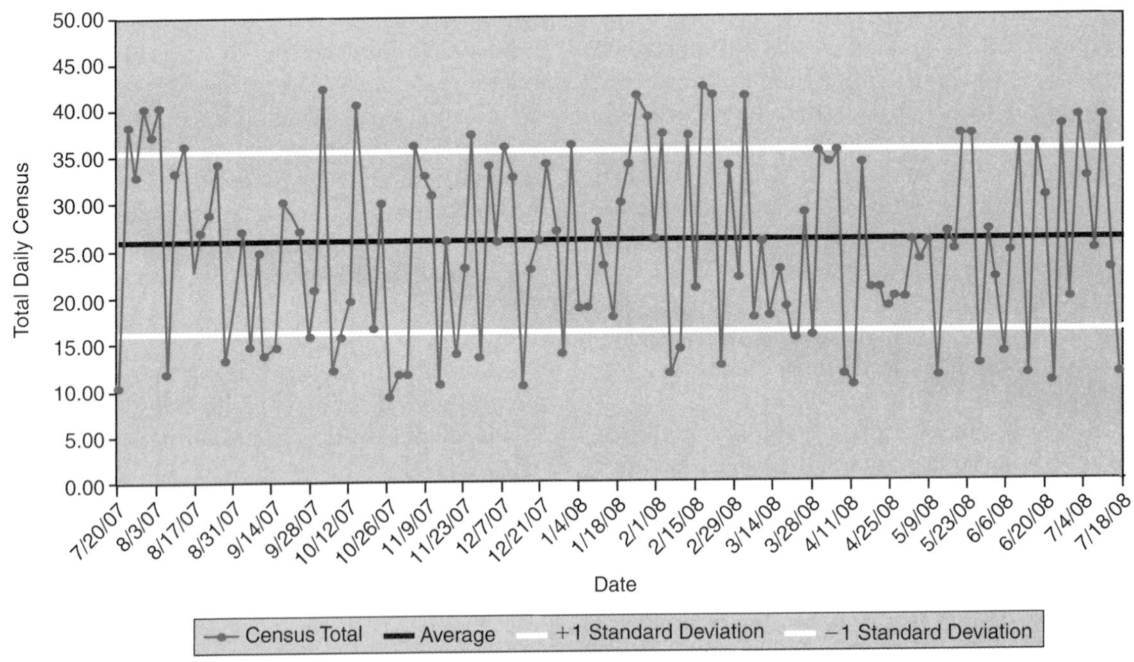

Figure 30.9
Actual workload compared with budget.

- Business constraints such as:
  - Work rules
  - Nurse-to-patient ratios
  - Scheduling policies

Nurses along with their managers are key participants in identifying the various parameters that affect staffing and scheduling. They can also apply systems theory in thinking about staffing and scheduling. Because all of the parameters such as patient volume, acuity, work rules, and staff preferences are interrelated, the problem requires a systematic approach, not unlike the systems approach used to resolve patients' needs. For example, administering certain medications may affect other physiological processes; therefore medication use is measured and monitored and action is taken to minimize that impact. This same systems approach can be applied to administrative processes as well, including staffing and scheduling. This is often referred to as the *creation of win-win solutions* or, in process improvement parlance, *optimizing the system as a whole.*

Technology solutions in isolation address only small pieces of this puzzle. In fact, multiple disjointed technologies may complicate the process and provide little incremental benefit. Although technology can be helpful in making portions of the process more efficient, such as scheduling, it is important to understand, document, and improve the entire system before implementing technology.

Many organizations are using staffing and scheduling strategies as an essential part of their recruitment and retention plan. By using an integrated and systematic approach, nurses can assist managers in the following:

- *Demand planning:* Understand and quantify workload patterns, and identify day-to-day and seasonal variation.
- *Analyzing processes and work rules:* Assess staff satisfaction with current staffing and scheduling processes, and make suggestions for improvements. This should also include suggestions for changes in work rules to support the changing demographic of the work force (e.g., the needs for more part-time opportunities, shorter shift lengths).

Understanding nursing workload and developing attractive staffing patterns that will retain nurses in the workforce are challenges for all nursing specialties. The determination of an inpatient nursing workload includes such elements as admission, discharge, and transfer activity, as well as the measurement of patient acuity. The methodologies used in the measurement of nursing workload, and specifically client acuity, must reflect the complexity of care and the setting in which that care is provided. Leaders in community health nursing use a unique approach to this analysis.

Community Health Staffing

Although nurse staffing for non-inpatient services may still be complex, it can incorporate different issues. For instance, community health nursing caseloads and workloads can also vary according to the client's complexity and the frequency and length of contact. In many community health programs, caseload management and continuity of care are key factors. For instance, chronic disease management requires that nurses develop a long-term relationship with clients, which promotes greater participation and self-care management.

Activity Cost Analysis

Understanding work activities and what causes them to take more or less time can become a powerful operational and financial management tool, especially when costs are included. Recent research has identified that acute care nurses spend more time on non–patient care activities. In fact, acute care nurses spend less time with patients than do home health nurses who travel between each patient contact. This fact, together with the fact that over one third of nursing unit time and wage costs are non–value added (NVA), provides a tremendous opportunity for improving the cost-effectiveness of nursing services. NVA time is time spent doing things that do not add value to the client, including searching for supplies, calling multiple times for a report, or documenting the same thing in several places. In acute care units, wage costs of NVA time amount to approximately $1 million per year (Storfjell et al., 2008; Storfjell et al., 2009). Doing an

Practical Tips

Tip # 1: Collaborate with Financial Specialists

Nurses should welcome financial specialists (e.g., accountants, data managers) as part of their financial management team. These experts can be invaluable in determining the financial impact of clinical and management decisions; and the more they understand about clinical issues, the better advice they will provide.

Tip # 2: Reduce Costs by Managing Activities

It is more effective to manage activities and processes than individuals in attempting to reduce costs. Inefficiencies and non–value added time are major contributors to high costs.

Tip # 3: Measure Workload to Optimize Staffing

Optimizing Staffing: To create schedules that not only mirror the workload within the department but also create opportunity for employee flexibility, workload must be measured in the smallest increment possible—hourly or at least at the shift level.

Tip # 4: Use a Dynamic Staffing Method

The Flaw of Averages: Staffing problems are dynamic; therefore resource planning and deployment approaches that are based on static averages will not solve the problem.

activity analysis can be quite simple. Have clinical staff estimate the percent of their work time they spend on four patient care activities (assessment, teaching, direct care [treat], psychosocial support) and two or more support activities (coordinate care, manage clinical records) (Figure 30.10). Have other staff identify their four to six major activities and the percent of time for each. Percent of time can also be verified by doing time studies or observations. Then, divide total wage costs by the percent of time assigned to each activity to determine the total cost per activity.

Finally, have staff estimate the percent of time spent doing NVA work for each activity and the "drivers" (causes) of this NVA work. These "drivers" can then become the targets for process improvement initiatives. This is the first step in an activity-based costing (ABC) process—one that can be done simply by using a spreadsheet and readily available financial data. It can also form the basis for more definitive ABC analyses—for instance, determining the true costs of specific processes, services, or procedures or the cost to serve specific clients or payers.

Revenue Enhancement

Beyond understanding costs, nurses need to understand how health care charges and prices are determined. Setting prices and rate-setting approaches are finance-type decisions that nurses may be able to influence with powerful data. Too often, prices are set based on tradition or the assumption that costs are a percentage of charges (ratio of costs to charges), rather than understanding the true costs of specific services. Traditionally, health care was paid on a fee-for-service basis—a flat fee for each type of service provided. This incentivizes the provision of high volumes of service units to increase revenue. This approach puts the entire financial risk with the payer. In the 1980s, Medicare led the way in changing reimbursement to a "prospective" payment approach by authorizing a set

NURSING ACTIVITY	*Value-added*	*NVA*	*Total*
Assess	$ 208,000	$ 68,000	$ 276,000
Teach	$ 123,000	$ 22,000	$ 145,000
Treat	$ 311,000	$ 145,000	$ 456,000
Psychosocial	$ 97,000	$ 12,500	$ 109,500
Coordinate	$ 300,000	$ 288,000	$ 588,000
Clinical record	$ 211,000	$ 155,000	$ 366,000
Totals	$1,250,000	$ 690,500	$1,940,500
	64%	36%	

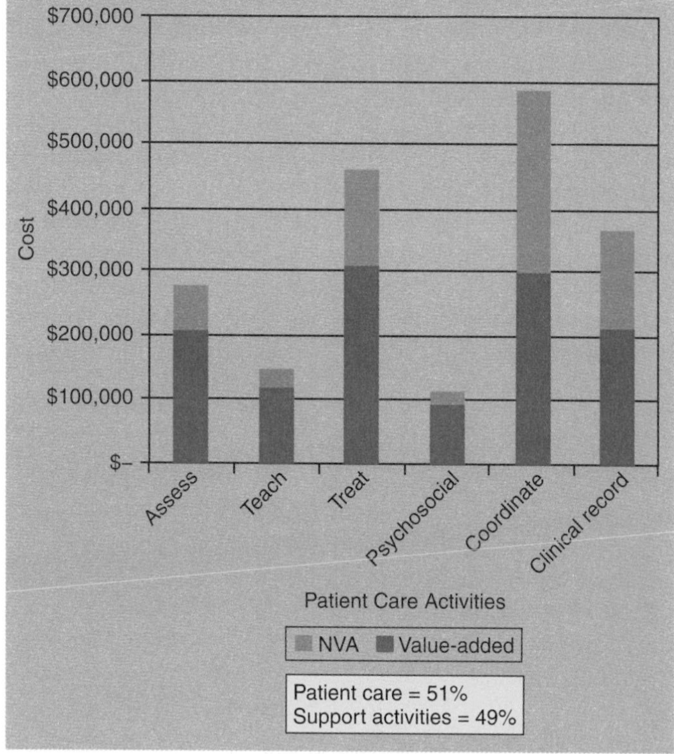

Figure 30.10
Nursing activity cost example. *NVA,* Non–value added.

fee for a specific illness or diagnosis, starting with diagnosis-related groups (DRGs) for inpatient care and extending to other health care services providers, thus sharing the risk with both health care providers and beneficiaries. Because revenue is stable, a prospective pay approach can incent providers to reduce the amount of services provided to decrease costs, thus increasing profit/gain. Another strategy has been "managed care." Under managed care, a "capitated" amount *per member per month (PMPM)* is paid to a provider or group of providers to manage the health care of enrolled individuals, generally called *members,* placing the financial risk squarely on the providers.

Nurses need to understand the various reimbursement types and the impact they may have on revenue, costs controls, and quality. Certain advantages and risks exist for all three approaches.

For instance, a capitated payment approach allows the provider to provide whatever services and supports are deemed necessary and could incent the provider to promote wellness over the long term. However, it could also promote a reduction in high-cost procedures if not managed well.

LEADERSHIP AND MANAGEMENT IMPLICATIONS

There is a saying that "no margin equals no mission." Nurses have the honorable mission of improving the health care status and functionality of their clients/patients. However, without adequate financial support (a positive financial "margin"), the viability of the highest quality program is in jeopardy. By using several simple financial management tools and partnering with financial experts, the dangerous chasm between finance and nursing can be eliminated.

With a trend toward decentralization of decision making, the nurse manager's role includes increasing accountability for financial management of the work unit. With a trend toward consolidation and the elimination of middle managers, individual nurses have to assume more of this accountability and responsibility.

Traditionally, in hospitals, nursing was included as part of the room charge and not separated from hospital-based hotel functions such as housekeeping, support services, and dietary. Thus the actual costs of care and the revenue captured from nursing effort were, in effect, "invisible." This approach hurt nursing by attributing costs incurred by the operations of other departments to nursing. Nursing was then seen as the costliest item in the organization's budget and was targeted first for budget reductions, restructuring, and layoffs. With the exception of home health services, in which nursing services are reimbursable, nurses have not been reimbursed for their services until recently. Now that advanced practice nurses (APNs) can bill for services and especially since APNs are a major provider of primary care, nursing is being

LEADERSHIP & MANAGEMENT **BEHAVIORS**

Leadership Behaviors

- Determines financial contributions of the group
- Guides a visionary identification of costs and resources
- Analyzes nursing costs and benefits
- Uses creativity to strategize and negotiate for the group's resource needs
- Motivates the group to increase financial knowledge
- Influences the group to find innovative ways to increase revenue
- Develops new resource streams
- Creates a financially savvy work environment
- Demonstrates basic skills in the analysis of financial statements, balance sheets, and cost report interpretation
- Demonstrates the basic skills required to educate and familiarize patient care team members on the financial implications of patient care decisions
- Understands the importance of establishing procedures to ensure accurate charging mechanisms

Management Behaviors

- Plans for financial management
- Organizes the needed resources
- Organizes financial data
- Implements the unit budget and financial processes
- Controls expenses
- Determines resource requirements within organizational constraints
- Evaluates technology
- Motivates subordinates to learn about financial elements

Overlap Areas

- Determines resource requirements
- Motivates expanded knowledge about financial aspects
- Manages expenditures

seen more positively as a revenue producer than as an expense. This, however, puts the burden on nurses to capture charges and monitor the cost-effectiveness of their services.

Overall, both nurses and nurse managers have seen their roles expand in scope and importance as empowerment, innovative change, shared governance, APN reimbursement, and cost containment have occurred. Leaders and managers can motivate personnel to expand their knowledge base and can model savvy financial management while planning, organizing, implementing, and controlling money and resources.

CURRENT ISSUES AND TRENDS

Ethical and Legal Issues

Budgeting and financial management involve intensive decision making about the allocation of scarce resources. Conflicts and ethical dilemmas easily arise in the balancing of competing needs and wants. For example, the organization has an advantage if labor budgets are tightly restricted. However, clients may incur greater wait times or diminished direct care time if nurses and other care providers are not readily available and accessible. Furthermore, nurses experience greater stress when workloads rise and clients' care needs are difficult to meet in the time available. Chronic stress saps nurses' energy and is reflected in their ability to deliver client-oriented service. In severe cases, patient safety is jeopardized and medical errors increase.

Money, personnel, space, and time are scarce resources in organizations, and they become the focal points for power, politics, and conflict. Ethical and moral problems occur as values clash. Ethical obligations of fidelity can be interpreted as promise keeping, an obligation to act in good faith, fulfilling agreements, maintaining relationships, and upholding trust and confidence. Professional fidelity or loyalty means upholding the clients' interests as a priority over the professional's self-interest or others' interests in any conflict. This is also called *advocacy.* Divided loyalties arise from the organizational and financial structures of health care. For example, issuing orders; assigning duties; or allegiance to other providers, employing agencies, funding sources, corporate structures, or governmental agencies may compel an ethical choice. Some examples include aggressiveness of treatment, impact of teaching and research functions in care delivery, and conflicts of interest with payer restrictions or denial of coverage when care needs still exist.

The Case Study at the end of this chapter illustrates a type of legal and ethical dilemma that may result from the changing structure of health care financing. The scenario described in the chart is simplified; in reality, the issues would probably be much more complex. The purpose of this example is to show the ethical and legal challenges that nurses and other health care providers may face as they decide whether to provide specific interventions for a client. The example given could affect the financial solvency of the neonatal intensive care unit within the larger institution. It is possible, if not likely, that there will be financial sanctions against the department or health care providers who work there when the department overspends its budget because of a decision to provide the additional services to the client even when there will be no reimbursement for them. Employment arrangements may create legal as well as ethical rights and obligations. Financial and budgeting implications arise from legal obligations. Malpractice and negligence place nurses and employers at financial risk. The employer is responsible for the acts of its employees. Under the doctrine of corporate negligence, health care organizations have a responsibility to monitor or supervise all personnel, including the quality of care given, and to investigate physicians' credentials (Aiken, 1994).

Although there are clear organizational liabilities for employment issues, the legal risks related to deployment issues are less clear. Short staffing, leading to inadequate care and medical errors, remains a major nursing management ethical problem (Corley & Raines, 1993). The requirement of the law is that the nurse's actions be reasonable under the circumstances. Reasonable in relationship to short staffing is a matter of judgment. Client safety, accepted professional standards and guidelines, and the language of organizational policies and procedures are major considerations. Budgeting and financial management are managerial decisions fraught with both ethical and legal ramifications.

Summary

- Financial management is a major nonclinical managerial task for nurses.
- The allocation of scarce resources is the focus of financial management.
- The four phases of financial management are budgeting, recording, reporting, and evaluating.
- Nurses have specific tools and strategies to facilitate proactive financial management.
- Strategic planning in nursing affects financial outcomes.
- A *charge* is the price asked for services; the *cost* is the amount required to cover direct production inputs.
- Staffing is optimized when the right number of the right type of staff are deployed at the right time to meet the workload demands of the unit.
- Nurses at all levels have a role in participating in financial management efforts.
- Financial management decisions may create legal and ethical dilemmas for nurses.

Case Study

Ethical Factors Created by Health Care Financing Restructuring

Scenario: An attending physician in the neonatal intensive care unit (NICU) of a major research hospital has determined that a premature infant (21 weeks' gestation) is of questionable viability. Because of the infant's underdeveloped lungs and other complications, the physician is considering issuing an order to not provide basic life support, including feeding, to the newborn. With the astronomical costs associated with prolonged NICU care and the likely reimbursement level, cost burdens become a consideration. Before finalizing the order, the physician consults with the NICU nurse in charge of the infant.

CRITICAL THINKING EXERCISE

Nurse Hiroshi Watanabe has been the director of a home health agency for 15 years. The agency has experienced some difficult times but has managed to survive. Now, however, with increased competition, rising client acuity, an increase in uncompensated care, and a drop in the major volume indicator (episodes of care), the agency is seriously threatened. Furthermore, the Centers for Medicare & Medicaid Services (CMS) has decided to adopt new rules that will severely reduce payments for Medicare home health visits and episodes. A close scrutiny of the financial projections indicates impending deficits. Nurse Watanabe has developed the following two options to present to the board of directors:

- Merge with the agency's largest competitor
- Reduce nursing staff and switch employees' health care benefits to a managed care contract that limits the choice of physicians and providers

1. What is/are the problem(s)?
2. How should Nurse Watanabe handle the situation?
3. What other options do Nurse Watanabe and the Board have?
4. What financial management strategies might work?
5. What creative strategies might be best suited to the situation?
6. What would motivate others to assist in this situation?

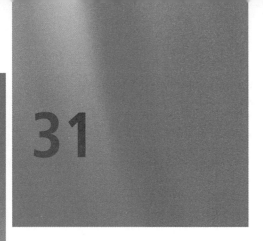

31

Budgeting

Heidi Nobiling

CHAPTER OBJECTIVES

- Define and describe a budget
- Categorize general types of budgets
- Define and differentiate traditional budgets, zero-based budgets, and flexible budgets
- Outline the stages of a typical budgetary process
- Distinguish between direct and indirect costs, and critique costing out nursing services
- Exercise critical thinking to conceptualize and analyze possible solutions to a practice exercise

The management of client care involves coordinating and integrating clinical care delivery, quality of care, human resources management, and financial management. Budgeting is focused on money as a strategic resource. The amount of money that is allocated to a nursing unit, service, or organization will have a significant impact on the amount and type of supplies, equipment, and human resources that will be used to deliver safe and effective patient care. Nurses carry responsibility and accountability for care management, program management, and service delivery. Therefore nurse managers and nurse administrators must understand the budget process so that they can effectively advocate for resources through the budgeting process and then appropriately monitor the use of allocated resources on an ongoing basis.

As professionals, nurses have a significant degree of discretion and decision making inherent in their work. Nurses play a major role in making decisions about care provision and related use of supplies and equipment that have significant financial ramifications. They evaluate equipment for purchase and use. They manage and have access to a significant inventory of patient care supplies. Nurses are a major element of the personnel budget of a health care facility. Charge nurses, nursing supervisors, and nurse managers make decisions about the use of available nursing personnel. All of these decisions have a direct financial impact on health care organizations.

Budgeting concepts are important to nursing practice but often are not fully understood or appreciated by nurses. A basic working familiarity with budgeting concepts can help nurses make better decisions, communicate with financial management staff, and negotiate more effectively for their share of the often scarce resources available to an organization (Gormley & Verdejo, 2000). Nurses will be involved in budgeting for nursing services in different ways and to different degrees, depending not only on their position within an institution but also on the institution. Nurse managers in any organization need to be involved in the development and ongoing monitoring of the budgets for their assigned units or services. In many organizations, staff nurses are also expected to be aware of their unit's financial performance and the impact their decisions may have on it. Staff nurses' involvement is essential to the ability to contain costs at the unit level because they make many decisions about supply and resource use.

Budgeting is a basic process of managing financial resources. Long-term forecasting (beyond the forecasting needed to develop a budget) and decision analysis are more advanced management tools that add to the organization's overall financial management. However, they are beyond the scope of this chapter.

BACKGROUND

Budgeting is a major aspect of an organization's or unit's planning processes (Figure 31.1). A budget is a plan that is specified in dollar amounts. Expressed in written or electronic form and quantified in dollar amounts, this plan becomes a guiding framework for organizational activities. It conveys management's intentions and financial expectations regarding revenues and expenditures. An organization-level budget compares expected revenues with expected expenses to forecast profit (surplus) or loss (deficit). Budgeting is a continuous process of preparing projections, implementing current budgets, and evaluating outcomes and performance related to the budget that was constructed. Preparing a budget entails forecasting the future (usually 1 year ahead) and anticipating the demand for services and how many units of service will need to be provided to meet that demand.

A specific budget timetable should be constructed to outline the activities and timelines of the annual budgeting decision process. A budget can be thought of as a roadmap. It is used as a guide to avoid crises, achieve goals and objectives, anticipate potential problems or develop potential solutions, encourage communication and coordination, and evaluate unit and managerial performance (Finkler & Ward, 1999). In thinking of the budget as a roadmap, it is important to remember that often more than one route exists to reach the intended destination. Budgets are designed to be planning documents. Individuals and organizations should not become so constrained by the approved budget that they hesitate to take appropriate actions or make appropriate decisions that vary from or were unanticipated in the budget process. The inclusion of contingency funds in the organization's overall master budget is one mechanism that can help ensure that funds are available throughout the fiscal year to address unexpected or emergency needs not planned for in the budget process. It is important to develop pre-established

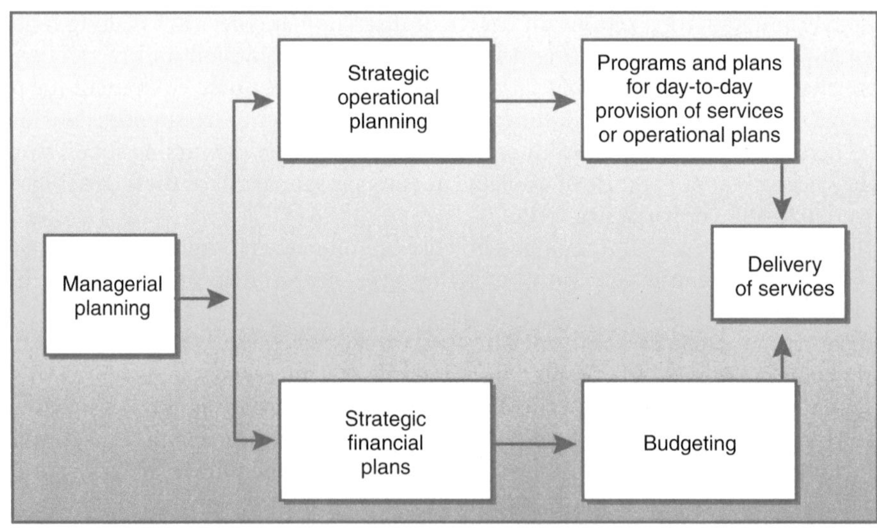

Figure 31.1
Process of managerial and strategic planning.

guidelines for requesting funding from a contingency budget so that managers and leaders in the organization are aware of the process and the associated guidelines and can better manage contingency funds.

DEFINITIONS

A **budget** is defined as a written financial plan aimed at controlling the allocation of resources. It functions as both a planning instrument and an evaluation tool useful for financial management. A budget is used to manage programs, plan for goal accomplishment, and control costs. **Expenses** are defined as the costs or prices of activities undertaken in the organization's operations. **Revenues** are defined as income or amounts owed for purchased services or goods. *Total operating expenses* are the result of summing the costs of all resources used to produce services. *Total operating revenues* are the result of multiplying the volume of services provided by the charges (rate) for the services. *Income* is the excess of revenues over expenses, or revenues minus expenses, for a given time (Johnson & Carpenter, 1990) (Box 31.1). A *variance* is the difference between the budgeted and the actual amounts. A budget becomes a financial timetable and plan for the organization that is translated into monetary terms. However, an alternative viewpoint sees a budget as a political document that results from a complicated bargaining process. The output is a financial document, although the budgetary process varies among organizations. Expenses, for example, may be program-based or may be itemized individually on a separate expense line as line items.

Organizational budgets actually include a variety of different types of budgets. The master budget is a set of all the organization's budgets from individual units, services, or cost centers. It is important to realize that multiple types of budgets are in simultaneous operation. Finkler and Kovner (2000) identified the following seven general types of budgets:

1. The **operating budget** is the plan for the unit's or organization's daily operating revenues and expenses and usually applies to a

Box 31.1

Calculating Total Operating Expenses, Revenues, Income

Total operating expenses = Cost of resources (1) + Cost of resources (2) + ...

Total operating revenues = Service provided (1) × Charge + Service provided (2) × Charge + ...

Income = Revenues − Expenses

LEADING & MANAGING DEFINED

Budget
A written financial plan aimed at controlling the allocation of resources.

Expenses
The costs of activities undertaken in an organization's operations.

Revenues
Income or amounts owed for purchased services or goods.

Operating Budget
The plan for the unit's or organization's daily operating revenues and expenses.

Expense Budget
Plan that tracks expenditure of resources or costs paid (e.g., wages, benefits, maintenance costs).

Capital Budget
Plan that tracks purchases of capital assets (e.g., buildings, land, equipment).

single year. The operating budget for a unit is the budget in which nurse managers tend to have the most involvement. Extensive information is needed to prepare the operating budget. Elements included in operational budgeting are (1) a workload budget with activity reports, units of service, and workload calculations; (2) **expense budgets** with personnel and staffing requirements and labor costs; (3) expense budgets for supplies, equipment, and overhead; and (4) a revenue budget.
2. A *long-range budget* is a plan, often called *a strategic plan*, that looks at goals and purposes over a span of 3, 5, and sometimes 10 years.
3. A *program budget* analyzes a specific program, one that is planned for the future or one that is in existence and requires evaluation. A budget often cuts across departments and years.
4. The **capital budget** tracks the acquisition of capital assets, or long-term investments (e.g., buildings, land, or equipment). Capital budget items provide useful service beyond the year they are first acquired or put in use. Expensive equipment generally is procured and replaced through the capital budget.
5. *Product-line budgets* look at the revenues and expenses associated with a defined group of clients, such as those with a common diagnosis. Product lines often are associated with disease groups or medical diagnoses, such as congestive heart failure or heart disease.
6. The *cash budget* tracks the monthly cash receipts and cash disbursements.
7. A *special purpose budget* is prepared for a program or activity that was not previously planned or budgeted.

In addition, a well-managed organization will have a set of all the major budgets in an organization, called the *master budget.*

THE BUDGETARY PROCESS

Each institution will establish standard budgetary formats and processes. Because the budget is actually implemented by all employees, the involvement of all employees in all aspects of budgeting is recommended (Finkler & Kovner, 2000).

The budgeting process is complex and requires the completion of several complicated documents. A typical budget process ties into overall strategic and managerial planning. The multiple steps of a budget process can be grouped into the following three phases (Finkler & Kovner, 2000):

1. *Establishing the basis for budget preparation:* Strategic plans and program budgets need to be prepared. Other data need to be gathered from an environmental scan; general goals, objectives, and policies; budget assumptions; program priorities; and a list of specific and measurable operating objectives.
2. *Preparing the first draft:* Unit and department managers use the gathered data to prepare budget documents for their areas. These documents are used at the organizational level to prepare cash budgets.
3. *Reviewing and re-budgeting:* As budget documents go through serial review and flow to top administration, requests tend to exceed the available resources. This necessitates review, adjustment, and appeal. There may be multiple iterations of re-budgeting before the final budget is approved.

It is at stage 3—reviewing and re-budgeting—that the art of negotiation is employed. At the top levels of management, budgetary requests are collated and coordinated. In many organizations, the final budget must be approved by the governing board or board of directors. Therefore managers and leaders need to prepare a strong defense for any item or program requested.

BUDGET FORMATS

Budgets and the budgeting process may be approached from a variety of strategies or perspectives. Common types of budget formats are traditional budgets, zero-based budgets, and flexible budgets.

Traditional budgets identify expenses to be tracked. In nursing, the most common expense items are salaries, benefits, supplies, and equipment. Traditional budgets may be called *incremental*

Practical Tips

Tip #1: Know the Process!

If you are a new nurse manager or even if you are an experienced nurse manager who has recently joined a new organization, be sure to familiarize yourself with the organization's budgeting process. Schedule an orientation session with someone from the organization's finance department early in your orientation so that you will understand the organization's financial reports. Ask your chief nurse executive to help you identify a colleague in the nursing department who is highly knowledgeable of the organization's budgeting methodology and who has had experience in successfully navigating the organization's budgeting process in the past. Ask that colleague for assistance as you prepare your first budget.

Tip #2: Plan Ahead

It is imperative that nurse managers and nurse executives obtain support for significant new budgetary initiatives as early as possible, well ahead of the budget development process. Review the pertinent literature, and conduct appropriate internal and external benchmarking. Share your ideas strategically with key leaders from departments or services that will be involved in approving the budget request to identify any major obstacles you may need to overcome to ensure the success of your proposal. Have a solid justification prepared well in advance, and be sure to include the impact on clinical quality and safety as part of your business plan or proposal.

budgets. Other expenses include overhead, administrative, and educational costs. Often negotiations are centered on the appropriate amount to increase the budget each year.

Zero-based budgets are rebuilt from zero each year or each budget cycle. The traditional approach takes the previous year's budget as the status quo and builds from there. With zero-based budgeting, all expenses are re-justified each year. This process uncovers exactly how money is being spent and avoids budgets becoming bloated over time. Zero-based budgets emphasize the consideration of alternative means of providing the same service or program. They provide a method for a sophisticated analysis of these alternatives (Finkler & Kovner, 2000).

Flexible budgets are budgets that are flexed or adjusted to reflect changes in variables (e.g., volume, labor costs) that may occur during the course of a budget cycle (Barr, 2005). With traditional and zero-based budgets, the manager or individual preparing the budget uses the information available at the time the budget is prepared to develop the budget forecast for the budget cycle. During the year, one of the variables may show a major change (e.g., an unanticipated but not uncommon significant increase in patient volume). If this occurs, the financial reports based on a traditional or zero-based budget will likely show a considerable budget variance because of the added resources required to care for the increased number of patients for the remainder of the budget cycle. In that case, the manager will spend much time and energy trying to account for and justify the budget variance. Using the flexible budgeting methodology in the same scenario would result in a midcycle adjustment of the expense projections based on the increased patient volume. The manager would then be expected to manage and monitor the financial performance for the remainder of the budget cycle based on those revisions. A primary advantage to the flexible budgeting methodology as compared with the traditional or zero-based budget approach is that the flexible budget can respond to the changes that affect health care systems over the course of a budget cycle.

Operating Budgets

The *operating* budget covers a specific period, called a *fiscal year,* and is the budget plan for day-to-day service delivery operations. It includes historical or trend data, expenses, and revenues. To prepare the annual operating budget, a variety of information is needed. Nurse managers typically prepare three major aspects of the operating budget: (1) the expense budget for personnel; (2) the expense budget for costs other than personnel; and (3) the revenue budget. Not all hospital nursing units prepare revenue budgets (Finkler & Kovner, 2000).

Development of the Operating Budget

The specific process used to develop operating budgets will vary considerably from one organization to another. Most organizations now use electronic means to develop and submit operating budgets. Although the budget development process will vary, the nurse manager's and/or nurse executive's role in developing operating budgets for nursing units and services will typically include input on or determination of volume projections, development of associated expense projections (including supplies, equipment, and salary/labor expenses), and some form of revenue projection. Many organizations develop and disseminate a set of budget assumptions that are to be used by managers and leaders in developing the operating budget. These assumptions may include such items as pre-established increases in labor or salary expenses based on contractual obligations, adjustments that must be made based on economic forecasts for supply charge changes (e.g., increased utility rates, increased cost of pharmaceuticals), or factors that will affect patient volume such as the addition of a new service line.

The foundation of the development of the operating budget at the unit level is based on the projected volume of work for the coming year. The workload aspect often is measured in units of service. Key units of service need to be identified, the number of units predicted, and expenses and staffing calculated accordingly. Activity reports, such as historical census and average length of stay, identify trends related to volume of activity. The unit of service often needs to be adjusted to the case or patient mix, which is a proxy for severity of illness or need (Finkler & Kovner, 2000).

Table 31.1 shows a sample volume budget flow sheet. Historical trend data are needed (e.g.,

Table 31.1

Volume Budget Flow Sheet

Month	Patient Days Budgeted	Patient Days Actual
January	268	272
February	310	315
March		
April		
May		
June		
July		
August		
September		
October		
November		
December		

occupancy percentages by time frames such as weekly or monthly) to determine growth projections and any impact of seasonality. The volume of services delivered for a year may be expressed as patient days, visits, procedures, or other units of service. Other effects on volume are environmental effects such as reimbursement changes, new programs, process improvements, new technology, and marketing. If volume projections depend on another service or department, it is important for the two departments to communicate closely so that similar assumptions are used in establishing volume projections.

Once the volume projection has been completed, the manager can determine the personnel services (or staffing budget) portion of the expense budget. Calculation of staffing is complex, and, given that staffing expenses generally are the largest portion of the nursing operating budget, nurse managers and nurse executives must have a consistent and well-defined approach to estimating staffing expenses. The methodology used will likely vary from organization to organization. Finkler & Kovner (2000) described the following method that may be used to estimate staffing expenses.

First, the average daily census and occupancy (or utilization) rate are calculated using volume projections that have been developed. Next, the number of full-time equivalents (FTEs)—that is, the mix of full-time and part-time staff—needed to provide care for the expected volume is determined based on the unit's staffing plan. The staffing plan should include any needed adjustments for nonproductive (benefits and knowledge work) hours based on benefit levels. The staffing plan should also specify the skill mix of direct care staff (registered nurse, licensed practical nurse/licensed vocational nurse, nursing assistant [RN, LPN/LVN, NA]) and the nursing hours per patient day appropriate for the patient population on the unit. Costs for administrative and other fixed staff members such as clerks need to be included. Other labor costs, such as overtime, shift or other differentials and premiums, and fringe benefit costs, must also be factored into the personnel budget.

Table 31.2 displays a sample budget expense sheet for salaries, and Table 31.3 demonstrates how personnel budgets might be displayed. Salary increases might also be included as another column.

Table 31.2

Budgeted Salary Expense Flow Sheet

Expense Item	Budgeted	Actual
Salaries		
Regular		
Overtime		
On-call		
Vacation		
Holiday		
Illness		
Other		
Total Salaries		

Table 31.3

Personnel Budget Sheet

Position	Name	FTE	Hourly Wage ($)	Yearly Salary ($)
RN	Smith	1.0		38,000
RN	Jones	1.0		38,000
LPN	Roe	0.5		29,000
NA	Ash	1.0		22,000
Clerk	Oak	1.0		20,000

LPN, Licensed practical nurse; *NA*, nurse assistant; *RN*, registered nurse.

Supply budgets are a major component of the operating budget. Many supply items are variable (the amount used will vary based on the volume of service provided). Other supply costs are fixed and will be incurred at the same level no matter the volume of service that is provided. Supply items such as office supplies, intravenous (IV) solutions, instruments, linen, gloves and other personal protective equipment, medical/surgical supplies, drugs, leases, maintenance contracts, staff education funds for travel to conferences or meetings, and books and subscriptions are all examples of line items that will likely be budgeted for. Dollar amounts are assigned based on historical projections and any known or anticipated adjustments resulting from inflation, contractual increases, or other factors as specified in the organization's budgetary assumptions. The operating budget will also need to include expenses for overhead, depreciation, utilities, telecommunications services, and other related facility expenses.

Revenue budgets are based on a set of calculations that determine expected receipts that will result from charging patients and payers for services. Nursing services are often not viewed as revenue-generating departments, but in many organizations, the patient days and related charges are used as a proxy for revenue. Revenue projections are based on volume projections. Factors such as payer mix and contractual rates will affect the overall revenue that is received. Contractual allowances (discounts), bad debt, and indigent care all become reductions of gross revenue and generally are not under the nurse manager's control (Finkler & Kovner, 2000).

Capital Budgets

The *capital* budget is the plan specific to major purchases that meet or exceed the organization's particular definition of a capital expense. The capital budget is prepared for large equipment, long-term investments, physical plant, or program expenditures. Examples of capital expenses are fixed assets, new or replacement equipment (e.g., new informatics technology), building renovation or unit relocation, or adding a new program (e.g., endoscopy suite). The specific process used to create a capital budget will vary from organization to organization. Most organizations require extensive background material to support capital budget requests. The background or supporting material required will probably include the vendor quotes for costs of purchase, installation, and staff education or training; a justification or explanation of the reasons that the capital expenditure is needed; and the relationship of the expenditure to the organization's strategic goals or objective. For capital construction projects, architectural plans, regulatory considerations, and other supporting materials may also be required as part of the capital budget preparation process.

TRACKING AND MONITORING OF BUDGETS

The budget process is often viewed as an event that occurs once a year and then ends until the next budget development process begins. This view needs to change in order for organizations to achieve financial success (Barr, 2005). Although the budget development process may occur once a year, the budget sets the stage for ongoing monitoring and evaluation of the organization's financial performance related to the budget projection. Regular budget analyses (e.g., quarterly or monthly) are used for monitoring, feedback, and managerial control. The variance (difference) between budgeted and actual revenue and expenses is determined to identify problem areas, enhance control, and ensure timely adjustments. In organizations that use flexible budgeting, some of the adjustments will be made automatically (Barr, 2005). Variances between actual and budgeted (planned) performance need to be analyzed to determine the cause so that nurses can take the appropriate action. Variances can be favorable or unfavorable. Most organizations now use electronic reporting formats that automatically calculate variance rates, but it is important that nurses understand the reasons for the variances. Variances can result from a single cause (e.g., volume of patients; a rate change such as salary, usage, or price) or from a combination of causes.

Nurse executives often require nurse managers to document their analysis of budget variances. Many nurse managers also find it is useful to share variance reports and the reasons for budget variances with their nursing staff. This will enhance the nursing staff's awareness of the unit's financial performance. Engaging unit staff in discussions about the unit's financial performance will also provide nursing staff the opportunity to suggest cost-saving strategies to control costs at the unit level.

LEADERSHIP AND MANAGEMENT IMPLICATIONS

Nursing services make up the single largest aggregate expense in most health care organizations because they represent a large personnel component and control a large share of supplies and equipment. This is both a strength and a weakness. It is a strength because nurses clearly manage the organization and system, especially at the operational unit level. With powerful and accurate data and analysis support, unit-level management becomes effective and efficient. However, many organizations simply do not provide a nurse-friendly support structure. It is a weakness to be the largest aggregate expense because quick, short-term economic gains can be made by ratcheting down on resources allocated to nursing services. This often occurs at the expense of long-term gains, staff morale, and group cohesion. Because health care generally faces strict fiscal constraints, both staff nurses and nurse managers must be knowledgeable and skilled in anticipating financial fluctuations and trends and in making bold decisions based on rapid analysis of information. Staff nurses often will be handling day-to-day budgetary decisions; thus they must be aware of the unit budget, the financial status of the unit and the organization, and the impact of their decisions about supply and resource (staff) utilization on the financial performance of the unit. Nurse managers are more involved with strategic or long-range financial planning and decision making.

The budgeting process requires a broad range of leadership and management skills. Resources are limited. This fact is difficult for some nurses, especially if they believe they should be able to do everything for every client under every circumstance. Some professionals think that their job is to provide the maximum quantity and quality of service and that cost-consciousness should not be a part of service provision. Nurses are familiar with managing clinical service delivery. These skills can be transferred into the management of money as a necessary adjunct to clinical service provision. However, the management of any scarce resource such as money includes balancing competing interests and making difficult decisions.

Leadership is involved in influencing others to achieve the group's goals within the constraints of scarce resources. Leaders need to be actively involved in setting the vision for how to accomplish goals through budget planning. Ethical

LEADERSHIP & MANAGEMENT BEHAVIORS

Leadership Behaviors

- Determines resource requirements for the group
- Guides a visionary justification of resources
- Analyzes expenditures
- Uses creativity to strategize and negotiate for the group's resource needs
- Motivates the group to increase budgetary knowledge
- Influences the group to find innovative ways to do things better
- Finds new sources for resources
- Creates a financially savvy work environment

Management Behaviors

- Plans the budget
- Organizes the needed resources
- Organizes budget justification
- Implements the unit budget and budget processes
- Controls expenses
- Determines resource requirements within organizational constraints
- Evaluates technology
- Motivates subordinates to learn about budgeting

Overlap Areas

- Determines resource requirements
- Motivates expanded knowledge about financial aspects
- Manages expenditures

considerations, such as fairness and reasonable targets, are part of leadership decision making. Leaders can influence employee morale and organizational culture through role modeling and the decision-making process. Organizational culture can be engaged to diminish the negative tone sometimes associated with budgeting.

Budgeting is a managerial responsibility. It involves skillful planning and projecting, mathematical analysis, and attention to detail in the preparation and interpretation of financial forms. The budgeting process also can be used as a tool for employee motivation, a chance to hone skills in negotiation, and an opportunity for quality improvement or program planning. For example, a break-even analysis was used to investigate the financial viability of a nurse-run community nursing center in the Chicago area. The results pointed to the opportunity for expanding into the market for Medicaid managed care enrollment (Ervin et al., 1998). In another study, activity-based costing and cost-driven analysis were used to develop a care requirements tool and to explore linkages among work-flow processes, time requirements, and resource consumption. Data were fed into benchmarking and quality improvement activities (Dodson et al., 1998).

Benchmarking figures are important for both budgeting and staffing. These figures can be generated by both internal and external data. Some external data estimates come from publicly reported databases. Comparisons based on risk-adjusted figures are needed. Resource consumption depends on client case mix and the severity of client illness. Factors such as client type, type and size of facility, services provided, and severity of illness are important for comparable external benchmarking. For internal benchmarking, actual versus budgeted costs; historical trend data on worked hours, client days, visits, or episodes; activity; and product costs are used. Some intervening factors skew data, such as restructuring, changes in client acuity, new programs or services, changes in physician practices, new therapies or treatments, and large changes in volume or census (Kenny, 1996).

Nurse managers and nurse executives must decide which budget-related variables are to be tracked and analyzed. Other leadership and management activities include keeping the boss informed, developing ways to increase revenues, emphasizing the return on the present investment, and looking for creative ways to fund what needs to be done (Starck & Bailes, 1996). In a successful budget, the money, staff, equipment, and materials available must be sufficient to meet the quantity and quality of anticipated and provided services (Bailey, 1996).

COST AWARENESS

Continuous change in the health care delivery and reimbursement systems has created a challenge to reducing costs while continually improving the quality of care. Nursing's attention has been drawn to cost-containment efforts. In trying to improve client care by improving managerial and clinical decisions in nursing, cost-consciousness is essential. The cost to clients from health care services is a social and professional concern. Cost and quality remain as two major themes for nursing practice. The questions that will be asked are: What is the cost? Will this provide high-quality care? What will the cost be (to the patient and to society) if the care is not provided or is not of high quality? The cost variable relates to decision making. Cost certainly is not the only consideration to use in decision making, but nurses must consider it as one element.

Reducing costs and capturing reimbursement are a part of a health care organization's goals that nurses are encouraged to incorporate into their practice. For example, in one facility a cost-containment work group consisting of staff nurses and other nonsupervisory employees was formed to develop cost-reduction strategies. The following five strategies were chosen:

1. Offering education to increase employees' awareness
2. Identifying and eliminating costly habits
3. Making cost-effective decisions
4. Recycling
5. Reducing unnecessary inventory

Specific cost-containment efforts were most effective with managing materials, choosing the least expensive alternatives, and recycling. Developing a unit-based cost-containment program was combined with quality improvement processes to garner significant cost savings (Brady et al., 1998). In another example, a multidisciplinary financial education research project was undertaken to assess effects on awareness and profit (Krugman et al., 2002).

What cost decisions do nurses control? What can nurses do to reduce costs? The following are suggestions to promote cost control:

- *Do the job efficiently.* The more efficiently the nursing care delivery is organized and run and the greater the contribution of individuals to the care provided, the less costly that care will be.
- *Remember that time is money.* For example, simple scheduling errors can increase the length of a client's stay. The time element is especially crucial in care coordination activities.
- *Help motivate clients to recover.* This approach improves their health status and reduces dependency costs.
- *Use supplies carefully.* Know the costs of those supplies. For example, posting a per-unit cost list that would include the cost of an alcohol swab or a roll of tape helps keep employees aware of the costs of the supplies they are using.

Knowing the costs will facilitate better substitution decisions (Striegel, 1986). For example, Chagares and Jackson (1987) compared price and performance of six pressure-relieving devices, and Smith and Amen (1989) compared the costs of IV drug delivery systems. Their results indicated potential alternatives. Such cost-comparison projects need to be an ongoing part of practice.

For a client with poor skin integrity, perhaps the most expensive tape should be used because the tape needs to stick and be waterproof. However, in a routine situation, can a lower-cost item be substituted adequately? Nurses cannot help reduce costs unless they know the per-item cost of the supplies they use and then use this information to evaluate substitutions. Even small cost reductions can be significant if they are applied to high-volume

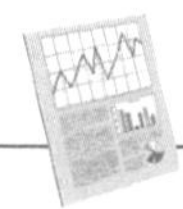

Research Note

Source: Beglinger, J.E. (2006). Quantifying patient care intensity: An evidence-based approach to determining staffing requirements. *Nursing Administration Quarterly 30*(3), 193-202.

Purpose

The purpose of this project was to provide data during the hospital budget process that would justify the increasing hours of nursing care to levels essential to providing the promise of the organizational mission: delivery of exceptional nursing care.

Method

The author identified drivers of intensity as follows: length of stay; admission, discharge, and transfer activity; age of patients; and complexity of patients (including alcohol withdrawal, confusion/disorientation, need for sitters or restraints, continuous oximetry, epidurals for pain management, tracheostomy outside critical care units, ventilators outside critical care units, euglycemia). These data were organized by patient care units, compared with external benchmarks, and trended over time. Staff experience was also incorporated into the unit level database. These data were then used to construct the nursing budget.

Discussion

The initial hospital budget was more than $20 million short of meeting essential profitability goals. Although some slight reductions were made in nursing units where possible, nurse leaders were firm in their commitment to require the resources necessary to provide safe, quality care.

Application to Practice

This study illustrates the use of nursing productivity data to inform financial decision making. Production process might be considered.

items. Immediately apparent is the costliness of inappropriate use of items (e.g., wiping up spills with a sterile pad; opening a sterile pack to use only one of the instruments; using preprinted forms as scratch pads). Convenience versus cost trade-off must be considered (e.g., bag baths may be convenient or necessary in a staffing shortage but are an expensive supply cost).

Nurses need to participate in organization-wide cost containment and take credit for the cost savings generated. A formal, documented way is needed in which nurses' decisions and the cost savings that result are visible and rewarded. Knowing the health care organization's costs and what the clients are charged for treatments and procedures (costs are not equal to charges) enables nurses to advocate for clients. Nurses need nursing cost data for analysis and evaluation, and they need the informatics and information support structure to accomplish this.

Nurses can identify inefficient or redundant activities and use decision-making abilities in certain areas of nursing practice. Serving on product committees gives nurses an opportunity to advocate for products that save nursing time and to influence vendors to create technology adaptations that decrease nursing workload. This will assist nurses to work intelligently and efficiently while still enjoying the work of nursing. Nurses should also serve on process improvement teams because they are key resources who can identify costly inefficiencies.

Nurses need to help control costs while using professional decision making. In other words, they need to allocate resources when it is appropriate and save money when it does not need to be spent. This is a key element of professional decision making.

CURRENT ISSUES AND TRENDS

Evaluation of Budget Expenditures

The public is becoming increasingly knowledgeable regarding the quality and safety of health care. Health care consumers and payers expect that money for new initiatives will be well invested and that a significant return on investment will be realized in terms of improved quality or safety of care. Business plans must include specific metrics that will be used to measure the impact of the expenditures on clinical outcomes, quality and safety, as well as on cost. Metrics should specify the impact on nurse-sensitive indicators when feasible to further validate the significant role that nurses play in improving the health status of patients.

Costing Out Nursing Services

Under a fee-for-service reimbursement system, the inequity among provider payment systems was a disadvantage to nursing. Nursing was seen as a cost but not a revenue generator. One strategy proposed to compensate for nursing's revenue disparity was to cost out nursing services. This idea became popular for a while but lost attraction as capitated reimbursement systems gained prominence. With a "per member per month" flat payment structure, conventional wisdom indicated that efforts to cost out for purposes of charging a fee for service were useless. Therefore costing out nursing services was cast aside. However, the unintended consequence was that the value of knowing precisely what it costs to deliver nursing services was lost. Whether the purpose is to establish a fee charge or to use the data for other strategic purposes, such as efficiently deploying resources or using data in contract negotiations, accurately determining the costs of nursing service is still an important budgetary function. Nurses need to know their costs to plan better and negotiate more effectively.

Costing out nursing services is defined as the determination of the costs of the services provided by nurses. By identifying the specific costs related to the delivery of nursing care to each client, nurses have data to identify the actual amount of services received. As a result, nursing will be in a much better position to autonomously monitor, justify, and control the costs of nursing care within a cost-conscious environment (Eckhart, 1993). Scherubel (1994) offered a warning, however. If nurses use costing out nursing care services to decrease costs, nursing budget requests may be reduced through decreased resource allocation to nursing departments. Thus it is important to capture incentives in return for cost-control efforts and to ensure that needed resources are actually spent on client service needs.

In reviews of the literature related to costing out nursing services, a variety of variables were examined, such as length of stay, nursing care costs, direct care costs, and DRG reimbursements. Most common was the extrapolation of nursing costs from a specific acuity system. Standardization of definitions and elements used to compute direct and indirect nursing care costs is lacking (Eckhart, 1993), which impedes comparisons across settings and sites.

The old health care system reimbursed mainly for medical services aimed at curing diseases. Despite reimbursement changes in a managed care environment, nursing costs still need to be determined. The usual model multiplies the amount of nursing time per intensity level (for a DRG) by the average nursing hourly salary and benefits and adds this to the indirect cost amount to arrive at the total nursing cost per DRG or intensity level. Nursing intensity usually is represented by a patient classification measure as a proxy. A serious flaw in this model is the inability to identify what nursing activities actually are delivered to clients. Patient classification or acuity systems tend to measure average or projected care needs, not actual needs and actual services delivered.

Another approach is to calculate nursing cost per nursing intervention or diagnosis. The amount of nursing time per nursing intervention can be multiplied by the nursing average hourly salary and benefits and added to equipment costs to determine direct costs. Direct costs plus indirect costs equal the total nursing cost. As nursing interventions replace intensity in the calculation, the actual nursing care delivered to clients is being measured more accurately. Dodson and colleagues (1998) presented yet another approach to costing by determining the cost drivers for an activity-based costing system. Cost-driver analysis, activity analysis, and performance analysis were employed to create an activity-based management system. The activities of the work processes, inputs, controls, outputs, and activity mechanisms combined to form a model of core processes, time requirements, and resource consumption useful for benchmarking and quality improvement.

Summary

- A budget is a plan designed to control the allocation of resources. It becomes a financial timetable.
- Seven types of budgets within the master budget are (1) operating, (2) long-range, (3) program, (4) capital, (5) product-line, (6) cash, and (7) special purpose.
- Traditional budgets, zero-based budgets, and flexible budgets are typical budgetary formats.
- The budgetary process is a financial planning and control system.
- It is imperative to involve nursing staff at all levels in appropriate aspects of budgeting to ensure successful financial management.

CASE STUDY

Helpful Community Hospital was in a tight squeeze. Of all revenue, payment from Medicare made up 70% of the hospital's income. The state was ranked dead-last in the Medicare payment fee schedule. The result was a squeezed-tight and ever-shrinking hospital operating margin. Hospitals in similar circumstances had closed. However, Helpful Community Hospital was the only acute care facility serving a wide geographic rural area. The chief nurse executive (CNE), Kathryn Gardner, decided to take bold action in one specific area over which nursing had control: supply chain management.

Nurse Gardner had read about the success of a Visiting Nurse Association (VNA) in patient-specific supply management (Maurano, 2004). Intrigued, she reviewed the supply budgets for the entire hospital. Costs were very high. Next, she met with her managers to discuss the issue. The managers reported high staff dissatisfaction with the "hassle factor" and the time wasted hunting for needed supplies. She asked the nurse managers to formally survey staff members. These results highlighted many opportunities for systems improvements.

Next, Nurse Gardner networked with her peers and looked for "best practice" trends in the field. This environmental scan led her to the Supply Sharpies Consulting group. She evaluated their proposal and completed the contract.

The consulting group began with a two-pronged initiative: a detailed analysis of the supply system and an educational initiative with the staff. Over the course of a year, barriers and resistance were overcome or worked through. A dramatic change in the way supplies were distributed and managed was proposed and accepted. A pretest and posttest evaluation design was implemented.

The new system was called *patient-specific supply management.* It involved purchasing and implementing an informatics technology that ordered supplies, tracked inventory, managed use, inserted management controls, and generated billing and other reports and documents. It also involved purchasing high-technology supply carts for each unit. Nurses identified needed supplies for each patient, which were then stocked in the supply cart on a daily exchange basis. Passwords were used to access the carts and remove supplies. If anything else was needed, the order was placed electronically and delivered to the unit.

The system had real-time delivery, individualized supplies, proactive monitoring of supplies, formulary compliance, and nurse convenience. Slippage and wastage, caused by such random events as physicians withdrawing supplies from bulk stocks and not using them for patients on that unit, were greatly reduced. Other positive effects were a dramatic drop in inventory, greater adherence to a standardized product formulary, and decreased waste of nurses' time tracking down and picking up supplies. Significant cost savings to the supply budgets translated into greater operating margin available for new program development. Nurse Gardner was considering using the freed-up resources for a disease management program using nurses to improve patient self-care management.

CRITICAL THINKING EXERCISE

Mariah Tokyandak is a relatively new nurse manager in the medical intensive care unit at a community hospital in a suburban location in the Pacific Northwest. Ms. Tokyandak has been preparing for her CCRN certification examination. In the course of her preparations, she came across an article describing the use of remote cardiac monitoring for patients in telemetry units. Ms. Tokyandak has a keen interest in this concept, also having heard about it from a colleague at a large academic medical center on the East Coast. Ms. Tokyandak's colleague claimed that the use of the remote cardiac monitors in the hospital in which she works has saved the salary expense for monitor technicians on every telemetry unit. In addition to her colleague's anecdotal report, the journal article states that patients who are monitored via the remote system have significantly improved clinical outcomes and shorter lengths of stay in the hospital.

Ms. Tokyandak is excited by the possibility of introducing this cutting-edge technology in her own hospital. She approached her chief nurse executive (CNE) to share her enthusiasm about this new technology and was told by the CNE that she should develop a formal proposal for the remote monitoring initiative as part of her capital budget development process for the coming fiscal year. The CNE also indicated that Ms. Tokyandak should include the other two monitored intermediate units in her proposal because the technology could then be used consistently across the organization.

Ms. Tokyandak is pleased that her CNE thinks her idea is a good one, but she is unsure about what to do next. Although Ms. Tokyandak completed the capital budget last year and was successful in obtaining a new overhead lift for bariatric patients on her unit, she has never prepared a capital budget proposal of this magnitude. She knows she will need to consider many factors, especially in light of the fact that capital budget requests are due in less than 2 months.

1. What should Ms. Tokyandak do next?
2. What strategies should Ms. Tokyandak use to increase the likelihood of successful approval of her capital budget proposal?
3. The finance director hears about this initiative and claims that he knows that these systems cannot save money. What actions should Ms. Tokyandak take to respond to his comments?
4. A staff nurse on Ms. Tokyandak's unit is concerned about this new initiative because she thinks that "nurses are being replaced by machines." What should Ms. Tokyandak do to address her concerns?

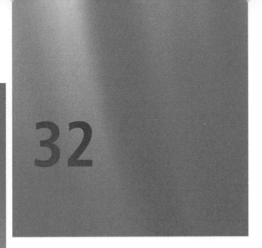

Productivity and Costing Out Nursing

Mary Ellen Murray

CHAPTER OBJECTIVES

- Describe the trends and projections for National Health Expenditures from 1998 to 2016
- Analyze productivity in nursing using the production process model
- Use a cost-analysis strategy to determine the cost of a good or service produced by nurses
- Analyze the leadership and management implications of the production process
- Differentiate among cost analysis, cost-effectiveness analysis, and cost-benefit analysis as methods of economic evaluation
- Analyze the challenges of managing a multigenerational workforce
- Exercise critical thinking to conceptualize and analyze possible solutions to a practice exercise

A "perfect storm" exists when conditions come together simultaneously to create an effect with greater impact than any single condition would have alone (Yoder-Wise, 2007). The simultaneous conditions of a worldwide nursing workforce shortage, the aging adult population, and managed care together have created what one nurse author calls "the perfect storm" (Curtin, 2007). Curtin described a growing demand for nurses that reflects the needs of an increasing geriatric population in the United States, placed within the context of the health insurance industry, which can be equated with managed care, a profit-maximizing business. This constellation, coupled with continuing increases in health care costs, has made it imperative that nurses be concerned with issues of productivity in all settings of clinical practice. Nursing is the largest health profession and the single most costly line item in hospital budgets, and the hospital is the most expensive setting of the health care system. Because nursing costs account for a major part of the labor costs in health care organizations, improving nursing productivity is a reasonable strategy for cost savings. However, given the nature of the work of nursing, it is essential to maintain the quality of care and provide for patient safety while considering issues of production.

DEFINITIONS

Productivity is a measurement of the output produced using a quantity of inputs. The **production process** is a representation of the relationship between outputs and the inputs used to produce them. The process is characterized by the following concepts (Jacobs & Rapoport, 2004):

1. *Marginal productivity:* additional output gained by adding additional input
2. *Economies of scale:* increasing the inputs to the production process, resulting in a volume increase such that the average cost per unit is decreased
3. *Short-run distinctions:* period in which there can be limited change to the inputs to the production process; inputs that cannot be changed are called *fixed*

LEADING & MANAGING DEFINED

Productivity

Output produced using a quantity of inputs.

Production Process

Relationships of outputs to inputs.

Costing Out Nursing Services

Methods to determine the actual costs of nursing services.

Economic Evaluation

Evaluating different programs or actions in terms of both costs and outcomes.

Cost Minimization

A common cost efficiency analysis concept that investigates what is the least costly alternative of two programs.

Charges

Dollar amount billed to a customer.

Price

Dollar value of each input to the production process.

Total Cost

Dollar value of the production process.

4. *Long-run distinctions:* period in which all of the inputs to the production process can be varied
5. *Substitution:* strategy of replacing a higher cost input with a lower cost input in the production process

Costing out nursing services refers to methods of determining the actual costs of nursing in any setting in which patients receive care.

Economic evaluation is defined by Drummond and colleagues (1997) as dealing with both the inputs and outputs to the production process or the costs and consequences of activities. This type of evaluation is concerned with the choices people make about the use of scarce resources—in this case, health care resources. Methods of economic evaluation include the following four basic techniques (Table 32.1):

1. *Cost analysis:* determining how much it costs to produce a good or service
2. *Cost-benefit analysis:* measuring the worth of a program, expressed in dollars
3. *Cost-effectiveness analysis:* comparing the costs of two (or more) methods of achieving the same outcome
4. *Cost-utility analysis:* considering the preferences of an individual for alternative types of treatment

In addition, **cost minimization** is a common cost efficiency analysis concept that investigates what is the least costly alternative of two programs. In all economic analyses, it is important to differentiate between **charges**, which is the dollar amount billed to a customer for a good or service before discounts are taken, and **price**, which is the dollar value of each of the inputs to the production process. **Total cost** is used here as the total dollar value of the production process. For any business to remain viable over time, charges must exceed costs.

BACKGROUND

National Health Expenditures (NHE) is a measure of spending for health care in the United States by type of service delivered (Heffler et al., 2003). In 1998, NHE exceeded $1 trillion for the first time. By 2016, NHE is projected to increase to $4.1 trillion (Poisal et al., 2007). Considered from another perspective, this amount of money in 1998 represented 13.1% of the gross domestic product (GDP), the value of all the goods and services produced in the United States in 1 year. By 2016, NHE is projected to represent 19.6% of the GDP. Although it is necessary to recognize the uncertainty of these

Table 32.1

Types of Economic Evaluation

Type of Study	Answers the Question
Cost analysis	What does it cost? *Example:* What is the cost of having a nurse practitioner conduct preoperative physical examinations before elective surgery?
Cost-benefit analysis	Is the program worthwhile, as measured in dollars? *Example:* Intervention A costs $300, has a benefit of $600, and can help 1000 people. Thus the benefit-cost (BC) ratio is 2:1. And the net benefit is $600,000 – $300,000 = Benefit of $300,000. Intervention B costs $4,000, has a benefit of $12,000, and helps only 10 people. Thus the BC ratio is 3:1. And the net benefit is $120,000 – $40,000 = Benefit of $80,000. Therefore A is preferred from the perspective of society.
Cost-effectiveness analysis	What is the cost of Method A versus Method B of achieving the same outcome? *Example:* What is the cost of renal dialysis versus renal transplant for 10 years of life gained?
Cost minimization	What is the least costly alternative of two programs? *Example:* Surgery for a modified mastectomy may be performed in an ambulatory surgical center or in the hospital requiring a 1-night stay. Both programs accomplish the same outcome, but which one is accomplished at least cost?
Cost-utility analysis	What is the incremental cost of the program compared with the health improvement attributed to the program? *Example:* There are multiple treatment programs for diabetes, but which program will improve both physical, social function, and psychological well-being (Drummond et al., 1997) of the patient?

projections, by analyzing the component parts of NHE, an understanding of the reasons for such increases is gained. Experts predict that out-of-pocket (OOP) expenditures—the amount of health care costs not covered by insurance—will grow more rapidly than other sectors because of efforts of employers and insurers to share costs with employees and patients. Hospital spending growth, largely driven by rising labor costs, is expected to remain the most important driver of health spending growth (Poisal et al., 2007).

The magnitude of these expenditure increases emphasizes the need for nurses, as members of the largest health care profession, to understand the implications of these data for clinical practice. As early as 1992, Davis (1992) indicated that, as nurses, "we are responsible for assuring that each dollar spent is spent wisely and that supplies and equipment are not wasted. Economic necessity dictates that even if we were to achieve a consensus about universal access to health care, we would need to couple this with economical nursing practice" (p. 217). Similarly, Hunt (2001) stated that clinical competency is not the only tool that nurses need in an era when economics dominates the health care arena. Nurses also need to have complex business skills.

Understanding the concept of productivity and relating it to the management of professional nursing is a leadership skill that will serve nursing in an era of accelerating health care expenditures. Based on this understanding, the nurse manager will be able to determine the costs associated with providing nursing care.

PRODUCTION PROCESS

The concept of a production process was first used in industrial applications (Murray & Henriques, 2003). For example, in the automotive industry, managers discuss the production process for manufacturing cars. The production process is a relationship between outputs and the inputs used to produce a given quantity of the output. The output of a production process in the automotive industry may be the production of 10,000 cars per month for a certain plant. The inputs would be, for example, the steel, rubber, person hours, and technology required to produce those cars. In this example, the output is a durable good. However, the output could also be a service, as it is in health care. Although the model may seem mechanistic and devoid of the caring that characterizes clinical nursing practice, cost awareness and associated cost-control practices are realities that are integral to the survival of the nursing profession. If nurses understand these concepts, they can more effectively participate in the decision-making process about the use of health care resources.

Transferring the concept of the production process to health care helps nurses understand the inputs required to produce the services associated with patient care. In the health care setting, the output of a production process could be as varied as a patient education program, a critical pathway, a specified number of units of family perinatal care, or a wound treatment procedure. Inputs in a health care setting could include laboratory tests, diagnostic procedures, registered nurse time, and medical equipment.

The generic representation of a production process is summarized in the following equation:

$$O_Q = f(I_1, I_2, I_3, Z\ldots)$$

In this equation, the output quantity *(O_Q)* is a specified amount of a good or service being produced. The output is a function *(f)* of all the inputs *(I)* used, beginning with the inception of the process and ending at the completion of the specified output. The inputs I_1, I_2, I_3, $Z\ldots$ represent all the inputs to the production process.

The following example transfers this model to health care:

QSNPC = f (time of registered nurses [RNs], time of licensed practical nurses/licensed vocational nurses[LPNs/LVNs], time of nursing assistants [NAs], computer hardware, equipment, Z...)

In this example, the output *(Q)* is a quantity of surgical nursing patient care *(SNPC)*. The inputs to the production of the care include the time of professional nurses and various assistive personnel, the technology and equipment required, and so forth *(Z...)*. *Z* represents all other inputs to the production process.

There are multiple possible inputs to the production process, which might include elements not usually considered, such as pharmacy time, nutritional services, and physical therapy. One approach to identifying the list of inputs to the production process is the use of the line items in the monthly budget reports that are routinely generated as part of the fiscal management process. These reports typically include wage and salary costs, fringe benefits, postage, mileage costs, telephone charges, and supplies that may be helpful in the identification of inputs. Specification of the inputs to the production process is a tedious but essential step that makes it possible to conduct cost analysis.

COST-ANALYSIS STRATEGY

After the inputs have been identified, it is now possible to conduct a cost analysis, the most basic form of economic evaluation that is fundamental to all other forms of economic evaluation. Cost analysis answers the question, "What did it cost to do a certain nursing intervention, to staff a patient care unit, or to produce nursing care for a certain population of patients?" Cost analysis consists of three steps: (1) the identification of the inputs (just discussed); (2) determination of total costs of the production process; and (3) determination of the average cost of each unit of output.

Total Cost of the Production Process

To determine the total cost of the production process, it is necessary to know both the price of each input and the amount of each input used. It also is necessary to define what is meant by "price" and "total cost." *Price* is defined as the dollar value of an input to the production process. *Total cost* is defined as the total dollar value of the production process. The total cost of the production process is equal to the price of the inputs multiplied by the quantity of the inputs used. This is represented by the following equation:

$$TC_{OQ} = (PI_1 \times QI_1) + (PI_2 \times QI_2) + (PI_3 \times QI_3) + (PZ\ldots \times QZ\ldots)$$

In this equation, the total cost *(TC)* of the production process is represented by TC_{OQ} or the total cost of the output quantity. Next, the cost of the first input (I_1) is calculated by multiplying the price of the input (PI_1) times the quantity of the input (QI_1). For example, if input I_1 is the time spent by the RN to care for a patient having a radical mastectomy and if 8 hours of time is used, the price of the input is 8 multiplied by the hourly salary of the nurse, which might be $26, for a total of $208.

When using the price of time as an input into the production process, it is necessary to include a proportion of the fringe benefits earned by that staff member. If this is omitted, the total cost calculation will be seriously understated. To add the input of fringe benefits to the cost of the production process, it is necessary to include a proportion of the costs of the benefits of the employee. Typically, an employer determines that fringe benefits are a percentage of salary. It may be, for example, that fringe benefits are 35% of an employee's salary. Thus in this calculation, the cost of the fringe benefits is an additional $72. The prices of all the inputs are added in this manner to determine the total cost of the production process.

Average Cost per Case

In the final step, the average cost per case is determined from the following equation:

$$ACC = \frac{TC}{OQ}$$

in which *ACC* represents the average cost per case, and *TC* represents the total cost (derived as just described) divided by the output quantity *(OQ)*. This last step is important because cost per unit of output may well determine the viability of the program or innovation. For example, if a health care system wishes to implement a day treatment program for adults with mental illness and a cost analysis reveals the operational costs to be $500 per day per patient but reimbursement is only $250 per patient, it is unlikely that the program will be viable.

LEADERSHIP AND MANAGEMENT IMPLICATIONS

Once the production process is defined and the cost analysis is complete, it is possible to use this information to analyze the following five characteristics of the production process:

1. Economic efficiency
2. Substitutability of inputs
3. Marginal productivity
4. Long-run and short-run distinctions
5. Economies of scale

These characteristics are important analysis tools for nurse leaders and managers to use in their clinical practice because they provide economic data to inform decision making.

Economic Efficiency

In the health care environment, the nurse manager is responsible for economic efficiency—that is, producing patient care at the lowest possible cost or, stated differently, minimizing the costs of production. It is essential that, concurrent with cost minimization strategies, nurses maintain high-quality patient care. In fact, poorly produced patient care is often *more* costly, since it results in adverse outcomes. Therefore although it may

LEADERSHIP & MANAGEMENT BEHAVIORS

Leadership Behaviors

- Plans strategy for productive use of resources
- Envisions a productive group output
- Enables followers to be productive
- Influences followers to increase productivity
- Enables release of followers' potential
- Creates a productive environment
- Communicates values that enhance productivity

Management Behaviors

- Plans resource allocation to improve productivity
- Organizes the environment to enhance productivity
- Calculates costs and productivity indices
- Monitors cost factors
- Controls resource expenditure
- Communicates the need for productivity
- Evaluates productivity patterns
- Influences subordinates to be productive
- Justifies departmental budget

Overlap Areas

- Plans for productivity
- Influences others toward productivity

be possible to decrease the amount of RN time in producing the output of patient care, this action may not produce the desired outcomes.

A comparison of several production processes that use different inputs may answer the question, "What is the least cost method for producing a good or service?" Within each production process, the combinations of inputs and their corresponding costs may be analyzed to determine economic efficiency. The nurse leader selects inputs into the production process with a consideration of the price associated with each input. For example, both certified nurse midwives and obstetricians produce maternity care for low-risk women, but research has shown that midwives produce the care using a lower cost combination of inputs (Oakley et al., 1996).

Substitutability of Inputs

The effect of substitution in the production process is another consideration. Substitution occurs when scarcity drives up the price of one good, or input (Input A). The result is that the quantity used of a second input (Input B) increases, because it is substituted for the more costly input. For example, as the price of RNs (Input A) has increased in the past decade, some hospitals have increased employment of LPNs/LVNs (Input B). This is the substitution of a less costly input (time of LPNs/LVNs) for a more costly input (time of RNs).

Substitution can be done safely when evidence shows that outcomes remain the same (Darmody et al., 2007). However, the manager must consider multiple factors before adopting such a practice. Is there an impact on patient outcomes from this substitution? What are state licensure laws that govern the scope of practice of LPNs/LVNs? Similar considerations apply when one considers the use of unlicensed assistive personnel (UAP) such as nursing assistants.

Marginal Productivity

Within the production process, *marginal productivity* is defined as the additional output achieved by increasing one input while keeping all other inputs constant. The manager might ask, "What would be the effect of adding an additional RN on each of three shifts?" Would such an addition increase the output of the patient care unit? It depends. It may be that the additional nurse will produce an increase in the number of hours available to care for patients who are increasingly acutely ill. In this case, output would not increase, which is the number of patients cared for, but the quality of patient care may be improved significantly. In another example in an ambulatory care setting, the manager considers adding additional staff but the number of examination rooms cannot be increased. Productivity, as measured by patient visits, may not increase by the

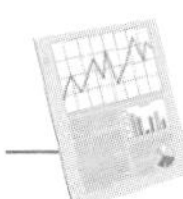

Research Note

Source: Darmody, J., Pawlak, R., Hook, M., Semeniuk, Y., Westphal, J., Murray, M.E., et al. (2007). Substitution of hospital staff in concurrent utilization review. *Journal of Nursing Care Quality, 22*(3), 239-246.

Purpose

Most hospitals employ registered nurses (RNs) to conduct concurrent utilization review (UR), a cost-containment strategy used by the managed care industry. The UR process requires that hospital providers communicate clinical information about patients to payers, who determine if the planned care is certified for payment. The purpose of the study was to determine the effect that substitution of different job classifications of hospital employees has on the outcomes of the UR process. There were two main effects of interest: (1) Was there a difference in the number of denials of certification of reimbursement when the function was performed by different types of employees? and (2) Is there a difference in the cost of conducting the UR process?

Four types of hospital staff conduct UR in the study hospital: case managers, case manager associates (non-clinical support position), RNs, and social workers.

Discussion

The authors reported that over a period of 2 years, 26,636 reviews were conducted. Fewer than 1% of the reviews resulted in a denial of certification of reimbursement. There was no significant difference in the proportion of denials across the four classifications of employees. In a part of the study previously reported by Murray and Henriques (2003), however, different costs per review by the four types of hospital employees were as follows: RN, $7.24; MS-prepared clinical social worker, $7.71; MS-prepared RN, $9.25; and assistive personnel, $4.78.

Application to Practice

This study illustrates the use of substitution in a production process for concurrent utilization review. The authors demonstrated that, in this institution, four categories of staff completed the reviews with similar results, though at different costs. This raises the question of the necessity of having RNs involved in the process. Given that the United States is experiencing a critical nursing shortage, is this a function that requires the expertise of RNs or could it be delegated to other personnel without a decrease in quality? A second issue is that the cost of having an advanced practice nurse case manager conduct the review is nearly twice the cost of a review completed by an assistive staff person. Though there are limitations to the study, it would appear that it may be possible to substitute ancillary personnel for RNs for this process.

addition of staff. In this situation, the manager may consider changing another input to the production process—specifically, additional examination rooms.

Long-Run and Short-Run Distinctions

A nurse manager also needs to consider the time context of the production process. It is not possible at all points in time to simultaneously vary all of the inputs to the production process. The "short-run" is usually defined as that period in which it is possible to vary only some of the inputs; in the "long-run," all inputs may be varied. For example, in the very short term, which might be considered the next 8-hour shift, it may not be possible to hire additional RNs or to increase the number of patient rooms on a given unit. But in the long term, both of these options are possible. The manager needs to be aware that when one input is fixed in the short-run, increasing another input may lead to decreased productivity or diminishing returns. This is the case when a hospital makes a decision to increase the number of patient beds in a facility but then cannot hire the staff to care for the additional patients. This results in a diminished return on the input of additional beds.

Economies of Scale

When all of the inputs to the production process increase and the output volume increases by a larger percentage, economies of scale are said to exist. The result is that the average cost per unit of output declines. The basic question becomes, Is it less expensive per case to produce a good or service in quantity? For example, when DVD players were first produced, they were quite expensive. With an increase in production, the cost per unit (i.e., cost per DVD) decreased substantially. The same concept applies to the production of nursing care. Many hospitals have chosen to employ diabetes nurse educators and develop extensive programs of care and teaching for patients with diabetes. Nurse managers found that it is less costly per patient to increase all of the inputs to the production process for diabetic care (e.g., nurse's time, physician's time, teaching tools, facilities) and produce this care for a larger number of patients than to produce the same care for a very small number of patients. This is an example of economies of scale. When considering such a venture, managers may be asked to determine the volume of patients they would have to serve to "break-even." The break-even level is the point at which the expense of the program equals the revenue to be generated. In the early implementation of such a project, a break-even level may be acceptable, but at some point, most programs will need to show revenues greater than costs (profit) to remain viable.

In general, too little effort has been devoted to determining the actual costs of nursing and the provision of nursing care. With actual data, nurses will be in a better position to demonstrate their economic value to health care and nurse managers will have appropriate information with which to accurately manage nursing services.

ALTERNATIVE MEASURES OF PRODUCTIVITY

Various measures of productivity exist, but all involve relationships between volume of inputs and cost. Nurses' time is the critical input in the production of nursing care. Home health agencies measure their productivity in patient home visits and hours of care; hospitals measure patients days; clinics measure the number of patient visits. The cost measure is the cost of the nursing time required to produce this care. Box 32.1 provides additional methods of calculating productivity.

> Box 32.1
>
> **Measures of Productivity**
>
> Productivity (P) = Cost per unit of output
>
> $$P = \frac{\text{Input}}{\text{Output}}$$
>
> $$P = \frac{\text{Cost}}{\text{Unit of output}}$$
>
> $$P = \frac{\$}{\text{Work hours}}$$
>
> $$P = \frac{\text{Nursing hours worked}}{\text{Number of hospital patient days}}$$
>
> $$P = \frac{\text{Number of nursing staff}}{\text{Census or patient days}}$$

The oldest method of measuring nursing productivity is the analysis of hours per patient day (HPPD). The input is the nursing hours worked. The number of hospitalized patient days is the output. This index is imprecise because of the wide variation in client acuity, with the result that the measure of patient days is not equivalent across cases.

A variety of data sources and productivity indices can also be considered. In nursing, productivity has been tightly linked to staffing numbers. For example, staffing, calculated as the total number of hours of a given staff for a given time period, can be compared with client volume or census. Using this method, if the output (patient days) increased while staffing remained the same, the productivity, strictly speaking, would be increased. This typically happens in hospitals when the influenza season is severe and a large number of geriatric patients are admitted to the hospital. In this short-term staffing crisis, the same numbers of staff are available to care for the high census and productivity temporarily increases. However, the gains may be short-lived, in that the short-staffing situation may result in nurse burnout and resignations.

No one measure of productivity adequately measures the knowledge-based work of nursing. Productivity measurement is complex because of the following (Edwardson, 1989):

- Measuring nursing care outcomes is difficult and controversial.
- The relationships between care processes and nursing outcomes are not well understood.
- The most efficient combination of resources for performing care processes is not known.

One solution has been to emphasize outcomes measurement. Research on outcomes measurement is accelerating and provides empirical data to support staffing decision making. Nurse researchers (Cho et al., 2003) demonstrated a relationship between staffing and adverse patient outcomes. They found that an increase in 1 hour worked by RNs per patient day was associated with an 8.9% decrease in the odds of patients acquiring pneumonia. These researchers also found that the occurrence of all adverse events (pneumonia, pressure ulcers, wound infections) was associated with a prolonged length of hospital stay, increased mortality, and increased hospital costs. This is an example of outcomes research that will aid managers' decision making in the future.

COSTING OUT NURSING SERVICES

Fundamentally, nurses need to have their own data on actual and specific costs of nursing care. These data are essential to developing an understanding of the relationship between the use of nursing resources and quality outcomes that are sensitive to direct nursing care (Pappas, 2007). Capturing these data has been difficult. In the era of diagnosis-related groups (DRGs) and fee-for-service reimbursement in the 1980s, costing out nursing services was seen as a strategy to capture reimbursement for nursing. However, under managed care and capitated reimbursement systems, service costing may need to be done by alternative methods. Activity-based costing is one approach to service costing that is quite different from traditional methods and may be useful in settings such as home health care. It can measure quality improvement efforts in relation to activity costs. The key advantage of activity-based costing is that it reflects what it costs to provide services and identifies why costs were incurred.

There are two steps to the activity-based cost assignment process. The *first* step is to identify activities that consume resources, such as provision of client services; the *second* step is to assign activities to cost categories such as service lines or programs. Costs tend to follow a four-level cost hierarchy of unit, batch, business, and enterprise levels. Underlying principles are that activities consume resources and that activities will be different based on payer, product line, program, and positioning in the cost hierarchy. Resource cost is then assigned to activities directly or with resource drivers. Assignment of resource cost to activities is based on actual time spent by activity. Activities with similar attributes can be aggregated. For example, all client care costs related to admission visits in home care would identify the total cost of admission visits. Dividing this figure by the number of clients admitted would result in the average cost of an admission visit, which can be used to benchmark outcomes and performance (McKeon, 1996).

Nursing has been unable to adequately address costs and efficiency insofar as data on the actual costs of nursing services are unavailable to nurses. Yet nurses have become interested in costing out nursing services for the purposes of productivity analysis and for purposes of being acknowledged as a revenue-generating component of the institution. Ideas about costing out nursing services arose in the mid-1980s, coinciding with the implementation of DRGs. The importance of determining costs is compelling. The purposes of costing out nursing services are to facilitate health policy and for reimbursement decisions. Costing out nursing services provides data for productivity comparisons. Acuity, or patient classification, is the most frequently used tool for collecting nursing's cost data. A variety of acuity tools are used.

The Medicare Cost Report (MCR) has been suggested as an information resource for costing out nursing services in hospitals. Hospitals being reimbursed by Medicare submit annual data on cost-to-charge ratios. To determine nursing costs, the nursing product needs to be defined in terms of output, process, or a combination. A patient classification system can be used to establish a productivity or relative value unit. Client care hours can be charged on a daily basis, a database developed, and daily charges entered as an outcome measure. Hospital bills can be unbundled and both a cost and price for nursing services set. Services are costed out as direct and indirect expenses, as extracted from the MCR. The costs of nursing care for clients of

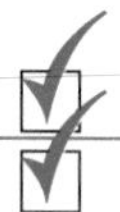

Practical Tips

*Tip #1: Listen and **Hear** Nursing Staff; Buy a lot of Coffee Breaks!*

As a nurse manager, it is crucial that you take the time to understand the workload of nurses on your patient care unit. This can be done in brief 1:1 coffee breaks at the manager's invitation or in small, informal group meetings. An opening remark may be as simple as, "How is it going?" When nurses tell their manager that they do not have time to give quality care, it is time to engage in problem solving and advocate for staff and their patients.

Tip #2: Provide Feedback and Data

As a nurse manager, you have access to data about the productivity of the unit—share it with nursing staff. They are the workers producing patient care and have a right to know how they are performing. If there has been a month of very high census and staff have filled the holes in the schedule, provide data in a bar or line graph. It is helpful to provide a benchmark comparison, such as a second line that shows "last year at this time." Teach staff the meaning of the terms "actual" and "budgeted."

Tip #3: Evaluate Productivity and Patient Satisfaction

When presenting productivity data to staff, simultaneously present patient satisfaction data. It may be that productivity increased in a given period, but if patients are not satisfied with the quality of the nursing care, productivity scores do not matter.

Tip #4: Monitor Turbulence

The activity on a patient care unit may be described as "turbulence"—the traffic patterns, change-of-shift activity, and extraneous commotion (e.g., filling supply cabinets, medication delivery, patient visitors) on a patient care unit. These activities tend to decrease productivity on the unit and interfere with patient care. Are there ways to minimize the impact of turbulence—ways to "keep the seatbelts on"?

Tip #5: Productivity Cannot Be Separated from Acuity, or "Acuity Trumps Volume"

The charge nurse on a patient care unit has the ultimate responsibility for deciding how many nurses are required to provide quality nursing care for the patients on the unit for that shift. The charge nurse needs to consider not only how many patients are currently on the unit but also how ill they are and the intensity of their care needs. This is a judgment of an expert clinician and cannot be forecasted by looking at the numbers alone. The nurse manager needs to communicate and support this clinical decision making.

all acuity types can be calculated from this model (Swansburg & Sowell, 1992).

Two models for costing out nursing services have been identified (McCloskey, 1989). The first model reflects the general trend of the literature: the amount of nursing time per intensity level as related to a specific DRG is multiplied by the nurse's average hourly salary/benefits and added to an indirect cost amount to determine the total nursing cost per DRG. Because the first model has some limitations and cannot define what nursing activities are provided for the cost, it yields only nursing cost per DRG or intensity level. A second model was developed to yield nursing cost per nursing intervention or nursing diagnosis. In the second model, medical diagnosis and nursing diagnosis both initiate nursing interventions. To measure the costs of nursing interventions, direct costs (nursing time multiplied by average salary, plus equipment) and indirect costs are added to derive total nursing costs. In general, too little effort has been devoted to isolating actual nursing costs. With actual data, nurses are in a better position to demonstrate value.

CURRENT ISSUES AND TRENDS

Four major issues related to productivity are the focus of nurse leaders today: (1) a national nursing shortage; (2) integration of economics into the practice of clinical nursing; (3) increasing acuity of hospitalized patients; and (4) a multigenerational nursing workforce.

National Nursing Shortage

Studies by the U.S. Department of Health and Human Services (National Center for Health Workforce Analysis, 2002) predicted a national nursing shortage of 800,000 nurses by the year 2020. A shortage is created when the demand for nurses exceeds the supply. A state-by-state analysis of the nursing shortage places the impact in a personal context. In 2020, for example, California is predicted to experience a nursing shortage in excess of 120,000 nurses. Florida will have a shortage of 61,000 and New York almost 45,000. Hospitals will continue to be the major employer of RNs (62%), but need for RNs in nursing homes and home health care will increase. Simultaneous with an increased demand is an increasing rate of nurses leaving the workforce, largely as a result of an aging RN workforce.

Although nursing educational institutions have attempted to increase the supply of RNs, they have not been entirely successful. Between 2006 and 2007, enrollment in baccalaureate programs increased by 4.98%; however, more than 30,000 qualified applicants were turned away from baccalaureate nursing programs primarily because of a shortage of nursing faculty (American Association of Colleges of Nursing [AACN], 2007).

These dire statistics point out the need to maximize the productivity of professional nurses. However, this productivity cannot be accomplished by decreasing staffing to levels that place patients in jeopardy. The research of Aiken and colleagues (2002) demonstrated that in hospitals with high nurse-patient ratios, surgical patients experienced higher risk-adjusted mortality and higher failure-to-rescue rates. Dr. Aiken also reported that nurses in these hospitals were more likely to experience burnout and job dissatisfaction.

It is possible that increased use of technology will be a partial solution to increasing nursing productivity. Computerized documentation and medication administration systems are widespread applications of technology that have resulted in time savings and subsequent increased productivity for nurses. Information technology is another enhancement to nurses' productivity. Medical records are easily accessed from multiple sites, results of diagnostics tests are communicated instantly, and monitoring devices detect deviations from normal limits and communicate these to the nurse as they occur.

Another responsibility of nurse leaders related to productivity is ensuring a future workforce by participating in the recruitment of future nurses. A telephone survey of 800 youths in grades 7 to 11 and adults ages 18 to 49 years revealed disturbing results (Erickson et al., 2004). Only 5% of the students in the sample group stated they would choose nursing; only 29% of the adults (deemed potential career switchers) think nurses are becoming more appreciated and respected in the workplace. Both groups believed that nursing does not offer the economic benefits that they desire. Fewer than 20% of both groups believed that nurses earn $45,000 per year, when in reality nurses earn that much or more. These results indicated that nurse leaders, and all nurses, have a heightened responsibility to present the profession in a favorable and honest way. In a recent conference, a speaker reported that as a colleague leaves her home for work each day, she tells her young children, "Mom is going to go to the hospital to save lives today." Although nursing does not *always* offer that level of drama, it certainly speaks of the importance of the work that nurses do. That importance needs to be communicated to the pool of persons who are potential nurses.

Integration of Economics into Clinical Practice

The incorporation of economic evaluation into clinical practice is important to productivity because health care resources are limited and choices must, and will, be made. In the years preceding managed care, health care providers acted as if health care resources were infinite, with the result that health care costs spun out of control. Today, providers are faced with difficult decisions about "who gets what." Although rationing health care is inherently unacceptable to most of the U.S. population, it is true that rationing is occurring. Today, rationing is done on the basis of the ability to pay for health care, with the uninsured receiving less health care. Well-educated nurses who understand economics and finance are in a unique position to bring the values of nursing to decision making about the allocation of health care resources.

Cost analysis is the foundation for all economic evaluation. Within the nursing literature, nurse leaders increasingly advocate for "cost-effective nursing practice" without defining what is meant by that term. The term "cost-benefit" is also loosely used without precise definition. It is necessary to make these distinctions to use appropriately the work of nurse researchers conducting these studies and to be able to conduct similar studies. See Table 32.1 for definitions and examples of these terms. On a cautionary note, it is important to remember that these analyses are not intended to be used as the sole tools for decision making. Economic analyses are one factor among many to be considered in decision making about health care programs and policies.

Recognizing the impact of the predicted national health expenditures, the National Institute for Nursing Research in the summer of 2004 partnered with the Agency for Healthcare Quality and Research and the Institute for Johns Hopkins Nursing to sponsor a workshop on the integration of cost-effectiveness analysis (CEA) into research. The conference brochure pointed out that in a time of constraints on health care resources, CEA studies are tools that help determine which intervention provides the highest health care benefit per dollar. This conference is recognition of the importance of economic evaluation by leaders in nursing. Study of health care economics may be required coursework in the future curricula of all baccalaureate nursing programs.

Increasing Acuity of Hospitalized Patients

Acuity is defined as a measure of the severity of illness of an individual patient or the aggregate patient population on a unit. Any nurse who has engaged in clinical practice in hospitals for 10 or more years can recount how much the acuity of patients has increased in the past decade. In the past, patients were admitted for diagnostic tests and for additional preparation before surgery. They typically remained in the hospital until they were able to care for themselves, often through a lengthy convalescence. A nurse was able to provide care to larger numbers of these patients because they required less care and assessment. Today these patients are receiving care in other settings and only very ill patients remain in the hospital. This increased acuity decreases the number of patients for whom a nurse may safely provide care. This results in what might look like, on paper, a decrease in productivity. Any measure of the productivity of nursing staff that does not consider the acuity level of patients is seriously flawed and would probably result in a gross underestimation of the output.

Various approaches are used to determine this acuity level and then relate it to staffing needs. Patient classification software is available for purchase. These systems attempt to categorize the levels of nursing care required by patients and then project appropriate nursing and ancillary staff. Such systems are often very expensive to purchase, to modify to meet the needs of a specific hospital, to install, and to maintain. Critics argue that such systems cannot capture the invisible knowledge work of nursing. The systems are often inadequate to adjust for the experience level and varied expertise of RNs. However, measures do exist to capture patient acuity and its impact on nurse staffing (Beglinger, 2006).

Multigenerational Nursing Workforce

For the first time, four generations of nurses are employed at once in the workforce: the Traditional, or Mature, Generation (born between 1922 and 1943); the Baby Boomers (born between 1943 and 1960); the Generation Xers (born between 1960 and 1980); and the Nexters (born between 1980 and 2000). Gerke (2001) described the impact of a multigenerational workforce in the selection of benefit plans. Baby Boomers wanted generous pension plans, whereas Xers wanted salary increases that would enable savings for future educational needs of children. Staff members around the age of 20 years (Nexters) wanted similar things but also valued more paid time off. The two younger generations wanted balance between leisure and work. Balancing pay, benefits, and related economic incentives for diverse age cohorts is a major economic challenge, especially in a cost-containment milieu. Nurse managers may need to construct a menu of economic and work-life reward options. Gerke (2001) described new management and motivational skills that will be needed to manage these diverse employees. For example, the Traditional Generation may not desire full-time employment but should be valued for their experience. Generation Xers need to hear in pre-employment interviews that the organization wants them to have a life outside of work. Nexters seek connections between their job and their personal goals. Each of these generations contributes to the productivity of nursing, and each is needed in the workforce despite the potential conflicts that might arise from their differing work ethics.

Clearly, raising the productivity of nursing while protecting the quality of patient care will continue to be a major challenge for nurse leaders. The use of the production process is one method to examine the productivity of nurses, comparing the relationship between the output (nursing care) and the inputs used to produce it. The characteristics of the production process (economic efficiency, substitution, marginal productivity, long-run/short-run distinctions, and economies of scale) are tools for managers to use in considering changes to the production process. Strategies of economic analysis are presented as ways to compare and evaluate interventions and programs of care.

Summary

- Issues of productivity are important in all clinical practice settings.
- Productivity is the measure of output produced using a quantity of inputs.
- Four basic techniques of economic evaluation are cost analyses, cost-benefit analyses, cost-effectiveness analyses, and cost-utility analyses. Cost minimization is used in efficiency analyses.
- Charges are different from price and costs.
- Nurses need to understand the concept of productivity.
- The production process applies to the inputs required to produce the services associated with patient care.
- Cost analyses can be performed after inputs are identified.
- Nurse managers need production-process and cost-analysis data to analyze economic decisions.
- Productivity measurement is complex.

- The incorporation of economic evaluation into clinical practice is important to productivity because of limited resources.

CASE STUDY

Nurse Manager Susan Lange, RN, MS, is responsible for an inpatient orthopedic surgical unit and the associated orthopedic surgical clinic. The inpatient hospital unit cares for an average of 8 patients each week who have had total hip replacement surgery and 12 patients per week who have had total knee replacement surgery. Most of these patients are older than 75 years and depend on either an elderly spouse or other family caregiver for assistance throughout the surgery and recovery. For elective surgery, patients are admitted to the hospital on the morning of surgery. They have had a preoperative physical and laboratory work within 4 days preceding the surgery.

Nurse Lange is aware of the inconsistency of the quality of the preoperative teaching that the patients receive. Some patients are well prepared, know what to expect, and have practiced ambulation techniques before the surgery. Other patients are confused about the plan of care and appear to have had little or no preparation. Nurse Lange has discussed this problem with the RNs who work in the clinic. The RNs acknowledge the problem and report that they "do the best that time allows." A second problem in the care of this patient population is the frequent need for temporary nursing home placement after the surgery. The difficulty in finding this type of posthospitalization placement often results in delays in discharge of 1 to 3 days.

Nurse Lange has conducted brainstorming sessions with her staff. They have designed a program whereby an RN would function in the dual role of educator/case manager for this group of patients. The person in the new role would be responsible for designing care plans that would begin in the clinic, follow the patient throughout the surgical experience, and even resume in the clinic at postsurgical follow-up. The person would also function as a patient educator. Now, Nurse Lange must "sell" the program to the chief nursing officer and gain funding for the additional position.

1. What data does Nurse Lange need to present to support the request for the new position?
2. What should be the educational requirements of a person in the new position?
3. What should be the experience requirements of the person in the new position?
4. Is any reimbursement possible to offset the costs of the new position? From what source?
5. What outcomes should be measured to demonstrate the impact of the new program?
6. How will the productivity of the person in the position be measured?
7. What other stakeholders in the care of the patient population should be consulted and have input into the program?

CRITICAL THINKING EXERCISE

Bill Ryan is a clinical nurse manager employed at a home health care agency associated with a large teaching hospital. He is frequently called on to provide home care for patients who are ventilator-dependent upon discharge from the hospital. It is a challenge for the agency to accept these patients because they require RN care for 16 to 24 hours per day. Nurse Ryan wants to conduct an economic analysis of keeping the patients in the hospital versus caring for them in their homes.

1. What is the economic question Nurse Ryan is asking?
2. What are the programs he is comparing?
3. What are the outcomes of interventions, and what are the units of measurement?
4. What method of economic analysis would you recommend? Why?

Performance Appraisal

Lynne S. Nemeth

CHAPTER OBJECTIVES

- Define and describe performance appraisal
- Explain factors that drive the need for effective nursing performance
- Describe how organizational culture can catalyze changes in performance
- Discuss the roles and expectations of interdisciplinary team members in the process of performance appraisal
- Review performance appraisal criteria critically, considering reliability and validity in measurement
- Relate the role of leadership in performance appraisal, contrasting the need for effective staff development with the process for performance appraisal
- Exercise critical thinking to conceptualize and analyze possible solutions to a practice exercise

Managing the performance of people is an important organizational strategy designed to exceed expectations of consumers in today's competitive health care environment. Many complex processes and strategies are involved in managing employee behavior. Managers need to clearly define the roles and expectations that are needed in the variety of settings in which individuals provide their efforts in return for compensation. Active engagement by managers in the process of setting standards of performance motivates the staff they employ to achieve goals. By communicating the important issues that affect performance and the problem-solving issues that arise with the individual who may experience conflict or difficulty following established procedures, managers can provide a fair appraisal of the individual's abilities, talents, and opportunities for improvement.

DEFINITIONS

Performance is defined as the execution of an action; something accomplished; the fulfillment of a promise, claim, or request (*Merriam-Webster's Collegiate Dictionary*, 1997). Leading staff to accomplish the goals and responsibilities inherent in a specific position requires clear communication, effective observation and feedback in a concurrent manner, coherent performance criteria, and the ability to reflect organizational mission, vision, and values.

Performance appraisal means evaluating the work of others. Albrecht (1972) defined **conventional performance appraisal** as a systematic, standardized evaluation of an employee by the supervisor, aimed at judging the perceived value of the employee's work contribution, quality of work, and potential for advancement. The employee's work is measured against standards, and in that sense it is very much like the quality improvement process. Standards, whether explicit or not, are applied to what ought to be or to what is superior, excellent, average, or unacceptable performance. **Peer review** in nursing is defined as the examination and evaluation of practice by a nurse's associates (Christensen, 1990). **Self-evaluation** is the aspect of performance appraisal whereby employees do self-assessments of their own perceptions about their performance as compared with stated objectives and expectations.

PERFORMANCE APPRAISAL PROCESS

Performance appraisal is a required process in organizations to help ensure that the quality of care is met and to provide a fair human resources management process. Feedback is needed by all staff employed in a designated role. Performance appraisals provide staff members with the information necessary to determine whether they are meeting expectations or can improve their performance to the required level.

The process of performance appraisal includes assessing needs and setting goals, establishing objectives and time frames, assessing progress and evaluating performance, and then starting over again (Figure 33.1). At the start of a new job, core competencies (knowledge and skills) of new hires need to be evaluated. Regulatory agencies such as The Joint Commission require organizations to verify and document staff qualifications to provide care, treatment, and services to patients (The Joint Commission [TJC], 2008). During the orientation program, progress should be tracked, and competence needs should be reassessed periodically throughout employment, at least every 3 years.

Performance appraisal is a cyclical process that begins when the employee is hired and ends when

LEADING & MANAGING DEFINED

Conventional Performance Appraisal

A systematic, standardized evaluation of an employee by the supervisor, aimed at judging the perceived value of the employee's work contributions, quality of work, and potential for advancement.

Peer Review

The examination and evaluation of practice by the employee's associate.

Self-Evaluation

A self-assessment of the employee's own perceptions regarding performance according to stated expectations.

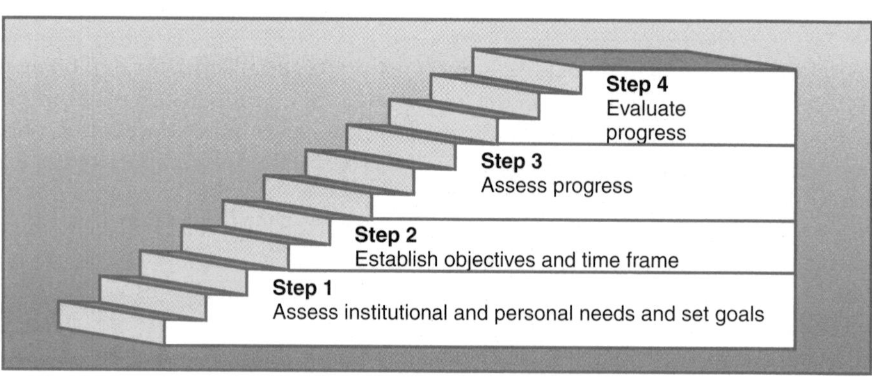

Figure 33.1
Four steps of a performance appraisal.

the employee leaves. Job analysis should identify competencies required for job performance. Next, the job description should identify work standards and the knowledge, skills, and abilities necessary for the job. The performance appraisal specifies employee behaviors and compares job performance with criteria. A variety of measurement methods may be used to ensure that reliable and valid appraisals are conducted. Using the performance appraisal interview, goals are set, corrective action may be taken, or training needs may be identified. Outcome criteria include equitable rewards and recognition that are objectively administered using valid tools (Frank, 1998).

The performance appraisal process is both informal and formal. The informal process includes day-by-day supervision or coaching to moderate, modulate, or refine small parts of performance. Coaching is an approach to developing people in an organization that falls somewhere between preceptoring and mentoring. The term *coach* invokes a sports metaphor. Every team relies on a coach to help the athlete(s) reach full potential. Coaching as a management tool is ongoing, face-to-face collaboration and influence to improve skills and performance. By contrast, the formal performance appraisal should include written documentation and a formal interview with follow-up.

The employee's work is measured against some standard for the purpose of determining the level of quality of the job performance. The guides to evaluation criteria include governmental standards such as Medicare/Medicaid regulations, professional standards published by the American Nurses Association or other specialty organization, nursing care audits, opinion polls, client feedback in various forms, and departmentally developed standards. Organizational standards are becoming increasingly more prevalent as systems undertake service and operational excellence initiatives to improve customer service, employee experience, quality, financial performance, and growth. Organizational pillars to "hardwire excellence" provide a platform for all employees to understand and buy into the mission, vision, and values of the organization (Studer, 2003).

Ideally, a performance appraisal measures performance and motivates the person. However, performance appraisal is not the only or major source of motivation for most nurses. Measuring performance is not at all easy, and motivating someone else is an art. Cultural sensitivity is important to consider as the nursing workforce becomes more diversified (Smith-Trudeau, 2008). The performance appraisal process can create a lot of stress for individuals if it is not managed well by both the manager and the employee (Duncan, 2007). Job satisfaction and organizational commitment have been found to be positively related to satisfaction with the feedback from performance appraisals (Jawahar, 2006). Integral components of a comprehensive performance appraisal system provide an overarching framework for the process. The tools and methods for a comprehensive performance appraisal system involve a clear determination of the abilities required for the position (job description); a match of the key requirements for the position with the individual's capabilities (personnel selection); development of the abilities of the employee (staff development); and using a motivational reward system to enhance employee performance (reward system) (Nauright, 1987). Box 33.1 outlines the key components of the performance appraisal process.

Performance attributes of an individual are determined by two elements: ability and motivation. Ability is made up of a collection of physical and mental capacities that enable a person to exhibit a skill or set of skills. Knowledge,

Box 33.1

Components of a Comprehensive Appraisal System

- Determine the ability required (job description)
- Match abilities of the employee with job requirements (personnel selection)
- Improve employee's abilities (staff development)
- Enhance employee's motivation (staff development and reward system)

experience, and skill form the ability to successfully complete a task (Hersey et al., 2008). Thus ability is an innate capacity that is molded by experience and training. Motivation is a willingness to work and a desire to achieve. Motivation influences the vigor and diligence with which an individual applies his or her capability to a task (Nauright, 1987).

Performance management includes processes of human resources management. There are several purposes for this system. For the employee, these include job productivity, compensation, job performance recognition, and planning for professional development. For the organization, they include worker requirements, job analysis, compensation administration, training needs analysis, and employee promotion or discipline evaluation. Performance management is focused on the job, involves continual evaluation, and is participative. As a major component of the system, performance appraisal is done for evaluation purposes (Frank, 1998).

ORGANIZATIONAL CULTURE AS A CATALYST TO IMPROVING PERFORMANCE

Given the national concerns about patient safety and quality of care, it is important to look at organizational culture as a factor influencing performance appraisal for change and improvement. The change of an error-prone health care system involves leadership and organizational learning, which requires significant strategic commitment and administrative direction. An environment that values and creates shared vision and purpose can lead to reflection and learning, which then enables and strengthens organizational culture toward creative and effective solutions in health care delivery (Carroll & Edmondson, 2002).

Culture consists of shared norms, behaviors, and values. Schein (1992) defined the culture of a group as "a pattern of shared basic assumptions that the group learned as it solved its problems of external adaptation and internal integration, that has worked well enough to be considered valid and, therefore, to be taught to new members as the correct way to perceive, think, and feel in relation to those problems" (p. 12). Culture is "the integrated pattern of human knowledge, belief and behavior that depends on man's capacity for learning and transmitting knowledge to the succeeding generations; the set of shared attitudes, values, goals and practices that characterizes a company or corporation" (*Merriam-Webster's Collegiate Dictionary*, 1997, p. 282). Culture consists of "the predominating attitudes and behavior that characterize the functioning of a group or organization" (*The American Heritage Dictionary of the English Language*, 2000). The learning that occurs within the system over time influences organizational culture.

The quality of care and the quality of work life are driven by the culture within a health care organization (Gershon et al., 2004). Culture is reflected in "the way things are done" in an organization (Stetler, 2003), and it surrounds all individuals and influences leadership. Characteristics of the culture are manifested differently in subgroups and by the various stakeholders within the organization, which warrant more in-depth assessment to fully understand (Nemeth, 2005).

SUBCULTURES AND STAKEHOLDERS

Socialization of new members into an organization is an important way to learn the rules and norms of a group. New members need to learn the assumptions of the group, which are not always transparent. Group behaviors and perceptions may reveal some elements of the culture, and some of the rituals and processes undertaken within the organization may reflect the assumptions that are held. Groups that are stable and have a history of shared learning are likely to have developed some degree of culture, but groups with significant turnover of members and leaders may lack shared assumptions (Schein, 1992). Organizational culture has been referred to as the *social glue that binds the organization,* in which the deeper meanings of the way things are done in the organization are learned (Cameron & Quinn, 1999; Detert et al., 2000).

Evaluation of organizational culture needs to consider both the larger organization and the smaller unit within which a member belongs. Exploring the microsystem within a health care system reveals the unique disciplinary focus of each department and treatment setting (Donaldson & Mohr, 2000). The performance characteristics of academic departments, clinics, and hospital units and departments highlight the different functions and shared assumptions that members bring to the patient care setting. These varying perspectives enrich the mix of the organization by enabling diverse contributions, attitudes, and skills to be developed.

Members of a larger organizational culture may also belong to subcultures within that organization, whose group learning over time may have generated very different sets of basic assumptions. Behavior and language of organizational members are subject to interpretation through the cultural biases of the subgroup. Conflict may be experienced when members of the subculture do not understand the biases within the larger culture or vice versa. Using an organizational cultural approach to conflict management would enable subcultures to examine the assumptions that underlie the behavior and reinterpret such conflict as the result of diverse experiences. Problem-solving issues that are based on different assumptions, with the intent to evaluate the utility of such differences, demonstrate an effective learning process (Nemeth, 2005).

The criteria for performance appraisals should include measures of key performance indicators that reflect the values of the organizational culture. With these characteristics embedded within appraisal tools, managers can craft the culture within the unit. If there is not an explicit organizational mission, vision, or value statement, managers must translate their vision and values into a clear framework that all can understand. This framework should provide the structure for staff to operationalize the required behaviors for successful performance. The scoring of the performance appraisal tool indicates the weight that these organizational culture characteristics contribute toward performance, which communicates the importance of those to the overall appraisal.

GOALS FOR PERFORMANCE APPRAISAL

The most direct goal of any performance appraisal system is the improvement of performance. Considering the process of performance appraisal systems, the outcome for the system should lead to positive organizational outcomes. Used effectively, the performance appraisal offers the opportunity for numerous organizational goals to be achieved. Box 33.2 provides an overview of the goals of the process of performance appraisal.

Roles and Expectations of Team Members

Numerous stakeholders are within the process of performance appraisal of nurses. Most important is the voice of the patient, who is the end consumer of the care provided and needs to be considered within the overall process that is used to evaluate the performance of nurses. The patient's voice can be obtained from patient satisfaction data that are formally used within the organization. Often, the patient or family member will offer direct verbatim comments that can be used to provide constructive support to individuals or groups. Nurse managers should seek out the comments of the patient regarding the patient's experience of care. Through this proactive process, the manager may find that the voice of the patient regarding specific exceptional staff members or those who may need to improve can provide useful input for managing staff behavior.

Box 33.2

Goals of Performance Appraisal

- Improve performance
- Improve communication
- Reinforce positive behavior
- Communicate about and ultimately correct negative or less-than-optimal behaviors
- Provide a basis for rewards, which also is a basis for motivation
- Provide a basis for termination if necessary
- Identify learning needs and develop personnel

The peers of the nurse, who are co-workers in the setting in which the nursing care is delivered, are individuals who have the greatest opportunity to know firsthand how well the individual meets patient care needs and how well the individual can meet his or her responsibilities as a member of the team. These peers include the staff members who may work on the same shift or alternate shifts or the nurses who may interact with the individual from the perspective of another unit's function. Those nurses generally have the experience of direct communication about the patient's status, and they know the specific expectations of care that are required in the individual setting. For example, a nurse may work on a unit that receives patients frequently from the emergency department or the recovery room, and there are bilateral communications and expectations that these staff members have of one another. These are key individuals who interact with the nurse and may be in an excellent position to provide input related to performance. Although this may not be a customary source of performance appraisal input, it may be a worthwhile source to consider. There is a caution here, however, because peers may be competitive or even adversarial.

The interdisciplinary team members who count on the nurse also have expectations for the nurse to communicate and collaborate regarding the plan of care and inform key members of the need to become involved in assisting the patient. For example, social workers or therapists may rely on referrals from the nurse who has made an initial assessment of the patient's needs. If key criteria for referrals are clearly identified but not implemented, then the interdisciplinary care plan for the patient may not be developed as effectively as is needed. Interdisciplinary team members need to work together on behalf of the patient's needs, not just within their own disciplinary silos. Nurse managers need to think about acquiring input from the perspective of the key interdisciplinary team members who provide services within the specific unit or department.

Physicians also have expectations that the nurse will follow through on the orders that are prescribed for patient care, observing the patient for critical changes in condition and communicating any changes that warrant more intensive physician interventions. Physicians thus can provide feedback in the process for performance appraisal of staff. Multiple levels of physicians and other medical staff members are in the hierarchy. The most effective clinical areas establish a collaborative and inclusive process so that all clinical care can be guided by a strong base of supportive relationships. To develop this level of support requires the mutual trust and respect among the physician teams that provide care within the specific area. This would include ongoing communication regarding opportunities for improved performance by staff and physicians alike.

Administrative members have expectations that are more global in nature, but essentially they require that individual staff have the knowledge of policies and procedures that must be implemented in the care of patients. The commitment of employees to organizational pillars of excellence is important to these stakeholders. With numerous stakeholders, it is important that systematic processes guide the nursing management function of performance appraisals. With data being collected from numerous sources in a systematic way, a more meaningful performance appraisal process can be achieved.

Manager's Role

The management style of the person in charge is frequently cited by nurses when asked why they are leaving the nursing profession (Parse, 1997). The performance appraisal process provides the opportunity for managers to articulate and identify individual staff values and talents that bring them to the team. Parse identified reverence for others as an essential concept that differentiates managers from leaders. *Reverence* is defined as "honor or respect felt or shown" (*Merriam-Webster's Collegiate Dictionary*, 1997, p. 1002). The manager who has learned to lead with reverence respects the talents of others and is proud to offer opportunities for others to advance without fear of being overshadowed (Parse, 2004).

Practical Tips

Tip #1: Keep an Up-to-Date File

When a manager is prepared with exemplars of positive performance criteria, as well as areas in which coaching and mentoring were needed, performance appraisals are evidence-based. When adding these exemplars, take the time to review individualized goals to see how the evidence collected fits with the plans made at the last performance appraisal.

Tip #2: Set the Stage for a Productive Exchange of Ideas

Relaxed and comfortable settings for those being appraised are important to increase their receptivity to the honest feedback and perceptions of the manager regarding opportunities for growth. The seating arrangements should be next to one another rather than across a desk, and the timing should be negotiated in advance with sufficient time allocated. This provides the opportunity for setting new plans and objectives to work on during the next period of review.

The nursing population is growing older. In 2003, the average age of a nurse was 44.5 years, and some predict the average age will be 50 years by 2020 (Letvak, 2003). The nursing profession must develop new leaders, and a powerful tool to accomplish this is the performance appraisal. Nurse managers who have learned to lead with reverence use the performance appraisal process as an opportunity to mentor and coach their staff into new experiences.

Ideally, upon filling a nursing position, the manager meets with the employee during a planning stage to discuss the tasks, objectives, competencies, and performance characteristics. The preparation of the planning stage is an integral step in the performance management process because it allows the manager to clearly communicate what is expected of the employee (McKirchy, 1998). Clarity is essential in the performance appraisal process, and the manager has the duty to provide this to all staff members. This process allows the individual to talk specifically about his or her performance goals and to come to agreement with the manager on reasonable performance expectations.

Many managers will include staff self-appraisal as an important component in the appraisal process. This is a valued aspect of the process because it promotes individual input, personal responsibility, and feedback regarding job performance. Appraisal is a structured process of facilitated self-reflection, which allows individuals to review their professional activities comprehensively and to identify areas of real strength and need for development (Conlon, 2003).

It is imperative to provide staff members with adequate time to participate in the performance appraisal process. A schedule for conducting performance appraisals must be consistent and clear. Managers who create a healthy work environment offer adequate time for feedback and input. If the concept of reverence is important for managers in the performance appraisal, the concept of self-esteem may shed some light on the perspective of the staff member. Audit and feedback are important mechanisms to provide objective data to the nurse regarding the quality of care provided. To improve clinical practice and motivate nurses to learn from the audit experience, individual self-esteem must be at a level that promotes motivation (Ward, 2003). The imperative for nurse managers is to recognize that the use of feedback in the performance appraisal process may influence an individual's self-esteem, which may affect practice. Providing feedback is a delicate art of nursing management, which should be managed to encourage and motivate the individual to improve his or her individual care provision. The Practical Tips box in this chapter highlights some tips for managing the performance appraisal process.

Melding Multiple Sources of Input

Incorporating the input of peers in the performance appraisal process also must be handled carefully because the opinions of peers often substantially influence a person's self-esteem (Ward, 2003). This allows managers to determine whether opinions are consistent regarding the employee's job performance. Objectivity can never be presumed in reviewing the input of others, and when perceptions differ, the manager is in the position of determining the final score for the performance appraisal. This process must be used judiciously to avoid creating conflict among staff members and management (Arnold & Pulich, 2003).

Individual self-appraisal, as well as peer and other stakeholder input, provides a mechanism for a 360-degree performance appraisal that enables a wider perspective beyond what the individual manager can provide to the staff member. Organizational cultures that encourage the use of 360-degree feedback do so to provide a learning opportunity for the individual. Financial rewards are not necessarily tied to 360-degree reviews, but development opportunities are to be gained through this method, which is a more important outcome. A key decision in the process of using 360-degree feedback is whether to keep the process as a confidential process or to have it be one in which the person being evaluated knows or selects peers and subordinates to participate in the review.

PERFORMANCE APPRAISAL AND RETENTION

Performance-based career advancement systems provide a means to recognize and reward clinical expertise in direct patient care roles. Differentiated practice models enable employee development and higher performance at a level consistent with individual interest and motivation. For those nurses who seek a higher level of professional contribution, these systems can provide a mechanism for compensation that is based on additional performance and effort. The Vanderbilt Professional Nursing Practice Program is an example of a program that was designed to attract, retain, and reward nurses (Robinson et al., 2003).

A supportive environment is one of the key factors related to the success of professional nursing practice models. In the 1990s, large system redesign and reengineering occurred in many hospital systems, which decreased the numbers of full-time equivalent (FTE) employees in many institutions. Many systems merged several units under the scope of responsibility of one nurse manager (NM), who often had to manage more than 80 employees. Nurse managers had a mixed reaction to this movement. On the one hand, they were flattered that the organization had increased the importance of the NM role. However, the overall result to the NM was a feeling of being pulled away from the bedside to focus on staffing issues and management problems. NMs believed that they should be more visible on the units to set direction and address issues and concerns for the staff members to come together as a team. Although NMs believed they were needed on the unit by their staff, their increased responsibilities made it difficult to be visible at the bedside. To address this issue, many institutions have decreased the scope of responsibility of the NM to enable a more consistent presence on the unit. This has enabled NMs to have the time to work with their staff and be able to evaluate staff members' performance in a more effective manner.

PERFORMANCE APPRAISAL CRITERIA

It is essential to set expectations regarding job criteria and performance as soon as the nurse begins employment. The organization should have the employee sign the performance tool as a planning stage for the performance criteria that are to be met and should provide a copy for the employee to refer to throughout the year. Armed with clear expectations, the employee should understand how he or she will be rated at the end of the evaluation year.

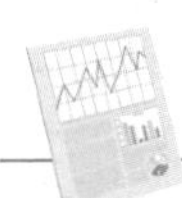

Research Note

Source: Drach-Zahavy, A. (2004). Primary nurses' performance: Role of supportive management. *Journal of Advanced Nursing, 45*(1), 7-16.

Purpose

Few studies have evaluated the outcomes of staff performance and the role of supportive management practices in primary nursing systems. This study evaluated how the role of the manager influences the performance of primary nurses; the study was conducted in a hospital in Haifa, Israel.

Discussion

A cross-sectional survey was designed to examine the impact of primary nursing on the performance of nurses and to evaluate the impact of supervisor support and the perceived costs of seeking support. The study aimed to develop a predictive model regarding the performance of primary nurses. Surveys (n = 520) were distributed in 56 nursing units from 6 major hospitals in Israel. Returned surveys totaled 368, indicating a response rate of 71%. Primary nursing was rated using a 5-point Likert scale, with the items representing different types of support. Supervisors rated nurses' performance using a 7-item measure to provide an overall evaluation of performance and professional competence. A moderating model was used in which the independent variable (primary nursing) was used to examine the effect of the dependent variable (nurses' performance), along with the moderating variables of supervisor support and the costs of seeking support. A hierarchical regression analysis was used to compute the predictors regarding nursing performance in primary nursing environments. Primary nursing was not associated with nurses' performance, but supervisor support was seen to be positively associated with it. The highest levels of primary nursing practice were seen in areas in which the supervisor's support was the highest.

Application to Practice

The study highlighted a model that used structure, process, and outcome variables to predict performance of nurses in a primary nursing professional model. The structure is the primary nursing model of care delivery, the processes are supervisor support and nurses' perceptions regarding the costs of seeking such support, and the outcomes are nursing performance in such a system. Supervisor support was seen as efficient in improving the performance of primary nurses. A social exchange framework helps explain the bilateral commitments that are made by both employees and supervisors in such a system. With the supervisor's support, stress can be reduced and the increased responsibility and accountability that are needed to be effective in a primary nursing system can be seen. When nursing models are changed, supportive interactions by nurse managers can lead to higher performance by nurses. This suggests that more autonomy and support provided by the nurse manager can lead to higher motivation and performance levels by nurses. Empowerment and support can be combined to augment the performance levels of nurses.

It is a challenge for a manager to maintain objectivity when conducting performance appraisals. Because of the wide variety of individuals in the workforce and the increased diversity of cultures, there may be instances of personality conflicts with the manager and the employee. Employees may feel that the manager dislikes them and therefore is biased about their performance (Arnold & Pulich, 2003).

Potential problems may impede a manager from performing a fair evaluation on an employee. Arnold and Pulich (2003) described the following potential problems, called *sources of error,* related to perception that may incorrectly influence managerial ratings on performance appraisals:

- *Recent behavior bias:* Occurs when the rater remembers behavior primarily from the most recent period of the employee's performance period as opposed to the entire rating period
- *Horn effect:* Occurs when a manager perceives one negative aspect about an employee or his or her performance and generalizes it into an overall poor appraisal rating
- *Halo effect:* Occurs when a manager perceives one positive characteristic about an employee or his or her performance and generalizes it into an overall high rating
- *Similar-to-me effect:* Occurs when a manager rates the employee performance higher when a person is accurately or inaccurately perceived to have the same characteristics as the manager

Developing skill in assessment and interview techniques is a key to effective performance appraisal. Asking questions can elicit important evaluative data. Using a coaching process means studying present behavior and developing planned, purposeful change strategies or intermediate multiple small steps to bring performance closer to what is desired. Coaching uses constant communication and clear consequences. Coaching becomes the management of consequences by praising, reprimanding, and redirecting (Hersey et al., 2008). A process of the employer and employee establishing mutual goals contributes to improved performance.

Distinction can be made between counseling, coaching, and mentoring. *Counseling* addresses problem performers such as employees whose work is consistently substandard, those who regularly miss deadlines, or those who are uncooperative, insubordinate, absent, or tardy. The problem needs to be brought to the employee's attention, the employee should be given time to respond, and specific actions to improve performance should be agreed on. *Coaching* involves all employees in improving their ability to do their job and increase potential. Activities include role modeling, hiring carefully, encouraging growth, creating a positive environment, using praise, and encouraging stretch goals. *Mentoring* is for employees who show promise and is used to shorten learning curves and increase productivity. Developmental needs demand a greater commitment. The closer the link between the employee's needs and the mentor's competencies, the more likely it is that the mentorship will be productive. Mentoring requires mutual trust and respect (Stone, 1999).

The more explicitly the performance criteria are stated, the less conflict is generally experienced in the scoring. Reliability of scoring on an institutional basis can be enhanced by stating the extent of the performance required to achieve specific ratings. In specific position descriptions, the behaviors that are needed to score a rating of "meets expectations," "exceeds expectations," or "substantially exceeds expectations" can be elaborated. This methodology sets a standard that is institution-wide and provides clarity and consistency among nurse managers on different units.

An example of evaluation criteria associated with each job task is shown in Figure 33.2 for the Registered Nurse II at the Medical University of South Carolina. These criteria were developed to enable employees to have a clear understanding of the expectations for performance, with specific criteria for the ratings that indicate what the employee will need to do to reach each level. These criteria explicitly define performance attributes so that a fair rating can be easily achieved. This is important when compensation is tied to performance.

ALTERNATIVE TYPES OF APPRAISAL

To minimize factors of bias in the performance appraisal, the manager should use other methods to perform a fair evaluation of performance on each employee. The following are some of these alternative methods:

- *360-Degree evaluation:* The 360-degree evaluation can be obtained by seeking input from approximately four sources: (1) a peer, (2) a physician, (3) a subordinate, and (4) a self-evaluation. Once all the input is obtained, the evaluating manager adds his or her input and merges the feedback to develop the final score.

Text continued on p. 735

<table>
<tr><td colspan="3">Job Purpose:

<u>Clinical Nurse Coordinator (CNC)</u>

The CNC on the _______________ Unit reports to the Manager. Under general supervision, the CNC provides individualized, goal-directed patient care to families and patients at the competent level utilizing the principles and practices of the nursing process, delivers safe and effective care, and interacts with other members of the health care team to achieve desired results.</td></tr>
<tr><td>Part A

JOB TASKS

Job Tasks and Objectives (optional) account for 70% of the performance evaluation rating.</td><td>% weight</td><td>Performance Level

S(4) E(3) M(2) B(1)

weight × rating = score

(use whole number, not percentage weight, in this calculation)</td></tr>
<tr><td>1. Job Task (E):

<u>Clinical Practice (Assessment)</u>

Manages comprehensive nursing care for patients (within specialty area) whose needs range from uncomplicated to complex and rapidly changing.

Success Criteria:

a. Based on holistic assessment, identifies relevant aspects of the situation and determines the appropriate course of action and reports abnormal findings to appropriate members of interdisciplinary team.
b. Assesses subtle changes in patient status; anticipates problems before they occur and implements measures to minimize risk.
c. Begins to become a resource person for case-specific procedures, positioning devices, sterilizers, and equipment.
d. Actively reports and troubleshoots discrepancies in patient care, equipment, and instruments.
e. Exhibits knowledge of sterilizers and functions.
f. Understands, implements, and monitors patient safety guidelines.</td><td>20%</td><td>Evaluation Criteria:

<u>1a.</u>
4. Always coordinates and follows through on completion of Perioperative Record. Demonstrates greater individualization of plans of care.
3. Demonstrates greater individualization of patient care. Regularly recognizes exceptions/additions; consistently revises plan of care.
2. Completes admission assessment and consistently updates plan of care. Prioritizes and follows through on patient needs.
1. Inconsistently completes assessment. Fails to identify all patient needs. Does not implement a complete standard of care. Cannot prioritize patient needs.

<u>1b.</u>
4. Adapts to rapidly changing complex needs and takes appropriate action. Consistently tailors plans to meet complex patient needs and follows through to desired outcomes.
3. Demonstrates greater age-appropriate individualization of plans; regularly notes exceptions/additions; consistently revises needs list.
2. Develops patient needs list; reflects both patient/family needs.
1. Does not implement standards of care.</td></tr>
</table>

Continued

Figure 33.2

Registered Nurse II evaluation criteria. (Adapted from Medical University of South Carolina—Charleston.)

		1c. 4. Independently works with interdisciplinary team. Documents all personal and positioning devices. A resource person. 3. Assists others to work with interdisciplinary team. Documents all personal and positioning devices. 2. Provides, identifies, and uses proper equipment, instruments, and positioning devices for case-specific procedures. 1. Consistently fails to identify, use, and provide proper equipment, instruments, and positioning devices for case-specific procedures.
		1d. 4. Excels in patient care and immediately recognizes any discrepancies and anticipates needs of team members to take corrective action. Knows the operation of most pieces of equipment/instruments in the operating room and can be a resource to others. 3. Monitors the patient and recognizes problems immediately and takes corrective actions. Consistently advocates for patient. Able to troubleshoot pieces of equipment/instruments within specialty and be a resource for others. 2. Recognizes discrepancies in patient care and reports to proper team member. Checks and/or tests equipment/instruments before time of use. Can identify problems and resources. 1. Does not report discrepancies in patient care. Unable to identify major problems with equipment/instrument malfunctions and unable to troubleshoot. **1e.** 4. Actively participates and assists in development of unit Quality Improvement Program. 3. Understands and initiates recall method for positive monitor indicator. Participates in unit Quality Improvement Program. 2. Understands, demonstrates, and documents appropriate methods of sterilization of instruments and completes appropriate biological testing as needed. 1. Inconsistently demonstrates, understands, or documents methods of sterilization. **1f.** 4. Recognizes the need for all team members to understand safety guidelines and is a resource to other Perioperative RNs.

Figure 33.2—cont'd

		3. Collaborates with the perioperative team about the importance of patient safety guidelines to patient outcomes. Always implements, monitors, and documents patient safety guidelines. 2. Identifies, implements, and monitors patient safety guidelines (and updates as needed). 1. Inconsistently implements, monitors, and documents patient safety guidelines.
2. Job Task (E): **Clinical Practice (Planning)** Organizes and prioritizes nursing care activities considering the needs of the patients and other staff members. **Success Criteria:** a. Provides leadership to develop, analyze, integrate complex data for, and update individualized plan of care. b. Utilizes the nursing process to facilitate the individualized plan of care using time and resources efficiently, and assumes accountability for plan's effectiveness. Coordinates care with the interdisciplinary members consistent with roles and responsibilities. c. Designs, implements, and evaluates a comprehensive, culturally sensitive patient plan of care. d. Uses professional judgment to appropriately delegate and follow through. e. Participates with service coordinators to individualize plans of care.	20%	**Evaluation Criteria:** **2a.** 4. Demonstrates the flexibility to adapt resources to the changing needs of the patient. 3. Coordinates and evaluates resources utilizing chain of command to provide needs of patient. 2. Utilizes personnel, supplies, and equipment to meet the needs of the patient. 1. Does not identify needs completely or does not utilize personnel, supplies, and equipment appropriately. **2b.** 4. Independently intervenes, follows through, and evaluates effectiveness of interdisciplinary team. 3. Consistently collaborates with interdisciplinary team. 2. Identifies and facilitates referral for services of other disciplines. 1. Fails to address needs of the patient and impedes function of other disciplines. **2c.** 4. Initiates in-services and/or projects to (increase) improve efficient staff resource utilization. Takes initiative to plan and follows through on complex patient needs in a timely manner. 3. Consistently collaborates with interdisciplinary team to evaluate patient's plan of care with regard to Cultural Sensitivity. Efficiently utilizes suitable resources, including people and materials. 2. Identifies appropriate problems and implements a care plan. Documents and evaluates patient's progress in the intraoperative setting. 1. Inconsistently plans and implements a comprehensive patient care plan.

Figure 33.2—cont'd

Continued

		2d. 4. Takes appropriate action related to failure of team members to perform delegated tasks. 3. Delegates and follows up on delegated activities to ensure plan is carried out. 2. Is consistently able to delegate safely and appropriately to other members of the health care team, including assistive personnel. 1. Fails to consistently delegate and/or uses ineffective interpersonal skills to delegate. **2e.** 4. Participates in identifying needs, creating tools, or revising existing tools to enhance knowledge and improve patient care. 3. Actively utilizes teaching/learning tools to improve patient outcomes. 2. Documents individualized plan of care. 1. Fails to participate with Service Coordinator to coordinate the individual plan of care.
3. Job Task (E): **Clinical Practice (Intervention)** Makes age-appropriate interventions based on individual patient needs. **Success Criteria:** a. Competently performs technical skills in area of practice. Demonstrates practice based on knowledge of hospital policies, procedures, nursing standards, and legal issues in areas of specialty. b. Coordinates and manages care by applying analytical reasoning, reflection, and problem-solving skills; using age-appropriate information; and incorporating patient safety initiatives. c. Participates in shared decision making and problem solving to promote effective collaboration with interdisciplinary partners and to enhance own practice.	20%	**Evaluation Criteria:** **3a.** 4. Consistently performs technical skills with little or no supervision and functions as a clinical resource in the specified area of practice. 3. Practice consistently reflects awareness of hospital and departmental policy changes as well as "Current Standards and Recommended Practices" of AORN. 2. Completes and demonstrates in practice unit-specific competencies. 1. Inconsistently complies with policies and procedures. **3b.** 4. Develops and implements a plan of care utilizing and coordinating appropriate resources. 3. Participates in plan of care and makes suggestions to enable a positive patient outcome utilizing appropriate resources. 2. Carries out plan of care consistently and safely. 1. Is unfamiliar with patient problems and needs. Requires additional assistance with implementing plan of care.

Figure 33.2—cont'd

		3c. 4. Is an active member of committee or task force, participating in development of tools for improvement of patient care. 3. Uses critical thinking and appropriate resources to identify and/or anticipate problems. Regularly provides input to Manager and colleagues to improve departmental concerns and/or positive patient outcomes. 2. Consistently obtains patient care data from multiple data sources to generate and implement feasible patient care solutions. Regularly attends and participates in staff meetings and other unit meetings. 1. Does not participate in data gathering. Inconsistently attends staff and unit meetings.
4. Job Task (E): **Clinical Practice (Evaluation)** Uses established outcome measures to evaluate effectiveness of care. **Success Criteria:** a. Promotes effective and efficient use of Perioperative Standards of Care to promote achievement of best clinical outcomes that are targeted to age-specific populations.	15%	**Evaluation Criteria:** **4a.** 4. Verbalizes and identifies all Perioperative Standards of Care, including criteria. Serves as a resource to other team members. 3. Utilizes all Standards of Care and documents appropriate outcomes. 2. Utilizes Standards of Care in daily practice. 1. Fails to utilize Standards of Care in daily practice.
5. Job Task (E): **Professional Development** Assumes personal responsibility for quality patient care, environment, and professional development.	10%	**Evaluation Criteria:** **5a.** 4. Obtains formal education, including conferences, workshop attendance, and formal classes and presents to staff, service groups, and/or orientees. On self-evaluation lists strengths, weaknesses, and goals. Utilizes Employee Performance Management System (EPMS) as a professional growth tool. Attends 100% of all staff and educational offerings.

Figure 33.2—cont'd

Continued

Success Criteria:		
a. Identifies own learning needs and seeks out resources to meet those needs, utilizing EPMS and self-evaluation. Demonstrates the insight and self-awareness necessary to recognize own impact on others and to change behavior accordingly. Accepts constructive feedback and uses it to improve performance. Attends and participates in staff meetings and Continuing Education opportunities. b. Shares knowledge with interdisciplinary team to improve patient care and to contribute to overall unit functions. c. Assists in the orientation of new staff members and students. d. Demonstrates effective use of computer-based information for decision support, continuous quality improvement, and professional development. e. Annually obtains six Continuing Education Units (CEUs) and provides documentation. f. Is able to communicate by hospital-based e-mail system.		3. Obtains formal education, including conferences, workshop attendance, and formal classes. Completes self-evaluation and lists strengths, weaknesses, and goals. Attends 95% of all staff and educational offerings. 2. Identifies and follows through with additional educational opportunities. Completes self-evaluation and goals in a timely manner. Accepts constructive feedback and develops appropriate objectives to improve practice. Attends 85% of all staff and educational offerings. 1. Does not complete self-evaluation and/or provide goals. Does not seek out learning needs. Does not accept constructive feedback. Fails to attend 85% of all staff educational offerings. **5b.** 4. Presents information or in-services on a yearly basis to staff and interdisciplinary team members. 3. Presents information at unit in-service. 2. Knows unit resources and administration personnel. Communicates problems and suggestions to appropriate personnel. Utilizes appropriate tools to document issues and concerns. Routinely participates in unit staff meetings. Arrives at staff meeting in a timely manner. 1. Fails to follow chain of command. Communicates problems to inappropriate persons and/or uses inappropriate manner. **5c.** 4. Actively assists in orientee assignments to meet learning needs of specific service group. Assists with learning needs of students related to aseptic technique and patient safety. 3. Seeks out learning needs for new employees. Actively evaluates orientee performance. Assists students in meeting learning needs and goals. 2. Demonstrates a positive attitude. Explains interdisciplinary team member roles and functions. Acts as a preceptor for new employees. 1. Demonstrates lack of a positive attitude in educating new staff members and students.

Figure 33.2—cont'd

		5d. 4. Utilizes additional computer resources to identify additional patient care resources (e.g., Picture Archiving Communication System [PACS]) 3. Notifies appropriate coordinator if changes are needed to computer-based preference cards/pick sheets. Utilizes computer programs to increase knowledge base. 2. Utilizes appropriate computer programs in daily practice, hospital-based e-mail and intranet, and Computerized Annual Training & Tracking System (CATTS). Updates surgeon preference books as necessary. 1. Does not utilize computer programs in daily practice. **5e.** 4. Obtains greater than 9 CEUs. 3. Obtains 7-8 CEUs. 2. Obtains 6 CEUs. 1. Fails to obtain 6 CEUs. **5f.** 4. Consistently communicates with interdisciplinary team by offering constructive unit improvements. 3. Communicates with interdisciplinary team members. 2. Utilizes hospital-based e-mail to check for education and/or unit updates. 1. Fails to communicate with hospital-based e-mail system.
6. Job Task (E): **Leadership** Actively and effectively assumes leadership role in unit. **Success Criteria:** a. Demonstrates high standards of patient care and is a role model for others. b. Knows the roles of the interdisciplinary team members and delegates appropriately to provide effective patient care. c. Communicates with team members, service coordinators, and charge nurse in proactive manner, orally and in writing, to promote patient care.	10%	**Evaluation Criteria:** **6a.** 4. Serves as a resource for staff, coaches others in decision making, and actively serves on a committee. 3. Follows through on issues and concerns. 2. Adheres to the standards of nursing practice. 1. Fails to practice according to standards of nursing practice. **6b.** 4. Prioritizes/delegates well in stressful situations. Able to function as a nurse coordinator. 3. Sets appropriate priorities; holds others accountable for their actions. 2. Delegates appropriately to others. 1. Delegates reluctantly and/or inappropriately.

Figure 33.2—cont'd

Continued

PART V

d. Promotes teamwork by facilitating positive group relationships. e. Demonstrates a spirit of service and cooperation in responding to needs of patients and co-workers, including ability to deal with stressful situations in a mature, positive manner. f. Participates in unit development by supporting change and offering suggestions; actions and decisions reflect an awareness of unit budget. g. Demonstrates a professional commitment to patients and staff by adhering to unit procedures, rules, and policies (including attendance and call). h. Follows through on meeting patient needs and requests by using appropriate mechanisms. i. Addresses problems and systems issues in a timely manner by contacting appropriate personnel through the proper chain of command. j. Demonstrates and practices fiscal accountability for one's own practice while providing quality care.		**6c.** 4. Discusses issues and identifies problem-solving solutions with appropriate surgical team members, utilizing communication skills. 3. Demonstrates assertive communication, independent problem solving, thorough documentation. 2. Demonstrates ability to communicate effectively. Utilizes resources to problem solve. 1. Does not communicate effectively. **6d.** 4. Confronts barriers to positive group relationships. 3. Acknowledges, utilizes, and promotes the abilities of others. 2. Is a positive team player. 1. Creates barriers to teamwork. **6e.** 4. Helps others effectively deal with stressful situations; demonstrates initiative and willingness to respond to the needs of others. 3. Is proficient in stressful situations (e.g., codes, multiple admissions, staffing issues, interpersonal conflicts); collaborates/delegates effectively, positively. 2. Handles stress appropriately; helps without hesitation. 1. Is unable to function effectively under stress; unwilling to help others. **6f.** 4. Takes initiative to implement and facilitate positive change. 3. Identifies need for change; supports it. 2. Adapts to change with a positive, cooperative attitude. 1. Creates barriers to change. **6g.** 4. Demonstrates exceptional flexibility with own schedule to meet unit needs. 3. Is willing to make adjustments to meet unit needs. 2. Adheres to unit Policies and Procedures expectations. 1. Is nonadherent with policies and schedule.

Figure 33.2—cont'd

		6h. 4. Evaluates effectiveness; changes strategies as needed. 3. Makes extra effort to ensure follow-through. 2. Meets patient needs in timely manner. 1. Fails to follow through on patient needs. **6i.** 4. Evaluates and reassesses problems for a new plan of action. 3. Takes steps to develop a plan of action to resolve problems. 2. Addresses issues and problems by utilizing the proper chain of command. 1. Fails to contact appropriate personnel to address problems. **6j.** 4. Researches, implements, and evaluates ideas for cost-saving changes in practice. 3. Demonstrates a heightened awareness of costs to patient and institution. Formulates cost-saving measures. 2. Provides quality patient care while demonstrating fiscal accountability. 1. Inconsistently demonstrates fiscal accountability for practice.
7. Job Task (E): **Research and Evaluation** Participates in Performance Improvement/Research activities designed to improve patient care and/or organizational processes. **Success Criteria:** a. Is knowledgeable of Unit's Performance Improvement Projects/Research Activities. b. Actively contributes and participates in Unit-Based Performance Improvement Projects. c. Demonstrates spirit of inquiry through ongoing and systematic evaluation of care given to patients.	5%	**Evaluation Criteria:** **7a.** 4. Leads and evaluates Process Improvement Project/Research Activity. 3. Uses individual and unit data to make changes in patient care delivery systems. 2. Independently completes required hospital/unit audits, mandatories, computer-based competencies, and license. 1. Fails to complete required hospital/unit audits, mandatories, computer-based competencies, and license. **7b.** 4. Assists committee member/chair; promotes Continuous Quality Improvement (CQI) to colleagues. Identifies and seeks resources for study. 3. Willingly participates in unit/hospital studies. Completes 95% of assigned monitors. 2. Adheres to clinical protocols in ongoing studies. Completes 85% of assigned monitors.

Figure 33.2—cont'd

Continued

	= 100%	1. Fails to consistently adhere to research protocols. Completes fewer than 85% of assigned monitors and chooses to not participate in projects and monitors. **7c.** 4. Initiates area for study, seeks resources, and challenges effectiveness of treatment/care based on investigation and evaluation. 3. Identifies a need for investigation of chosen specific project (specify) and willingly participates in unit/hospital-wide studies. 2. Adheres to clinical protocols of ongoing projects/studies and explores reasons for perioperative care. 1. Fails to consistently adhere to clinical protocols and does not question perioperative care for its cause and effect.
	SECTION III, Part A Sum of Tasks (and OBJECTIVES SCORES) ÷ 100 = Total Tasks Score ________	

Figure 33.2—cont'd

The 360-degree evaluation tends to be more applicable in evaluating advanced practice roles or for management positions because of the diverse interactions that staff in these roles have. For evaluation of the staff nurse role, the 360-degree process may not be as effective because the expectations may be for a more uniform standard of performance.

- *Peer review:* In this process, employees rate the performance of others in the same job classification, using objective criteria that have been established. Input is provided to the manager by a peer review committee. The manager then incorporates the feedback into the person's evaluation along with the manager's comments. The negative aspect of this process is that staff may feel that members of the peer review committee are not fair in their assessment of other staff members' abilities. Peer review is most applicable for evaluating staff positions in which a common set of expectations and performance standards exists, because the staff members who work with one another are best suited to having the core knowledge about the quality and nature of the work performed by the individual. An effective peer review system may offer the individual honest and specific feedback that allows that person to make specific adjustments in his or her role to better meet objectives and performance standards.
- *Management by objectives:* In this method, the employee and manager establish performance goals for the upcoming appraisal year. This process is difficult for evaluating the entry-level nurse. As the nurse develops and gains more experience, management by objectives may be helpful in defining goals and objectives for the next year and providing the manager with a specific set of goals to follow up with the individual at regular intervals.

RELIABILITY AND VALIDITY IN MEASUREMENT

Reliability and validity are important considerations in any system of measurement. Tools must be constructed so that the score one rater would give would be consistent with another person's rating. If the criteria are developed in a manner that is clear and observable, they are more likely to lead to increased inter-rater reliability. Performance appraisal tools should be tested by several raters who, using the same criteria on the same person, would rate observable performance consistently. If two raters were recording their observations on the same person using the same tool, results should be equivalent. This would indicate a highly reliable tool.

Testing the reliability of a tool involves examining the amount of random error. The characteristics of the tool must be dependable, consistent, accurate, and comparable (Burns & Grove, 2001). Stability of the performance criteria demonstrates consistency with repeated measures of the same tool. Nurse managers who are comfortable with a performance appraisal tool should be able to measure the same person at multiple intervals in a stable and consistent manner. This is referred to as *test-retest reliability.*

Establishing equivalence is a more complex process that involves direct observation of specific processes at the same time by different individuals. The percentage of agreement is computed to derive inter-rater reliability. Perfect inter-rater reliability would be demonstrated if two individuals rated all performance criteria consistently. The lowest acceptable coefficient for reliability would be 0.80 (Burns & Grove, 2001).

The validity of a tool is the determination of the extent that the tool is measuring the construct that is under evaluation. Evaluation tools must capture the critical behaviors and outcomes that result from effective nursing care. The term *construct validity* is used to establish that the criteria are appropriate, meaningful, and useful in measuring what they are intending to measure. Perfect validity is not guaranteed, and to define validity in a specific tool often takes many years.

To provide objective measures to ensure that staff members are evaluated fairly, both the reliability and validity of the evaluation tool must be established. Drawing from recent research regarding performance appraisal and variance in measurement, generalizability theory (GT) has been used to describe the variability that is associated with multisource ratings (Greguras et al., 2003). As more employment settings undertake the use of multiple raters providing feedback for performance appraisal systems, it is important to understand the nature of the feedback and consider the reliability of the sources used to provide this feedback. It has been demonstrated that when ratings are used for administrative purposes, the scores have tended to be less reliable than those scores used for development of the person being rated.

Generalizability theory provides a framework for examining the dependability of behavioral measurements of raters. As the information that has been obtained for the performance appraisal is compiled, the final rater must consider the variance due to the person being evaluated, the items being evaluated, and the interaction of the rater with the person being evaluated. For peers and subordinates, amount of variance may be substantial (Greguras et al., 2003).

When compiling the information that is used to complete the performance appraisal, the rater must consider the following factors affecting the reliability and validity of the ratings:

- The way the information is communicated, either verbally or in writing
- How the information is organized
- The potential influence of the relationship the rater has with the person being rated
- The cognitive ability of the rater

LEADERSHIP AND MANAGEMENT IMPLICATIONS

Developing Staff Members Through Performance Appraisal

For managers, the performance appraisal process is an opportunity to gather insight about their staff. This is more than just a piece of paper that is addressed yearly; it is a process in discovering the individual's perception of his or her job. Managers who are leaders consider the performance appraisal an opportunity to identify what motivates their staff members and also to identify their values and interest.

Managers use the performance appraisal process as a way to translate organizational goals into concrete objectives for the individual employee to fulfill. Through a process of communication, coaching, and development, employees are provided with feedback regarding how their performance fits with the expectations for the organization and the manager's vision regarding the culture of the individual microsystem. The manager identifies the strengths and weaknesses of the employee and provides recognition and support of positive behavior, as well as encouragement and specific recommendations regarding opportunities for improvement. The appraisal should show both the employee and the manager what the employee's possibilities for growth and development are. All of the developmental activities that a manager provides to an individual employee needs to be aimed at helping the individual better utilize his or her skills and improve performance on the current position or develop toward desired future opportunities for advancement. Leaders, supervisors, and managers who model preferred organizational behaviors, identified through the performance appraisal process, inevitably motivate staff to adapt desired outcomes.

The prevailing purpose of performance appraisal is to improve and motivate the staff, which in turn will enhance organizational effectiveness. This clearly identifies the performance appraisal process as a means to addresses institutional needs, as well as individual staff needs and abilities. The manager who uses the performance appraisal process effectively will become more capable in supporting, coaching, and managing the development of his or her staff members.

CURRENT ISSUES AND TRENDS

The appraisal of performance occurs at multiple levels. There appears to be a hierarchy of performance evaluation targets. At the individual level, performance is measured by a performance appraisal. At the unit level, performance may be estimated using budget or quality criteria. At the organizational level, performance is appraised by

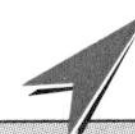

LEADERSHIP & MANAGEMENT BEHAVIORS

Leadership Behaviors

- Enables high-level performance
- Inspires high performance in individuals
- Models desirable performance characteristics
- Evaluates performance
- Counsels followers with performance problems
- Motivates followers to improve knowledge and skills

Management Behaviors

- Evaluates performance
- Conducts performance appraisals
- Coaches subordinates
- Analyzes performance problems
- Corrects performance problems
- Disciplines employees
- Validates clinical competence

Overlap Areas

- Evaluates performance
- Takes corrective actions

accreditation review by such entities as the National Committee for Quality Assurance (NCQA) Healthcare Effectiveness Data and Information Set (HEDIS) or The Joint Commission accreditation. Thus performance review ranges from individual employee evaluations through unit and organizational quality reviews to the level of political accountability performance appraisals done by the United States Department of Health and Human Services (USDHHS). In fact, the analysis can be carried on to include performance appraisal of the USDHHS and its Inspector General by the President of the United States and the Congress. Ultimately, their performance is appraised by the U.S. voters. Within an organization, performance appraisal of individuals and teams forms the core of management process control.

Performance appraisal is an activity that individuals do informally all the time. For example, restaurants and hotels solicit client feedback. For employees in an organization, part of a manager's job is to formally appraise the performance of employees. The process of managerial control includes doing evaluations. These are done for multiple purposes. For example, managers need to assess and determine the competency of staff personnel as one element of quality care. It is not sufficient to assume that because nurses are licensed, they are competent. Certainly to payers and consumers, the quality of caregivers is an issue. Regulatory agencies also are requiring proof of competency evaluation. They look for evidence of staff in-service and the range of nursing skills attained. The overall reason for the management step of evaluating and controlling is to measure the quality and effectiveness of nursing performance.

The current processes for appraising staff performance in health care environments need to be revisited. With the increased concern for patient safety exposed by the Institute of Medicine (IOM) (2000, 2001, 2003, 2004), the drive for a blame-free culture of safety, and current research regarding nursing-sensitive outcomes and nurse staffing (Aiken et al., 2002; IOM, 2004; Needleman et al., 2002), nurse managers and administrators have much to consider regarding how this process can best be crafted.

Considering the multitude of system errors and the current emphasis by regulatory agencies for improvements in system performance and patient safety (The Joint Commission, 2009), nurses are in an extremely visible position at the forefront of health care delivery. The 44,000 to 98,000 deaths per year in American hospitals that were presented as evidence in *To Err Is Human: Building a Safer System* (IOM, 2000) provide the impetus for health care leaders to redesign safer systems of care. Errors occur when planned actions fail or when wrong plans are used, resulting in unintended outcomes. Health care interventions that injure patients are adverse events and are considered preventable (IOM, 2004).

Health systems managers and administrators need to consider that to reduce errors that harm patients, a systems approach is needed. Recognition of the fact that human error is to be expected in all organizations (Reason, 2000), combined with diligence to uncover the root causes of events that result in patient harm, is a management responsibility. Multiple factors in health care systems increase the vulnerability of the nurse to errors. The experience and educational background of the nurse, the supervision and feedback that the individual nurse receives daily in the process of care, and the maturity of the nurse to raise issues in the environment that pose a risk to safe patient care are factors to be considered. Nursing performance can be enhanced in an environment in which open and honest feedback to individuals is valued, shared leadership and decision making are encouraged, and a system is created whereby errors are discussed or risky situations are analyzed by all participants. Nurse managers and leaders need to develop their staff members as critical "systems thinkers" who explore issues that negatively affect patient outcomes, as well as job satisfaction. Critical "systems thinkers" can see the bigger context than their individual perspective within the subculture to which they belong. Individual goals and performance should be viewed within the context of how one interacts within a system; but, clearly, the competencies of the individual, as well as the behaviors that are enacted, must be developed and strengthened for optimal performance. Performance appraisal is one component of a performance management system used by organizations to motivate employees.

Summary

- Conventional performance appraisal systems are designed to measure performance and motivate personnel.
- Peer review is an examination and evaluation of practice by a nurse's associates.
- Performance is determined by two elements: (1) ability and (2) motivation.
- The most direct goal of any performance appraisal system is the improvement of performance.
- In health care, performance appraisal is done as a part of overall quality assessment.
- Performance appraisal may be conducted through personal, peer, or administrative/managerial evaluation.
- The process of performance appraisal includes assessing the needs and setting goals, establishing the objective and the time frame, assessing the progress and evaluating the performance, and then starting over again.
- Performance appraisal can have positive outcomes.
- Performance is measured from collected data. Various methods and tools are used.
- A number of evaluator rating errors should be considered.
- To be effective, a performance appraisal system needs to provide objective assessment of the knowledge, skills, and abilities of employees; it also needs to enhance staff development.

Interactive Group Exercise

A useful method to promote creative group interaction and discussion is role playing. Role playing allows participation in actual challenging situations. For this exercise, the readers are asked to conduct a mock performance appraisal. One participant will portray the role of employee and one will portray the role of manager. In preparation for this exercise, the employee will complete a self-evaluation and the manager will complete an evaluation; Figure 33.2 can be used for this exercise. Role playing will provide participants the opportunity to present different employee and management styles in a creative manner. This interaction should occur in a setting that promotes open dialogue regarding the performance appraisal process.

Case Study

Julie Henderson, RN, BSN, was a nurse manager of PICU/Pediatrics at the Cleveland Clinic Foundation Children's Hospital in Cleveland, Ohio. She described her techniques for managing staff performance appraisal:

"For a nurse manager, annual staff evaluations are a natural part of the job. Nurse managers, however, cannot always identify the positive and negative attributes of all members of the staff. I found this out in my first year as a nurse manager, when I had to write the annual evaluations for the entire staff.

The difficulty I encountered was in being able to describe the individual's performance throughout the year. I kept a log in which, every 2 to 3 weeks, I would write down my observations of staff members' performance. I would also note any comments from patients or families and feedback from peers. Nurses, however, can sometimes be overly critical of their co-workers. Whenever something went wrong, as when a nurse did not follow a doctor's order, someone would make sure I was the first to know. If something positive happened, as when a nurse acted as a patient advocate or handled a difficult situation, I was usually the last to be informed. Thus, when it came time to write the evaluation, I had the data to write constructive criticism but was unable to include positive feedback or cite that special incident with a patient or family. Pointing out where a nurse excels is necessary so that the positive feedback can promote a healthy and hopeful work environment.

The following year I tried a different approach, peer evaluation, which I found to be more reliable. I gave each staff member two blank evaluations with a peer's name on each, so that each nurse evaluated two other nurses. Each nurse also received a blank evaluation form for self-evaluation. Guidelines for evaluation were provided and posted in the unit. Performance ratings were *Exceeds Expectations, Achieves Expectations,* or *Needs Improvement.* Staff members were instructed to cite examples of their peer's performance to support one of the three ratings. Matching up those being evaluated with those doing the evaluation required much planning on my part to avoid the bias that might arise from two nurses who were close friends.

As the staff turned in the evaluations, I reviewed the self-evaluation along with the two peer evaluations. I also continued to maintain my own log of observations and incidents. I used these to write my final evaluation for each staff member for the annual performance appraisal. Confidentiality was essential for the peer evaluations and self-evaluations so that the feedback could be as honest and constructive as possible.

In the administration of the annual evaluations, the staff would ask me what others thought of their performance. This would give me the opportunity to relay the positive qualities that their peers identified, which really helped create a better team by clarifying everyone's expectations. Peer evaluations also helped identify suggestions for improvement and strategies for achieving it, such as a seminar on how to deal with difficult people.

The self-evaluations and peer evaluations often had similar comments. For example, one nurse had difficulty communicating with physicians. Both the nurse herself and her peers identified this problem, and her peers suggested how she might improve this skill. Together the nurse and I set goals for the upcoming year and focused on her communication skills. Throughout the year, the rest of the staff and I worked with this nurse and noticed a marked improvement.

Peer evaluations and self-evaluations seem to have been successful in our unit by giving the staff a chance to think about the quality of performance and to critique their peers on a professional level."

CRITICAL THINKING EXERCISE

Nurse Linda Gero has completed her first year as a nurse on a 17-bed orthopedic floor. During her first year, she has worked 40 hours per week at a day-night position and has begun to assume charge nurse duties. She arrives to work in a timely fashion and completes her tasks. Because she is shy, she avoids personal conversations. Her co-workers described her as quiet and a bit distant.

One evening, Nurse Gero's nurse manager hands her the self-appraisal form that is part of her performance appraisal and asks her to complete it by the end of her shift. Her nurse manager will be back in the morning to discuss the performance appraisal with her. Two of Nurse Gero's co-workers, picked by her manager, have already completed peer evaluations. This is the first time Nurse Gero had seen or heard about a performance appraisal. She attempts to finish her evaluation but is unclear about how to complete the form. In the morning, at the end of Nurse Gero's shift, her nurse manager asks her to come to her office to discuss her performance appraisal. During their discussion, her manager identifies that Nurse Gero has been described as distant and unapproachable by her co-workers. The manager continues by telling Nurse Gero that immediate improvement is necessary for her to remain in her position. Nurse Gero is stunned. She has never had a conversation with her manager regarding job performance before this moment. She signs the appraisal at her manager's request because she does not want to appear difficult. Nurse Gero leaves her unit distraught and confused.

1. What is the problem?
2. Why is it a problem?
3. Whose problem is it?
4. What should Nurse Gero do?
5. How should the problem be handled?
6. Describe the management and leadership style of Nurse Gero's nurse manager.
7. What parts of the performance appraisal process could be improved? How?

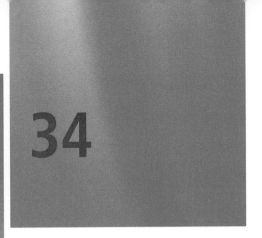

34 Prevention of Workplace Violence

L. Jean Henry   Gregory O. Ginn

CHAPTER OBJECTIVES

- Explain why violence in the workplace is a particular concern for nurses
- Define the various terms associated with workplace violence
- Discuss the legal, ethical, and economic costs of workplace violence in health care organizations
- Identify the sources of and risk factors for violence
- Give an overview of regulatory actions and NIOSH and OSHA recommendations to prevent workplace violence
- Explain the relationship of various management frameworks and leadership in mitigating and preventing workplace violence
- Explain the role of human resource management policies and procedures in preventing workplace violence
- Identify the legal issues concerning workplace violence
- Discuss management actions necessary to provide a legal defense against claims arising from workplace violence
- Exercise critical thinking and inquiry to conceptualize and analyze possible solutions to a practice exercise

Violence in the workplace is a salient issue for nurses and others in the health care industry. The Department of Labor reported a workplace violence rate of 38 cases per 10,000 workers for nursing and personal care facilities. This is much higher than the rate of 3 cases per 10,000 workers in private industry. The majority of nonfatal assaults that were reported occurred in service industries such as health care. Of those assaults, 27% occurred in nursing homes, 13% in social services, and 11% in hospitals. Health care and social service workers have the highest incidence of injuries from workplace assaults (National Institute for Occupational Safety and Health [NIOSH], 1996).

Assaults and threats of violence against nurses are prevalent throughout the world. Studies in the United Kingdom, Canada, and Australia also reported high rates of violence against nurses. The Australian Institute of Criminology cited the health care industry as the most violent industry in Australia (Henry & Ginn, 2002). In Britain, according to the National Audit Office (2003), violence and aggression accounted for 40% of health and safety incidents in the National Health Service.

Violence in hospitals is caused by a combination of internal and external factors. External conditions include an increasingly violent society, the availability of handguns, and high-crime neighborhoods. Many health care facilities are located in inner cities where crime rates are higher than average. Internal factors include inadequate staffing levels, larger numbers of dangerous patients, poor security for drugs and money, staff members working alone, poorly lit facilities, and unsecured, continuous access to health care facilities. Furthermore, the turbulent nature of the health care industry makes working conditions increasingly stressful. Health care workers are often required to work in shifts that result in their coming and going at odd hours of the day and night, when they are more vulnerable to crime (Bruser, 1998). The very nature of the jobs that nurses perform places them at high risk for workplace violence, and circumstances inherent in health care work increase workers' susceptibility to homicide or assault. Nurses often deal with people who are ill or injured. Staffs in nursing home/long-term care facilities, intensive care, psychiatric/behavioral or emergency departments, and geriatric facilities appear to be the most at risk. In one study, patients/clients accounted for 97% of physical violence perpetrated against nurses (Gerberich et al., 2004). Many patients are in pain, emotionally disturbed, or cognitively impaired, and often their families are experiencing strong emotions brought on by grief, catastrophic injuries, criminal victimization, or severe psychiatric disturbances (Edwards, 1999; Smith-Pittman & McKoy, 1999). Finally, because approximately one third of nurses report a history of sexual abuse, they may be more vulnerable to violence in the workplace. Childhood abuse may result in developing and carrying maladaptive beliefs, behaviors, and attitudes throughout adulthood (Anderson, 2002). Thus for a number of reasons, violence in the workplace is a particular concern for nurses.

From a public health perspective, it makes sense to approach workplace violence prevention in much the same way as other types of illnesses or injuries. However, from the perspective of an organization, the connection between workplace violence prevention and the attainment of broader organizational objectives such as financial performance may seem very tenuous. At the same time, the organization is uniquely situated to exert a powerful influence over the environment of the workplace and, because of its position, has far more ability to effectively reduce both the incidence and severity of incidents of workplace violence. Thus the issue is to convince organizations that (1) they can be effective in accomplishing a public health objective such as workplace violence prevention and (2) the attainment of broader organizational objectives is very much facilitated by success in workplace violence prevention programs (Ginn & Henry, 2002).

DEFINITIONS

Violence may be defined narrowly to include only obvious acts of violence such as assault, battery, manslaughter, or homicide. The National Institute for Occupational Safety (NIOSH) (1996) defined **workplace violence** as violent acts, including physical assaults and threats of assault, directed toward persons at work or on duty. The Center for Violence Prevention and Control (1996) identified violence as the intentional use of physical force that results in or has a high likelihood of resulting in injury or death.

Violence may be defined broadly to include aggressive behavior such as verbal abuse, threats, and harassment (Carroll & Morin, 1998). Speaking in a hostile manner or adopting a threatening posture can be considered an assault. For workplace policies and procedures, it is important to define violence broadly (Elliot, 1997). Consequences appear to be greater for non-physical than for physical violence (Gerberich et al., 2004).

The cost of violence is significant. When broadly defined, violence can be enormously dysfunctional to an organization in terms of lost productivity because of absenteeism, low morale, emotional pain, anxiety, and turnover (Murray & Synder, 1991; Smith-Pittman & McKoy, 1999). One source estimates that the eradication of bullying in the workplace may increase productivity and profits by as much as 10% ("Violence Threatens the Workplace," 1998). When combined with other costs, such as lawsuits, lost productivity, higher insurance costs, and workers' compensation claims, the bottom line of workplace violence is an estimated $36 billion annually (Jossi, 1999).

Sources of violence vary. One source of violence is from criminals who have no other connection with the workplace but simply intend to commit a crime. Indeed, the findings of one study showed that violent crime in the area where an organization was located predicted workplace violence in that organization (Dietz et al., 2003). A second source of violence is from customers, clients, patients, or students; this is regarded as the most prevalent source of violence against nurses. A third source is from a current or former employee. A fourth source of violence is from someone who is not employed at the workplace but has a personal relationship with an employee, such as a spouse or domestic partner (Rugala & Isaacs, 2004).

Risk factors for violence in health care organizations include working with volatile people, understaffing, long waits, poor environmental design, lack of training, inadequate security, substance abuse, access to firearms, poor lighting, and unrestricted access by the public (NIOSH, 2002). Working in hospitals may be dangerous because of the availability of drugs or money in the pharmacy area, the necessity of working evening or night shifts in high-crime areas, and the availability of furniture or medical equipment that could be used as weapons (Occupational Safety and Health Administration [OSHA], 2004).

LEADING & MANAGING DEFINED

Violence

Narrowly defined: assault, battery, manslaughter, or homicide; broadly defined: ranging from verbal abuse, threats, and unwanted sexual advances to physical assault and homicide.

Workplace Violence

Violent acts directed toward persons at work or on duty.

Sources of Violence

Violent acts committed by (1) criminals who have no connection with the workplace; (2) customers, clients, patients; (3) current or former co-workers; or (4) persons not employed at the workplace but who have a personal relationship with an employee.

Risk Factors for Violence

Things that predispose a workplace to violence, including interpersonal elements, environmental characteristics and design, and organizational culture.

Environmental Designs

Provisions that include signaling systems, alarm systems, monitoring systems, security devices, security escorts, lighting, and architectural and furniture modifications to improve worker safety.

Administrative Controls

Measures that include (1) adequate staffing patterns to prevent personnel from working alone and to prevent long waiting times, (2) controlled access, and (3) development of systems to alert security personnel when violence is threatened.

Behavior Modifications

Changes in behavior that provide all workers with training in recognizing and managing assaults, resolving conflicts, and maintaining hazard awareness.

Violence Prevention Programs

Programs that are available to all employees that track progress in reducing work-related assaults, reduce severity of injuries sustained by employees, decrease the threat to worker safety, and reflect the level and nature of threat faced by employees.

Violence Prevention Written Plans

Plans that demonstrate management commitment by disseminating a policy that no type of violence will be tolerated, ensure that no reprisals are taken against employees who report or experience workplace violence, encourage prompt reporting of all violent incidents, and establish a plan for maintaining security in the workplace.

Worksite Analysis

A common-sense look at the workplace to find existing or potential hazards for workplace violence.

Continued

LEADING & MANAGING **DEFINED**—cont'd

Hazard Prevention and Control

The implementation of work practices to prevent and control identified hazards.

Safety and Health Training

Education designed to make all staff members aware of security hazards and ways to protect themselves through established policies, procedures, and training.

Recordkeeping and Evaluation of Programs

Systems designed to provide the data to track progress in reducing work-related assaults.

Risk Management

An integrated effort across all disciplines and functional areas to protect the financial assets of an organization from loss by focusing on the prevention of problems that can lead to untoward events and lawsuits.

Total Quality Management (TQM)

The general processes of setting standards, collecting information, assessing outcomes, and adjusting policies; and evaluation of all systems to improve the quality of goods or services by reducing costs in ways that ensure customer satisfaction.

Threat Assessment

The evaluation of the threat itself and an evaluation of the threatener.

Threat Management

The course of action to be taken after conducting a threat assessment.

Employee Assistance Programs (EAPs)

Programs that provide a range of services to help employees cope with stressors that occur at home and at work.

Damage Control

An aspect of risk management that refers to the organizational actions taken in response to untoward events in an effort to mitigate damages.

Managerial factors have implications for workplace violence. Organizations should be particularly careful regarding employees' perceptions of procedural fairness concerning layoffs, performance, and conflict resolution. Another managerial factor is whether organizations take a control and monitoring approach to prevent injurious actions from being fully executed. Last, levels of workplace violence may vary depending on how much organizations focus on the root causes of workplace violence such as individual characteristics and organizational environment factors (O'Leary-Kelly et al., 1996).

REGULATORY BACKGROUND

Workplace violence has received increasing attention over the past three decades as a substantial contributor to occupational injury and death. NIOSH reported that homicide has become the second leading cause of occupational injury and death. Assaults represent a serious safety and health hazard for American workers, and violence against employees continues to increase (NIOSH, 1996).

Acknowledging that workplace violence was a pervasive and growing problem, the Occupational Safety and Health Act of 1970 declared that employers had a general duty to provide safe and healthy working conditions. Through this act, NIOSH was charged with drafting and recommending occupational safety and health standards (OSHA, 2004).

OSHA followed up on the general duty requirement in 1989 with voluntary generic safety and health program management guidelines for all employers to use as a foundation for their safety and health programs. The guidelines were not regulations; however, under the OSHA act, employers face fines if an incident of workplace violence occurs. The agency made it clear that safety and health programs could include workplace violence prevention programs (OSHA, 2004).

In 1998, OSHA built on the 1989 generic workplace safety and health guidelines by announcing guidelines specifically targeted at the health care and social services industry. The new guidelines identify common risk factors and include policy recommendations and practical corrective methods to help prevent and mitigate the effects of workplace violence (OSHA, 2004).

In summary, managers of health care organizations have an ethical obligation to protect the safety of workers. Managers also have a general legal duty to prevent workplace violence. Last, given the significant economic costs of workplace violence and the potential legal liability, managers have a fiscal responsibility to prevent workplace violence.

NIOSH Recommendations

NIOSH is located within the Centers for Disease Control and Prevention (CDC). NIOSH recognizes that workplace violence is a particular issue in the health care industry and recommends the following violence prevention strategies for employers: environmental designs, administrative controls, and behavior modifications. **Environmental designs** include signaling systems, alarm systems, monitoring systems, security devices, security escorts, lighting, and architectural and furniture modifications to improve worker safety. **Administrative controls** include (1) adequate staffing patterns to prevent personnel from working alone and to reduce waiting times, (2) controlled access, and (3) development of systems to alert security personnel when violence is threatened. **Behavior modifications** provide all workers with training in recognizing and managing assaults, resolving conflicts, and maintaining hazard awareness (NIOSH, 2002).

OSHA Guidelines

The Occupational Safety and Health Administration (OSHA) is an agency in the U.S. Department of Labor. OSHA suggests that all health care organizations should have a violence prevention program. Ideally, **violence prevention programs** are available to all employees, track progress in reducing work-related assaults, reduce severity of injuries sustained by employees, decrease the threat to worker safety, and reflect the level and nature of threat faced by employees (OSHA, 2004). The main components in a violence prevention program are (1) a written plan, (2) worksite analysis, (3) hazard prevention and control, (4) safety and health training, and (5) recordkeeping and evaluation of program (Box 34.1 and Figure 34.1). **Violence prevention written plans** demonstrate management commitment by disseminating a policy that all types of violence will not be tolerated, ensure that no reprisals are taken against employees who report or experience workplace violence, encourage prompt reporting of all violent incidents, and establish a plan for maintaining security in the workplace. **Worksite analysis** is a common-sense look at the workplace to find existing or potential hazards for workplace violence. **Hazard prevention and control** implements work practices to prevent and control identified hazards. **Safety and health training** makes all the staff aware of security hazards and how to protect themselves through established policies, procedures, and training. **Record keeping and evaluation of programs** provide the data to track progress in reducing work-related assaults.

LEADERSHIP AND MANAGEMENT IMPLICATIONS

Management Frameworks

The implications for management of the threat of workplace violence vary depending somewhat on the source of violence. With regard to the first source of violence (criminals with no connection to the employer), a risk management approach is appropriate. With the second source of violence (patients), a total quality management approach may be effective. Concerning the third source of violence (current or former workers), good human resource management policies are essential. In dealing with the fourth source of violence (someone who has a personal relationship with an employee), employee assistance programs can be especially useful.

Box 34.1

Environmental Analysis

Hazard Prevention and Control

Identify hazards found in the worksite analysis and then provide administrative and work practice controls to make hospitals a safer workplace. For example, the following measures may increase safety:

- Provide better visibility and good lighting, especially in high-risk areas such as the pharmacy or isolated treatment areas.
- Implement safety measures to deter handguns inside facility—for example, using metal detectors.
- Install Plexiglas in the payment window in the pharmacy area.
- Use security devices such as panic buttons, beepers, surveillance cameras, alarm systems, two-way mirrors, card-key access systems, and security guards.
- Place curved mirrors at hallway intersections or concealed areas.
- Control access to work areas.
- Provide training for staff in recognizing and managing hostile and assaultive behavior.
- Provide adequate staffing even during night shifts. Increase staffing in areas in which assaults by patients are likely (e.g., emergency department).
- Increase worker safety during arrival and departure by encouraging car pools and by providing security escorts and shuttle service to and from parking lots and public transportation.
- Ensure accurate reporting of all violent behavior.
- Make patients aware of zero-tolerance policy for violence.
- Establish liaison with police authorities, and contact them when indicated.
- Obtain previous records of patients to learn of any past violent behaviors.
- Establish a system to chart or track and evaluate possible assaultive behaviors, including a way to pass on information from one shift to another.
- Implement a violence prevention plan to develop strategies to deal with possibly violent patients.

A safer room for a possibly violent patient features the following:

- Has furniture arranged to prevent entrapment of staff; furniture should be minimal, lightweight, without sharp corners, and/or affixed to the floor
- Is free from clutter, with nothing available on countertops to throw at workers or use as weapons
- Is provided with a secondary door for escape in case main door is blocked by patient
- Is one entered with a buddy; do not be alone with patient

Modified from Occupational Safety and Health Administration [OSHA]. [2004]. *Guidelines for preventing workplace violence for health care and social service workers.* Washington, DC: OSHA, U.S. Department of Labor. Retrieved May 26, 2009, from http://www.osha.gov/Publications/OSHA3148/osha3148.html.

Risk management is an integrated effort across all disciplines and functional areas to protect the financial assets of an organization from loss by focusing on the prevention of problems that can lead to untoward events and lawsuits. A wide variety of measures are appropriate to prevent violence from criminal activity. Among these measures are the posting of security guards, the restriction of access to the general public, adequate lighting, escort services for those coming or going from parking lots, and the installation of alarm systems and systems to call for emergency assistance. If efforts at prevention fail, insurance is available to cover the specific costs of workplace violence (Law & Pettit, 2007). All of these actions can help prevent or mitigate losses from actions by criminals with no connection to the workplace.

Workplace Violence Checklist

The following items serve merely as an example of what might be used or modified by employers to help identify potential workplace violence problems.

This checklist helps identify present or potential workplace violence problems. Employers also may be aware of other serious hazards not listed here.

Designated competent and responsible observers can readily make periodic inspections to identify and evaluate workplace security hazards and threats of workplace violence. These inspections should be scheduled on a regular basis; when new, previously unidentified security hazards are recognized; when occupational deaths, injuries, or threats of injury occur; when a safety, health and security program is established; and whenever workplace security conditions warrant an inspection.

Periodic inspections for security hazards include identifying and evaluating potential workplace security hazards and changes in employee work practices that may lead to compromising security. Please use the following checklist to identify and evaluate workplace security hazards. **TRUE** notations indicate a potential risk for serious security hazards:

____T ____F This industry frequently confronts violent behavior and assaults of staff.

____T ____F Violence has occurred on the premises or in conducting business.

____T ____F Customers, clients, or coworkers assault, threaten, yell, push, or verbally abuse employees or use racial or sexual remarks.

____T ____F Employees are **NOT** required to report incidents or threats of violence, regardless of injury or severity, to employer.

____T ____F Employees have **NOT** been trained by the employer to recognize and handle threatening, aggressive, or violent behavior.

____T ____F Violence is accepted as "part of the job" by some managers, supervisors, and/or employees.

____T ____F Access and freedom of movement within the workplace are **NOT** restricted to those persons who have a legitimate reason for being there.

____T ____F The workplace security system is inadequate—i.e., door locks malfunction, windows are not secure, and there are no physical barriers or containment systems.

____T ____F Employees or staff members have been assaulted, threatened, or verbally abused by clients and patients.

____T ____F Medical and counseling services have **NOT** been offered to employees who have been assaulted.

____T ____F Alarm systems such as panic alarm buttons, silent alarms, or personal electronic alarm systems are **NOT** being used for prompt security assistance.

____T ____F There is no regular training provided on correct response to alarm sounding.

____T ____F Alarm systems are **NOT** tested on a monthly basis to ensure correct function.

____T ____F Security guards are **NOT** employed at the workplace.

____T ____F Closed circuit cameras and mirrors are **NOT** used to monitor dangerous areas.

____T ____F Metal detectors are **NOT** available or **NOT** used in the facility.

____T ____F Employees have **NOT** been trained to recognize and control hostile and escalating aggressive behaviors and to manage assaultive behavior.

____T ____F Employees **CANNOT** adjust work schedules to use the "Buddy system" for visits to clients in areas where they feel threatened.

____T ____F Cellular phones or other communication devices are **NOT** made available to field staff to enable them to request aid.

____T ____F Vehicles are **NOT** maintained on a regular basis to ensure reliability and safety.

____T ____F Employees work where assistance is **NOT** quickly available.

Figure 34.1

Checklist for violence in the workplace. (From Occupational Safety and Health Administration [OSHA]. [2003]. *Guidelines for preventing workplace violence for health care and social service workers* [rev. 2003]. Washington, DC: OSHA, U.S. Department of Labor. Retrieved November 28, 2008, from www.osha.gov/SLTC/etools/hospital/hazards/workplaceviolence/checklist.html.)

Total quality management (**TQM**) comprises the general processes of setting standards, collecting information, assessing outcomes, and adjusting policies. TQM and risk management share the goals of problem elimination, performance enhancement, and eliciting total organizational commitment. Under TQM, the organization uses all available resources, builds long-term relationships with both employees and patients, and remains open to ways in which processes can be improved to enhance the quality of operations. Teamwork is an integral part of TQM, along with a system for tracking violent incidents (Smith, 2001; Wagner et al., 2001). All levels of the organization are expected to be involved in decision making and employee training. Training topics should impart skills that support the strategic goals of the organization and could include the following: prevalence, incidence, and warning signs of violence; policies and procedures; critical incident response; and availability of services associated with violence in the workplace (Smith-Pittman & McKoy, 1999). Health care organizations can expand the team concept to include providers outside the organization by engaging staff with local police in security planning and education (Hoag-Appel, 1999).

Essential to establishing a safe working environment is developing systems for reporting and documenting incidents of assaults and acts of aggression, as well as taking prompt action when a report is made. The reporting system should include the creation of special forms to report violent incidents, as well as the establishment of a hotline and confidential procedures for employees, to encourage timely and accurate reporting of all forms of violence (McKoy & Smith, 2001; Smith-Pittman & McKoy, 1999). The principles of TQM are manifested in OSHA's guidelines for violence prevention programs in health care; Henry and Ginn (2002) illustrated and discussed this relationship in more depth.

Human Resource Management Policies

A comprehensive violence prevention policy and procedural manual should be developed to guide organizational violence prevention efforts. Violence prevention occurs on three levels: primary, secondary, and tertiary. *Primary* refers to lowering the risk of occurrence; *secondary* refers to containing or limiting the violence; and *tertiary* refers to retrospective assistance and support to the injured (Hogh & Viitasara, 2005).

A number of management policy recommendations in the literature can be applied to the prevention of workplace violence. For example, explaining to employees how or why certain events such as layoffs have occurred will lessen the likelihood of workplace aggression due to highly emotionally charged events. Further, organizations can train employees on how to handle situations of unfairness and how to create fair working environments. Organizations can implement zero-tolerance policy

LEADERSHIP & MANAGEMENT **BEHAVIORS**

Leadership Behaviors

- Envisions a violence prevention program
- Creates a zero-tolerance environment
- Inspires the commitment to a safe work environment
- Collaborates to secure the work environment

Management Behaviors

- Plans a worksite analysis of threats
- Analyzes workplace security trends
- Takes action to modify areas of concern
- Collaborates on strategies to minimize violence
- Manages violence risks
- Develops systems of documentation and reporting
- Structures a violence prevention policy

Overlap Areas

- Takes prompt and appropriate action regarding potential and actual violence
- Collaborates with others for safety and security

toward aggression to lessen the possibility of work groups encouraging an individual to act aggressively (Beugre, 2005).

In the area of personnel, some suggest that organizations have policies to require thorough screening of applicants to weed out those who may have a propensity for violence. Such procedures may eliminate some violence from co-workers because a history of violence is the best indicator of future violence (Corbo & Siewers, 2001). One possibility is to include screening for domestic violence in new employee screening (Anderson, 2002). Thorough employee screening and appropriate termination policies will, at least, contribute to a legal defense that reasonable action to prevent violence has been taken.

In dealing with potential violence from co-workers, threat assessment and threat management are important concepts to consider. **Threat assessment** consists of the evaluation of the threat itself and an evaluation of the threatener. Health care managers must make some effort to determine whether the person making threats was serious about inflicting harm or just verbalizing frustration; however, this is not to diminish the seriousness of verbal assaults. **Threat management** refers to the course of action to be taken after conducting a threat assessment. Health care managers might want to investigate the person making threats and admonish, reprimand, counsel, or terminate the employee, as well as provide post-incident counseling for the victim of the threats (Rugala & Isaacs, 2004). Still another procedural approach is to circulate generalized information such as typical profiles of workplace killers (violent employees), characteristics of disgruntled employees, motivations for violent actions, and factors that contribute to the problem. Furthermore, established disciplinary responses should be flexible enough to consider situational circumstances (Litke, 1996) (Boxes 34.2 and 34.3).

An essential issue for human resource management is accurate reporting of violent incidents. Nurses often fail to report threats or other verbal assaults because institutional policies fail to classify them as violence (Harulow, 2000). Nurses frequently encounter acts of intimidation—an implied threat when someone hits a wall, throws an object, or glares at someone in the immediate area—as a form of violence (Carroll & Morin, 1998). Unfortunately, the toleration of hostile or threatening behavior can result in escalation that results in physical harm (Hoag-Apel, 1999). Health care organizations can train nurses to identify

Box 34.2

Questions to Ask in a Threat Assessment

1. Is there evidence of substance abuse or mental illness/depression?
2. Has the subject shown an interest in violence through movies, games, books, or magazines?
3. Is the subject preoccupied with violent themes; interested in publicized violent events; or fascinated with and/or recently acquired weapons?
4. Has the subject identified a specific target and communicated with others his thoughts or plans for violence?
5. Is the subject obsessed with others or engaged in any stalking or surveillance activity?
6. Has the offender spoken of homicide or suicide?
7. Does he have a criminal history or history of past violent behavior?
8. Does the offender have a plan for what he would do?
9. Does the plan make sense; is it reasonable; is it specific?
10. Does the offender have the means, knowledge, and wherewithal to carry out his plan?

From Rugala, E.R., & Isaacs, A.R. (Eds.). (2004). *Workplace violence: Issues in response.* Washington, DC: U.S. Department of Justice, Federal Bureau of Investigation (FBI). Retrieved May 27, 2009, from http://www.fbi.gov/publications/violence.pdf.

Box 34.3

Threat Assessment: A True-Life Example

The following is an account of a threat assessment conducted jointly by a criminal investigator and a mental health professional as reported at the NCAVC's Violence in the Workplace Symposium.

During a training session, the 46-year-old subject made comments regarding his alcoholism, causing such a disturbance that he was subsequently referred to the Employee Assistance Counseling Program. On two other occasions, he displayed inappropriate behavior by storming around the office, cursing, and throwing objects. In another training workshop, he made verbally abusive comments, disturbing the class.

After a month's leave, he had a verbal outburst during a meeting on his first day back in the office and requested a transfer due to stress. The request was denied. He then requested more leave, which was granted. The subject was noticeably withdrawn and his performance declined. Supervisors documented a pattern of unusual agitation over minor issues, unreasonable complaints, unacceptable work, and allegations that co-workers were conspiring against him. The subject was voluntarily hospitalized twice for homicidal ideations. He was treated for psychosis and suicidal and paranoid delusions associated with his co-workers. His physician recommended a disability retirement.

A month before his disability pension was approved, he began to leave harassing voice-mail messages on a co-worker's telephone. An example of the messages is: "Hi Darlene, it's Stan, Just wanted to say Happy Thanksgiving. And, you give this message to Yvonne. Tell her if she had been off the property the day she hollered at me, I would have beat her [obscenity deleted]. Bye Darlene." He was diagnosed with delusional disorder, paranoid type. This information was also provided to law enforcement during the investigation.

His retirement papers contained disturbing comments. For example, recalling a meeting with a Human Resources staff member, he said: "I started to grab her by the throat and choke her, until the top part of her head popped off. Then I was going to step on her throat and pluck her bozo hairdo bald. Strand by strand ..."

Some months later, the subject told a former co-worker that he was following a former supervisor and her family. He provided specific information, stating that he knew where some of the targets lived and the types and colors of vehicles they drove. The subject also made comments about the target's family members and stated that he had three guns for each of his former supervisors.

At this point, law enforcement was notified. While the police investigation was under way, the subject made threats against five former female co-workers. A threat assessment was conducted analyzing letters, voice mails, reports from EAP, and interviews with various individuals. The subject's communications were organized and contained specific threats. For example, he wrote "Don't let the passage of time fool you, all is not forgotten or forgiven," and "I will in my own time strike again, and it will be unmerciful." The material suggested that he was becoming increasingly fixated on the targets and his communications articulated an action imperative that suggested that the risk was increasing. After obtaining additional information, the investigators informed the subject of specific limits and consequences that would occur if he continued his threatening behavior and communications.

The subject assured law enforcement agents that his intent was to pursue legal reparations. Four months later, however, he mailed letters to his five targets stating that he wanted to "execute" one of them. The letters indicated that he was close to committing an attack. Based on the foregoing assessment and insight into his thinking and behavior over several months, the threat assessment team, consisting of an investigator and a mental health professional, initiated a conference call with the district attorney. In the conference, the mental health professional provided an assessment of the subject's potential for violence, and the investigator presented evidence regarding the laws violated and law enforcement actions taken to date.

The threat assessment report, along with other evidence, was used by the district attorney in obtaining an arrest warrant and a search warrant. The final recommendation by the team was that the subject should be arrested and held without bond. Six months later, he was found not guilty by reason of insanity.

From Rugala, E.R., & Isaacs, A.R. (Eds.). (2004). Workplace violence: Issues in response. Washington, DC: U.S. Department of Justice, Federal Bureau of Investigation (FBI). Retrieved May 27, 2009 from www.fbi.gov/publications/violence.pdf.

potentially aggressive patients and treat them appropriately. Staff training is recognized as a key preventive measure. Numerous regulatory bodies and agencies (e.g., OSHA, National Health Service [NHS]) advocate for training to meet the needs of different types of staff groups. At a minimum, staff should be trained in basic violence behavior prevention and correct emergency response procedures (Beech & Leather, 2005). Training programs should emphasize the broad definition of violence and the importance of reporting all incidents of violence (Sheehan, 2000).

Human resource management policies are essential for the prevention of violence from current or former workers in health care organizations. Policies on hiring, discipline, counseling, training, threat assessment, threat management, and reporting can prevent or mitigate loss caused by violence from co-workers.

Employee assistance programs (EAPs) provide a range of services to help employees cope with stressors that occur at home and at work. Family counseling might be useful in reducing domestic violence that can spill over into the workplace. Programs that counsel both the victim and the abuser could be instrumental in initiating needed interventions to defuse domestic violence situations that could impact the worksite. Furthermore, individual counseling can help employees cope with personal stressors that might contribute to unpredictable or violent behaviors. In short, EAPs can be very useful in preventing or mitigating loss caused by domestic violence that spills over into the workplace.

Leadership

It is important to establish and maintain a corporate culture that is serious about protecting employees from violence. Similar to safety climate, a perceived violence climate exists that correlates to both physical and verbal aggression. Depending on the choices that are made, organizations can create a violent climate or nonviolent climate (Spector et al., 2007). Employees often perceive the failure of management to prevent violent incidences or to respond quickly and appropriately when incidents do occur as lack of organizational commitment and loyalty. Ensuring a nonviolent workplace may require culture change, and alterations in practice may be necessary in such areas as labor relations, injury management, and other human resource procedures (McKoy & Smith, 2001). Consistent with the principles of quality improvement, leadership for such tasks as worksite analysis, threat assessment, and development of organizational policies and procedures would be provided by multidisciplinary teams composed of representatives of all aspects of the organization.

LEGAL IMPLICATIONS

Although the levels of threat vary among the issues (Matchulat, 2007), several *legal issues* surround workplace violence, as follows (Dolan, 2000):

- Employers may be faced with paying higher workers' compensation rates after injuries are sustained from workplace violence.
- Employers may be subject to claims that they were negligent with regard to the security provided.
- Employers may be subject to claims concerning negligent hiring, retention, and supervision.
- Employers may be subject to claims that they failed to warn subsequent employers about the criminal propensities of former employees.
- Threat management is complicated in that disability discrimination legislation restricts employers from taking action against employees solely because of their psychological disabilities and requires that action be taken only when the employee poses a direct threat.
- Sexual discrimination laws make employers liable in some instance for sexual harassment.
- Employers may be liable for citations, fines, and even criminal penalties.

Legal defense can be based on a variety of proactive actions by management, including conducting a risk assessment to determine what would be reasonable and appropriate action (Egger, 2000). Developing written antiviolence policies and procedures is the first step in reducing workplace violence. Policies should address factors such as employees, patients, non-hospital employee providers, and visitors (Smith-Pittman & McKoy, 1999). The following policies are useful in both preventing workplace violence and providing a legal defense if violence should occur: policies forbidding weapons, alcohol, drug use, bullying, and sexual harassment; and policies requiring pre-employment screening and appropriate termination procedures. Similarly, policies clearly defining violence, requiring the reporting of violent acts, and specifying appropriate disciplinary actions for committing violence are essential (Ginn & Henry, 2002). Although no program can guarantee violent acts will not occur, the existence of a program can provide evidence in court that the health care organization has taken appropriate and reasonable action.

Last, there is **damage control** if all prevention efforts fail. Health care organizations can assemble an emergency response team staffed appropriately to respond at the times of day when the threat is greatest (Sheehan, 2000). The literature suggests specific steps to respond to workplace incidents such as the following (Litke, 1996):

- Remain calm.
- Evaluate facts objectively.
- Call in additional resources.

Furthermore, after a violent incident, employers must address the emotions of employees and notify family members. Employers must also take steps to preserve the company image, quash rumors, prepare for ancillary incidents, ward off lawsuits, and return to normal operations (Botting, 2001). EAPs can also serve as a valuable tool in debriefing employees after involvement in a violent incident, reducing the potential negative impact on both the employees and the organization.

CURRENT ISSUES AND TRENDS

Violence appears to be inherent in modern U.S. society and increasing in all aspects of society. Thus it is understandable that violence will continue to be present in the nursing profession. Reducing the impact of violence on the profession will require an expansive view of the problem that objectively explores all potential factors and pursues broad-based, collaborative efforts at resolution. In recent years, violence in the workplace has come to be viewed in the same light as other occupational hazards, allowing some measure of controllability by health and safety professionals.

Publicized violent incidents against nurses and the evidence in the literature that violence against nurses continues to rise have prompted increased emphasis on prevention of violence in the health care workplace. In response, government agencies have published voluntary guidelines for preventive measures, the health care community has launched several initiatives aimed at prevention, and some states have passed legislation requiring training in prevention. The following violence prevention topics have been determined in the literature to warrant discussion as critical or new perspectives: improving prediction of violence, environmental design, collaboration among organizations and agencies, and increasing government oversight.

In responding to violence, it is easy to focus attention strictly on individual responses and behaviors; however, there is growing emphasis on evaluation of the contribution of the physical environment. Clearly, physical aspects could enable or contribute to the perpetration of violent incidents. NIOSH (2002) presented a variety of suggestions for designing a safe work environment, including the following: emergency signaling alarms and monitoring systems; metal detectors at entrances and security cameras in hallways; appropriate design of waiting areas for patients and families; adequate lighting and security escorts in parking lots; and design of triage and other public areas to minimize risk for assault.

Organizational culture is also considered an aspect of environment in a systems approach. The health care delivery environment is turbulent and evolving rapidly (Kreitzer et al., 1997). In order to evolve, the U.S. health care industry is experiencing substantial restructuring through ownership consolidation and development of new forms of interorganizational relationships.

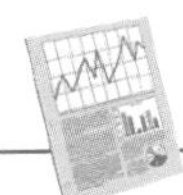

Research Note

Source: Lowe, T., Wellman, N., & Taylor, R. (2002). Limit-setting and decision-making in the management of aggression. *Journal of Advanced Nursing, 41*(2), 154-161.

Purpose

Previous research has suggested that inpatient aggression toward nursing staff is influenced by characteristics of the nurse-patient interaction. This study examined mental health nurses' judgments in conflict situations. Nurses' perceptions of the relative importance of different aspects of interaction with patients in potentially aggressive situations were measured.

Discussion

The rise in incidence of violence and aggression by patients is a growing concern in the nursing profession and is of particular note in mental health nursing. Nurses experience considerable internal conflict in making decisions regarding interaction with patients in potentially aggressive situations. This study used a case scenario approach, presenting nurses with 10 conflict situations and 10 possible nursing responses to each event. Nurses were asked to rate the response statements for appropriateness. The results suggest that imposing limits and boundaries in patient behavior (limit-setting) and giving clear guidelines and expectations of patients (use of structure) are regarded as highly important; however, these must be considered concurrently with a sense of respect for patients and their autonomy (confirming). The relative importance of confirming interventions suggests that moral judgments are being made and that assumptions about blame or accountability are involved. Results showed that nurses with the most experience tended to make less restrictive judgments. Among the proposed explanations for this are the following: mental health training could have an effect on individual judgments about the appropriateness of interventions; greater understanding of mental illness leads to less blaming of patients; and increased knowledge leads to greater confidence and a more relaxed view of patient behaviors. Clearly, there is evidence of a need for more research and discussion regarding effective nurse responses in potentially critical situations, as well as the role of the organization in eliciting and reinforcing positive responses.

Application to Practice

The management of patients in potentially aggressive situations clearly presents a challenge to nurses. Many nursing practices are firmly based in history and law; thus nurses find it difficult to see alternatives to traditional modes of intervention. The results of this study carry implications for nursing administration and policy in terms of standardizing procedures for dealing with potentially aggressive patients, emphasizing nurse training in recognition and management of violence, establishing post-incident reviews, and reviewing ethical dilemmas and dimensions of decision making among nurses.

Organizational changes, such as restructuring, mergers, and downsizing, create significant levels of uncertainty and anxiety in employees, which can eventually lead to stress-related consequences, possibly including violence.

Among the recommendations of OSHA and TQM approaches in the area of environmental design is to have a worksite analysis conducted by a threat assessment team or similar taskforce or coordinator. Such an effort analyzes records, trends, workplace security, physical characteristics, operating policies, and screening surveys of staff to provide an overview of the work environment. Based on the results of this assessment, direct action should be taken to resolve any identified areas of concern.

Practical Tips

Tip # 1: Create a Nonviolent Organizational Culture

Define and establish a just, fair, and ethical culture of nonviolence in the workplace. Enforce zero-tolerance for aggressive or violent behavior from any source; ensure supportive, non-punitive responses to the reporting of violent or potentially violent acts.

Tip # 2: Use Evidence-Based Policies and Interventions

Establish strong policies against workplace violence that are imbedded in the mission and values of the organization. Implement evidence-based intervention systems that impose behavioral expectations that preclude violent or maladaptive behaviors.

Tip # 3: Implement Rigorous Risk Management

Implement a rigorous risk management plan for prevention of violence. Take a proactive systems approach to violence prevention; conduct a thorough needs assessment, including threat assessment and environmental assessment, and implement strategies to reduce risk in all aspects of the organization.

Tip # 4: Develop a Proactive Post-Incident Response Plan

Proactively plan for post-incident response. Respond quickly and appropriately to violent incidents, providing adequate support to affected individuals, with the first priority being safety and well-being of victims. A strong employee assistance program is key.

Gaps Between Legal Theory and Workplace Practices

For workplace violence, significant gaps exist between legal theory and workplace practices. Most research focuses on issues within the realm of social psychology such as stress, justice, and social cognition theory. The large legal questions revolve around negligent employment, workplace harassment, and the Americans with Disabilities Act accommodation issues. Thus most of the gaps would fall in the realm of psychology. Research is needed that would identify people who would likely be aggressive in a way that was a genuine threat to others. Research is needed that would establish the effectiveness of anti-harassment policies. Last, research is needed that would establish the relationships between various mental illnesses and genuine threats to co-workers (Paetzold et al., 2007).

Collaboration

Nursing care occurs in many different settings, involves both professionals and laypersons, and exposes nurses to unacceptably high levels of many different types of violence. Thus there is the potential for various organizations and agencies to work together to develop strategies to minimize violence against nurses. McPhaul and Lipscomb (2004) explored the application of three theoretical perspectives in the approach to workplace violence prevention in academic, union, and employer partnerships. Based on their reviews, they advocated that any effective intervention needs to use a collaborative, systemic approach. When necessary, advice and assistance should be sought from resources outside the health care facility, such as threat-assessment psychologists, psychiatrists, and other professionals; social service agencies; and law enforcement agencies. Rugala and Isaacs (2004) offered a number of suggestions for strengthening the relationship between health care organizations and local law enforcement for preventing workplace violence.

Increased Government Oversight

OSHA is the only regulatory agency that directly oversees the safety and health of health care workers, although several health care oversight agencies attempt to provide industry self-regulation of the safety of health care workers. At this time, OSHA's guidelines are voluntary, thus lacking in power of enforcement. The Joint Commission (TJC) (formerly Joint Commission on Accreditation of Healthcare Organizations [JCAHO]) provided clear standards for support of patient safety but does not offer the same guidance with regard to the safety of health care workers. The American Nurses Association (ANA) supports the establishment of the OSHA recommendations as mandatory requirements.

New perspectives are also offered in the literature to shed light on the problem of violence in nursing, including horizontal violence (nurse against nurse), the potential impact of terrorism on nursing, and post-incident response. In addition, one nursing setting that was noted in the literature as becoming of more concern regarding violence is that of schools.

Horizontal Violence

The literature reveals that nurses are the most common perpetrators of some forms of violence, such as bullying. Some researchers (McMillan, 1995) suggested that the workplace environment and nursing culture allow this horizontal violence to occur unimpeded and actually accept it as a normal part of workplace culture. This seems to be particularly evident in regard to nursing experience; bullying is most often reported to be directed toward new nurses by more seasoned nurses. This type of violence usually manifests as psychological harassment rather than physical aggression, involves a series of incidents, and often creates hostility and discomfort among staff. These acts often seem to be precipitated by staffing shortages and increasing workloads.

The impact of horizontal violence is in some ways greater that that of other types. In addition to dealing with the violent episode itself, the victim also has to deal with the ramifications of poor working relationships—a situation that affects all co-workers, as well. A number of consequences have been found to accompany horizontal violence, including demoralization, feelings of vulnerability, a changed-to-negative attitude to work, loss of confidence, and impaired work performance (McKenna et al., 2003). Some nurses report that such incidents have led to consideration of leaving the profession (Wheeler, 1998). Taking the problem of horizontal violence beyond the direct impact on personal work performance, research also indicates that nurses' lack of satisfaction with the job will lead to reduced patient satisfaction (Tzeng & Ketefian, 2002). Violence in the form of bullying and harassment may be so endemic that it is taken for granted and dismissed as inconsequential. Nurses are urged to confront this underreported form of workplace violence, become a source of support for colleagues, and work as change agents in calling for managerial support for workplace safety.

Terrorism

The threat of terrorism has captured the attention of the world, and the workplace is no exception. The most notable terrorist attacks in the United States have occurred in settings that qualify them as occupational violence: the World Trade Center and the Oklahoma City Federal Building. Since the attack on the World Trade Center, America's workplaces have recognized the need to be prepared to handle not only the traditional threats of violence but also the external threat of terrorism. Terrorist activity can be motivated by political, social, issue-oriented, and religious views. For some militant groups, Western civilization represents evil and thus anything in Western civilization could be a target. However, some organizations may have characteristics that make them particularly salient to terrorists. By considering the motivations of some terrorist groups and attempting to view one's organization through the eyes of a potential terrorist, one may conclude that the profile of an organization should be altered in subtle ways to make it a less egregious symbol to terrorists (Brown, 1998). Certainly, health care providers will be pivotal responders in the event of major terrorist incidents, and the violence itself may spill into the health care workplace.

Post-Incident Response

Post-incident response is becoming recognized as a critical element in reducing both the short-term and the long-term impact of workplace violence. Health care workers who do not receive adequate support after an incident may quit or be fearful of returning to work. Failure to respond quickly and appropriately to violent incidents is perceived by employees as lack of management commitment and concern for the workforce. OSHA (2004) and the Federal Bureau of Investigation (FBI) (Rugala & Isaacs, 2004) have recommended that employers set up trained response teams and provide post-incident response that includes such measures as prompt medical treatment, psychological evaluation, counseling, support groups, stress debriefing, trauma crisis counseling, and employee assistance programs. The first responsibility of the response team is to ensure the safety and well-being of the victim(s) of violence. Response team members may be called in at any stage of a violent incident—to defuse an escalating situation, intervene in an event, or respond to the aftermath of a traumatic event. Consequently, response teams should receive special training in evaluation, threat assessment, and conflict resolution, as well as procedures to monitor, document, and respond to situations. Teams should also have plans for dealing with other issues, such as news media and public reaction to a major incident. Post-incident response should involve an integrated system of services and procedures to reduce the potential impact of a violent incident on employees. Incident debriefing should be offered to all employees, not just to those involved in the event (Henry & Ginn, 2002).

Clearly, violence in the workplace has an impact that goes beyond what is done to a particular victim. It damages trust, community, and the sense of security that every employee has a right to feel while at work. Employing agencies need to show a commitment to safety for nurses, providing protection against acts of violence in all clinical areas and especially in high-risk settings. Educational institutions and employers need to share responsibility for properly preparing nurses to deal with potentially violent situations.

Summary

- Employers have legal and ethical obligations to promote a work environment free from violence.
- Workplace violence exacts an economic cost through lost productivity, low morale, increased workers' compensation, medical claims, and possible lawsuit and liability costs.
- The four sources of violence are (1) person with no connection to the organization, (2) patient or family of patient, (3) current or former employee, and (4) someone with a personal relationship with an employee.
- Management philosophy and practice influence the potential for violence in an organization.
- NIOSH recommended three violence prevention strategies: environmental design, administrative controls, and behavior modifications.
- The main components of a violence prevention program as set forth by OSHA are a written plan, worksite analysis, hazard prevention and control, safety and health training, and record keeping and evaluation.
- Human resources departments should develop comprehensive violence prevention policies and procedures manuals to include such issues as pre-employment screening, threat assessment, and threat management.

- EAP programs can help employees and their families cope with stressors that might contribute to unpredictable or violent behaviors.
- Leadership should be provided by multidisciplinary teams composed of representatives of all areas of the health care organization and appropriate community representatives.
- Legal defensibility should be grounded in proactive actions by management, starting with written antiviolence policies and procedures.
- Research is warranted in improving the prediction of violence, including consideration of lowering the level of confidence for statistical prediction.
- Efforts at environmental design should include both the physical environment and the organizational culture.
- Horizontal violence has a greater impact on the organization than do other types and contributes to reduced morale, increased turnover, nurses leaving the profession, and reduced quality of patient care.
- Effective violence prevention collaborations will include representatives from within and outside of the health care organization.
- The first responsibility of the post-incident response team is to ensure the safety and well-being of the victims of violence.

CASE STUDY

Nurse Juanita Evans is in her first nursing job. She was assigned to the emergency department (ED) 4 months ago, as a last-minute assignment, without any prior ED training. Ms. Amy Jones has been waiting in the ED for 3 hours to receive care for abdominal pain. Amy's brother, John, becomes agitated, begins to pace the waiting area, and chastises several staff members as they pass by. As Nurse Evans passes, John tries to grab her arm; she pulls away and tells him that there are other people in worse shape and that he will just have to wait his turn. He continues to chastise and to make verbal threats of retaliation against the hospital and staff if his sister is not cared for soon. The staff ignore him and dismiss his threats as just the stress of the situation. Amy eventually receives the care she needs and is released. Four days later, Nurse Evans is walking to her car in a far corner of the parking garage when she is attacked by John and left unconscious on the ground.

1. What are the warning signs of a potential problem?
2. Why is each a problem?
3. Apply the five components of OSHA's Violence Prevention Plan to identify what should be done to ensure that such a situation does not happen again.
4. How could Nurse Evans have handled the situation differently?

CRITICAL THINKING EXERCISE

Nurse Millie Adams is a nursing administrator at Good Care Hospital, a facility that serves as an educational training hospital. Nurse Adams has noticed several trends recently: nurse turnover has been higher than usual; sick leave has increased; student nurses frequently request transfers to other facilities. In searching for answers, she hears a lot of talk about nurses being threatened or verbally confronted by other nurses; however, the number of reports of violent incidents has not increased.

1. What are the problems?
2. What are the potential sources for these problems?
3. What are some possible explanations for the problems?
4. What information does Nurse Adams need, and how should she gather this information?
5. What could be done to resolve the problems?

All-Hazards Disaster Preparedness

Karen N. Drenkard Gene S. Rigottii

CHAPTER OBJECTIVES

- Present an overview of all-hazards preparedness
- Define and discuss multiple facets of all-hazards preparedness
- Analyze planning for a comprehensive all-hazards preparedness strategy for health care
- Discuss strategies to resolve implementation issues
- Critique nursing leadership and management implications
- Identify all-hazards preparedness resources
- Explore emerging issues related to allocation of scarce resources
- Exercise critical thinking to conceptualize and analyze possible solutions to a practice exercise

TRANSITIONING THEORY INTO PRACTICE FOR ALL-HAZARDS PREPAREDNESS

September 11, 2001, was a tragic day that touched everyone's lives and changed Americans' perception of a "safe" world forever. Since that time, people of all backgrounds have been scrambling to prepare significant others and themselves, their homes, and their workplaces for what might happen. A list of terrorism possibilities is endless: biological mishaps, chemical spills, radiological exposures, nuclear blasts, conventional bombings, agricultural contamination, cyber viruses, and other unforeseen cataclysmic events. Thus disaster and bioterrorism preparedness is most appropriately termed **all-hazards disaster preparedness.**

Since September 11, people in every community have been gathering information from a variety of resources, reevaluating personal perspectives about preparing for an inevitable disaster, and planning what they would do in the event of a disaster (Ashcroft, 2001; Myers, 2001; Richter, 2004; Vecchio, 2000). But how does one go about preparing for an event in the workplace, and more specifically, the hospital environment? Traditionally the community hospital is a place of refuge for the sick and wounded. How does all that change in the event of a disaster?

Health care executives across the country are continuing to focus on dedicating resources to effectively participate in all-hazards preparedness. The Health Insurance Portability and Accountability Act (HIPAA) and the Joint Commission Resources (JCR) require all health care facilities to have detailed all-hazard preparedness plans. Nursing leaders are an integral part of this planning because they know best that the measure of success is based on the degree of effective planning. Nurse leaders possess the necessary skills, competencies, and experience that serve them well in taking on a primary role in disaster preparedness (Lindholm & Uden, 2001). In addition, sustainability of attention and focus becomes a key role of the nurse executive in ensuring a constant state of readiness for the organization.

Effective planning for all-hazards preparedness is an important process, and skill in planning is an essential management competency for nurse leaders. This chapter describes how to orchestrate a multilevel plan for a health care facility. A comprehensive all-hazards preparedness plan will assist in establishing the following: (1) an organized hospital-based plan for both internal and external disasters at the department/unit level, (2) an interhospital plan for effectively collaborating with other hospitals within a health care system and within the local vicinity, (3) a community plan that will integrate the hospital plan with other external community plans, and (4) a national plan that will guide nurse leaders in accessing financial assistance from federal and state all-hazards preparedness resources.

DEFINITIONS

From a health care perspective, a **disaster** is an unforeseen and often sudden event that causes great damage, destruction, and human suffering. Although often caused by nature, disasters can have human origins. Wars and civil disturbances that destroy homelands and displace people are included among the causes of disasters. Other causes can be a building collapse, blizzard, drought, epidemic, earthquake, explosion, fire, flood, hazardous material transportation incident (e.g., chemical spill), hurricane, nuclear incident, tornado, or volcano (Disaster Relief Library, 2004).

There are a wide variety of types and causes of disasters. Disasters can be *internal,* such as a catastrophic event that occurs within a facility and is usually handled within the facility, depending on the size of the event; or *external,* a catastrophic event that affects the community, which may or may not affect the facility. Causes of natural disasters include such things as earthquakes, forest fires, floods, or hurricanes, such as the devastation caused by Hurricane Katrina in New Orleans in 2005. Disasters also can be caused by human acts; these can include biological, chemical, radiological, nuclear, cyber, or conventional terrorist events.

Other disaster-related definitions are as follows:

- *All-hazards:* A general term that is descriptive of all types of natural and/or human terrorist events.
- *All-hazards disaster preparedness:* Multifaceted internal and external disaster preparedness that establishes action plans for every type of disaster or combination of disaster events.
- *Altered standards of care:* The term "altered standards" definition has not reached national consensus but generally is assumed to mean a shift to providing care and allocating scarce equipment, supplies, and personnel in a way that saves the largest number of lives in contrast to the traditional focus on saving individuals (Agency for Healthcare Research and Quality [AHRQ], 2005a).
- *Biological disaster:* An incident involving a natural or deliberate outbreak of a pathogen affecting large numbers of adults and children (Inova Health System, 2001a).
- *Chemical disaster:* Exposure to hazardous chemically toxic materials that may produce a wide range of adverse health effects (Inova Health System, 2001b).
- *Conventional disaster:* A catastrophic event caused by the use of weapons such as guns, bombs, missiles, or grenades.
- *Cyber disaster:* A catastrophic event affecting large numbers of people and lasting more than a few hours that affects the ability to use information technology.
- *Mass casualty event (MCE):* A catastrophic public health or terrorism-related event that results in the community's health care system being overwhelmed by the needs of victims (AHRQ, 2007). MCEs can be organized into two categories: (1) immediate or sudden impact; and (2) events resulting in ongoing or sustained impact (AHRQ, 2007).
- *Radiological/nuclear disaster:* A radiological or nuclear emergency that may result from accidents occurring within a facility (e.g., the departments of nuclear medicine and radiation oncology) or from external sources involving vehicles transporting radioactive materials (RAM) or caused by terrorism events involving nuclear weapons or radiologically contaminated conventional weapons (Inova Health System, 2001c).
- *Surge capacity:* "Health care facility surge capacity is the term that should be applied to the ability of each and every hospital to discharge existing patients to make those

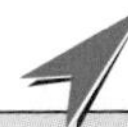

LEADING & MANAGING **DEFINED**

All-Hazards Disaster Preparedness	Disaster
Action plans for every type of disaster or combination of disaster events.	An unforeseen and often sudden event that causes great damage, destruction, and human suffering.

hospital beds available for incoming hospital patients. This term should be applied to the creative use of available space by a healthcare facility for the initial management of disaster victims" (Hanfling, 2006, p. 1233).

GETTING STARTED: FIRST STEPS

Starting any complex systems project can be confusing and difficult. Beginning the work of establishing a comprehensive all-hazards preparedness plan is no exception. Historically, most hospitals have had some sort of disaster plan in place. Being the leader in the evaluation of the hospital's current disaster plan, in light of the nation's current focus on maintaining a state of constant readiness, can be a complicated process. One of the first steps to gaining participation from appropriate stakeholders and moving the evaluation process forward is the creation of an oversight committee, or all-hazards preparedness task force (AHPTF, referred to as *Task Force*). The nursing executive, often called a *chief nurse officer (CNO)*, will play a pivotal role in facilitating the initial Task Force.

Creating an All-Hazards Preparedness Task Force

As nurses know, effective projects that create lasting change start with the basic nursing process: assessment, planning, implementation, evaluation, and modification. The AHPTF will similarly follow this process. It is essential to get administrative support regarding the need for an all-hazards preparedness plan. This is best accomplished by establishing a high-level administrative Task Force whose purpose will be oversight of the multilevel all-hazards preparedness plan development. Whether the hospital is part of a larger health care system or is a freestanding, independent hospital, the Task Force will function similarly.

Health care systems with multiple facilities are very familiar with the complexity and intricacies of trying to establish a standardized system-wide approach to care needs. In organizations such as these, system-wide executive administrators need to be part of the Task Force. Having a senior executive administrator of the health care system serve as the chairperson of the Task Force will provide the leadership needed to communicate the importance of all-hazards preparedness as a system priority. A representative CNO and emergency care physician, serving as co-chairs with the senior executive administrator, will create a dynamic team that is uniquely prepared to tackle any issues that arise. A project facilitator is also helpful in getting the Task Force started and operational.

Establishing the Task Force requires that all departments be committed to the tasks at hand and cognizant of the need for consensus building and standardization of processes. Bidirectional communication is imperative. Coordination of the work of the Task Force members also needs to be addressed. Fortunately, most of the work will be broken down into step-by-step pieces that allow each member to play a vital role and have control over his or her department's contribution to the plan as a whole. The standing membership should be composed of stakeholders representing all areas of the organization. Because not all departments can logistically be on the Task Force, the members will have large areas of oversight and communication. The Task Force membership might typically look like that outlined in Table 35.1.

Table 35.1

All-Hazards Preparedness Task Force Membership Responsibilities

Responsibility Area(s)	Position Title	Detail of Area Covered
Executive owner (Chair)	Executive administrator	Leads the All-Hazards Preparedness Task Force as chair. If the hospital is part of a health care system, this person will be a system-wide senior administrator. If the hospital is a freestanding, independent facility, this person will be the hospital's chief operating officer.
Clinical operations (Co-chair)	Chief nurse officer	Represents all nursing and clinical departments. Co-chairs the Task Force.
Chemical/ radiological/ conventional threats (Co-chair)	Emergency department/ air care medical director	Represents all aspects of emergency medicine and physician needs related to all-hazards preparedness. This person also will co-chair the Task Force.
Physician liaison(s)	Department chiefs	Serve as spokespersons for physician needs with regard to disaster preparedness. Facilitate communication of timely information should an event occur. Have oversight for physician credentialing in times of a disaster. Assist in approval of medical standards established for various types of disasters.
Chief operating officers (COOs) from health care system facilities	Chief operating officer(s)	Represent the needs of their facilities in establishing an effective all-hazards preparedness plan. Facilitate system-wide collaboration in standardizing practices and communicate essential information to employees.
Security	Safety and security director	Serves as liaison for system-wide safety and security departments in the system. Coordinates and synchronizes efforts of all departments as related to all-hazards preparedness. Responsible for rapid "lockdown" of all entrances and flow of people in the event of a disaster.
Communications	Chief information technology officer	Oversees successful operation of the integrated information system, including telephones, radios, and computers and satellite technology, during times of instability. Creates and maintains redundant systems to ensure an ability to communicate within facilities, outside to other hospitals, and partners with community.
Messages/media	Marketing director	Plays an active role in communicating the "All-Hazards Preparedness" message to all employees, patients, and community. Acts on behalf of the health care system or hospital in speaking with press about impending or actual disaster situations.

Courtesy Inova Health System, Falls Church, VA.

Note: This assessment tool was developed by Inova Health System based on a bioterrorism preparedness survey created by a committee consisting of representatives from Baylor University's Graduate Program in Healthcare Administration, the U.S. Army Center for Healthcare Education and Studies, and the University of Texas Health Science Center at San Antonio. (For more information, see Drenkard et al., 2002.)

Table 35.1

All-Hazards Preparedness Task Force Membership Responsibilities—cont'd

Responsibility Area(s)	Position Title	Detail of Area Covered
Human resources	Human resources director	Serves as the staff's voice in meeting the needs of employees during a disaster. Creates manuals to guide staff in preparing for and responding to a disaster.
Financial reimbursement	Chief financial officer	Leads efforts in monitoring financial expenses related to establishing an effective all-hazards preparedness plan. Seeks out state/federal reimbursement opportunities for planning.
Government funding	Government affairs director	Serves as a vital link to local, state, and federal boards representing the system financial and operational needs regarding all-hazards preparedness. Advocates for funding related to all-hazards preparedness.
Biological threats	Infectious disease medical director	Serves as the liaison for all infection control (IC) departments in the system.
	Infection control nurse	Coordinates and synchronizes efforts of all IC departments as related to all-hazards preparedness. Responsible for development, dissemination, and understanding of procedures related to biological events.
Legal	Executive attorney	Advises All-Hazards Preparedness task force in legal matters related to establishing an effective All-Hazards Preparedness plan.
Education planning	Education director	Has oversight for planning and implementing educational efforts for staff and patients. As needed, coordinates "just in time" training for any arising incident. Is an integral partner in planning and implementing internal and external disaster drills.
Logistics	Pharmacy director	Serves as the liaison for all system pharmacies. Has oversight for stockpiling medications for use in a disaster. Establishes par levels of drugs for use in "patient surge" situations. Establishes contracts with pharmaceutical vendors to ensure adequate supply of medications in the event of a disaster. Has oversight for any medical supply trucks ready for deployment in times of a disaster (e.g., stocking par level of drugs used in a chemical disaster).

Continued

Table 35.1

All-Hazards Preparedness Task Force Membership Responsibilities—cont'd

Responsibility Area(s)	Position Title	Detail of Area Covered
Logistics	Materials management director	Serves as an active participant on the task force. This liaison is the system representative for all materials management departments. Is very involved in setting par levels for supplies and equipment on the units at the time of a disaster. Establishes contracts with materials management vendors to ensure adequate supply of medications in the event of a disaster (e.g., stocking a supplemental supply truck for use in a disaster).
Logistics	Engineering	Directs any operational building redesign needed to prepare hospital for handling a disaster (e.g., decontamination showers).

Courtesy Inova Health System, Falls Church, VA.
Note: This assessment tool was developed by Inova Health System based on a bioterrorism preparedness survey created by a committee consisting of representatives from Baylor University's Graduate Program in Healthcare Administration, the U.S. Army Center for Healthcare Education and Studies, and the University of Texas Health Science Center at San Antonio. (For more information, see Drenkard et al., 2002.)

As the team evolves in its work, ad hoc members can be added as needed. Internal ad hoc members might include medical radiology, facility engineering, telecommunications, volunteer support, chaplain services, physician chairs, social work, case management, and dietary, respiratory, and laboratory services. External ad hoc members might include public health administrators, government liaison support, police force liaison, public school system liaison, community church representatives, community physicians, and even vendor representatives, who can be contracted to provide such things as oxygen, ice, food, cots, and linens in the event of a disaster.

For the first year, the system-wide Task Force will probably need to meet every other week. During this period, the Task Force will perform a gap analysis based on the JCR standards and other regulations and start a working action plan to correct any deficiencies. Nursing leaders will play key roles in creating aggressive timelines, often 1 to 2 weeks, for resolving issues on the action plan. The goal should be to have resolutions that are correct but not necessarily perfect. Most resolutions will be modified and enhanced over time as the Task Force gains more knowledge about all-hazards planning.

From the gap analysis assessment, the Task Force will establish high-level, multifaceted standards of practice and system-wide goals for all-hazards preparedness. These standards and goals will be implemented at the facility level and department level as directed by the chief operating officer (COO), CNO, and emergency department medical director. At this point, there is latitude for departments to design and implement the standards and goals based on the unique needs of each area. Annual review and evaluation of goals is an effective project management activity, with new goals being created based on the needs of the organization, the changing requirements, and the results of gaps identified during drills.

Performing an Effective Gap Analysis

There are many ways to perform an all-hazards preparedness gap analysis so that leaders have a good starting point. A multitude of online reference websites exist, including, but not limited to, the following examples: Office of National Preparedness, Health and Human Services, Health and Medical Services Support Plan, the American Hospital Association (AHA), the Centers for Disease Control and Prevention (CDC), Agency for Healthcare Research and Quality (AHRQ), and the Hospital Emergency Incident Command System (HEICS) (Pletz et al., 1998).

The guiding principle for creating a hospital-specific all-hazards gap analysis is to "keep it simple!" One example of a simple way to assess the current state is to create an emergency preparedness survey that is easy to read and requires the department directors to answer in simple checklists one of two ways: (1) "Yes, we have it" or (2) "No, we don't have it." Survey questions need to be concise and clear. The goal is to begin by identifying the areas in which gaps in the facility's preparedness plans exist. Questions should be addressed to appropriate departments, who then assess the items and determine the current state. A review of the literature and online web searches will assist the team in identifying the areas of assessment (English et al., 1999; Macintyre et al., 2000; McLaughlin, 2001; Wetter et al., 2001). Examples of questions to ask in the survey might include those listed in Box 35.1.

Box 35.1

Hospital Gap Analysis Survey: Sample Questions

General

- Does your hospital have an internal disaster plan addressing what to do if an emergency occurs only in your facility?
- Does your hospital have an external disaster plan addressing what to do if an emergency occurs in the community and you need to be prepared to respond?
- Do the directors know where to find facility internal and external disaster plans?
- Do the directors know who is in charge of the command center in a disaster?
- Does your department staff know the chain of command in an emergency?
- Does your department know their role in a disaster?
- Does your hospital know their role in the community in an emergency situation?
- Are those in charge identified by a vest or have some sort of distinction?
- Are there specific plans for biological, chemical, nuclear, and conventional emergencies? Does all staff in your department know their role in each emergency?
- Is there a bed and staffing plan for surge capacity for 50 patients? 100 patients? 250 patients? Do you have portable cots contracted for use in a surge situation?
- Does your facility have an operational command center to coordinate the hospitals response in the event of a disaster?
- Is there a central command center phone number to use in the event of a disaster?

Human Resources

- Does your department staff know how to prepare themselves, their significant others, and pets in the event of a disaster?
- Is there a credentialing plan for health care professionals who come to the nearest facility in a disaster to volunteer their services?

Safety and Security

- Does your facility:
  - Have a lockdown plan in case of an emergency?

Courtesy Inova Health System. From Drenkard, K., & Rigotti, G. (2002, updated 2008). *Inova Health System survey 2001.* Falls Church, VA: Inova Health System.

Continued

Box 35.1

Hospital Gap Analysis Survey: Sample Questions—cont'd

- Have a plan for allowing staff to get to work and be allowed entry to hospital during an emergency?
- Have a plan for facility traffic flow during an emergency?
- Have multilanguage signage to direct people as to where to go during an emergency?

Communication

- Does your hospital have emergency-powered phones in case of a disaster?
- Does your facility have a backup radio system and volunteer staff to run it?
- Does your facility have a tiered paging system that can reach multiple staff simultaneously?
- Does your department know the central command center number (if there is one)?
- Is there an on-call procedure for notifying the administrator on-call and opening the command center in the event of a disaster?
- Are there established linkages to the external community (e.g., other hospitals in the region, fire department, police, emergency medical system, public schools, public health)?
- Do the telephone operators know how to link patients and families both in your facility and in the community should a disaster occur?
- Is there an on-call list for administrative coverage of the command center? If so, do the telephone operators know how to contact the administrator on-call for the command center?
- Is there a plan for contacting essential employees and administrators in a disaster?

Logistics

- Does your facility have:
  - Backup emergency supplies, pharmaceuticals, and equipment?
  - The ability to release and send pharmaceuticals, medical supplies, and equipment such as respirators to the areas in need in the event of a chemical or biological emergency?
  - Prearranged plans with physicians, ambulances, nearby churches, and nursing homes to clear beds in an emergency? (What sites can take patients?)
  - Contracts with vendors to bring in food, ice, oxygen, etc.?
- Is there an established written psychosocial role for social work, chaplains, psychiatry, employee health, and case management in the event of a disaster?
- Are there contingency plans for 3 to 5 days for no power, no water, no computers and/or no food?
- Are there contingency plans for staff to report to nearest facility to work?
- Are there contingency plans for childcare during an emergency so that parents can work?
- Is there common nomenclature used during an emergency so that everyone understands what is happening and who has what responsibility?

Clinical Operations

- Does your facility have:
  - Procedures established to maximize staff safety in the event of a disaster?
  - Procedures for fit testing of respiratory masks for staff?
  - Procedures and training for using protective equipment?

Box 35.1

Hospital Gap Analysis Survey: Sample Questions—cont'd

- The ability to track patients until discharge, admission, or death using HIPAA guidelines?
- Clear established policies and procedures to respond to biological, chemical, nuclear, and conventional emergencies?
- A decontamination area and detailed step-by-step procedures on how to work in this area?
- A backup staff to assist with people/patients arriving to the hospital?

- Does your facility have procedures for how to:
  - Open and operate the command center?
  - Track available beds?
  - Track staff working and direct them to a designated area?
  - Track volunteer staff and direct them to a designated area?
  - Track arriving patients and direct them to a designated area?
  - Operate every department of the hospital during an emergency?
  - Track discharged patients and direct them to a designated area?
  - Handle surge capacity situations?
  - Handle OR cases in the event of an emergency?
  - Track biological, chemical, or nuclear events and report them to authorities?

Financial

- Is there an established plan to tracking costs during an emergency?
- Is there an established plan for submitting for disaster reimbursement?

Messages/Media

- Is there an established communication plan in case of an emergency?
- Is there an established communication script in the event of an emergency?
- Is there an alternative communication plan if power, telephones, and radios are not working?

Courtesy Inova Health System. From Drenkard, K., & Rigotti, G. (2002, updated 2008). *Inova Health System survey 2001.* Falls Church, VA: Inova Health System.

Once the survey is created, it should be distributed to all stakeholders. Directors should be challenged to complete and return it in 5 working days so that work can be initiated to address outstanding issues. The Task Force should review the survey results and start an issues list to address deficiencies.

Keeping the Momentum Going

Once the gap analysis is completed and the issues are identified, a critical time in development of the comprehensive plan occurs. The work can appear daunting, and it is hard to know where to start. It is at this point that nursing leadership has the opportunity to take a lead. Nurses are experts at creating workable action plans for seemingly impossible obstacles and helping others to see the steps to take, because they do this every day in caring for patients. So even though the gap analysis may show multitudes of areas for improvement, issues are solvable one step at a time. The CNO and nurse leaders can help focus the Task Force and department directors. Focused effort on creating a streamlined, comprehensive internal all-hazards preparedness plan will set the foundation for later steps when the hospital begins to work externally with the community.

Working the Issues List

Over the next phase, the development of an issues list will become the working action plan used to prioritize and organize work to be done. Subgroups made up of members from the Task Force can be assigned to lead efforts to resolve issues. Issues need to be constantly added and resolved so that the work will be ongoing as the facility refines plans. Reports from subgroup progress should be relayed to the Task Force every 2 weeks or monthly, depending on the meeting schedule of the Task Force. The Task Force should have oversight for the subgroups and should strive to "clear the road" for subgroup progress as needed. Hospitals may need to address some common issues.

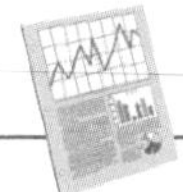

Research Note

Source: Christian, M.D., Hawryluck, L., Wax, R.S., Cook, T., Lazar, N.M., Herridge, M.S., et al. (2006). Development of a triage protocol for critical care during an influenza pandemic. *Canadian Medical Association Journal, 175*(11), 1377-1381.

Purpose

The development of a protocol for use in determining which patient should receive care is a necessary tool, but this is one that is subject to interpretation in a crisis situation. Planning in advance and creating a method for distributing potentially scarce resources, such as ventilators and antivirals, is a key activity that needs to occur by health care organizations. The purpose of this research process was to develop a protocol that could be used to prioritize access to critical care resources.

Discussion

The researchers applied a collaborative process including expert panels, consultation, and ethical principles application to create a triage protocol for prioritizing access to resources that might be needed during a pandemic, including mechanical ventilation and antiviral medications. The triage protocol describes an assessment tool called the *Sequential Organ Failure Assessment (SOFA)* score and has four main components: inclusion criteria, exclusion criteria, minimum qualifications for survival, and a prioritization tool. Basically, a patient is assessed based on clinical parameters and receives a score in each of the key clinical indicators, including respiratory status, hemodynamic status (i.e., blood pressure and shock symptoms), kidney function, end-organ function, and cardiac function. If a patient meets exclusion criteria (e.g., metastatic malignant disease), then he or she is excluded from treatment. Patients arriving at treatment centers would be assigned a SOFA score, which would then guide clinical triage decision making. Training results indicated 36% of staff had received training. Only 3.2% of facilities reported meeting all 10 of the readiness criteria.

Application to Practice

"This protocol is intended to provide guidance for making triage decisions during the initial days to weeks of an influenza pandemic if the systems and resources for providing critical care become overwhelmed. Although the authors designed this protocol for use during an influenza pandemic, the triage protocol would apply to patients both with and without influenza, since all patients must share a single pool of critical care resources" (Christian et al., 2006). A key practice application will be planning well in advance about how to apply a tool such as the SOFA scale. Once the scale is available for use, a plan needs to be developed to ensure that a process exists for initiating the protocol as well as for identifying key clinical decision makers who have the challenge of putting the protocol into action.

Establishing a Common Nomenclature, Structure, and Role Definition for Writing All-Hazards Preparedness Plans

Often the disaster plan on file at the hospital relates specifically to safety and security preparedness. The primary responsibility of the safety and security department, in conjunction with nursing leadership, will be to develop or refine the hospital's internal disaster plan for incidents occurring at the facility. In addition, the external all-hazards preparedness plan, for incidents involving two or more facilities or disaster events occurring in the community, should be addressed as well. The safety and security department should have assigned oversight for facility security, quick lockdown, and management of people flowing into and out of the hospital. Nursing leadership should lead efforts to ensure that all facility departments have a plan for what they will do in a disaster situation. Nurse leaders are the coordinators in synchronizing department plans so that everything fits together to meet the staff's, patients', and hospital's essential needs. Once the disaster plans are complete, every department should have an identified written role.

Helping Staff Overcome Fear Associated with Disaster and All-Hazards Preparedness

It is important to know that the first rule of disaster preparedness is to keep staff safe. In a disaster, the paradigm of keeping the patient safe first needs to change its focus so that the staff members (and their families) feel as safe as possible. This may be a shift in thinking, but the reality is that if staff members do not feel comfortable coming to work, then the patients' needs cannot be met at all.

Nursing leadership, in partnership with the human resources and education department leadership, will be needed to develop educational tools to assist staff in creating personal disaster preparedness plans for themselves, significant others, their families, and even their pets. Many websites are available to assist in developing educational tools, such as the Federal Emergency Management Agency (FEMA) and the America Red Cross websites. Tools such as personal disaster preparedness plans should be effectively communicated so that employees know that the facility will "keep staff safe" as their first priority in a disaster. Then when a disaster occurs, the staff will feel as comfortable as possible coming to work. Arrangements will need to be made for 24-hour childcare somewhere close to the hospital or on-site. Employee assistance programs need to be available on an ongoing basis for coping with fear related to a disaster. Having personal protective equipment (PPE) for staff available on-site is also critical.

Creating Procedural Addendums to All-Hazards Preparedness Plans

In addition to the overall all-hazards preparedness plans, the hospital will need to define procedures regarding what will be done in any biological, chemical, nuclear/radiological, or conventional disaster, and the surge capacity needs to be related to any of the events. *Surge capacity* refers to a health care system's ability to rapidly expand or flex up beyond normal capacity to meet an increased demand for qualified personnel, beds, and medical care services in the event of a large-scale emergency or disaster (Agency for Healthcare Research and Quality [AHRQ], 2005b). The Task Force can assign the creation of each of these procedures to a subgroup. The time frame for completing the initial plans should be about 3 weeks. These teams are often led by nursing leadership and the emergency medicine director with appropriate ad hoc participation. For example, the infectious disease department, in partnership with public health, can co-lead the biological and chemical planning efforts; the radiology department can co-lead the nuclear/radiological efforts, partnering closely with local authorities; and nursing and emergency medicine can co-lead the conventional and surge capacity efforts, partnering closely with police, fire, and rescue. The goal with these procedural addendums is to create easy, step-by-step action plans, fact sheets, and algorithms for identifying, intervening, and notifying the appropriate authorities. As with most all-hazards preparedness literature, the most current references will be online. Some essential websites to assist in writing specific hospital procedures include the CDC, the Department of Homeland Security (DHS), and the U.S. Department of Labor's Occupational Safety and Health Administration (OSHA).

In establishing procedural addendums and the overall all-hazards disaster preparedness plan, the general thought in the literature is to plan to be "on your own without external help" for at least 72 hours should an external disaster occur that impacts the region (Kaji, 2004). Lessons learned from Hurricane Katrina illustrate just how long it can take before assistance is available. Hospital leadership needs to make sure every operating unit and department is prepared. In general, the following are only a few examples of what hospitals will need:

- A conservative stockpile of essential antibiotics for biological threats
- Antidotes for chemical exposures
- Basic food and bottled water surpluses for environmental contamination events
- Preplanned contracts with local supply companies and businesses for ice, oxygen and gases, and emergency power
- Alternate communication methods and plans, both internally and externally, in case of power outage
- Staff and volunteer credentialing and identification procedures
- Established entrances for staff during lockdowns
- Patient identification systems for families in search of loved ones
- Downtime procedures for cyber threats (these need to be able to extend up to 5 days)
- Accommodations for staff to bring in their children for care while they are working

Creating an All-Hazards Planning Subgroup

Even with comprehensive all-hazards preparedness plans and procedural addendums, the unexpected will happen, as in recent threats and incidents involving anthrax, severe acute respiratory syndrome (SARS), monkey pox, and smallpox. Initially, no one will know whether these are true terrorist threats or just isolated spontaneous incidents. At all times, the hospital will need to be ready to respond. An ongoing all-hazards planning subgroup needs to be formed and chaired by a nurse leader who sits on the Task Force, along with key stakeholder membership (including emergency department, infection control, and employee health staff). Based on the changing needs of the events, this planning subgroup will enable the facility to respond quickly to the "just in time" educational needs of the staff, allow for rapid procedural planning to occur related to community needs, and ensure appropriate authority notification in the event of a disaster. For example, the staff will be expected to recognize the symptoms and presentation of smallpox and respond by critical thinking, as follows:

- Triaging and isolating the patient on admission to the emergency department (ED) and placing the patient in the hospital or facility negative pressure room if available
- Obtaining and having the staff wear appropriate PPE
- Locking down the department and determining whether the entire hospital should be on lockdown
- Identifying (name, address, telephone number) all patient contacts, transport services (EMS) staff, and patients in the waiting room
- Notifying the infection control practitioner, hospital/facility infectious disease physician or epidemiologist, public health officials, and police

Developing a Command Center

Should a disaster occur, the hospital would need a dedicated centralized command center where all department directors can report for direction. The four essential elements of a command center, explained in more detail in the following sections, are as follows:

1. Setting up the room
2. Developing processes in the command center
3. Establishing the hospital's role in the community
4. Testing the all-hazards preparedness plans and command center

Practical Tips

Tip # 1: Read the Disaster Plan

Take the time to read your organization's disaster plan. Identify your role. When a disaster occurs, there will likely not be enough time to read the plan and sort out roles.

Tip # 2: Run a Mock Drill

Communications often are the first to go in a disaster (consider what happens when power goes out and cell towers become overwhelmed). Run a mock drill to uncover communication strengths and weaknesses. Make plans for improvements.

Tip # 3: Network with Colleagues

Network with health care organizations similar to yours around the country that have experienced a large-scale disaster. Compare notes. What specific actions can your organization take to be more rapidly responsive should disaster strike.

Setting Up the Room

This center is often located near the safety and security department and is commanded by the on-call administrator along with the CNO, the ED medical director, and the safety and security director. Present in the room are the following:

- Multiple telephones/telephone lines with speed dial for frequently called numbers
- Computer access (with both intranet and Internet capabilities)
- Printing capability
- Batch fax and copying capabilities
- Alternative phone options (e.g., 800 MHz radio technology and/or voice-over Internet protocol technology—a phone system that operates over Internet lines with functioning antenna) and people trained to use them
- Tiered paging capability
- Television access
- Office-related supplies such as paper, pens, easels, dry erase boards, work tables, and phone books

The command center should be available at a moment's notice and fully functional within minutes. The usual scenario will be that the call comes into the ED. Nursing leadership staff in the ED, along with medical staff, will determine the gravity of the situation and decide whether the incident can be handled in the ED or whether the hospital administrator needs to be contacted. If it is deemed appropriate to contact the hospital administrator, there will be dialogue among nursing leadership, medical leadership, and the administrator to decide whether the command center should be opened. If the command center is to be opened, the hospital administrator will start the process to open the command center and notify any on-call additional staff to come in and assist in the operations of the command center. In the event that the disaster involves the area where the command center is located, hospitals may want to establish a back-up command center in another location. In the case of a multifacility system, the alternate command center could be another hospital.

Developing Processes in the Command Center

Because several of the rotating on-call administrators may be the person who needs to open the command center, the creation of a simple, step-by-step, short (1- to 2-page) document of how to open, operate, and close down the command center is important. A more extensive manual can also be created, but in times of a disaster, the short "How to Open the Command Center" document is crucial: "EMS transported casualties will start arriving at the nearest hospitals within 30 minutes of the event and the numbers will peak over the next 60 to 90 minutes. Additionally hospitals will experience waves of self-transporting victims and the worried well arriving at facilities" (Kaji, 2004).

If the facility does not have an on-call administrator list, one should be established; and staff must know how to reach the on-call person(s). A clear decision matrix should be in place, outlining when to open the command center and who needs to be notified. It may be helpful to create a communication tree identifying the process for notifying administrative team and AHPTF members quickly. Techniques such as using vests to identify people in charge during a disaster with generic nomenclature for roles and a 1-page role and responsibility sheet in each vest pocket are essential in a crisis situation. Color-coded vests may also be useful in identifying roles. All hospital and department all-hazards preparedness plans must be on hand and clearly labeled in the command center, along with in-house phone and pager directories.

Establishing the Hospital's Role in the Community

Once the hospital's internal all-hazards preparedness plans are in place, members of the Task Force can take a step back and begin to assess their role. More than likely, the hospital will play an important role in the community in the case of a disaster. Knowing how the hospital fits into the disaster response plan from the perspective of such entities as the police and fire departments, the local school system, area physician practices, public health department, and emergency medical systems will be important in coordinating efforts. When working with the community, recognizable nomenclature becomes especially important for communication in crisis situations. More and more hospitals have adopted the Hospital Emergency Incident Command System (HEICS) (Pletz et al., 1998), for their all-hazards preparedness plans, because it allows logical standardization with common nomenclature that is understood both in the hospital environment and in the community setting.

The Task Force will be instrumental in defining the hospital's role locally in the community, as well as nationally concerning federal government expectations. On a local level, the chairperson of the Task Force will partner with public health, local police and fire departments, local school systems, community physicians, regional alliances with other health care facilities, and local emergency management agencies/councils. It will be important to define the hospital's role and the community's role in the emergency situation. Testing of plans using local disaster drills, on a biannual basis, is essential to continually improve processes. The hospital may wish to test its internal all-hazards preparedness plans, along with any planned community drills, to get a full picture of its ability to respond in a disaster.

Nationally, each hospital will play an important role in the political arena by helping local and federal government personnel understand that hospitals, like police and fire departments, are first responders in a disaster. The materials, equipment, and training required for hospitals to prepare adequately for their role in responding to disasters are very expensive. Capital expenditures will be required to create decontamination facilities; purchase PPE; train and educate staff on effective all-hazards preparedness; stockpile emergency equipment, supplies, and pharmaceuticals; ensure adequate isolation rooms; and outfit a hospital command center. Hospitals need financial assistance to do this well, and the AHPTF members can all be advocates for federal and state funding. It is helpful to establish a financial subgroup whose mission will be to establish a set plan for capturing costs related to the event as the disaster unfolds. This will enable the hospital to submit immediately for any reimbursement funding that becomes available after the event.

Testing the All-Hazards Preparedness Plans and Command Center

Having comprehensive all-hazards preparedness plans requires frequent (at least biannual) drills to work through problems and allow for a streamlined preparedness plan. There are many types of drills, including the following:

- *Internal drills* to test specific department and/or hospital responses (e.g., setting up and operating the command center; recognizing a biological event both in the emergency department and on the units; lockdown of the hospital entrances; simulating decontamination processes; operating using downtime procedures during a communications or cyber disaster event; handling various surge capacity situations)
- *External drills* in collaboration with community agencies and departments involving patients (police, fire, and rescue, public health); table-top drills simulating an unknown biological, nuclear/radiological, or chemical scenario and prioritizing the response by departments; and surge capacity drills, testing a community's ability to respond to overwhelming demand

All of these drills offer great insight into the merit of the all-hazards preparedness plan and allow facilities the opportunity to modify plans to improve processes.

LEADERSHIP AND MANAGEMENT IMPLICATIONS

Moving into the Future with Confidence

Nursing leaders can effect change within 6 to 12 months and can ensure that an effective all-hazards preparedness plan is developed for the hospital. The journey toward preparedness is ongoing and constant. Nursing leadership and competencies in disaster planning and crisis management will prove invaluable as health care organizations face a changing future that requires skills of collaboration, outreach, and negotiation (Ehrat, 2001). Clearly, nurse executives are in a position to take a greater role in the planning process for their organizations. Nurse leaders are called upon to take charge, make decisions, implement successfully, and then evaluate and modify their action plans. Emotional competencies include good interpersonal skills, excellent and clear communication skills, and calm, controlled delegation (Fahlgren & Drenkard, 2002). In addition, being willing to take risks is an important attribute of the nursing leader. Nurse leaders are in a unique position to forge new pathways in the arena of disaster preparedness because of their combination of clinical skills, strong organizational ability, networking expertise, and training in clinical crises. With strong nursing leadership at the managerial and executive level, the management of disasters can be proactively addressed. With proactive planning, a constant state of readiness can be obtained and maintained.

CURRENT ISSUES AND TRENDS

As we continue in the "new world order," in which all-hazards preparedness is a way of life and knowledge about the level of alertness (low = green; guarded = blue; elevated = yellow; high = orange; severe = red [The White House, 2002]) is an everyday expectation, hospital staff and leadership have begun to settle in at a heightened state of preparedness. If the AHPTF is not diligent in its efforts to keep everyone focused on preparedness, there may even be a sense of complacency around refining all-hazard preparedness plans on an ongoing basis.

Current nursing and medical literature is focused on specific departments and how they are establishing their unique roles and responsibilities in a disaster. Nurse leaders can use these benchmark articles to springboard units and departments forward in fully assessing and defining their roles in all-hazards preparedness. As the CNO explores the breadth of disaster nursing within his or her facility, care can be enhanced in many ways during a disaster. For instance, making decisions about consolidating care sites may require closing clinics, emergency care centers, and community health programs during a disaster to free up clinical staff to assist in a hospital's surge capacity planning in a disaster, provide staff for vaccination teams in a biological event, or help with decontamination in a chemical exposure event. Allocation of staff may be required to build capacity in outpatient and community arenas depending on the disaster threat. Decisions about alternate care sites should be considered well ahead of an event and often require regional collaboration across many disciplines and agencies.

LEADERSHIP & MANAGEMENT BEHAVIORS

Leadership Behaviors

- Demonstrates calm
- Commands the environment
- Keeps open communication channels
- Develops strategic long-term plans to protect staff and patients
- Influences policy makers about financial requirements to ensure readiness
- Demonstrates decision-making skills
- Serves as a role model for directors in times of crisis
- Seeks creative alternatives when problem solving
- Demonstrates emotional intelligence by being emotionally self-aware and self-managed
- Builds partnerships through networking
- Allocates resources in times of crisis

Management Behaviors

- Stays calm
- Demonstrates controlled delegation
- Communicates clearly
- Leads drills to ensure preparation
- Implements the plans
- Works well on the team
- Thinks critically
- Takes appropriate risks
- Ensures plans are up-to-date
- Shares critical information with upper levels of leadership to aid in good decision making

Overlap Areas

- Remains calm
- Ensures communication

One area of all-hazards preparedness that has not been fully developed in many areas but has great potential is the role of long-term care (LTC) facilities in disaster planning. The nurse leader can lead the way in establishing a partnership between the hospital and the LTC facility. If the CNO can work with the LTC facility in establishing plans for moving patients out of LTC to receive stable patients from the hospital, then surge capacity stress could be dramatically reduced as more inpatient beds would be made available for the influx of victims during a disaster event.

To effectively manage large-scale events, networking beyond the hospital will be critical to create partnerships with other facilities, hospitals, community agencies, and local, state, and federal departments. A trend is underway, evidenced by a growing alliance between regional hospitals and the community at large throughout the United States, to strategically plan for allocation and sharing of federal and state resources in the event of a disaster.

As an example, in Virginia, a Regional Hospital Command Center (RHCC) has been established in which 14 northern Virginia hospitals have been networked to more effectively respond in a disaster. This is accomplished via radio communication and a shared web-based bed availability tracking system, displaying each hospital's ability to take varying levels of patient acuities. These hospitals can directly link with Washington, D.C., hospitals to coordinate efforts during an event and communicate effectively with fire, police, EMS, schools, public health, the emergency operating center (a local command center for overseeing the event), and the field incident commander in coordinating the disaster response and effectively assisting victims. Cohorts of hospitals, firefighters, EMS, law enforcement, schools, public health, and businesses, similar to the Virginia RHCC just mentioned, are joining together to form regional alliances and collaborations to leverage their capability to respond in a coordinated manner.

On a national level, the U.S. Department of Homeland Security Secretary at the time, Tom Ridge, created a National Incident Management System (NIMS) that will further standardize

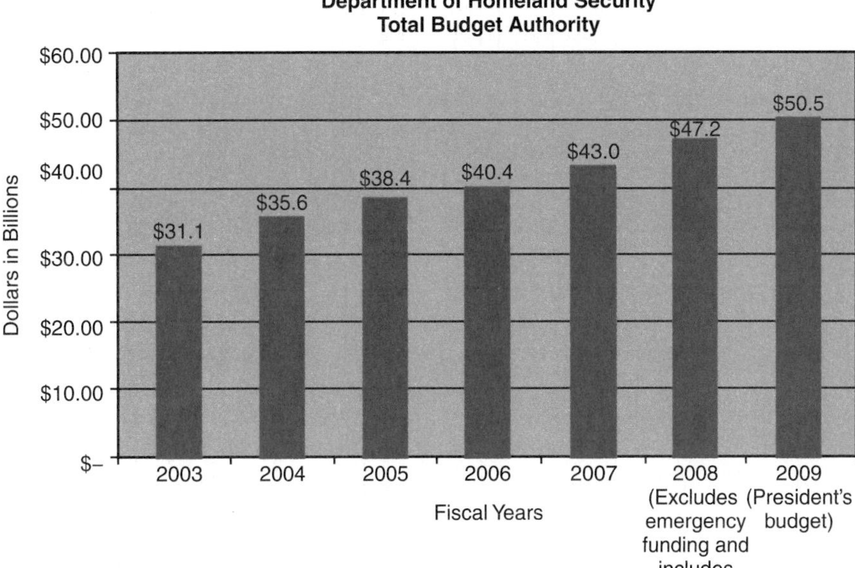

Figure 35.1
Department of Homeland Security total budget authority. (Data from Testimony of Secretary Chertoff, U.S. Department of Homeland Security, before the U.S. House of Representatives Committee on Homeland Security. [November 29, 2008, release date]. *FY 2009 Budget Request.* Cannon House Office Building. www.dhs.gov/xnews/testimony/testimony_1203008767192.shtm.)

and integrate response practices nationally (U.S. Department of Homeland Security, 2004):

> NIMS incorporates incident management best practices developed and proven by thousands of responders and authorities across America. These practices, coupled with consistency and national standardization, will now be carried forward throughout all incident management processes: exercises, qualification and certification, communications interoperability, doctrinal changes, training, and publications, public affairs, equipping, evaluating, and incident management. All of these measures unify the response community as never before. (p. 1)

Under the direction of NIMS, incident management assistance teams (IMATs) are being created to send supplemental assistance to the region affected by a disaster. These teams consist of "trained personnel from different departments, organizations, agencies, and jurisdictions within a state or DHS Urban Area Security Initiative region, activated to support incident management at major or complex emergency incidents or special events that extend beyond one operational period" (American-Firefighter.com, 2004, p. 1). It is likely that hospital leadership, with nursing in the forefront, will learn from this benchmark program and partner with other area hospitals and departments to create IMATs—teams ready to assist one another at the site most affected by a disaster.

In 2008, disaster preparedness was a top national issue. The then Secretary of Homeland Security, Michael Chertoff, outlined the newest plan to promote all-hazards preparedness ("Testimony of Secretary Chertoff", 2008). Secretary Chertoff testified on the President's 2009 budget request for $50.5 billion before the House Committee on Homeland Security on February 13, 2008, and before the Senate Committee on Homeland Security and Governmental Affairs on February 14, 2008. This is a 7% increase over the FY 2008 enacted level excluding emergency funding (Figure 35.1).

In pursuit of the five priorities that were established in 2007, the Department continues to work to align resources to lead a unified national effort in securing America. Those five priorities are as follows:

- Goal 1. Protect our nation from dangerous people
- Goal 2. Protect our nation from dangerous goods
- Goal 3. Protect critical infrastructure
- Goal 4. Build a nimble, effective emergency response system and a culture of preparedness
- Goal 5. Strengthen and unify DHS operations and management

Across the nation, political leaders are readily acknowledging the vital role that hospitals are filling in establishing a reliable plan for all-hazards preparedness. As never seen before, CNOs and the entire nursing management team are being called to assume difficult but rewarding leadership roles. These roles involve partnering with various community frontline professionals to establish viable first-line response strategies that ensure the safety of the communities they serve.

One other emerging issue that challenges care during a disaster is allocation of scarce resources when the system is overwhelmed. This need was demonstrated during the Hurricane Katrina event, and as a result of those lessons learned, both the state and the national disaster preparedness leaders are examining planning needs for response strength when scarce resources need to be allocated. These efforts also include substantial planning efforts to address pandemic influenza needs, including ethical considerations and planning assumptions, as well as management issues regarding staff prophylaxis to protect the health care workforce. In recommendations of the Ethics Subcommittee of the Advisory Committee to the Director of the Centers for Disease Control and Prevention, ethical guidelines were outlined for pandemic planning. To maximize the level of national and regional preparedness, these principles included the identification of clear overall goals, principles of transparency in decision making, public engagement and involvement in the process, use of sound scientific evidence for decision making, and thinking in a global context. The guidelines recommended early planning efforts that balance utilitarian concepts with respect of persons, nonmaleficence, and justice. The recommendations gave examples of distribution criteria that will need to be considered well ahead of the time of an actual event. The development of triage criteria for allocation of scarce resources has been documented in several articles (Hick, & O'Laughlin, 2006; Kraus et al., 2007). Also, adopting standards of care under altered conditions has been described and addressed in numerous documents from states and associations seeking to offer guidelines to care providers (American Nurses Association, 2007; New York State Department of Health Task Force on Life and the Law, 2007; Phillips & Knebel, 2007). Each nursing leader and team needs to understand these guidelines and begin the planning process at both a local and a regional level for developing a plan for allocation of scarce resources and the implementation of triage criteria for care in overwhelming events. Implementing periodic table-top discussions regarding how to allocate resources in a time of scarcity will prove to be a powerful tool in setting the stage for what to do if such an event occurs. Collaborative professional staff and hospital leadership discussions about scarce resource allocation will present ethical dilemmas that need to be thoughtfully considered in a planning time that is devoid of emotion. Questions to be discussed at the tabletop include (1) Which hospital and clinical leaders will make the final decisions about ventilator allocation and other scarce resource distribution? (2) What are the criteria used to determine which patients receive aggressive treatment and which will receive palliative care? (3) How are prophylactic pharmaceutical dissemination plans going to be activated to protect staff and their families? Knowing the hospital's approach to handling these types of scenarios will be a critical precursor in implementing an effective plan in the event of a disaster that is compounded by a shortage of resources.

Summary

- All-hazards disaster preparedness is essential in strategic planning for hospitals.
- Nursing leaders play a significant role in the successful implementation of a hospital's all-hazards disaster plan.
- Keeping the staff safe is the most important element in the implementation of an effective all-hazards disaster plan.
- Using the nursing process of assessing, planning, implementing, evaluating, and modifying will result in a comprehensive all-hazards disaster preparedness plan.
- It is important to use accepted, standardized terminology when writing the all-hazards disaster plan.
- Having a multidisciplinary hospital-wide team led by a nurse leader, hospital administrator, and medical leader is essential in creating an effective and workable all-hazards disaster plan.
- Comprehensive all-hazards disaster planning includes internal and external disaster plans, a surge capacity plan, and addendums for biological, chemical, nuclear/radiological, and conventional disasters.
- Emerging issues such as pandemic influenza, allocation of scarce resources, and alteration in standards of care will need to be addressed increasingly by nursing and health care leaders to successfully plan and implement care during a crisis. Ethical considerations and frameworks for planning need to be considered.
- Collaboration with community resources in a partnership is a requirement of effective all-hazards disaster preparedness.
- All-hazards disaster preparedness is never complete; the plan keeps evolving and expanding to link all facets of effective coordination of care internally, externally, locally, statewide, and nationwide during a disaster event.

CASE STUDY

Patients had arrived first at hospitals in Oklahoma, Pennsylvania, and Georgia, states that are far removed from your hospital in Virginia. These patients had presented complaining of aches and fevers and exhibiting unusual rashes. Each patient had visited one of three shopping centers, and laboratory tests confirmed that they did not have influenza or measles. They had all contracted variola (smallpox).

The federal government began to deploy what was left of the nation's smallpox vaccine stockpile to the states that were first affected. A television news station reported that an epidemiologist projected 3 million cases and a million deaths within 90 days unless everyone was inoculated. Hysteria spread. Then Reuters reported that a variola case was confirmed in Maryland, a state in proximity to your hospital.

Because the stock of vaccine was nearly depleted, the remaining vaccine would be rationed and health care providers would be inoculated first, according to the CDC. Vaccine delivery was scheduled to arrive on Monday, 2 days from now.

The press had leaked news of the vaccine distribution, and by Monday morning, people began arriving at your hospitals and emergency care centers, first requesting, and then demanding the vaccine. The decision was made to restrict entry to the hospital until the crisis passed. Total hospital lockdown of entrances and exits began at 11 AM.

What Happens Next

The safety and security department issues the lockdown notice to your hospital after consulting with the ED charge nurse, the ED medical director, the hospital administrator, and the chief nurse officer. Entrance to the hospital for patients is restricted to the main ED entrance with a double-door alcove entrance area for triage. Signs in multiple languages are posted on windows and locked doors to direct patients on campus. Security staff wearing protective masks are stationed strategically outside to direct patients already on the campus.

Local police are called in to work at the hospital road entrances and to reroute traffic away from the hospital. Only local ambulances and staff with hospital identification are allowed entrance onto the hospital campus. People in the hospital desiring to leave the facility are escorted out after giving their name and contact information to the ED. This information is gathered as a precautionary measure in the event that smallpox is identified in the facility. Staff reporting to work are directed to a separate hospital entrance away from the ED, where they report from and to work in a designated general personnel pool area, which will be operational for as long as the lockdown remains in effect. There, staff receive instruction about any personal protective equipment needed at that time, assignment of staffing for shift, and general updates on the situation. ED staff also receive a 1-page fact sheet on smallpox signs, symptoms, and treatment, along with instructions as to isolation procedures for any high-risk patients arriving either by ambulance or by walk-in.

The general personnel pool is a function of the all-hazards disaster preparedness plan and is set up as needed by the command center. Designated departments should know in advance whether they have responsibility for staffing this function. In this case, the nursing education staff has the responsibility for setting up and operating the general personnel pool; they assess staffing needs and allocate resources. Constant contact is maintained between the general personnel pool area and the command center regarding any staffing needs.

As soon as the lockdown is initiated, the command center is activated. A mandatory 30-minute management meeting is held outlining the internal and external lockdown plan, as well as the communication plan for staff, patients, and the media. Handouts with frequently asked questions and answers are given to managers. Managers are instructed about where to obtain additional N95 masks. Ongoing management briefings are established at set intervals throughout the event to keep everyone informed. The clinical management staff is given a 1-page fact sheet on smallpox and is asked to assess patients in their departments/units who might be at risk and to immediately report findings back to the medical director in the command center. They are asked to assess bed availability in case this is needed. Clinical and support departments such as pharmacy, respiratory therapy, materials management, and nutrition are asked to inventory their supplies and equipment and report back to the command center with this information.

The psychosocial needs of everyone (staff, patients, visitors) need to be supported. Social workers, clergy, and clinical nurse specialists are reassigned in designated roles to assist with the support needs throughout the hospital. Visitors to the hospital are moved to a designated area of the hospital where they can be counseled and receive information about the situation and their loved ones. It is important to keep visitors away from the patients to reduce exposure to high-risk patients.

Externally, the command center staff is working with public health, the local police department, the media, and the external operating center for the county to coordinate next steps. The goal is to lift the lockdown as soon as reasonably possible. Information is disseminated on an ongoing basis as the event unfolds.

Once the lockdown is terminated and the situation has deescalated to the point of closing the command center, it is important to have the key stakeholders involved in a debriefing. The following questions could be used in the debriefing:

- Overall, how effective was the lockdown, the operations of the command center, and the communication flow? What could have gone more smoothly, and how could this have been accomplished?
- Was there a clear chain of command? Did communications flow logically? Were they helpful?
- What parts of the all-hazards disaster plan helped staff handle this situation? What parts were not helpful and why?
- How were staff and visitors notified about the lockdown (e.g., PA announcement, e-mail, media, signs)? Was it effective or not? Why?
- How were the police notified? What was their role? Did their participation work well?

- What entrances were locked, and who was stationed at each entrance? What were the pros and cons of this effort?
- How were persons who arrived at locked entrances informed? Did this work effectively? What could have been done better?
- How did the general personnel pool area work for staff reporting and leaving work? Any suggestions for improvements with this process?
- What precautions should be adopted right now to ensure that no patients with smallpox are admitted to the hospital without detection?
- *Internal notifications:* What security measures, if any, should have been taken before a lockdown?
- *External notifications:* Were local and state agencies involved appropriately? Who was called? Who was missed? What worked and did not work?
- How should the all-hazards disaster preparedness plan and addendums be enhanced to better meet the needs in a disaster like this one?
- What staff safety procedures should be implemented based on this disaster?
- How can the planning for vaccinations in an event like this one be better organized so that this scenario does not happen again?
- If hospital workers were quarantined until they received the vaccine, how did this go? What worked and did not work well in this situation?
- How well were "external" agencies integrated? Was communication effective or not? What would make that more effective?
- How did communications with the media go? What were the learning opportunities with this?
- Was surge capacity an issue with this scenario? If so, what worked well and what needed improvement?
- If more ventilators, linens, and protective masks had been needed, could they have been obtained?
- Were staff members all fitted for a protective mask before the event? What were the learning opportunities here?
- Was the ED able to treat ill patients with conditions unrelated to the current emergency? What worked well, and what needs to be improved with this process?
- Were resources sufficient to meet the hospital needs?
- If a suspect case was being transported by EMS, where did the patient go? Were alternate locations identified?
- How were inpatients being triaged to make room for admissions? Were they discharged home? Were alternate locations identified?
- *Morgue:* Was capacity and capability enough to house contaminated patients?
- What were the plans if staff did not—or could not—report for duty?
- What processes were in place to address the emotional and supportive needs of the staff?

CRITICAL THINKING EXERCISE

The All-Hazards Preparedness Task Force has reviewed the current literature on altered standards of care, determining alternate care sites and the need for pandemic influenza planning. The team decides that a planning session is needed and that the planning process for how your hospital is going to respond should begin at this time.

Planning process: Readiness preparation for influenza pandemic.

Purpose: To prepare for a pandemic influenza wave and be prepared with plans for allocation of resources, prophylaxis for staff, and triage criteria for mass patient response.

Background information: You are the chief nurse officer of a 500-bed hospital that serves as the leader of the community for acute care response. You are leading the effort to develop a pandemic influenza response plan.

1. What planning framework should you use to develop the plan for addressing a pandemic influenza outbreak?
2. What ethical considerations need to be addressed in the planning process?
3. What triage considerations need to be included in the plan? What considerations will you include to identify those most likely to live and those most likely to die?
4. Who will be the decision makers (clinical and administrative) for determining when triage criteria of plans for allocation of scarce human, equipment, and pharmaceutical resources need to be put in place? How will the decision be made? How and to whom will it be communicated?
5. What is the chain of command in notification of a contagious disease event both internally and externally?
6. What training needs exist for the staff that can be completed pre-event? What "just in time" training needs are evident? How will this training be delivered during an emerging event?
7. What is the staff prophylaxis plan? What are the plans to conduct a drill on the prophylaxis plan?
8. What will the staffing requirements be in the event of a pandemic influenza event?
9. What pharmaceuticals and equipment will be needed, and what is the plan to prepare in advance?
10. What alternate care sites or re-arrangement of care settings (e.g., setting up a palliative care unit within the hospital) has been determined?
11. What should be done to secure the area, keep staff safe, and keep patients safe?

36 Data Management and Informatics

Jacqueline Moss

CHAPTER OBJECTIVES

- Highlight the importance of data management for decision making
- Define and describe computer applications in nursing, nursing informatics, and management information systems
- Analyze information needs in health care
- Classify nursing's data needs
- Appraise the implementation of a computerized patient record
- Explore nursing informatics
- Describe a Nursing Minimum Data Set for administrative practice
- Integrate effectiveness research and nursing informatics
- Analyze the need for a standardized and retrievable management data set
- Speculate about future informatics trends
- Exercise critical thinking to conceptualize and analyze possible solutions to a practice exercise

The information age has truly arrived. In the past 30 years, society has seen the widespread adoption of personal computers, cell phones with camera and electronic mail capabilities, personal digital assistants, podcasting, wireless computing, global positioning systems, and satellite and cable television. Information can now be transmitted across the world, immediately, in a variety of formats. Information technology has changed the way people work, play, learn, manage their personal lives, and view the world. Consequently, information has become a commodity to be bought, sold, and managed.

The business of health care information management is growing rapidly. Management of the health care industry and care delivery relies extensively on the collection and analysis of data. Data can provide information about the patient, provider, outcomes, and processes of care delivery (Mills et al., 1996). These data are collected from many individuals practicing in different specialties and must be integrated, coordinated, and managed. In addition, the increasing demand to use these data for performance measurement and reporting to managed care customers, regulators, and accrediting bodies comes at a time when payment of providers and health care institutions is being linked with patient outcome measures (Petersen et al., 2006). Reimbursement for health care services can be increased, decreased, or denied based on the patient's response to treatment. Beginning in 2008, Medicare did not pay claims for eight hospital-acquired patient conditions deemed preventable, including objects left in the patient during surgery, air embolisms, urinary tract infections, and pressure ulcers (O'Brien & Anderson, 2007). Regulatory and governmental agencies require the collection of data to measure performance (e.g., The Joint Commission [TJC]), the organization of these data into specific formats (e.g., Medicare/Medicaid), and adequate protections to ensure the confidentiality of these data (e.g., Health Insurance Portability and Accountability Act [HIPAA]). To meet these demands, administrators need data that can be compared across multiple settings, both geographically and clinically.

DEFINITIONS

Computer applications in nursing administration can be understood best as arising from the intersection of three areas: nursing administration, informatics, and effectiveness research or research on client outcomes. The computer is a tool for collecting, organizing, and analyzing vast amounts of complex data. Having these data in an accessible format increases nursing administrators' ability to make informed decisions regarding the organization and delivery of patient care. Not finding the information needed in a timely manner can force us to make decisions without considering key elements.

As a part of the larger domain of technology, informatics is a combination of computer science, cognitive science, and information science. **Nursing informatics** is defined as the management and processing of nursing data, information, and knowledge to support the practice of nursing and the delivery of nursing care (Graves & Corcoran, 1989). **Effectiveness research** is defined as the study of relationships among health care problems, interventions, outcomes, and costs, generally by analyzing large databases or using epidemiological methods.

A **management information system (MIS)** is defined as an integrated system for collecting, storing, retrieving, and processing a collective set of data. Management information systems can be paper-based, but more and more tend to be automated through the use of computers. An MIS organizes and processes information to monitor the quality of care and to manage human resources, physical resources, and fiscal resources (Hannah et al., 2006). An MIS is essentially a system that provides information that managers use in decision-making processes. The 10 criteria, or desirable characteristics, for a good MIS are (1) informative, (2) relevant, (3) sensitive, (4) unbiased, (5) comprehensive, (6) timely, (7) action-oriented, (8) uniform, (9) performance-targeted, and (10) cost-effective (Austin, 1979). An example of a component of an MIS is a nursing workload management system (NWMS), also called a *patient classification system (PCS).* These systems automate the collection of patient acuity data to calculate the number of patient care hours needed to provide care to the same group of patients (Hannah et al., 2006).

Automated information systems also are used for the collection of clinical data related to the direct care of clients and managing care processes. Information systems support clinical data gathering in areas such as laboratory test results, medication administration, and nursing documentation. Nursing documentation systems generally include structured entry using drop-down menus and checklists. They also allow the documentation of unstructured narrative documentation that is not included in the structured portion of the system (Moss et al., 2007). Information collected through the use of clinical information systems can be used to evaluate the effectiveness of nursing care and track adverse events. Integrating these data with other information systems can facilitate safe medication administration practice and adherence to evidence-based practice protocols (Brokel, 2007).

LEADING & MANAGING DEFINED

Nursing Informatics

The management and processing of nursing data, information, and knowledge to support the practice of nursing and the delivery of nursing care.

Effectiveness Research

The study of relationships among health care problems, interventions, outcomes, and costs, generally by analyzing large databases or using epidemiological methods.

Management Information System (MIS)

An integrated system for collecting, storing, retrieving, and processing a collective set of data; the data are transformed from storage into knowledge that is directly useful and applicable in the process of directing and controlling resources and their application to the achievement of specific management objectives.

NURSING'S DATA NEEDS

Nursing's data needs fall into four domains—client care, provider staffing, administration of care and the organization, and knowledge-based research for evidence-based practice. The first three are distinct areas; but research, the fourth domain, interacts with all of the other three. The four areas and the sources for the data are as follows:

1. *Client:* Client care/clinical care and its evaluation, clinical data, and client outcomes. Source: the client's health care record.
2. *Provider:* Professional data, caregiver outcomes, and decision maker variables. Source: personnel records, national data banks, and links to client records.
3. *Administrative:* Management and resource oversight, administrative data, system outcomes, and contextual variables. Source: administrative, fiscal, and regulatory data.
4. *Research:* Knowledge base development. Source: existing and newly gathered data and relational databases.

Table 36.1 displays examples of outcomes and variables to be measured in relation to the three distinct domains of nursing's data needs. For example, in the client domain, the cost of care to the client is an important outcome for which data are needed to manage care. Intensity of nursing care is one variable that may be measured to monitor and control costs.

The collection and analysis of data is a critical thrust of current health services research. Data analysis is aimed at cost, quality, and effectiveness outcomes. Collecting data that describe the processes and outcomes of nursing care electronically has the potential to provide evidence for the design of care protocols and delivery models. The formal process of using these patient data for providing

Table 36.1

Outcomes and Variables in Three Domains of Nursing Data Needs

Domain	Outcomes	Variables
Client	Client satisfaction Achieved care outcomes Costs Access to care	Attitudes/beliefs Diagnosis, gender, age Marital status Support system Satisfaction Level of dependency Severity of illness Intensity of nursing care
Provider	Job enrichment Job/work satisfaction Physician satisfaction Job stress Intent to leave	Attitudes/beliefs Education Years of experience Age Work excitement
Administrative	Costs Productivity Turnover Income	Agency philosophy Priorities Organizational structure Fiscal data Climate Policies and procedures Conflict

this evidence is termed *practice-based evidence* (DeJong, 2007). Although both are used to inform the delivery of practice with evidence, practice-based evidence and evidence-based practice are derived from different sources. Deriving evidence for informing practice from research is termed *evidence-based practice,* informing practice from the analysis of patient data collected during the delivery of care is termed *practice-based evidence.* However, this contribution rests on structuring the input logically, providing adequate processing and memory, and ensuring valid and reliable output. Clear definition, valid linkage between datasets, and clear coding of input are essential in securing meaningful output that has utility. The aggregation of information over time and how this aggregation affects the quality of information are especially important to uniform datasets. Using practice-based evidence requires the compilation of clinical data into a *clinical data repository.* This compilation may also be called an *information warehouse* or simply a *data repository.* Data are stored longitudinally over multiple episodes of care. These data can then be accessed to provide continuity of care to the individual patient, to measure care effectiveness and productivity, to provide evidence for care delivery, or to inform public policy.

NURSING INFORMATICS

Recognized by the American Nurses Association (ANA) as a nursing specialty in 1992, informatics is one of the fastest growing practice areas in health care. As defined by Graves and Corcoran, "nursing informatics is a combination of computer science, information science and nursing science designed to assist in the management and processing of nursing data, information and knowledge to support the practice of nursing and the delivery of nursing care" (1989, p. 227). *Data* is defined as discrete, objective entities, without interpretation; *information* as data that are structured, organized, or interpreted; and *knowledge* as synthesized information with identified relationships.

The focus of nursing informatics practice is the organization, analysis, and dissemination of information, not the computer itself (Abbott & Lee, 2001). Nursing informatics specialists assist practitioners by providing information to enhance decision making and the delivery of safe patient care. Although these specialists may not be directly involved with care delivery, their work is integrally related to clinical and administrative practice. Nursing informatics specialists participate in analysis, design, and implementation of information and communication systems; effectiveness and informatics research; and education of nurses in informatics and information technology.

The first master's degree in nursing informatics was offered by the University of Maryland in 1989. In 1992, that same university followed with the first doctoral program in nursing informatics. Now, programs in nursing informatics can be found throughout the United States. These programs offer a variety of educational options, including master's degrees, post-master's certificates, and doctoral degrees. Nurses prepared at the master's level in nursing informatics are titled *informatics nursing specialists (INSs)* (Hannah et al., 2006). Nurses prepared at the baccalaureate or master's level can obtain certification in nursing informatics from the American Nurses Credentialing Center (ANCC).

ELECTRONIC HEALTH RECORD

In 1965, El Camino Hospital in Mountain View, California, was one of the first to attempt to develop an electronic health record (EHR). Along with Technicon Medical Information Systems and Lockheed Missiles and Space Company, an information system was created that communicated physicians' orders, retrieved laboratory results, and supported the documentation of nursing care (Staggers et al., 2001). The development of early information systems designed to support an EHR was confined to large tertiary care centers and federal agencies such as the U.S. Department of Veterans Affairs (VA) and the National Institutes of Health (NIH). The high cost of these systems and the fee-for-service reimbursement structure for health care costs provided little incentive for most health care institutions to change the way they were managing health care data.

The shift from a retrospective fee-for-service to a prospective managed care financial structure for the payment of medical services changed the way patient data were perceived and shared (Staggers et al., 2001). Currently, patient data are of interest not only to health care providers but also to managed care organizations and governmental payers, who want to ensure that their money is spent in the most effective way to produce the best patient outcomes. These data are also scrutinized by health care providers to ensure that patient needs are being met in the most efficient and cost-effective manner.

Harvesting these data from traditional paper documentation systems is expensive and inefficient. Those conducting chart reviews to collect data are frequently confronted with incomplete and inconsistent documentation. Using standards for data collection, an EHR could be accessed across health networks, linking clinical and business processes,

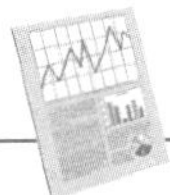

Research Note

Source: Vogelsmeier, A., Halbesleben, J., & Scott-Cawiezell, J. (2008). Technology implementation and workarounds in the nursing home. *Journal of the American Medical Informatics Association, 15,* 114-119.

Purpose

Medication administration errors are a serious safety issue in health care. Errors in medication administration can occur at multiple points along the process of preparing, administering, and/or monitoring medications. Technological solutions such as computerized provider order entry, electronic medication administration records, and decision support have the potential to decrease medication error. However, technological solutions that do not fit nursing work processes can force nurses to develop methods to work around the technology. The purpose of this study was to explore the relationship of workarounds related to the implementation of an electronic medication administration record and medication safety practices in five Midwestern nursing homes.

Discussion

Nurses developed workarounds to two types of process blocks imposed by the implemented electronic medication administration record and medication safety practices—intentional technology blocks and unintentional technology blocks. Intentional technology blocks were those purposely integrated into the system to prevent an error, and unintentional technology blocks were those blocks to work processes that were not intended by the system design. Working around the system-induced blocks negates the system safeguards that the system is intended to provide. These workarounds can result in an increased number of medication administration errors. Unintentional system blocks can also result in an increased number of medication errors caused by the unintended consequences of system implementation.

Application to Practice

Workarounds to technology implementation occur because the system design is not congruent with nursing work processes. Before system implementation, current practices must be clearly defined and the proposed system customized to conform to these processes where feasible. In addition, a thorough understanding of current processes will uncover those that could be improved or may need to be redesigned with the implementation of the information system. Another analysis of nursing processes related to the system must also be conducted after implementation to determine what practices have been affected and may need to be altered. Information systems are transformed by the environment in which they are implemented; also, the environment is transformed by the system.

reducing data replication, and increasing the availability and accessibility of information. Well-designed computerized information systems can facilitate the collection of complete and accurate data in a form that is easily accessible to enhance clinical practice, analyze patient outcomes, or manage institutional resources.

The purpose of an EHR is to document patient care in a single repository as a clinical, financial, and legal record. The electronic format makes the record available as a communication device among health care members regardless of their location. The EHR is a virtual record. It does not originate from one place. It is a compilation of information from a variety of integrated systems.

In 2004, President George W. Bush announced the creation of the position of National Health Information Technology Coordinator at the Department of Health and Human Services (HHS). The coordinator's role is to provide the leadership to develop the standards and infrastructure necessary to harness the use of information technology to improve patient care and reduce health care costs (Phoenix Health Systems, 2004). The central focus of the President's Consolidated Health Informatics Initiative (CHI) is for each American to have an EHR by 2014. The HHS and other federal agencies will adopt 15 standards for the exchange of electronic information across the federal government. To facilitate the development of interoperable EHR systems across the country, the standardized vocabulary, Systematized Nomenclature of Medicine Clinical Terms (SNOMED CT), has been made available for free download through the National Library of Medicine (U.S. Department of Health and Human Services [USDHHS], 2004).

Much of the recent push for the development of an EHR has been related to the public's awareness regarding the frequency of medical errors in health care. An estimated 23,000 hospital patients die each year as a result of an adverse drug event (Kimmel & Sensmeier, 2002). Most errors (49%) that result in adverse drug events occur when the drug is ordered. Ordering errors identified include the following: wrong dose, wrong choice of drug, known allergy, wrong frequency, and drug-drug interaction (Bates et al., 1995). Handwritten medication orders are often incomplete or contain illegible penmanship. A study of handwritten medication orders in three hospital units found that, over a 48-hour period, 20% of medication orders and 78% of signatures were either illegible or legible only with effort. In this same study, 24% of medication orders were found to be incomplete (Winslow et al., 1997).

In a description of errors by stage of medication process, Kopp and colleagues (2006) reported that lack of drug knowledge was the cause of 10% of errors and that slips and memory lapses were responsible for 40% of errors at the administration stage. Because health care work occurs in an interruption-driven environment, it is not surprising that some medication administration errors are attributable to slips and memory lapses. Integrating an EHR with pharmacy, laboratory, and clinical information systems allows the implementation of computerized provider order entry (CPOE), decision support systems (DSSs), and medication administration systems (MASs) designed to reduce errors in health care systems.

Implementing technological solutions in health care is extremely expensive, and it has been difficult to show a return on investment (ROI) for these expenditures. However, an estimated $12.7 to $36 billion could be saved annually from the national implementation of an EHR through the associated reduction in adverse events, unnecessary clinical procedures, and staff time, along with more rapid record retrieval (Staggers et al., 2001). The growing trend is to regard these expenditures as part of the cost of institutional infrastructure and to tie them to the cost savings gained by improving patient outcomes. The Leapfrog Group, a coalition of major employers, is requiring that health care organizations have CPOE in place if they want to continue to provide care to their employees. Partly because of the documented cost of medication errors, 67% of health care organizations plan to add CPOE in the next few years (Ball, 2003).

EFFECTIVENESS

The first person to analyze patient outcomes associated with nursing care delivery was Florence Nightingale in the nineteenth century. After that, research into patient outcomes was not emphasized until health care cost and quality became social and policy issues (Maas et al., 1996). Health care systems are struggling to contain costs and determine effectiveness for their survival in a managed care environment. Current measures that focus solely on reduced mortality, length of stay, and hospital costs provide little information about the quality of health care provided. Computer technology and the development of nursing classification systems have made the measurement and evaluation of nursing-sensitive outcomes feasible.

Nurses spend approximately 50% of their time coordinating and documenting patient information (Meadows, 2002). Unfortunately, these data are generally documented in a format that is difficult to access and analyze. Nursing informatics specialists work to organize and aggregate these data for decision making in care delivery management and the analysis of patient outcomes. These activities require data that are organized in nursing outcomes databases. Without clinical outcomes databases that reflect nursing care, data available in current billing systems will be used for generic outcome evaluation. Nursing outcome databases are critical for two reasons: (1) nurses must be able to measure and document how nurses influence patient outcomes; and (2) the study of nursing-sensitive outcomes will allow comparisons among interventional strategies and advance the science of nursing care delivery (Iowa Intervention Project, 1997).

Formulation of the Nursing Minimum Data Set (NMDS) was an effort to standardize the collection of essential nursing information for comparison of nursing data across patient populations. The NMDS identifies the data essential for inclusion in clinical information systems necessary to support decision making in clinical and administrative nursing practice (Brokel, 2007). Three categories of data elements are included in the NMDS: nursing care, demographic, and service. Data elements related to nursing care include nursing diagnosis, intervention, outcome, and intensity of nursing care (Werley & Lang, 1988). Using the NMDS as a guide helps ensure that data are collected regarding institutional structure (having the right things), process (doing things right), and outcomes (having the right things happen). Linking structure, process, and outcomes is necessary for the accurate evaluation of efficiency and effectiveness (Donabedian, 1986).

Practical Tips

Tip #1: Implement Change with New Technology

When planning to implement a new technological system, involve others in the design and deployment of the system from the beginning stages of development. This not only will help ensure that the system meets the needs of individual users but also will increase acceptance and user satisfaction.

Tip #2: Design Data Collection Databases

When designing a database for measuring nursing administrative or clinical outcomes, first determine what questions you would like the collected data to answer. Determining output in advance of design will ensure that the right data elements are included in the database and that time and energy are not wasted in the collection of data that will never be used.

Tip #3: Plan for Intensive Education

Build into any informatics initiative ample time for educational strategies. Make it easy and fun to build everyone's proficiency.

STANDARDIZED CLINICAL TERMINOLOGY

Nurses spend a great deal of their time collecting and documenting information related to patient care delivery. Vast amounts of data are compiled, describing every detail of the patient's encounter with the health care system. Unfortunately, these data are rarely recorded in a way that makes them amenable to analysis. When charting the description of the same surgical incision, five different nurses may chart five different entries. They may describe the size of the wound in centimeters or inches. The wound color could be depicted as pink, slightly reddened, or slightly inflamed. When different terms are used to describe the same observable fact, it is difficult to know that everyone is referring to the same phenomenon.

Norma Lang, a pioneer in nursing informatics, once wrote "If we cannot name it, we cannot control it, practice it, research it, teach it, finance it, or put it into public policy" (Clark & Lang, 1992, p. 109). For nearly 30 years, nurses have been striving to develop classification systems that itemize the diagnoses, interventions, and most recently, outcomes of the professional domain. Often, this process has been fraught with controversy and disagreement, resulting in multiple approaches to classification. These disagreements usually were viewed as divisive and disruptive to the profession. However, the result has been a richer, more inclusive representation of "what nurses do" in different practice environments. Currently, the ANA recognizes 13 standardized terminologies. These include terminologies for nursing administration, home health care, perioperative nursing, acute care, and a terminology for describing nursing care internationally. The ANA-recognized terminologies for nursing are as follows: North American Nursing Diagnosis Association International (NANDA International), Nursing Interventions Classification (NIC) system, Nursing Outcomes Classification (NOC) system, Nursing Management Minimum Data Set (NMMDS), Clinical Care Classification (CCC), Omaha System, Patient Care Data Set (PCDS), SNOMED CT, NMDS, International Classification for Nursing Practice (ICNP), ABC codes, and Logical Observation Identifier Names & Codes (LOINC) (American Nurses Association [ANA], 2007).

Terminology structures most commonly used in health care are classification systems. Classification systems are non-combinatorial hierarchical languages designed to categorize objects (Ingenerf, 1995). In health care classification systems, objects classified are generally patient diagnoses and care interventions. Nursing classifications, also referred to as *interface terminologies,* are generally implemented at the point of care to describe clinical practice (Coenen et al., 2001).

However, most classification terminologies lack the conceptual structure necessary for their direct incorporation in modern object-oriented computer database systems (Button et al., 1998). Concept-oriented or reference terminologies have the potential to provide the necessary structure for documentation in modern computer database systems. On the other hand, concept-oriented terminologies require the user to combine terms, making them awkward for their direct use as a documentation tool (Hardiker & Rector, 2001). Therefore recent efforts have centered on the development of reference terminologies that can serve as intermediaries between standardized nursing documentation and computer database systems. Classification systems can help provide the terms used in documenting practice, and the reference terminology model can provide the structure for their organization in the computer database.

A reference terminology model (RTM) depicts the system of concepts that provide the structure for the organization of documentation terms (Bakken et al., 2001). In recent years, progress has been made in the development of reference terminology models that represent the domain concepts of diagnoses and interventions in nursing. Prominent in these efforts is the work of the European Standardization Committee (CEN TC 251). The CEN combined the efforts of groups working on the ICNP and TeleNurse ID projects, producing a proposed categorical structure for nursing diagnosis and intervention. This work was continued by the International Standards

Organization (ISO) Technical Committee ISO/TC 215 Health Informatics, Working Group 3 Health Concept Representation (ISO/TC 215/WG 3). The efforts of the ISO working group focused specifically on the conceptual structure required by a nursing reference terminology model (International Organization for Standardization [ISO], 2002). The resulting conceptual structure for nursing diagnoses and interventions were designed to integrate with evolving multidisciplinary terminology standards. Through the use of these terminology models, diagnosis and intervention terms contained within existing clinical classification systems can be mapped for harmonization across medical and nursing terminologies.

The ISO RTM for Nursing Action is composed of six categories designed to describe nursing interventions in a modern object-oriented computer database. The six categories are action, target, recipient of care, means, route, and site (ISO, 2002). By using these categories to guide the decomposition and mapping of nursing documentation, the ability of the model to support nursing documentation can be evaluated (Moss et al., 2003), the ability of the documentation to meet regulatory requirements can be evaluated (Moss, 2003), and the structure of formal terminology systems can be enhanced (Hardiker, 2003).

NURSING MANAGEMENT MINIMUM DATA SET

Awareness of the need for standardized, uniformly collected, retrievable, and comparable service-related management data elements, combined with the awareness of their unavailability in practice, was the impetus for the research to develop and test a Nursing Management Minimum Data Set (NMMDS) (Huber et al., 1992; Huber et al., 1997) (Figure 36.1).

Building on the NMDS, the NMMDS specifically identified variables essential to nurse managers for decision making about nursing care effectiveness. For example, the NMMDS can be linked to the nursing care elements of intensity/staff mix to provide an enhanced assessment of the consumption of health care resources to produce specific client care outcomes for a specific age cohort, racial/ethnic group, or geographical region. Linkage to the NMDS service elements, specifically the expected payer of the bill, would assist in isolating budgetary elements. Therefore the NMDS and NMMDS can complement each other to provide data useful for the financial and clinical management of patient care (Delaney & Huber, 2001).

The NMMDS identified 18 elements potentially critical to evaluating the impact of nursing interventions on client outcomes. The NMMDS work has the potential of facilitating the linking and augmenting of the other minimum health data sets by providing information uniquely important to nursing administrative decisions and thus to the evaluation of nursing services for cost and quality outcomes of care delivery.

The NMMDS work helps clarify and expand the data points that tap contextual variables, which intervene between provider actions and client outcomes. Despite the use of the NMDS in nursing research and practice, the fourth element of intensity is often ignored. The focus of the NMDS is limited to the first three nursing variables of diagnosis, interventions, and outcomes. For example, Blewitt and Jones (1996) reported a pilot study using elements of the NMDS in a sample of clients undergoing parathyroidectomy. After reviewing the four elements of the NMDS, they noted that their study focused on diagnosis, intervention, and outcomes. This strategy ignores the important impact of contextual variables. To fully capture outcomes for quality and effectiveness determinations, multiple domains need to be included (Huber & Oermann, 1999). This is especially important because "the effectiveness of nursing interventions is especially sensitive to the influences of organizational structures and processes" (Maas et al., 1999, p. 4).

Nursing needs a standardized data set that will facilitate decision making and policy development in such areas as job satisfaction, turnover, cost of nursing services, allocation of nursing personnel, and comparison of nursing care delivery models. Such a data set would foster data collection,

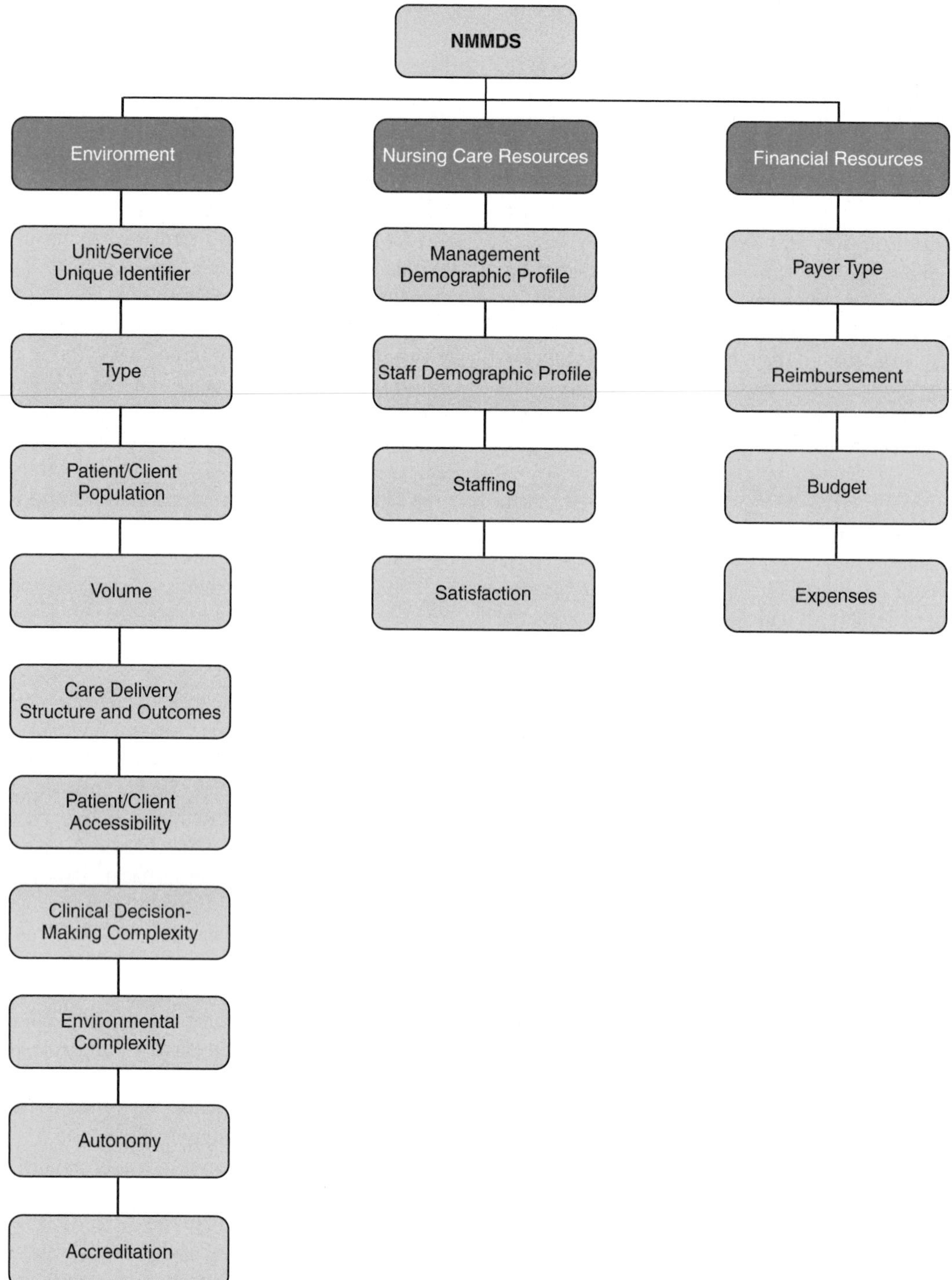

Figure 36.1

Nursing Management Minimum Data Set (NMMDS) variables. These elements are at the unit-of-service level.

retrieval, analysis, and comparison of nursing management outcomes across settings, populations, time intervals, and geographical regions. Using a core of variables captured by computerized information systems, data essential to nursing care delivery management can be analyzed and used to meet nursing's goals and objectives. Management information systems join large database development efforts and other information software applications to enhance nursing leadership and management. The future points to further developments and refinements to augment the practice of nursing. The future will hold more computer power, portable computers and hand-held terminals, voice input, videodisk technology, expert systems, artificial intelligence, and more advanced decision support and modeling systems. Connectedness and outreach linkages will be greater. Computing is the medium of communication in the future; information is the message that needs to be delivered (Ball & Douglas, 1988).

LEADERSHIP AND MANAGEMENT IMPLICATIONS

The Institute of Medicine's (IOM) landmark report on medical errors in the United States was based, in part, on the landmark study of medical errors conducted by Lucian Leape. Leape found that all seven of the most frequent medical errors cited resulted from impaired access to information. These errors were primarily the result of system design faults and accounted for 78% of the total errors uncovered (Leape et al., 1995).

Technological applications have the capability to change system processes to improve communication and information access and thereby decrease errors and adverse events (Moss et al., 2002). However, inadequate information system design can actually *increase* rather than decrease the risk for medical errors. In January of 2003, Cedars-Sinai Medical Center suspended the use of a $43 million computerized system for physician order entry because physicians complained that the system endangered patient safety and required too much work (Ornstein, 2003). In another case, poor information system design resulted in a transplant patient receiving organs from a donor of another blood type (Stenson, 2003). Although information regarding the donor's blood type was listed in a computerized database, no system was in place for cross-checking this information with that of the recipient's blood type.

It is implicitly acknowledged that collecting, sharing, and analyzing information will positively affect the quality of care delivered. However, too often in the past, the documentation of nursing care has not been included in the collection of organizational data. The result of this has been that nursing practice and its contribution to institutional effectiveness have not been visible in the analysis of organizational data. Nurse leaders are in the position of ensuring that information systems are selected that collect nursing data and support the way nurses work. Effective information system structure requires the determination of the appropriate information system requirements for the specific users' needs (Moss & Xiao, 2004). Successful information systems are those with the ability to accurately measure and analyze the efficiency and effectiveness of care.

Implementation of technology to improve the documentation and delivery of health care services will require organizational change in a technical, structural, and behavioral sense (Ball, 2003). Strategically planning for the design and implementation of health care information systems requires the participation and collaboration of all stakeholders within the organizational system. Implementing information systems designed without the involvement and buy-in of representatives from all user groups often results in poorly designed systems that fail to gain acceptance and fail to meet institutional needs.

Increasingly, nurse managers are being asked to participate in the selection, design, and implementation of institutional information systems. Managers will need a combination of technical skills (both computer and clinical), project management skills, and organizational skills (Lorenzi & Riley, 2003). During this process, managers will serve as change agents to overcome resistance from

LEADERSHIP & MANAGEMENT BEHAVIORS

Leadership Behaviors

- Envisions a structure to capture data needs
- Projects data needs
- Enables followers to use data and information
- Models knowledge-based practice
- Uses electronic data management resources
- Uses data and information for power and political advantage

Management Behaviors

- Identifies needed data
- Plans for the collection of data
- Organizes data collection
- Uses electronic resources
- Analyzes data
- Uses information strategically

Overlap Areas

- Identifies data and information needs

unit nurses and other members of the health care team. A basic understanding of the dynamics of the change process will be essential for successful adoption of these systems (Jones & Moss, 2006). Successful implementation of these systems will require nurse managers with leadership, vision, and commitment.

CURRENT ISSUES AND TRENDS

Nursing and health care organizations are calling for the redesign of the existing work environment to improve clinician and client satisfaction, client outcomes, and the profitability of all health care organizations. The American Organization of Nurse Executives (AONE) has called for the redesign of work through the use of technology to augment nursing practice during this period of a decreasing and aging workforce (Kennedy, 2003). The purpose of this mandate is twofold: (1) to improve the work environment and attract more individuals to the profession; and (2) to use technology to enable aging nurses to remain active in direct-care roles.

Another goal of nursing work redesign is to build systems and safeguards to decrease error and to enhance patient safety. In 2004, the Institute of Medicine (IOM, 2004) published the report *Keeping Patients Safe: Transforming the Work Environment of Nurses*. In this report, the IOM noted that inherent risks to patient safety are imbedded in many work processes and proposed a combination of technological and system interventions to support these processes.

Toward this goal, system designers are focusing on how to communicate information for the automation and coordination of health care work. According to Stetson and colleagues (2001), there is no instance in which coordination of care takes place in the absence of communication and there is no instance in which clinical information exchange occurs in the absence of clinical communication. Technological solutions to enable this goal exist to enhance the communication of information through voice, video, imaging, or text. In the past, tasks supported by computers have been classified as *information tasks* and those supported by telephones as *communication tasks* (Coiera, 2000). With the use of telephones for information processing and computers for distance conferencing, these distinctions have tended to blur. It is now possible to integrate cell phones, hand-held devices, global positioning systems, barcode scanners, and medication administration systems with traditional information systems through a wireless intranet for the immediate communication of information to the correct person, at the correct time, in the correct format. For example, it is now possible to link laboratory systems with nursing call systems to alert a patient's nurse when laboratory values fall outside of set limits.

The integration of these systems can also enhance the efficiency of the collection and aggregation of clinical data for use in the management of workload and staffing. Calculating acuity data directly from nursing documentation and treatment plans can more accurately reflect scheduling needs for immediate online retrieval (Kennedy, 2003). This documentation can also be used to determine the quality of care delivered on an institutional, unit, or individual basis. Efficiency and effectiveness can be compared between units, or the data can be used for an individual nurse's performance evaluation.

Summary

- Critical data and information to support nursing decision making are essential.
- Computerized data make real-time analysis possible and swift.
- Computer applications in nursing administration can be understood best as arising from nursing administration, informatics, and effectiveness research.
- Nursing informatics is the management and processing of nursing data, information, and knowledge to support the practice of nursing and the delivery of nursing care.
- A management information system (MIS) is an integrated system for collecting, storing, retrieving, and processing a collective set of data from storage into knowledge.
- The information collected in health care is used to establish reimbursement, determine access to health care, define services, monitor the quality of care, direct health care policy, and affect the standard of care delivered.
- Information systems that support nursing administrative practice and provide essential decision support are being developed and used.
- Nursing's data needs lie in the areas of the client, the provider, administration, and research.
- Nursing's data have been described as being "invisible."
- Computerized nursing management information, standardized language, and the development of and access to uniform nursing management data sets would enhance the collection, retrieval, analysis, and comparison of nursing's "invisible" data.

CASE STUDY

Dennis Fowler is the vice president for nursing at a busy university hospital. The hospital is in the process of determining documentation requirements for a proposed clinical information system. Mr. Fowler has asked each unit manager to identify his or her nursing documentation needs. Sandy Jones is the manager of the hospital's nephrology unit. Ms. Jones formed a committee consisting of clinical leaders on her unit and requested that the nursing informatics specialist for their area, Jill Ross, be a member of this committee.

Ms. Ross suggested using the categories of the Nursing Minimum Data Set (NMDS) as a guide to the collection and organization of data requirements for documentation. Using these categories helped guide their evaluation of data for the examination of nursing process, patient demographics, organizational structure, and outcomes of care.

The committee started by reviewing all current documentation tools used by nurses on the unit and reviewing the literature related to computerized nursing documentation. Next, they visited several similar nursing units at other hospitals in the area that had already implemented computerized nursing documentation. Then they identified the patient outcomes that were important for their unit to track on their particular patient group and what data were needed to analyze these outcomes. Finally, they observed nurses as they provided and documented patient care and questioned them regarding their documentation practices. This work provided them with a list of data point categories they thought were necessary to document and analyze patient care on their unit.

Mr. Fowler has compiled all of the documentation requirements collected from each unit in the hospital. He has asked hospital nursing informatics specialists and nursing leaders to assist in the selection of a nursing documentation system. The documentation system selected not only must meet the general documentation needs of the hospital but also must be adaptable to different nursing contexts. The committee's first task is to create a document that identifies specific data, nursing language, and organizational requirements for the proposed information system.

CRITICAL THINKING EXERCISE

No nurse wants to make a mistake. However, the nurses on this busy and short-staffed medical-surgical floor of an acute care tertiary-level hospital know that medication errors frequently happen. The nurse manager meets with the Nurse Manager Council from time to time to discuss this problem of high rates of medication errors. The discussion focuses on the extent and causes of the problem. Crisis management allows little time for systematic problem analysis. Short-staffing leaves nurses exhausted from running from task to task. Now the administration has announced the purchase of a new computer system for the hospital. Nurses will enter all the data, including medication orders handwritten by physicians. The nurse managers are afraid that the nurses will rebel over another burdensome duty.

1. What problem(s) can you identify in this scenario?
2. What makes this (or these) problematic?
3. What should the nurse manager do?
4. What factors do the nurses and the nurse manager need to assess and analyze?
5. What data needs might the nurses anticipate?
6. What can the nurse manager do to form a persuasive data management plan?

37 Strategic Management

Belinda E. Puetz

CHAPTER OBJECTIVES

- Draw conclusions about the importance of strategic management
- Define and describe strategic management, organizational vision or mission, strategy, tactics, strategic plan, business or action plan, and objectives
- Examine the elements of strategic planning
- Analyze the strategic planning process
- Compare strategic planning with the nursing process
- Exercise critical thinking to conceptualize and analyze possible solutions to a practice exercise

Strategic management is an approach to doing business that involves assessing the environment, knowing the competition, establishing successful performance, achieving targets, and evaluating success. This approach has long been used in business to ensure a competitive advantage over similar enterprises. Because of the changes in health care over the past decades, it has become imperative for health care organizations, as well, to function as businesses. Those that do not do so fail to remain viable for long.

Reimbursement, shortages of health care workers, particularly nurses, and the proliferation of health care ventures have necessitated the use of strategic management to obtain and maintain a competitive advantage. The success of an enterprise depends on its competitive advantage—that is, how well it does something compared with similar efforts and how well it is able to continuously achieve superior performance. Examples abound: Nordstrom is known for its customer service; McDonalds for its fast, friendly service and consistent food; Starbuck's for its custom-made coffee served in a pleasant atmosphere (Collins & Porràs, 1994). More recently, these same authors (2004) studied companies such as Boeing, Disney, Marriott, and 3M and identified elements of strategic management approaches that these companies used that set them apart from their competition and allowed them to dominate the market.

Strategic management involves strategic planning and implementation. It provides a "blueprint" for operating a business, establishing a competitive position, ensuring customer satisfaction, and reaching strategic objectives or goals. Although most strategic management occurs at the "macro" level (i.e., the executive levels of the health care institution), it can benefit the "micro" level as well, such as the nursing division, department, or unit. Strategic management prepares nurses to adapt to the ever-changing and demanding environment in which they practice as they respond to the changes in the external environment in which the health care institution is located. Strategic management helps nurses achieve their goals, whether those goals relate to the workplace or to the profession.

DEFINITIONS

Thinking and behaving strategically are prime methods for nurses to be proactive in a complex, fast-changing, rapid-cycle environment. The overarching concept is strategic management, which includes strategic planning and also focuses on strategy implementation. The terms associated with an organization's use of strategy include *strategic management, organizational vision or mission, strategy, strategic plan*, and *objectives*. **Strategic management** is defined as the management of an organization based on its vision or mission. **Organizational vision or mission** is a guiding framework that describes what the organization views as its business and future direction. **Core values** define the characteristics or values that underlie the organization's activities. The **core purpose** is the reason the organization is in business. **Strategy** is a competitive move or business approach designed to produce a successful outcome. **Tactics** are operational choices for action that are made to implement a strategy. A **strategic plan** is a document that specifies a plan for actualizing the mission. A strategic plan may also involve a *business plan* or an *action plan* (either as part of the strategic plan or as an adjunct to it) that consists of the who, what, by when, where, and in general terms, the costs involved in implementing the activities identified as objectives in the strategic plan. **Objectives** are defined as the targets an organization wants to achieve. These can be financial or performance-based and short-range or long-range targets.

STRATEGIC PLANNING PROCESS

Strategic management generally begins with a strategic planning process, triggered by recognition of the need for an organization to establish its competitive position in the marketplace or to address some other believed need (e.g., seeking Magnet™ recognition, applying for the Malcolm Baldrige award, or simply to establish future directions). The following are questions to be answered in the strategic planning process:

- Where are we currently?
- Where do we want to go?
- How will we get there?

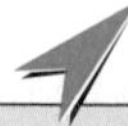

LEADING & MANAGING DEFINED

Strategic Management

Management of an organization based on its vision or mission.

Organizational Vision or Mission

A guiding framework that describes what the organization views as its business and future direction.

Core Values

Those values that are central to the organization and how it conducts its business.

Core Purpose

The reason that the organization exists.

Strategy

Competitive move or business approach designed to produce a successful outcome.

Tactics

Choices for action that are made to implement a strategy.

Strategic Plan

Document specifying the plan for actualizing the organization's mission.

Objectives

The financial or performance-based, short-range or long-range targets that an enterprise wishes to achieve.

The components of the nursing process—assessment, planning, implementation, and evaluation—are similar to those employed in strategic management, as follows:

- Developing a strategic mission or vision
- Setting objectives
- Developing strategies to achieve the objectives
- Implementing the strategies
- Evaluating the results

The strategic plan provides a framework for strategic management, considering both external and internal environmental factors.

Developing a Mission and Vision

The first step of the strategic planning process is to identify the organization's vision or mission. This requires a determination of what the organization is, what business it is in and for whom, and where the business seeks to be in the future. The mission statement reflects the vision of what the organization seeks to do and to become; it provides a clear view of what the organization is trying to accomplish, and it indicates its intent to carve out a particular position in the industry or field. For instance, Baptist Health Care in Pensacola, Florida, a recipient of the Malcolm Baldrige award, has as its mission "To provide superior service based on Christian values to improve the quality of life for people and communities served" (Baptist Health Care, 2004, p. 20). Thus the organization sees providing superior service based on Christian values as what it is trying to accomplish. Baptist Health Care's vision is "to be the best health system in America" (Baptist Health Care, 2004, p. 1). This statement clearly reflects what the organization seeks to become, and it certainly describes Baptist Health Care's intent to stake out a particular position in the health care industry.

The core values of an organization and its core purpose inform its mission statement. The core values held by an organization are those that are held whether or not circumstances (either internal or external) change. These core values are so embodied in the culture of the organization that even if they were seen as a liability, they would not be abandoned. These core values do not change even if the industry in which the organization operates changes. Thus, in health care, the organization that has as its core values excellent customer service, integrity, and social responsibility would retain those core values despite internal changes (e.g., changes in chief executive officers [CEOs]) or external changes (e.g., reimbursement, the nursing shortage).

The organization's core purpose is the reason the organization exists. The core purpose, like the core values, is relatively unchanging. The core purpose provides direction to the organization and contributes to the articulation and implementation of its mission.

In the strategic planning process, a facilitator or the planners themselves address questions that assist the planners to arrive at a specific vision and mission including the following:

- What business are we in now?
- What business do we want to be in?
- What do our customers expect of us now?
- What will be the customers' expectations in the future?
- Who are our customers now?
- Who will be our customers in the future?
- Who are our current stakeholders (other than customers)?
- How will those stakeholders change in the future? What about their expectations?
- Who are our primary competitors currently?
- Who will be our competitors in the future?
- What about partners, now and in the future?
- What will be the effect of technology?
- What are the available and the needed resources, both human and financial?
- What is happening in the environment both internally and externally now and in the future that may affect us?

It is assumed that the core values and the core purpose of the organization have been defined previously, but if not, planners should develop these using questions such as the following:

- What are the values on which we base our work?
- How central or essential are these to the organization?

- Would these values be supported if circumstances changed? If the industry in which we currently operate changes?

The core purpose can be explicated by asking and answering questions such as what business are we in and what business do we want to be in? The core purpose can be refined by asking "why," so that the initial response "We are in the business of health care" may be further refined to "We want to contribute to the community in which we exist." Thus asking "why" may result in the core value of social responsibility and the core purpose of providing needed health care services to the community in which the organization exists.

Generally, addressing the strategic planning process questions involves considering both external environmental factors (e.g., activities of regulatory bodies) and internal environmental factors (e.g., financial and human resources). The assessment of future environmental impact takes the form of assumptions. These assumptions encompass the socio-demographic, political, economic, and technological aspects of the external environment. Of course, these assumptions are merely "best guesses," because it is impossible to predict the future with any certainty.

Responses to these questions by the principals involved in an organization (e.g., executive management, supervisory staff, department heads) will shape an organization's strategic plan and, as a result, its strategic management. Involving individuals at all levels of the organization (e.g., staff nurses, clerical workers) in addition to those at the top of the hierarchy will ensure a variety of perspectives and more "buy-in" to the final product. In fact, experts in strategic planning recommend that the process occur from the "bottom up" and involve everyone in the organization (Peters, 1987).

Crafting a vision with the input of many individuals has the advantage of being a result of many perspectives, and it also engages those individuals in helping make the vision a reality. When everyone involved in an institution shares the vision, then individuals know where the organization is going and can be instrumental in helping get it there through their daily activities. As the old saying goes, "If you don't know where you're going, then any path will take you there." Conversely, if all of the individuals in the institution know where they are going, they will all take the same path.

Setting Objectives

Once the organization's mission and vision have been established, the next step in strategic planning is to develop the ways and means to get there. Thus strategic goals and objectives are crafted. These objectives generally define the "who," "what," and "where" of the strategies to be implemented. Focusing the objectives allows individuals to recognize where the organization currently is, where it wants to go, and what time it will take to get there. Absence of strategic objectives results in individuals trying to move in too many directions without a coordinated plan or not moving at all because of confusion about the organization's direction.

The strategic objectives provide a way of converting the rather abstract mission of an organization into concrete terms—targets of performance that, taken together, will achieve the mission. Objectives also offer a way of measuring progress toward achieving the organization's mission. These objectives generally are written to reflect not what *is* but what *should be*—activities that encourage the individuals implementing them to be creative, to stretch beyond their current limits, and to challenge themselves to improve their performance. These objectives must be achievable, however, lest individuals lose faith that they can accomplish them. If the strategic objectives are challenging but achievable, they will prevent employees of an institution from becoming complacent or from settling only for the status quo.

Objectives generally are written in terms of financial outcomes that relate to improvements in an organization's fiscal health and those that will result in a stronger position for the institution in the industry. For example, a for-profit hospital may set a financial objective to increase earnings growth by a specific percentage each year. A specific strategic objective might be to achieve lower overall costs than competitors or to attain technological advantage.

Developing an Implementation Strategy

The third step in the strategic planning process is to decide how to achieve the financial and strategic objectives that were established, how to obtain a competitive advantage over rivals in the field or industry, how to respond to changing conditions both externally and internally, how to defend against adverse conditions, and how to grow the business to increase market share. The strategies that are developed must be planned in advance and must also be adaptable to outside influences. Thus objectives are the targeted results and outcomes, and the strategy is how to achieve that outcome. The strategy must be deliberate and purposeful (planned and intentional) and also flexible enough to be responsive to events that are unanticipated when the strategy is developed. For example, new opportunities may arise that were unknown at the time a strategic objective was developed; these opportunities could greatly increase an organization's competitive position. Changes in a product line or service provided by an organization may necessitate a change in a strategic objective.

Basically, an organization's strategy consists of how it treats its customers and stakeholders; how it responds to changes in the industry and marketplace; how it capitalizes on new opportunities; how it manages its operations; how it grows and develops; and how it achieves its financial and strategic objectives. The challenge is to involve key people in the organization in developing this strategy so that these individuals can champion the implementation of the strategy. The desired outcome is to ensure that the strategy is timely, responsive, innovative, creative, and designed to take advantage of opportunities as they arise.

The benefits of strategic management cannot be overemphasized. In today's business climate, particularly in the health care environment, survival is tenuous and success is fraught with difficulty. A good management strategy helps an organization remain strong enough to withstand competition, overcome obstacles, and achieve peak performance. The organization's strategy must be flexible to respond appropriately to the following:

- Evolving needs and preferences of customers and stakeholders
- Advances in technology
- Changes in political climate and regulatory requirements
- New opportunities
- Altered market conditions
- Disasters and crises

The organization's strategic plan must include these aspects: where the organization is currently and where it is headed, how it plans to get to its desired future through short-term and long-term performance targets (i.e., strategic objectives), and what will be done to achieve these outcomes. The strategic plan encompasses the organization's mission and vision, strategic and financial objectives, and a strategy for achieving the objectives.

Implementing the Strategy

Once the strategy has been explicated, the next step is to implement it. Implementation involves trying out the activities in a way that determines how best to close the gap between how things are done and what it takes to achieve the strategy. For example, given an objective related to improvement of the financial bottom line, the first step is to determine current cost and then compare it with desired cost to decide what needs to be changed to reach the desired lower cost.

Strategy must be implemented proficiently and efficiently, as well as in a timely manner, if it is to be effective. For this to occur, the organization must attend to its capabilities, the reward structure, available support systems, and the organizational culture. If any of these characteristics are not in place, implementation of the strategy will surely fail. If, for example, employees are not rewarded in ways that are meaningful to them to implement a strategy, it is highly unlikely that they will initiate or maintain efforts to implement the strategy. If the organizational culture does not support innovation or risk taking or if the prevailing attitude is "if it's not broke, don't fix it," efforts to improve performance or outcomes will be doomed.

Implementing strategy is closely linked to an organization's operations; it involves managing, budgeting, motivating, changing culture, supervising, and leading. Strategic planning and implementation are managerial processes that perform the following functions:

Practical Tips

Tip # 1: Read the Organization's Strategic Plan

Obtain a copy of the organization's strategic plan. Review it carefully for implications/applications to your work setting. You may wish to ask others in the institution, both from your work area and outside of it, to participate in this review and discussion. Then set some objectives and strategies that you can implement in your work setting to complement the organization's goals. Share these with others in the institution, particularly those involved in developing the strategic plan so they are aware of your efforts to implement the plan.

Tip # 2: Identify Core Values

Learn the organization's core values and help disseminate them in your work area. Post them on the area bulletin boards. Hold a discussion in a staff meeting or change-of-shift report about what the institution's core values mean to you, and ask your co-workers what they mean to them and how they apply them in their practice. Then use these examples in an article for the institution's newsletter or in performance appraisals. Or consider displaying a poster in the lobby of the institution to inform patients and their families and others from the community about these core values and how they are being used in practice. Be certain you communicate your efforts to your supervisor and other executives in the institution.

Tip # 3: Use SWOT Analysis Techniques

Apply the principles of SWOT analysis to your own career. Knowing your core values and personal philosophy of nursing provides self-analysis that you can apply to career-related decision making.

- Demonstrate leadership in implementation of strategy
- Reward those who carry out strategy successfully
- Allocate necessary resources to activities critical to strategy
- Formulate policies and procedures that support identified strategy
- Initiate continuous quality improvement activities
- Develop and reward best practices
- Maintain a culture that supports strategy

Evaluating Effectiveness

The final step in strategic management is to evaluate the outcomes of the strategic planning process and the implementation of strategy. This evaluation component is an ongoing process; it is not a static endeavor. Because of the nature of health care environments, things change and it is necessary to constantly evaluate performance and strategy, use the data collected to decide how things are going, and make changes as indicated. Changes that may need to be made range from adjusting the organization's long-term direction, raising or lowering performance expectations, or modifying a strategy, depending on what the situation requires.

It may be—and often is—necessary to make midcourse corrections to the strategic plan, the strategic objectives, or the strategy. The evaluation process should facilitate identification of the areas in which changes need to be made. The need for changes should not be interpreted as failure of the process; rather, elements of the plan may flounder for a variety of reasons, such as diminished focus on the strategic plan, lack of commitment on the part of employees (who may not have initially been part of the process of developing the plan), and the inability to create a balance between staying the course and making corrections in midcourse.

Part of the evaluative process of a strategic plan is an annual review of the plan, of the assumptions underlying it, and of the feedback received from performance data, activity reports, market indications, and customer surveys. Also, an environmental scan and analysis should be undertaken to ensure that the conditions that affect the organization, its mission, vision, and strategic plan have not changed to a level sufficient to necessitate change in the organization itself.

Environmental analysis incorporates an internal analysis such as a review of the mission statement and value system, as well as an external analysis. The analysis needs to review four areas: strengths, weaknesses, opportunities, and threats (SWOT). The key principle is that the more systematically and carefully environmental factors and key trends are assessed, the greater the likelihood that the impact of change will be accurately gauged (Fidellow & Hogan, 1998). The following four questions can be explored (Martin, 1998):

1. For threats and opportunities, what might we do?
2. For internal competencies, what can we do?
3. For values of key implementers, what do we want to do?
4. For societal responsibilities, what should we do?

The SWOT method is one of the most popular ways to develop strategic plans for an organization. In this approach, strengths and weaknesses internal to the organization are identified. These strengths and weaknesses generally are related to resources, programs, and operations in key areas of the organization, examples of which are the following:

- *Operations:* efficiency, capacity, processes
- *Management:* systems, expertise, resources
- *Products:* quality, features, prices
- *Finances:* resources, performance

Once identified, these components are analyzed for the purpose of drafting a picture of the critical features of the organization, its achievements and failures, and its good points and bad points.

The external components are described as opportunities and threats, and they are identified in the same manner as the internal factors. Opportunities and threats may include changes in the following:

- Industry
- Marketplace
- Economy
- Political climate
- Technology
- Competition

The external factors, or the "macro" environment, in which the organization is located may also be assessed using the PEST (or STEP) analysis. This framework is expressed in terms of the following factors:

- **P**olitical (e.g., stability, pricing regulations, antitrust laws, safety regulations)
- **E**conomic (e.g., exchange rates, inflation rates, labor costs, unemployment rate)
- **S**ocial (e.g., demographics, culture, entrepreneurial spirit, health consciousness, lifestyle changes, education)
- **T**echnological (e.g., recent developments, government research spending, impact on cost, automation, rate of technological diffusion)

Once identified, these strengths, weaknesses, opportunities, and threats must be analyzed for their impact on the organization. Questions from the analysis include the following (Below et al., 1987):

- Have we identified the critical issues facing the organization?
- Do we have sufficient information to select the critical issues?
- Are we using adequate judgment to agree on these critical issues?
- Have we sufficiently discussed the root causes of the critical issues?
- Are we able to arrive at conclusions about the causes of these critical issues?
- Can we defend our conclusions both inside and outside of the organization?

Once satisfied with the responses to these questions, priorities must be established for the critical issues so that strategies are based on the priority issues. For example, a change in the market for the organization's services may be a threat but a low priority, so the organization determines it is not essential to target resources (e.g., human, financial) to deal with the threat when a higher priority is to take advantage of an opportunity involving technology. The SWOT analysis often leads to future strategies in which the organization determines to do the following:

- Build on strengths
- Resolve or minimize weaknesses
- Exploit opportunities
- Avoid threats

The strategies identified through the SWOT analysis can be shaped into a strategic plan on which strategic management is based. The more carefully the analysis is done, the more reliable the strategic plan. A plan based on faulty assumptions or careless analysis will not serve the organization well and, indeed, may lead eventually to its demise.

ELEMENTS OF A STRATEGIC PLAN

Most strategic plans result in a written document. This document can be written by the individuals involved in the strategic planning process or, more likely, by the individual who facilitated the strategic planning process (e.g., consultant, employee). Generally, strategic plan documents contain the following sections:

- *Executive summary:* A two- to three-page encapsulation of the essence of the plan, written in language understandable by all potential readers, since many will not venture beyond the first few pages of the document
- *Background:* A description of the institution, its history, and current state, including its accomplishments, as well as the situation that prompted the strategic planning process
- *Mission, vision, and values:* Should describe the philosophy of the organization
- *Goals and strategies:* Should describe the target objectives and the strategies identified to ensure achievement of the objectives
- *Appendixes:* Includes all the documentation related to the strategic planning process so that the reader obtains a sense of the background information used by the strategic planners in order to arrive at the strategic plan

Appendix materials can include the following elements:

- Annual reports of the institution
- SWOT analysis results
- Financial information
- Environmental scan (PEST analysis) results
- Staffing information
- Current and projected programs and services

Other materials can be included as desired. Caution should be exercised, however, to not include confidential data that should not be viewed by individuals outside of the organization.

The strategic plan should be disseminated widely throughout the institution. It is not necessary to reproduce the document in its entirety for distribution to everyone in the institution. A decision needs to be made about which parts of the strategic plan are appropriate for the individuals who will receive them. Some will need the entire plan; others may need only the executive summary; and still others perhaps need only the goals and strategies.

In any case, the strategic plan should be communicated to stakeholders: board members, management, and staff. Copies should be included in orientation programs for new employees. The institution's vision and mission, including the core values, should be displayed in public areas (e.g., waiting rooms, cafeteria), as well as in areas reserved for employees. The core values can be listed on employee identification badges and printed in all marketing materials for the organization. The strategic plan tenets should be incorporated into all of the institution's policies and procedures.

Copies of the plan can also be provided to trade or professional organizations with which the institution is associated. The public relations or community outreach department in the institution can use the strategic plan as the basis for a media campaign to educate the community and other stakeholders and audiences about the institution's vision and mission. Patients can be provided with a condensed summary of the strategic plan on admission, particularly those sections related to their care. Patients should be informed of the institution's core values as well.

IMPLEMENTATION OF THE STRATEGIC PLAN

At this point, strategic management often fails. Strategic plans are developed and then allowed to languish as the necessary commitment to implementation is not realized for whatever reason. Often the reason is conflicting priorities. Executives and staff in health care organizations have a myriad of tasks facing them, and implementing strategic objectives adds another burden to an already overwhelming workload. To overcome this obstacle, the strategic plan must be integrated into the organization's daily activities. Everyone must be committed to implementing the strategic plan, from the leaders to the staff at all levels and in all departments. Focusing on the strategic plan and its meaning to the viability and future of the institution is imperative.

As mentioned, it also is necessary to develop an action plan based on the strategic plan. Those individuals who will be responsible for implementing the strategic objectives need to develop this plan. The action plan should include the following elements:

- A priority order for achieving the strategic objectives or outcomes
- The determination of who (individual or group) will be responsible for achieving these objectives
- An indication of available or necessary financial support
- A timetable outlining when achievement of the objectives can be expected

It may also be advisable to include interim activities and time frames if the strategic objective is long-term or complex, so that progress can be monitored.

The action plan breaks the strategic plan into manageable components, particularly for those individuals who were not directly involved in crafting the strategic plan. The action plan, then, must become a living document so that it is constantly referenced, consulted, and discussed. The action plan should be reviewed and updated at intervals. Actions that have been completed or those that do not move the organization toward achievement of its goals should be deleted, and new actions based on existing environmental conditions should be added. It may also be necessary to readjust the time line for completion of some activities in response to external or internal factors that affect the ability to accomplish the desired activities.

Ensuring that the action plan remains at the forefront of daily activities, whether in an institution as a whole, a department, or a unit, often requires a "champion." This is an individual who is passionate and committed to the process and who can inspire others also to be. Often, a champion appears as the strategic planning process unfolds; generally, this individual contributes freely, is engaged in the work groups, and expresses interest in the process. Champions can be selected as well, but those who volunteer are usually more enthusiastic about the work than those who are "drafted."

LEADERSHIP AND MANAGEMENT IMPLICATIONS

Strategic management is useful for nursing leaders and managers because it can be used to analyze the environment for opportunities and threats; to set measurable, achievable goals and plans; and to help determine the future of the nursing area, such as a department or unit. Success in strategic planning and implementing that strategic plan will position nursing well in an institution. The process provides an opportunity for nursing to shine, because the similarities between the nursing process and the strategic planning process allow nurses to shortcut the learning curve and begin to move forward with the implementation phase while others may still be grappling with the planning process. Nursing skills and abilities make it relatively easy to plan strategically; and nurses, as 24-hour workers, can approach implementation as an ongoing, continuous, and seamless process. Nurses' involvement with continuous quality improvement and performance improvement systems provides a basis for participation in strategic planning that is systematic and thorough.

Implementation of the organization's strategic plan can be useful in unifying staff on a nursing unit or in a department. Collaboration and

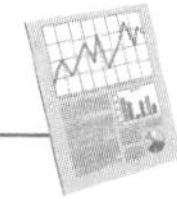

Research Note

Source: Roderer, C.A. (2001). Strategic planning for the recruitment and retention of health care professionals. *Oncology Issues, 16*(5), 31-34.

Purpose

The purpose of this article was to describe strategies hospitals can use to recruit and retain health care professionals, including nurses.

Discussion

The strategies employed were incorporated in categories such as managing and mentoring, recognizing and rewarding employees, compensation and benefit strategies, recruiting strategies, and "growing your own." Managing and mentoring includes managers being sensitive to a culturally diverse staff and managing with respect rather than with authority. The author cautioned that the institution's mission statement must be clear and valued by all employees. Recognition and rewards for employees encompassed equitable and competitive compensation but also flexible scheduling, childcare centers, stress reduction programs, and financial planning for employees. Compensation and benefits described bonuses for referral, weekend work and project completion, and profit sharing, as well as financial incentives for certification or degree completion. Recruitment programs extended beyond the typical classified ads to direct-mailing campaigns, billboards, and cinema advertising. "Growing your own" involved tuition reimbursement, internship programs, and scholarship programs for employees' children. The author concluded that employers need to use a strategic plan to ensure that their employment practices are competitive in this era of critical labor shortages.

Application to Practice

This article demonstrated the process of strategic planning to achieve a goal: sufficient individuals to staff hospitals. The author described the strategic objectives and the tactics that can be used to achieve this goal. Not all of the objectives and tactics will be relevant to each institution. Regardless of the applicability of the objectives, it is apparent that strategically planning and managing to avert a shortage of employees will produce a better result than leaving recruitment and retention to chance.

cooperation among staff generally are required to accomplish strategic objectives. Working together to accomplish a strategic objective keeps staff engaged. Involvement in decisions that ultimately will affect them is essential and often results in positive spin-offs; for example, staff members feel a sense of ownership in the process and pride in their accomplishments.

Involvement in strategic planning at the institution-wide level provides an opportunity for nurses to actualize practice autonomy, be recognized for their contributions, and lessen the feelings of being disenfranchised. Although admittedly a lot of work, the benefits of engaging in strategic planning and then implementing that plan far outweigh the disadvantages.

A strategic plan should be realistic and make sense to nurses at all levels. Participation and input help shape the organization's future and that of the nurses employed in the institution.

CURRENT ISSUES AND TRENDS

The focus on the nursing shortage underscores the need to retain nurses in the workplace, and strategic planning is an integral component of efforts in

LEADERSHIP & MANAGEMENT BEHAVIORS

Leadership Behaviors

- Involves subordinates in the strategic planning process
- Inspires a vision
- Develops strategic plans and tactics
- Creates new or unique products or services
- Assesses current market position
- Establishes organizational priorities
- Forecasts resource requirements
- Analyzes key vision implications
- Creates the environment to encourage participation in the development of strategic plans

Management Behaviors

- Develops operational and action plans and tactics
- Develops control and evaluation plans
- Monitors implementation of strategy and tactics
- Organizes the strategic planning committee
- Conducts surveys and data collection
- Ensures that strategies are sound operationally

Overlap Areas

- Participates in the strategic planning process
- Ensures strategic plan implementation
- Involves all employees in the strategic planning process

recruitment and retention of nurses. Those institutions that successfully retain nurses are more often those that have obtained Magnet™ recognition from the American Nurses Credentialing Center (ANCC). Institutions generally seek Magnet™ status to demonstrate excellence in the delivery of nursing services to patients, promote quality in an environment that supports professional practice, and provide a mechanism for the dissemination of "best practices" in nursing services (ANCC, 2009). Nurses seek out these institutions for their employment; and students look to them for clinical experiences and, after graduation, for employment. Increasingly, schools and colleges of nursing choose Magnet™ hospitals as sites for clinical affiliations of students.

Aiken and colleagues (2000) reported that nurses in Magnet™ organizations are more satisfied with their jobs, and patients in Magnet™ hospitals rate the care they receive more favorably. These authors also reported patient outcomes that ranged from increased satisfaction to shorter length of stay and lower disease-specific mortality rates. McClure and Hinshaw (2002) reported on the impact and promise of Magnet™ hospitals and provided evidence for these superior outcomes. These authors further described strategies for creating "magnet environments" in health care facilities.

This process of becoming a Magnet™-recognized health care institution is similar to that of strategic planning. The assessment, goal setting, implementation, and evaluation phases are the basis of the application and site visit processes required for Magnet™ recognition (ANCC, 2009).

Strategic planning is not reserved for activities such as seeking Magnet™ recognition, however. Any business venture will benefit from having a strategic plan. The plan provides for assessment of the environment, including current and future opportunities, and identification of specific, measurable, realistic ways of taking advantage of those opportunities. Most important, perhaps, the strategic plan answers the question, "What business are we in?" In many instances, nurses have found themselves in businesses other than nursing. Clearly defining a mission and vision will help a nursing unit or department focus its efforts on its core business.

Woods (2001) described how evidence-based methods were used to create a strategic plan for recruitment and retention of staff. Crossan (2003) described the process of strategic management and called for nurses to employ strategic management in their institutions, particularly in the area of policy development.

Nurses in entrepreneurial roles benefit from a clearly defined business plan, which provides direction and often serves as a vehicle for obtaining outside funding for the venture. Puetz and Shinn (1997) called for nurses who sought to become consultants in their area of expertise to develop a business plan before proceeding.

Nurses in all areas of practice and in all employment settings can use strategic planning principles to explore programs, projects, and services. Whether those are new or the strategic planning process is used to determine which programs, projects, and services to discontinue, the process of assessment, setting objectives, implementation, and evaluation guides these activities.

Strategic planning and strategic management are necessary components of business in today's competitive and highly unstable environment. Strategic planning is a process similar to the nursing process, with defined and specific steps to be taken to ensure a comprehensive and thorough process. Strategic management involves implementation of the strategic plan to ensure that the organization is responsive to changes in its environment, as well as to internal events.

Strategic planning and strategic management are not reserved exclusively for organizations. Individuals, such as nurses, can use these techniques to determine their own direction and establish objectives to ensure that they meet the goals they have set for themselves.

Summary

- Competition and competitive advantage are pressures that can be helped with strategic management.
- Strategic management includes both strategic planning and strategy implementation.
- Strategic planning prepares the nurse for readiness to respond.
- A strategy is an integrated plan of action.
- Tactics are choices used to implement strategy.
- Strategic planning is a continuous process of making decisions.
- A strategic plan is a written document.
- Strategic planning is a systematic approach to meeting goals and objectives.
- The strategic management process has five components.
- Strategic planning can be a vehicle for nurse participation and input.

CASE STUDY

Nurse Kory Danielson is the director of an adolescent substance abuse comprehensive assessment clinic affiliated with a university health care center. This clinic was developed and has been operating for 4 years based on financing from a federal government grant. The grant funding will expire in 1 year. Although a grant resubmission is underway, continued funding from the federal government is uncertain. The other employees are becoming anxious about their job options. A formal program evaluation is underway, but the data will not be analyzed for 9 months.

Nurse Danielson calls a whole clinic staff meeting to begin the strategic planning process. First, a set of questions are posed and discussed: Where are we currently? Where do we want to go? How will we get there? The group has been provided with the clinic's mission, vision, and purpose statements along with current goals and objectives. A number of unanswered questions arise, such as, Do we need to start charging for services and billing insurance carriers?

The meeting is productive but exhausting. Nurse Danielson knows that closure of this initial planning segment needs to be facilitated. The question "So what do we do next?" has generated many fruitful ideas. The following are the top three suggestions:

- Do a formal SWOT analysis
- Investigate whether a professor from the College of Business or a representative from

the Service Corps of Retired Executives (SCORE) can work with the group on a business plan

- Form an outreach team that will present and promote the clinic within the community by means of presentations and personal liaison

The group divides into three groups to tackle the three suggestions, gather information, and formulate a plan for the group. Nurse Danielson begins to plan for a formal strategic planning session within a month.

CRITICAL THINKING EXERCISE

Nurse Martha Smith serves on the board of directors of the local chapter of her specialty nursing organization. One of the chapter's activities is to establish a high school–to–nursing school program to recruit youngsters into nursing. Nurse Smith wishes to use the unit on which she is manager as the location where the high school students can "shadow" nurses. Because of clinical affiliations by local colleges and universities and preceptorship programs for new orientees, nursing staff on the unit are overloaded already. Nurse Smith is convinced of the value of the chapter's program and believes that it is her responsibility as a chapter leader to help implement this program in her setting.

1. What are the issues that are present in this situation?
2. How should Nurse Smith approach the problem?
3. What are the elements of strategic planning and strategic management that might be helpful?
4. Why might these particular elements of strategic planning and strategic management be helpful here?

38 Marketing

Dana Woods

CHAPTER OBJECTIVES

- Frame marketing in the context of health care delivery
- Define and describe a market, marketing, marketing mix, marketing orientation, market share, and market research
- Examine marketing exchanges
- Illustrate marketing strategy and its place in strategic planning
- Analyze the marketing process
- Describe elements of marketing mix
- Interpret leadership and management implications in marketing
- Illustrate current trends in marketing in nursing and health care
- Exercise critical thinking to conceptualize and analyze possible solutions to a practice exercise

Marketing is a business administration concept related to the activities of product development, sales, influence, positioning, persuasion, and image projection. As an offshoot of capitalism, marketing is concerned with paying attention to stimulating and meeting consumer demand. In the most basic business terms, marketing is defined as "meeting needs profitably." In a societal context, marketing involves "identifying and meeting human and social needs" (Kotler, 2000, p. 2).

Understanding and satisfying buyer wants and needs is a critical part of successful business marketing. Because nurses are at the center of care delivery—the primary product of health care organizations—they are in a unique position to understand what customers need. This is true regardless of which of its multiple customers (e.g., patients, physicians, payers) a health care organization may serve (Woods, 2002).

Marketing a service such as health care may be dramatically different, from an implementation standpoint, from marketing a consumer product such as a soft drink. However, the underlying concepts are universal. The business goal of a for-profit company is to maximize value so that shareholders will eventually benefit from their financial investment. The business goal of a non-profit, or social sector, organization, which includes many health care organizations, is to fulfill its mission of meeting consumer needs. To achieve its business goal, either type of organization must be financially viable, because without sustaining infrastructures and investing in new technologies, neither a hospital nor a soft drink company will be able to satisfy its customer needs for very long. "No money, no mission" is a maxim for both.

The operation of free market economies provides a perspective on how the principles of marketing apply to nursing and health care. However, marketing health care services has its challenges because the traditional rules of an efficient free market often do not apply. Supply and demand, foundational elements of a free market, are significantly distorted in the health care market for several reasons. First, because of the third-party payer system, the end customer—the patient or potential patient—rarely acts like a typical consumer. In fact, the patient is but one of several customers that a health care service provider must satisfy.

Furthermore, the seller of services (e.g., a hospital) does not have the same control over the market price of its product that a typical product provider enjoys. Add to this a nearly unlimited demand for services, and health care presents itself as an industry that is neither efficient nor compliant with the rules of free market economy (Alward & Camunas, 1991; Woods, 2002). Is it any wonder that the American health care system is often described as broken and in disarray?

In this turbulent market, it is imperative that a health care organization be deliberate when scanning its environment, setting relevant strategic objectives, and planning effectively to achieve those objectives, no matter which of several possible scenarios plays out in the future. Organizations no longer develop separate organization-wide strategic and marketing plans. Without a marketing orientation that ensures customers' needs are met, the most impressive-looking strategic plans are worthless (Schnaars, 1991).

Although formerly marketing was seen as a for-profit business strategy, it has become more widely used and vital in social sector organizations as well. Highly competitive, resource-constrained environments set up conditions necessitating effective marketing. Marketing theory can be used and applied to enhance patient care, nursing, and organizations (Alward & Camunas, 1991). This is because marketing can be thought of as the art of finding, developing, and profiting from opportunities (Kotler, 1999). In times of fiscal crisis or financial uncertainty, marketing is an especially critical survival strategy. For example, in the early 1980s, hospitals turned to marketing strategies when diagnosis-related groups (DRGs) became the basis for reimbursement (Alward & Camunas, 1991).

Although nurses experience the impact of a marketing orientation in their daily lives as consumers, they are unlikely to be exposed to it as an essential ingredient of their professional practice. Because of its for-profit roots, the term *marketing* often carries a negative connotation when applied to health care. Critics have described marketing in a variety of negative ways: a waste of scarce health care dollars; intrusive; associated with high-pressure sales, manipulation, and the promotion of low-quality products; stimulating competition; and creating unnecessary demand (Alward & Camunas, 1991). Some nurses may think that marketing does not have a legitimate place in nursing. However, Kotler's simple but profound definition of marketing, "meeting needs profitably," makes it consistent with, not contrary to, nursing practice (Kotler, 2000, p. 2). Marketing's primary benefits are improved satisfaction of customers—the target market; improved attraction of marketing resources such as nurses, physicians, and funding; and improved efficiency in marketing activities, which contributes to better stewardship of financial and human resources (Kotler & Clarke, 1987).

Whether or not they realize it, nurses, as essential providers of the health care product, are engaged in marketing every day. A health care organization dedicated to achieving excellence realizes this and works hard to see that all caregivers and support staff are informed and thoughtful about what it takes to meet customer needs. In excellence-driven organizations, marketing is more than a department; it is at the core of the organizational business framework.

DEFINITIONS

Marketing is a process that relates to transactions when goods and services are exchanged in a market. It seeks to achieve an organization's strategic goals through the analysis, planning, implementation, and control of systematically developed programs that generate voluntary exchanges of values with target markets (Kotler & Clarke, 1987).

A **market** can be defined broadly or narrowly. Originally, a market was the physical place where buyers and sellers assembled. Economists now see a market as a collection of buyers and sellers who transact (in person, by phone, by mail, or electronically) around a specific product group. From a marketer's perspective, the "industry" sells and the "market" buys (Kotler, 2003). Thus **marketing** is a social and managerial process in which individuals or groups obtain what they need and want by creating, offering, and exchanging products and services of value with others (Kotler, 2000). *Exchange* is the act of getting a desired product from someone by offering something in return (Kotler, 2000). Exchange is the defining concept that underlies marketing. By extension, "marketing comprises the set of activities that facilitate transactions in an exchange economy" (Graham, 1993, p. 2).

Marketing mix is an individualized blend of marketing tools or tactics an organization uses to achieve its objectives (Kotler, 2000). A **marketing orientation**, also called a *customer orientation*, is the focusing of energy on the identification of the needs and wants of customers and on the delivery of services that create satisfaction (Alward & Camunas, 1991). **Market share** is the percentage of the total available market for a product or service that is captured by an organization or producer. **Market research** is the systematic process for studying marketing problems or opportunities by designing a study, collecting and analyzing the data, and using information from the findings to refine strategic and/or operational plans (Alward & Camunas, 1991).

The marketing process is similar to the nursing process—a framework designed to identify, analyze, and solve problems. Skillful marketing is carefully structured. It uses analysis, planning, implementation, and control of programs designed to create voluntary exchanges of values between an organization and target markets to achieve objectives. Organizations need to design offerings to match the target market's needs and wants, using communication, price, and distribution to effectively inform, motivate, and deliver services to the market (Kotler & Clarke, 1987).

LEADING & MANAGING DEFINED

Market

A set of actual or potential buyers and users of goods, services, and ideas.

Marketing

A social and managerial process in which individuals or groups obtain what they need and want by exchanging products and values with others.

Marketing Mix

An individualized blend of marketing tools and tactics implemented to achieve goals.

Marketing Orientation

The focusing of energy on the identification of the needs and wants of customers and on the delivery of services that create satisfaction.

Market Share

The percentage of the total market for a product or service that is captured by an organization or producer.

Market Research

The systematic process for studying a marketing problem by designing a study, collecting and analyzing the data, and using information from the findings.

Needs

Individuals' basic biological, psychological, and social requirements.

Wants

Individuals' desires or preferences satisfied by specific goods and services as influenced by external cues.

Service

Any act or performance that one party can offer to another that is essentially intangible and does not result in the ownership of anything.

Product

Anything that can be offered to a market to satisfy a want or need.

The marketing process is designed to manage relationships. It is important to determine who the key customers *are* and who they *should be.* The primary markets for most nurses are patients and their families, physicians, and the employing organization. For hospitals and other health care organizations, patients, payers, employees, and physicians are the primary markets. The basis for a marketing orientation is assessment of the needs and wants of customers in an organization's markets. The needs and wants of every party to the exchange must be considered.

Needs can be basic biological, psychological, and social. For example, a hospital patient may require safety, pain management, compassionate care, sterile conditions, and prevention of complications. These are needs. **Wants** are desires or preferences satisfied by specific goods and **services** as influenced by external cues. A hospital patient's wants may include a quiet and spacious room, good food, and cable television. Wants and needs can be satisfied through goods, services, or ideas that are collectively called **products** (Alward & Camunas, 1991). "A *product* is anything that can be offered to a market to satisfy a want or need" (Kotler, 2000, p. 394).

BACKGROUND

Marketing occurs within the framework of a voluntary exchange, which in health care is often complex. When an employer selects a third-party payer, the result can make it difficult for a patient to connect with a hospital or a physician. In managed care, the exchange is multidimensional, requiring appropriate physician-hospital-payer contracts. Therefore health care organizations must be thoughtful and savvy about each dimension of the exchanges in which they seek to engage. Careful monitoring of the market environment and shrewd contracting are essential if a health care organization seeks to achieve significant market share.

Terms and phrases such as *patient-centered care, staying close to the customer,* and *an obsession with service* reflect a marketing or customer orientation. Organizational culture, philosophy, and values all need to align for true customer-centeredness. A marketing orientation contains five attributes: a customer-oriented philosophy, an integrated marketing organization, adequate marketing information, strategic orientation, and operational efficiency (Alward & Camunas, 1991; Kotler & Clarke, 1987). A marketing orientation is the foundation for the marketing process. A successful marketing orientation means that energy is devoted to identifying customers' needs and wants and delivering satisfying services.

MARKETING STRATEGY

Strategy and research are key elements of marketing. Organizational strategy evolves from setting the mission and deliberate planning to further that mission by "developing and maintaining a strategic fit between the organization's goals and capabilities and its changing marketing opportunities" (Kotler & Armstrong, 2008, p. 36). Research uncovers, analyzes, and monitors the needs and preferences of target markets. Strategic planning sets the overall frame for an organization. Defining the business, determining the mission, and formulating long-term objectives form the basis of an organization's strategic plan. Marketing strategies and programs must be aligned and guided by the organization-wide strategic plan (Kotler & Armstrong, 2008). This cannot be done effectively without investing adequate time and resources in evaluating the environment in which an organization is competing for customers. Environmental scanning is a critical step in both the strategic and marketing planning processes. A formal environmental scan includes systematic review of the external and internal factors that are likely to have a significant impact on the organization's performance factors. These include the following:

- Demographic and societal trends relevant to the business
- The organization's position in the market compared with its competitors
- Internal business performance indicators—for example, financial results, utilization trends, quality indicators, and customer characteristics
- Market and customer research
- The strength of suppliers and partners

To be most effective, compilation, review, and analysis of the environmental scan should involve every functional area in an organization, including its nurse leaders. Not only must this information be shared, but also all key stakeholders must participate in the planning process. What good is accurate market and customer information when only a handful of people have access to it?

Marketing strategy is based on how target markets are defined. Markets are both broad and narrow. Mass marketing offers a product to an entire market. Niche marketing focuses on capturing a small but important part of the market. Consider the difference between a full-service community hospital and a children's hospital. The former serves a broad market, the latter targets very specific customers—children and their families. Three critical concepts—product differentiation, segmentation, and positioning—are essential to become fluent in the language of marketing. Table 38.1 gives the definitions of these terms, along with an example of each.

Segmentation is a foundational practice in marketing that involves identifying pieces of the total market that contain potential customers with distinguishable characteristics such as age, gender, geographic location, or ethnicity. The essence of segmentation is to break down the mass market into submarkets of individuals with similar needs (Harvard Business School Press, 2006). Segmentation cannot be achieved without differentiation; yet differentiation does not require segmentation (Schnaars, 1991). A product offering's differentiation is typically what cements its position in the market against competitors.

By analyzing the competitive market, a hospital can determine key strategies to meet the unmet needs in its service area. A small rural community hospital in a market 200 miles from any other hospital will adopt strategies for defining and serving its market that are very different from the strategies of a large suburban hospital in a market with four other hospitals within a 25-mile radius. The rural hospital would likely position itself as a full-service facility capable of meeting the most frequently occurring needs of the mass population. For example, its profile of services is likely to include women's services, emergency care, diagnostic care, and general surgery. On the other hand, the large suburban hospital in a highly competitive market might seek to differentiate itself from competitors by creating a specialty center for heart disease or cancer. However, product or service lines are not the only way to differentiate. Differentiation based on quality measures and other

Table 38.1

Critical Marketing Concepts

Definition	Example
Product differentiation is "the act of designing a set of meaningful differences to distinguish the company's offering from competitors' offerings" (Kotler, 2000, p. 287).	*Example:* Nordstrom differentiates itself from other department stores by offering highly personalized and excellent customer service.
Segmentation is described as "a merchandising strategy by which products are adjusted to serve a particular group of users" (Schnaars, 1991, p. 101).	*Example:* Nike makes and promotes different shoe products for specific customer groups—for example, runners, hikers, basketball players.
Positioning "is the act of designing the company's offering and image to occupy a distinctive place in the target market's mind" (Kotler, 2000, p. 298).	*Example:* Rolls Royce designs, prices, and promotes cars to achieve a desired position in the small extreme luxury market, compared with Saturn, which strives to appeal to a broader market of economy-minded buyers.

distinctions such as The Joint Commission (TJC) accreditation, the Malcolm Baldrige National Quality Award, the AACN Beacon Award for Critical Care Excellence, and the Magnet Recognition Program® is becoming more prevalent. Heightened patient and regulatory scrutiny, fueled by more frequent accounts in the media of medical errors, has motivated hospitals to refocus on patient care excellence and seek ways to promote this excellence to the public to gain a competitive advantage.

Setting marketing strategy is a shared responsibility within a health care organization. This critical activity must be guided by the strategic plan with input from every key stakeholder group—and especially nursing—who is engaged in meeting customer needs. Likewise, the organization's marketing team must be engaged from the start when new products and services are planned. With multiple perspectives represented at the planning table, an organization will respond more effectively to the needs and challenges of its market.

THE MARKETING PROCESS: IMPLEMENTING STRATEGY

Effective marketing evolves from a five-step linear process that includes (1) research, (2) segmentation, (3) mix, (4) implementation, and (5) control. The process is represented visually as follows (Kotler, 1999, pp. 60-61):

$$R \rightarrow STP \rightarrow MM \rightarrow I \rightarrow C$$

where
R = research (i.e., market research)
STP = segmentation, targeting, and positioning
MM = marketing mix
I = implementation
C = control (getting feedback, evaluating results, and revising or improving STP strategy and MM tactics)

The process begins with a thorough market analysis, usually employing rigorous marketing research (R) to uncover opportunities and provide strategic planning data. Target segments (STP) are determined, and a positioning of the product or service is strategized. Then the optimal tactical marketing mix (MM) is established. The marketing plan is implemented (I) and controlled (C) for effectiveness (Kotler, 1999).

Determining a marketing mix is one aspect of the marketing process. In this stage, specific tactics are custom-designed to influence the buyer's decision to purchase the product or service. The tactics chosen for the marketing mix become the basis for operational marketing activities. From the seller's point of view, the marketing mix emerges as a unique combination of the four *P's* of (1) product, (2) price, (3) place, and (4) promotion. From the customer's point of view, the marketing mix emerges from the four *C's* of (1) customer solution, (2) cost, (3) convenience, and (4) communication (Kotler & Armstrong, 2008). Table 38.2 displays the marketing mix applied to health care.

A product is the basis of any business. It is whatever is offered to satisfy a market's need, desire, or preference. Products generally include objects, services, and ideas. They can be at the core, tangible, or augmented levels in relation to the market. A core product is what the client seeks in order to satisfy a basic need. A tangible product has characteristics such as style, quality, packaging, added features, and brand name. Augmented products include added services and benefits (Alward & Camunas, 1991; Kotler, 1999).

A *service* "is any act or performance that one party can offer to another that is essentially intangible and does not result in the ownership of anything. Its production may or may not be tied to a physical product" (Kotler, 2000, p. 428). Services are differentiated from products that are goods by four characteristics: (1) intangibility, (2) inseparability, (3) variability, and (4) perishability. Services are actions. Their performance varies according to circumstances related to both the provider and the recipient. They are sold first and then simultaneously produced and consumed. Services cannot be saved, stored, resold, or returned (Kotler, 2000).

Healing and palliation (intangible products, hence a service) are the ultimate outcomes desired from the health care industry. Nursing is a service within the industry. To successfully market itself, nursing must define and clearly articulate the features of

Table 38.2

The Fours *P's* and *C's* of the Marketing Mix Applied to Health Care

Four *P's*	Four *C's*	General Description	Health Care Applications
Product	Customer solution	Product variety Quality Design Features Packaging Brand name	Product/service lines Patient outcomes Service quality Physical plant design/décor Hospital "name" Health care system "name" and reputation
Price	Customer cost	List price Discounts Allowances Payment period Credit terms	Cash prices Contract prices/reimbursement PPO HMO Medical groups
Place	Convenience	Location Coverage Assortments Inventory Channels Transport	Health care system location, including clinics or other service branches Adjacent medical offices Ancillary services on site Referral relationship with physicians, medical groups, insurance providers, etc. External patient transportation such as vans, taxi vouchers, etc.
Promotion	Communication	Sales promotion Advertising Sales force Public relations Direct marketing	Physician relations Advertising Community events and outreach Media relations Direct mail

From Woods, D. (2002). Realizing your marketing influence. Part 1. Meeting patient needs through collaboration. *Journal of Nursing Administration, 32*(4), 189-195.
HMO, Health Maintenance Organization; *PPO,* Preferred Provider Organization.

its service. Yet articulating the unique contribution of nurses has long been a struggle for individual nurses and for the profession. Quality care is one ideal and intangible product of nursing services. Kramer and Schmalenberg (1988) noted that the product of a hospital is a high-quality, accessible, cost-effective service called *client-centered care.* Zander (1992) identified nursing as a business with a product of enhanced client outcomes and contained costs.

The eternal question lingers: What is nursing? One way to formulate an answer that best communicates a vision of professional nursing is to describe the process and product of nursing as the use of expertise to solve problems for patients and their families. How often do nurses explain the value of what they have done? Are patients and families—for that matter, even hospital administrators or physician colleagues—aware of the contribution of nursing, especially when that contribution may be invisible (except in its absence), such as in the case of preventing an adverse outcome? To convey the importance of the content of nursing, experts advise that nurses describe the complexity of the care they provide and the clinical judgments they use, being deliberate in differentiating their role from other caregivers (Buresh & Gordon, 2006).

Nurses must capitalize on their unique service attributes when planning a health care marketing strategy or mix. Some specific nursing-related service benefits for patients include competence and technical ability in care, compassion and caring, support of family members, comfort and amenities, convenience, and coping augmentation. These attributes need to be balanced by cost considerations in order to promote value positioning. In the case of hospitals, it has long been understood that the primary criterion for hospitalizing a patient is determining what level of nursing care and intervention he or she requires (Woods, 2002). So, if nursing care is the essence of the hospital product, aligning this care with patient needs is a vital part of the organization's success.

The marketing process includes deliberate steps taken to design an effective marketing plan for specific products or services that are aligned with and extensions of the organization-wide strategic plan (Kotler & Armstrong, 2008). Creating total value is one way to differentiate and position a product or service. Translating a product or service into a benefits package and effectively promoting those benefits can help advance marketing objectives (Alward & Camunas, 1991; Kotler, 1999).

Ensuring that nursing is provided with the necessary resources to, in turn, ensure positive patient outcomes is one of the most critical features that the health care product can offer to meet customer needs. For nursing, the core of patient care, marketing strategy should be analyzed and employed so that nursing services and strategic organizational goals are aligned.

Practical Tips

Tip #1: Learn What Is Most Important to Patients

Familiarize yourself with your organization's customer research. Pay close attention to those areas that patients report as highly important to their satisfaction. If the issues are highly influenced by nurses, assess your own practice against what is being rated. For example, are you able to respond to patient concerns effectively and promptly? If you find that improvement is warranted, work with your manager and other colleagues to identify barriers to providing the level of service you desire and participate in developing solutions to remove the barriers.

Tip #2: Establish Priorities

With the rapidly increasing barrage of initiatives being implemented at U.S. hospitals and the continuing shortage of professional staff, especially nurses, it can be impossible to focus equal attention on all that is demanded of you. Work with your manager to identify the highest priorities in your particular role, and come to agreement on the measurable outcomes you will track to affirm that the priorities have been appropriately aligned.

Tip #3: Influence Your Environment

Truly excellent organizations understand that every individual must know what is important to customers and be able to deliver on what is important. Take stock of what you can personally affect in the patient experience—whether by changing your individual behaviors, learning a new skill, or collaborating with others to identify and address issues that get in the way of delivering safe, high-quality patient care. Engage, and stay engaged, in systems designed to improve care.

LEADERSHIP AND MANAGEMENT IMPLICATIONS

Marketing comprises "the analysis, planning, and control of exchanges in order to develop and hold relationships with priority clients, suppliers, partners, and relevant publics, such as employers, other health care providers, and the media" (Harvey, 1998, p. 189). Thus understanding the motivations and reasons for transactions between organizations and clients is central to the practice of marketing in health care.

Adopting a marketing orientation has both leadership and management implications for nurses. An analysis of the internal and external landscape helps identify primary markets for nursing services. Patients are the first obvious market. However, other health care providers and even the pool of potential nurse employees can be primary markets for nursing. Nurse leaders are responsible for developing ways to articulate the value of the nursing product to purchasers and partners. Nurse leaders can also develop nursing internally with an eye toward marketing to prospective employees and retaining current ones—a critical consideration with the prolonged nursing shortage that lies ahead.

Profound ethical issues and controversies abound in health care. End-of-life care, organ procurement, reproductive technology and parenting, human gene therapy, and health care costs are but a few examples (Alward & Camunas, 1991). A unique layer of ethical issues may arise around the marketing of health care, one in which marketing ethics is also amplified. Non-profit and other social sector organizations, like hospitals, have a higher ethical standard to meet because they serve the greater public benefit and are often afforded special rights, privileges, and financial support that for-profit organizations do not receive (Andreasen & Kotler, 2008).

There is an inherent order to things in marketing. If a health care system or provider has not developed a product or service to conform to industry standards, promoting the product or service can present an ethical challenge. For example, can a hospital, in good conscience, promote the opening of a state-of-the-art cancer facility when it has not invested in recruiting and orienting competent specialized nurses, physicians, and other caregivers? This is an example in which the product is not just the building, the equipment, and the beds. In fact, here, the caregivers are the product's primary feature. Attaching an elegant sign to a building and filling the building with the latest equipment do not make it a cancer center (Woods & Cardin, 2002). These issues challenge nurse leaders and managers who may envision effective marketing strategies yet confront ethical dilemmas when seeking to implement them.

In the marketing context, nurse leaders contribute vision for meeting current and future customer needs and creating and supporting the systems that maximize nurses' contributions to excellent patient care. Leaders analyze and translate environmental data to support and inspire good decision making at all levels in the organization. Managers contribute further by actively participating in the delivery of services, providing and communicating data that support day-to-day decision making, and ensuring that optimal systems and resources are present to meet patient care standards.

CURRENT ISSUES AND TRENDS

Change is such a pervasive characteristic of the health care industry that achieving or sustaining market leadership over competitors in this turbulent market may seem daunting. However, environmental turbulence and rapid change can also clarify the difference between competitors' resources and capabilities. This can lead to greater dispersion of profitability in the health care industry (Grant, 1991). Making good strategic decisions in the face of industry turbulence can set an organization apart from competitors far more rapidly than in a stable market. The key is to be ready with the services or products that consumers need to help them cope with the change. Helpful strategies include analyzing the business in five categories: (1) outputs, (2) personnel, (3) resources, (4) operations, and (5) customers. A series of questions then can be asked, as follows (Zell, 2002):

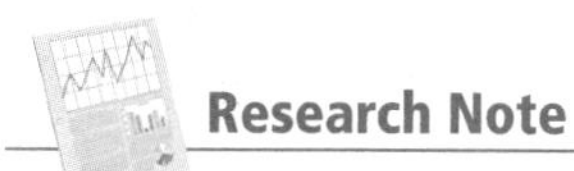

Research Note

Source: Press Ganey Associates, Inc. (2007). *Hospital pulse report 2007: Patient perspectives on American health care*. South Bend, IN: Author.

Purpose

To examine the experiences and perceptions of patients treated at U.S. acute care hospitals in 2006.

Discussion

Press Ganey is a leading provider of patient satisfaction research services for individual hospitals and health care systems. This Pulse Report reflects the aggregate patient satisfaction findings for more than 1700 acute care hospitals. The report provides national patient perspectives regarding the quality of hospital care.

Among the key findings from the research are the following:

- Surprisingly, patients were very complimentary when writing comments on their surveys. Almost half of the comments were positive. Patients were three times more likely to write a positive comment about their nurse or physician than a negative comment.
- Patients are more critical of their physical surroundings than they are about their care—57% of their comments about their hospital room were negative versus only 25% positive.
- Communication between hospital staff and patients needs improvement. From the patient perspective, the top priority for improving hospitals is responding better to patient concerns and complaints.
- Patients report higher safety ratings when they are presented with more information regarding their rights and end-of-life issues.

The researchers concluded that, "patients want care that is safe, complete, and delivered in a manner that respects their personhood. Communication is a key driver of satisfaction. Patients want more attention and credence given to their personal needs. Responding to concerns with compassion and sensitivity is essential to providing quality patient care. Even clinical care can be affected when the patient's personal needs are not met. The bottom line is, if hospitals listen to what patients are saying they can offer them better quality health care."

Application to Practice

Beginning with discharges in July 2007, the Centers for Medicare and Medicaid Services (CMS) now requires hospitals to participate in HCAHPS®, Hospital Consumer Assessment of Healthcare Providers and Systems, to be eligible to receive full CMS reimbursement. The major goals of the program are the following:

- To provide comparable data on patient perspectives that give consumers an "apples to apples" comparison among hospitals
- To encourage hospitals to improve their quality of care by publicly reporting scores
- To improve transparency and accountability of health care quality through public reporting

Press Ganey identified five questions on the Hospital Pulse survey that they concluded are the best predictors of how patients will rate hospitals on the HCAHPS® survey. The questions focus on these five areas:

- Attention to personal needs
- Response to concerns/complaints
- Nurses treating the patient with courtesy/respect
- Doctors listening carefully to the patient
- Staff doing everything to relieve pain

By concentrating on these five issues, a hospital could achieve a higher Overall Rating of the Hospital score on HCAHPS®. Because scores will be publicly reported and therefore influence patients' choices on where they go for care, achieving this high rating is especially important to hospitals. There are many marketing implications to this new public reporting system. Nurses have primary or significant influence over most of the focus areas of highest importance to the patient.

LEADERSHIP & MANAGEMENT BEHAVIORS

Leadership Behaviors

- Envisions new and innovative ways to meet customers' needs and wants
- Anticipates customer expectations based on environmental scanning data
- Inspires others to identify and meet customers' needs and wants
- Provides leadership in strategic marketing planning process
- Role-models effective communication, collaboration, and relationship building; inspires these behaviors in others
- Finds and develops new opportunities

Management Behaviors

- Analyzes and reports on markets and market segments
- Plans marketing mix and tactics
- Monitors performance and market share
- Allocates marketing resources
- Coordinates marketing staffing

Overlap Areas

- Promotes healthy work environments that sustain marketable nursing services of high quality
- Contributes to the marketing process
- Recognizes and promotes the value of the contribution that nurses make
- Links nursing to the organization's marketing plan and activities
- Communicates with staff and customers

- Can we adapt to the change?
- How are we going to do this?
- What can we add to meet our customers' needs under the change scenario?
- Who will be responsible for this development?
- How will it integrate into our present products and services?

Gathering and analyzing information will lay the foundation for proactive capitalization on change opportunities. Change may open the door to new products, services, or ventures.

A multitude of entrenched trends have emerged that affect the marketing of nursing and health care services—none more concerning than the protracted nursing shortage that is predicted to linger for decades. There is growing evidence that insufficient nurse staffing in hospitals is one of the greatest dangers to patient safety the hospital industry has ever faced (Joint Commission on Accreditation of Healthcare Organizations [JCAHO], 2002; Needleman et al., 2002). Hospitals that can preserve and optimize this scarce resource will benefit with a distinct advantage over competitors that fail to optimize their nursing resources. As the public becomes further educated about the dangers of the nursing shortage and the related problem of medical errors, hospitals are increasingly promoting the experience and skill of nursing staff as a point of differentiation.

With increasing scrutiny from regulators, payers, and consumers, hospitals increasingly showcase national recognition to differentiate themselves from their competitors—not only in the eyes of patients but also to attract nurses, physicians, and other employees. National recognition programs gaining momentum include the following:

- American Association of Critical-Care Nurses Beacon Award for Critical Care Excellence
- American Nurses Credentialing Center Magnet Recognition Program®
- Malcolm Baldrige National Quality Award
- *U.S. News & World Report's* list of "America's Best Hospitals"

Quality and patient safety have emerged as a focal point for health care organizations, regulators, and the patients they serve. Increasingly, quality statistics on hospitals and physicians are available to the public. At the same time, the pay-for-performance movement has resulted in the Centers for Medicaid and Medicare Services (CMS) providing financial incentives for hospitals to report quality measures and for physicians who improve their quality scores. To further drive improved patient safety and quality of care, CMS now imposes penalties, in the form of lower or no reimbursement, for those hospitals that do not comply or that have preventable errors. The implications and outcomes of these new strategies are not yet known. Should the strategies prove effective, patients stand to gain tremendously. Hospitals with strong patient safety and quality scores also stand to gain by attracting more patients and receiving higher reimbursements from payers.

Summary

- Marketing is a business concept related to the activities of determining and meeting customer wants and needs.
- Marketing is a social and managerial process.
- Marketing capitalizes on opportunities.
- Changes in health care create market opportunities for nurses.
- Nurse leaders and managers need to adopt a marketing orientation. A marketing orientation is a focus on customers.
- Marketing is widely employed in competitive and resource-constrained environments like health care.
- Marketing must be central to and included in organizational strategic planning.
- A marketing mix is a blend of tools and tactics to elicit the desired response from the target markets.
- A marketing mix is based on product, price, place, and promotion; otherwise known as *customer solution, cost, convenience, and communication.*
- Marketing results in voluntary transactions and exchanges in a market.
- The marketing process uses research, segmentation, mix, implementation, and control.
- The primary elements of marketing are strategy and research. Marketing strategies, and the tactics that support the strategies, help position organizations to reach their goals. Market research is the systematic study of markets.

Case Study

A regional hospital system in a highly competitive suburban market has decided to purchase a very small community hospital. The hospital currently offers limited services and has a questionable reputation but is seen as an opportunity to stake a claim in a part of the region that is experiencing rapid population growth because of aggressive real estate development. The community has a very high proportion of affluent young professionals with small children. There are no full-service hospitals within 20 miles of this burgeoning community where the small hospital is located. Competing hospital systems do not have any satellite centers or clinics in the area yet.

Rather than incurring the significant capital expense associated with renovating and expanding the small 70-bed community hospital, the system is considering keeping the hospital as it is and attaching it to the same license as their nearest full-service hospital, which has 500 beds and is 25 miles away. In addition to evaluating the small hospital's offered services against the changing needs of the community, leaders in the health care system are considering placing one or more satellite centers, such as a women's health center, near the small hospital to appeal to very specific needs in the community. It is thought that the satellite centers and the small community hospital will act as feeders to the large full-service hospital, which is in tight competition with another hospital that is 5 miles closer to the growing community the small hospital has been serving. If, for example, women are able to get their wellness examinations and prenatal care at the satellite center in their community, they will likely be admitted to the large hospital for surgery and childbirth.

Which elements of the marketing mix are at play in this scenario? What are the implications from the customer's perspective, including physicians? What role could nursing play in helping the hospital system determine its positioning, differentiation, and segmentation strategies?

CRITICAL THINKING EXERCISE

Luisa Herrera is a nurse in a community hospital maternity center. She is at the end of her rope and is considering leaving her job. As one of a handful of nurses in her hospital who speak fluent Spanish, she is frequently asked to interpret for other nurses' patients and their families. Herrera's growing concern is that her own patients and families are not receiving quality care because of her added duties as an interpreter.

The hospital has expended significant financial and human resources promoting itself as the market leader in specialized maternity services for the Latino community. Full-page newspaper advertisements and attractive brochures proclaim in Spanish and English: "With our full complement of bilingual physicians and nurses, we ensure that you and your family will be active participants in every decision affecting your care."

1. What is the problem?
2. What marketing strategy is the hospital trying to adopt?
3. What might have led to the implementation problems Herrera and her colleagues are experiencing?
4. What can Herrera do to become part of a solution?
5. What steps might the hospital take to ensure successful implementation of its strategy?
6. What could prevent this problem from occurring when another new service or feature is launched?

References

Chapter 1

Alvesson, M., & Sveningsson, S. (2003). Managers doing leadership: The extra-ordinarization of the mundane. *Human Relations, 56*(12), 1435–1459.

American Nurses Credentialing Center (ANCC). (2008). Modifying the Magnet™ model: The shape of things to come. *American Nurse Today, 3*(7), 22.

American Organization of Nurse Executives (AONE). (2005). AONE nurse executive competencies. *Nurse Leader, 3*(1), 15–21.

Anderson, R. (1997). Future organizational leadership. *Journal of Professional Nursing, 13*(6), 334.

Aroskar, M. (1994). The challenge of ethical leadership in nursing. *Journal of Professional Nursing, 10*(5), 270.

Barker, A. (1990). *Transformational nursing leadership: A vision for the future.* Baltimore: Williams & Wilkins.

Barker, A. (1991). An emerging leadership paradigm: Transformational leadership. *Nursing & Health Care, 12*(4), 204–207.

Bass, B. (1982). *Stogdill's handbook of leadership.* New York: The Free Press.

Bass, B. (1985). *Leadership and performance beyond expectations.* New York: The Free Press.

Bass, B., & Avolio, B. (1990). *Transformational leadership development: Manual for the Multifactor Leadership Questionnaire.* Palo Alto, CA: Consulting Psychologists Press.

Bass, B., Waldman, D., Avolio, B., & Bibb, M. (1987). Transformational leadership and the falling dominos effect. *Group and Organizational Studies, 12*(1), 73–87.

Bennis, W. (1994). *On becoming a leader.* Reading, MA: Addison-Wesley.

Bennis, W., & Nanus, B. (1985). *Leaders: The strategies for taking charge.* New York: Harper & Row.

Bennis, W. G. (2004). The seven ages of the leader. *Harvard Business Review, 82*(1), 46–53.

Bennis, W. G., & Thomas, R. J. (2002). Crucibles of leadership. *Harvard Business Review, 80*(9), 39–45.

Blake, R., & Mouton, J. (1964). *The managerial grid.* Houston: Gulf Publishing.

Blake, R. R., & McCanse, A. A. (1991). *Leadership dilemmas—Grid solutions.* Houston: Gulf Publishing.

Brakey, M. (1991). Are you a good follower? *Nursing 91, 21*(12), 78–81.

Burns, J. (1978). *Leadership.* New York: Harper & Row.

Cartwright, D., & Zander, A. (Eds.). (1960). *Group dynamics: Research and theory* (2nd ed.). Evanston, IL: Row, Peterson.

Clancy, T. R. (2003). Courage and today's nurse leader. *Nursing Administration Quarterly, 27*(2), 128–132.

Collins, J. (2001). *Good to great.* New York: HarperCollins, Publishers.

Curtin, L. (1989). Things unattempted yet. *Nursing Management, 20*(7), 7–8.

Drucker, P. F. (1994). *The post-capitalist society.* New York: Harper & Row.

Drucker, P. F. (1996). Foreword. In F. Hesselbein, M. Goldsmith, & R. Beckhard (Eds.), *The leader of the future: New visions, strategies, and practices for the next era.* San Francisco: Jossey-Bass.

Dunham, J., & Klafehn, K. (1990). Transformational leadership and the nurse executive. *Journal of Nursing Administration, 20*(4), 28–34.

Fiedler, F. (1967). *A theory of leadership effectiveness.* New York: McGraw-Hill.

Fiedler, F., & Chemers, M. (1984). *Improving leadership effectiveness: The leader match concept* (2nd ed.). New York: John Wiley & Sons.

Fiedler, F., & Garcia, J. (1987). *New approaches to effective leadership: Cognitive resources and organizational performance.* New York: John Wiley & Sons.

Goleman, D. (1997). *Emotional intelligence.* New York: Bantam Books.

Goleman, D. (2000). *Working with emotional intelligence.* New York: Bantam Books.

Goleman, D. (2007). *Social intelligence: The new science of social relationships.* New York: Bantam Dell Publishing Group.

Grant, A. (1994). *The professional nurse: Issues and actions.* Springhouse, PA: Springhouse.

Greenleaf, R. K. (2002). *Servant leadership: A journey into the nature of legitimate power and greatness* (25th anniversary ed.). Mahwah, NJ: Paulist Press.

Guidera, M., & Gilmore, C. (1988). In defense of followership. *American Journal of Nursing, 88*(7), 1017.

Hagenow, N. R. (2001). Care executives: Organizational intelligence for these times. *Nursing Administration Quarterly, 25*(4), 30–35.

Heifetz, R. A., & Laurie, D. L. (1997). The work of leadership. *Harvard Business Review, 75*(1), 124–134.

Helgeson, S. (1995a). *The web of inclusion: A new architecture for building organizations.* New York: Doubleday.

Helgeson, S. (1995b). *The female advantage: Women's ways of leadership* (2nd ed.). New York: Doubleday.

Hersey, P., Blanchard, K. H., & Johnson, D. E. (2008). *Management of organizational behavior: Leading human resources* (9th ed.). Upper Saddle River, NJ: Pearson Education.

Huber, D. L., Maas, M., McCloskey, J., Scherb, C. A., Goode, C. J., & Watson, C. (2000). Evaluating nursing administration instruments. *Journal of Nursing Administration, 30*(5), 251–272.

Huber, D. L., & Watson, C. A. (2001). *Effective leadership in health care organizations.* Indianapolis: The College Network.

Institute of Medicine (IOM). (2004). *Keeping patients safe: Transforming the work environment of nurses.* Washington, DC: National Academies Press.

Kelley, R. (1988). In praise of followers. *Harvard Business Review, 66*, 142–148.

Kison, C. (1989). Leadership: How, who and what? *Nursing Management, 20*(11), 72–74.

Kleinman, C. (2004). The relationship between managerial leadership behaviors and staff nurse retention. *Hospital Topics, 82*(4), 2–9.

Knickman, J. R., & Snell, E. K. (2002). The 2030 problem: Caring for aging baby boomers. *Health Services Research, 37*(4), 849–884.

Kotter, J. (2001). What leaders really do. *Harvard Business Review, 79*(11), 85–96.

Kouzes, J., & Posner, B. (1987). *The leadership challenge.* San Francisco: Jossey-Bass.

Kouzes, J., & Posner, B. (1988). *The leadership practices inventory.* San Diego: Pfeiffer & Company.

Kouzes, J., & Posner, B. (1990). *Leadership practices inventory (LPI): A self-assessment and analysis.* San Diego: Pfeiffer & Company.

Kramer, M. (1990). The Magnet hospitals: Excellence revisited. *Journal of Nursing Administration, 20*(9), 35–44.

Likert, R. (1961). *New patterns of management.* New York: McGraw-Hill.

Longest, B. B., Jr. (1998). Managerial competence at senior levels of integrated delivery systems. *Journal of Healthcare Management, 43*(2), 115–133.

Malloch, K. (2002). Trusting organizations: Describing and measuring employee-to-employee relationships. *Nursing Administration Quarterly, 26*(3), 12–19.

Marchionni, C., & Ritchie, J. (2008). Organizational factors that support the implementation of a nursing Best Practice Guideline. *Journal of Nursing Management, 16*(3), 266–274.

Mathena, K. A. (2002). Nursing manager leadership skills. *Journal of Nursing Administration, 32*(3), 136–142.

McCauley, G. (2004). *Leadership in a quantum age.* Ottawa, Ontario, Canada: ProGenerations, a division of the WEL Systems Institute. Retrieved September 6, 2004, from www.progenerations.com/articles/Leadership.htm

McClure, M., Poulin, M., Sovie, M., & Wandelt, M. (1983). *Magnet hospitals: Attraction and retention of professional nurses.* Kansas City, MO: American Nurses Association.

McDaniel, C., & Wolf, G. (1992). Transformational leadership in nursing service: A test of theory. *Journal of Nursing Administration, 22*(2), 60–65.

Mintzberg, H. (1998). Covert leadership: Notes on managing professionals. *Harvard Business Review, 76*(6), 140–147.

Murphy, D. (1990). Followers for a new era. *Nursing Management, 21*(7), 68–69.

Murphy, M., & DeBack, V. (1991). Today's nursing leaders: Creating the vision. *Nursing Administration Quarterly, 16*(1), 71–80.

O'Connor, M. (2008). The dimensions of leadership: A foundation for caring competency. *Nursing Administration Quarterly, 32*(1), 21–26.

O'Neil, E., Morjikian, R. L., Cherner, D., Hirschkorn, C., & West, T. (2008). Developing nursing leaders: An overview of trends and programs. *Journal of Nursing Administration, 38*(4), 178–183.

Pagonis, W. (1992). The work of the leader. *Harvard Business Review, 70*(6), 118–126.

Pipe, T. B. (2008). Illuminating the inner leadership journey by engaging intention and mindfulness as guided by caring theory. *Nursing Administration Quarterly, 32*(2), 117–125.

Porter-O'Grady, T. (2003). A different age for leadership, Part 1. *Journal of Nursing Administration, 33*(2), 105–110.

Rosenfeld, P. (1994). *Profiles of the newly licensed nurse: Historical trends and future implications* (2nd ed.) (Publication No. 19-2530). New York: National League for Nursing Press.

Shirey, M. R. (2006). Building authentic leadership and enhancing entrepreneurial performance. *Clinical Nurse Specialist, 20*(6), 280–282.

Shirey, M. R. (2007). Leadership and organizational strategies to increase innovative thinking. *Clinical Nurse Specialist, 21*(4), 191–194.

Smola, B. (1988). Refinement and validation of a tool measuring leadership characteristics of baccalaureate nursing students. In O. Strickland, & C. Waltz (Eds.), *Measurement of nursing outcomes* (Vol. 2, pp. 314–366). New York: Springer.

Stodgill, R. (1963). *Manual for the Leader Behavior Description Questionnaire—Form XII: An experimental revision.* Columbus, OH: Ohio State University.

Tannenbaum, R., & Schmidt, W. (1973). How to choose a leadership pattern. *Harvard Business Review, 51*(3), 162–180.

Tornabeni, J. (2001). The competency game: My take on what it really takes to lead. *Nursing Administration Quarterly, 25*(4), 1–13.

Ulrich, D., Zenger, J., & Smallwood, N. (1999). *Results-oriented leadership*. Boston: Harvard Business School Press.

Upenieks, V. (2003a). Nurse leaders' perceptions of what compromises successful leadership in today's acute inpatient environment. *Nursing Administration Quarterly, 27*(2), 140–152.

Upenieks, V. (2003b). What constitutes effective leadership? *Journal of Nursing Administration, 33*(9), 456–467.

U.S. Census Bureau. (2001). *Age: 2000. Census 2000 brief.* Washington, DC: Author.

U.S. Census Bureau. (2008). *2006 American Community Survey Data Profile Highlights*. Washington, DC: Author. Retrieved July 12, 2008, from http://factfinder.census.gov/servlet/ACSSAFFFacts?_event=Search&geo_id=&_geoContext=&_street=&_county=United+States&_cityTown=United+States&_state=&_zip=&_lang=en&_sse=on&pctxt=fph&pgsl=010

U.S. Department of Health and Human Services (USDHHS). (1997). *The registered nurse population*. Rockville, MD: Author.

U.S. Department of Health and Human Services (USDHHS). (2002). *The registered nurse population, March 2000: Findings from the national sample survey of registered nurses*. Rockville, MD: Author. Retrieved July 5, 2004, from www.bhpr.hrsa.gov/healthworkforce/reports/rnsurvey/rnss1.htm

U.S. Department of Health and Human Services (USDHHS), Health Resources and Services Administration (HRSA). (2008). *The registered nurse population*. Washington, DC: Author. Retrieved July 12, 2008, from http://bhpr.hrsa.gov/healthworkforce/rnsurvey04/

Wheatley, M. J. (1992). *Leadership and the new science: Learning about organization from an orderly universe*. San Francisco: Berrett-Koehler.

Wilson, C. K., & Porter-O'Grady, T. (1999). *Leading the revolution in health care: Advancing systems, igniting performance* (2nd ed.). Gaithersburg, MD: Aspen.

Yukl, G. (1981). *Leadership in organizations*. Englewood Cliffs, NJ: Prentice-Hall.

Chapter 2

Ackoff, R. (1981). *Creating the corporate future*. New York: John Wiley & Sons.

Aiken, T. (1994). *Legal, ethical, and political issues in nursing*. Philadelphia: F.A. Davis.

American Nurses Association (ANA). (2004). *Scope and standards for nurse administrators* (2nd ed.). Washington, DC: Author.

American Nurses Credentialing Center (ANCC). (2004). *ANCC certification: Specialty nursing, nursing administration (basic, advanced), clinical nurse specialist (community health and home health)*. Washington, DC: Author.

American Nurses Credentialing Center (ANCC). (2008). *Overview of ANCC Magnet Recognition Program® new model*. Silver Spring, MD: Author.

Bass, B., & Avolio, B. (1990). *Transformational leadership development: Manual for the Multifactor Leadership Questionnaire*. Palo Alto, CA: Consulting Psychologists Press.

Crowell, D. M. (1998). Organizations are relationships: A new view of management. *Nursing Management, 29*(5), 28–29.

Curtin, L. L. (2000). The first ten principles for the ethical administration of nursing services. *Nursing Administration Quarterly, 25*(1), 7–13.

Drucker, P. F. (1954). *The practice of management*. New York: Harper & Row.

Drucker, P. F. (1988). The coming of the new organization. *Harvard Business Review, 68*(1), 45–53.

Drucker, P. F. (2004). What makes an effective executive. *Harvard Business Review, 82*(6), 58–63.

Fayol, H. (1949). *General and industrial management*. London: Pitman & Sons.

Foust, J. (1994). Creating a future for nursing through interactive planning at the bedside. *Image, 26*(2), 129–131.

Genovich-Richards, J., & Carissimi, D. (1986). Developing nurses' managerial competence. *Nursing Management, 17*(3), 36–38.

Gosling, J., & Mintzberg, H. (2003). The five minds of a manager. *Harvard Business Review, 81*(11), 54–63.

Hayes-Roth, B., & Hayes-Roth, F. (1979). A cognitive model of planning. *Cognitive Science, 3*, 275–310.

Hersey, P., Blanchard, K. H., & Johnson, D. E. (2008). *Management of organizational behavior: Leading human resources* (9th ed.). Upper Saddle River, NJ: Pearson Education.

Herzliner, R. E. (1998). The managerial revolution in the U.S. health care sector: Lessons from the U.S. economy. *Health Care Management Review, 23*(3), 19–29.

Jennings, B. M., Scalzi, C. C., Rodgers, J. D., III, & Keane, A. (2007). Differentiating nursing leadership and management competencies. *Nursing Outlook, 55*, 169–175.

Kanter, R. M. (1989). The new managerial work. *Harvard Business Review, 69*(6), 85–92.

Katz, R. (1955). Skills of an effective administrator. *Harvard Business Review, 33*(1), 33–42.

Kepler, T. (1980). Mastering the people skills. *Journal of Nursing Administration, 10*(11), 15–20.

Koontz, H. (1961). The management theory jungle. *Academy of Management Journal*, (December), 174–188.

Levenstein, A. (1985). *Planning. Nursing Management, 16*(9), 54–55.

Lewin, K. (1947). Frontiers in group dynamics: Concept, method, and reality in social science; social equilibria and social change. *Human Relations, 1*(1), 5–41.

McClure, M. (1991). Introduction. In I. Goertzen (Ed.), *Differentiating nursing practice: Into the twenty-first century* (pp. 1–11). Kansas City, MO: American Academy of Nursing.

McNamara, C. (1999a). *Skills and practices in organizational management.* Minneapolis, MN: Carter McNamara. Retrieved July 6, 2004, from www.managementhelp.org/mgmnt/skills.htm

McNamara, C. (1999b). *Basic guidelines for successful planning process.* Minneapolis, MN: Carter McNamara. Retrieved July 6, 2004, from www.managementhelp.org/plan_dec/gen_plan/gen_plan.htm

McNamara, C. (1999c). *Management function of organizing: Overview of methods.* Minneapolis, MN: Authenticity Consulting, LLC. Retrieved July 6, 2004, from www.mapnp.org/library/orgnzing/orgnzing.htm

McNamara, C. (1999d). *Management function of coordinating/controlling: Overview of basic methods.* Minneapolis, MN: Authenticity Consulting, LLC. Retrieved July 6, 2004, from www.mapnp.org/library/cntrllng/cntrllng.htm

McNamara, C. (1999e). *Introduction to management.* Minneapolis, MN: Authenticity Consulting, LLC. Retrieved July 6, 2004, from www.managementhelp.org/mng_thry/mng_thry.htm

McNamara, C. (1999f). *New paradigm in management.* Minneapolis, MN: Carter McNamara. Retrieved July 6, 2004, from www.managementhelp.org/mgmnt/paradigm.htm

McNamara, C. (1999g). *Brief overview of contemporary theories in management.* Minneapolis, MN: Authenticity Consulting, LLC. Retrieved July 6, 2004, from www.managementhelp.org/mgmnt/cntmpory.htm

Metts, L. (2008). The emotionally intelligent case manager. *Case In Point*, (April/May), 11–13.

Mintzberg, H. (1973). *The nature of managerial work.* New York: Harper & Row.

Mintzberg, H. (1975). The manager's job: Folklore and fact. In M. Matteson, & J. Ivancevich (Eds.), *Management classics* (3rd ed., pp. 63–85). Plano, TX: Business Publications.

Mintzberg, H. (1994). Managing as blended care. *Journal of Nursing Administration, 24*(9), 29–36.

Morse, J. J., & Wagner, F. R. (1978). Measuring the process of managerial effectiveness. *Academy of Management Journal, 21*(1), 23–35.

Organizational Dynamics. (1975). *The evolution of management theory. Part I* (Videotape). Burlington, MA: Organizational Dynamics.

Porter-O'Grady, T. (1997). Process leadership and the death of management. *Nursing Economic$, 15*(6), 286–293.

Rosenhead, J. (1998). Complexity theory and management practice. *The Human Daily Review.* Retrieved July 6, 2004, from www.human-nature.com/science-as-culture/rosenhead.html

Stacey, R. D. (1993). *Strategic management and organizational dynamics.* London: Pitman.

Steiner, G. (1962). Making long-range company planning pay off. *California Management Review, 4*(2), 28–41.

Sull, D. N. (2003). Managing by commitments. *Harvard Business Review, 81*(6), 82–91.

Thomas, L. (1983). *The youngest science: Notes of a medicine watcher.* New York: Viking Press.

von Bertalanffy, L. (1968). *General systems theory.* New York: George Braziller.

Wheatley, M. J. (1999). *Leadership and the new science: Discovering order in a chaotic world* (2nd ed.). San Francisco: Berrett-Koehler Publishers.

Zaleznik, A. (1992). Managers and leaders: Are they different? *Harvard Business Review, 70*(2), 126–135.

Chapter 3

Alas, R. (2007). Organizational change from learning perspective. *Problems and Perspectives in Management, 5*(2), 43–50.

American Organization of Nurse Executives (AONE). (2005). AONE nurse executive competencies. *Nurse Leader, 3*(1), 15–21.

Balfour, M., & Clarke, C. (2001). Searching for sustainable change. *Journal of Clinical Nursing, 10*, 44–50.

Balogun, J. (2006). Managing change: Steering a course between intended strategies and unanticipated outcomes. *Long Range Planning, 39*, 29–49.

Bennis, W., Benne, K., Chin, R., & Corey, K. (1976). *The planning of change.* New York: Holt, Rinehart & Winston.

Bennis, W. G., Benne, K. D., & Chin, R. (Eds.). (1961). *The planning of change: Readings in the applied behavioral sciences.* New York: Holt, Rinehart & Winston.

Bhola, H. S. (1994). The CLER model: Thinking through change. *Nursing Management, 25*(5), 59–63.

Bonalumi, N., & Fisher, K. (1999). Healthcare change: Challenge for nurse administrators. *Nursing Administration Quarterly, 23*(2), 69–73.

Burnes, B. (2004). Kurt Lewin and complexity theories: Back to the future? *Journal of Change Management, 4*(4), 309–325.

Burns, J. M. (1978). *Leadership.* New York: Harper & Row.

Cambridge Advanced Learner's Dictionary. (2008). Retrieved July 28, 2008, from http://dictionary.cambridge.org/define.asp?key=84436&dict=CALD

Copnell, B., & Bruni, N. (2006). Breaking the silence: Nurses' understandings of change. *Journal of Advanced Nursing, 55*(3), 301–309.

Davidhizar, R. (1996). Surviving organizational change. *Health Care Supervisor, 14*(4), 19–24.

Drucker, P. (1985). *Innovation and entrepreneurship: Practice and principles.* New York: Harper & Row.

Drucker, P. (1992). *Managing for the future: The 1990s and beyond.* New York: Truman Talley Books/Plume.

Falk-Rafael, A. R. (2000). Nurses' orientations to change: Debunking the resistance to change myth. *Journal of Professional Nursing, 16*(6), 336–344.

Fagin, C. (2001). *When care becomes a burden: Diminishing access to adequate nursing.* New York: Milbank Memorial Fund.

Gilmartin, M. J. (1999). Creativity: The fuel of innovation. *Nursing Administration Quarterly, 23*(2), 1–8.

Gustafson, D. H., Sainfort, F., Eichler, M., Adams, L., Bisognano, M., & Steudel, H. (2003). Developing and testing a model to predict outcomes of organizational change. *Health Services Research, 38*(2), 751–776.

Havelock, R. (1973). *The change agent's guide to innovation in education.* Englewood Cliffs, NJ: Educational Technology Publications.

Hayman, B., Cioffi, J., & Wilkes, L. (2006). Redesign of the model of nursing practice in an acute care ward: Nurses' experiences. *Collegian (Royal College of Nursing, Australia), 13*(1), 31–36.

Hersey, P., Blanchard, K. H., & Johnson, D. E. (2008). *Management of organizational behavior: Leading human resources* (9th ed.). Upper Saddle River, NJ: Pearson Education.

Hughes, F. (2006). Nurses at the forefront of innovation. *International Nursing Review, 53,* 94–101.

Issel, L. M., & Anderson, R. A. (1996). Take charge: Managing six transformations in healthcare delivery. *Nursing Economic$, 14*(2), 78–85.

Johnson, S. (1998). *Who moved my cheese?* New York: G.P. Putnam's Sons.

Jones, J. E., & Bearley, W. L. (1996). *Organizational change-readiness scale.* Amherst, MA: HRD Press.

Kanter, R. M. (1983). *The change masters: Innovation and entrepreneurship in the American corporation.* New York: Simon & Schuster.

Kerfoot, K. (1998). Leading change is leading creativity. *Nursing Economic$, 16*(2), 98–99.

Leeman, J., Baernholdt, M., & Sandelowski, M. (2007). Developing a theory-based taxonomy of methods for implementing change in practice. *Journal of Advanced Nursing, 58*(2), 191–200.

Lewin, K. (1947). Frontiers in group dynamics: Concept, method, and reality in social science; social equilibrium and social change. *Human Relations, 1*(1), 5–41.

Lewin, K. (1951). *Field theory in social science: Selected theoretical papers.* New York: Harper & Row.

Lippitt, G. (1973). *Visualizing change: Model building and the change process.* La Jolla, CA: University Associates.

Lippitt, R., Watson, J., & Westley, B. (1958). *The dynamics of planned change: A comparative study of principles and techniques.* New York: Harcourt, Brace & World.

Manion, J. (1995). Understanding the seven stages of change. *American Journal of Nursing, 95*(4), 41–43.

McCloskey, J., Maas, M., Huber, D., Kasparek, A., Specht, J., Ramler, C., et al. (1994). Nursing management innovations: A need for systematic evaluation. *Nursing Economic$, 12*(1), 35–44.

Perlman, D., & Takacs, G. (1990). The 10 stages of change. *Nursing Management, 21*(4), 33–38.

Pettigrew, A. M. (1990). Longitudinal field research on change: Theory and practice. *Organizational Science, 3*(1), 267–292.

Porter-O'Grady, T., & Malloch, K. (2007). *Quantum leadership: A resource for health care innovation* (2nd ed.). Boston, MA: Jones and Bartlett.

Robbins, B., & Davidhizar, R. (2007). Transformational leadership in healthcare today. *The Health Care Manager, 26*(3), 234–239.

Rogers, E. M. (2003). *Diffusion of innovations* (5th ed.). New York: Free Press.

Romano, C. (1990). Diffusion of technology innovation. *Advances in Nursing Science, 13*(2), 11–21.

Rost, J. (1991). *Leadership for the 21st century.* New York: Praeger Publishers.

Senge, P. M., Kleiner, A., Roberts, C., Ross, R. B., & Smith, B. J. (1994). *The fifth discipline fieldbook: Strategies and tools for building a learning organization.* New York: Doubleday.

Shanley, C. (2007). Management of change for nurses: Lessons from the discipline of organizational studies. *Journal of Nursing Management, 15,* 538–546.

Shirey, M. R. (2007). Competencies and tips for effective leadership: From novice to expert. *Journal of Nursing Administration, 37*(4), 167–183.

Tiffany, C., Cheatham, A., Doornbos, D., Loudermelt, L., & Momadi, G. (1994). Planned change theory: Survey of nursing periodical literature. *Nursing Management, 25*(7), 54–59.

Tiffany, C. R., & Lutjens, L. R. J. (1998). *Planned change theories for nursing: Review, analysis, and implications.* Thousand Oaks, CA: Sage.

Watzlawick, P., Weakland, J., & Fisch, R. (1974). *Change: Principles of problem formation and resolution.* New York: Norton.

Wakefield, M. (2003). Change drivers for nursing and health care. *Nursing Economic$, 21*(3), 150–151.

Wheatley, M. J. (2007). *Finding our way: Leadership for an uncertain time.* San Francisco, CA: Berrett-Koehler.

Chapter 4

Agency for Healthcare Research and Quality. (2002). *National Healthcare Quality Report: Update.* Fact Sheet. AHRQ Publication No. 02-P028. Rockville, MD: Author.

Aiken, L. H., Clarke, S. P., Sloane, D. M., Sochalski, J. A., Busse, R., Clarke, H., et al. (2001). Nurses' reports on hospital care in five countries. *Health Affairs, 20*(3), 43–53.

Aiken, L. H., & Fagin, C. M. (1997). Evaluating the consequences of hospital restructuring. *Medical Care, 35*(10), OS1–OS4.

Aiken, L. H., Lake, E. T., Sochalski, J., & Sloane, D. M. (1997). Design of an outcomes study of the organization of hospital AIDS care. *Research in the Sociology of Health Care, 14,* 3–26.

Aiken, L. H., Sochalski, J., & Lake, E. T. (1997). Studying outcomes of organizational change in health services. *Medical Care, 35*(11), NS6–NS18.

Aiken, L. H., Sloane, D. M., & Lake, E. T. ((1997). Satisfaction with inpatient acquired immunodeficiency syndrome care: A national comparison of dedicated and scattered-bed units. *Medical Care, 35*(9), 948–962.

Aiken, L. H., Smith, H. L., & Lake, E. T. (1994). Lower Medicare mortality among a set of hospitals known for good nursing care. *Medical Care, 32*, 771–785.

Alderfer, C. P. (1980). *Consulting to underbounded systems* (Vol. 2). New York: Wiley.

American Nurses Association (ANA). (1997). *Implementing nursing's report card: A study of RN staffing, length of stay and patient outcomes.* Washington, DC: American Nurses Publishing.

American Nurses Association (ANA). (2004). *American Nurses Association's scope and standards for nurse administrators.* Silver Spring, MD: Author.

American Nurses Credentialing Center (ANCC). (2004). *Magnet Recognition Program®, Forces of Magnetism.* Silver Spring, MD: Author. Retrieved February 22, 2008, from www.nursecredentialing.org/magnet/forces.html

American Nurses Credentialing Center (ANCC). (2008). *Magnet Recognition Program®.* Silver Spring, MD: Author. Retrieved July 30, 2008, from http://nursecredentialing.org/Magnet.aspx

Anthony, M. K., Standing, T. S., Glick, J., Duffy, M., Paschall, F., Sauer, M., et al. (2005). Leadership and nurse retention: The pivotal role of nurse managers. *Journal of Nursing Administration, 35*, 146–155.

Blegen, M. A., Pepper, G. A., & Rosse, J. (2005). *Safety climate on hospital units: A new measure.* Retrieved February 1, 2008, from http://ahrq.gov/downloads/pub/advances/vol4/Blegen.pdf

Boyle, D. K., Bott, M. J., Hansen, H. E., Woods, C. Q., & Taunton, R. L. (1999). Managers' leadership and critical care nurses' intent to stay. *American Journal of Critical Care, 8*, 361–371.

Boyle, S. M. (2004). Nursing unit characteristics and patient outcomes. *Nursing Economic$, 22*, 111–119.

Brennan, P. F., & Anthony, M. K. (2000). Measuring nursing practice models using multiattribute utility theory. *Research in Nursing and Health, 23*, 372–382.

Clarke, S., Rockett, J., Sloane, D., & Aiken, L. (2002). Organizational climate, staffing, and safety equipment as predictors of needlestick injuries and near-misses in hospital nurses. *American Journal of Infection Control, 30*(4), 207–216.

Clarke, S., Sloane, D., & Aiken, L. (2002). Effects of hospital staffing and organizational climate on needlestick injuries to nurses. *American Journal of Public Health, 92*(7), 1115–1119.

Coeling, H., & Simms, L. (1993). Facilitating innovation at the nursing unit level through cultural assessment. Part 1. *Journal of Nursing Administration, 23*, 46–52.

Connor, M., Duncombe, D., Barclay, E., Bartel, S., Borden, C., Gross, E., et al. (2007). Creating a fair and just culture: One institution's path toward organizational change. *The Joint Commission Journal on Quality and Patient Safety, 33*, 617–624.

Daft, R. L. (2001). *Organizational theory and design* (7th ed.). New York: West Publishing.

DeJoy, D. M., Schaffer, B. S., Wilson, M. G., Vandenbert, R. J., & Butts, M. M. (2004). Creating safer workplaces: Assessing the determinants and role of safety climate. *Journal of Safety Research, 35*, 81–90.

Diers, D. K. (2001). *Between practice and ... Unpublished dissertation.* Sidney, Australia: University of Technology.

Duchscher, J. E., & Cowin, L. (2004). Multigenerational nurses in the workplace. *Journal of Nursing Administration, 34*, 493–501.

Hart, K., & Moore, M. (1989). The relationship among organizational climate variables and nurse stability in critical care units. *Journal of Professional Nursing, 5*(3), 124–131.

Hemingway, M., & Smith, C. (1999). Organizational climate and occupational stressors as predictors of withdrawal behaviors and injuries among nurses. *Journal of Occupational and Organizational Psychology, 72*, 285–299.

Hinshaw, A. S. (2008). Navigating the perfect storm: Balancing a culture of safety with workforce challenges. *Nursing Research, 57*, S4–S10.

Institute of Management Administration. (2000). Harvard Business School's 5 point quiz tells if your organization can learn. In *Management and Training Development.* Harvard Business School Press.

Institute of Medicine (IOM). (2001). *Crossing the quality chasm.* Washington, DC: National Academies Press.

Kimball, B., & O'Neill, E. (2002). *Health care's human crisis: The American nursing shortage.* Princeton, NJ: Robert Wood Johnson Foundation.

Koerner, J. G. (1996). Congruency between nurses' values and job requirements: A call for integrity. *Holistic Nursing Practice, 10*, 69–77.

Kohn, L. T., Corrigan, J. M., & Donaldson, M. S. (Eds.). (2000). *To err is human: Building a safer health system.* Washington, DC: National Academies Press.

Kramer, M., & Hafner, L. P. (1989). Shared values: Impact on staff nurse job satisfaction and perceived productivity. *Nursing Research, 38*, 172–177.

Litwin, G., & Stringer, R. (1968). *Motivation and organizational climate.* Boston: Division of Research, Graduate School of Business Administration, Harvard University.

Manojlovich, M. (2005). The effect of nursing leadership on hospital nurses' professional practice behavior. *Journal of Nursing Administration, 35*, 366–374.

Mark, B. A. (1996). Organizational culture. In J. J. Fitzpatrick, & J. Norbeck (Eds.), *Annual review of nursing research* (Vol. 14, pp. 145–163). New York: Springer Publishing.

Mark, B. A., Hughes, L. C., Belyea, M., Chang, Y., Hoffman, D., Jones, C. B., et al. (2007). Does safety climate moderate the influence of staffing adequacy and work condition on nurse injuries? *Journal of Safety Research, 38,* 431–446.

Marx, D. (2001). *Patient safety and the "Just Culture": A primer for health care executives.* New York: Columbia University.

McClure, M., Poulin, M., Sovie, M., & Wandelt, M. (1982). *Magnet hospitals: Attraction and retention of professional nurses.* Kansas City, MO: American Nurses Association.

Mitchell, P. H., & Shortell, S. M. (1997). Adverse outcomes and variations in organization of care delivery. *Medical Care, 35,* NS19–NS32.

Needleman, J., Buerhaus, P. I., Mattke, S., Stewart, M., & Zelevinsky, K. (2001). *Nurse staffing and patient outcomes in hospitals* (Contract No. 230-99-0021). Boston: Health Resources Services Administration.

Peters, T., & Waterman, R. H. (1982). *In search of excellence.* New York: Warner Communications.

Schein, E. H. (1996). Culture: The missing concept in organization studies. *Administrative Science Quarterly, 41*(2), 220–240.

Schmalenberg, C., & Kramer, M. (2008). Essentials of a productive work environment. *Nursing Research, 57,* 2–13.

Scott, T., Mannion, R., Davies, H., & Marshall, M. (2003). The quantitative measurement of organizational culture in health care: A review of the available instruments. *Health Services Research, 38,* 923–945.

Seago, J. A. (2001). Nurse staffing, models of care delivery, and interventions. In K. G. Shojania, B. W. Duncan, K. M. McDonald, & R. M. Wachter (Eds.), *Making health care safer: A critical analysis of patient safety practices* (Vol. 43, pp. 427–450). Rockville, MD: Agency for Healthcare Research and Quality.

Sleutel, M. R. (2000). Climate, culture, context, or work environment? Organizational factors that influence nursing practice. *Journal of Nursing Administration, 30,* 53–58.

Snow, J. (2002). Enhancing work climate to improve performance and retain valued employees. *Journal of Nursing Administration, 33*(2), 111–117.

Sochalski, J., Estabrooks, C. A., & Humphrey, C. K. (1999). Nurse staffing and patient outcomes: Evolution of an international study. *Canadian Journal of Nursing Research, 31,* 69–88.

Sorrentino, E., Nalli, B., & Schriesheim, C. (1992). The effect of head nurse behaviors on nurse job satisfaction and performance. *Hospital and Health Services Administration, 37,* 103–113.

Sovie, M. D., & Jawad, A. F. (2001). Hospital restructuring and its impact on outcomes. *Journal of Nursing Administration, 31,* 588–600.

Stone, P. W., Harrison, M. I., Feldman, P., Linzer, M., Peng, T., Roblin, D., et al. (2005). *Organizational climate of staff working conditions and safety: An integrative model.* Retrieved February 1, 2008, from www.ahrq.gov/downloads/pub/advances/vol2/Stone.doc

Stone, P. W., Larson, E. L., Mooney-Kane, C., Smolowitz, J., Lin, S. X., & Dick, A. W. (2006). Organizational climate and intensive care nurses' intention to leave. *Critical Care. Medicine, 34,* 1907–1912.

Taunton, R. L., Boyle, D. K., Woods, C. Q., Hansen, H. E., & Bott, M. J. (1997). Manager leadership and retention of hospital staff nurses. *Western Journal of Nursing Research, 19,* 205–226.

Upenieks, V. (2003). What constitutes effective leadership? Perceptions of Magnet and nonmagnet nurse leaders. *Journal of Nursing Administration, 33,* 456–467.

U.S. Department of Health and Human Services, Health Resources and Services Administration. *The registered nurse population: Findings from the 2004 National Sample Survey of Registered Nurses.* Retrieved February 28, 2008, from http://bhpr.hrsa.gov/healthworkforce/rnsurvey04/appendixa.htm

Uttal, B. (1983). The corporate culture vultures. *Fortune Magazine,* (October).

Wolf, G. (2006). A road map for creating a magnet work environment. *Journal of Nursing Administration, 36,* 458–462.

Wooten, L. P., & Crane, P. (2003). Nurses as implementers of organizational culture. *Nursing Economic$, 21,* 275–279.

Chapter 5

Ackermann, A. D., Kenny, G., & Walker, C. (2007). Simulator programs for nurses' orientation: A retention strategy. *Journal for Nurses in Staff Development, 23*(3), 136–139.

Adams, B. L. (1999). Nursing education for critical thinking: An integrative review. *Journal of Nursing Education, 38*(3), 111–119.

Albarran, J. W. (2004). Creativity: An essential element of critical care nursing practice. *Nursing in Critical Care, 9*(2), 47–49.

American Association of Colleges of Nursing. (1998). *Essentials of baccalaureate education for professional nursing practice.* Retrieved May 18, 2008, from www.aacn.nche.edu/education/pdf/BaccEssentials98.pdf

American Nurses Association (ANA). (2008). *ANA principles on safe staffing.* Retrieved May 18, 2008, from www.safestaffingsaveslives.org/WhatisSafeStaffing/SafeStaffingPrinciples.aspx

Belsky, G., & Gilovich, T. (1999). *Why smart people make money mistakes and how to correct them.* New York: Simon & Schuster.

Benner, P. (1984). *From novice to expert: Excellence and power in clinical practice.* Menlo Park, CA: Addison-Wesley.

Benner, P. (2003). Beware of technological imperatives and commercial interests that prevent best practices! *American Journal of Critical Care, 12*(5), 469–471.

Buhler, P. M. (2004). Managing in the new millennium—The talent search: Every manager's responsibility. *Supervision, 65*(4), 20–22.

Burke, D. S., Epstein, J. M., Cummings, D. A. T., Parker, J. I., Cline, K. C., Singa, R. M., et al. (2006). Individual computational modeling of smallpox epidemic control strategies. *Academic Emergency Medicine, 13*(11), 1142–1149.

Campbell, E. M., Sittig, D. F., Ash, J. S., Guappone, K. P., & Dykstra, R. H. (2006). Types of unintended consequences related to computerized provider order entry. *Journal of the American Medical Informatics Association, 13*(5), 547–556.

Cannon, S., Boswell, C., & Robinson, M. (2007). Making research come alive at the bedside. *Nursing Management, 38*(10), 16–17.

Chambers, C. C. (2009). *Creative nursing leadership and management.* Sudbury, MA: Jones and Bartlett.

Choo, C. W. (2006). *The knowing organization* (2nd ed.). New York: Oxford University Press.

Chu, D., Strand, R., & Fjelland, R. (2003). Theories of complexity. *Complexity, 8*(3), 19–30.

Clancy, T. R., & Delaney, C. W. (2005). Complex nursing systems. *Journal of Nursing Management, 13*, 192–201.

Clancy, T. R., Delaney, C. W., Morrison, B., & Gunn, J. K. (2006). The benefits of standardized nursing languages in complex adaptive systems such as hospitals. *Journal of Nursing Administration, 36*(9), 426–434.

Cohen, S. (2002). Don't overlook creative thinking. *Nursing Management, 33*(8), 9–10.

Cox, S. A. (2005). It's all about ownership. *Nursing Management, 36*(3), 57.

Coyle, G. A., Sapnas, K. G., & Ward-Presson, K. (2007). Dealing with disaster. *Nursing Management, 38*(7), 24–29.

Currie, K., Tolson, D., & Booth, J. (2007). Helping or hindering: The role of nurse managers in the transfer of practice development learning. *Journal of Nursing Management, 15*, 585–594.

Davidhizar, R., & Bowen, M. (1999). There are solutions to problems. *Health Care Manager, 18*(1), 14–19.

De Bleser, L., DePreitere, R., De Waele, K., Vanhaecht, K., Vlayen, J., & Sermeus, W. (2006). Defining pathways. *Journal of Nursing Management, 14*(7), 553–563.

deChesnay, M. (1983). Problem solving in nursing. *Image, 15*(1), 8–11.

del Bueno, D. (2005). A crisis in critical thinking. *Nursing Education Perspectives, 26*(5), 278–282.

Drummond, H. (2001). *The art of decision making.* Chichester, England: John Wiley & Sons.

Dunbar, B., Park, B., Berger-Wesley, M., Cameron, T., Lorenz, B. T., Mayes, D., et al. (2007). Shared governance: Making the transition in practice and perception. *Journal of Nursing Administration, 37*(4), 177–183.

Elder, L., & Paul, R. (n.d.). *Becoming a critic of your thinking.* Retrieved May 12, 2008, from www.criticalthinking.org/page.cfm?PageID=478&CategoryID=68

Ellermann, C. R., Katoka-Yahiro, M. R., & Wong, L. C. (2006). Logic models to enhance critical thinking. *Journal of Nursing Education, 45*(6), 220–227.

Emmanuel, E. (2002). Health care reform: Still possible. *Hastings Center Report, 32*(2), 33–34.

Etheridge, S. A. (2007). Learning to think like a nurse: Stories from new nurse graduates. *Journal of Continuing Education in Nursing, 38*(1), 24–30.

Etzioni, A. (1989). Humble decision making. *Harvard Business Review, 67*(4), 122–126.

Facione, P. (2007). *2007 Update—Critical thinking: What it is and why it counts.* Retrieved May 11, 2008, from www.insightassessment.com/pdf_files/what&why2007.pdf

Ferrario, C. G. (2004). Developing clinical reasoning strategies. *Journal for Nurses in Staff Development, 20*(5), 229–234.

Finkelman, A. W. (2001). Problem-solving, decision-making, and critical thinking: How do they mix and why bother? *Home Care Provider, 6*(6), 194–197.

Forman, H. (2006). Never-ending problems. *Journal of Nursing Administration, 36*(11), 518–521.

Gladwell, M. (2005). *Blink.* New York: Little, Brown and Company.

Grossman, S. (2007). Assisting critical care nurses in acquiring leadership skills. *Dimensions of Critical Care Nursing, 26*(2), 57–65.

Hader, R. (2005). Carve out time to think—yes, think. *Nursing Management, 36*(4), 4.

Hammond, J. S., Keeney, R. L., & Raiffa, H. (1998). The hidden traps in decision making. *Harvard Business Review, 76*(5), 47–58.

Hammond, J. S., Keeney, R. L., & Raiffa, H. (1999). *Smart choices: A practical guide to making better decisions.* Boston: Harvard Business School Press.

Holden, L. M. (2005). Complex adaptive systems: Concept analysis. *Journal of Advanced Nursing, 52*(6), 651–657.

Ignatavicius, D. D. (2008). *Critical thinking skills in the clinical setting.* Message posted to Nursing Educators Discussion List, archived at https://lists.uvic.ca/mailman/private/nrsinged/

Insight Assessment. (2008a). *California critical thinking skills test—Form 2000.* Milbrae, CA: Insight Assessment/California Academic Press, LLP. Retrieved May 18, 2008, from www.insightassessment.com/test-cctst.html

Insight Assessment. (2008b). *The health sciences reasoning test manual.* Retrieved May 18, 2008, from www.insightassessment.com/pdf_files/HSRT%20manual.pdf

Institute of Medicine (IOM). (2001). *Crossing the quality chasm: A new health system for the 21st century.* Washington, DC: National Academies Press.

Institute of Medicine (IOM). (2003). *Health professions education: A bridge to quality.* Washington, DC: National Academies Press. Retrieved August 4, 2008, from http://books.nap.edu/openbook.php?record_id=10681&page=4

Janis, I., & Mann, L. (1977). *Decision making: A psychological analysis of conflict, choice, and commitment.* New York: Free Press.

Junttila, K., Meretoja, R., Seppala, A., Tolppanen, E., Ala-Nikkola, T., & Silvennoinen, L. (2007). Data warehouse approach to nursing management. *Journal of Nursing Management, 15*, 155–161.

Kane, R. L., Shamliyan, T. A., Mueller, C., Duval, S., & Wilt, T. J. (2007). The association of registered nurse staffing levels and patient outcomes: Systematic review and meta-analysis. *Medical Care, 45*(12), 1195–1204.

Kennedy, C. (2002). The decision making process in a district nursing assessment. *British Journal of Community Nursing, 7*(10), 505–513.

Kerfoot, K. (2006). Reliability between nurse managers: The key to the high-reliability organization. *Nursing Economic$, 24*(5), 274–275.

Keynes, M. (2008). Making good decisions, Part 1. *Nursing Management-UK, 14*(9), 32–34.

Kirton, M. (1994). *Adaptors and innovators: Styles of creativity and problem solving.* London: Routledge.

Lemire, J. A. (2002). Leader as critical thinker. *Nursing Leadership Forum, 7*(2), 69–76.

Le Storti, A. J., Cullen, P. A., Hanzlik, E. M., Michiels, J. M., Piano, L. A., Ryan, P. L., et al. (1999). Creative thinking in nursing education: Preparing for tomorrow's challenges. *Nursing Outlook, 47*(2), 62–66.

McNichol, E. (2002). Thinking outside the box. *Nursing Management-UK, 9*(4), 19–22.

Menkes, J. (2006). The leadership difference: Executive intelligence. *Leader to Leader, 2006*(40), 51–56.

Minas, H. (2005). Leadership for change in complex systems. *Australasian Psychiatry, 13*(1), 33–39.

Morgan, S. P., & Cooper, C. (2004). Shoulder work intensity with Six Sigma. *Nursing Management, 35*(3), 29–32.

Newell, A., & Simon, H. A. (1972). *Human problem solving.* Englewood Cliffs, NJ: Prentice Hall.

Perrow, C. (1984). *Normal accidents: Living with high risk technologies.* New York: Basic Books.

Pesut, D. J., & Herman, J. (1999). *Clinical reasoning: The art and science of critical and creative thinking.* Albany, NY: Delmar Publishers.

Peters, R. M. (2002). Nurse administrators' role in health policy: Teaching the elephant to dance. *Nursing Administrative Quarterly, 26*(4), 1–8.

Pew Health Professions Commission. (1998). *Twenty-one competencies for the twenty-first century.* San Francisco: Center for the Health Professions. Retrieved May 18, 2008, from www.futurehealth.ucsf.edu/pewcomm/competen.html

Pidgeon, N., & Gregory, R. (2004). Judgment, decision making, and public policy. In D. J. Koehler, & N. Harvey (Eds.), *Blackwell handbook of judgment and decision making* (pp. 604–623). Malden, MA: Blackwell Publishing.

Porter-O'Grady, T. (2003). A different age for leadership, Part 2. *Journal of Nursing Administration, 33*(3), 173–178.

Porter-O'Grady, T., Igein, G., Alexander, D., Blaylock, J., McComb, D., & Williams, S. (2005). Critical thinking for nursing leadership. *Nurse Leader, 3*(4), 28–31.

Rubenfeld, M. G., & Scheffer, B. K. (2006). *Critical thinking tactics for nurses.* Sudbury, MA: Jones and Bartlett Publishers.

Saulo, M. (1996). Quality problem-solving, decision-making, type theory, and case managers. *Nursing Case Management, 1*(5), 201–208.

Scheffer, B. K., & Rubenfeld, M. G. (2000). A consensus statement on critical thinking in nursing. *Journal of Nursing Education, 39*(8), 352–359.

Sengstack, P. P., & Gurerty, B. (2004). CPOE systems: Success factors and implementation issues (electronic version). *Journal of Healthcare Information Management, 18*, 36–45. Retrieved May 18, 2008, from www.himss.org/content/files/jhim/18-1/focus_success.pdf

Shenk, D. (1997). *Data smog: Surviving the information edge.* San Francisco: Harper Edge.

Sherman, R. O., Bishop, M., Eggenberger, T., & Karden, R. (2007). Development of a leadership competency model. *Journal of Nursing Administration, 37*(2), 85–94.

Shirey, M. R. (2007). Competencies and tips for effective leadership: From novice to expert. *Journal of Nursing Administration, 37*(4), 167–170.

Smith-Trudeau, P. (2006). Culturally creative problem solving. *Vermont Nurse Connection, 9*(3), 1, 4.

Tan, J., Wen, H. J., & Awad, N. (2005). Health care and services systems as complex adaptive systems. *Communications of the ACM, 48*(5), 36–44.

Tanner, C. A. (2000). Critical thinking: Beyond nursing process. *Journal of Nursing Education, 39*(8), 338–339.

Tanner, C. A. (2006). Thinking like a nurse: A research-based model of clinical judgment in nursing. *Journal of Nursing Education, 45*(6), 204–211.

Taylor, C. (1997). Problem solving in clinical nursing practice. *Journal of Advanced Nursing, 26*, 329–336.

The Critical Thinking Community. (2008). *A brief history of the idea of critical thinking.* Retrieved May 12, 2008, from www.criticalthinking.org/aboutCT/briefHistoryCT.cfm

Thomas, J., & Herrin, D. (2008a). The executive master of science in nursing program: Competencies and learning experiences. *Journal of Nursing Administration, 38*(1), 4–7.

Thomas, J., & Herrin, D. (2008b). Executive master of science in nursing program: Incorporating the 14 Forces of Magnetism. *Journal of Nursing Administration, 38*(2), 64–67.

Toofany, S. (2008). Critical thinking among nurses. *Nursing Management-UK, 14*(9), 28–31.

Van de Ven, A., & Delbecq, A. (1974). The effectiveness of nominal, Delphi, and interacting group decision making processes. *Academy of Management Journal, 17*(4), 605–621.

Vanhaecht, K., De Witte, K., DePreitere, R., & Sermeus, W. (2006). Clinical pathway audit tools: A systematic review. *Journal of Nursing Management, 16*(7), 529–537.

Vroom, V., & Yetton, P. (1973). *Leadership and decision making.* Pittsburgh: University of Pittsburgh Press.

Waldrop, M. (1992). *Complexity, the emerging science at the edge of order and chaos*. New York: Simon & Schuster.

Walsh, C. M., & Seldomridge, L. A. (2006). Critical thinking: Back to square two. *Journal of Nursing Education, 45*(6), 212–219.

Watson, G. B., & Glaser, E. M. (1994). *Watson-Glaser critical thinking appraisal form S manual*. San Antonio, TX: Harcourt Brace.

Wheatley, M. (1999). *Leadership and the new science*. San Francisco: Bennett-Koehler Publishers.

Chapter 6

American Hospital Association (AHA). (April 2002). *In our hands: How hospital leaders can build a thriving workforce*. Chicago: Author.

American Nurses Association (ANA). (2001). *Code of ethics for nurses with interpretive statements*. Silver Spring, MD: Author. Retrieved August 4, 2004, from www.nursingworld.org/ethics/ecode.htm

Arnold, E., & Pulich, M. (2004). Improving productivity through more effective time management. *Health Care Manager, 23*(1), 65–70.

Aurelio, J. (1993). An organizational culture that optimizes stress: Acceptable stress in nursing. *Nursing Administration Quarterly, 18*(1), 1–10.

Bailey, J. T. (1980). Stress and stress management: An overview. *Journal of Nursing Education, 19*(6), 5–8.

Benson, H., & Allen, R. L. (1980). How much stress is too much? *Harvard Business Review, 58*(5), 86–92.

Bratt, M. M., Broome, M., Kelber, S., & Lostocco, L. (2000). Influence of stress and nursing leadership on job satisfaction of pediatric intensive care unit nurses. *American Journal of Critical Care, 9*(5), 307–317.

Business Town.com. (2004). *Five reasons why we procrastinate and five strategies to put off putting off*. Retrieved August 4, 2004, from www.businesstown.com/time/time-5reasons.asp

CBS Broadcasting Inc. (2006). *The Sandwich Generation*. Broadcast on CBS News, May 8, 2006.

Centers for Medicare and Medicaid Services (CMS). (2008). *State Medicaid Director letter*. Baltimore: Author.

Charnley, E. (1999). Occupational stress in the newly qualified staff nurse. *Nursing Standard, 13*(29), 32–37.

Conway, M. (1988). Theoretical approaches to the study of roles. In M. E. Hardy, & M. E. Conway (Eds.), *Role theory: Perspectives for health professionals* (2nd ed., pp. 63–72). Norwalk, CT: Appleton & Lange.

Covey, S., Merrill, A., & Merrill, R. (1994). *First things first*. New York: Simon & Schuster.

Cox, K. S. (2002). Inpatient nurses and their work environment. *Nursing Leadership Forum, 7*(1), 34–37.

Department of Labor. (2007). *The Family and Medical Leave Act (FMLA) of 1993*. Public Law 103-3, Enacted February 5, 1993. Retrieved December 2007, from www.dol.gov/esa/regs/statutes/whd/fmla.htm

Dewe, P. J. (1987). Identifying the causes of nurses' stress: A survey of New Zealand nurses. *Work & Stress, 1*(1), 15–24.

Dietz, M. (1991). Stressors and coping mechanisms of older rural women. In A. Bushy (Ed.), *Rural nursing* (Vol. 1, pp. 267–280). Newbury Park, CA: Sage.

Elliott, G., & Eisdorfer, C. (1982). *Stress and human health*. New York: Springer.

Ferner, J. D. (1995). *Successful time management: A self-teach ing guide* (2nd ed.). New York: John Wiley & Sons.

Getzels, J. W. (1958). Administration as a social process. In A. W. Halpin (Ed.), *Administrative theory in education* (pp. 150–165). Chicago: University of Chicago Press.

Grant, P. (1993). Manage nurse stress and increase potential at the bedside. *Nursing Administration Quarterly, 18*(1), 16–22.

Hahn, H. (2008). *A monochronic/polychronic self test*. Salt Lake City, UT: The Harley Hahn Experience. Retrieved August 3, 2008, from www.innovint.com/downloads/mono_poly_test.php

Hardy, M. E. (1978). Role stress and role strain. In M. E. Hardy, & M. E. Conway (Eds.), *Role theory: Perspectives for health professionals*. Norwalk, CT: Appleton-Century-Crofts.

Hardy, M. E., & Conway, M. E. (1988). *Role theory: Perspectives for health professionals* (2nd ed.). Norwalk, CT: Appleton & Lange.

Hardy, M. E., & Hardy, W. L. (1988). Role stress and role strain. In M. E. Hardy, & M. E. Conway (Eds.), *Role theory: Perspectives for health professionals* (2nd ed., pp. 159–239). Norwalk, CT: Appleton & Lange.

Harris, R. (1989). Review of nursing stress according to a proposed coping adaptation framework. *Advances in Nursing Science, 11*(2), 12–28.

Hartl, D. (1989). Stress management and the nurse. *Advances in Nursing Science, 11*(2), 91–100.

Health Resources and Services Administration (HRSA), Bureau of Health Professions (BHPr). (2002). *Projected supply, demand, and shortages of Registered Nurses: 2000–2020*. Rockville, MD: Author.

Hinshaw, A. S. (1989). Programs of nursing research for nursing administration. In B. Henry, C. Arndt, M. Di Vincenti, & A. Marriner-Tomey (Eds.), *Dimensions of nursing administration* (pp. 251–266). Boston: Blackwell.

Hinshaw, A. S., & Atwood, J. R. (1983). Nursing staff turnover, stress, and satisfaction: Models, measures, and management. *Annual Review of Nursing Research, 1*, 133–153.

Hinshaw, A. S., Smeltzer, C. H., & Atwood, J. R. (1987). Innovative retention strategies for nursing staff. *Journal of Nursing Administration, 17*(6), 8–16.

Huber, D. (1994). What are the sources of stress for nurses. In J. McCloskey, & H. Grace (Eds.), *Current issues in nursing* (4th ed., pp. 623–631). St. Louis: Mosby.

Huber, D., Maas, M., McCloskey, J., Scherb, C. A., Goode, C. J., & Watson, C. (2000). Evaluating nursing administration instruments. *Journal of Nursing Administration, 30*(5), 251–272.

Huckabay, L. M. D., & Jagla, B. (1979). Nurses' stress factors in the intensive care unit. *Journal of Nursing Administration, 9*(2), 21–26.

Iaffaldano, M. T., & Muchinsky, P. M. (1985). Job satisfaction and job performance: A meta-analysis. *Psychological Bulletin, 97*(2), 251–273.

Irvine, D. M., & Evans, M. G. (1995). Job satisfaction and turnover among nurses: Integrating research findings across studies. *Nursing Research, 44*(4), 246–253.

Kane, R. L., Shamliyn, T., Mueller, C., Duval, S., & Wilt, T. (2007). *Nursing staffing and quality of patient care.* Evidence report/technology assessment No. 151 (Prepared by the Minnesota Evidence-based Practice Center under Contract No. 290-02-0009.) AHRQ Publication No. 07-E005. Rockville, MD: Agency for Healthcare Research and Quality.

Kanter, R. M. (1977). *Work and family in the United States: A critical review and agenda for research and policy.* New York: Sage.

Kanter, R. M. (1993). *Men and women of the corporation* (2nd ed.). New York: Basic Books.

Keenan, M., Hurst, J., & Olnhausen, K. (1993). Polarity management for quality care: Self-direction and manager direction. *Nursing Administration Quarterly, 18*(1), 23–29.

Kobasa, S. C., Maddi, S. R., & Kahn, S. (1982). Hardiness and health: A prospective study. *Journal of Personality & Social Psychology, 42*(1), 168–177.

Kramer, M. (1974). *Reality shock: Why nurses leave nursing.* St. Louis: Mosby.

Kramer, M., & Schmalenberg, C. (1977). *Path to biculturalism.* Wakefield, MA: Contemporary Publishing.

Lancaster, L. C., & Stillman, D. (2002). *When generations collide.* New York: HarperCollins.

Landstrom, G. L., Biordi, D. L., & Gillies, D. A. (1989). The emotional and behavioral process of staff nurse turnover. *Journal of Nursing Administration, 19*(9), 23–28.

Laschinger, H. K., Almost, J., & Tuer-Hodes, D. (2003). Workplace empowerment and Magnet hospital characteristics. *Journal of Nursing Administration, 33*(7/8), 410–422.

Laschinger, H. K., Finegan, J., & Shamian, J. (2001). Promoting nurses' health: Effect of empowerment on job strain and work satisfaction. *Nursing Economic$, 19*(2), 42–52.

Laschinger, H. K., Finegan, J., Shamian, J., & Almost, J. (2001). Testing Karasek's demands-control model in restructured healthcare settings: Effects of job strain on staff nurses' quality of work life. *Journal of Nursing Administration, 31*(5), 233–243.

Lazarus, R. (1966). *Psychological stress and the coping process.* New York: McGraw-Hill.

Lazarus, R., & Folkman, S. (1984). *Stress, appraisal and coping.* New York: Springer.

Leatt, P., & Schneck, R. (1980). Differences in stress perceived by head nurses across nursing specialties in hospitals. *Journal of Advanced Nursing, 5,* 31–46.

Lowery, B. (1987). Stress research: Some theoretical and methodological issues. *Image, 19*(1), 42–46.

Lyon, B. L., & Werner, J. S. (1987). Stress. *Annual Review of Nursing Research, 5,* 3–22.

Maslach, C., & Jackson, S. (1981). The measurement of experienced burnout. *Journal of Occupational Behaviour, 2,* 99–113.

McCloskey, J. C., & McCain, B. E. (1987). Satisfaction, commitment, and professionalism of newly employed nurses. *Image, 19,* 20–24.

McClure, M., Poulin, M., Sovie, M., & Wandelt, M. (1983). *Magnet hospitals: Attraction and retention of professional nurses.* Kansas City, MO: American Nurses Association.

McCranie, E., Lambert, V., & Lambert, C. (1987). Work stress, hardiness, and burnout among hospital staff nurses. *Nursing Research, 36,* 374–378.

McGrath, J. E. (1976). Stress and behavior in organizations. In M. D. Dunnette (Ed.), *Handbook of industrial and organizational psychology* (pp. 1351–1395). Chicago: Rand McNally.

McVicar, A. (2003). Workplace stress in nursing—A literature review: Integrative literature reviews and meta-anal yses. *Journal of Advanced Nursing, 44*(6), 633–642.

Miller, J. (1971). The nature of living systems. *Behavioral Science, 16,* 278.

Mills, A. C., & Blaesing, S. L. (2000). A lesson from the last nursing shortage: The influence of work values on career satisfaction with nursing. *Journal of Nursing Administration, 6,* 309–315.

Morgenstern, J. (2004). *Never check e-mail in the morning: And other unexpected strategies for making your work life work.* New York: Simon & Schuster.

Narasi, B. (1994). A tool for living through stress. *Nursing Management, 25*(9), 73–75.

Norbeck, J. S. (1985). Perceived job stress, job satisfaction, and psychological symptoms in critical care nursing. *Research in Nursing & Health, 8,* 253–259.

Noreiko, P. (1996). Time management: Getting the most out of the day. *Occupational Health: A Journal for Occupational Health Nurses, 48*(5), 172–174.

Pagana, K. D. (1994). Teaching students time management strategies. *Journal of Nursing Education, 33*(8), 381–383.

Perlman, B., & Hartman, E. (1982). Burnout: Summary and future research. *Human Relations, 35*(4), 283–305.

Pollock, S. (1984). The stress response. *Critical Care Quarterly, 3,* 1–13.

Price, J. L., & Mueller, C. W. (1981). *Professional turnover: The case of nurses.* New York: Spectrum.

Rich, L., & Rich, A. R. (1987). Personality hardiness and burnout in female staff nurses. *Image, 19,* 63–66.

Robert Wood Johnson Foundation (RWJF). (2006). *Wisdom at work: The importance of the older and experienced nurse in the workplace.* Princeton, NJ: Author.

Rocchiccioli, J. T., & Tilbury, M. S. (1998). *Clinical leadership in nursing.* Philadelphia: Saunders.

Rocco, T. S., Stein, D., Munn, S. L., & Ginn, G. (2006). *From social policies to organizational practice: Do national policies translate into organizational policies to retain, retrain, or rehire older workers?* Presented at the Midwest Research-to-Practice Conference in Adult, Continuing, and Community Education, University of Missouri—St. Louis, St. Louis, MO.

Santos, S. R., Carroll, C. A., Cox, K. S., Teasley, S. L., Simon, S. D., Bainbridge, L., et al. (2003). Baby boomer nurses bearing the burden of care. *Journal of Nursing Administration, 33*(4), 243–250.

Santos, S. R., & Cox, K. (2000). Workplace adjustment and intergenerational differences between Matures, Boomers and Xers. *Nursing Economic$, 18*(1), 7–13.

Sawatzky, J. V. (1998). Understanding nursing students' stress: A proposed framework. *Nurse Education Today, 18*(2), 108–115.

Scalzi, C. (1988). Role stress and coping strategies of nurse executives. *Journal of Nursing Administration, 18*(3), 34–38.

Schmalenberg, C., & Kramer, M. (1979). *Coping with reality shock: The voices of experience.* Wakefield, MA: Nursing Resources.

Schumacher, L., & Larson, K. (1993). Thriving and striving on the turbulence of rural health care. *Nursing Administration Quarterly, 18*(1), 11–15.

Schwab, L. (1996). Individual hardiness and staff satisfaction. *Nursing Economic$, 14*(3), 171–173.

Selye, H. (1965). *The stress of life.* Toronto: McGraw-Hill.

Selye, H. (1976). *Stress in health and disease.* Boston: Butterworth.

Severance, J. S., & Cervantes, E. (1996). Time management training for home care workers. *Caring: National Association for Home Care magazine, 15*(5), 58–61.

Sherry, D. (1996). Time management strategies for the new home care nurse. *Home Healthcare Nurse, 14*(9), 718–720.

Simoni, P. S., & Paterson, J. J. (1997). Hardiness, coping, and burnout in the nursing workplace. *Journal of Professional Nursing, 13*(3), 178–185.

Smythe, E. (1984). Burn-out: From caring to apathy. In E. Smythe (Ed.), *Surviving nursing* (pp. 46–57). Menlo Park, CA: Addison-Wesley.

Sovie, M. D., & Jawad, A. F. (2001). Hospital restructuring and its impact on outcomes. *Journal of Nursing Administration, 31*(12), 588–600.

Stehle, J. L. (1981). Critical care nursing stress: The findings revisited. *Nursing Research, 30,* 182–186.

Tarolli-Jager, K. (1994). Personal hardiness: Your buffer against burnout. *American Journal of Nursing, 94*(2), 71–72.

Thomas, E. J., & Biddle, B. J. (1966). Basic concepts for classifying the phenomena of role. In B. J. Biddle, & E. J. Thomas (Eds.), *Role theory: Concepts and research* (pp. 23–45). New York: John Wiley & Sons.

Tucker, A. L. (2004). The impact of operational failures on hospital nurses and their patients. *Journal of Operations Management, 22,* 151–169.

Wagnild, G., & Young, H. M. (1991). Another look at hardiness. *Image, 23*(4), 257–259.

Weisman, C. S., Alexander, C. S., & Chase, G. (1981). Determinants of hospital staff nurse turnover. *Medical Care, 19*(4), 431–443.

Welton, J. M., Zone-Smith, L., & Fischer, M. H. (2006). Adjustment of inpatient care reimbursement for nursing intensity. *Policy, Politics and Nursing Practice, 7*(4), 270–280.

Woodhouse, D. (1993). The aspects of humor in dealing with stress. *Nursing Administration Quarterly, 18*(1), 80–89.

Chapter 7

Agency for Healthcare Research and Quality (AHRQ). (2004). *Hospital nurse staffing and quality of care. Research in Action Issue #4.* Washington, DC: U.S. Department of Health and Human Services. Retrieved December 1, 2007, from www.ahrq.gov/research/nursestaffing/nursestaff.pdf

Agency for Healthcare Research and Quality (AHRQ). (2007). *Nurse staffing and quality of patient care.* Retrieved December 1, 2007, from www.ahrq.gov/downloads/pub/evidence/pdf/nursestaff/nursestaff.pdf

Aiken, L. H., Clarke, S. P., Sloane, D. M., Sochalski, J., & Silber, J. H. (2002). Hospital nurse staffing and patient mortality, nurse burnout, and job dissatisfaction. *Journal of the American Medical Association, 288*(16), 1987–1993.

Aiken, T. D. (2004). *Legal, ethical, and political issues in nursing* (2nd ed.). Philadelphia: F.A. Davis.

American Hospital Association (AHA). (2002). *In our hands: How hospital leaders can build a thriving workforce.* Chicago: Author.

American Medical Association (AMA). (1994). *Withholding or withdrawing life-sustaining medical treatment. Opinion on social policy issues E-2.20.* Chicago: Author. Retrieved December 1, 2007, from www.ama-assn.org/ama/pub/category/8457.html

American Medical Association (AMA). (2000). *Organizational ethics in health care.* Chicago: Author.

American Nurses Association (ANA). (1980). *Nursing: A social policy statement.* Kansas City, MO: Author.

American Nurses Association (ANA). (2001). *Code of ethics for nurses: With interpretive statements.* Washington, DC: Author. Retrieved December 1, 2007, from nursingworld.org/ethics/code/protected_nwcoe813.htm

Andrews, D. R. (2004). Fostering ethical competency: An ongoing staff development process that encourages professional growth and staff satisfaction. *The Journal of Continuing Education in Nursing, 35*(1), 27–33.

Auerbach, D. I., Buerhaus, P. I., & Staiger, D. O. (2007). Better late than never: Workforce supply implications of late entry into nursing. *Health Affairs, 26*(1), 178–185.

Austin, W. (2007). The ethics of everyday practice: Healthcare environments as moral communities. *Advances in Nursing Science, 30*(1), 81–88.

Beauchamp, T., & Childress, J. (2001). *Principles of biomedical ethics* (5th ed.). New York: Oxford University Press.

Blake, D. C. (1999). Organizational ethics: Creating structural and cultural change in health care organizations. *Journal of Clinical Ethics, 10*(3), 187–193.

Brothers, D. (2005). *A practical guide to legal issues: Skills for nurse managers.* Marblehead, MA: HCPro, Inc.

Buerhaus, P. I., Clifford, J., Erickson, J. I., Fay, M. S., Miller, J. R., Sporing, E. M., et al. (1997). Executive nursing leadership: Summary of the Harvard Nursing Research Institute's follow-up conference. *Journal of Nursing Administration, 27*(4), 12–20.

Buerhaus, P. I., Donelan, K., Ulrich, B. T., DesRoches, C., & Dittus, R. (2007). Trends in the experiences of hospital-employed registered nurses: Results from three national surveys. *Nursing Economic$, 25*(2), 69–80.

Buerhaus, P. I., Donelan, K., Ulrich, B. T., Norman, L., & Dittus, R. (2006). State of the registered nurse workforce in the United States. *Nursing Economic$, 24*(1), 6–12.

Buerhaus, P. I., Donelan, K., Ulrich, B. T., Norman, L., Williams, M., & Dittus, R. (2005). Hospital RNs' and CNOs' perceptions of the impact of the nursing shortage on the quality of care. *Nursing Economic$, 23*(5), 214–221.

Cooper, R. W., Frank, G. L., Gouty, C. A., & Hansen, M. C. (2002). Key ethical issues encountered in health care organizations: Perceptions of nurse executives. *Journal of Nursing Administration, 32*(6), 331–337.

Cooper, R. W., Frank, G. L., Gouty, C. A., & Hansen, M. C. (2003). Ethical helps and challenges faced by nurse leaders in the health care industry. *Journal of Nursing Administration, 33*(1), 17–23.

Cooper, R. W., Frank, G. L., Hansen, M. M., & Gouty, C. A. (2004). Key ethical issues encountered in health care organizations: The perceptions of staff nurses and nurse leaders. *Journal of Nursing Administration, 34*(3), 149–156.

Croke, E. M. (2003). Nurses, negligence, and malpractice. *American Journal of Nursing, 103*(9), 54–63. Retrieved December 3, 2007, from www.nursingcenter.com/library/journalarticle.asp?article_id=423284

Curtin, L. L. (2000). The first ten principles for the ethical administration of nursing services. *Nursing Administration Quarterly, 25*(1), 7–13.

Dodd, S., Jansson, B. S., Brown-Saltzman, K., Shirk, M., & Wunch, K. (2004). Expanding nurses' participation in ethics: An empirical examination of ethical activism and ethical assertiveness. *Nursing Ethics, 11*(1), 15–27.

Douglas, M. R. (2007). Encourage corporate compliance and disclosure. *Nursing Management, 38*(1), 16–17.

Eskreis, T. R. (1998). Seven common legal pitfalls in nursing. *American Journal of Nursing, 98*(4), 34–41.

Frank-Stromborg, M., & Christensen, A. (2001a). Nurse documentation: Not done or worse, done the wrong way, Part I. *Oncology Nursing Forum, 28*(4), 697–702.

Frank-Stromborg, M., & Christensen, A. (2001b). Nurse documentation: Not done or worse, done the wrong way, Part II. *Oncology Nursing Forum, 28*(5), 841–846.

Goodstein, J. D., & Carney, B. (1999). Actively engaging organizational ethics in health care: Four essential elements. *Journal of Clinical Ethics, 10*(3), 224–229.

Gordon, S. (2005). *Nursing against the odds: How health care cost-cutting, media stereotypes, and medical hubris undermine nursing and patient care.* Ithaca, NY: Cornell University Press.

Guido, G. W. (2006). *Legal and ethical issues in nursing* (4th ed.). Upper Saddle River, NJ: Pearson Prentice-Hall.

Hassmiller, S. B., & Cozine, M. (2006). Addressing the nurse shortage to improve the quality of patient care. *Health Affairs, 25*(1), 268–274.

Johnson, R. (2005). Shifting patterns of practice: Nurse practitioners in a managed care environment. *Research and Theory for Nursing Practice: An International Journal, 19*(4), 323–340.

Joint Commission on Accreditation of Healthcare Organizations (JCAHO). (1996). *Standards for organizational ethics: 1996 comprehensive accreditation manual for hospitals.* Oakbrook Terrace, IL: Author.

Lachman, V.D. (2002). Organizational ethics need not be an oxymoron. *Patient Care Management, 18*(3), 1, 4–5.

Lachman, V.D. (2007a). Moral courage: A virtue in need of development? *MEDSURG Nursing, 16*(2), 131–133.

Lachman, V.D. (2007b). Moral courage in action: Case studies. *MEDSURG Nursing, 16*(4), 275–277.

Miller, J. (2006). Opportunities and obstacles for good work in nursing. *Nursing Ethics, 13*(5), 471–487.

Miller, J., & Glusko, J. (2003). Standing up to the scrutiny of medical malpractice. *Nursing Management, 34*(10), 20.

Mohr, W. K., & Mahon, M. M. (1996). Dirty hands: The underside of marketplace health care. *Advances in Nursing Science, 19*(1), 28–37.

Nurses Service Organization (NSO). (2007). *Nurse's Guide to Malpractice.* Hatboro, PA: Author. Retrieved December 3, 2007, from www.nsohomestudy.com/intro.swf

O'Neil, E., & Seago, J. A. (2002). Meeting the challenge of nursing and the nation's health. *Journal of the American Medical Association, 288*(16), 2040–2041.

O'Neill, O. (2001). Practical principles and practical judgment. *Hastings Center Report, 31*(4), 15–23.

Pentz, R. D. (1999). Beyond case consultation: An expanded model for organizational ethics. *Journal of Clinical Ethics, 10*(1), 34–41.

Porter-O'Grady, T. (2003). A different age for leadership, Part 2. *Journal of Nursing Administration, 33*(3), 173–178.

PricewaterhouseCoopers' (PWC) Health Research Institute. (2007). *What works: Healing the healthcare staffing shortage.*

New York, NY: Author. Retrieved December 1, 2007, from www.pwc.com/extweb/pwcpublications.nsf/docid/674D1E79A678A0428525730D006B74A9

Shirey, M. R. (2005). Ethical climate in nursing practice: The leader's role. *JONA'S Healthcare Law, Ethics, and Regulation, 7*(2), 59–67.

Silverman, H. (2000). Organizational ethics in health care organizations: Proactively managing the ethical climate to ensure organizational integrity. *Hospital Ethics Committee Forum, 12*, 202–215.

Spencer, E. M. (1997). A new role for institutional ethics committees: Organizational ethics. *Journal of Clinical Ethics, 8*(4), 372–376.

Trott, M. C. (1998). Legal issues for nurse managers. *Nursing Management, 29*(6), 38–41.

Upenieks, V. (2003). Nurse leaders' perceptions of what compromises successful leadership in today's acute care inpatient environment. *Nursing Administration Quarterly, 27*(2), 140–152.

Wetter, D. (2007). *The best defense is a good documentation offense (Online course)*. Wilmington, DE: Corexcel. Retrieved December 3, 2007, from www.corexcel.com/html/body.documentation.title.ceus.htm

Zuzelo, P. R. (2007). Exploring the moral distress of registered nurses. *Nursing Ethics, 14*(3), 344–359.

Chapter 8

Aiken, L. H., Clarke, S. P., Sloane, D. M., Sochalski, J. A., Busse, R., Clarke, H., et al. (2001). Nurses' reports on hospital care in five countries. *Health Affair, 20*(3), 43–53.

American Nurses Association (ANA). (2005). *Documents on spiritual assessment*. Retrieved March 1, 2009, from http://nursingworld.org/Books/pdescr.cfm?CNum=29

Anthony, M. K., & Preuss, G. (2002). Models of care: The influence of nurse communication on patient safety. *Nursing Economic$, 20*(5), 209–215, 248.

Apker, J., & Fox, D. H. (2002). Communication: Improving RNs' organizational and professional identification in managed care hospitals. *Journal of Nursing Administration, 32*(2), 106–114.

Argenti, P. A. (2002). *Corporate communication* (3rd ed.). Burr Ridge, IL: Richard D. Irwin.

Argyris, C. (1962). *Interpersonal competence and organizational effectiveness*. Homewood, IL: Irwin, Dorsey Press.

Baldacchino, D. R. (2006). Nursing competencies for spiritual care. *Journal of Clinical Nursing, 15*(7), 885–896.

Battey, B. W. (2006). *Spiritual assessment in health care: Guidelines for providing the third dimension of holistic health care (a workshop for nursing staff and other health care providers)*. Antioch, CA: Author.

Battey, B. W. (2007). *The practice of faith community (parish) nursing: A computer assisted instructional program with instructor's manual and student handbook*. Antioch, CA: Author. Computer assisted instructional tools are available from A.S.K. Data Systems, Inc. (www.askdatasystems.com)

Battey, B.W. (in press). *Spiritual assessment for nurses and other health care professional: A computer assisted instructional program with instructor's manual and student handbook*. Antioch, CA: Author. Computer assisted instructional tools are available from A.S.K. Data Systems, Inc. (www.askdatasystems.com)

Bavelas, A. (1953). Communication patterns in task-oriented groups. In D. Cartwright, & A. Zander (Eds.), *Group dynamics: Research and theory*. Evanston, IL: Row, Peterson.

Bettinghaus, E. P. (1968). *Persuasive communication*. New York: Holt, Rinehart & Winston.

Berman, A., Snyder, S. J., Lozier, B., & Erb, G. (2007). *Kozier & Erb's fundamentals of nursing: Concepts, process, and practice* (8th ed.). Upper Saddle River, NJ: Prentice Hall Health.

Boyle, D. K., & Kochinda, C. (2004). Enhancing collaborative communication of nurse and physician leadership in two intensive care units. *Journal of Nursing Administration, 34*(2), 60–70.

Brann, M., & Mattson, M. (2004). Toward a typology of confidentiality breaches in health care communication: An ethic of care analysis of provider practices and patient perceptions. *Health Communications, 16*(2), 231–251.

Buerhaus, P. I., Donelan, K., Norman, L., & Dittus, R. (2005). Nursing student's perceptions of a career in nursing and impact of a national campaign designed to attract people into the nursing profession. *Journal of Professional Nursing, 21*(2), 75–83.

Buerhaus, P. I., Donelan, K., Ulrich, B. T., Norman, L., DesRoches, C., & Dittus, R. (2007). Impact of the nurse shortage on hospital patient care: Comparative perspectives. *Health Affairs, 26*(3), 853–862.

Carson, S. (2000). *Mental health nursing: The nurse-patient journey* (2nd ed.). Philadelphia: Saunders.

Childers, L. (2004). Nurses in hostile work environments must take action against abusive colleagues. *Nurse Week*. Retrieved March 1, 2009, from http://workplacebullying.org/press/nw042604.html

DeMarco, R., Roberts, S. J., Norris, A. E., & McCurry, M. (2007). Refinement of the silencing the self scale: Work for registered nurses. *Journal of Nursing Scholarship, 39*(4), 375–378.

de Shazer, S. (1985). *Keys to solution in brief therapy*. New York: W.W. Norton.

Dombeck, M. (2002). Chaos and self-organization as a consequence of spiritual disequilibrium. *Clinical Nurse Specialist: The Journal for Advanced Nursing Practice, 16*(1), 42–47.

Duldt, B. W. (1980). *Job communication-satisfaction-importance instruction manual*. Springfield, VA: Duldt & Associates, Inc. (Battey, B.W.; Revised & reprinted, 1997, and available from the author.)

Duldt, B. W. (1989). *Nursing communication observation tool (NCOT) instruction manual*. Springfield, VA: Duldt &

Associates, Inc. (Battey, B.W.; Revised & reprinted, 2008, and available from the author.)

Duldt, B. W. (1991). "I-Thou": Research supporting Humanistic Nursing Communication Theory. *Perspectives of Psychiatric Care, 27*(3), 5–12.

Duldt, B. W. (2002). The spiritual dimension of holistic care. *Journal of Nursing Administration, 32*(1), 20–24.

Duldt, B. W., & Giffin, K. (1985). *Theoretical perspectives for nursing*. Boston: Little Brown.

Duldt, B. W., Giffin, K., & Patton, B. R. (1984). *Interpersonal communication in nursing*. Philadelphia: F.A. Davis.

Farley, M. (1989). Assessing communication in organizations. *Journal of Nursing Administration, 19*(12), 27–31.

Gardner, M. (2008). Happiness is a warm "thank you": Seven things that workers want. *Christian Science Monitor*, Monday, January 28, pp. 13, 16. Retrieved October 4, 2008, from www.csmonitor.com/2008/0128/p13s03-wmgn.html

Haigh, C. (2002). Using Chaos Theory: The implications for nursing. *Journal of Advanced Nursing, 37*(5), 462–469.

Harvey, K. (1990). The power of positive questioning. *Nursing Management, 21*(5), 94–96.

Hersey, P. H., Blanchard, K. H., & Johnson, D. E. (2008). *Management of organizational behavior: Leading human resources* (9th ed.). Upper Saddle River, NJ: Prentice Hall.

Hitchcock, J. E., Schubert, P. E., & Thomas, S. H. (2003). *Community health nursing: Caring in action*. Albany, NY: Delmar.

Institute for Safe Medication Practices (ISMP). (2008). Huntingdon Valley, PA. Retrieved October 4, 2008, from www.ismp.org

Johnson, J. (2000). The nursing shortage: A difficult conversation. *Journal of Nursing Administration, 30*(9), 401–402.

Keefe, S. (2007). Bullying among nurses. *Advance for Nursing, 9*(16), 34–36.

Kramer, M., & Schmalenberg, C. (2003). Securing "good" nurse/physician relationships. *Nursing Management, 34*(7), 34–38.

Kraus, P., & Holmes, W. (in press). *Pastoral care: A computer assisted instruction program*. St. Louis: A.S.K. Data Systems.

Leininger, M. (1978). *Transcultural nursing: Concepts, theories, and practices*. New York: John Wiley & Sons.

Lemmer, C. (2002). Teaching the spiritual dimension of nursing care: A survey of U.S. baccalaureate nursing programs. *Journal of Nursing Education, 41*(11), 482–490.

Lindeke, L. L., & Sieckert, A. M. (2004). *Nurse-Physician workplace collaboration*. American Nurses Association. *Online Journal of Issues in Nursing*.

Lorenz, E. N. (1993). *The essence of chaos*. Seattle: University of Washington Press.

Lowenstein, A. J. (2003). Vision for the future of nursing (editorial). *ICUS & Nursing Web Journal, 16*, 1–2. Retrieved October 2, 2008, from www.nursing.gr/editorialLowenstein.pdf

McClung, E., Grossoehme, D. H., & Jacobson, A. F. (2006). Collaborating with chaplains to meet spiritual needs. *MEDSURG Nursing, 15*(3), 147–156.

McEwen, B. S. (2000). Allostasis and allostatic load: Implications for neuropsychopharmacology. *Neuropsychopharmacology: Official Publication of the American College of Neuropsychopharmacology, 22*, 108–124.

McEwen, M. (2004). Analysis of spirituality content in nursing textbooks. *Journal of Nursing Education, 43*(1), 20–30.

McEwen, B. S., & Seaman, T. (1999). Protective and damaging effects of mediators of stress: Elaborating and testing the concepts of allostasis and allostatic load. *Annals of the New York Academy of Sciences, 896*, 30–37.

McSherry, W., & Cash, K. (2004). The language of spirituality: An emerging taxonomy. *International Journal of Nursing Studies, 41*, 151–161.

Mitchell, D. L., Bennett, M. J., & Manfrin-Ledet, L. (2006). Spiritual development of nursing students: Developing competence to provide spiritual care to patients at the end of life. *Journal of Nursing Education, 45*(9), 365–370.

Moss, J., & Xiao, Y. (2004). Improving operating room coordination: Communication pattern assessment. *Journal of Nursing Administration, 34*(2), 93–100.

Namie, R., & Namie, G. (2008). *The Workplace Bullying Institute, WBI*. Retrieved January 27, 2008, from www.bullyinginstitute.org/

Neuman, B. (1982). *The Neuman systems model: Applications to nursing education and practice*. Norwalk, CT: Appleton Lange.

Nightingale, F. (1959). *Notes on nursing: What it is, and what it is not* (5th ed.). London: Harrison, 59, Pall Mall, 1959 A facsimile reproduced from the copy in the Rare Book Room from the Library of Congress, Washington, DC, published by J.B. Lippincott, Philadelphia, 1946.

North American Nursing Diagnosis Association (NANDA). (2008). *Nursing diagnoses: Definitions and classification, 2009–2011*. Indianapolis, IN: Wiley-Blackwell.

Patterson, K., Grenny, J., McMillan, R., & Switzler, A. (2002). *Crucial conversations: Tools for talking when stakes are high*. New York: McGraw-Hill.

Patton, B. R., & Giffin, K. (1977). *Interpersonal communication in action*. New York: Harper & Row.

Patton, B. R., & Giffin, K. (1981). *Interpersonal communication in action: Basic text and readings*. New York: Harper & Row.

Pediani, R. (1996). Chaos and evolution in nursing research. *Journal of Advanced Nursing, 23*(4), 645–646.

Pincus, J. (1986). Communication: Key contributor to effectiveness—The research. *Journal of Nursing Administration, 16*(9), 19–25.

Power, J. (2006). Spiritual assessment: Developing an assessment tool. *Nursing Older People, 18*(2), 16–18.

Puchalski, C. M. (2004). Restoring the heart and humanity of medicine: Integrating spirituality into healthcare.

In *Spirituality and healing in medicine: The enhanced importance of the integration of mind/body practices and prayer.* (A continuing education course sponsored by the Harvard Medical School and the Mind/Body Medical Institute, and George Washington University and the George Washington Institute for Spirituality and Health.). Boston. For additional information, go to http://cme.med.harvard.edu/

Rosenhead, J. (1998). *Complexity theory and management practice. Science as culture.* Retrieved January 28, 2008, from www.human-nature.com/science-as-culture/rosenhead.html

Sanford, F. H. (1950). *Authoritarianism and leadership.* Philadelphia: Institute for Research in Human Relations.

Sherer, J. (1994). Resolving conflict (the right way). *Hospitals and Health Networks, 68*(8), 52–55.

Taylor, E. J. (2002). *Spiritual care: Nursing theory, research and practice.* Prentice-Hall: Upper Saddle River, NJ.

The Joint Commission (TJC). (2008). *Comprehensive accreditation manual for hospitals.* Oakbrook Terrace, IL. Retrieved September 28, 2008, from www.jointcommission.orgStandards/Manuals/

Troupin, B. (2001). *16th WONCA World Conference of Family Doctors Conference Summary,* June 2001. Retrieved July 21, 2009, from http://medscape.com/viewarticle/403641.

Ulrich, B. (2004). Fear factor: Management must stay on top of hostile behavior for nurses'—and patients'—sake. *California NurseWeek: A Nursing Spectrum Publication. 17*(9), 4. Website: www.nurseweek.com

U.S. Department of Health and Human Services, Health Resources and Services Administration. (2008). *The registered nurse population: Findings from the 2004 national sample survey of registered nurses.* Retrieved October 4, 2008, from bhpr.hrsa.gov/healthworkforce/rnsurvey04/

U.S. Department of Labor, Bureau of Labor Statistics. Retrieved October 4, 2008, from www.bls.gov/oco/ocos083.htm

Velde, B. P., Greer, A. G., Lynch, D. C., & Escott-Stump, S. (2002). Chaos Theory as a planning tool for community based educational experiences for health students. *Journal of Allied Health.* Retrieved January 28, 2008, from http://findarticles.com/p/articles/mi_qa4040/is_200210/ai_n9123126/pg_4

Waldrop, M. M. (1992). *Complexity: The emerging science at the edge of order and chaos.* New York: Simon & Schuster Paperbacks.

Walsh, M. (2000). Chaos, complexity and nursing. *Nursing Standard, 14*(3), 39–42.

Chapter 9

Alderfer, C. (1969). A new theory of human needs. *Organizational Behavior and Human Performance,* 4, 142–175.

Amabile, T. M. (1997). Motivating creativity in organizations: On doing what you love and loving what you do. *California Management Review, 40*(1), 39–58.

Ambrose, M. L., & Kulik, C. T. (1999). Old friends, new faces: Motivation research in the 1990s. *Journal of Management, 25*(3), 231–292.

Apter, M. (2007). *Reversal theory: The dynamics of motivation, emotion, and personality* (2nd ed.). Oxford, England: Oneworld Publications.

Batson, C. D., Ahmad, N., Lishner, D. A., & Tsang, J. (2002). Empathy and altruism. In C. R. Snyder, & S. J. Lopez (Eds.), *Handbook of positive psychology* (pp. 485–498). New York: Oxford University Press.

Blanchard, K., Edington, D. W., & Blanchard, M. (1999). *The one minute manager balances work and life.* New York: W. Morrow.

Carver, C. S., & Scheier, M. F. (2002). Optimism. In C. R. Snyder, & S. J. Lopez (Eds.), *Handbook of positive psychology* (pp. 231–243). New York: Oxford University Press.

Collins, J. (2001). *Good to great.* New York: Harper Business.

D'Aunno, T. A., Fottler, M. D., & O'Connor, S. J. (2000). Motivating people. In S. M. Shortell, & A. D. Kaluzny (Eds.), *Health care management: Organization design and behavior.* Albany, NY: Delmar.

Hackman, J., & Oldham, G. (1979). *Work redesign.* Reading, MA: Addison-Wesley.

Heine, S. J. (2007). Culture and motivation: What motivates people to act in the ways that they do. In S. Kitayama, & D. Cohen (Eds.), *Handbook of cultural psychology* (pp. 714–733). New York: The Guilford Press.

Henderson, M. (1993). Measuring managerial motivation: The power management inventory. *Journal of Nursing Measurement, 1*(1), 67–80.

Herzberg, F. (2003). One more time: How do you motivate employees? *Harvard Business Review, 81*(1), 87–96.

Herzberg, F., Mausner, B., & Snyderman, B. (1959). *The motivation to work.* New York: John Wiley & Sons.

Hofstede, G. (1993). Cultural constraints in management theories. *Academy of Management Executive, 7*(1), 81–94.

Kane, K., & Montgomery, K. (1998). A framework for understanding disempowerment in organizations. *Human Resource Management, 37*(3-4), 263–275.

Laamanen, R., Broms, U., Happola, A., & Brommels, M. (1999). Changes in the work and motivation of staff delivering home care services in Finland. *Public Health Nursing, 16*(1), 60–71.

Lachman, R. (1997). Taking another look at the elephant: Are we still (half) blind? Comments on the crosscultural analysis of achievement motivation. *Journal of Organizational Behavior, 18*(7), 317–321.

Laschinger, H. K., Finegan, J., & Shamian, J. (2001). The impact of workplace empowerment, organizational trust on staff nurses' work satisfaction and organizational commitment. *Health Care Management Review, 26*(3), 7–23.

Lawler, E. III. (1973). *Motivation in work organizations.* Monterey, CA: Brooks/Cole Publishing.

Lewin, K. (1935). *A dynamic theory of personality.* New York: McGraw-Hill.

Locke, E., & Latham, G. P. (2004). What should we do about motivation theory? Six recommendations for the 21st century. *Academy of Management Review, 29*(3), 388–403.

Maslow, A. (1954). *Motivation and personality*. New York: Harper & Row.

McClelland, D. (1961). *The achieving society*. Princeton, NJ: Van Nostrand.

McClelland, D. (1976). Power is the great motivation. *Harvard Business Review, 54*(2), 100–110.

McClelland, D., & Boyatzis, R. (1982). Leadership motive patterns and long-term success in management. *Journal of Applied Psychology, 67*, 737–743.

McClure, M. L., & Hinshaw, A. S. (2002). *Magnet hospitals revisited: Attraction and retention of professional nurses*. Washington, DC: American Nurses Publishing.

McConnell, C. R. (1998). Employee involvement: Motivation or manipulation? *Health Care Supervisor, 16*(3), 69–85.

McGregor, D. (1960). *The human side of enterprise*. New York: McGraw-Hill.

Miner, J. B. (2002). *Organizational behavior: Foundations, theories and analyses*. New York: Oxford University Press.

Mitchell, T., & Daniels, D. (2003). Observations and commentary on recent research in work motivation. In L. W. Porter, G. A. Bigley, & R. M. Steers (Eds.), *Motivation and work behavior* (7th ed., pp. 26–44). Boston: McGraw-Hill/Irwin.

Moore, S. C., & Hutchison, S. A. (2007). Developing leaders at every level: Accountability and empowerment actualized through shared governance. *Journal of Nursing Administration, 37*(12), 564–568.

Morse, G. (2003). Why we misread motives: We think other people are more mercenary than they really are. *Harvard Business Review, 81*(1), 18–19.

Nicholson, N. (2003). How to motivate your problem people. *Harvard Business Review, 81*(1), 57–65.

O'Reilly, C. A., & Chatman, J. A. (1999). Working smarter and harder: A longitudinal study of managerial success. In L. W. Porter, G. A. Bigley, & R. M. Steers (Eds.), *Motivation and work behavior* (7th ed., pp. 603–627). Boston: McGraw-Hill/Irwin.

Petri, H. L. (1996). *Motivation: Theory, research and applications* (4th ed.). New York: Brooks/Cole Publishing.

Pinder, C. C. (1998). *Work motivation in organizational behavior*. Upper Saddle River, NJ: Prentice-Hall.

L. Porter, G. A. Bigley, & R. M. Steers (Eds.). (2003). *Motivation and work behavior* (7th ed.). Boston: McGraw-Hill/Irwin.

Porter, L., & Lawler, E. (1968). *Managerial attitudes and performance*. Homewood, IL: Dorsey Press.

Price, J., & Mueller, C. (1986). *Handbook of organizational measurement*. Marshfield, MA: Pitman.

Rainey, H. G. (2001). Work motivation. In R. T. Golembiewski (Ed.), *Handbook of organizational behavior* (2nd ed., pp. 19–42). New York: Marcel Dekker.

Rantz, M. J., Scott, J., & Porter, R. (1996). Employee motivation: New perspectives of the age-old challenge of work motivation. *Nursing Forum, 31*(3), 29–36.

Redman, R. W., & Ketefian, S. (1995). Conceptual and methodological issues in work redesign. In K. Kelly, & M. Maas (Eds.), *Series on nursing administration: Health care work redesign* (Vol. VII). Thousand Oaks, CA: Sage Publications.

Rousseau, D. M. (2004). Psychological contracts in the workplace: Understanding the ties that motivate. *Academy of Management Executive, 18*(1), 120–127.

Sanchez-Runde, C. J., & Steers, R. M. (2001). Cultural influences on work motivation and performance. In L. W. Porter, G. A. Bigley, & R. M. Steers (Eds.), *Motivation and work behavior* (7th ed., pp. 357–374). Boston: McGraw-Hill/Irwin.

Schweiger, J. (1980). *The nurse as manager*. New York: John Wiley & Sons.

Steers, R., & Porter, L. (1987). *Motivation and work behavior* (4th ed.). New York: McGraw-Hill.

Steers, R. M., Mowday, R. T., & Shapiro, D. L. (2004). The future of work motivation theory. *Academy of Management Review, 29*(3), 379–387.

Tzeng, H. M. (2002). The influence of nurses' working motivation and job satisfaction on intention to quit: An empirical investigation in Taiwan. *International Journal of Nursing Studies, 39*(8), 867–878.

Vroom, V. (1964). *Work and motivation*. New York: John Wiley & Sons.

Chapter 10

Aguayo, R. (1990). *Dr. Deming: The American who taught the Japanese about quality*. New York: Carol Publishing Group.

Beachy, P., & Biester, D. (1986). Restructuring group meetings for effectiveness. *Journal of Nursing Administration, 16*(12), 30–33.

Blegen, M. (1993). Nurses' job satisfaction: A meta-analysis of related variables. *Nursing Research, 42*(1), 36–41.

Book, C., & Galvin, K. (1975). *Instruction in and about small group discussion*. Falls Church, VA: Speech Communication Association.

Brown, B. (1998). 10 trends for the new year: Nurse managers predict the skills, technology, and mind-set you'll need to prosper in 1999. *Nursing Management, 29*(2), 33–36.

Cherniss, C., & Goleman, D. (2001). *The emotionally intelligent workplace: How to select for, measure, and improve emotional intelligence in individuals, groups, and organizations*. San Francisco: Jossey-Bass.

Dabney, D. (1995). Workplace deviance among nurses: The influence of work group norms on drug diversion and/or use. *Journal of Nursing Administration, 25*(3), 48–55.

Darr, K. (1989). Applying the Deming method in hospitals, Part 1. *Hospital Topics, 67*(6), 4–5.

Deveau, B. J., & McCabe, D. U. (1996). Results-oriented committee restructuring. *Journal of Nursing Administration, 26*(10), 35–46.

DiMeglio, K., Padula, C., Piatek, C., Korber, S., Barrett, A., Ducharme, M., et al. (2005). Group cohesion and nurse satisfaction: Examination of a team-building approach. *Journal of Nursing Administration, 35*(3), 110–120.

Drucker, P. F. (1993). *Post capitalist society.* New York: Harper Business Publishers.

Farley, M., & Stoner, M. (1989). The nurse executive and interdisciplinary team building. *Nursing Administration Quarterly, 13*(2), 24–30.

Gage, M. (1998). From independence to interdependence: Creating synergistic healthcare teams. *Journal of Nursing Administration, 28*(4), 17–26.

Goldratt, E. M., & Cox, J. (2004). *The goal.* Great Barrington, MA: North River Press.

Hersey, P., Blanchard, K. H., & Johnson, D. E. (2008). *Management of organizational behavior: Leading human resources* (9th ed.). Upper Saddle River, NJ: Pearson Education.

Jacobs, B., & Rosenthal, T. (1984). Managing effective meetings. *Nursing Economic$, 2*(2), 137–141.

Jay, A. (1982). How to run a meeting. *Journal of Nursing Administration, 12*(1), 22–28.

Katzenbach, J., & Smith, D. (1993). *The wisdom of teams: Creating the high-performance organization.* New York: Harper Collins.

Kohn, L. T., Corrigan, J. M., & Donaldson, M. S. (Eds.). (2000). *To err is human: Building a safer health system.* Washington, DC: National Academies Press.

Lancaster, J. (1981). Making the most of meetings. *Journal of Nursing Administration, 11*(10), 15–19.

Laramee, A. (1999). The building blocks of successful relationships. *The Journal of Care Management, 5*(4), 40, 42, 44–45.

Lassen, A. A., Fosbinder, D. M., Minton, S., & Robins, M. M. (1997). Nurse/physician collaborative practice: Improving health care quality while decreasing cost. *Nursing Economic$, 15*(2), 87–91, 104.

Lencioni, P. (2002). *The five dysfunctions of a team.* San Francisco: Jossey-Bass.

Lencioni, P. (2004). *Death by meeting.* San Francisco: Jossey-Bass.

Lencioni, P. (2006). *Silos, politics and turf wars.* San Francisco: Jossey-Bass.

Leppa, C. J. (1996). Nurse relationships and work group disruption. *Journal of Nursing Administration, 26*(10), 23–27.

Manion, J. (2004). Strengthening organizational commitment: Understanding the concept as a basis for creating effective workforce retention strategies. *The Health Care Manager, 23*(2), 167–176.

Manion, J. (2005). *Create a positive healthcare workplace: Practical strategies to retain today's workforce and find tomorrow's.* Chicago: AHA Press.

Manion, J., & Bartholomew, K. (2003). Community in the workplace: A proven retention strategy. *Journal of Nursing Administration, 34*(1), 46–53.

Manion, J., Lorimer, W., & Leander, W. J. (1996). *Team-based health care organizations: Blueprint for success.* Gaithersburg, MD: Aspen.

Page, C. (1998). Pathway leadership: A mature framework for teams. *Seminars for Nurse Managers, 6*(4), 195–198.

Ponte, P. R., Fay, M. S., Brown, P., Doyle, M., Perron, J., Zizzi, L., et al. (1998). Factors leading to a strike vote and strategies for reestablishing relationships. *Journal of Nursing Administration, 28*(2), 35–43.

Schmeiding, N. (1990). A model for assessing nurse administrators' actions. *Western Journal of Nursing Research, 12*(3), 293–306.

Sheafor, M. (1991). Productive work groups in complex hospital units: Proposed contributions of the nurse executive. *Journal of Nursing Administration, 21*(5), 25–30.

Sorrells-Jones, J. (1997). The challenge of making it real: Interdisciplinary practice in a "seamless" organization. *Nursing Administration Quarterly, 21*(2), 20–30.

Sorrells-Jones, J., & Weaver, D. (1999). Knowledge workers and knowledge-intense organizations. I. A promising framework for nursing and healthcare. *Journal of Nursing Administration, 29*(7/8), 12–18.

Sovie, M. (1992). Care and service teams: A new imperative. *Nursing Economic$, 10*(2), 94–100.

Spitzer, R. (1998). Teams and teamwork. *Seminars for Nurse Managers, 6*(4), 169.

Van de Ven, A., & Delbecq, A. (1974). The effectiveness of nominal, Delphi, and interacting group decision making processes. *Academy of Management Journal, 17*(4), 605–621.

Veninga, R. (1982). *The human side of health administration: A guide for hospital, nursing, and public health administrators.* Englewood Cliffs, NJ: Prentice-Hall.

Wilson, R. D., Mateo, M. A., & Brumm, S. K. (1999). Revitalizing a departmental committee. *Journal of Nursing Administration, 29*(3), 45–48.

Chapter 11

American Association of Critical-Care Nurses (AACN). (2004). *AACN delegation handbook* (2nd ed.). Aliso Viejo, CA: Author.

American Journal of Nursing (AJN). (1996a). $3 million suit exposes "de-skilling." *American Journal of Nursing, 96*(11), 70.

American Journal of Nursing (AJN). (1996b). Pennsylvania lawmakers probe RN cuts, grill hospitals on UAP use. *American Journal of Nursing, 96*(11), 71–72.

American Nephrology Nurses' Association (ANNA). (2008). The role of unlicensed assistive personnel in dialysis therapy. *Nephrology Nursing Journal.* Retrieved March 28, 2009, from http://findarticles.com/p/articles/mi_m0ICF/is_3_35/ai_n27927978

American Nurses Association (ANA). (1992). *Joint statement on maintaining professional and legal standards during a shortage of nursing personnel.* Washington, DC: Author.

American Nurses Association (ANA). (1996). *Registered professional nurses & unlicensed assistive personnel.* Washington, DC: Author.

American Nurses Association (ANA). (1999). *Principles for nurse staffing.* Washington, DC: Author.

American Nurses Association (ANA). (2001). *Code of ethics for nurses with interpretive statements.* Washington, DC: Author.

American Nurses Association (ANA). (2003). *ANA applauds federal legislation to mandate safe nurse-to-patient ratios.* Retrieved February 14, 2008, from www.aacn.org/aacn/practice.nsf/vwdoc/ns?opendocument

Anthony, M. K., Standing, T., & Hertz, J. E. (2000). Factors influencing outcomes after delegation to unlicensed assistive personnel. *Journal of Nursing Administration, 30*(10), 474–480.

Association of Operating Room Nurses (AORN). (2004). *Official statement on unlicensed assistive personnel.* Denver: Author.

Barter, M., & Furmidge, M. (1994). Unlicensed assistive personnel: Issues relating to delegation and supervision. *Journal of Nursing Administration, 24*(4), 36–40.

Bureau of Labor and Statistics. (2006). *Occupational outlook handbook.* Washington, DC: Author: Retrieved October 13, 2008, from www.bls.gov/oco/ocos083.htm

Department for Professional Employees, AFL-CIO. (2007). *The costs and benefits for staffing ratios fact sheet.* Retrieved February 14, 2008, from www.dpeaflcio.org/programs/factsheets/fs_2007_staffratio.htm

Fisher, M. (2000). Do you have delegation savvy? *Nursing, 30*(12), 58–59.

Global Insight. (2006). *Does nurse-to-patient ratio legislation help patients or harm hospitals in the United States?* Retrieved October 13, 2008, from www.globalinsight.com/Perspective/PerspectiveDetail6099.htm

Hansten, R. (1991). Delegation: Learning when and how to let go. *Nursing, 21*(2), 126–133.

Hodge, M. B., Romano, P. S., Harvey, D., & Samuels, S. J. (2004). Licensed caregiver characteristics and staffing in California acute care hospital units. *Journal of Nursing Administration, 34*(3), 125–133.

Hudspeth, R. (2007). Understanding delegation is a critical competency for nurses in the new millennium. *Journal of Nursing Administration Quarterly, 32*(2), 183–184.

Institute for Healthcare Improvement (IHI). (2008). *Failure modes and effects analysis (FMEA) tool (IHI tool).* Boston, MA. Retrieved February 12, 2008, from www.ihi.org/IHI/Topics/PatientSafety/SafetyGeneral/Tools/Failure+Modes+and+Effects+Analysis+%28FMEA%29+Tool+%28IHI+Tool%29.htm

Institute of Medicine (IOM). (2003). *Patient safety: Achieving a new standard for care.* Washington, DC: National Academies Press.

Iowa Board of Nursing. (2003). *Nursing practice for registered nurses/licensed practical nurses.* Des Moines, IA: The State of Iowa. Retrieved September 23, 2004, from www.state.ia.us/nursing/nursing_practice.html

Kleinman, C. S. (2004). Leadership strategies in reducing staff nurse role conflict. *Journal of Nursing Administration, 34*(7/8), 322–324.

Kraus, K., & Cameron, M. E. (2004). Legal and ethical issues: Communication and malpractice lawsuits. *Journal of Nursing Administration, 34*(1), 3.

Marthaler, M. (2003). Delegation of nursing care. In P. Kelly-Heidenthal (Ed.), *Nursing leadership and management* (pp. 266–279). Clifton Park, NY: Delmar.

Martin, J., & Cain, S. K. (2003). Legal aspects of patient care. In P. Kelly-Heidenthal (Ed.), *Nursing leadership and management* (pp. 266–279). Clifton Park, NY: Delmar.

McIntosh, J. (2003). Questions we should ask about community nursing practice. *Primary Health Care Research and Development, 4,* 137–145.

McIntosh, J., Moriarty, D., Lugton, J., & Carney, O. (2000). Evolutionary change in the use of skills within the district nursing team: A study in two Health Board areas in Scotland. *Journal of Advanced Nursing, 32,* 783–790.

National Council of State Boards of Nursing (NCSBN). (1990). *Concept paper on delegation.* Chicago: Author.

National Council of State Boards of Nursing (NCSBN). (1995). *Delegation: Concepts and decision-making process.* Chicago: Author.

National Council of State Boards of Nursing (NCSBN). (1997a). *Delegation decision-making tree.* Chicago: Author.

National Council of State Boards of Nursing (NCSBN). (1997b). *Delegation decision-making grid.* Chicago: Author.

National Council of State Boards of Nursing (NCSBN). (1998a). *Diagram to illustrate roles of nurse and AP.* Chicago: Author. Retrieved from www.ncsbn.org/340.htm

National Council of State Boards of Nursing (NCSBN). (1998b). *The continuum of care framework.* Chicago: Author. Retrieved from www.ncsbn.org/contcaregrid.pdf

National Council of State Boards of Nursing (NCSBN). (1998c). *The continuum of care: A regulatory perspective.* Chicago: Author. Retrieved from www.ncsbn.org/contcarepaper.pdf

National Council of State Boards of Nursing (NCSBN). (2006). *NCSBN model nursing practice act and model nursing administrative rules.* Retrieved February 12, 2008, from www.ncsbn.org/Model_Nursing_Act_and_Rules.pdf

National Council of State Boards of Nursing (NCSBN) Bylaws. (2007). *NCSBN bylaws.* Chicago: Author. Retrieved October 13, 2008, from www.ncsbn.org/

National Council of State Boards of Nursing (NCSBN) Research Brief. (2002). *Report of findings from the Practice and Professional Issues Survey.* Chicago, IL: Author. Retrieved October 13, 2008, from www.ncsbn.org/

National Council of State Boards of Nursing (NCSBN) and the American Nurses Association (ANA). (2006). *Joint statement on nursing delegation.* Retrieved February 2008, from www.ncsbn.org/1056.htm

Nightingale, F. (1859). *Notes on nursing: What it is and what it is not.* London: Harrison & Sons.

Niven, C., & Scott, P. (2003). The need for accurate perception and informed judgment in determining the appropriate use of the nursing resource: Hear the patient's voice. *Nursing Philosophy, 4*, 201–210.

Poteet, G. (1989). Nursing administrators and delegation. *Nursing Administration Quarterly, 13*(3), 23–32.

Potter, P., & Grant, E. (2004). Understanding RN and unlicensed assistive personnel working relationships in designing care delivery strategies. *Journal of Nursing Administration, 34*(1), 19–25.

Richards, A., Carley, J., Jenkins-Clarke, S., & Richards, D. (2000). Skill mix between nurses and doctors working in primary care-delegation or allocation: A review of the literature. *International Journal of Nursing Studies, 37*, 185–197.

Rivers, F., Wertenberger, D., & Lindgren, K. (2006). U.S. Army professional filler system nursing personnel: Do they possess competency needed for deployment? *Military Medicine, 171*(2), 144–149.

Rushton, H. C. (2007). Respect in critical care: A foundational ethical principle. *AACN Advanced Critical Care, 18*(2), 149–156.

The Joint Commission. (2004). *Staffing effectiveness standard.* Oakbrook Terrace, IL: Author. Retrieved October 11, 2004, from www.jcaho.org/accredited+organizations/hospitals/standards/draft+standards/staffingeffectivenessstandard0804.pdf

The Joint Commission. (2007). *National patient safety goals.* Retrieved February 12, 2008, from www.jointcommission.org/PatientSafety/NationalPatientSafetyGoals/

Zerwekh, J., & Claborn, J. C. (2003). *Nursing today: Transition and trends* (4th ed.). Philadelphia: Saunders.

Chapter 12

Abood, S. (2007). Influencing health care in the legislative arena. *Online Journal of Issues in Nursing, 12*(1), Retrieved October 15, 2008, from www.nursingworld.org/MainMenuCategories/ANAMarketplace/ANAPeriodicals/OJIN/TableofContents/Volume122007/No1Jan07/tpc32_216091.aspx

Adlersberg, M., & Ottem, P. (2004). *Managing conflict.* Vancouver, BC: Registered Nurses Association of British Columbia. Retrieved June 3, 2004, from www.rnabc.bc.ca/registrants/nursing_practice/articles/conflpg1.htm

Agency for Healthcare Research and Quality (AHRQ). (2008). *2007 National healthcare disparities report.* Rockville, MD: U.S. Department of Health and Human Services, Agency for Healthcare Research and Quality; AHRQ Publication No. 08-0041. Retrieved October 15, 2008, from www.ahrq.gov/qual/qrdr07.htm

Almost, J. (2005). Conflict within nursing work environments: Concept analysis. *Journal of Advanced Nursing, 53*(4), 444–453.

Amason, A. (1996). Distinguishing effects of functional and dysfunctional conflict on strategic decision making: Resolving a paradox for top management teams. *Academy of Management Journal, 39*, 123–148.

Amason, A., & Sapienza, H. (1997). The effects of top management team size and interaction norms on cognitive and affective conflict. *Journal of Management, 23*, 496–516.

Bacharach, S. B., & Lawler, E. J. (1980). *Power and politics in organizations.* San Francisco: Jossey-Bass.

Barki, H., & Hartwick, J. (2001). Interpersonal conflict and its management in information system development. *MIS Quarterly, 25*, 195–228.

Barki, H., & Hartwick, J. (2004). Conceptualizing the construct of interpersonal conflict. *International Journal of Conflict Management, 15*(3), 216–244.

Bartol, G., Parrish, R. S., & McSweeney, M. (2001). Effective conflict management begins with knowing your style. *Journal of Nursing Staff Development, 17*(1), 34–40.

Barton, A. (1991). Conflict resolution by nurse managers. *Nursing Management, 22*(5), 83–86.

Benner, P. (1984). *From novice to expert: Excellence and power in clinical nursing practice.* Menlo Park, CA: Addison-Wesley.

Bennis, W., & Nanus, B. (1985). *Leaders: The strategies for taking charge.* New York: Harper & Row.

Bierstedt, R. (1950). An analysis of power. *American Sociological Review, 15*, 730–738.

Blake, R., & Mouton, J. S. (1964). *The managerial grid.* Houston, TX: Gulf Publishing.

Blau, P. M. (1964). *Exchange and power in social life.* New York: Wiley.

Booth, R. (1993). Dynamics of conflict and conflict management. In D. Mason, S. Talbott, & J. Leavitt (Eds.), *Policy and politics for nurses: Action and change in the workplace, government, organizations, and community* (2nd ed., pp. 149–165). Philadelphia: Saunders.

Boswell, C., Cannon, S., & Miller, J. (2005). Nurses' political involvement: Responsibility versus privilege. *Journal of Professional Nursing, 21*(1), 5–8.

Brown, L. D. (1983). *Managing conflict at organizational interfaces.* Reading, MA: Addison-Wesley Publishing.

Cavanagh, S. (1991). The conflict management style of staff nurses and nurse managers. *Journal of Advanced Nursing, 16*, 1254–1260.

Centers for Disease Control and Prevention (CDC). (2008). *Chronic disease prevention.* Atlanta, GA: CDC. Retrieved March 28, 2009, from www.cdc.gov/nccdphp/

Cohen, L. B. (1992). Power and change in health care: Challenge for nursing. *Journal of Nursing Education, 31*, 113–116.

Cohen, R. A., Martinez, M. E., & Free, H. L. (2008). *Health insurance coverage: Early release of estimates from the National Health Interview Survey.* National Center for Health Statistics. Retrieved October 15, 2008, from www.cdc.gov/nchs/nhis.htm

Conrad, C. (1990). *Strategic organizational communication: An integrated perspective* (2nd ed.). Fort Worth, TX: Holt, Rinehart & Winston.

Coser, L. A. (1956). *The functions of social conflict*. Glencoe, IL: Free Press.

Cox, K. B. (2004). The intragroup conflict scale: Development and psychometric properties. *Journal of Nursing Measurement, 12*(2), 133–146.

Crozier, M. (1964). *The bureaucratic phenomenon*. Chicago: University of Chicago Press.

Daft, R. L. (2006). *Organization theory and design* (9th ed.). Cincinnati, OH: South-Western Publishing.

Dahl, R. A. (1957). The concept of power. *Behavioral Science, 2*, 202–210.

DeDreu, C. K. W., & Weingart, L. R. (2003). Task versus relationship conflict, team performance, and team member satisfaction: A meta-analysis. *Journal of Applied Psychology, 88*(4), 741–750.

Dennis, K. E. (1983). Nursing's power in the organization: What research has shown. *Nursing Administration Quarterly, 8*, 47–57.

Deutsch, M. (1973). *The resolution of conflict: Constructive and destructive processes*. New Haven, CT: Yale University Press.

Emerson, R. M. (1957). Power-dependence relations. *American Sociological Review, 27*(1), 31–40.

Filley, A. C. (1975). *Interpersonal conflict resolution*. Glenview, IL: Scott, Foresman.

Fisher, R., Ury, W., & Patton, B. (1992). *Getting to yes: Negotiating agreement without giving in* (2nd ed.). New York: Penguin Books.

Folger, J. P., Poole, M. S., & Stutman, R. K. (1997). *Working through conflict: Strategies for relationships, groups, and organizations*. New York: Longman.

French, J., & Raven, B. (1959). The bases of social power. In D. Cartwright (Ed.), *Studies in social power* (pp. 150–167). Ann Arbor, MI: University of Michigan, Institute for Social Research.

Gardner, D. L. (1992). Conflict and retention of new graduate nurses. *Western Journal of Nursing Research, 14*, 76–85.

Gerardi, D. (2004). Using mediation techniques to manage conflict and create healthy work environments. *AACN Clinical Issues, 15*(2), 182–195.

Hampton, D. R., Summer, C. E., & Webber, R. A. (1987). *Organization behavior and the practice of management*. Glenview, IL: Scott, Foresman.

Hardy, C., & Leiba-O'Sullivan, S. (1998). The power behind empowerment: Implications for research and practice. *Human Relations, 51*(4), 451–483.

HealthGrades. (2008). *The fifth annual HealthGrades patient safety in American hospitals study*. Retrieved June 19, 2008, from www.healthgrades.com/media/dms/pdf/HealthGradesPatientSafetyRelease2008.pdf

Hersey, P., Blanchard, K. H., & Johnson, D. E. (2008). *Management of organizational behavior: Leading human resources* (9th ed.). Upper Saddle River, NJ: Pearson Education.

Hersey, P., Blanchard, K. H., & Natemeyer, W. E. (1979). Situational leadership, perception, and the impact of power. *Group and Organization Studies, 4*, 418–428.

Hickson, D. J., Hinings, C. R., Lee, C. A., Schneck, R. E., & Pennings, J. M. (1971). A strategic contingencies theory of intraorganizational power. *Administrative Science Quarterly, 16*, 216–229.

Hightower, T. (1986). Subordinate choice of conflict handling modes. *Nursing Administration Quarterly, 11*(1), 29–34.

Hinings, C. R., Hickson, D. J., Pennings, J. M., & Schneck, R. E. (1974). Structural conditions of intraorganizational power. *Administrative Science Quarterly, 19*, 22–44.

Hodges, L. C., Williams, B. G., & Carman, D. D. (2002). Taking political responsibility for nursing's future. *MEDSURG Nursing, 11*(1), 15–24.

Jehn, K. A. (1995). A multimethod examination of the benefits and detriments of intragroup conflict. *Administrative Science Quarterly, 40*, 256–282.

Jehn, K. A. (1997). A qualitative analysis of conflict types and dimensions in organizational groups. *Administrative Science Quarterly, 42*, 530–557.

Jehn, K. A., Northcraft, G., & Neale, M. (1999). Why differences make a difference: A field study of diversity, conflict, and performance in workgroups. *Administrative Science Quarterly, 44*, 741–763.

Kane, R. L., Shamliyan, T., Mueller, C., Duvai, S., & Wilt, T. (2007). *Nursing staffing and quality of patient care. Evidence report/technology Assessment No. 151* (prepared by the Minnesota Evidence-based Practice Center under Contract No. 290-0009). AHRQ Publication No. 07-E005. Rockville, MD: Agency for Healthcare Research and Quality.

Kanter, R. M. (1977). *Men and women of the corporation*. New York: Basic Books.

Kaplan, A. (1964). Power in perspective. In R. L. Kahn, & E. Boulding (Eds.), *Power and conflict in organizations* (pp. 11–32). London: Tavistock.

Kelly, J. (2006). An overview of conflict. *Dimensions of Critical Care Nursing, 25*(1), 22–28.

King, I. M. (1981). *A theory for nursing: Systems, concepts, process*. New York: Wiley & Sons.

Kipnis, D., Schmidt, S. M., Swaffin-Smith, C., & Wilkinson, I. (1984). Patterns of managerial influence: Shotgun managers, tacticians, and bystanders. *Organizational Dynamics, 12*(3), 58–67.

Kipnis, D., Schmidt, S. M., & Wilkinson, I. (1980). Intraorganizational influence tactics: Explorations in getting one's way. *Journal of Applied Psychology, 65*(4), 440–452.

Kohn, L. T., Corrigan, J. M., & Donaldson, M. S. (Eds.), Committee on quality of healthcare in America. Institute of Medicine of the National Academies. (2000). *To err is human: Building a safer health system*. Washington, DC: National Academies Press.

Kotter, J. P. (1979). *Power in management: How to understand, acquire, and use it*. New York: AMACOM.

Kouzes, J., & Posner, B. (1987). *The leadership challenge: How to get extraordinary things done in organizations.* San Francisco: Jossey-Bass.

Kramer, M., & Schmalenberg, C. (1990). Fundamental lessons in leadership. In E. Simendinger, T. Moore, & M. Kramer (Eds.), *The successful nurse executive: A guide for every nurse manager* (pp. 5–21). Ann Arbor, MI: Health Administration Press.

Laschinger, H. K., Finegan, J., & Shamian, J. (2001). The impact of workplace empowerment, organizational trust on staff nurses' work satisfaction and organizational commitment. *Health Care Management Review, 26*(3), 7–23.

Laschinger, H. K., Finegan, J., Shamian, J., & Casier, S. (2000). Organizational trust and empowerment in restructured healthcare settings: Effects on staff nurse commitment. *Journal of Nursing Administration, 30*(9), 413–425.

Laschinger, H. K., Finegan, J., Shamian, J., & Wilk, P. (2001). Impact of structural and psychological empowerment on job strain in nursing work settings: Expanding Kanter's model. *Journal of Nursing Administration, 31*(5), 260–272.

Laschinger, H. K., & Havens, D. S. (1997). The effect of workplace empowerment on staff nurses' occupational mental health and work effectiveness. *Journal of Nursing Administration, 27*(6), 4–50.

Laschinger, H. K., Purdy, N., & Almost, J. (2007). The impact of leader-member exchange quality, empowerment, and core self-evaluation on nurse manager's job satisfaction. *Journal of Nursing Administration, 37*(5), 221–229.

Laschinger, H. K., Sabiston, J. A., & Kutszcher, L. (1997). Empowerment and staff nurse decision involvement in nursing work environments: Testing Kanter's theory of structural power in organizations. *Research in Nursing and Health, 20,* 341–352.

Liberatore, P., Brown-Williams, R., Brucker, J., Dukes, N., Kimmey, L., McCarthy, K., et al. (1989). A group approach to problem-solving. *Nursing Management, 20*(9), 68–72.

Mallory, G. (1981). Believe it or not: Conflict can be healthy once you understand it and learn to manage it. *Nursing, 11*(6), 97–101.

Manojlovich, M. (2007). Power and empowerment in nursing: Looking back to inform the future. *The Online Journal of Issues in Nursing, 12*(1). Retrieved June 5, 2008, from www.nursingworld.org/MainMenuCategories/ANAMarketplace/ANAPeriodicals/OJIN/TableofContents/Volume122007/No1Jan07/LookingBackwardtoInformtheFuture.aspx

Mechanic, D. (1962). Sources of power in lower participants in complex organizations. *Administrative Science Quarterly, 7,* 349–364.

Moore, C. (2003). *The mediation process: Practical strategies for resolving conflict* (3rd ed.). New York: John Wiley & Sons.

Nagle, L. (1999). A matter of extinction or distinction. *Western Journal of Nursing Research, 21*(1), 71–82.

National Nursing Centers Consortium. (2008). *The nurse-managed health clinic investment act.* Retrieved February 1, 2008, from www.nncc.us/policy/NMHCAct.pdf

Oetzel, J. G., & Ting-Toomey, S. (2003). Face concerns in interpersonal conflict: A cross-cultural empirical test of the face negotiation theory. *Communication Research, 30*(6), 599–624.

Oetzel, J. G., Ting-Toomey, S., Masumoto, T., Yokochi, Y., Pan, X., Takai, J., et al. (2001). Face and facework in conflict: A cross-cultural comparison of China, Germany, Japan, and the United States. *Communication Monographs, 68,* 235–258.

Pfeffer, J. (1981). *Power in organizations.* Boston: Pitman Books.

Pinkley, R. (1990). Dimensions of the conflict frame: Disputant interpretations of conflict. *Journal of Applied Psychology, 75*(2), 117–128.

Poisal, J. A., Truffer, C., Smith, S., Sisko, A., Cowan, C., Keehan, S., et al. (2007). Health spending projections through 2016: Modest changes obscure part D's impact. *Health Affairs, 26*(2), 242–253.

Pondy, L. R. (1967). Organizational conflict: Concepts and models. *Administrative Science Quarterly, 12,* 296–320.

Ponte, P. R., Glazer, G., Dann, E., McCollum, K., Gross, A., Tyrrell, R., et al. (2007). The power of professional nursing practice: An essential element of patient and family centered care. *The Online Journal of Issues in Nursing, 12*(1). Retrieved October 15, 2008, from www.nursingworld.org/MainMenuCategories/ANAMarketplace/ANAPeriodicals/OJIN/TableofContents/Volume122007/No1Jan07/tpc32_316092.aspx

Putnam, L. L., & Poole, M. S. (1987). Conflict and negotiation. In F. M. Jablin, L. L. Putnam, K. Roberts, & L. W. Porter (Eds.), *Handbook of organizational communication* (pp. 549–599). Newbury Park, CA: Sage.

Rahim, M. A. (1983a). A measure of styles of handling interpersonal conflict. *Academy of Management Journal, 26,* 368–376.

Rahim, M. A. (1983b). Measurement of organizational conflict. *The Journal of General Psychology, 109,* 189–199.

Rahim, M. A. (1983c). *Rahim organizational conflict inventories: Experimental edition: Professional manual.* Palo Alto, CA: Consulting Psychologists Press.

Rahim, M. A. (2001). *Managing conflict in organizations* (3rd ed.). Westport, CT: Quorum.

Rahim, M. A., & Bonoma, T. V. (1979). Managing organizational conflict: A model for diagnosis and intervention. *Psychological Reports, 44,* 1323–1344.

Raven, B., & Kruglanski, W. (1975). Conflict and power. In P. Swingle (Ed.), *The structure of conflict* (pp. 177–219). New York: Academic Press.

Rebmann, T. (2006). Defining disaster preparedness for nurses: Concept analysis. *Journal of Advanced Nursing, 54*(5), 623–632.

Robbins, S. P. (2003). *Organizational behavior* (10th ed.). Englewood Cliffs, NJ: Prentice-Hall.

Robbins, S. P., & Judge, T. A. (2008). *Organizational behavior* (13th ed.). Upper Saddle River, NJ: Pearson Prentice Hall.

Robbins, S. P., & Langton, N. (1999). *Organizational behavior, concepts, controversies, applications* (Canadian ed.). Scarborough, ON: Prentice-Hall Canada.

Sabiston, J. A., & Laschinger, H. K. (1995). Staff nurse empowerment and perceived autonomy: Testing Kanter's theory of structural power in organizations. *Journal of Nursing Administration, 25*(9), 42–50.

Salancik, G. R., & Pfeffer, J. (1974). Organizational decision making as a political process: The case of a university budget. *Administrative Science Quarterly, 19*(1), 453–473.

Schira, M. (2004). Reflections on "about power in nursing." *Nephrology Nursing Journal, 31*(5), 583.

Sieloff, C. L. (2003). Measuring nursing power within organizations. *Journal of Nursing Scholarship, 32*, 183–187.

Sportsman, S., & Hamilton, P. (2007). Conflict management styles in the health professions. *Journal of Professional Nursing, 23*(3), 157–166.

Stokowski, L. (2004). Trends in nursing: 2004 and beyond. *Topics in Advanced Practice Nursing eJournal, 4*(1). Retrieved June 15, 2004, from www.medscape.com/viewarticle/466711 (online access granted after free registration).

Thomas, K. W. (1976). Conflict and conflict management. In M. D. Dunnette (Ed.), *The handbook of industrial and organizational psychology* (pp. 889–935). Chicago: Rand McNally.

Thomas, K. W. (1992). Conflict and negotiation processes in organizations. In M. D. Dunnette, & L. M. Hough (Eds.), *The handbook of industrial and organizational psychology* (2nd ed., Vol. 3, pp. 651–717). Palo Alto, CA: Consulting Psychologist Press.

Thomas, K. W., & Kilmann, R. H. (1974). *Thomas-Kilmann conflict mode instrument.* Tuxedo, NY: Xicom.

Thorman, K. (2004). Nursing leadership in the boardroom. *Journal of Obstetric, Gynecologic, and Neonatal Nursing, 33*, 381–387.

Ting-Toomey, S. (1988). Intercultural conflict styles: A face-negotiation theory. In Y. Y. Kim, & W. Gudykunst (Eds.), *Theories in intercultural communication* (pp. 213–235). Newbury Park, CA: Sage.

Ting-Toomey, S. (2005). The matrix of face: An updated face-negotiation theory. In W. B. Gudykunst (Ed.), *Theorizing about intercultural communication* (pp. 71–92). Thousand Oaks, CA: Sage.

Ting-Toomey, S., & Kurogi, A. (1998). Facework competence in intercultural conflict: An updated face-negotiation theory. *International Journal of Intercultural Relations, 22*, 187–225.

Ulrich, B. (2001). A matter of trust. *NurseWeek*, December 17, p. 1. Retrieved June 15, 2004, from www.nurseweek.com/ednote/01/121701a_print.html

U.S. Department of Health and Human Services, Health Resources and Services Administration, Bureau of Health Professions (USDHHS, HRSA, BHPr). (2003). *Changing demographics: Implications for physicians, nurses, and other health workers.* Washington, DC: Author. Retrieved June 15, 2004, from www.bhpr.hrsa.gov/healthworkforce/reports/changedemo/Content.htm

Wall, J. A., & Callister, R. R. (1995). Conflict and its management. *Journal of Management, 21*, 515–558.

Walton, R. E. (1966). Theory of conflict in lateral organizational relationships. In J. R. Lawrence (Ed.), *Operational research and the social sciences* (pp. 409–426). London: Tavistock Publications.

Weber, M. (1947). *The theory of social and economic organization* (A. M. Henderson, & T. Parsons, Trans.)New York: Oxford University Press (Original work published 1923).

Whitehead, D. (2003). The health-promoting nurse as a health policy career expert and entrepreneur. *Nurse Education Today, 23*(8), 585–592.

Woodtli, A. O. (1987). Deans of nursing: Perceived sources of conflict and conflict handling modes. *Journal of Nursing Education, 26*, 272–277.

Yukl, G., & Falbe, C. M. (1991). Importance of different power sources in downward and lateral relations. *Journal of Applied Psychology, 76*(3), 416–423.

Yukl, G., Falbe, C., & Joo, Y. Y. (1993). Patterns off influence behavior for managers. *Group and Organization Management, 18*(1), 5–28.

Yukl, G., Lepsinger, R., & Lucia, T. (1992). Preliminary report on development and validation of the Influence Behavior Questionnaire. In K. E. Clark, M. B. Clar, & D. P. Campbell (Eds.), *The impact of leadership* (pp. 417–427). Greensboro, NC: Center for Creative Leadership.

Chapter 13

Agency for Healthcare Research and Quality (AHRQ). (2003). *What is cultural and linguistic competence?* Rockville, MD: Author. Retrieved September 27, 2004, from www.ahrq.gov/about/cods/cultcompdef.htm

Alexander, C. (2001). Understanding generational differences helps you manage a multi-age workforce. In *The digital edge* (p. 3). Vienna, VA: New Media Federation, Newspaper Association of America. Retrieved June 17, 2004, from www.digitaledge.org/monthly/2001_07/gengap1.html

Alexander, G. R. (2002). A mind for multicultural management. *Nursing Management, 33*(10), 30–33.

American Association of Colleges of Nursing (AACN). (2008). *Enhancing Diversity in the Nursing Workforce.* Fact sheet. Washington, DC: Author. Retrieved March 31, 2009, from www.aacn.nche.edu/Media/FactSheets/diversity.htm

American Hospital Association (AHA) Commission on Workforce for Hospitals and Health Systems. (2002). *In our hands: How hospital leaders can build a thriving workforce.* Chicago: Author.

American Hospital Association (AHA). (2003). *Unequal treatment: Confronting racial and ethnic disparities in health care*. Chicago: AHA news.com.

Betancourt, J. R., Carrillo, J. E., & Green, A. R. (2002). *Cultural competence in health care: Emerging frameworks and practical approaches*. New York: The Commonwealth Fund.

Brett, J., Behfar, K., & Kern, M. C. (2006). Managing multicultural teams. *Harvard Business Review*, 84–91.

California Newsreel. (2003). *Race: The power of an illusion*. San Francisco: Author. Retrieved June 4, 2004, from www.pbs.org/race

Campinha-Bacote, J., Yahle, T., & Langenkamp, M. (1996). The challenge of cultural diversity for nurse educators. *The Journal of Continuing Education in Nursing, 27*(2), 59–64.

Center for the Health Professions. (2002). *Toward culturally competent care: A tool box for teaching communication strategies*. San Francisco: University of California.

Crow, K., Matheson, L., & Steed, A. (2000). Informed consent and truth telling: Cultural directions for health care providers. *Journal of Nursing Administration, 30*(3), 148–152.

Dantley, S. J. (2004). Leaving no child behind in science education. *Black Issues in Higher Education, 21*(8), 114.

Davidhizar, R., Bechtel, G., & Giger, J. (1998). Model helps CMS deliver multicultural care. *Case Management Advisor, 9*(6), 97–100.

Galanti, G. (1999). Caring for culturally diverse patients at home. *Home Health Care Consultant, 6*(1), 33–34.

Gazmararian, J. A., Baker, D. W., Williams, M. V., Parker, R. M., Scott, T. L., Green, D. C., et al. (1999). Health literacy among Medicare enrollees in a managed care organization. *Journal of the American Medical Association, 281*(6), 545–551.

Grossman, D., & Taylor, R. (1995). Cultural diversity on the unit. *American Journal of Nursing, 95*(2), 64–67.

Habayeb, G. L. (1995). Cultural diversity: A nursing concept not yet reliably defined. *Nursing Outlook, 43*(5), 224–227.

Hall, E. T., & Hall, M. R. (1990). *Understanding cultural differences*. Yarmouth, ME: Intercultural Press.

Health Resources and Services Administration (HRSA). (2001). *The registered nurse population: Findings from the 2000 national sample survey*. Rockville, MD: Author, U.S. Department of Health and Human Services.

Health Resources and Services Administration (HRSA). (2002). *Projected supply, demand, and shortages of registered nurses: 2000–2020*. Rockville, MD: Author, U.S. Department of Health and Human Services.

Health Resources and Service Administration (HRSA). (2003). *Changing demographics: Implications for physicians, nurses, and other health workers*. Rockville, MD: Author, U.S. Department of Health and Human Services.

Hecker, D. E. (2004). Occupational employment projections to 2012. *Monthly Labor Review Online, 127*(2). Retrieved March 31, 2009, from www.bls.gov/opub/mlr/2004/02/art5abs.htm

Institute of Medicine (IOM). (2003). *Unequal treatment: Confronting racial and ethnic disparities in health care*. Washington, DC: National Academies Press.

ISCOPES. (2003). *Cultural competence. ISCOPES*. Washington, DC: The George Washington University.

Joint Commission on Accreditation of Healthcare Organizations (JCAHO). (2005). *JCAHOnline. New requirement for language, communication needs*. Oakbrook Terrace, IL: Author.

Kotlikoff, L. J., & Burns, S. (2004). The perfect demographic storm: Entitlements imperil America's future. *The Chronicle of Higher Education, LI*(3), B6–B10.

Leininger, M. (1997). Transcultural nursing research to transform nursing education and practice: 40 years. *Image, 29*(4), 341–347.

Loustaunau, M. O., & Sobo, E. J. (1997). *The cultural context of health, illness, and medicine*. Westport, CT: Bergin & Garvey.

Murphy Leadership Institute. (2004). *National conference on transforming the work environment of nurses. February 25–26*. Washington, DC: Author.

Office of Minority Health. (2001). *Assuring cultural competence in health care: Recommendations for national standards and an outcomes-focused research agenda*. Rockville, MD: Author, Public Health Service, U.S. Department of Health and Human Services. Retrieved October 24, 2004, from www.omhrc.gov/clas/cultural1a.htm

Pew Health Professions Commission. (1998). *Recreating health professional practice for a new century*. San Francisco: Author.

Pew Research Center. (2008). *Immigration to play lead role in future U.S. growth*. Retrieved February 19, 2008, from http://pewresearch.org/pibs/729/united-states-population-projections

U.S. Census Bureau. (1996). *Population projections of the United States by age, sex, race, and Hispanic origin: 1995 to 2050* (Current Population Reports, Series P25–1130). Washington, DC: Author, U.S. Department of Commerce.

Wendover, R. W. (2002). *The corrosion of character*. Aurora, CO: The Center for Generational Studies.

Chapter 14

Agency for Healthcare Research and Quality (AHRQ). (2004). Optimizing surge capacity: Hospital assessment and planning. *Bioterrorism and Health System Preparedness Issue Brief*, No. 3. Retrieved June 12, 2004, from www.ahrq.gov/news/ulp/btbriefs/btbrief3.htm

America's Health Insurance Plans (AHIP). (2009). *America's health insurance plans*. Washington, DC: Author. Retrieved March 31, 2009, from http://www.ahip.org/content/default.aspx?bc=36

American Health Information Management Association. (2004). *The state of HIPAA privacy and security compliance*. Chicago: Author.

American Hospital Association (AHA). (2002). *Cracks in the foundation: Averting a crisis in America's hospitals*. Chicago: Author.

American Hospital Association (AHA). (2004a). *Hospital statistics: 2004 edition*. Chicago: Author.

American Hospital Association (AHA). (2004b). The economic contributions of hospitals. *TrendWatch*, *6*(1), 5.

Anderson, G., Reinhart, U., Hussey, P., & Petrosyan, V. (2003). It's the prices, stupid: Why the United States is so different from other countries. *Health Affairs*, *22*(3), 89–105.

Baicker, K., & Chandra, A. (2004). Medicare spending, the physician workforce, and beneficiaries' quality of care. *Health Affairs: Web Exclusive*, 184–197. Retrieved August 20, 2004, from www.content.healthaffairs.org/webexclusives/index.dtl?year=2004

Barnes, P. M., Powell-Griner, E., McFann, K., & Nahin, R. L. (2004). *Complementary and alternative medicine use among adults: United States, 2002*. Advance data from vital and health statistics (No. 343). Washington, DC: Centers for Disease Control and Prevention. Retrieved August 20, 2004, from www.cdc.gov/nchs/data/ad/ad343.pdf

Berk, M., & Monheit, A. (2001). The concentration of health care expenditures, revisited. *Health Affairs*, *20*(2), 9–18.

Birnbaum, J. (2001). Fat & happy in D.C. *Fortune*, *143*(11), 94–97.

Blank, R. (1997). *The price of life: The future of American health care*. New York: Columbia University Press.

Blumenthal, D. (2004). New steam from an old cauldron: The physician supply debate. *The New England Journal of Medicine*, *350*(17), 1780–1787.

Brooks, C. (2003). Healthcare organizations. In P. Yoder-Wise (Ed.), *Leading and managing in nursing* (3rd ed., pp. 91–105). St. Louis, MO: Mosby.

Buerhaus, P., Staiger, D., & Auerbach, D. (2003). Is the current shortage of hospital nurses ending? *Health Affairs*, *22*(6), 191–198.

Clancy, T. R. (2008). Directing: A complex systems perspective. *Journal of Nursing Administration*, *38*(2), 61–63.

Cooper, R. A., Getzen, T. E., McKee, H. J., & Laud, P. (2002). Economic and demographic trends signal an impending physician shortage. *Health Affairs*, *21*(1), 140–154.

Council on Graduate Medical Education (COGME). (2004). *Physician workforce report*. Rockville, MD: COGME/BHP/HRSA/USDHHS.

Department of Homeland Security (DHS). (2004). *A better prepared America: A year in review (Fact sheet)*. Washington, DC: Author. Retrieved June 12, 2004, from www.dhs.gov

Dickler, R., & Shaw, G. (2000). The Balanced Budget Act of 1997: Its impact on U.S. teaching hospitals. *Annals of Internal Medicine*, *132*(10), 820–824.

Dobias, M. (2007). Medicare up and up. *Modern Healthcare*, *38*(2), 6–7.

Donabedian, A. (1980). *The definition of quality and approaches to its assessment* (Vol. I). Ann Arbor, MI: Health Administration Press.

Draper, D. A., & Claxton, G. (2004). *Managed care redux: Health plans shift responsibilities to consumers (Issue Brief No. 79)*. Washington, DC: Center for Studying Health System Change. Retrieved August 20, 2004, from www.hschange.org/CONTENT/666/?topic=topic03

Ehringhaus, S. (2004). *AAMC project to document the effects of HIPAA on research*. Presentation at the Association of American Medical Colleges Government Relations Representatives meeting, Washington, DC.

Families USA. (2004a). *Sticker shock: Rising prescription drug prices for seniors* (Publication No. 04-103). Washington, DC: Author.

Families USA. (2004b). *One in three: Non-elderly Americans without health insurance, 2002–2003* (Publication No. 04-104). Washington, DC: Author.

Families USA. (2009). *Americans at risk: One in three uninsured*. Washington, DC: Author. Retrieved, April 1, 2009, from http://www.familiesusa.org/resources/publications/reports/americans-at-risk.html

Feldstein, P. (1994). *Health policy issues: An economic perspective on health reform*. Ann Arbor, MI: AUPHA Press/Health Administration Press.

Findlay, S. (2001). Direct-to-consumer promotion of prescription drugs. *Pharmacoeconomics*, *19*(2), 109–119.

Firshein, J., Schadelbauer, C., & Milder, M. (2007). *Pay for performance improving health care quality and changing provider behavior: But challenges persist*. Robert Wood Johnson Foundation. Retrieved October 18, 2008, from www.rwjf.org/newsroom/newsreleasesdetail.jsp?productid=21847

Frank-Stromborg, M. (2004). They're real and they're here: The new federally regulated privacy rules under HIPAA. *Dermatology Nursing*, *16*(1), 13–14, 17–18, 22–24.

Fyffe, K. (2004). *National health information infrastructure (NHII): Overview*. Presentation at the Association of American Medical Colleges Government Relations Representatives meeting, Washington, DC.

Gabel, J., Claxton, G., Holve, E., Pickreign, J., Whitmore, H., Dhont, K., et al. (2003). Health benefits in 2003: Premiums reach thirteen-year high as employers adopt new forms of cost sharing. *Health Affairs*, *22*(5), 117–126.

General Accounting Office (GAO). (2003). *Medical malpractice insurance: Multiple factors have contributed to increased premium rates* (GAO-03-702). Washington, DC: Author.

General Accounting Office (GAO). (2004). *Health care: Unsustainable trends necessitate comprehensive and fundamental reforms to control spending and improve value* (GAO-04-793SP). Washington, DC: Author.

Geyman, J. (2002). *Health care in America: Can our ailing system be healed?* Boston: Butterworth/Heinemann.

Haugh, R. (2003). Surviving medical malpractice madness. *Hospitals & Health Networks, 77*(5), 47–50.

Hewitt Associates. (2004). *HMO rates continue double-digit increases, but begin to moderate.* Lincolnshire, IL: Hewitt Associates. Retrieved August 20, 2004, from www.was4.hewitt.com/hewitt/resource/newsroom/pressrel/2004/06-03-04.htm

Hobbs, F., & Stoops, N. (2002). *Demographic trends in the 20th century* (Census 2000 Special Reports Series CENSR-4). Washington, DC: U.S. Census Bureau.

Institute of Medicine (IOM). (2000). *To err is human: Building a safer health system.* Washington, DC: National Academies Press.

Institute of Medicine (IOM). (2001). *Crossing the quality chasm: A new health system for the 21st century.* Washington, DC: National Academies Press.

Institute of Medicine (IOM). (2004a). *Insuring America's health: Principles and recommendations.* Washington, DC: National Academies Press.

Institute of Medicine (IOM). (2004b). *Keeping patients safe: Transforming the work environment of nurses.* Washington, DC: National Academies Press.

Johnson, N. (2007). *Two's company, three is complexity.* Oxford, UK: Oneworld.

Jolly, P., & Hudley, D. (Eds.). (1998). *AAMC data book: Statistical information related to medical education.* Washington, DC: Association of American Medical Colleges.

Kaiser Family Foundation. (2008). *Medicare spending and financing, fact sheet.* Menlo Park, CA: Author. Retrieved March 31, 2009, from http://www.kff.org/medicare/upload/7305_03.pdf

Kalisch, P., & Kalisch, B. (2004). *American nursing: A history* (4th ed.). Philadelphia: Lippincott Williams & Wilkins.

Lavizzo-Mourey, R. (2003). President's message. In *The Robert Wood Johnson Foundation Report 2003* (pp. 1–6). Princeton, NJ: Robert Wood Johnson Foundation.

Lee, T., Meyer, G., & Brennan, T. (2004). A middle ground on public accountability. *The New England Journal of Medicine, 350*(23), 2409–2412.

Litman, T. (1997). The relationship of government and politics to health care: A sociopolitical overview. In T. Litman, & L. Robins (Eds.), *Health politics and policy* (3rd ed., pp. 3–45). Albany, NY: Delmar Publishers.

Longest, B., Rakich, J., & Darr, K. (2000). *Managing health services organizations and systems* (4th ed.). Baltimore: Health Professions Press.

Lubell, J. (2007). *DRG proposal part of payment system overhaul.* Retrieved February 22, 2008, from www.modernhealthcare.com/apps/pbcs.dll/article?AID=/20070424/FREE/70424001/0/FRONTPAGE

Mariner, W. (1996). State regulation of managed care and the Employee Retirement Income Security Act. *The New England Journal of Medicine, 335*(26), 1986–1990.

McMahon, G. (2004). Coming to America: International medical graduates in the United States. *The New England Journal of Medicine, 350*(24), 2435–2437.

Medicare Payment Advisory Commission (MedPAC). (2004). *Report to the congress: Medicare payment policy, March 2004.* Washington, DC: Author.

Miller, M., & Zhan, C. (2004). Pediatric patient safety in hospitals: A national picture in 2000. *Pediatrics, 113*(6), 1741–1746.

Mokdad, A., Marks, J., Stroup, D., & Gerberding, J. (2004). Actual causes of death in the United States, 2000. *Journal of the American Medical Association, 291*(10), 1238–1245.

National Center for Complementary and Alternative Medicine (NCCAM). (2004). *The use of complementary and alternative medicine in the United States.* Bethesda, MD: Author. Retrieved August 20, 2004, from www.nccam.nih.gov/news/camsurvey_fsl.htm

National Center for Health Statistics (NCHS). (2003). *Health, United States, 2003* (Publication No. 2003-1232). Hyattsville, MD: U.S. Department of Health and Human Services.

National Center for Health Workforce Analysis. (2003). *Changing demographics: Implications for physicians, nurses, and other health workers.* Washington, DC: U.S. Department of Health and Human Services.

National Coalition on Health Care. (2009). *Health insurance costs.* Washington, DC: Author. Retrieved March 31, 2009 from http://www.nchc.org/facts/cost.shtml

National Committee for Quality Assurance (NCQA). (2003a). *NCQA Overview.* Washington, DC: Author.

National Committee for Quality Assurance (NCQA). (2003b). *The state of health care quality: 2003.* Washington, DC: Author.

National Governors Association. (2004). *The fiscal survey of states.* Washington, DC: National Governors Association and National Association of State Budget Officers.

National Institutes of Health (NIH). (2004). *Overview of the NIH roadmap.* Bethesda, MD: Author. Retrieved March 31, 2009, from http://nihroadmap.nih.gov/overview.asp

Osheroff, J., Teich, J., Middleton, B., Steen, E., Wright, A., & Detmer, D. (2006). *A roadmap for national action on clinical decision support.* Retrieved March 31, 2009, from http://www.amia.org/files/cdsroadmap.pdf

Pharmaceutical Research and Manufacturers of America (PhRMA). (2004). *The issues: Research & development.* Washington, DC: Author. Retrieved June 6, 2004, from www.phrma.org/issues/researchdev/

Raffel, M., & Barsukiewicz, C. (2002). *The U.S. health system origins and functions* (5th ed.). Australia: Delmar.

Runy, L. A. (2008). The aging workforce. *Hospitals & Health Networks, 82*(1), 48–57.

Sanmartin, C., Ng, E., Blackwell, D., Gentleman, J., Martinez, M., & Simile, C. (2004). *Joint Canada/United States survey of health, 2002–2003* (Catalogue 82M00220-XIE). Ottawa, ON: Statistics Canada.

Schorr, T., & Kennedy, M. (1999). *100 years of American nursing: Celebrating a century of caring.* Philadelphia: Lippincott.

Shi, L., & Singh, D. (2001). *Delivering health care in America: A systems approach* (2nd ed.). Gaithersburg, MD: Aspen Publishers.

Staiti, A., Katz, A., & Hoadley, J. (2003). Has bioterrorism preparedness improved public health? *Center for Studying Health System Change, Issue Brief No. 65.*

Starfield, B. (2000). Is U.S. health really the best in the world? *Journal of the American Medical Association, 284*(4), 483–485.

Starr, P. (1982). *The social transformation of American medicine.* New York: Basic Books.

States Health Access Data Assistance Center. (2004). *Characteristics of the uninsured: A view from the states.* Minneapolis, MN: University of Minnesota. Retrieved May 31, 2004, from www.covertheuninsuredweek.org/media/research/brffs.pdf

Steinbrook, R. (2004). The cost of admission: Tiered copayments for hospital use. *The New England Journal of Medicine, 350*(25), 2539–2542.

Studdert, D., Mello, M., & Brennan, T. (2004). Medical malpractice. *The New England Journal of Medicine, 350*(3), 283–292.

Sultz, H., & Young, K. (2004). *Health care USA: Understanding its organization and delivery* (4th ed.). Sudbury, MA: Jones and Bartlett Publishers.

Taylor, M. (2008). Working through the frustrations of clinical integration. *Hospitals & Health Networks, 82*(1), 35–40.

The Joint Commission (TJC). (2009). *Facts about The Joint Commission.* Oakbrook Terrace, IL: Author. Retrieved March 31, 2009, from http://www.jointcommission.org/AboutUs/Fact_Sheets/joint_commission_facts.htm

Thomas, R. (2003). *Society and health: Sociology for health professionals.* New York: Kluwer Academic/Plenum Publishers.

Thompson, E., & Propst, S. (2004). *2002 investment in U.S. health research.* Alexandria, VA: Research!America. Retrieved June 1, 2004, from www.researchamerica.org/publications/appropriations/healthdollar2002.pdf

Torrens, P. R. (2002). Historical evolution and overview of health services in the United States. In S. Williams, & G. Torrens (Eds.), *Introduction to health services* (6th ed., pp. 2–17). Albany, NY: Delmar Publishers.

Tripp Umbach Healthcare Consulting, Inc. (2003). *The economic impact of medical college and teaching hospital members of the Association of American Medical Colleges (2002).* Washington, DC: Association of American Medical Colleges.

U.S. Census Bureau. (2003). *Statistical abstract of the United States: 2003.* Washington, DC: U.S. Government Printing Office.

U.S. Department of Health and Human Services (USDHHS). (2003). *National healthcare quality report* (p. 1). Washington, DC: Author. Retrieved August 20, 2004, from www.qualitytools.ahrq.gov/qualityreport/download_report.aspx

Wachter, R., & Goldman, L. (1996). The emerging role of "hospitalists" in the American health care system. *The New England Journal of Medicine, 335*(7), 514–517. PMID 8672160.

Weinberg, D. (2004). *Evidence from census 2000 about earnings by detailed occupation for men and women.* Census 2000 Special Reports Series CENSR-15. Washington, DC: U.S. Census Bureau.

Whitted, G. (1999). Private health insurance and employee benefits. In S. Williams, & G. Torrens (Eds.), *Introduction to health services* (5th ed.). Albany, NY: Delmar Publishers.

Zaneski, C. T. (2004, June 17). Medical sales reps arrive bearing gifts. Pharmaceuticals: The medical profession is taking a closer look at inducements for doctors to prescribe certain drugs. *Baltimore Sun*, p. 1A.

Chapter 15

Algase, D. L., Beel-Bates, C., & Ziemba, R. (2004). Lead, link, and learn: A policy/research fellowship program in aging. *Policy, Politics, & Nursing Practice, 5*(2), 116–124.

Allred, C. A., Arford, P. H., Mauldin, P. D., & Goodwin, L. K. (1998). Cost-effectiveness analysis in the nursing literature, 1992–1996. *Image, 30*(3), 235–242.

Anderson, J. E. (1990). *Public policymaking.* Boston: Houghton-Mifflin.

Block, L. E. (2008). Health policy: What it is and how it works. In C. Harrington, & C. L. Estes (Eds.), *Health policy: Crisis and reform in the U.S. health care delivery system* (5th ed., pp. 4–14). Boston: Jones and Bartlett Publishers.

Bowers-Lanier, R. (2007). Coalitions: A powerful political strategy. In D. Mason, J. K. Leavitt, & M. W. Chaffee (Eds.), *Policy and politics in nursing and health care* (5th ed., pp. 135–144). Philadelphia: Saunders.

Buchholz, R. A. (1994). *Business environment and public policy: Implications for management and strategy formulation* (5th ed.). Englewood Cliffs, NJ: Prentice Hall.

Buerhaus, P. I. (1998). Milton Weinstein's insights on the development, use, and methodologic problems in cost-effectiveness analysis. *Image, 30*(3), 223–228.

Buresh, B., & Gordon, S. (2000). *From silence to voice: What nurses know and must communicate to the public.* Ottawa, ON: Canadian Nurses Association.

Cohen, S., Mason, D., Kovner, C., Leavitt, J., Pulcini, J., & Sochalski, J. (1996). Stages of nursing's political development: Where we've been and where we ought to go. *Nursing Outlook, 44*(6), 259–266.

Cohen, S., & Milone-Nuzzo, P. (2001). Advancing health policy in nursing education through service learning. *Advances in Nursing Science, 23*(3), 28–40.

Cooksey, J. A., McLaughlin, W., Russinof, H., Martinez, L. I., & Gordon, C. (2004). Active state-level engagement with the nursing shortage: A study of five Midwestern states. *Policy, Politics, & Nursing Practice, 5*(2), 102–122.

Cramer, M. E. (2002). Factors influencing organized political participation in nursing. *Policy, Politics, & Nursing Practice, 3*(2), 97–107.

Daniels, N., & Sabin, J. E. (2002). *Setting limits fairly: Can we learn to share medical resources?* New York: Oxford University Press.

Dunn, W. N. (1994). *Public policy analysis: An introduction.* Englewood Cliffs, NJ: Prentice-Hall.

Dye, T. R. (1992). *Understanding public policy.* Englewood Cliffs, NJ: Prentice-Hall.

Fawcett, J. (2007). A comment on integrating nursing and health policy. *Nursing Outlook, 56*(1), 41–43.

French, J. R. P., & Raven, B. (1959). The basis of social power. In D. Cartwright (Ed.), *Studies in social power* (pp. 150–167). Ann Arbor, MI: The University of Michigan.

Furlong, E. A. (2008). Agenda setting. In J. A. Milstead (Ed.), *Health policy and politics: A nurse's guide* (3rd ed., pp. 41–63). Boston: Jones and Bartlett Publishers.

Grudzen, C. R., & Brook, R. H. (2007). High-deductible health plans and emergency department use. *Journal of the American Medical Association, 297*(10), 1126–1127.

Hanley, B., & Falk, N. L. (2007). Policy development and analysis: Understanding the process. In D. J. Mason, J. K. Leavitt, & M. W. Chaffee (Eds.), *Policy and politics in nursing and health care* (5th ed., pp. 75–93). Philadelphia: Saunders.

Hersey, P., Blanchard, K. H., & Johnson, D. E. (2008). *Management of organizational behavior: Leading human resources* (9th ed.). Upper Saddle River, NJ: Pearson Education.

Hudson, J., & Lowe, S. (2004). *Understanding the policy process.* Bristol: The Policy Press.

International Council of Nurses (ICN). (2001). *Guidelines on shaping effective health policy.* Geneva, Switzerland: Author.

Jones, K. R., Jennings, B. W., Moritz, P., & Moss, M. T. (1997). Policy issues associated with analyzing the outcomes of care. *Image: Journal of Nursing Scholarship, 29*(3), 261–267.

Kelly, K. (2003). Power, politics, and influence. In P. Yoder-Wise, (Ed.), *Leading and managing in nursing* (3rd ed., pp. 431–448). St. Louis, MO: Mosby.

Keys, B., & Case, T. (1990). How to become an influential manager. *The Executive, 4,* 38–51.

Kingdon, J. W. (2003). *Agendas, alternatives and public policies* (2nd ed.). New York: Longman.

Kronenfeld, J., Whicker, J., & Lynn, M. (1984). *U.S. national health policy: An analysis of the federal role.* New York: Praeger.

Leavitt, J. K., Chaffee, M. W., & Vance, C. (2007). Learning the ropes of policy, politics, and advocacy. In D. J. Mason, J. K. Leavitt, & M. W. Chaffee, (Eds.), *Policy and politics in nursing and health care* (5th ed., pp. 34–46). Philadelphia: Saunders.

Lineberry, R. L., Edwards, G. C., & Wattenberg, M. P. (1995). *Government in America* (2nd ed.). New York: HarperCollins College Publishers.

Longest, B. B., Jr. (1997). *Seeking strategic advantage through health policy analysis.* Chicago: Health Administration Press.

Longest, B. B., Jr. (1998). *Health policymaking in the United States* (2nd ed.). Chicago: Health Administration Press.

Longest, B. B., Jr. (2001). *Contemporary health policy.* Chicago: Health Administration Press.

Longest, B. B., Jr. (2002). *Health policy making in the United States* (3rd ed.). Chicago: Health Administration Press.

Longest, B. B., Jr. (2004). An international constant: The crucial role of policy competence in the effective strategic management of health services organizations. *Health Services Management Research, 17*(2), 71–78.

Malone, R. (1999). Policy as product: Morality and metaphor in health policy discourse. *Hastings Center Report, 29,* 16–22.

Mason, D. J., Leavitt, J. K., & Chaffee, M. W. (2007). Policy and politics: A framework for action. In D. J. Mason, J. K. Leavitt, & M. W. Chaffee (Eds.), *Policy and politics in nursing and health care* (5th ed., pp. 1–16). Philadelphia: Saunders.

Mazmanian, D., & Sabatier, P. (1983). *Implementation and public policy.* Dallas, TX: Scott, Foresman.

McLaughlin, C. P., & McLaughlin, C. D. (2008). *Health policy analysis: An interdisciplinary approach.* Boston: Jones & Bartlett Publishers.

Milio, N. (1984). The realities of policymaking: Can nurses have an impact? *Journal of Nursing Administration, 14*(3), 18–23.

Milstead, J. A. (2008). Advanced practice nurses and public policy, naturally. In J. A. Milstead (Ed.), *Health policy and politics: A nurses' guide* (3rd ed., pp.1–39). Gaithersburg, MD: Aspen.

Morgan, I., & Marsh, G. (1998). Historic and future health promotion contexts for nursing. *Image: Journal of Nursing Scholarship, 30,* 379–383.

National Conference of State Legislatures (NCSL). (2001). *State health priorities survey.* Washington, DC: Author.

Odom-Ferren, J., & Hahn, E. J. (2006). Mandatory reporting of health care–associated infections: Kingdon's multiple streams approach. *Policy, Politics, & Nursing Practice, 7*(1), 64–72.

Reutter, L. (2000). Socioeconomic determinants of health. In M. J. Stewart (Ed.), *Community nursing: Promoting Canadians' health* (2nd ed., pp. 174–193). Toronto, ON: Harcourt Canada.

Reutter, L., & Duncan, S. (2002). Preparing nurses to promote health-enhancing public policies. *Policy, Politics, & Nursing Practice, 3*(4), 294–305.

Reutter, L., & Williamson, D. L. (2000). Advocating healthy public policy: Implications for baccalaureate nursing education. *Journal of Nursing Education, 39*, 21–26.

Ripley, R. B. (1985). *Policy analysis in political science.* Chicago: Nelson-Hall.

Ripley, R. B. (1996). Stages of the policy process. In D. C. McCool (Ed.), *Public policy theories, models, and concepts: An anthology* (pp. 157–162). Englewood Cliffs, NJ: Prentice-Hall.

Rosenthal, M., & Daniels, N. (2006). Beyond competition: The normative implications of consumer-driven health plans. *Journal of Health Policy, Politics, and Law, 31*(3), 671–685.

Smart, P. (2008). Policy design. In J. A. Milstead (Ed.), *Health policy and politics: A nurse's guide* (3rd ed., pp. 129–141). Boston: Jones and Bartlett Publishers.

Soumerai, S. (2003). Unintended outcomes of Medicaid drug cost-containment policies on the chronically mentally ill. *Journal of Clinical Psychiatry, 64*(Suppl. 17), 19–22.

Stone, D. A. (1997). *Policy paradox: The art of political decision-making.* New York: Norton.

Stone, P. W. (1998). Methods for conducting and reporting cost-effectiveness analysis in nursing. *Image, 30*(3), 229–234.

Wakefield, M. (2001). Linking health policy to nursing and health care scholarship: Points to consider. *Nursing Outlook, 49*(4), 111–113.

Wakefield, M. (2008). Government response: Legislation. In J. A. Milstead (Ed.), *Health policy and politics: A nurse's guide* (3rd ed., pp. 65–88). Gaithersburg, MD: Aspen.

Weissert, C. S., & Weissert, W. G. (2002). *Governing health: The politics of health policy* (2nd ed.). The Johns Hopkins University Press.

Wharam, J. F., & Daniels, N. (2007). Toward evidence-based policy making and standardized assessment of health policy reform. *Journal of the American Medical Association, 298*(6), 676–679.

Wilken, M. (1999). Policy implementation. In J. A. Milstead (Ed.), *Health policy and politics. A nurse's guide* (pp. 187–218). Gaithersburg, MD: Aspen.

Wilken, M. (2008). Policy implementation. In J. A. Milstead (Ed.), *Health policy and politics: A nurse's guide* (3rd ed., pp. 157–164). Gaithersburg, MD: Aspen.

Chapter 16

Aarons, G. A. (2006). Transformational and transactional leadership: Association with attitudes toward evidence-based practice. *Psychiatric Services, 57*(8), 1162–1169.

Aldridge, M. D. (2004). Writing and designing readable patient education materials. *Nephrology Nursing Journal, 31*(4), 373–377.

Andresen, H., Higgins, T. S., & Schuring, L. T. (2008). Ear. In L. L. Harris & M. B. Huntoon (Eds.), *Core curriculum for otorhinolaryngology and head-neck nursing* (2nd ed., pp. 81–151). New Smyrna Beach, FL: SOHN.

Asch, S. M., Kerr, E. A., Keesey, J., Adams, J., Setodji, C., Malik, S., et al. (2006). Who is at greatest risk for receiving poor-quality health care? *The New England Journal of Medicine, 354*(11), 2617–2619.

Avorn, J., & Soumerai, S. B. (1983). Improving drug-therapy decisions through educational outreach: A randomized controlled trial of academically based "detailing". *The New England Journal of Medicine, 318*(24), 1457–1463.

Berwick, D. (2003). Disseminating innovations in health care. *Journal of the American Medical Association, 289*(15), 1969–1975.

Bloom, B. (2005). Effects of continuing medical education on improving physician clinical care and patient health: A review of systematic reviews. *International Journal of Technology Assessment in Health Care, 21*(3), 380–385.

Boström, A. M., Wallin, L., & Nordström, G. (2007). Evidence-based practice and determinants of research use in elderly care in Sweden. *Journal of Evaluation in Clinical Practice, 13*, 665–673.

Bowman, A., Greiner, J., Doerschug, K., Little, S., Bombei, C., & Comried, L. (2005). Implementation of an evidence-based feeding protocol and aspiration risk reduction algorithm. *Critical Care Nursing Quarterly, 28*(4), 324–333.

Brewer, B. B. (2006). Relationships among teams, culture, safety and cost outcomes. *Western Journal of Nursing Research, 28*(6), 641–653.

Burns, N., & Grove, S. K. (2005). *The practice of nursing research: Conduct, critique, and utilization.* Philadelphia: Saunders.

Clark, A. (2005). Measuring quality of care nationwide. *Caring, 24*(3), 42–45.

Cooke, L., Smith-Idell, C., Dean, G., Gemmill, R., Steingass, S., Sun, V., et al. (2004). Research to practice: A practical program to enhance the use of evidence-based practice at the unit level. *Oncology Nursing Forum, 31*(4), 825–832.

Cullen, L. (2006). Educational strategies to promote use of evidence-based practices. *Perioperative Nursing Clinics, 1*(3), 289–298.

Cullen, L. (2007). *Moving nursing's agenda forward into the 21st century: Sigma Theta Tau International's position on evidence-based practice and translational research.* Paper presented at the Sigma Theta Tau International 39th Biennial Convention, Baltimore, MD.

Cullen, L., Greiner, J., Greiner, J., Bombei, C., & Comried, L. (2005). Excellence in evidence-based practice: An organizational and MICU exemplar. *Critical Care Nursing Clinics of North America, 17*(2), 127–142.

Cullen, L., & Titler, M. G. (2004). Promoting evidence-based practice: An internship for staff nurses. *Worldviews on Evidence-Based Nursing, 1*(4), 215–223.

Cummings, G. G., Estabrooks, C. A., Midodzi, W. K., Wallin, L., & Hayduk, L. (2007). Influence of organizational characteristics and context on research utilization. *Nursing Research, 56*(Suppl. 4), S24–S39.

Davies, B., Edwards, N., Ploeg, J., Virani, T., Skelly, J., & Dobbins, M. (2006). *Determinants of the sustained use of research evidence in nursing: Final report.* Ottawa, ON: Canadian Health Services Research Foundation & Canadian Institutes for Health Research.

Davies, D. A., Thomson, M. A., Oxman, A. D., & Haynes, R. B. (1995). Changing physician performance: A systematic review of the effect of continuing medical education strategies. *Journal of the American Medical Association, 274*(9), 700–705.

Dobbins, M., Ciliska, D., Cockerill, R., Barnsley, J., & DiCenso, A. (2002). A framework for the dissemination and utilization of research for health-care policy and practice. *Online Journal of Knowledge Synthesis for Nursing, 9*(7).

Dopson, S., FitzGerald, L., Ferlie, E., Gabbay, J., & Locock, L. (2002). No magic targets! Changing clinical practice to become more evidence based. *Health Care Management Review, 27*(3), 35.

Doumit, G., Gattellari, M., Grimshaw, J., & O'Brien, M. A. (2007). Local opinion leaders: Effects on professional practice and health care outcomes. (1), CD000125. DOI: 10.1002/14651858.CD000125.pub3.

Estabrooks, C. A., Midodzi, W. K., Cummings, G. G., & Wallin, L. (2007). Predicting research use in nursing organizations. *Nursing Research, 56*(Suppl. 4), S7–S23.

Ferlie, E. B., & Shortell, S. M. (2001). Improving the quality of health care in the United Kingdom and the United States: A framework for change. *Milbank Quarterly, 79*, 281.

Fink, R., Thompson, C. J., & Bonnes, D. (2005). Overcoming barriers and promoting the use of research in practice. *Journal of Nursing Administration, 35*(12), 517–518.

Fleuren, M., Wiefferink, K., & Paulussen, T. (2004). Determinants of innovation within health care organizations. *International Journal for Quality in Health Care, 16*(2), 107–123.

Funk, S. G., Champagne, M. T., Wiese, R. A., & Tornquist, E. M. (1991a). BARRIERS: The barriers to research utilization scale. *Applied Nursing Research, 4*(1), 39–45.

Funk, S. G., Champagne, M. T., Wiese, R. A., & Tornquist, E. M. (1991b). Barriers to using research findings in practice: The clinician's perspective. *Applied Nursing Research, 4*(2), 90–95.

Gifford, W. (2006). Nursing research: Leadership strategies to influence the use of clinical practice guidelines. *Canadian Journal of Nursing Leadership, 19*(4), 72–88.

Gifford, W., Davies, B., Edwards, N., Griffin, P., & Lybanon, V. (2007). Managerial leadership for nurses' use of research evidence: An integrative review of the literature. *Worldviews on Evidence-Based Nursing, 4*(3), 126–145.

Goode, C. J., & Piedalue, F. (1999). Evidence-based clinical practice. *Journal of Nursing Administration, 29*(6), 15–21.

Green, L. A., Wyszewianski, L., Lowery, J. C., Kowalski, C. P., & Krein, S. L. (2007). An observational study of the effectiveness of practice guideline implementation strategies examined according to physicians' cognitive styles. *Implementation Science, 2*, 41.

Greenhalgh, T., Robert, G., Bate, P., Macfarlane, F., & Kyriakidou, O. (2005). *Diffusion of innovations in health service organizations.* Danvers, MA: Blackwell Publishing.

Hagedorn, H., Hogan, M., Smith, J. L., Bowman, C., Curran, G. M., Espadas, D., et al. (2006). Lessons learned about implementing research evidence into clinical practice: Experience from the VA QUERI. *Journal of General Internal Medicine, 21*(Suppl. 2), S21–S24.

Harrill, W. C., Jenkins, H. A., & Coker, N. J. (1996). Barotrauma after stapes surgery: A survey of recommended restrictions and clinical experiences. *The American Journal of Otology, 17*, 835–846.

Hinds, P., Gattuso, J., & Morrell, A. (2000). Creating a hospital-based nursing research fellowship program for staff nurses. *Journal of Nursing Administration, 30*(6), 317–324.

Hogan, D. L., & Logan, J. (2004). The Ottawa model of research use: A guide to clinical innovation in the NICU. *Clinical Nursing Specialist, 18*(5), 255–261.

House, J. W., Toh, E. H., & Perez, A. (2001). Diving after stapedectomy: Clinical experience and recommendations. *Otolaryngology—Head and Neck Surgery, 125*, 356–360.

Hudak, M., & Bond-Domb, A. (1996). Postoperative head and neck cancer with artificial airways: The effect of saline lavage on tracheal mucus evacuation and oxygen saturation. *ORL-Head and Neck Nursing, 14*(1), 17–21.

Hutchinson, A., & Johnston, L. (2006). Beyond the BARRIERS scale. *Journal of Nursing Administration, 36*(4), 189.

Hysong, S. J., Best, R. G., & Pugh, J. A. (2006). Audit and feedback and clinical practice guideline adherence: Making feedback actionable. *Implementation Science, 1*, 9.

Jiang, H. J., Fieselmann, J. F., Hendryx, M. S., & Bock, M. J. (1997). Assessing the impact of patient characteristics and process performance on rural intensive care unit hospital mortality rates. *Critical Care Medicine, 25*(5), 773–778.

Kirchhoff, K. (2004). State of the science of translation research: From demonstration projects to intervention testing. *Worldviews on Evidence-Based Nursing, 1*(Suppl. 1), S6–S12.

Kitson, A., Harvey, G., & McCormack, B. (1998). Enabling the implementation of evidence based practice: A conceptual framework. *Quality in Health Care, 7*(3), 149–158.

Lacey, E. (1995). Facilitating research-based practice by educational interventions. *Nurse Education Today, 16*, 296–301.

Logan, J., Harrison, M. B., Graham, I. D., Dunn, K., & Bissonnette, J. (1999). Evidence-based pressure-ulcer practice: The Ottawa model of research use. *Canadian Journal of Nursing Research, 31*(1), 37–52.

Lundman, L., Mendel, L., Bagger-Sjoback, D., & Rosenhall, U. (1999). Hearing in patients operated unilaterally for otosclerosis: Self-assessment of hearing and audiometric results. *Acta Oto-laryngolica, 119*, 453–458.

Madsen, D., Sebolt, T., Cullen, L., Folkdahl, B., Mueller, T., Richardson, C., et al. (2005). Listening to bowel sounds: An evidence-based practice project. *American Journal of Nursing, 105*(12), 40–50.

Majumdar, R., Tsuyuki, F., & McAlister, F. A. (2007). Impact of opinion leader-endorsed evidence summaries on the quality of prescribing for patients with cardiovascular disease: A randomized controlled trial. *American Heart Journal, 153*(1), 22.

Mangione-Smith, R., DeCristofaro, A., Setodji, C., Keesey, J., Klein, D. J., Adams, J., et al. (2007). The quality of ambulatory care delivered to children in the United States. *The New England Journal of Medicine, 357*(15), 15–23.

Marinopoulos, S. S., Dorman, T., Ratanawongsa, N., Wilson, L. M., Ashar, B. H., Magaziner, J. L., et al. (2007). *Effectiveness of continuing medical education.* Evidence report/technology assessment No. 149. Rockville, MD: Agency for Healthcare Research and Quality.

McCormack, B., Rycroft-Malone, J., Cullen, L., Griffith, R., & DiCenso, A. (under development). *Sigma Theta Tau International's position on evidence-based practice.*

McGlynn, E. A., Asch, S. M., Adams, J., Keesey, J., Hicks, J., DeCristofaro, A., et al. (2003). The quality of health care delivered to adults in the United States. *The New England Journal of Medicine, 348*(26), 35–45.

McInerny, T. K., Cull, W. L., & Yudkowsky, B. K. (2005). Physician reimbursement levels and adherence to American Academy of Pediatrics well-visit and immunization recommendations. *Pediatrics, 115*(4), 833–838.

Nagy, S., Lumby, J., McKinley, S., & Macfarlane, C. (2001). Nurses' beliefs about the conditions that hinder or support evidence-based nursing. *International Journal of Nursing Practice, 7,* 314–321.

Newhouse, R. P. (2007). Creating infrastructure supportive of evidence-based nursing practice: Leadership strategies. *Worldviews on Evidence-Based Nursing, 4*(1), 21–29.

Newman, K., Pyne, T., Leigh, S., Rounce, K., & Cowling, A. (2000). Personal and organizational competencies requisite for the adoption and implementation of evidence-based health care. *Health Services Management Research, 19,* 97–110.

O'Brien, M. A., Freemantle, N., Oxman, A. D., Wolf, F., Davis, D. A., & Herrin, J. (2001). Continuing education meetings and workshops: Effects on professional practice and health care outcomes. *Cochrane Database of Systematic Review,* (1), CD003030. DOI: 10.1002/14651858.CD003030.

O'Brien, M. A., Rogers, S., Jamtvedt, G., Oxman, A. D., Odgaard-Jensen, J., Kristoffersen, D. T., et al. (2007). Educational outreach visits: Effects on professional practice and health care outcomes. *Cochrane Database of Systematic Review,* (4), CD000409. DOI: 10.1002/14651858.CD000409.pub2.

Oxman, A. D., Thomson, M. A., Davis, D. A., & Haynes, R. B. (1995). No magic bullets: A systematic review of 102 trials of interventions to improve professional practice. *Canadian Medical Association Journal, 153*(10), 1423–1431.

Pepler, C. J., Edgar, L., Frisch, S., Rennick, J., Swidzinski, M., White, C., et al. (2006). Strategies to increase research-based practice. *Clinical Nursing Specialist, 20*(1), 23–31.

Peterson, E. D., Roe, M. T., Mulgond, J., DeLong, E. R., Lytle, B. L., Brindis, R. G., et al. (2006). Association between hospital process performance and outcomes among patients with acute coronary syndromes. *The Journal of the American Medical Association, 295*(16), 1912–1920.

Pippalla, R. S., Riley, D. A., & Chinburapa, V. (1995). Influencing the prescribing behavior of physicians: A metaevaluation. *Journal of Clinical Pharmacy and Therapeutics, 20,* 189–198.

Pravikoff, D. S., Tanner, A. B., & Pierce, S. T. (2005). Readiness of U.S. nurses for evidence-based practice. *American Journal of Nursing, 105*(9), 40–51, quiz 52.

Ramsey, H., Kärkkäinen, J., & Palva, T. (1997). Success in surgery for otosclerosis: Hearing improvement and other indicators. *American Journal of Otolaryngology, 18,* 23–28.

Reeleder, D., Goel, V., Singer, P. A., & Martin, D. K. (2006). Leadership and priority setting: The perspective of hospital CEOs. *Health Policy, 79*(1), 24–34.

Ring, N., Malcolm, C., Coull, A., Murphy-Black, T., & Watterson, A. (2005). Nursing best practice statements: An exploration of their implementation in clinical practice. *Journal of Clinical Nursing, 14,* 1048–1058.

Rogers, E. (2003). *Diffusion of innovations* (5th ed.). New York: Simon & Schuster.

Rosswurm, M., & Larrabee, J. (1999). Clinical scholarship. A model for change to evidence-based practice. *Image: The Journal of Nursing Scholarship, 31*(4), 317–322.

Rubenstein, L. V., & Pugh, J. A. (2006). Strategies for promoting organizational and practice change by advancing implementation research. *Journal of General Internal Medicine, 21*(Suppl. 2), S58–S64.

Rycroft-Malone, J., Harvey, G., Kitson, A., McCormack, B., & Titchen, A. (2002). Getting evidence into practice: Ingredients for change. *Nursing Standard, 16*(37), 38–43.

Sackett, D. L., Strauss, S. E., Richardson, W. S., Rosenberg, W., & Haynes, R. B. (2000). *Evidence-based medicine: How to practice and teach EBM.* London: Churchill Livingstone.

Sakagami, M., Sone, M., Fukazawa, K., Tsuji, K., & Mishiro, Y. (2003). Rate of recovery of taste function after preservation of chorda tympani nerve in middle ear surgery with special reference to type of disease. *Annals of Otology, Rhinology, and Laryngology, 112,* 52–56.

Schimizu, Y., & Shimanouchi, S. (2006). Effective components of staff and organizational development for client outcomes by implementation of action plans in home care. *International Medical Journal, 13*(3), 175–183.

Schoenbaum, S., Sundwall, D. N., Bergman, D., Buckle, J. M., Chernov, A., George, J., et al. (1995). *Using clinical practice guidelines to evaluate quality of care (Vol. 2: Methods).* Rockville, MD: U.S. Department of Health and Human Services, Public Health Service, Agency for Healthcare Research and Quality.

Scott-Findlay, S., & Golden-Biddle, K. (2005). Understanding how organizational culture shapes research use. *Journal of Nursing Administration, 35*(7–8), 359–365.

Shirey, M. R. (2006). Evidence-based practice: How nurse leaders can facilitate innovation. *Nursing Administration Quarterly, 30*(3), 252–265.

Shortell, S. M. (2004). Increasing value: A research agenda for addressing the managerial and organizational challenges facing health care delivery in the United States. *Medical Care Research and Review, 61*(Suppl. 3), S12–S30.

Shrank, W. H., Asch, S. M., Adams, J., Setodji, C., Kerr, E. A., Keesey, J., et al. (2006). The quality of pharmacologic care for adults in the United States. *Medical Care, 44*(10), 936–945.

Sohn, W., Ismail, A., & Tellez, M. (2004). Efficacy of educational interventions targeting primary care providers' practice behaviors: An overview of published systematic reviews. *Journal of Public Health Dentistry, 64*(3), 164–172.

Stebral, L., & Steelman, V. (2006). Double-gloving for surgical procedures: An evidence-based practice project. *Perioperative Nursing Clinics, 1*(3), 251–260.

Stetler, C. (2001). Updating the Stetler Model of Research Utilization to facilitate evidence-based practice. *Nursing Outlook, 49*(6), 272–279.

Stevens, K. R. (2004). *ACE Star Model of EBP: Knowledge transformation.* San Antonio: Academic Center for Evidence-Based Practice, The University of Texas Health Science Center.

Titler, M. G. (2002). *Toolkit for promoting evidence-based practice.* Iowa City, IA: University of Iowa Hospitals and Clinics.

Titler, M. (2004). Methods in translation science. *Worldviews on Evidence-Based Nursing, 1*(1), 38–48.

Titler, M. G. (2005). *Moving evidence-based practice forward: Priorities for translation.* Paper presented at the 12th National Evidence-Based Practice Conference. Iowa City, IA: University of Iowa Hospitals and Clinics.

Titler, M. (2007). *Moving nursing's agenda forward into the 21st century: Sigma Theta Tau International's position on translation research.* Paper presented at the Sigma Theta Tau International 39th Biennial Convention, Baltimore, MD.

Titler, M. (2008). The evidence for evidence-based practice implementation. In R. Hughes (Ed.), *Advances in patient safety & quality: An evidence-based handbook for nurses* (Vol. 1, Chapter 7). Rockville, MD: Agency for Healthcare Research and Quality.

Titler, M., & Everett, L. Q. (2001). Translating research into practice: Considerations for critical care investigators. *Critical Care Nursing Clinics of North America, 13*(4), 587–604.

Titler, M., Kleiber, C., Steelman, V., Rakel, B. A., Budreau, G., Everett, L. Q., et al. (2001). The Iowa Model of Evidence-Based Practice to Promote Quality Care. *Critical Care Nursing Clinics of North America, 13*, 497–509.

Titler, M., Cullen, L., & Ardery, G. (2002). Evidence-based practice: An administrative perspective. *Reflections on Nursing Leadership, 28*(2), 26–27, 45, 46.

Tranmer, J. E., Kisilevsky, B. S., & Muir, D. W. (1995). A nursing research utilization strategy for staff nurses in the acute care setting. *Journal of Nursing Administration, 25*(4), 21–29.

Udod, S. A., & Care, W. D. (2004). Innovation in leadership. Setting the climate for evidence-based nursing practice: What is the leader's role? *Canadian Journal of Nursing Leadership, 17*(4), 64–75.

Vaughn, T. E., McCoy, K. D., BootsMiller, B. J., Woolson, R. F., Sorofman, B., Tripp-Reimer, T., et al. (2002). Organizational predictors of adherence to ambulatory care screening guidelines. *Medical Care, 40*(12), 1172–1185.

Wallin, L., Boström, A., Wikblad, K., & Ewald, U. (2003). Sustainability in changing clinical practice promotes evidence-based nursing care. *Journal of Advanced Nursing, 41*(5), 509–518.

Wallin, L., Ewald, U., Wikblad, K., Scott-Findlay, S., & Arnetz, B. B. (2006). Understanding work context factors: A short-cut to evidence-based practice? *Worldviews on Evidence-Based Nursing, 3*(4), 153–164.

Wallin, L., Rudberg, A., & Gunningberg, L. (2005). Staff experiences in implementing guidelines for Kangaroo Mother Care: A qualitative study. *International Journal of Nursing Studies, 42*, 61–73.

Wells, N., Free, M., & Adams, R. (2007). Nursing research internship: Enhancing evidence-based practice among staff nurses. *Journal of Nursing Administration, 37*(3), 135–143.

Williams, K. (2006). *Stapedectomy: Development of a patient education brochure—an evidence-based practice approach.* Paper presented at the Society of Otorhinolaryngology—Head and Neck Surgery Annual Congress Symposium, Toronto, ON.

Woolf, S. H., & Atkins, D. (2001). The evolving role of prevention in health care. Contributions of the U.S. Preventive Services Task Force. *American Journal of Preventive Medicine, 20*(Suppl. 1), 13–20.

World Health Organization. (2007). *Practical guidance for scaling up health service innovations.* Switzerland: Author.

Zhan, C., Friedman, B., Mosso, A., & Pronovost, P. (2006). Medicare payment for selected adverse events: Building the business case for investing in patient safety. *Health Affairs, 25*(5), 1386–1393.

Zohar, D., Livine, Y., Tenne-Gazit, O., Admi, H., & Donchin, Y. (2007). Healthcare climate: A framework for measuring and improving patient safety. *Critical Care Medicine, 35*(5), 1312–1317.

Zuckerman, B., Stevens, G. D., Inkelas, M., & Halfon, N. (2004). Prevalence and correlates of high-quality basic pediatric preventive care. *Pediatrics, 114*, 1522–1529.

Zwarenstein, M., & Reeves, S. (2006). Knowledge translation and interprofessional collaboration: Where the rubber of evidence-based care hits the road of teamwork. *The Journal of Continuing Education in Health Professions, 26*(1), 46–54.

Chapter 17

Adams, D. (2004). *The pillars of planning: Mission values, vision.* Washington, DC: National Endowment for the Arts. Retrieved October 20, 2008, from www.arts.endow.gov/resources/Lessons/ADAMS.HTML

Appenzeller, L. (1993). Merging nursing departments: An experience. *Journal of Nursing Administration, 23*(12), 55–60.

Benner, P., & Wrubel, J. (1988). Caring comes first. *American Journal of Nursing, 88*(8), 1072–1075.

Brown-Stewart, P. (1987). Thinly disguised contempt: A barrier to excellence. *Journal of Nursing Administration, 17*(4), 14–18.

Cody, B. (1990). Shaping the future through a philosophy of nursing. *Journal of Nursing Administration, 20*(10), 16–22.

Drenkard, K. N. (2001). Creating a future worth experiencing: Nursing strategic planning in an integrated healthcare delivery system. *Journal of Nursing Administration, 31*(7/8), 364–376.

Drucker, P. (1973). *Management: Tasks, responsibilities, practices.* New York: Harper & Row.

Foley, B. J., Minick, M. P., & Kee, C. C. (2002). How nurses learn advocacy. *Journal of Nursing Scholarship, 34*(2), 181–186.

Gaut, D. (1983). Development of a theoretically adequate description of caring. *Western Journal of Nursing Research, 5*, 313–324.

Getzels, J. (1958). Administration as a social process. In A. Halpin (Ed.), *Administrative theory in education* (pp. 150–165). Chicago: University of Chicago Press.

Graham, P., Constantini, S., Balik, B., Bedore, B., Hooke, M., Papin, D., et al. (1987). Operationalizing a nursing philosophy. *Journal of Nursing Administration, 17*(3), 14–18.

Kramer, M. (1974). *Reality shock: Why nurses leave nursing.* St. Louis, MO: Mosby.

Kramer, M., & Schmalenberg, C. (1988a). Magnet hospitals: Institutions of excellence: Part 1. *Journal of Nursing Administration, 18*(1), 13–24.

Kramer, M., & Schmalenberg, C. (1988b). Magnet hospitals: Institutions of excellence: Part 2. *Journal of Nursing Administration, 18*(2), 11–19.

Kreitzer, M. J., Wright, D., Hamlin, C., Towey, S., Marko, M., & Disch, J. (1997). Creating a healthy work environment in the midst of organizational change and transition. *Journal of Nursing Administration, 27*(6), 35–41.

McCloskey, J. (1991). Creating an environment for success with fun, hope, and trouble. *Journal of Nursing Administration, 21*(4), 5–6.

McNamara, C. (2008a). *Strategic planning (in nonprofit or for-profit organizations).* St. Paul, MN: Free Management Library: Authenticity Consulting, LLC. Retrieved October 20, 2008, from www.managementhelp.org/plan_dec/str_plan/str_plan.htm

McNamara, C. (2008b). *Basics of developing mission, vision and values statements.* St. Paul, MN: Free Management Library: Authenticity Consulting, LLC. Retrieved October 20, 2008, from www.managementhelp.org/plan_dec/str_plan/stmnts.htm

Minnick, A., Roberts, M., Curran, C., & Ginzberg, E. (1989). What do nurses want? Priorities for action. *Nursing Outlook, 37*, 214–218.

Nickols, F. (2000). *The goals grid: A tool for clarifying goals and objectives.* Howard, OH: Distance Consulting. Retrieved October 20, 2008, from http://home.att.net/ nickols/goals_grid.htm

Park, E. J., & Huber, D. L. (2009). Case management workforce in the United States. *Journal of Nursing Scholarship, 41*(2), 175–183.

Pepin, J. (1992). Family caring and caring in nursing. *Image, 24*(2), 127–131.

Poteet, G., & Hill, A. (1988). Identifying the components of a nursing service philosophy. *Journal of Nursing Administration, 18*(10), 29–33.

Swanson, K. (1991). Empirical development of a middle range theory of caring. *Nursing Research, 40*(3), 161–166.

Trexler, B. (1987). Nursing department purpose, philosophy, and objectives: Their use and effectiveness. *Journal of Nursing Administration, 17*(3), 8–12.

Wilson, D. M. (1996). Highlighting the role of policy in nursing practice through a comparison of "DNR" policy influences and "No CPR" decision influences. *Nursing Outlook, 44*(6), 272–279.

Zander, K. (1992). Nursing care delivery methods and quality. *Series on Nursing Administration, 3*, 86–104.

Chapter 18

Academy of Canadian Nurse Executives, & Association of Canadian Academic Healthcare Organizations. (2005). Patient safety culture and leadership in Canada's Academic Health Science Centres. *Healthcare Quarterly, 8*(1), 36–38.

Alidina, S., & Funke-Furber, J. (1988). First line nurse managers: Optimizing the span of control. *Journal of Nursing Administration, 18*(5), 34–39.

Altaffer, A. (1998). First-line managers: Measuring their span of control. *Nursing Management, 29*(7), 36–39.

Ashkenas, R. (1999). Creating the boundaryless organization. *Business Horizons, 42*(5), 5–10.

Balkundi, P., & Kilduff, M. (2006). The ties that lead: A social network approach to leadership. *The Leadership Quarterly, 17*, 419–439.

Birch, S., O'Brien-Pallas, L., Alksnis, C., Tomblin Murphy, G., & Thomson, D. (2003). Beyond demographic change in health human resources planning: An extended framework and application to nursing. *Journal of Health Services Research and Policy, 8*(4), 225–229.

Blau, P. M. (1968). The hierarchy of authority in organizations. *American Journal of Sociology, 73*(4), 453–467.

Blau, P. M. (1970). A formal theory of differentiation in organizations. *American Sociological Review, 35*(2), 201–218.

Canadian Nursing Advisory Committee. (2002). *Our health, our future: Creating quality workplaces for Canadian nurses.* Ottawa, ON: Advisory Committee on Health Human Resources.

Carter, N. M., & Cullen, J. B. (1984). A comparison of centralization/decentralization of decision making concepts and measures. *Journal of Management, 10*(2), 259–268.

Charnes, M., & Tewksbury, L. (1993). The continuum of organization structures. In *Collaborative management in health care: Implementing the integrative organization* (pp. 20–43). San Francisco: Jossey-Bass.

Clegg, S. R. (1990). *Modern organizations: Organization studies in the postmodern world.* London: Sage Publications.

Clegg, S. R., & Hardy, C. (Eds.). (1999). *Studying organization: Theory and method* (1st ed.). London: Sage Publications.

Covell, C. L. (2008). The middle-range theory of nursing intellectual capital. *Journal of Advanced Nursing, 63*(1), 94–103.

Curtin, L. (1994). Restructuring: What works and what does not! *Nursing Management, 25*(10), 7–8.

Donaldson, L. (1996). The normal science of structural contingency theory. In S. R. Clegg, & C. Hardy (Eds.), *Studying organization: Theory and method* (pp. 51–70). London: Sage Publications.

Doran, D., McCutcheon, A. S., Evans, M. G., MacMillan, D., McGillis Hall, L., Pringle, D., et al. (2004). *Impact of the manager's span of control on leadership and performance.* Ottawa, ON: Canadian Health Services Research Foundation.

Duffield, C., & Franks, H. (2001). The role and preparation of first-line nurse managers in Australia: Where are we going and how do we get there? *Journal of Nursing Management, 9,* 87–91.

Eisenstein, H. (1995). The Australian femocratic experiment: A feminist case for bureaucracy. In M. M. Ferree, & P. Y. Martin (Eds.), *Feminist organizations: Harvest of the new women's movement* (pp. 69–83). Philadelphia: Temple University Press.

Farmer, D. J. (1997). The postmodern turn and the Socratic gadfly. In H. T. Miller, & C. J. Fox (Eds.), *Postmodernism "reality" and public administration* (pp. 105–117). Burke, VA: Chatelaine Press.

Feldman, M. S., & Pentland, B. T. (2003). Reconceptualizing organizational routines as a source of change and flexibility. *Administrative Science Quarterly, 48,* 94–118.

Filerman, G. (2003). Closing the management competence gap. *Human Resources for Health, 1*(7), 1–3.

Galbraith, J. R. (1974). Organization design: An information processing view. *Interfaces, 4*(3), 28–36.

Galbraith, J., Downey, D., & Kates, A. (2002). How networks undergird the lateral capability of an organization: Where the work gets done. *Journal of Organizational Excellence, 21*(2), 67–78.

Gittell, J. H. (2002). Coordinating mechanisms in care provider groups: Relational coordination as a mediator and input uncertainty as a moderator of performance effects. *Management Science, 48*(11), 1408–1426.

Gittell, J. H. (2003). A theory of relational coordination. In K. S. Cameron, J. E. Dutton, & R. E. Quinn (Eds.), *Positive organizational scholarship: Foundations of a new discipline* (pp. 279–435). San Francisco: Berrett-Koehler Publishing.

Gittell, J. H. (2004). Achieving focus in hospital care: The role of relational coordination. In R. E. Herzlinger (Ed.), *Consumer-driven health care: Implications for providers, payers, and policymakers* (pp. 683–695). San Francisco: Jossey-Bass.

Gittell, J. H., & Weiss, L. (2004). Coordination networks within and across organizations: A multi-level framework. *Journal of Management Studies, 41*(1), 127–153.

Gulick, L. (1937). Notes on the theory of organization. In L. Gulick, & L. Urwick (Eds.), *Papers on the science of administration* (pp. 1–46). New York: Institute of Public Administration, University of Columbia.

Hammer, M., & Champy, J. (1993). *Reengineering the corporation: A manifesto for business revolution.* New York: HarperCollins.

Hatch, M. J., & Cunliffe, A. L. (2006). *Organization theory: Modern, symbolic, and postmodern perspectives* (2nd ed.). New York: Oxford University Press.

Hoffman, C., Beard, P., Greenall, J. U. D., & White, J. (2006). *Canadian Root Cause Analysis Framework: A tool for identifying and addressing the root causes of critical incidents in health care.* Edmonton, AB: Canadian Patient Safety Institute.

House, R. J., & Miner, J. B. (1969). Merging management and behavioral theory: The interaction between span of control and group size. *Administrative Science Quarterly, 14*(3), 451–464.

Institute of Medicine of the National Academies. (2004). *Keeping patients safe: Transforming the work environment of nurses.* Washington, DC: National Academies Press.

Jaques, E. (1990). In praise of hierarchy. *Harvard Business Review, 68*(1), 127–133.

Kanter, R. M. (1977). *Men and women of the corporation.* New York: Basic Books.

Katz, D., & Kahn, R. L. (1978). *The social psychology of organizations* (2nd ed.). New York: John Wiley and Sons.

Kimberly, J. R. (1976). Organizational size and the structuralist perspective: A review, critique, and proposal. *Administrative Science Quarterly, 21*(4), 571–597.

Kramer, M., Maguire, P., Schmalenberg, C., Brewer, B., Burke, R., Chmielewski, L., et al. (2007). Nurse manager support: What is it? Structures and practices that promote it. *Nursing Administration Quarterly, 31*(4), 325–340.

Laschinger, H. K. S. (1996). A theoretical approach to studying work empowerment in nursing: A review of studies testing Kanter's theory of structural power in organizations. *Nursing Administration Quarterly, 20*(2), 25–41.

Laschinger, H. K. S., & Finegan, J. (2005). Using empowerment to build trust and respect in the workplace: A strategy for addressing the nursing shortage. *Nursing Economic$, 23*(1), 6–13.

Laschinger, H. K. S., Wong, C., McMahon, L., & Kaufmann, C. (1999). Leader behavior impact on staff nurse empowerment, job tension, and work effectiveness. *Journal of Nursing Administration, 29*(5), 28–39.

Lawrence, P. R., & Lorsch, J. W. (1967). *Organization and environment: Managing differentiation and integration.* Boston: Graduate School of Business Administration, Harvard University.

Leape, L. L., & Berwick, D. M. (2005). Five years after To Err Is Human: What have we learned? *JAMA, 293*(19), 2384–2390.

Leatt, P., Lemieux-Charles, L., & Aird, C. (1994). Program management: Introduction and overview. In L. Lemieux-Charles, P. Leatt, & C. Aird (Eds.), *Program management and beyond: Management innovations in Ontario hospitals* (pp. 1–10). Ottawa, ON: Canadian College of Health Service Executives.

Likert, R. (1961). *New patterns of management.* New York: McGraw Hill.

Little, L., & Buchan, J. (2007). *Nursing self sufficiency/sustainability in the global context.* Geneva: International Centre on Nurse Migration.

Lorenz, H. L. (2008). Service line leadership. *Nurse Leader, 6*(1), 42–43.

Mahon, A., & Young, R. (2006). Health care managers as a critical component of the health care workforce. In C. Dubois, M. McKee, & E. Nolte (Eds.), *Human resources for health in Europe* (pp. 116–139). Berkshire: Open University Press.

March, J. G., & Simon, H. A. (1958). *Organizations.* New York: John Wiley & Sons.

Mark, B. A., Sayler, J., & Smith, C. S. (1996). A theoretical model for nursing systems outcomes research. *Nursing Administration Quarterly, 20*(4), 12–27.

Matthews, S., Laschinger, H. K. S., & Johnstone, L. (2006). Staff nurse empowerment in line and staff organizational structures for chief nurse executives. *Journal of Nursing Administration, 6*(11), 526–533.

McCutcheon, A. S. (2004). *Relationships between leadership style, span of control and outcomes.* Unpublished doctoral dissertation. Toronto, ON: University of Toronto.

McGillis Hall, L., & Donner, G. J. (1997). The changing role of hospital nurse managers: A literature review. *Canadian Journal of Nursing Administration, 10*(2), 14–39.

Meier, K. J., & Bohte, J. (2003). Span of control and public organizations: Implementing Luther Gulick's research design. *Public Administration Review, 63*(1), 61–70.

Meyer, R. M. (2008). Span of management: Concept analysis. *Journal of Advanced Nursing, 63*(1), 104–112.

Mintzberg, H. (1983). *Structure in fives: Designing effective organizations.* Englewood Cliffs, NJ: Prentice-Hall.

Morash, R., Brintnell, J., & Rodger, G. L. (2005). A span of control tool for clinical managers. *Canadian Journal of Nursing Leadership, 18*(3), 83–93.

Moss, M., Eagen, M., & Russell, M. (1994). Service integration in the reform era. *Nursing Economic$, 12*(5), 256–260, 286.

Nedd, N. (2006). Perceptions of empowerment and intent to stay. *Nursing Economic$, 24*(1), 13–19.

O'Connor, E. S. (1999). The politics of management thought: A case study of the Harvard Business School and the Human Relations School. *Academy of Management Review, 24*(1), 117–131.

Pabst, M. K. (1993). Span of control on nursing inpatient units. *Nursing Economic$, 11*(2), 87–90.

Porter-O'Grady, T. (2003). A different age for leadership, Part 1. *Journal of Nursing Administration, 33*(2), 105–110.

Porter-O'Grady, T. (2007). The CNE as entrepreneur: Innovation leadership for a new age. *Nurse Leader, 5*(1), 44–47.

Prins, G. (2000). *Testing theories on structure and strategy: An assessment of organizational knowledge.* Delft, The Netherlands: Eburon.

Redman, R. W., & Jones, K. R. (1998). Effects of implementing patient centered care models on nurse and non-nurse managers. *Journal of Nursing Administration, 28*(11), 46–53.

Reed, M. I. (1992). *The sociology of organizations: Themes, perspectives and prospects.* New York: Harvester Wheatsheaf.

Registered Nurses' Association of Ontario (RNAO). (2006). *Developing and sustaining nursing leadership.* Toronto, ON: Author.

Scott, W. R. (1992). *Organizations: Rational, natural, and open systems* (3rd ed.). Englewood Cliffs, NJ: Prentice-Hall.

Shaffer, F. A. (2003). Stepping beyond "yesterday thinking": Preparing nurse managers for a new world order. *Nurse Leader, 1*, 33–37.

Simon, H. (1946). Proverbs of administration. *Public Administration Review, 6*(1), 53–67.

Taylor, F. W. (2003). Scientific Management. In K. Thompson (Ed.), *Early sociology of management and organizations* (Vol. 1). New York: Taylor & Francis. (on-line). Retrieved March 13, 2008, from www.myilibrary.com.myaccess.library.utoronto.ca/Browse/open.asp?ID=9994&loc=235

Taylor, M. (2008). Working through the frustrations of clinical integration. *H&HN: Hospitals & Health Networks, 82*(1), 34–40.

Thielst, C. B. (2007). Regional health information networks and the emerging organizational structures. *Journal of Healthcare Management, 52*(3), 146–150.

Tichy, N. M., Tushman, M. L., & Fombrun, C. (1979). Social network analysis for organizations. *Academy of Management Review, 4*(4), 507–519.

Van de Ven, A. H., Delbecq, A. L., & Koenig, R. (1976). Determinants of coordination modes within organizations. *American Sociological Review, 41*(3), 322–338.

Venkatraman, N. (1994). IT-enabled business transformation: From automation to business scope redefinition. *Sloan Management Review, 35*(2), 73–87.

Weber, M. (1978). *Economy and society: An outline of interpretive sociology* (E. Fischoff, H. Gerth, A. M. Henderson, F. Kolegar, C. W. Mills, T. Parsons, M. Rheinstein, G. Roth, E. Shils, & C. Wittich, Trans., Vol. 2). Berkeley, CA: University of California Press.

Wenger, E. (2008). *Communities of practice: A brief introduction.* Retrieved March 12, 2008, from www.ewenger.com/theory/communities_of_practice_intro_WRD.doc

West, E., & Barron, D. N. (2005). Social and geographical boundaries around senior nurse and physician leaders: An application of social network analysis. *Canadian Journal of Nursing Research, 37*(3), 132–148.

Willem, A., Buelens, M., & De Jonghe, I. (2007). Impact of organizational structure on nurses' job satisfaction: A questionnaire survey. *International Journal of Nursing Studies, 44*, 1011–1020.

Young, G. J., Charnes, M. P., & Heeren, T. C. (2004). Product-line management in professional organizations: An empirical test of competing theoretical perspectives. *Academy of Management Journal, 47*(5), 723–734.

Young-Ritchie, C., Laschinger, H. K. S., & Wong, C. (2007). The effects of emotionally intelligent leadership behaviour on emergency staff nurses' workplace empowerment and organizational commitment. *Outlook, 30*(2), 24.

Chapter 19

Aiken, L. H., Clarke, S. P., Sloane, D. M., Sochalski, J., & Silber, J. H. (2002). Hospital nurse staffing and patient mortality, nurse burnout, and job dissatisfaction. *Journal of the American Medical Association, 288*(16), 1987–1993.

Aiken, L. H., Lake, E. T., Sochalski, J., & Sloane, D. M. (1997). Design of an outcomes study of the organization of hospital AIDS care. *Research in the Sociology of Health Care, 14*, 3–26.

American Nurses Association. (2002). *Nursing's agenda for the future: A call to the nation.* Washington, DC: American Nurses Publishing.

Argyris, C. (1994). Good communication that blocks learning. *Harvard Business Review, 72*(4), 77–85.

Beyers, M. (1999). The management of nursing services. In L. F. Wolper (Ed.), *Health care administration: Planning, implementing, and managing organized delivery systems* (3rd ed., pp. 349–370). Gaithersburg, MD: Aspen.

Brooks, B. A. (2004). Measuring the impact of shared governance. *Online Journal of Issues in Nursing, 9*(1), Manuscript la. Retrieved October 23, 2008, from www.nursingworld.org/MainMenuCategories/ANAMarketplace/ANAPeriodicals/OJIN/TableofContents/Volume92004/No1Jan04/MeasuringtheImpact.aspx

Bush, G. W. (2006). *State of the Union Address—2006.* Retrieved October 23, 2008, from www.whitehouse.gov/stateoftheunion/2008/index.html

David, F. R. (1987). *Concepts of strategic management.* Columbus, OH: Merrill.

DeBaca, V., Jones, K., & Tornabeni, J. (1993). A cost-benefit analysis of shared governance. *Journal of Nursing Administration, 23*(7/8), 50–57.

Drucker, P. F. (1999). *Management challenges for the 21st century.* New York: Harper Collins.

Finkler, S. A., Kovner, C. T., Knickman, J. R., & Hendrickson, G. (1994). Innovation in nursing: A benefit/cost analysis. *Nursing Economic$, 12*(1), 18–27.

Frith, K., & Montgomery, M. (2006). Perceptions, knowledge, and commitment of clinical staff to shared governance. *Nursing Administration Quarterly, 30*(3), 273–284.

George, V., Burke, L. J., Rodgers, B., Duthie, N., Hoffmann, M. L., Koceja, V., et al. (2002). Developing staff nurse shared leadership behavior in professional nursing practice. *Nursing Administration Quarterly, 26*(3), 44–59.

Golanowski, M., Beaudry, D., Kurz, L., Laffey, W. J., & Hook, M. L. (2007). Interdisciplinary shared decision-making: Taking shared governance to the next level. *Nursing Administration Quarterly, 31*(4), 341–353.

Green, A., & Jordan, C. (2004). Common denominators: Shared governance and workplace advocacy—Strategies for nurses to gain control over their practice. *Online Journal of Issues in Nursing, 9*(1), Manuscript 6. Retrieved October 23, 2008, from www.nursingworld.org/MainMenuCategories/ANAMarketplace/ANAPeriodicals/OJIN/TableofContents/Volume92004/No1Jan04/SharedGovernanceandWorkPlaceAdvocacy.aspx

Hatcher, B. J., Bleich, M. R., Connolly, C., Davis, K., O'Neill Hewlett, P., & Hill, K. S. (2006). Retaining older nurses in bedside practice. *Nurse Educator, 31*(5), 206.

Havens, D. S. (1998). An update on nursing involvement in hospital governance: 1990–1996. *Nursing Economic$, 16*(1), 6–11.

Herrick, L. M. (1998). Shared governance in an academic health center. In J. A. Dienemann (Ed.), *Nursing administration: Managing patient care* (2nd ed., pp. 417–424). Stamford, CT: Appleton & Lange.

Herrin, D. M. (2004). Shared governance: A nurse executive response. *Online Journal of Issues in Nursing, 9*(1),

Manuscript 1b. Retrieved October 23, 2008, from www.nursingworld.org/MainMenuCategories/ANAMarketplace/ANAPeriodicals/OJIN/TableofContents/Volume92004/No1Jan04/ANurseExecutiveResponse.aspx

Hess, R., Jr. (1994). Shared governance: Innovation or imitation? *Nursing Economic$, 12*(1), 28–34.

Hess, R. G. (2004). From bedside to boardroom: Nursing shared governance. *Online Journal of Issues in Nursing, 9*(1), Manuscript 1. Retrieved October 23, 2008, from www.nursingworld.org/MainMenuCategories/ANAMarketplace/ANAPeriodicals/OJIN/TableofContents/Volume92004/No1Jan04/FromBedsidetoBoardroom.aspx

Institute of Medicine (IOM). (2004). *Keeping patients safe: Transforming the work environment of nurses.* Washington, DC: The National Academies Press.

Johnson, S. (1998). *Who moved my cheese?* New York: G.P. Putnam's Sons.

Jones, C., Stasiowski, S., Simons, B., Boyd, N., & Lucas, M. (1993). Shared governance and the nursing practice environment. *Nursing Economic$, 11*(4), 208–214.

Kanter, R. (1993). *Men and women of the corporation* (2nd ed.). New York: Basic Books.

Kouzes, J. M., & Posner, B. Z. (1993). *Leadership Practices Inventory (LPI): Participant's workbook and LPI form.* San Francisco: Jossey-Bass.

Ludemann, R. S., & Brown, C. (1989). Staff perceptions of shared governance. *Nursing Administration Quarterly, 13*(4), 49–56.

Maas, M., & Specht, J. (1990). Nursing professionalization and self-governance: A model from long-term care. In G. Mayer, M. Madden, & E. Lawrenz (Eds.), *Patient care delivery models* (pp. 151–168). Rockville, MD: Aspen.

McClure, M. L., & Hinshaw, A. S. (2002). *Magnet hospitals revisited: Attraction and retention of professional nurses.* Washington, DC: American Nurses Publishing.

Miller, G. J. (1992). *Managerial dilemmas: The political economy of hierarchy.* New York: Cambridge University Press.

Moore, S. C., & Hutchison, S. A. (2007). Developing leaders at every level: Accountability and empowerment actualized through shared governance. *Journal of Nursing Administration, 37*(12), 564–568.

North, D. C. (1990). *Institutions, institutional change and economic performance.* New York: Cambridge University Press.

Porter-O'Grady, T. (1987). Shared governance and new organizational models. *Nursing Economic$, 5*(6), 281–286.

Porter-O'Grady, T. (2001). Is shared governance still relevant? *Journal of Nursing Administration, 31*(10), 468–473.

Porter-O'Grady, T. (2003a). Of hubris and hope: Transforming nursing for a new age. *Nursing Economic$, 21*(2), 59–64.

Porter-O'Grady, T. (2003b). Researching shared governance: A futility of focus. *Journal of Nursing Administration, 33*(4), 251–252.

Porter-O'Grady, T., Hawkins, M. A., & Parker, M. L. (1997). *Whole-systems shared governance: Architecture for integration.* Gaithersburg, MD: Aspen.

Porter-O'Grady, T., & Malloch, K. (2002). *Quantum leadership: A textbook of new leadership.* Gaithersburg, MD: Aspen.

Prince, S. B. (1997). Shared governance: Sharing power and opportunity. *Journal of Nursing Administration, 27*(3), 28–35.

Robert Wood Johnson Foundation. (2002). *Health care's human crisis: The American nursing shortage.* Princeton, NJ: Author.

Scott, J. G., Sochalski, J., & Aiken, L. (1999). Review of magnet hospital research: Findings and implications for professional nursing practice. *Journal of Nursing Administration, 29*(1), 9–19.

Straub, J. T., & Attner, R. F. (1994). *Introduction to business* (5th ed.). Belmont, CA: Wadsworth.

The Joint Commission (TJC). (2007). *Improving America's hospitals: The Joint Commission's Annual Report on Quality and Safety.* Retrieved March 2, 2008, from www.jointcommissionreport.org

Thompson, B., Hateley, P., Molloy, R., Fernandez, S., Madigan, A. L., Thrower, C., et al. (2004). A journey, not an event: Implementation of shared governance in a NHS trust. *Online Journal of Issues in Nursing, 9*(1), Manuscript 3. Retrieved October 23, 2008, from www.nursingworld.org/MainMenuCategories/ANAMarketplace/ANAPeriodicals/OJIN/TableofContents/Volume92004/No1Jan04/ImplementationofSharedGovernance.aspx

Tourangeau, L. A., Cranley, L. A., & Jeffs, L. (2006). Impact of nursing on hospital patient mortality: A focused review and related policy implications. *Quality and Safety in Health Care, 15*, 4–8.

U.S. Department of Health and Human Services (USDHHS). (2005). *Preliminary findings: 2004 National Sample Survey of Registered Nurses.* Retrieved March 2, 2008, from http://bhpr.hrsa.gov/healthworkforce/reports/rnpopulation/preliminaryfindings.htm

U.S. General Accounting Office. (2001). *Nursing workforce: Emerging nurse shortages due to multiple factors.* Report to the Chairman, Subcommittee on Health, Committee on Ways and Means, House of Representatives, No. GAO-01-944.

Westrope, R. A., Vaughn, L., Bott, M., & Taunton, R. L. (1995). Shared governance: From vision to reality. *Journal of Nursing Administration, 25*(12), 45–54.

Chapter 20

Abts, D., Hofer, M., & Leafgreen, P. (1994). Redefining care delivery: A modular system. *Nursing Management, 25*(2), 40–46.

Aiken, L. H., Clarke, S. P., Sloane, D. M., Sochalski, J., & Silber, J. H. (2002). Hospital nurse staffing and patient mortality, nurse burnout, and job dissatisfaction. *Journal of the American Medical Association, 288*(16), 1987–1993.

Aiken, L. H., & Patrician, P. A. (2000). Measuring organizational traits of hospitals: The Revised Nursing Work Index. *Nursing Research, 49*(3), 146–153.

Altman, D. E., Clancy, C., & Blendon, R. J. (2004). Improving patient safety: Five years after the IOM report. *The New England Journal of Medicine, 351*(20), 2041–2043.

American Nurses Association (ANA). (1988). *Nursing case management* (Publication No. NS-32). Kansas City, MO: Author.

American Nurses Association (ANA). (1997). *Definitions related to ANA 1992 position statements on unlicensed assistive personnel.* Washington, DC: Author.

American Nurses Association (ANA). (2005). *ANA principles for delegation.* Washington, DC: Author. Retrieved October 28, 2008, from www.safestaffing-saveslives.org//WhatisSafeStaffing/SafeStaffingPrinciples/PrinciplesforDelegationhtml.aspx#Definitions

Anderson, C., & Hughes, E. (1993). Implementing modular nursing in a long-term care facility. *Journal of Nursing Administration, 23*(6), 29–35.

Anthony, M. K., Brennan, P. F., O'Brien, R., & Suwannaroop, N. (2004). Measurement of nursing practice models using multiattribute utility theory: Relationship to patient and organizational outcomes. *Quality Management in Health Care, 13*(1), 40–52.

Atencio, B. L., Cohen, J., & Gorenberg, B. (2003). Nurse retention: Is it worth it? *Nursing Economic$, 21*(6), 262–268, 299.

Bard, J., Jimenez, F., & Tornack, R. (1994). An outcome-focused, community-based health support program. *Journal of Nursing Administration, 24*(3), 48–54.

Barnum, B. (1990). Cycles of nursing. *Nursing and Health Care, 11*(8), 395.

Barry-Walker, J. (2000). The impact of systems redesign on staff, patient, and financial outcomes. *Journal of Nursing Administration, 30*(2), 77–89.

Bower, K. A. (2004). Patient care management as a global nursing concern. *Nursing Administration Quarterly, 28*(1), 39–43.

Case Management Society of America (CMSA). (2002). *Standards of practice for case management* (2nd ed.). Little Rock, AR: Author.

Cohen, E. L., & Cesta, T. G. (2005). *Nursing case management: From essentials to advanced practice applications* (4th ed.). St. Louis, MO: Mosby.

Cole, L., & Houston, S. (1999). Structured care methodologies: Evolution and use in patient care delivery. *Outcomes Management for Nursing Practice, 3*(2), 53–59.

Comack, M., Paech, G., & Porter-O'Grady, T. (1999). From structure to culture: A journey of transformation. In S. P. Smith, & D. L. Flarey (Eds.), *Process-centered health care organizations* (pp. 45–67). Gaithersburg, MD: Aspen.

Deutschendorf, A. L. (2003). From past paradigms to future frontiers: Unique care delivery models to facilitate nursing work and quality outcomes. *Journal of Nursing Administration, 33*(1), 52–59.

Duffy, J. R., Baldwin, J., & Mastorovich, M. J. (2007). Using the Quality-Caring Model to organize patient care delivery. *Journal of Nursing Administration, 37*(12), 546–551.

Eastaugh, S. R., & Regan-Donovan, M. (1990). Nurse extenders offer a way to trim staff expenses. *Healthcare Financial Management, 44*(4), 58–60, 62.

Fox, R. T., Fox, D. H., & Wells, P. J. (1999). Performance of first-line management functions on productivity of hospital unit personnel. *Journal of Nursing Administration, 29*(9), 12–18.

Fuszard, B. (1988). What is case management? *The Facilitator, 4*(1), 3–4.

Gardner, K. (1991). A summary of findings of a five-year comparison study of primary and team nursing. *Nursing Research, 40*(2), 113–117.

Gerardi, T. (2005). The managed care market. In E. L. Cohen, & T. G. Cesta (Eds.), *Nursing case management: From essentials to advanced practice applications* (4th ed., pp. 210–218). St. Louis, MO: Mosby.

Gittell, J. H., Fairfield, K. M., Bierbaum, B., Head, W., Jackson, R., Kelly, M., et al. (2000). Impact of relational coordination on quality of care, postoperative pain and functioning, and length of stay: A nine-hospital study of surgical patients. *Medical Care, 38*(8), 807–819.

Glandon, G., Colbert, K., & Thomasma, M. (1989). Nursing delivery models and RN mix: Cost implications. *Nursing Management, 20*(5), 30–33.

Grimaldi, P. L. (1996). A glossary of managed care terms. *Nursing Management, 24*(10, Spec Suppl.), 5–7.

Guild, S., Ledwin, R., Sanford, D., & Winter, T. (1994). Development of an innovative nursing care delivery system. *Journal of Nursing Administration, 24*(3), 23–29.

Haase-Herrick, K. S., & Herrin, D. M. (2007). The American organization of nurse executives' guiding principles and American Association of Colleges of Nursing's clinical nurse leader: A lesson in synergy. *Journal of Nursing Administration, 37*(2), 55–60.

Hall, L. M. (1997). Staff mix models: Complementary or substitution roles for nurses. *Nursing Administration Quarterly, 21*(2), 31–39.

Hall, L. M., & Doran, D. (2004). Nurse staffing, care delivery model, and patient care quality. *Journal of Nursing Care Quality, 19*(1), 27–33.

Hardin, S. R., & Kaplow, R. (2005). *Synergy for clinical excellence: The AACN synergy model for patient care.* Sudbury, MA: Jones & Bartlett.

Hegyvary, S. (1977). Foundations of primary nursing. *Nursing Clinics of North America, 12*(6), 187–196.

Higginbotham, P. (1999). Teams: The essential work unit. In S. P. Smith, & D. L. Flarey (Eds.), *Process-centered health care organizations* (pp. 113–117). Gaithersburg, MD: Aspen.

Hoffart, N., & Woods, C. Q. (1996). Elements of a nursing professional practice model. *Journal of Professional Nursing, 12*(6), 354–364.

Ingersoll, G. L., Cook, J. A., Fogel, S., Applegate, M., & Frank, B. (1999). The effect of patient-focused redesign on midlevel nurse managers' role responsibilities and work environment. *Journal of Nursing Administration, 29*(5), 21–27.

Jennings, B. M. (2008). Care models. In R. G. Hughes (Ed.), *Patient safety and quality: An evidence-based handbook for nurses.* (Prepared with support from the Robert Wood Johnson Foundation.) AHRQ Publication No. 08–0043. Rockville, MD: Agency for Healthcare Research and Quality.

Jones-Schenk, J., & Hartley, P. (1993). Organization for communication and integration. *Journal of Nursing Administration, 23*(10), 30–33.

Kalisch, P., & Kalisch, B. (1978). *The advance of American nursing.* Boston: Little, Brown.

Kane, R. L., Shamliyan, T. A., Mueller, C., Duval, S., & Wilt, T. J. (2007). The association of registered nurse staffing levels and patient outcomes: Systematic review and meta-analysis. *Medical Care, 45*(12), 1195–1204.

Kimball, B., Joynt, J., Cherner, D., & O'Neil, E. (2007). The quest for new innovative care delivery models. *Journal of Nursing Administration, 37*(9), 392–398.

Kohn, L. T., Corrigan, J., & Donaldson, M. S. (2000). *To err is human: Building a safer health system.* Washington, DC: National Academies Press.

Koloroutis, M. (Ed.). (2004). *Relationship-based care: A model for transforming practice.* Minneapolis, MN: Creative Health Care Management.

Lambrinos, J., LaPosta, M. J., & Cohen, A. (2004). Increasing nursing hours without increasing nurses: A natural experiment at an academic medical center. *Journal of Nursing Administration, 34*(4), 195–199.

Lang, N., & Clinton, J. (1984). Assessment of quality of nursing care. *Annual Review of Nursing Research, 2*, 135–163.

Leape, L. L., & Berwick, D. M. (2005). Five years after *To Err Is Human:* What have we learned? *Journal of the American Medical Association, 293*(19), 2384–2390.

Lee, J. (1993). A history of care models in nursing. *Series on Nursing Administration, 5*, 20–38.

Lengacher, C., Mabe, P., Bowling, C., Heinemann, D., Kent, K., & Cott, M. (1993). Redesigning nursing practice: The partners in patient care model. *Journal of Nursing Administration, 23*(12), 31–37.

Lookinland, S., Tiedeman, M. E., & Crosson, A. E. (2005). Nontraditional models of care delivery: Have they solved the problems? *Journal of Nursing Administration, 35*(2), 74–80.

Lyon, J. (1993). Models of nursing care delivery and case management: Clarification of terms. *Nursing Economic$, 11*(3), 163–169.

Maehling, J. A. S. (1995). Process reengineering: Strategies for analysis and redesign. In S. S. Blancett, & D. L. Flarey (Eds.), *Reengineering nursing and health care: The handbook for organizational transformation* (pp. 61–74). Gaithersburg, MD: Aspen.

Magargal, P. (1987). Modular nursing: Nurses rediscover nursing. *Nursing Management, 18*(11), 98–104.

Manthey, M. (1989). Of bandwagons and partnerships. *Nursing Management, 20*(8), 22–23.

Manthey, M. (1990). Definitions and basic elements of a patient care delivery system with an emphasis on primary nursing. In G. Mayer, M. Madden, & E. Lawrenz (Eds.), *Patient care delivery models* (pp. 201–211). Rockville, MD: Aspen.

Manthey, M. (1991). Delivery systems and practice models: A dynamic balance. *Nursing Management, 22*(1), 28–30.

Mark, B. (1992). Characteristics of nursing practice models. *Journal of Nursing Administration, 22*(11), 57–63.

McCloskey, J., Blegen, M., & Gardner, D. (1991). Who helps you with your work? *American Journal of Nursing, 91*(4), 43–46.

Mikulencak, M. (1993). Public health stands as a proven model for future delivery systems. *The American Nurse, 25*(6), 18.

Minnick, A. F., Mion, L. C., Johnson, M. E., & Catrambone, C. (2007). How unit level nursing responsibilities are structured in U.S. hospitals. *Journal of Nursing Administration, 37*(10), 452–458.

Morjikian, R. L., Kimball, B., & Joynt, J. (2007). Leading change: The nurse executive's role in implementing new care delivery models. *Journal of Nursing Administration, 37*(9), 399–404.

Needleman, J., Buerhaus, P. I., Mattke, S., Stewart, M., & Zelevinsky, K. (2001). *Nurse staffing and patient outcomes in hospitals* (Contract No. 230–99–0021). U.S. Department of Health and Human Resources, Health Resources and Services Administration.

Neidlinger, S., & Miller, M. (1990). Nursing care delivery systems: A nursing administration practice perspective. *Journal of Nursing Administration, 20*(10), 43–49.

O'Rourke, M. W. (2003). Rebuilding a professional practice model: The return of role-based practice accountability. *Nursing Administration Quarterly, 27*(2), 95–105.

Parkman, C., & Loveridge, C. (1994). From nursing service to professional practice. *Nursing Management, 25*(3), 63–68.

Person, C. (2004). Patient care delivery. In M. Koloroutis (Ed.), *Relationship-based care: A model for transforming practice.* Minneapolis, MN: Creative Health Care Management.

Poulin, M. (1985). Configuration of nursing practice. In American Nurses Association (Ed.), *Issues in professional practice* (pp. 1–14). Kansas City, MO: ANA.

Powers, P. H., Dickey, C. A., & Ford, A. (1990). Evaluating an RN/co-worker model. *Journal of Nursing Administration, 20*(3), 11–15.

Reverby, S. (1987). *Ordered to care: The dilemma of American nursing 1850–1945.* Cambridge, MA: Cambridge University Press.

Ritter-Teitel, J. (2002). The impact of restructuring on professional nursing practice. *Journal of Nursing Administration, 32*(1), 31–41.

Seago, J. A. (1999). Evaluation of a hospital work redesign: Patient-focused care. *Journal of Nursing Administration, 29*(11), 31–38.

Smith, D. S., & Dabbs, M. T. (2007). Transforming the care delivery model in preparation for the clinical nurse leader. *Journal of Nursing Administration, 37*(4), 157–160.

Tiedeman, M. E., & Lookinland, S. (2004). Traditional models of care delivery: What have we learned? *Journal of Nursing Administration, 34*(6), 291–297.

Unruh, L. (2003). Licensed nurse staffing and adverse events in hospitals. *Medical Care, 41*(1), 142–152.

Unruh, L. (2008). Nurse staffing and patient, nurse, and financial outcomes. *American Journal of Nursing, 108*(1), 62–71; quiz 72.

Vlasses, F. R., & Smeltzer, C. H. (2007). Toward a new future for healthcare and nursing practice. *Journal of Nursing Administration, 37*(9), 375–380.

Watson, J., & Foster, R. (2003). The attending nurse caring model: Integrating theory, evidence and advanced caring-healing therapeutics for transforming professional practice. *Journal of Clinical Nursing, 12*(3), 360–365.

Wiggins, M. S. (2006). The Partnership Care Delivery Model. *Journal of Nursing Administration, 36*(7–8), 341–345.

Wolf, G. A., & Greenhouse, P. K. (2007). Blueprint for design: Creating models that direct change. *Journal of Nursing Administration, 37*(9), 381–387.

Wolf, G., Boland, S., & Aukerman, M. (1994). A transformational model for the practice of professional nursing. Part 2. Implementation of the model. *Journal of Nursing Administration, 24*(5), 38–46.

Zander, K. (1990). Case management: A golden opportunity for whom? In J. McCloskey, & H. Grace (Eds.), *Current issues in nursing* (3rd ed., pp. 199–204). St. Louis, MO: Mosby.

Zander, K. (1992). Nursing care delivery methods and quality. *Series on Nursing Administration, 3*, 86–104.

Zander, K., & Warren, C. (2005). Converting case managers from MD/service to unit-based assignments: A before and after comparison. *Lippincott's Case Management, 10*(4), 180–184.

Chapter 21

Allen, J. K., Blumenthal, R. S., Margolis, S., Young, D. R., Miller, E. R., III, & Kelly, K. (2002). Nurse case management of hypercholesterolemia in patients with coronary heart disease: Results of a randomized clinical trial. *American Heart Journal, 144*(4), 678–686.

American Nurses Association (ANA). (1988). *Nursing case management* (Publication No. NS-32). Kansas City, MO: Author.

American Nurses Credentialing Center (ANCC). (2009). *ANCC certification: Nursing case management*. Baltimore, MD: Author.

Aubert, R. E., Herman, W. H., Waters, J., Moore, W., Sutton, D., Peterson, B. L., et al. (1998). Nurse case management to improve glycemic control in diabetic patients in a health maintenance organization: A randomized, controlled trial. *Annals of Internal Medicine, 129*(8), 605–612.

Beilman, J. P., Sowell, R. L., Knox, M., & Phillips, K. D. (1998). Case management at what expense? A case study of the emotional costs of case management. *Nursing Case Management, 3*(2), 89–95.

Birmingham, J. (1996). How to apply CMSA's standards of practice for case management in a capitated environment. *Journal of Care Management, 2*(5), 9–10, 12, 14, 16–18, 20, 22.

Birmingham, J. (2007). Case management: Two regulations with coexisting functions. *Professional Case Management, 12*(1), 16–24.

Bower, K. A. (2004). Patient care management as a global nursing concern. *Nursing Administration Quarterly, 28*(1), 39–43.

Braden, C. J. (2002). *State of the science paper #2: Involvement/participation, empowerment and knowledge outcome indicators of case management*. Little Rock, AR: Case Management Society of America.

Case Management Society of America (CMSA). (2002). *Standards of practice for case management*. Little Rock, AR: Author.

Case Management Society of America (CMSA). (2008a). *History of CMSA*. Little Rock, AR: Author. Retrieved November 7, 2008, from www.cmsa.org/Home/CMSA/OurHistory/tabid/225/Default.aspx

Case Management Society of America (CMSA). (2008b). *Definition of case management*. Little Rock, AR: Author. Retrieved November 8, 2008, from www.cmsa.org/Home/CMSA/WhatisaCaseManager/tabid/224/Default.aspx

Centers for Medicare & Medicaid Services (CMS). (2003). Medicare program; demonstration: Capitated disease management for beneficiaries with chronic illnesses. *Federal Register, 68*(40), 9673–9680.

Cesta, T. G., & Tahan, H. A. (2003). *The case manager's survival guide: Winning strategies for clinical practice* (2nd ed.). St. Louis: Mosby.

Chan, F., Leahy, M. J., McMahon, B. Y., Mirch, M., & DeVinney, D. (1999). Foundational knowledge and major practice domains of case management. *Journal of Care Management, 5*(1), 10–30.

Clark, K. A. (1996). Alternate case management models. In D. L. Flarey, & S. S. Blancett (Eds.), *Handbook of nursing case management* (pp. 295–304). Gaithersburg, MD: Aspen.

Cline, B. G. (1990). Case management: Organizational models and administrative methods. *Caring: National Association for Home Care Magazine, 9*(7), 14–18.

Cole, L., & Houston, S. (1999). Structured care methodologies: Evolution and use in patient care delivery. *Outcomes Management for Nursing Practice, 3*(2), 53–59.

Coleman, J. R. (1999). Integrated case management: The 21st century challenge for HMO case managers, Part 1. *The Case Manager, 10*(5), 28–34.

Commission for Case Manager Certification (CCMC). (2004). *About case management.* Rolling Meadows, IL: Author. Retrieved May 6, 20089 from http://www.ccmcertification.org/download/backgrounder.pdf

Commission for Case Manager Certification (CCMC). (2008). *CCM certification guide for certified case manager.* St. Paul, MN: Author. Retrieved November 7, 2008, from www.ccmcertification.org/pages/14frame_set.html

Cook, T. H. (1998). The effectiveness of inpatient case management: Fact or fiction? *Journal of Nursing Administration, 28*(4), 36–46.

Dzyacky, S. C. (1998). An acute care case management model for nurses and social workers. *Nursing Case Management, 3*(5), 208–215.

Erkel, E. E. (1993). The impact of case management in preventive services. *Journal of Nursing Administration, 23*(1), 27–32.

Falk, C., & Bower, K. (1994). Managing care across department, organization, and setting boundaries. *Series on Nursing Administration, 6*, 161–176.

Fitzgerald, J. F., Smith, D. M., Martin, D. K., Freedman, J. A., & Katz, B. P. (1994). A case manager intervention to reduce readmissions. *Archives of Internal Medicine, 154*(15), 1721–1729.

Forbes, M. A. (1999). The practice of professional nurse case management. *Nursing Case Management, 4*(1), 28–33.

Goodwin, D. R. (1994). Nursing case management activities: How they differ between employment settings. *Journal of Nursing Administration, 24*(2), 29–34.

Goodwin, J. S., Satish, S., Anderson, E. T., Nattinger, A. B., & Freeman, J. L. (2003). Effect of nurse case management on the treatment of older women with breast cancer. *Journal of the American Geriatrics Society, 51*(9), 1252–1259.

Grimaldi, P. L. (1996). A glossary of managed care terms. *Nursing Management, 27*(10, Spec. Suppl.), 5–7.

Hampton, D. (1993). Implementing a managed care framework through care maps. *Journal of Nursing Administration, 23*(5), 21–27.

Harrison, J. P., Nolin, J., & Suero, E. (2004). The effect of case management on U.S. hospitals. *Nursing Economic$, 22*(2), 64–70.

Hawkins, J. W., Veeder, N. W., & Pearce, C. W. (1998). *Nurse–social worker collaboration in managed care.* New York: Springer.

Hicks, L., Stallmeyer, J., & Coleman, J. (1992). Nursing challenges in managed care. *Nursing Economic$, 10*(4), 265–276.

Hinitz-Satterfield, P., Miller, E., & Hagan, E. (1993). Managed care and new roles for nursing: Utilization and case management in a health maintenance organization. *Series on Nursing Administration, 5*, 83–99.

Howe, R. (1999). Case management in managed care: Past, present, future. *The Case Manager, 10*(5), 37–40.

Huber, D. L. (2005). The diversity of service delivery models. In D. Huber (Ed.). *Disease management: A guide for case managers.* Philadelphia: Saunders.

Improving Chronic Illness Care. (2008). *The chronic care model.* Seattle, WA: Author. Retrieved November 8, 2008, from www.improvingchroniccare.org/index.php?p=The_Chronic_Care_Model&s=2

Kelly, K. (1992). Managing care: A search for role clarity. *Journal of Nursing Administration, 22*(3), 9–10.

Laramee, A. S., Levinsky, S. K., Sargent, J., Ross, R., & Callas, P. (2003). Case management in a heterogeneous congestive heart failure population: A randomized controlled trial. *Archives of Internal Medicine, 163*(7), 809–817.

Levitt, D. A., Starz, T. W., & Higgins, R. (1998). Disease state case management in an academic medical center utilizing osteoarthritis-of-the-knee model. *Journal of Care Management, 4*(5), 45, 48, 51–52, 54, 56.

Lu, C. Y., Ross-Degnan, D., Soumerai, S. B., & Pearson, S. (2008). Interventions designed to improve the quality and efficiency of medication use in managed care: A critical review of the literature—2001–2007. *BMC Health Services Research, 8*, 1–12.

Mark, B. (1992). Characteristics of nursing practice models. *Journal of Nursing Administration, 22*(11), 57–63.

McClure, M. (1991). Introduction. In I. E. Goertzen (Ed.), *Differentiating nursing practice: Into the twenty-first century* (pp. 1–11). Kansas City, MO: American Academy of Nursing.

MedicineNet.com. (2008). *Definition of managed care.* Retrieved November 8, 2008, from www.medterms.com/script/main/art.asp?articlekey=4270

MediLexicon. (2008). *Medical dictionary—'Critical Pathway'.* Retrieved November 8, 2008, from www.medilexicon.com/medicaldictionary.php?t=66241

Mikulencak, M. (1993). Public health stands as a proven model for future delivery systems. *The American Nurse, 25*(6), 18.

National Association of Social Workers (NASW). (2008). *NASW standards for social work case management.* Washington, DC: Author. Retrieved November 7, 2008, from www.socialworkers.org/practice/standards/sw_case_mgmt.asp

Norris, S. L., Nichols, P. J., Caspersen, C. J., Glasgow, R. E., Engelgau, M. M., Jack, L. Jr., et al. (2002). The effectiveness of disease and case management for people with diabetes: A systematic review. *American Journal of Preventive Medicine, 22*(Suppl. 4), 1–25.

Park, E. J., Huber, D. L., & Tahan, H. A. (2009). The evidence base for case management practice. *Western Journal of Nursing Research.* First published on April 6, 2009 as doi:10.1177/0193945909332912.

Raiff, N. R., & Shore, B. K. (1993). *Advanced case management: New strategies for the nineties.* Newbury Park, CA: Sage.

Renholm, M., Leino-Kilpi, H., & Suominen, T. (2002). Critical pathways: A systematic review. *Journal of Nursing Administration, 32*(4), 196–202.

Rheaume, A., Frisch, S., Smith, A., & Kennedy, C. (1994). Case management and nursing practice. *Journal of Nursing Administration, 24*(3), 30–36.

Ridgely, M. S., & Willenbring, M. C. (1992). Application of case management to drug abuse treatment: Overview of models and research issues. *NIDA Monograph, 127*, 12–33.

Riegel, B., Carlson, B., Kopp, Z., LePetri, B., Glaser, B., & Unger, A. (2002). Effect of a standardized nurse case-management telephone intervention on resource use in patients with chronic heart failure. *Archives of Internal Medicine, 162*(6), 705–712.

Sesperez, J., Wilson, S., Jalaludin, B., Seger, M., & Sugrue, M. (2001). Trauma case management and clinical pathways: Prospective evaluation of their effect on selected patient outcomes in five key trauma conditions. *The Journal of Trauma, 50*(4), 643–649.

Shortell, S. M., Anderson, D. A., Gilles, R. R., Mitchell, J. B., & Morgan, K. L. (1993). The holographic organization. *Healthcare Forum Journal, 36*(2), 20–26.

Siefker, J. M., Garrett, M. B., Van Genderen, A., & Weis, M. J. (1998). *Fundamentals of case management: Guidelines for practicing case managers*. St. Louis: Mosby.

Simpson, R. (1993). Case-managed care in tomorrow's information network. *Nursing Management, 24*(7), 14–16.

Tahan, H. A. (1996). A ten-step process to develop case management plans. *Nursing Case Management, 1*(3), 112–121.

Tahan, H. A. (1998). Case management: A heritage more than a century old. *Nursing Case Management, 3*(2), 55–60.

Tahan, H. A., Downey, W. T., & Huber, D. L. (2006). Case managers' roles and functions: Commission for Case Manager Certification's 2004 research, Part II. *Lippincott's Case Management, 11*(2), 71–87.

Tahan, H. A., & Huber, D. L. (2006). The CCMC's national study of case manager job descriptions: An understanding of the activities, role relationships, knowledges, skills, and abilities. *Lippincott's Case Management, 11*(3), 127–144.

Tahan, H. A., Huber, D. L., & Downey, W. T. (2006). Case managers' roles and functions: Commission for Case Manager Certification's 2004 research, Part I. *Lippincott's Case Management, 11*(1), 4–22.

Wagner, E. H. (1998). Chronic disease management: What will it take to improve care for chronic illness? *Effective Clinical Practice, 1*, 2–4.

Wagner, E. H., Austin, B. T., Davis, C., Hindmarsh, M., Schaefer, J., & Bonomi, A. (2001). Improving chronic illness care: Translating evidence into action. *Health Affairs, 20*(6), 64–78.

Ward, M. D., & Rieve, J. A. (1997). The role of case management in disease management. In W. E. Todd, & D. Nash (Eds.), *Disease management: A systems approach to improving patient outcomes* (pp. 235–259). Chicago: American Hospital Publishing.

Weil, M., & Karls, J. M. (1985). *Case management in human service practice: A systematic approach to mobilizing resources for clients*. San Francisco: Jossey-Bass.

Weiman, M. G. (1995). Case management. A means to improve quality and control the costs of cure in children with acute myelogenous leukemia. *Journal of Pediatric Hematology and Oncology, 17*(3), 248–253.

Zander, K. (1990). Case management: A golden opportunity for whom? In J. McCloskey, & H. Grace (Eds.), *Current issues in nursing* (3rd ed., pp. 199–204). St. Louis: Mosby.

Zander, K. (1991). Case management in acute care: Making the connections. *The Case Manager, 2*(1), 39–43.

Zander, K. (1992). Nursing care delivery methods and quality. *Series on Nursing Administration, 3*, 86–104.

Zander, K. (1994). Nurses and case management: To control or collaborate? In J. McCloskey, & H. Grace (Eds.), *Current issues in nursing* (4th ed., pp. 254–260). St. Louis: Mosby.

Zander, K. (2002). Nursing case management in the 21st century: Intervening where margin meets mission. *Nursing Administration Quarterly, 26*(5), 58–67.

Chapter 22

Aikman, P., Andress, I., Goodfellow, C., LaBelle, N., & Porter-O'Grady, T. (1998). System integration: A necessity. *Journal of Nursing Administration, 28*(2), 28–34.

Alexander, J., & Kroposki, M. (1999). Outcomes for community health nursing practice. *Journal of Nursing Administration, 29*(5), 49–56.

Aliotta, S. (1999). Patient adherence outcome indicators and measurement in case management and health care. *Journal of Care Management, 5*(4), 24, 26, 29–31, 81–82.

Aliotta, S. L. (1996). Components of a successful case management program. *Managed Care Quarterly, 4*(2), 38–45.

Anderson, M. A., & Helms, L. B. (1998). Comparison of continuing care communication. *Image, 30*(3), 255–260.

Anderson, M. A., & Tredway, C. A. (1999). Communication: An outcome of case management. *Nursing Case Management, 4*(3), 104–111.

Aurora Health Care. (2004). *Aurora's continuum of care*. Milwaukee, WI: Author. Retrieved November 8, 2008, from www.aurorahealthcare.org/aboutus/continuum/index.asp

Berger, J., Slezak, J., Stine, N., McStay, P., O'Leary, B., & Addiego, J. (2001). Economic impact of a diabetes disease management program in a self-insured health plan: Early results. *Disease Management, 4*(2), 65–73.

Bryan, Y. E., Bayley, E. W., Grendel, C., Kingston, M. B., Tuck, M. B., & Wood, L. J. (1997). Preparing to change from acute to community-based care: Learning needs of hospital-based nurses. *Journal of Nursing Administration, 27*(5), 35–44.

Burgess, C. S. (1999). Managed care: The driving force for case management. In E. L. Cohen, & V. DeBack (Eds.),

The outcomes mandate: Case management in health care today (pp. 13–19). St. Louis: Mosby.

Carroll, P. L. (2004). *Community health nursing: A practical guide*. Clifton Park, NY: Thomson Delmar Learning.

Case Management Society of America (CMSA). (2002). *Definition of case management*. Little Rock, AR: Author. Retrieved November 8, 2008, from www.cmsa.org/Home/CMSA/WhatisaCaseManager/tabid/224/Default.aspx

Case Management Society of America (CMSA). (2004). The case report. *The Case Manager, 15*(3), 37.

Centers for Disease Control and Prevention (CDC). (2008). *Chronic disease prevention and health promotion*. Atlanta, GA: Author. Retrieved November 8, 2008, from www.cdc.gov/nccdphp/

Centers for Medicare & Medicaid Services (CMS). (2004). *National Health Care expenditures: Historical overview*. Baltimore: Author. Retrieved November 8, 2008, from www.cms.hhs.gov/NationalHealthExpendData/02_NationalHealthAccountsHistorical.asp#TopOfPage

Coggeshall Press. (2008). *Care for the total population*. Coralville, IA: Author.

Coleman, J. R. (1999). Integrated case management: The twenty-first century challenge for HMO case managers, Part I. *The Case Manager, 10*(5), 28–34.

Commission for Case Manager Certification (CCMC). (2008). *CCM certification guide for certified case manager*. St. Paul, MN: Author. Retrieved November 8, 2008, from www.ccmcertification.org/pages/14frame_set.html

Cousins, M. S., & Liu, Y. (2003). Cost savings for a preferred provider organization population with multi-condition disease management: Evaluating program impact using predictive modeling with a control group. *Disease Management, 6*(4), 207–217.

DMAA: The Care Continuum Alliance (DMAA). (2008a). *DMAA definition of disease management*. Washington, DC: Author. Retrieved November 8, 2008, from www.dmaa.org/dm_definition.asp

DMAA: The Care Continuum Alliance (DMAA). (2008b). *Population health*. Washington, DC: Author. Retrieved November 8, 2008, from www.dmaa.org/phi_definition.asp

Gillespie, J. L. (2002). The value of disease management. Part 3. Balancing cost and quality in the treatment of asthma. *Disease Management, 5*(4), 225–232.

Glick, D. F., Hale, P. J., Kulbok, P. A., & Shettig, J. (1996). Community development theory: Planning a community nursing center. *Journal of Nursing Administration, 26*(7/8), 44–50.

Goldstein, R. (1998). The disease management approach to cost containment. *Nursing Case Management, 3*(3), 99–103.

Hall, P. J. (1998). Planning an integrated population-based program. *Journal of Nursing Administration, 28*(10), 40–47.

Health Canada. (2004). *What is population health?* Ottawa, Ontario, Canada: Author. Retrieved November 8, 2008, from www.phac-aspc.gc.ca/ph-sp/approach-approche/index-eng.php#What

Ho, S. (2003). The emerging role for health plans: Info-Mediary. *Disease Management, 6*(Suppl. 1), 4–10.

Huber, D. L. (2005). Overview of disease management. In D. L. Huber (Ed.), *Disease management: A guide for case managers*. Philadelphia: Saunders.

Huston, C. J. (2001). The role of the case manager in a disease management program. *Lippincott's Case Management, 6*(5), 222–227.

Improving Chronic Illness Care. (2008). *The Chronic Care Model*. Seattle: MacColl Institute for Healthcare Innovation. Retrieved November 8, 2008, from www.improvingchroniccare.org/change/model/components.html

Institute of Medicine (IOM). (2001). *Crossing the quality chasm: A new health system for the 21st century*. Washington, DC: National Academies Press.

Institute of Medicine (IOM). (2004). *Crossing the quality chasm: The IOM health care quality initiative*. Washington, DC: National Academies Press.

Javors, J. R., Laws, D., & Bramble, J. E. (2003). Uncontrolled chronic disease: Patient non-compliance or clinical mismanagement? *Disease Management, 6*(3), 169–178.

Johnson, A. (2003). Why we can't wait to implement disease management. *Business and Health Archive, October 15*, 21.

Kindig, D. A. (1999). Purchasing population health: Aligning financial incentives to improve health outcomes. *Nursing Outlook, 47*(1), 15–22.

Kramer, M. S. (2004). Predictive models make smart purchasers. *Business and Health Archive*, January 10, 1–4.

Lewis, A. (2004). Savings opportunities through Medicaid disease management. *Disease Management, 7*(1), 35–46.

Lipold, A. G. (2002). Disease management comes of age, not a moment too soon. *Business and Health Archive*, June 19, 7.

Lynn, M. R., & Kelly, B. (1997). Effects of case management on the nursing context: Perceived quality of care, work satisfaction, and control over practice. *Image, 29*(3), 237–241.

Martin, D. C., Berger, M. L., Anstatt, D. T., Wofford, J., Warfel, D., Turpin, R. S., et al. (2004). A randomized controlled open trial of population-based disease and case management in a Medicare Plus Choice Health Maintenance Organization. *Preventing Chronic Disease, 1*(4). Retrieved November 8, 2008, from www.cdc.gov/pcd/issues/2004/oct/04_0015.htm

Misener, T. R., Alexander, J., Blaha, A. J., Clarke, P. N., Cover, C. M., Felton, G. M., et al. (1997). National Delphi study to determine competencies for nursing leadership in public health. *Image, 29*(1), 47–51.

Nobel, J. J., & Norman, G. K. (2003). Emerging information management technologies and the future of disease management. *Disease Management, 6*(4), 219–231.

Pareto Law. (2008). *Pareto's Law, a management principle/technique*. Retrieved November 8, 2008, from http://home.alltel.net/mikeric/Misc/Pareto.htm

Qudah, F. J., & Brannon, M. (1996). Population-based case management. *Quality Management in Health Care, 5*(1), 29–41.

Schuster, G. F., & Goeppinger, J. (1996). Community as client: Using the nursing process to promote health. In M. Stanhope, & J. Lancaster (Eds.), *Community health nursing: Promoting health of aggregates, families, and individuals* (4th ed., pp. 289–314). St. Louis: Mosby.

Smith, D. S., Auerbach, L. P., & Hamill, C. T. (2003). Case management return on investment. *Care Management, 9*(6), 24–48, 42.

Storfjell, J. L., Mitchell, R., & Daly, G. M. (1997). Nurse-managed health care: New York's community nursing organization. *Journal of Nursing Administration, 27*(10), 21–27.

Strohschein, S., Shaffer, M. A., & Lia-Hoagberg, B. (1999). Evidence-based guidelines for public health nursing practice. *Nursing Outlook, 47*(2), 84–89.

Todd, W. E., & Nash, D. (Eds.). (1997). *Disease management: A systems approach to improving patient outcomes.* Chicago: American Hospital Publishing.

U.S. Census Bureau. (2001). *Age: 2000. Census 2000 brief.* Washington, DC: Author.

Wagner, E. H. (1998). Chronic disease management: What will it take to improve care for chronic illness? *Effective Clinical Practice, 1*, 2–4.

Welch, W. P., Bergsten, C., Cutler, C., Bocchino, C., & Smith, R. I. (2002). Disease management practices of health plans. *The American Journal of Managed Care, 8*(4), 353–361.

Williams, C. A. (1996). Community-based population-focused practice: The foundation of specialization in public health nursing. In M. Stanhope, & J. Lancaster (Eds.), *Community health nursing: Promoting health of aggregates, families, and individuals* (4th ed., pp. 21–33). St. Louis: Mosby.

Wilson, T., & MacDowell, M. (2003). Framework for assessing causality in disease management programs: Principles. *Disease Management, 6*(3), 143–158.

Ziguras, S. J., & Stuart, G. W. (2000). A meta-analysis of the effectiveness of mental health case management over 20 years. *Psychiatric Services, 51*, 1410–1421.

Zitter, M. (1997). A new paradigm in health care delivery: Disease management. In W. E. Todd, & D. Nash (Eds.), *Disease management: A systems approach to improving patient outcomes* (pp. 1–25). Chicago: American Hospital Publishing.

Chapter 23

Aiken, L., Clarke, S., Sloane, D., Sochalski, J., & Silber, J. (2002). Hospital nurse staffing and patient mortality, nurse burnout, and job dissatisfaction. *Journal of the American Medical Association, 288*(16), 1987–1993.

Armola, R., & Topp, R. (2001). Variables that discriminate length of stay and readmission within 30 days among heart failure patients. *Lippincott's Case Management, 6*(6), 246–255.

Balstad, A., & Springer, P. (2006). Quantifying case management workloads, development of the PACE tool. *Lippincott's Case Management, 11*(6), 291–302.

Bolin, J., Phillips, C., & Hawes, C. (2006). Differences between newly admitted nursing home residents in rural and nonrural areas in a national sample. *The Gerontologist, 46*, 33–41.

Bradley, V. (2005). Placing emergency department crowding on the decision agenda. *Nursing Economic$, 23*(1), 14–24.

Butler, R., Johnson, W., & Gray, B. (2007). Timing makes a difference: Early nurse case management intervention and low back pain. *Professional Case Management, 12*(6), 316–327.

Clark, J. C., Snyder, J., Meek, R., Stutz, L., & Parkin, C. (2001). A systematic approach to risk stratification and intervention within managed care environment improves diabetes outcomes and patient satisfaction. *Diabetes Care, 24*(6), 1079–1086.

Clarke, S., & Aiken, L. (2006). More nursing, fewer deaths. *Quality and Safety Health Care, 15*, 2–3.

Claudio, T. (2004). Questioning workload resources. *Nurse Manager, 35*(10), 30–35.

Craig, K., & Huber, D. L. (2007). Acuity and case management: A healthy dose of outcomes, Part II. *Professional Case Management, 12*(4), 199–210.

Cusack, G., Jones-Wells, A., & Chisholm, L. (2004). Patient intensity in an ambulatory oncology research center: A step forward for the field of ambulatory care. *Nursing Economic$, 22*(2), 58–63.

Detwiler, C., & Clark, M. (1995). Acuity classification in the urgent care setting. *Journal of Nursing Administration, 25*(2), 53–61.

Fagerstrom, L., & Rauhala, A. (2007). Benchmarking in nursing care by the RAFAELA patient classification system: A possibility for nurse managers. *Journal of Nursing Management, 15*(7), 683–692.

Gallagher, R. M., Kany, K. A., Rowell, P. A., & Peterson, C. (1999). ANA's nurse staffing principles. *American Journal of Nursing, 99*(4), 50–51.

Griffin, K., & Swan, B. (2006). Linking nursing workload and performance indicators in ambulatory care. *Nursing Economic$, 24*(1), 41–44.

Haas, S., & Hackbarth, D. (1995). Dimensions of the staff nurse role in ambulatory care. Part IV. Developing nursing intensity measures, standards, clinical ladders, and QI programs. *Nursing Economic$, 13*(5), 285–294.

Huber, D., & Craig, K. (2007a). Acuity and case management: A healthy dose of outcomes, Part I. *Professional Case Management, 12*(3), 132–144.

Huber, D., & Craig, K. (2007b). Acuity and case managment: A healthy dose of outcomes, Part III. *Professional Case Management, 12*(5), 254–269.

Huber, D., Hall, J., & Vaugh, T. (2001). Dose of case management interventions. *Lippincott's Case Management, 6*(3), 119–126.

Huber, D., Sarrazin, M., Vaughn, T., & Hall, J. (2003). Evaluating the impact of case management dosage. *Nursing Research, 52*(5), 276–288.

Johnson, W. (2006). CI (computer informatics) for a DSS to predict nursing coverage in a geriatric care facility. *Student Health Technology Informatics, 23*(4), 86–90.

Kane, D., & Issel, L. (2005). Estimating Medicaid prenatal case management costs: The provider's perspective. *Nursing Economic$, 23*(4), 181–188.

Keene, R., & Cullen, D. (1983). Therapeutic interventions scoring system, update 1983. *Critical Care Medicine, 11*, 1–3.

King, R., Meadows, G., & LeBas, J. (2004). Compiling a caseload index for mental health case management. *Australian and New Zealand Journal of Psychiatry, 38*, 455–462.

Malloch, D., & Conovaloff, A. (1999). Patient classification systems. Part 1. The third generation. *JONA, 29*(7/8), 49–56.

Milliman. (2007). *Milliman Care Guidelines® Q&A: Advertisement materials.* Milliman Care Guidelines, LLC.

O'Brien-Pallas, L., Irvine, D., Peereboom, E., & Murray, M. (1997). Measuring nursing workload: Understanding the variability. *Nursing Economic$, 15*(4), 171–182.

O'Leary, D. (2002). *Staffing effectiveness.* Retrieved December 2007, from www.jointcommission.org/NewsRoom/OnCapitalHill/Testimony_112002.htm

Peters, R., Benkert, R., Dinardo, E., & Templin, T. (2007). Assessing quality of care for African Americans with hypertension. *Journal of Healthcare Quality, 29*(3), 10–20.

Phillips, C., Castorr, A., Prescott, P., & Soeken, K. (1992). Nursing intensity: Going beyond patient classification. *Journal of Nursing Administration, 22*(4), 46–52.

Prescott, P. (1991). Nursing intensity: Needed today for more staffing. *Nursing Economic$, 9*(6), 409–414.

Prescott, P., Ryan, J., Soeken, K., Castorr, A., Thompson, K., & Phillips, C. (1991). The Patient Intensity for Nursing Index: A validity assessment. *Research Nursing Health, 14*(3), 213–221.

Prescott, P., & Soeken, K. (1996a). Measuring nursing intensity in ambulatory care. Part I. Approaches to and uses of patient classification systems. *Nursing Economic$, 14*(1), 14–21, 33.

Prescott, P., & Soeken, K. (1996b). Measuring nursing intensity in ambulatory care. Part II. Developing and testing PINAC. *Nurse Economic$, 14*(2), 86–91, 116.

Prescott, P., Soeken, K., & Ryan, J. (1989). Measuring patient intensity. A reliability study. *Evaluative Health Professional, 12*(3), 255–269.

Ream, R., Mackey, K., Leet, T., Green, M., Andreone, T., Loftis, L., et al. (2007). Association of nursing workload and unplanned extubations in a pediatric intensive care unit. *Pediatric Critical Care Medicine, 8*(4), 366–371.

Saake, L. (1986). *Patient classification: Evaluating a system.* Thesis. St. Louis, MO: Saint Louis University.

Shaha, S., & Bush, C. (1996). Fixing acuity: A professional approach to patient classification and staffing. *Nursing Economic$, 14*(6), 346–356.

Swan, B. (2005). Measuring nursing workload in ambulatory care. *Nursing Economic$, 23*(5), 253–260.

The Joint Commission (TJC) (SI). (2008). *2008 National Patient Safety Standards.* Retrieved Dec 25, 2007, fromwww.jointcommission.org/PatientSafety/NationalPatientSafetyGoals/

Werley, H., Devine, E., Zorn, C., Ryan, P., & Westra, B. (1991). The Nursing Minimum Data Set: Abstraction tool for standarized, comparable, essential data. *American Journal of Public Health, 81*(4), 413–414.

Yeh, T. S., Pollack, M. M., Ruttimann, U. E., Holbrook, P. R., & Fields, A. I. (1984). Validation of a physiologic stability index for use in critically ill infants and children. *Pediatrics Research, 18*(5), 445–451.

Zhang, N., Unruh, L., Liu, R., & Wan, T. (2006). Minimum nurse staffing ratios for nursing homes. *Nursing Economic$, 24*(2), 78–85, 93.

Chapter 24

American Nurses Association (ANA). (2005). *Code of ethics for nurses with interpretive statements.* Retrieved January 21, 2008, from www.nursingworld.org/MainMenuCategories/ThePracticeofProfessionalNursing/EthicsStandards/CodeofEthics/AboutTheCode.aspx

American Nurses Association (ANA). (2009). *The national database.* Silver Spring, MD: Author. Retrieved May 15, 2009, from http://nursingworld.org/MainMenuCategories/ThePracticeofProfessionalNursing/PatientSafetyQuality/NDNQI/NDNQI_1.aspx

American Nurses Credentialing Center. (2009). *Program overview.* Silver Spring, MD: Author. Retrieved May 15, 2009, from http://www.nursecredentialing.org/Magnet/ProgramOverview.aspx

American Society for Quality (ASQ). (2007). *Basic concepts: Glossary.* Retrieved January 21, 2008, from www.asq.org/glossary/c.html

Berwick, D. M., Godfrey, A. B., & Roessner, J. (1990). *Curing health care: New strategies for quality improvement.* San Francisco: Jossey-Bass.

Chassin, M. R. (1997). Assessing strategies for quality improvement. *Health Affairs, 16*, 151–161.

Chrvala, C. A., & Bulger, R. J. (Eds.). (1999). *Leading health indicators for Healthy People 2010: Final Report.* Washington, DC: National Academies Press.

Commonwealth of Pennsylvania, Pennsylvania Health Care Cost Containment Council (HCCCC). (2004). *About the council: Mission.* Harrisburg, PA: Pennsylvania HCCCC. Retrieved June 30, 2004, from www.phc4.org/council/aboutthe.htm

Corrigan, J. M., Eden, J., & Smith, B. M. (Eds). (2002). *Leadership by example: Coordinating government roles in improving health care quality*. Washington, DC: National Academies Press.

Deming, W. E. (2000a). *The new economics for industry, government, education*. Cambridge, MA: MIT Center for Advanced Engineering Studies.

Deming, W. E. (2000b). *Out of the crisis*. Cambridge, MA: MIT Center for Advanced Engineering Studies.

Donabedian, A. (1980). *Explorations in quality assessment and monitoring: The definition of quality and approaches to its assessment* (Vol. 1). Ann Arbor, MI: Health Administration Press.

Donaldson, M. S., & Mohr, J. J. (Eds.). (2000). *Exploring innovation and quality improvement in health care microsystems*. Washington, DC: National Academies Press.

Durch, J. S., Bailey, L. A., & Stoto, M. A. (Eds.). (1997). *Improving health in the community: A role for performance monitoring*. Washington, DC: National Academies Press.

Foundation for Accountability (FACCT). (2002). *Supporting quality-based decisions*. New York: FACCT (now The Markle Foundation.) Retrieved March 7, 2002, from www.facct.org/

Frost, R. (2006). New, improved ISO 9000 guidelines for the health care sector. *ISO Management Systems*, (January/February). Retrieved January 21, 2008, from www.iso.org/iso/ims_en_2006_01_health.pdf

Harmon, F. G. (1997). Future present. In F. Hesselbein, M. Goldsmith, & R. Beckhard (Eds.), *The organization of the future* (pp. 239–247). San Francisco: Jossey-Bass.

Harry, M., & Schroeder, R. (2000). *Six Sigma: The breakthrough strategy revolutionizing the world's top corporations*. New York: Currency/Doubleday.

Hesselbein, F., & Johnston, R. (2002). *A leader-to-leader guide: On high-performance organizations*. San Francisco: Jossey-Bass.

His Holiness the Dalai Lama, & Cutler, H. C. (1998). *The art of happiness*. New York: Riverhead Books.

Hussey, P. S., Mattke, S., Morse, L., & Ridgely, M. S. (2007). *Evaluation of the use of AHRQ and other quality indicators* (Contract No. WR-426 HS to RAND Health). AHRQ Publication No. 08-M012-EF. Rockville, MD: Agency for Healthcare Research and Quality.

Hyde, P. S., Falls, K., Morris, J. A., & Schoenwald, S. A. (2003). *Turning knowledge into practice: A manual for behavioral health administrators and practitioners about understanding and implementing evidence-based practices*. Boston: The Technical Assistance Collaborative.

Institute for Healthcare Improvement (IHI). (2004). *About IHI*. Boston: Author. Retrieved June 30, 2004, from www.ihi.org/about/

Institute of Medicine (IOM), Committee on Enhancing Federal Healthcare Quality Programs (CEFHQP). (2002). *Project description*. Washington, DC: National Academies Press. Retrieved October 30, 2002, from www.iom.edu/iom/iomhome.nsf/pages/Fed + Qual + Home?OpenDocument

Institute of Medicine (IOM), Committee on Quality of Health Care in America (CQHCA). (2001). *Crossing the quality chasm: A new health system for the 21st century*. Washington, DC: National Academies Press.

Institute of Medicine (IOM), Committee on the National Quality Report on Health Care Delivery. (2001). In M. P. Hurtado, E. K. Swift, & J. M. Corrigan (Eds.), *Envisioning the national health care report*. Washington, DC: National Academies Press.

Jones, D., & Womack, J. (2003). *Lean thinking: Banish waste and create wealth in your corporation, revised and updated*. New York: Free Press.

Juran, J. M. (1989). *Juran on leadership for quality: An executive handbook*. New York: The Free Press.

Juran Institute. (2007). *Quality planning*. Retrieved January 21, 2008, from www.juran.com/quality_planning.asp

Katz, J. M., & Green, E. (1997). *Managing quality: A guide to system-wide performance management in healthcare* (2nd ed.). St. Louis: Mosby.

Kohn, L. T., Corrigan, J. M., & Donaldson, M. S. (Eds.). (2000). *To err is human: Building a safer health care system*. Washington, DC: National Academies Press.

Lohr, K. (Ed.). (1990). *Medicare: A strategy for quality assurance* (Vol. 2). Washington, DC: National Academies Press.

Maas, M. L., & Kerr, P. (1999). Risk adjustment in nursing effectiveness research. *Outcomes Management for Nursing Practice*, *3*(2), 50–52.

Marcus, L. J., Dorn, B. C., Kritek, P. B., Miller, V. G., & Wyatt, J. B. (1995). *Renegotiating health care: Resolving conflict to build collaboration*. San Francisco: Jossey Bass.

Martin, K. (2003). On Lean Enterprise and its potential health care applications (Editorial). *Journal for Healthcare Quality*, *25*(5), 2, 43.

Mayo Clinic. (2008). *Mayo's mission, primary value, core principles*. Retrieved January 22, 2008, from www.mayoclinic.org/about/missionvalues.html

National Committee for Quality Assurance (NCQA). (2000). *Desirable attributes of HEDIS measures (HEDIS 2001, vol. 1)*. Washington, DC: Author. Retrieved January 11, 2005, from www.ncqa.org/Programs/HEDIS/desirable%20attibutes.html

National Institute of Standards and Technology. (2007). Press release—Presidential award for excellence honors five U.S. organizations: Two nonprofits recognized in first year of category. Retrieved January 18, 2008, from www.nist.gov/public_affairs/releases/2007baldrigerecipients.htm

National Quality Forum (NQF). (2009). *"Patient safety can't wait": NQF calls for faster spread of safe practices*. Washington, DC: Author. Retrieved May 15, 2009, from http://www.qualityforum.org/news/releases/03102009.asp

Omenn, G. (2002). *Public briefing: Opening statement—Leadership by example: Coordinating government roles in improving health care quality*. Presented at the Institute of Medicine, Washington, DC, October 30, 2002.

O'Neil, E. H., & the Pew Health Professions Commission (PHPC). (1998). *Recreating health professional practice for a new century: The fourth report of the Pew Health Professions Commission*. San Francisco: PHPC.

Palmer, S., & Torgerson, D. J. (1999). Definition of efficiency. *British Medical Journal, 318*, 1136.

Pelletier, L. R. (1998). Guest editorial. *Journal of Nursing Care Quality, 13*(1), vii.

Pelletier, L. R. (1999a). On strategic planning (Editorial). *Journal for Healthcare Quality, 21*(3), 2, 17.

Pelletier, L. R. (1999b). On values and achievements (Editorial). *Journal for Healthcare Quality, 21*(6), 2, 10–11.

Pelletier, L. R. (2000). On error-free health care: Mission possible! (Editorial). *Journal for Healthcare Quality, 22*(3), 2, 9.

Pelletier, L. R., & Hoffman, J. A. (2002). A framework for selecting performance measures for opioid treatment programs. *Journal for Healthcare Quality, 24*(3), 24–35.

Plsek, P., & Omnias, A. (1989). *Juran Institute quality improvement tools: Problem solving/glossary*. Wilton, CT: Juran Institute.

President's Advisory Commission on Consumer Protection and Quality in the Health Care Industry. (1998). *Quality first: Better health care for all Americans*. Washington, DC: Government Printing Office.

Quality Interagency Coordination (QuIC) Task Force. (2000). *Doing what counts for patient safety: Federal actions to reduce medical errors and their impact. Report of the Quality Interagency Task Force (QuIC) to the President of the United States*. Rockville, MD: QuIC. Retrieved May 15, 2009), from www.quic.gov/report/errors6.pdf

Quality Interagency Coordination Task Force (QuIC). (2001). *Fact Sheet. Quality Interagency Coordination Task Force (QuIC)*. Rockville, MD: Author. Retrieved May 15, 2009, from http://www.quic.gov/about/quic-fact.htm

Sackett, D. L., Rosenberg, W. M. C., Gray, J. A. M., Haynes, R. B., & Richardson, W. S. (1996). Evidence-based medicine: What it is and what it isn't. *British Medical Journal, 312*(7023), 71.

Sharp HealthCare. (2008). *Mission, vision, and values*. Retrieved January 21, 2008, from www.sharp.com/generalinfo/index.cfm?id = 8718

Shojania, K. G., Duncan, B. W., McDonald, K. M., & Wachter, R. M. (Eds.). (2001). *Making health care safer: A critical analysis of patient safety practices*. Evidence Report/Technology Assessment No. 43 (Prepared by the University of California at San Francisco–Stanford Evidence-based Practice Center). (AHRQ Publication No. 01-E058.) Rockville, MD: Agency for Healthcare Research and Quality.

Shojania, K. G., McDonald, K. M., Wachter, R. M., & Owens, D. K. (2004). *Closing the quality gap: A critical analysis of quality improvement strategies* (vol. 1—Series overview and methodology. Technical Review 9). Contract No. 290–02–0017 to the Stanford University–UCSF Evidence-based Practice Center. (AHRQ Publication No. 04–0051–1.) Rockville, MD: Agency for Healthcare Research and Quality.

Smith, G. R., Manderscheid, R. W., Flynn, L. M., & Steinwachs, D. M. (1997). Principles of assessment for patient outcomes in mental health care. *Psychiatric Services, 48*, 1033–1036.

Sower, V. E., Duffy, J. A., & Kohers, G. (2008). *Benchmarking for hospitals: Achieving best-in-class performance without having to reinvent the wheel*. Milwaukee, WI: American Society for Quality, Quality Press.

2007 State Quality Awards Directory. (2007). *Quality Digest*. 3, 57–60. Retrieved January 18, 2008, from www.qualitydigest.com/pdfs/statedir.pdf

The Commonwealth Fund. (2004). *First report and recommendations of The Commonwealth Fund's International Working Group on Quality Indicators*. New York: Author. Retrieved June 8, 2004, from www.cmwf.org

The Joint Commission (TJC). (2007). *Looking at the ORYX data: Glossary*. Retrieved January 21, 2008, from www.jointcommission.org/AccreditationPrograms/Hospitals/ORYX/looking_at_oryx_data.htm#4

The Joint Commission (TJC). (2008a). *Current specification manual for national hospital quality measures*. Retrieved June 2, 2008, from www.jointcommission.org/PerformanceMeasurement/PerformanceMeasurement/Current+NHQM+Manual.htm

The Joint Commission (TJC). (2008b). *Glossary for measure information form B*. Retrieved January 21, 2008, from www.jointcommission.org/NR/rdonlyres/9B31EDE2-B7CF-4927–88EE-FAB24BE03541/0/glossary.pdf

The Joint Commission (TJC). (2008c). *2008 National Patient Safety Goals, hospital program*. Retrieved June 2, 2008, from www.jointcommission.org/PatientSafety/NationalPatientSafetyGoals/08_hap_npsgs.htm

The Joint Commission (TJC). (2008d). *Performance measure initiatives*. Retrieved June 2, 2008, from www.jointcommission.org/PerformanceMeasurement/PerformanceMeasurement/

The Joint Commission (TJC). (2008e). *Sentinel event policy and procedure*. Retrieved June 15, 2008, from www.jointcommission.org/SentinelEvents/PolicyandProcedures/se_pp.htm

The Joint Commission (TJC). (2009). *Sentinel event*. Retrieved May 16, 2009, from http://www.jointcommission.org/SentinelEvents/

The Leapfrog Group for Patient Safety. (2004). *About us*. Washington, DC: Author. Retrieved June 30, 2004, from www.leapfroggroup.org/

The White House. (2000). *Clinton-Gore Administration announces new actions to improve patient safety and assure health care quality (press release)*. Washington, DC: Author. Retrieved January 11, 2005, from www.clinton5.nara.gov/WH/New/html/20000222_1.html

U.K. Department of Health. (2002). *NHS performance indicators: February 2002*. London: Author. Retrieved March 7, 2002, from www.doh.gov.uk/nhsperformanceindicators/2002/index.html

U.S. Department of Health and Human Services (USDHHS), Centers for Medicare and Medicaid Services (CMS). (2004b). *Medicare quality improvement organization program: Summary of proposed 8th scope of work: May 13, 2004*. Baltimore: CMS. Retrieved June 30, 2004, from www.cms.hhs.gov/qio/2s.pdf

U.S. Department of Veterans Affairs. (2004). *The VA National Center for Patient Safety*. Ann Arbor, MI: VA National Center for Patient Safety. Retrieved June 30, 2004, from www.patientsafety.gov/index.html

Velianoff, G. D., & Hobbs, D. K. (1998). Designing a patient care risk management system. In J. A. Dienemann (Ed.), *Nursing administration: Managing patient care* (2nd ed., pp. 91–99). Stamford, CT: Appleton & Lange.

Visiting Nursing Service of New York. (2008). *Mission statement*. Retrieved January 21, 2008, from www.vnsny.org/mainsite/about/a_mission.html

Ward, B. (2004). *The five key facets of high performance leadership*. Edmonton, Alberta, Canada: Affinity Consulting. Retrieved June 30, 2004, from www.affinitymc.com/Five_Facets_of_Leadership.htm

White, S. V. (2003). Interview with a quality leader: Sister Mary Jean Ryan on the first Baldrige award in health care. *Journal for Healthcare Quality, 25*(3), 24–25.

Chapter 25

Agency for Healthcare Research and Quality. (2004). *Bioterrorism and health system preparedness* (Issue Brief No. 4). (AHRQ Publication No. 04-P009.) Rockville, MD: Author.

Aiken, L. H., Clarke, S. P., Sloane, D. M., Sochalski, J., & Silber, J. H. (2002). Hospital nurse staffing and patient mortality, nurse burnout, and job dissatisfaction. *JAMA: The Journal of the American Medical Association, 288*(16), 1987–1993.

American Nurses Association (ANA). (1996). *Nursing quality indicators: Definitions and implications*. Washington, DC: American Nurses Publishing.

American Nurses Association (ANA). (2004). *National database of nursing quality indicators*. Retrieved January 25, 2008, from www.nursingworld.org/quality

American Nurses Association (ANA). (2007). *Nurse staffing plans and ratios*. Retrieved August 23, 2007, from www.nursingworld.org/mainmenucategories/ANAPoliticalPower/State/StateLegislativeAgenda/StaffingPlansandRatios_1.aspx

Burritt, J. E., Wallace, P., Steckel, C., & Hunter, A. (2007). Achieving quality and fiscal outcomes in patient care: The clinical mentor care delivery model. *Journal of Nursing Administration, 37*(12), 558–563.

California Department of Health Services. (2002). *Hospital nursing staff ratios and quality of care: Final report on evidence, administrative data, an expert panel process, and a hospital staffing survey*. Davis, CA: Prepared by UC Davis Center for Health Services Research in Primary Care and UC Davis Center for Nursing Research.

California Department of Health Services. (2003). *Final statement of reasons, R-37–01*. Retrieved September 1, 2007, from www.dhs.ca.gov/lnc/pubnotice/NTPR/R-37–01_FSOR.pdf

Campbell, D. T., & Stanley, J. C. (1963). *Experimental and quasi-experimental designs for research*. Boston: Houghton Mifflin.

Clarke, S. P. (2005). The policy implications of staffing-outcomes research. *Journal of Nursing Administration, 35*(1), 17–19.

Donabedian, A. (1985). *The methods and findings of quality assessment and monitoring: An illustrated analysis* (Vol. 3). Ann Arbor, MI: Health Administration Press.

Donabedian, A. (2005). Evaluating the quality of medical care. 1966. *Milbank Quarterly, 83*(4), 691–729.

Elixhauser, A., Steiner, C., Harris, D. R., & Coffey, R. M. (1998). Comorbidity measures for use with administrative data. *Medical Care, 36*(1), 8–27.

Ellwood, P. M. (1988). Shattuck lecture—outcomes management: A technology of patient experience. *The New England Journal of Medicine, 318*(23), 1549–1556.

Gallagher, R. M., & Rowell, P. A. (2003). Claiming the future of nursing through nursing-sensitive quality indicators. *Nursing Administration Quarterly, 27*(4), 273–284.

Hall, L. M., Doran, D., Laschinger, H. S., Mallette, C., Pedersen, C., & O'Brien-Pallas, L. (2003). A balanced scorecard approach for nursing report card development. *Outcomes Management, 7*(1), 17–22.

Huber, D., & Oermann, M. (1998). The evolution of outcomes management. In D. L. Flarey, & S. S. Blancett (Eds.), *Cardiovascular outcomes: Collaborative, path-based approaches* (pp. 3–12). Gaithersburg, MD: Aspen.

Iezzoni, L. I. (2003a). Reasons for risk adjustment. In L. I. Iezzoni (Ed.), *Risk adjustment for measuring health care outcomes* (3rd ed., pp. 1–15). Chicago: Health Administration Press.

Iezzoni, L. I. (Ed.). (2003b). *Risk adjustment for measuring health care outcomes* (3rd ed.). Chicago: Health Administration Press.

Jennings, B. M., Staggers, N., & Brosch, L. R. (1999). A classification scheme for outcome indicators. *Image—the Journal of Nursing Scholarship, 31*(4), 381–388.

Kalisch, P. A., & Kalisch, B. J. (1978). *The advance of American nursing*. Boston: Little, Brown.

Kane, R. L. (2006a). Introduction. In R. L. Kane (Ed.), *Understanding health care outcomes research* (2nd ed., pp. 3–22). Boston: Jones and Bartlett Publishers.

Kane, R. L. (2006b). Introduction: an outcomes approach. In R. L. Kane (Ed.), *Understanding health care outcomes research* (2nd ed., pp. 3–22). Boston: Jones and Bartlett Publishers.

Kane, R. L., Shamliyan, T., Mueller, C., Duval, S., & Wilt, T. (2007). *Nursing staffing and quality of patient care.* Evidence report/technology assessment No. 151. (Prepared by the Minnesota Evidence-based Practice Center under Contract No. 290–02–0009.) (No. 07-E005.) Rockville, MD: Agency for Healthcare Research and Quality.

Lake, E. T. (2002). Development of the practice environment scale of the Nursing Work Index. *Research in Nursing & Health, 25*(3), 176–188.

Lang, N. M., & Marek, K. D. (1990). The classification of patient outcomes. *Journal of Professional Nursing, 6*(3), 158–163.

Mitchell, P. H., Ferketich, S., & Jennings, B. M. (1998). Quality health outcomes model. American Academy of Nursing Expert Panel on Quality Health Care. *Image—The Journal of Nursing Scholarship, 30*(1), 43–46.

National Quality Forum. (2004). *National voluntary consensus standards for nursing-sensitive care: An initial performance measure set—A consensus report* (No. NQFCR-08–04). Washington, DC.

Naylor, M. D. (2007). Advancing the science in the measurement of health care quality influenced by nurses. *Medical Care Research & Review, 64*(Suppl. 2), S144–S169.

Oermann, M. H., & Huber, D. (1997). New horizons. *Outcomes Management for Nursing Practice, 1*(1), 1–2.

Oermann, M. H., & Huber, D. (1999). Patient outcomes: A measure of nursing's value. *American Journal of Nursing, 99*(9), 40–47.

Park, E. J., & Huber, D. L. (2007). Balanced scorecards for performance management. *Journal of Nursing Administration, 37*(1), 14–20.

Peters, D. A. (1995). Outcomes: The mainstay of a framework for quality of care. *Journal of Nursing Care Quality, 10*(1), 61–69.

Tunis, S. R., Stryer, D. B., & Clancy, C. M. (2003). Practical clinical trials: Increasing the value of clinical research for decision making in clinical and health policy. *JAMA: The journal of the American Medical Association, 290*(12), 1624–1632.

Chapter 26

Administration on Aging. (2002). *Profile of older Americans: 2002.* Retrieved November 20, 2008, from www.aoa.gov/PROF/Statistics/profile/2002/profiles2002.aspx

Aiken, L. H., Clarke, S. P., Sloane, D. M., Sochalski, J., & Silber, J. H. (2002). Hospital nurse staffing and patient mortality, nurse burnout, and job dissatisfaction. *Journal of the American Medical Association, 288*(16), 1987–1993.

Alliance for Aging Research. (2002). *Medical never-never land: Ten reasons why America is not ready for the coming age boom.* Washington, DC: Author. Retrieved November 20, 2008, from www.agingresearch.org/content/article/detail/698/

American Association of Colleges of Nursing (AACN). (2001). *Older adults: Recommended baccalaureate competencies and curricular guidelines for geriatric nursing care.* Washington, DC: Author. Retrieved November 20, 2008, from www.aacn.nche.edu/Education/pdf/Gercomp.pdf

American Association of Colleges of Nursing (AACN). (2007). *2007 Survey on faculty vacancies.* Washington, DC: Author. Retrieved November 20, 2008, from www.aacn.nche.edu/ids/pdf/vacancy07.pdf

American Association of Colleges of Nursing (AACN). (2008a). *2007–2008 Enrollment and graduations in baccalaureate and graduate programs in nursing.* Washington, DC: Author.

American Association of Colleges of Nursing (AACN). (2008b). *2007–2008 Salaries of instructional and administrative nursing faculty in baccalaureate and graduate programs in nursing.* Washington, DC: Author.

American Association of Colleges of Nursing (AACN). (2008c). *Nursing shortage fact sheets.* Washington, DC: Author. Retrieved November 20, 2008, from www.aacn.nche.edu/Media/FactSheets/NursingShortage.htm

American Association of Colleges of Nursing (AACN). (2009). *Fact sheet: Accelerated baccalaureate and master's degrees in nursing.* Washington, DC: Author. Retrieved May 18, 2009, from http://www.aacn.nche.edu/Media/pdf/AccelProgs.pdf

American Hospital Association (AHA), Commission on Workforce for Hospitals and Health Systems. (2002). *In Our hands: How hospital leaders can build a thriving workforce* (AHA Product No. 210101). Chicago, IL: Author.

American Nurses Association (ANA). (2008). *Legislative updates.* Retrieved March 10, 2008, from http://bhpr.hrsa.gov/nursing/NACNEP/reports/third/default.htm

Andrews, D. R., & Dziegielewski, S. F. (2005). The nurse manager: Job satisfaction, the nursing shortage and retention. *Journal of Nurse Management, 13*(4), 286–295.

Anthony, M. K., Standing, T. S., Glick, J., Duffy, M., Paschall, F., Sauer, M. R., et al. (2005). Leadership and nurse retention: The pivotal role of nurse managers. *Journal of Nurse Administration, 35*(3), 146–155.

Apker, J., Zabava Ford, W., & Fox, D. (2003). Predicting nurses' organizational and professional identification: The effect of nursing roles, professional autonomy, and supportive communication. *Nursing Economic$, 21*(5), 226–233.

Bakker, B., Killmer, C., Siegriest, J., & Schaufeli, W. (2000). Effort-reward imbalance and burnout between nurses. *Journal of Advanced Nursing, 31*, 884–891.

Bass, B. (1998). *Transformational leadership: Industrial, military, and educational impact.* Mahwah, NJ: Lawrence Erlbaum Associates.

Blegen, M. (1993). Nurses' job satisfaction: A meta-analysis of related variables. *Nursing Research, 42*, 36–41.

Buerhaus, P. I., Auerbach, D., & Staiger, D. (2007). Recent trends in the registered nurse labor market in the U.S.: Short-run swings on top of long-term trends. *Nursing Economic$, 25*(2), 59–66.

Buerhaus, P. I., Donelan, K., Ulrich, B. T., Norman, L., & Dittus, R. (2005). Is the shortage of hospital registered nurses getting better or worse? Findings from two recent national surveys of RNs. *Nursing Economic$, 23*(2), 61–71, 96.

Buerhaus, P. I., Staiger, D., & Auerbach, D. (2000). Implications of an aging registered nurse workforce. *Journal of the American Medical Association, 283*(22), 2948–2954.

Buerhaus, P. I., Staiger, D., & Auerbach, D. (2003). Is the current shortage of hospital nurses ending? *Health Affairs, 22*(6), 191–200.

Buerhaus, P. I., Staiger, D., & Auerbach, D. (2008). *The future of the nursing workforce in the United States: Data, trends and implications.* Sudbury, MA: Jones and Bartlett Publishers.

Bureau of Health Professions (BHPr). (2002). *Authorizing legislation: Nursing workforce development* (Public Health Service Act, Title VIII). Rockville, MD: U.S. Department of Health and Human Services, Health Resources and Services Administration. Retrieved November 20, 2008, from http://bhpr.hrsa.gov/nursing/legislation.htm

Bureau of Health Professions (BHPr). (2004). *What is behind the Health Resources and Services Administration's projected supply, demand, and shortage of registered nurses?* Rockville, MD: U.S. Department of Health and Human Services, Health Resources and Services Administration. Retrieved November 20, 2008, from http://bhpr.hrsa.gov/healthworkforce/reports/nursing/rnbehindprojections/index.htm

Bureau of Health Professions (BHPr). (2006). *The registered nurse population: Findings from the 2004 National Sample Survey of Registered Nurses.* Rockville, MD: U.S. Department of Health and Human Services, Health Resources and Services Administration. Retrieved November 20, 2008, from http://bhpr.hrsa.gov/healthworkforce/rnsurvey04/

Bureau of Labor Statistics (BLS). (2007). Employment outlook: 2006–16. Occupational employment projections into 2016. In *Monthly Labor Review.* Washington, DC: U.S. Bureau of Labor Statistics. Retrieved November 20, 2008, from www.bls.gov/opub/mlr/2007/11/art5full.pdf

Carlson, S. M., Cowart, M. E., & Speaker, D. L. (1992). Perspectives of nursing personnel in the 1980s. In M. E. Cowart, & W. J. Serow (Eds.), *Nurses in the workplace* (pp. 1–27). Newbury Park, CA: Sage.

Colin-Thomé, D., & Belfield, G. (2004). *Improving chronic disease management.* London, UK: Department of Health. Retrieved May 18, 2009, from http://www.dh.gov.uk/en/Publicationsandstatistics/Publications/PublicationsPolicyAndGuidance/DH_4075214

Cooksey, J. A., McLaughlin, W., Russinof, H., Martinez, L. I., & Gordon, C. (2004). Active state-level engagement with the nursing shortage: A study of five midwestern states. *Policy, Politics & Nursing Practice, 5*(2), 102–112.

Cooper, R. A., & Aiken, L. H. (2006). Health services delivery: Reframing policies for global migration of nurses and physicians—A U.S. perspective. *Policy, Politics & Nursing Practice, 7*(Suppl. 3), S66–S70.

Davidson, H., Folcarelli, P., Crawford, S., Duprat, L., & Clifford, J. (1997). The effects of health care reforms on job satisfaction and voluntary turnover among hospital-based nurses. *Medical Care, 35,* 634–645.

Drucker, R. (1999). *Management challenges for the 21st century.* New York: HarperBusiness.

Duffield, C., Roche, M., O'Brien-Pallas, L., Diers, D., Aisbett, C., King, M., et al. (2007). *Glueing it together: Nurses, their work environment and patient safety.* Australia: University of Technology Sydney, Centre for Health Services Management.

First Consulting Group. (2001). *The healthcare workforce shortage and its implications for America's hospitals.* Long Beach, CA: Author. Retrieved November 20, 2008, from www.aha.org/aha/content/2001/pdf/Ioh03Crisis.pdf

Flynn, L. (2005). Importance of work environment: Evidence-based strategies for enhancing nurse retention. *Home Health Nurse, 23*(6), 366–371; quiz 385–387.

General Accounting Office Report (GAO-03-460). (2003). *Hospital emergency departments: Crowded conditions vary among hospitals and communities.* Washington, DC: U.S. General Accounting Office.

Gittell, J. (2001). Supervisory span, relational coordination and flight departure performance: A reassessment of post-bureaucracy theory. *Organization Science, 12,* 468–483.

Good, M. L. (2003). Patient simulation for training basic and advanced clinical skills. *Medical Education, 37*(Suppl. 1), S14–S21.

Grando, V. T. (1998). Making do with fewer nurses in the United States, 1945–1965. *Image, 30*(2), 147–149.

Green, S., Anderson, S., & Shivers, S. (1996). Demographic and organizational influences on leader-member exchange and related work attitudes. *Organizational Behavior and Human Decision Processes, 66,* 203–214.

Hartz, A., Krakauer, H., Kuhn, E., & Young, M. (1989). Hospital characteristics and mortality rates. *The New England Journal of Medicine, 321*(25), 1720–1725.

Hattrup, G., & Kleiner, B. (1993). How to establish the proper span of control for managers. *Industrial Management, 35,* 28–30.

Hayes, J. H., & Scott, A. S. (2007). Mentoring partnerships as the wave of the future for new graduates. *Nursing Education Perspectives, 28*(1), 27–29.

Health Resources and Services Administration. (2007). *Methods for identifying facilities and communities with shortages of nurses, technical report.* Rockville, MD: Author. Retrieved May 15, 2009, from http://bhpr.hrsa.gov/healthworkforce/nursingshortage/tech_report/default.htm

Health Resources and Services Administration. (2009). *Nursing.* Rockville, MD: Author. Retrieved May 18, 2009, from http://bhpr.hrsa.gov/nursing/

Herrin, D., & Spears, P. (2007). Using nurse leader development to improve nurse retention and patient outcomes: A framework. *Nursing Administration Quarterly, 31*(3), 231–243.

Huston, C. J. (2003). Quality health care in an era of limited resources: Challenges and opportunities. *Journal of Nursing Care Quality, 18*(4), 295–302.

International Council of Nurses. (2003). *Global issues in the supply and demand of nurses. SEW news January-March 2003.* Geneva, Switzerland: Author. Retrieved November 20, 2008, from www.icn.ch/sewjan-march03.htm

Irvine, D., & Evans, M. (1995). Job satisfaction and turnover between nurses: Integrating research findings across studies. *Nursing Research, 44,* 246–253.

Issenberg, S. B., McGaghie, W. C., Petrusa, E. R., Lee Gordon, D., & Scalese, R. J. (2005). Features and uses of high fidelity simulations that lead to effective learning: A BEME systematic review. *Medical Teacher, 27*(1), 10–28.

Johnson & Johnson. (2002). *The Campaign for Nursing's Future awards first scholarships to encourage new nurses.* Retrieved November 20, 2008, from www.jnj.com/news/jnj_news/20020418_1532.htm

Joint Commission on Accreditation of Healthcare Organizations (JCAHO). (2002). *Health care at the crossroads: Strategies for addressing the evolving nursing crisis.* Oakbrook Terrace, IL: Author. Retrieved November 20, 2008, from www.jointcommission.org/NR/rdonlyres/5C138711-ED76-4D6F-909F-B06E0309F36D/0/health_care_at_the_crossroads.pdf

Kane, R., Shamliyan, T., Mueller, C., Duval, S., & Wilt, T. (2007). *Nurse staffing and quality of patient care.* Report No. 151 prepared for U.S. Department of Health and Human Services, Agency for Healthcare Research and Quality. Retrieved November 20, 2008, from www.ahrq.gov/downloads/pub/evidence/pdf/nursestaff/nursestaff.pdf

Kimball, B. (2004). Health care's human crisis: RX for an evolving profession. *Online Journal of Issues in Nursing, 9*(2), 2.

Kimball, B., & O'Neil, E. (2002). *Health care's human crisis: The American nursing shortage.* RW Johnson Report. Princeton, NJ: Robert Wood Johnson Foundation: Retrieved November 20, 2008, from www.rwjf.org/pr/product.jsp?id=15647

King, M. G. (1989). Nursing shortage, circa 1915. *Image, 21*(3), 124–127.

Kovner, C., & Gergen, P. J. (1998). Nurse staffing levels and adverse events following surgery in U.S. hospitals. *Image, 30*(4), 315–321.

Kovner, C. T., Brewer, C., Fairchild, S., Poornima, S., Kim, H., & Djukic, M. (2007). Newly licensed RNs' characteristics, work attitudes, and intentions to work. *American Journal of Nursing, 107*(9), 58–70.

Kovner, C. T., Jones, C., Zhan, C., Gergen, P., & Basu, J. (2002). Nurse staffing and post-surgical adverse events: An analysis of administrative data from a sample of U.S. hospitals, 1990–1996. *Health Services Research, 37,* 611–629.

Larabee, J., Janney, M., Ostrow, C., Withrow, M., Hobbs, G., & Burant, C. (2003). Predicting registered nurse job satisfaction and intent to leave. *Journal of Nursing Administration, 33*(5), 271–283.

Leveck, M., & Jones, C. (1996). The nursing practice environment, staff retention, and quality of care. *Research in Nursing & Health, 19,* 331–343.

Little, L. (2007). Nurse migration: A Canadian case study. *Health Services Research, 42*(3 Pt 2), 1336–1353.

Loke, J. (2001). Leadership behaviours: Effects on job satisfaction, productivity and organizational commitment. *Journal of Nursing Management, 9,* 191–204.

Maran, N. J., & Glavin, R. J. (2003). Low-to-high fidelity simulation: A continuum of medical education. *Medical Education, 37*(Suppl. 1), 22–28.

May, J. H., Bazzoli, G. J., & Gerland, A. M. (2006). Hospitals' responses to nurse staffing shortages. *Health Affairs, 25*(4), W316–W323.

McCutcheon, A. (2005). Span of control. In L. McGillis Hall (Ed.), *Quality work environments: For nurse and patient safety* (pp. 93–104). Toronto, Ontario, Canada: Jones and Bartlett Publishers.

McCutcheon, A., Doran, D., Evans, M., McGillis-Hall, L., & Pringle, D. (2004). *The impact of the manager's span of control on leadership and performance.* Ottawa, Canada: Canadian Health Services Research Foundation. Retrieved May 15, 2009, from www.chsrf.ca/final_research/ogc/pdf/doran2_e.pdf

Medley, F., & Larochelle, D. (1995). Transformational leadership and job satisfaction. *Nursing Management, 26*(9), 64JJ–LL.

Moos, R. (1994). *Work environment scale manual—A social climate scale: Development, applications, research* (3rd ed.). Palo Alto, CA: Consulting Psychologists Press.

National Advisory Council on Nurse Education and Practice. (2003). *Third report to the Secretary of the Department of Health and Human Services on the basic registered nurse workforce.* Retrieved November 20, 2008, from http://bhpr.hrsa.gov/nursing/NACNEP/reports/third/default.htm

National Center for Health Workforce Analysis. (2002). *Projected supply, demand, and shortages of registered nurses: 2000–2020.* Rockville, MD: U.S. Department of Health and Human Services, Health Resources and Services Administration: Retrieved November 20, 2008, from www.ahcancal.org/research_data/staffing/Documents/Registered_Nurse_Supply_Demand.pdf

Needleman, J., Buerhaus, P., Mattke, S., Stewart, M., & Zelevinsky, K. (2002). Nurse-staffing levels and the quality of care in hospitals. *The New England Journal of Medicine, 346*(22), 1715–1722.

Nooney, J. G., & Lacey, L. M. (2007). Validating HRSA's nurse supply and demand models: A state-level perspective. *Nursing Economic$, 25*(5), 270–278.

Nurses for a Healthier Tomorrow (NHT) Coalition. (2005). Retrieved November 20, 2008, from www.nursesource.org/mission.html

PricewaterhouseCoopers. (2007). *What works: Healing the healthcare staffing shortage.* PricewaterhouseCoopers Health Research Institute. Retrieved November 20, 2008, from www.pwc.com/extweb/pwcpublications.nsf/docid/674D1E79A678A0428525730D006B74A9

Reid Ponte, P. (2004). The American health care system at a crossroads: An overview of the American Organization of Nurse Executives monograph. *Online Journal of Issues in Nursing, 9*(2), Manuscript 2. Retrieved November 20, 2008, from www.nursingworld.org/MainMenuCategories/ANAMarketplace/ANAPeriodicals/OJIN/TableofContents/Volume92004/No2May04/NurseExecutivesMonograph.aspx

Richardson, S. (2002). President's update. Alberta's nursing shortage: Consistent findings point to solutions. *Alberta RN, 58*(9), 3.

Robert Wood Johnson Foundation & AARP Foundation. (2007). *Center to Champion Nursing in America.* Retrieved November 20, 2008, from www.rwjf.org/pr/product.jsp?id=23991

Scalese, R. J., Obeso, V. T., & Issenberg, S. B. (2008). Simulation technology for skills training and competency assessment in medical education. *Journal of General Internal Medicine, 23*(Suppl. 1), 46–49.

Seago, J. A., Spetz, J., Alvarado, A., Keane, D., & Grumbach, K. (2006). The nursing shortage: Is it really about image? *Journal of Healthcare Management, 51*(2), 96–108; discussion 109–110.

Shader, K., Broome, M., Broome, C., West, M., & Nash, M. (2001). Factors influencing satisfaction and anticipated turnover for nurses in an academic medical center. *Journal of Nursing Administration, 31,* 210–216.

Stordeur, S., Vandenberghe, C., & D'Hoore, W. (2000). Leadership styles across hierarchical levels in nursing departments. *Nursing Research, 49,* 37–43.

Stordeur, S., D'Hoore, W., & Vandenberghe, C. (2001). Leadership, organizational stress, and emotional exhaustion between hospital nursing staff. *Journal of Advanced Nursing, 35,* 533–542.

Tri-Council for Nursing. (2004). *Strategies to reverse the new nursing shortage: A policy statement from Tri-Council members.* New York: National League for Nursing. Retrieved November 20, 2008, from www.aacn.nche.edu/Publications/positions/tricshortage.htm

University of Virginia. (2006). *The Darden MBA Program.* Charlottesville, VA. Retrieved November 20, 2008, from www.darden.virginia.edu/html/programs.aspx

U.S. Department of Labor. (2005). *The President's High Growth Job Training Initiative.* Washington, DC: Employment and Training Administration. Retrieved November 20, 2008, from www.doleta.gov/BRG/JobTrainInitiative/

Wieck, K. (2003). Faculty for the millennium: Changes needed to attract the emerging workforce into nursing. *Journal of Nursing Education, 42*(4), 151–159.

Williams, K. A., Stotts, R. C., Jacob, S. R., Stegbauer, C. C., Roussel, L., & Carter, D. (2006). Inactive nurses: A source for alleviating the nursing shortage? *Journal of Nursing Administration, 36*(4), 205–210.

Wolff, J. L., Starfield, B., & Anderson, G. (2002). Prevalence, expenditures, and complications of multiple chronic conditions in the elderly. *Journal of the American Medical Association, 162*(20), 2269–2276.

Chapter 27

Acree, C. M. (2006). The relationship between nurse leadership practices and hospital nursing retention. *Newborn and Infant Nursing Reviews, 6*(1), 34–40.

Aiken, L. H., Clarke, S. P., Sloane, D. M., Sochalski, J. A., Busse, R., Clarke, H., et al. (2001). Nurses' reports on hospital care in five countries. *Health Affairs, 20*(3), 43–53.

Aiken, L. H., Clarke, S. P., Sloane, D. M., Sochalski, J., & Sibler, J. H. (2002). Hospital nurse staffing and patient mortality, nurse burnout, and job dissatisfaction. *Journal of American Medical Association, 288,* 1987–1993.

Aiken, L. H., Sloane, D. M., & Klocinski, J. L. (1997). Hospital nurses' occupational exposure to blood: Prospective, retrospective, and institutional reports. *American Journal of Public Health, 87*(1), 103–107.

American Hospital Association (AHA). (2001). *Workforce supply for hospitals and health systems: Issues and recommendations.* Chicago: Author. Retrieved November 23, 2008, from www.hospitalconnect.com/ahapolicyforum/resources/workforce010123.html

American Hospital Association (AHA). (2002). *In our hands: How hospital leaders can build a thriving workforce.* Chicago: Author.

American Nurses Association (ANA). (2001). *Nursing organizations to hold summit to address quality of care, staffing issues and the emerging shortage* (ANA press release). Washington, DC: Author.

American Nurses Association (ANA). (2002). *Nursing's agenda for the future. A call to the nation.* Washington, DC: Author.

American Nurses Association (ANA). (2003). *Magnet recognition program: Recognizing excellence in nursing service.* Washington, DC: American Nurses Credentialing Center.

Anthony, M. K., Standing, T. S., Glick, J., Duffy, M., Paschall, F., Sauer, M. R., et al. (2005). Leadership and nurse retention: The pivotal role of nurse managers. *Journal of Nursing Administration, 35*(3), 146–155.

Atencio, B. L., Cohen, J., & Gorenberg, B. (2003). Nurse retention: Is it worth it? *Nursing Economic$, 21*(6), 262–268, 299.

Auerbach, D. I., Buerhaus, P. I., & Staiger, D. O. (2007). Better late than never: Workforce supply implications of later entry into nursing. *Health Affairs, 26*(1), 178–185.

Bower, F. L., & McCullough, C. (2004). Nurse shortage or nursing shortage: Have we missed the real problem? *Nursing Economic$, 22*(4), 200–203.

Buerhaus, P., Staiger, D., & Auerbach, D. (2000). Why are shortages of hospital RNs concentrated in specialty care units? *Nursing Economic$, 18*(3), 111–116.

Casey, K., Fink, R., Krugman, M., & Propst, J. (2004). The graduate nurse experience. *Journal of Nursing Administration, 34*(6), 303–311.

Cunningham, L. (2005). Ten ways to nurture your nurses and create a high-performance organization. *Nurse Leader, 3*(5), 38–40.

Curran, C. R. (2003). Nurse recruitment: A waste of postage, paper, and people. *Nursing Economic$, 21*(1), 5–32.

Daniel, P., Chamberlain, A., & Gordon, F. (2000). Expectations and experiences of newly recruited Filipino nurses. *British Journal of Nursing, 10*(4), 256–265.

Davidhizar, R. (2005). Joining the ranks: Nurses as role models. *Caring: National Association for Home Care Magazine, 24*(1), 50–51.

DDI. (1997). *LearningLinks: Your guide to using DDI technology to enhance performance.* Pittsburgh: Development Dimensions International.

DDI. (2004). *Targeted Selection®: Access®.* Pittsburgh: Development Dimensions International.

Dictionary.com. (2004a). *Recruitment definition.* Los Angeles: Lexico Publishing Group. Retrieved May 24, 2004, from http://dictionary.reference.com/browse/recruitment

Dictionary.com (2004b). *Retention definition.* Los Angeles: Lexico Publishing Group. Retrieved January 8, 2005, from http://dictionary.reference.com/browse/retention

Donelan, K., Buerhaus, P. I., Ulrich, B. T., Norman, L., & Dittus, R. (2005). Awareness and perceptions of Johnson & Johnson campaign for nursing's future: Views from nursing students, RNs, and CNOs. *Nursing Economic$, 23*(4), 150–156, 180.

Dumpel, H. (2005). Contemporary issues facing international nurses: Adopting a CAN/NNOC code of practice for international nursing recruitment. *California Nurse, November,* 18–22.

Erickson, J. I., Holm, L. J., & Chelminiak, L. (2004). Keeping the nursing shortage from becoming a nursing crisis. *Journal of Nursing Administration, 34*(2), 83–87.

Flynn, L., & Aiken, L. H. (2002). Does international nurse recruitment influence practice values in U.S. hospitals? *Journal of Nursing Scholarship, 34*(1), 67–73.

Force, M. V. (2005). The relationship between effective nurse managers and nursing retention. *Journal of Nursing Administration, 35*(7/8), 336–341.

Gamble, D. A. (2002). Filipino nurse recruitment as a staffing strategy. *Journal of Nursing Administration, 32*(4), 175–177.

Goodin, H. J. (2003). The nursing shortage in the United States of America: An integrative review of literature. *Journal of Advanced Nursing, 43*(4), 335–350.

Halfer, D., & Graf, E. (2006). Graduate nurse perceptions of the work experience. *Nursing Economic$, 24*(3), 150–155.

Hare, K. (2007). Recruit, retain, and recognize with a professional nurse ambassador program. *Journal of Nursing Administration, 37*(4), 171–173.

Hart, S. M. (2006). Generational diversity: Impact on recruitment and retention of registered nurses. *Journal of Nursing Administration, 36*(1), 10–12.

Health Resources and Services Administration (HRSA). (2004). *What is behind HRSA's projected supply, demand and shortage for registered nurses?* Retrieved November 23, 2008, from http://bhpr.hrsa.gov/healthworkforce/reports/behindrnprojections/

Henriksen, C., Page, N. E., Williams, R. I. I., & Worral, P. S. (2003). Responding to nursing's agenda for the future: Where do we stand on recruitment and retention? *Nursing Leadership Forum, 8*(2), 78–84.

Hoffman, P. M. (1984). *Financial management for nurse managers.* Norwalk, CT: Appleton-Century-Crofts.

HR Solutions, Inc. (2007). Onboarding new employees: Everything matters. *New Solutions, 40*(3), 3–4.

Institute of Medicine (IOM). (2001). *Crossing the quality chasm: A new health care system for the 21st century.* Washington, DC: National Academies Press.

International Council of Nurses (ICN). (1999). *Nurse retention, transfer and migration.* Geneva, Switzerland: Author. Retrieved June 21, 2004, from www.icn.ch/psretention.htm

International Council of Nurses (ICN). (2001). *Ethical nurse recruitment: Position statement.* Geneva, Switzerland: Author. Retrieved May 23, 2004, from www.icn.ch/psrecruit01.htm

International Council of Nurses (ICN). (2006). *ICN on healthy ageing: A public health and nursing challenge.* Retrieved March 3, 2008, from www.icn.ch/matters_aging.htm

Johnson & Johnson (J&J). (2008). *Support to nursing: The campaign for nursing's future.* Retrieved February, 28, 2008, from www.jnj.com/community/contributions/programs/support.htm

Jones, C. B. (2004a). The costs of nurse turnover. Part 1. An economic perspective. *Journal of Nursing Administration, 34*(12), 562–570.

Jones, C. B. (2004b). The costs of nurse turnover. Part 2. Application of the nursing turnover cost calculation methodology. *Journal of Nursing Administration, 35*(1), 41–49.

Kleinman, C. S. (2004). Leadership: A key strategy in staff nurse retention. *The Journal of Continuing Education in Nursing, 35*(3), 128–132.

Kramer, M., & Hafner, L. (1989). Shared values: Impact on staff nurse job satisfaction and perceived productivity. *Nursing Research, 38*(3), 172–177.

Kuhar, P. A., Miller, D., Spear, B. T., Ulreich, S. M., & Mion, L. C. (2004). The meaningful retention strategy inventory: A targeted approach to implementing retention strategies. *Journal of Nursing Administration, 34*(1), 10–18.

Laschinger, H. K. S., & Wong, C. (1999). Staff nurse empowerment and collective accountability: Effect on perceived productivity and self-rated work effectiveness. *Nursing Economic$*, *17*(6), 308–316.

Lee, D. (2008). *Successful onboarding: How to get your new employees started off right*. Retrieved March 3, 2008, from www.humannatureatwork.com/successfulonboarding.htm

Lipsey, J. (2004). *Targeted selection*. Omaha, NE: Leadership Solutions. Retrieved June 28, 2004, from www. leadsolutions.com/ts_article.htm

Manion, J. (2004). Nurture a culture of retention. *Nursing Management*, *35*(4), 29–39.

Manion, J., & Bartholomew, K. (2004). Community in the workplace: A proven retention. *Journal of Nursing Administration*, *34*(1), 46–53.

McClure, M. L., Poulin, M. A., Sovie, M. D., & Wandelt, M. A. (1983). *Magnet hospitals: Attraction and retention of professional nurses*. Kansas City, MO: American Nurses Association.

Mion, L. C., Hazel, C., & Cap, M. (2006). Retaining and recruiting mature experienced nurses: A multicomponent organizational strategy. *Journal of Nursing Administration*, *36*(3), 148–154.

Needleman, J., Buerhaus, P., Mattke, S., Stewart, M., & Zelevinsy, K. (2002). Nurse-staffing levels and the quality of care in hospitals. *The New England Journal of Medicine*, *346*, 1715–1722.

Nevidjon, B., & Erickson, J. I. (2001). The nursing shortage: Solutions for the short and long term. *Journal of Issues in Nursing*, *6*(1), Manuscript 4. Retrieved June 28, 2004, from www.nursingworld.org/ojin/topic14/tpc14_4.htm

Northwestern University. (2008). *New employee onboarding checklist*. Retrieved March 3, 2008, from www.northwestern.edu/hr/training/NewEmployeeOnboardingChecklist.doc

Nursing Executive Center. (2001). *Destination nursing: Recommitting to health care's greatest profession*. Washington, DC: The Advisory Board Company.

Orsini, C. H. (2005). A nurse transition program for orthopaedics: Creating a new culture for nurturing graduate nurses. *Orthopaedic Nursing*, *24*(4), 240–248.

Parsons, M. L., & Stonestreet, J. (2004). Staff nurse retention: Laying in groundwork by listening. *Nursing Leadership Forum*, *8*(3), 107–113.

Peterson, C. (2001). Nursing shortage: Not a simple problem—No easy answer. *Journal of Issues in Nursing*, *6*(1), Manuscript 1. Retrieved June 28, 2004, from www.nursingworld.org/ojin/topic14/tpc14_1.htm

Platz, B. (2008). Employee onboarding: One chance for a positive new employee experience. Retrieved March 3, 2008, from http://humanresources.about.com/od/orientation/a/onboarding.htm

Prescott, P. (2000). The enigmatic nursing workforce. *Journal of Nursing Administration*, *30*(2), 59–65.

Rosenstein, A. H. (2002). Nurse-physician relationships: Impact on nurse satisfaction and retention. *American Journal of Nursing*, *102*(6), 26–34.

Runy, L. A. (2008). The nurse and patient safety. *Hospitals & Health Networks*, *82*(11), 43, 45–48.

Shermont, H., & Krepcio, D. (2006). The impact of culture change on nurse retention. *Journal of Nursing Administration*, *36*(9), 407–415.

Sparacio, D. C. (2005). Winged migration: International nurse recruitment—Friend or foe to the nursing crisis? *Journal of Nursing Law*, *10*(2), 97–114.

The HMS Group. (2002). Acute care hospital survey of RN vacancy and turnover rates in 2000. *Journal of Nursing Administration*, *32*(9), 437–439.

Upenieks, V. (2003). Recruitment and retention strategies: A Magnet hospital strategies prevention model. *Nursing Economic$*, *21*(1), 7–13, 23.

Ward-Smith, P., Hunt, C., Smith, J. B., Teasley, S. L., Carroll, C. A., & Sexton, K. (2007). Spotlight on: Issues and opportunities for retaining experienced nurses at the bedside. *Journal of Nursing Administration*, *37*(11), 485–487.

Chapter 28

Abdoo, Y. M. (2000). Nurse staffing and scheduling. In L. M. Simms, S. A. Price, & N. E. Ervin (Eds.), *Professional practice of nursing administration* (pp. 264–280). Albany, NY: Delmar.

Aiken, L. H., Clarke, S. P., Cheung, R. B., Sloane, D. M., & Silber, J. H. (2003). Education level of hospital nurses and patient mortality. *Journal of the American Medical Association*, *290*, 1617–1623.

Aiken, L. H., Clarke, S. P., Sloane, D. M., Sochalski, J. A., Busse, R., Clarke, H., et al. (2001). Nurses' report on hospital care in five countries. *Health Affairs*, *20*(3), 43–53.

Aiken, L. H., Clarke, S. P., Sloane, D. M., Sochalski, J., & Silber, J. H. (2002). Hospital nurse staffing and patient mortality, nurse burnout, and job dissatisfaction. *Journal of the American Medical Association*, *288*(16), 1987–1993.

Aiken, L. H., Xue, Y., Clarke, S. P., Sloane, D. M. (2007). Supplemental nurse staffing in hospitals and quality of care. *Journal of Nursing Administration*, *37*(7–8), 335–342.

American Academy of Ambulatory Care Nursing (AAACN). (2005). *Ambulatory care nurse staffing: An annotated bibliography*. Pitman: NJ: Author. Retrieved May 23, 2009, from http://www.aaacn.org/cgi-bin/WebObjects/AAACNMain.woa/1/wo/qSOC44qaFPkC2Tv2yaX6fv6h-GHX/0.4.17.5.1.2.0.5.5.1.18?53,7

American Academy of Pediatrics (AAP) and the American College of Obstetricians and Gynecologists (ACOG). (2007). *Guidelines for perinatal care*. Washington, DC: March of Dimes.

American Association of Colleges of Nursing (AACN). (2003). *White paper on the role of the Clinical Nurse Leader™*. Washington, DC: Author.

American Association of Colleges of Nursing (AACN) (2007). *White paper on the education and role of the Clinical Nurse Leader™*. Washington, DC: Author.

American Nurses Association (ANA). (1999). *Principles for nurse staffing*. Silver Spring, MD: Author.

American Nurses Association (ANA). (2003). *Nursing's social policy statement* (2nd ed.). Silver Spring, MD: Author.

American Nurses Association (ANA). (2004). *Scope and standards for nurse administrators*. Silver Spring, MD: Author.

American Nurses Association (ANA). (2005). *Utilization guide for the ANA principles for nurse staffing*. Silver Spring, MD: Author.

American Nurses Association (ANA). (2008). *Safe staffing saves lives*. Retrieved February 17, 2008, from www.safestaffingsaveslives.org

American Organization of Nurse Executives (AONE). (2000). *Staffing management and methods: Tools and techniques for nurse leaders*. Chicago: Author. Retrieved May 19, 2009, from http://www.josseybass.com/WileyCDA/WileyTitle/productCd-0787955361.html

American Organization of Nurse Executives (AONE). (2008). *AONE 2008 Legislative Agenda*. Chicago: Author. Retrieved February 16, 2008, from www.aone.org/aone/advocacy/advagenda.html

Aydelotte, M. K. (1973). *Nurse staffing methodology: A review and critique of selected literature*. U.S. Department of Health, Education and Welfare, Division of Nursing. Publication No. (NIH) 73–433. Washington, DC: Government Printing Office.

Barnum, B., & Mallard, C. (1989). *Essentials of nursing management: Concepts and context of practice*. Rockville, MD: Aspen.

Bennett, T. (1981). Operations research and nurse staffing. *International Journal of Biomedical Computing, 12*, 433–438.

Beyers, M. (2000). Foreword. In M. Fralic (Ed.), *Staffing management and methods: Tools and techniques for nursing leaders* (pp. xxi–xxii). San Francisco: Jossey-Bass.

Brooten, D., & Youngblut, J. M. (2006). Nurse dose as concept. *Journal of Nursing Scholarship, 38*(1), 94–99.

Brown, B. (1999). How to develop a unit personnel budget. *Nursing Management, 30*(6), 34–35.

Buerhaus, P. (1997). What is the harm in imposing mandatory hospital nurse staffing regulations? *Nursing Economic$, 15*(2), 66–72.

Case Management Society of America (CMSA). (2002). *Standards of practice for case management*. Little Rock, AR: Author.

Centers for Medicare & Medicaid Services (CMS). (2009). *Overview: Medicaid and CHIP-quality practices: General information*. Baltimore, MD: Author. Retrieved May 24, 2009, from http://www.cms.hhs.gov/MedicaidCHIPQualPrac/

Cho, S. H. (2001). Nurse staffing and adverse patient outcomes: A systems approach. *Nursing Outlook, 49*(2), 78–85.

Cipriano, P., & Cutruzzula, J. (2007). Over-recruiting: Breaking the short staffing and turnover cycle. *Nurse Leader, 5*(6), 28–32.

Clarke, S. P. (2005). The policy implications of staffing-outcomes research. *Journal of Nursing Administration, 35*(1), 17–19.

Dalton, K. (2007). *A study of charge compression in calculating DRG relative weights*. Center for Medicaid and Medicare Services: Contract No. 500–00–0024-TO18.

Department of Veterans Affairs. (2002). *Glossary of terms*. Washington, DC: Author. Retrieved May 23, 2009, from http://www1.va.gov/lmr/page.cfm?pg=16#C_Terms

Deutschendorf, A. (2006). Models of care delivery. In D. Huber (Ed.), *Leadership and nursing care management* (3rd ed., pp. 315–336). Philadelphia: Saunders.

Donabedian, A. (1966). Evaluating the quality of medical care. *Milbank Memorial Fund Quarterly, 44*(3), 166–206.

Donaldson, N., Bolton, L., Aydin, C., Brown, D., Elashoff, J., & Sandhu, M. (2005). Impact of California's licensed nurse-patient ratios on unit-level nurse staffing and patient outcomes. *Policy, Politics, & Nursing Practice, 6*(3), 198–210.

Eck, S. A. (1999). *The effect of a change in skill mix on patient and organizational outcomes in one teaching hospital*. PhD dissertation. New Haven, CT: Yale University.

Edwardson, S. (2007). Conceptual frameworks used in funded nursing health services research projects. *Nursing Economic$, 25*(4), 222–227.

Finkler, S. A., Kovner, C. T., & Jones, C. B. (2007). *Financial management for nurse managers and executives*. (3rd ed.). Philadelphia: Saunders.

Fried, B. J., & Johnson, J. A. (2002). *Human resources in healthcare: Managing for success*. Washington, DC: AUPHA Press.

Haas, S., & Hastings, C. (2001). Staffing and workload. In J. Robinson (Ed.), *Core curriculum for ambulatory care nursing* (pp. 133–145). Philadelphia: Saunders.

Haase-Herrick, K. S., & Herrin, D. M. (2007). The American Organization of Nurse Executives' guiding principles and American Association of Colleges of Nursing's clinical nurse leader. *Journal of Nursing Administration, 37*(2), 55–60.

Hardin, S. R., & Kaplow, R. (2005). *Synergy for excellence: The AACN Synergy Model for patient care*. Sudbury, MA: Jones and Bartlett Publishers.

Havens, D., & Vasey, J. (2003). Measuring staff nurse decisional involvement: The decisional involvement scale. *Journal of Nursing Administration, 33*(6), 331–336.

Hinshaw, A. (2006). Keeping patients safe: A collaboration among nurse administrators and researchers. *Nursing Administrative Quarterly, 30*(4), 309–320.

Hung, R. (2002). A note on nurse self-scheduling. *Nursing Economic$, 20*(1), 37–38.

Institute of Medicine (IOM). (2004). *Keeping patients safe: Transforming the work environment of nurses.* Washington, DC: National Academies Press.

Jones, C. B. (2004). The costs of nurse turnover. Part 1. An economic perspective. *Journal of Nursing Administration, 34*(12), 562–570.

Jones, C. B. (2005). The costs of nurse turnover. Part 2. Application of the nursing turnover cost calculation methodology. *Journal of Nursing Administration, 35*(1), 41–49.

Jones, C. B., & Gates, M. (2007). The costs and benefits of nurse turnover: A business case for nurse retention. *The Online Journal of Issues in Nursing, 12*(3).

Jones, C. B., & Mark, B. A. (2005). The intersection of nursing and health services research: An agenda to guide future research. *Nursing Outlook, 53*(6), 324–332.

Jones, C. B., Mark, B. A., Gates, M., & Eck, S. A. (2005). *Manager and staff nurse perceptions of vacancy tolerance.* Paper presentation at the National Nursing Administration Research Conference, October, Tucson, AZ.

Kane, R., Shamliyan, T., Mueller, C., Duval, S., & Wilt, T. (2007a). *Nurse staffing and quality of patient care.* U.S. Department of Health and Human Services. AHRQ Publication No. 07-E005.

Kane, R., Shamliyan, T., Mueller, C., Duval, S., & Wilt, T. (2007b). The association of registered nurse staffing levels and patient outcomes. *Medical Care, 45*(12), 1195–1204.

Kaplow, R., & Reed, K. D. (2008). The AACN Synergy Model for patient care: A nursing model as a force of magnetism. *Nursing Economic$, 26*(1), 17–25.

Kirby, K., & Wiczai, L. (1985). Budgeting for variable staffing. *Nursing Economic$, 3*(3), 160–166.

Koloroutis, M. (Ed.). (2004). *Relationship-based care: A model for transforming practice.* Minneapolis: Creative Health Care Management.

Kovner, C., & Gergen, P. (1998). Nurse staffing levels and adverse events following surgery in U.S. hospitals. *Image: The Journal of Nursing Scholarship, 30*(4), 315–321.

Lauw, C., & Gares, D. (2005). Resource management: What's right for you? *Nursing Management, 36*(12), 46–49.

Litvak, E., Buerhaus, P., Davidoff, F., Long, M., McManus, M., & Berwick, D. (2005). Managing unnecessary variability in patient demand to reduce nursing stress and improve patient safety. *Journal on Quality and Patient Safety, 31*(6), 330–338.

Manthey, M. (1990). Definitions and basic elements of a patient care delivery system with an emphasis on primary nursing. In G. Mayer, M. Madden, & E. Lawrenz (Eds.), *Patient care delivery models* (pp. 201–211). Aspen. Rockville, MD.

Mark, B. (1992). Characteristics of nursing practice models. *Journal of Nursing Administration, 22*(11), 57–63.

Mark, B. A., Harless, D. W., & Berman, W. F. (2007). Nurse staffing and adverse events in hospitalized children. *Policy, Politics, and Nursing Practice, 8*(2), 83–92.

Mark, B. A., Harless, D. W., McCue, M., & Xu, Y. (2004). A longitudinal examination of hospital registered nurse staffing and quality of care. *Health Services Research, 39*(2), 279–300.

McKinley, J., & Cavouras, C. (2000). Evolving staffing measures. In American Organization of Nurse Executives (AONE), *Staffing management and methods: Tools and techniques for nurse leaders* (pp. 1–33). San Francisco: Jossey-Bass.

Moore, M., & Hastings, C. (2006). The evolution of an ambulatory nursing intensity system: Measuring workload in a day hospital setting. *Journal of Nursing Administration, 36*(5), 241–248.

Nash, M., Kniphfer, K., Kuklinski, S., & Sparks, D. (2000). In American Organization of Nurse Executives (AONE), *Staffing management and methods: Tools and techniques for nurse leaders* (pp. 35–57). San Francisco: Jossey-Bass.

National Association of Neonatal Nurses (NANN). (1999a). *Minimum staffing in NICU's.* NANN Position Statement No. 3009. Glenview, IL: Author.

National Association of Neonatal Nurses (NANN). (1999b). *Use of assistive personnel in providing care to the high-risk infant.* NANN Position Statement No. 3013. Glenview, IL: Author.

Needleman, J., Buerhaus, P., Mattke, S., Stewart, M., & Zelevinski, K. (2002). Nurse-staffing levels and the quality of care in hospitals. *The New England Journal of Medicine, 346*(22), 1715–1722.

Needleman, J., Buerhaus, P. I., Stewart, M., Zelevinsky, K., & Mattke, S. (2006). Nurse staffing in hospitals: Is there a business case for quality? *Health Affairs, 25*, 204–211.

Norrish, B. R., & Rundall, T. G. (2001). Hospital restructuring and the work of registered nurses. *Milbank Quarterly, 79*, 55–79.

Pappas, S. H. (2007). Describing cost related to nursing. *Journal of Nursing Administration, 37*(1), 32–40.

Person, C. (2004). Patient care delivery. In M. Koloroutis (Ed.), *Relationship-based care: A model for transforming practice* (pp. 159–182). Minneapolis: Creative Health Care Management.

Pickard, B., & Warner, M. (2007). Demand Management: A methodology for outcomes-driven staffing and patient flow management. *Nurse Leader, 4*(2), 30–34.

Potter, P., Barr, N., McSweeney, M., & Sledge, J. (2003). Identifying nurse staffing and patient outcome relationships: A guide for change in care delivery. *Nursing Economic$, 21*(4), 158–166.

PricewaterhouseCoopers Health Research Institute. (2007). *What works: Healing the healthcare staffing shortage.* Retrieved March 7, 2008, from www.pwc.com/extweb/pwcpublications.nsf/docid/674D1E79A678A0428525730D006B74A9

Robertson, R., & Samuelson, C. (1996). Should nurse patient ratios be legislated? Pros and cons. *Georgia Nursing, 56*(5), 2.

Seago, J. A., & Ash, M. (2002). Registered nurse unions and patient outcomes. *Journal of Nursing Administration, 32*(3), 143–151.

Seago, J. A., Spetz, J., Coffman, J., Rosenoff, E., & O'Neil, E. (2003). Minimum staffing ratios: The California workforce initiative survey. *Nursing Economic$, 21*(2), 65–70.

Sherman, R. (2005). Don't forget our charge nurses. *Nursing Economic$, 23*(3), 125–130, 143.

Smith, M. (1994). Staffing and scheduling: A systems approach. In R. Spitzer-Lehmann (Ed.), *Nursing management desk reference: Concepts, skills & strategies* (pp. 178–197). Philadelphia: Saunders.

Sullivan, J., Bretschneider, J., & McCausland, M. P. (2003). Designing a leadership development program for nurse managers: An evidence-driven approach. *Journal of Nursing Administration, 33*(10), 544–549.

The Joint Commission (TJC). (2006). *Management of human resources*. Oakbrook Terrace, IL: Author.

Thompson, J. D., & Diers, D. (1985). DRG's and nursing intensity. *Nursing and Healthcare*, 6, 434–439.

Unruh, L. (2003). The effect of LPN reductions on RN patient load. *Journal of Nursing Administration, 33*(4), 201–208.

Unruh, L. (2008). Nurse staffing: Patient, nurse, financial outcomes. *American Journal of Nursing, 108*(1), 62–71.

Unruh, L., & Fottler, M. D. (2004). *Patient turnover and nursing staff adequacy*. San Diego: AcademyHealth Annual Research meeting. Retrieved May 24, 2009, from www.ahsrhp.org/2004/ppt/unruh.ppt

Unruh, L., & Fottler, M. D. (2006). Patient turnover and nursing staff adequacy. *Healthcare Services Research, 41*(2), 599–612.

Unruh, L., & Hassmiller, S. (2007). Legislative: Economics of nursing invitational conference addresses quality and payment issues in nursing care. *The Online Journal of Issues in Nursing, 13*(1).

Warner, M. (2006). Personnel staffing and scheduling. In R. Hall (Ed.), *Patient flow: Reducing delay in healthcare delivery* (pp. 189–209). Los Angeles: Springer.

Watson, J. (1988). New dimensions of human caring theory. *Nursing Science Quarterly, 1*(4), 75–181.

Watson, J. (2002). *Assessing and measuring caring in nursing and health science*. New York: Springer.

Welton, J. (2007). Mandatory hospital nurse to patient staffing ratios: Time to take a different approach. *The Online Journal of Issues in Nursing, 12*(3).

Welton, J. M., & Harris, K. (2007). Hospital billing and reimbursement: Charging for inpatient nursing care. *Journal of Nursing Administration, 30*(6), 309–315.

Welton, J. M., Zone-Smith, L., & Fischer, M. H. (2006). Adjustment of inpatient care reimbursement for nursing intensity. *Policy, Politics, & Nursing Practice, 7*(4), 270–280.

White, K. M. (2006). Policy spotlight: Staffing plans and ratios. *Nursing Management, 37*(4), 18–22, 24.

Chapter 29

Aiken, L. H., Clarke, S. P., Sloane, D. M., Sochalski, J., & Sieber, J. H. (2002). Hospital nurse staffing and patient mortality, nurse burnout, and job dissatisfaction. *Journal of the American Medical Association, 288*(16), 1987–1993.

Headlines, A. J. N. (1993). Staff cuts are sparking unionization drives. *American Journal of Nursing, 93*(9), 9.

American Nurses Association and United American Nurses, AFL-CIO (ANA, UAN). (2003). *Brief of amici curiae American Nurses Association and United American Nurses, AFL-CIO*. Silver Spring, MD: Author. Retrieved May 24, 2009, from http://www.nursingworld.org/MainMenuCategories/ThePracticeofProfessionalNursing/workplace/Work-Environment/RightsofNurses/TheRESPECTAct/KentuckyRiverBrief.aspx

Auerbach, D. I., Buerhaus, P. I., & Staiger, D. O. (2007). Better late than never: Workforce supply implications of later entry into nursing. *Health Affairs, 26*(1), 178–185.

Bacon, N., & Blyton, P. (2007). Conflict for mutual gains? *Journal of Management Studies, 44*, 814–834.

Bernat, R. T. (2001). New management opportunities and the Kentucky River case. *The Physician Executive, 27*(6), 48–50.

Bodley, A. L., Carson-Smith, W., Winston, J., Davis, S., & Paster, R. S. (2003). *Brief of amici curiae American Nurses Association and United American Nurses, AFL-CIO*. Retrieved May 5, 2008, from www.nursingworld.org/MainMenuCategories/ThePracticeofProfessionalNursing/workplace/RightsofNurses/TheRESPECTAct/KentuckyRiverBrief.aspx

Breda, K. (1997). Professional nurses in unions: Working together pays off. *Journal of Professional Nursing, 13*(2), 99–109.

Budd, K. W., Warino, L. S., & Patton, M. E. (2004). Traditional and non-traditional collective bargaining: Strategies to improve the patient care environment. *Online Journal of Issues in Nursing, 9*(1), Retrieved January 3, 2008, from www.nursingworld.org/MainMenuCategories/ANAMarketplace/ANAPeriodicals/OJIN/TableofContents/Volume92004/Number1January31/CollectiveBargainingStrategies.aspx/

Buerhaus, P. I., Donelan, K., Ulrich, B. T., Norman, L., DesRochas, C., & Dittus, R. (2007). Impact of the nurse shortage on hospital patient care: Comparative perspectives. *Health Affairs, 26*, 853–862.

Caverley, N., & Cunningham, B. (2006). Reflections on public sector-based integrative collective bargaining: Conditions affecting cooperation within the negotiation process. *Employee Relations, 28*(1), 62–75.

Clark, P. F., & Clark, D. A. (2006). Union strategies for improving patient care: The key to nurse unionism. *Labor Studies Journal, 31*(1), 51–70.

Clark, P. F., Clark, D. A., Day, D. V., & Shea, D. G. (2000). The relationship between health care reform and nurses' interest in union representation: The role of workplace climate. *Journal of Professional Nursing, 16*, 92–96.

Congress May Determine Definition of "Supervisor." (2007). *RN, 70*(7), 14.

Cutcher-Gershenfeld, J., Kochan, T., Ferguson, J. P., & Barrett, B. (2007). Collective bargaining in the twenty-first century: A negotiations institution at risk. *Negotiation Journal, 3*, 249–265.

DeMoro, R. A. (2007). The roads we've taken: Revisiting our successes of the last two years, and looking toward the many challenges ahead. *Registered Nurse*, 15–28. Retrieved February 29, 2008, from www.calnurses.org/publications/registered-nurse-magazine/registered-nurse-october-2007.pdf

Department of Labor. (2007). *Handy reference guide to the Fair Labor Standards Act.* Washington, DC: U.S. Department of Labor. Retrieved March 3, 2008, from www.dol.gov/esa/regs/compliance/whd/hrg.htm

Flanagan, L. C. (1976). *One strong voice: The story of the American Nurses Association.* Kansas City, MO: American Nurses Association.

Forman, H. (1989). *Descriptive analysis of the effects of union and non-union affiliation on perceived role conflict, conflict resolution modes, leader behavior styles, and leadership effectiveness of head nurses.* New York: Columbia University Teachers College.

Genovese, M. (2006). RNs working together: A national coalition for unionized RNs. *Report: The Official Newsletter of the New York State Nurses Association.* Retrieved March 20, 2008, from www.nysna.org/publications/report/2006/apr/coalition.htm

Heumann, M., & Hyman, J. M. (1997). Negotiation methods and litigation settlement methods in New Jersey: You can't always get what you want. *Ohio State Journal on Dispute Resolution, 12*, 253–310.

Hirsch, B. T., & Macpherson, D. A. (2008). *Union membership and coverage database from the 2007CPS posted February 8, 2008.* An internet data resource retrieved March 30, 2008, from www.unionstats.com/

Institute of Medicine. (2004). *Keeping patients safe: Transforming the work environment of nurses.* Washington, DC: National Academies Press.

Iowa Public Employment Relations Act. (1999). 20 Iowa Code 20.9. *Scope of negotiations*, Supp. Retrieved March 8, 2008, from www.sos.state.ia.us/usefulLinks/frameIACode.asp?c=496C.20

Jacox, A. (1971). Collective action and control of practice by professionals. *Nursing Forum, 10*(3), 239–257.

Ketter, J. (1994). Ruling questions NLRA protection for nurses. *The American Nurse, 26*(6), 10–13.

Ketter, J. (1996). *A seat at the table: 50 years of progress.* Washington, DC: American Nurses Association E&GW Program. Retrieved March 6, 2008, from www.uannurse.org/who/historyBook/A%20Seat%20at%20the%20Table-%2050%20years.pdf

LaTourneau, B., & Hybben, L. (1990). Nurses' strikes: A profession maturing. *Physician Executive.* Retrieved March 15, 2008, from http://findarticles.com/p/articles/mi_m0843/is_/ai_8788175

Lavigna, R. J. (2002). Best practices in public-sector human resources: Wisconsin state government. *Human Resource Management, 41*, 369–384.

Legal Information Institute (LII): Wex. (2007a). *Collective bargaining and labor arbitration: An overview.* Ithaca, NY: LII, Cornell University Law School. Retrieved February 24, 2008, from www.law.cornell.edu/topics/collective_bargaining.html

Legal Information Institute (LII): Wex. (2007b). *Labor law: An overview.* Ithaca, NY: LII, Cornell University Law School. Retrieved February 24, 2008, from www.law.cornell.edu/topics/labor.html

Lovell, V. (2006). *Solving the nursing shortage through higher wages.* Washington, DC: Institute for Women's Policy Research. Retrieved February 24, 2008, from www.iwpr.org/pdf/c363.pdf

Madden, G. (1969). A theoretical basis for differentiating forms of collective bargaining in education. *Educational Administration Quarterly, 5*(2), 76–90.

Malmgren, J. (2008). Business and lobbying: Business, labor bring familiar fight over union rights to campaign trail. *The Hill, 15.* Retrieved June 1, 2008, from http://thehill.com/business--lobby/business-labor-bring-familiar-fight-over-union-rights-to-campaign-trail-2008–04–15.html

McAndrew, I., & Phillips, V. (2005). Documenting play: Using videotaped interviews to debrief collective bargaining games. *Human Resource Management Review, 15*, 214–225.

McKersie, R. B., Sharpe, T., Kochan, T. A., Eaton, A. E., Strauss, G., & Morgenstern, M. (2008). Bargaining theory meets interest-based negotiations: A case study. *Industrial Relations, 47*, 66–96.

McNeese-Smith, D. (2006). Nurses need to step up and speak for themselves. *UCLA Today ONLINE.* UCLA's Faculty and Staff Newsletter. Retrieved March 22, 2008, from www.today.ucla.edu/voices/donna-mcneese-smith_nurses/

Michigan Nurses Association. (2007). *Nurses and collective bargaining: Basic facts and considerations. Organizing.* Michigan Nurses Association: www.minurses.org. Retrieved March 23, 2008, from www.minurses.org/Labor/nursescollectgbn.shtml

Minnesota Nurses Association. (2008). *Diary of destiny: A 100 year chronicle of Minnesota Nurses Association.* Minnesota Nurses Association: www.mnnurses.org. Retrieved April 21, 2008, from http://nursesrev.advocateoffice.com/index.asp?Type = B_BASIC&SEC = {5C01F403-A061–4BBD-ABFD-F416E7ADC97F}

National Labor Relations Board (NLRB). (1997). *Basic guide to the National Labor Relations Act: General principles of law and procedures of the National Labor Relations Board.* Washington, DC: U.S. Government Printing Office.

National Labor Relations Board (NLRB). (2006). *NLRB issues lead case addressing supervisory status in response to Supreme Court's decision in Kentucky River.* Press Release retrieved May 20, 2008, from www.lawmemo.com/nlrb/kyrivercases.htm

Needleman, J., Buerhaus, P., Mattke, S., Stewart, M., & Zelevinski, K. (2002). Nurse staffing levels and the quality of care in hospitals. *The New England Journal of Medicine, 346*(22), 1715–1722.

Nyman, T. (1981). *A guide to the teaching of collective bargaining.* Geneva: International Labor Office.

Patton, M. E. (1998). The value of unity. *American Journal of Nursing, 98*(2), 80.

Porter-O'Grady, T. (1992). Of rabbits and turtles: A time of change for unions. *Nursing Economic$, 10*(3), 177–182.

Rainsberger, P. K. (2006a). *Collective bargaining: Effective negotiations.* University of Missouri—Columbia, Labor Education Program. Retrieved February 19, 2008, from http://labored.missouri.edu/Effective%20Negotiations.htm

Rainsberger, P. K. (2006b). *Collective bargaining: Historical models of collective bargaining in the U.S.* University of Missouri—Columbia, Labor Education Program. Retrieved February 19, 2008, from http://labored.missouri.edu/Historic%20Models%20of%20Collective%20Bargaining%20in%20the%20U.S.htm

Roberts, K., & Lundy, C. (2003). IX. Employment relations for health care workers: Does collective bargaining make a difference in nursing agreements? *Proceedings of The Industrial Relations Research Association.* Retrieved March 22, 2008, from www.press.uillinois.edu/journals/irra/proceedings2003/toc.html

Shepard, G. (2004). Ohio Nurses Association and collective bargaining. In L. S. Baas (Ed.), *100 Years of caring* (pp. 49–51). Columbus, OH: Ohio Nurses Foundation Press.

Spangler, B. (2003). Integrative or interest-based bargaining. In G. Burgess, & H. Burgess (Eds.), *Beyond intractability.* Boulder: Conflict Research Consortium, University of Colorado. Retrieved February 29, 2008, from www.beyondintractability.org/essay/interest-based_bargaining/

Stepp, J. R., & Bergel, G. I. (2008). Moving from interest-based to results-focused bargaining. *Perspectives on Work, 11*(2), 34–38.

U.S. Army CPOL. (2005). *Collective bargaining.* Washington, DC: U.S. Department of Defense: Retrieved February 24, 2008, from www.cpol.army.mil/library/permiss/4131.html

U.S. Army CPOL. (2006). *Bargaining unit.* Washington, DC: U.S. Department of Defense. Retrieved February 24, 2008, from www.cpol.army.mil/library/permiss/411.html

Wagner, S. (2002). How did the Taft-Hartley Act come about? *History News Network.* Retrieved February 2, 2008, from http://hnn.us/articles/1036.html

Walton, R. E., & McKersie, R. B. (1965). *A behavioral theory of labor negotiations: An analysis of a social interaction system.* New York: McGraw-Hill.

Wertheim, E. (n.d.). *Negotiations and resolving conflicts: An overview.* Study guide retrieved January 15, 2008 from http://web.cba.neu.edu/~ewertheim/interper/negot3.htm

Chapter 30

Aiken, L. H., Clarke, S. P., Sloane, D. M., Sochalski, J., & Silber, J. H. (2002). Hospital nurse staffing and patient mortality, nurse burnout, and job dissatisfaction. *The Journal of the American Medical Association, 288*(16), 1987–1993.

Aiken, T. (1994). *Legal, ethical, and political issues in nursing.* Philadelphia: F.A. Davis.

Amendment to the Illinois Hospital Licensing Act. (2008). *Nurse staffing by patient acuity.* SB 0867, Section 10.10. LRB095–05612-DRJ 25702b.

Buerhaus, P. I., Donelan, K., Ulrich, B. T., DesRoches, C., & Dittus, R. (2007). Trends in the experiences of hospital-employed registered nurses: Results from three national surveys. *Nursing Economic$, 25*(2), 69–79.

Cleverly, W. O., & Cameron, A. E. (2002). *Essentials of health care finance* (5th ed.). Gaithersburg, MD: Aspen Publishers.

Colosi, M. L. (2007). Nurses: When supply fails demand, a patient care catastrophe looms. *Nurse Leader, 5*(6), 46–53.

Corley, M., & Raines, D. (1993). An ethical practice environment as a caring environment. *Nursing Administration Quarterly, 17*(2), 68–74.

Cyr, J. P. (2005). Retaining older hospital nurses and delaying their retirement. *Journal of Nursing Administration, 35*(12), 563–567.

Jones, C. B. (2005). Nurse turnover: Why is it such a tough problem to solve? *Nurse Leader, 3*(3), 43–47.

Jones, C. B. (2008). Revisiting nurse turnover costs: Adjusting for inflation. *Journal of Nursing Administration, 38*(1), 11–18.

Kaplan, R. S., & Norton, D. P. (2006). *Alignment.* Boston: Harvard Business School Press.

Lang, T. A., Hodge, M., Olson, V., Romano, P. S., & Kravitz, R. L. (2004). Nurse-patient ratios: A systematic review on the effects of nurse staffing on patient, nurse employee, and hospital outcomes. *Journal of Nursing Administration, 34*(7–8), 326–337.

Mion, L. C., Hazel, C., Cap, M., Fusilero, J., Podmore, M. L., & Szweda, C. (2006). Retaining and recruiting mature experienced nurses. *Journal of Nursing Administration, 36*(3), 148–154.

O'Brien-Pallas, L. (2006). The impact of nurse turnover on patient, nurse, and system outcomes: A pilot study and focus for a multicenter international study. *Policy, Politics, & Nursing Practice, 7*(3), 169–179.

Spetz, J. (2004). California's minimum nurse-to-patient ratios: The first few months. *Journal of Nursing Administration, 34*(12), 571–578.

Storfjell, J. L., Ohlson, S., & Omoike, O. (2008). The balancing act: Patient care time vs. cost. *Journal of Nursing Administration, 38*(5), 244–249.

Storfjell, J. L., Allen, C. E., & Easley, C. E. (2009). Analysis and management of home health nursing caseloads and workloads. In M. Harris (Ed.), *Handbook of home health care administration* (5th ed., Chapter 35). Boston: Jones and Bartlett Publishers.

Storfjell, J. L., Ohlson, S., Omoike, O., Fitzpatrick, T., & Wetasin, K. (2009). Non-value-added time: The million dollar nursing opportunity. *Journal of Nursing Administration, 39*(1), 38–45.

Ward-Smith, P., Hunt, C., Smith, J. B., Teasley, S. L., Carroll, C. A., & Sexton, K. (2007). Issues and opportunities for retaining experienced nurses at the bedside. *Journal of Nursing Administration, 37*(11), 485–487.

Welton, J. M., Unruh, L., & Halloran, E. J. (2006). Nurse staffing, nurse intensity, staff mix, and direct nursing care costs across Massachusetts hospitals. *Journal of Nursing Administration, 36*(9), 416–425.

Young, C. M., Albert, N. M., Paschke, S. M., & Meyer, K. H. (2007). The "parent shift" program: Incentives for nurses, rewards for nursing teams. *Nursing Economic$, 25*(6), 339–344.

Chapter 31

Bailey, D. (1996). Budgeting skills. *Nursing Standard, 10*(19), 43–48.

Barr, P. (2005). Flexing your budget: Experts urge hospitals, systems to trade in their traditional budgeting process for a more dynamic and versatile model. *Modern Healthcare, 35*(37), 24, 26.

Brady, D. J., Cornett, E., & DeLetter, M. (1998). Cost reduction: What a staff nurse can do. *Nursing Economic$, 16*(5), 273–274, 276.

Chagares, R., & Jackson, B. (1987). Sitting easy: How six pressure-relieving devices stack up. *American Journal of Nursing, 87*(2), 191–193.

Dodson, G. M., Sinclair, G., Miller, M., Charping, C., Johnson, B., & Black, M. (1998). Determining cost drivers for pediatric home health services. *Nursing Economic$, 16*(5), 263–271.

Eckhart, J. (1993). Costing out nursing services: Examining the research. *Nursing Economic$, 11*(2), 91–98.

Ervin, N. E., Chang, W., & White, J. (1998). A cost analysis of a nursing center's services. *Nursing Economic$, 16*(6), 307–312.

Finkler, S. A., & Ward, D. M. (1999). *Essentials of cost accounting for health care organizations* (2nd ed.). Gaithersburg, MD: Aspen.

Finkler, S. A., & Kovner, C. T. (2000). *Financial management for nurse managers and executives* (2nd ed.). Philadelphia: Saunders.

Gormley, K. K., & Verdejo, T. (2000). A systems approach—Budgeting for the 21st century: Turning challenges into triumphs. *Nursing Administration Quarterly, 24*(4), 51–59.

Johnson, M., & Carpenter, C. (1990). Financial management for nursing executives. In E. Simendinger, T. Moore, & M. Kramer (Eds.), *The successful nurse executive: A guide for every nurse manager* (pp. 91–106). Ann Arbor, MI: Health Administration Press.

Kenny, M. P. F. (1996). Ask the experts. *Critical Care Nurse, 16*(4), 103.

Krugman, M., MacLauchlan, M., Riippi, L., & Grubbs, J. (2002). A multidisciplinary financial education research project. *Nursing Economic$, 20*(6), 273–278.

Maurano, L. (2004). The results are in: The financial impact of changing supply processes. *Remington Report, 12*(3).

Scherubel, J. (1994). Costing out nursing services: Is it happening. In J. McCloskey, & H. Grace (Eds.), *Current issues in nursing* (4th ed., pp. 483–489). St. Louis: Mosby.

Smith, C., & Amen, R. (1989). Comparing the costs of IV drug delivery systems. *American Journal of Nursing, 89*(4), 500–501.

Starck, P. L., & Bailes, B. (1996). The budget process in schools of nursing: A primer for the novice administrator. *Journal of Professional Nursing, 12*(2), 69–75.

Striegel, E. (1986). Cost-effective use of supplies in the NICU. *Neonatal Network, 4*(6), 46–48.

Chapter 32

Aiken, L. H., Clarke, S., Sloane, D., Sochalski, J., & Silber, J. H. (2002). Hospital nurse staffing and patient mortality, nurse burnout, and job dissatisfaction. *Journal of the American Medical Association, 288*(16), 1987–1993.

American Association of Colleges of Nursing (AACN). (2007). *Press release.* Retrieved February 28, 2007, from www.aacn.nche.edu/Media/NewsReleases/2007/enrl.htm

Beglinger, J. E. (2006). Quantifying patient care intensity: An evidence-based approach to determining staffing requirements. *Nursing Administration Quarterly, 30*(3), 193–202.

Cho, S., Ketefian, S., Barkauskas, V., & Smith, D. (2003). The effects of nurse staffing on adverse events, morbidity, mortality, and medical costs. *Nursing Research, 52*(2), 71–79.

Curtin, L. (2007). The perfect storm. *Nursing Administration Quarterly, 31*(2), 105–114.

Darmody, J., Pawlak, R., Hook, M., Semeniuk, Y., Westphal, J., Murray, M. E., et al. (2007). Substitution of hospital staff in concurrent utilization review. *Journal of Nursing Care Quality, 22*(3), 239–246.

Davis, C. K. (1992). Who will pay? The economic realities of health care reform. *Scholarly Inquiry for Nursing Practice, 6*(3), 217–219.

Drummond, M. F., O'Brien, B., Stoddart, G. L., & Torrance, G. W. (1997). *Methods of economic evaluation of health care programmes* (2nd ed.). New York: Oxford University Press.

Edwardson, S. (1989). Productivity measurement. In B. Henry, C. Arndt, M. Di Vincenti, & A. Mariner-Tomey (Eds.),

Dimensions of nursing administration: Theory, research, education, and practice (pp. 371–385). Boston: Blackwell.

Erickson, J. I., Holm, L. J., & Chelminiak, L. (2004). Keeping the nursing shortage from becoming a nursing crisis. *Journal of Nursing Administration, 34*(2), 83–87.

Gerke, M. L. (2001). Understanding and leading in the quad matrix—Four generations in the workplace: The Traditional Generation, Boomers, Gen-X, Nexters. *Seminars for Nurse Managers, 9*(3), 173–181.

Heffler, S., Smith, S., Keehan, S., Clemens, M. K., Won, G., & Zezza, M. (2003). Health spending projections for 2002–2012 [Online exclusive]. *Health Affairs: The Policy Journal of the Health Sphere.* Retrieved November 28, 2008, from http://content.healthaffairs.org/cgi/content/full/hlthaff.w3.54v1/DC1?maxtoshow=&HITS=10&hits=10&RESULTFORMAT=&author1=Heffler&fulltext=Health+Spending&andorexactfulltext=and&searchid=1&FIRSTINDEX=0&resourcetype=HWCIT

Hunt, P. S. (2001). Speaking the language of finance. *AORN Journal, 73*(4), 774–787.

Jacobs, P., & Rapoport, J. (2004). *The economics of health care* (5th ed.). Boston: Jones and Bartlett Publishers.

McCloskey, J. (1989). Implications of costing out nursing services for reimbursement. *Nursing Management, 20*(1), 44–49.

McKeon, T. (1996). Performance measurement: Integrating quality management and activity-based cost management. *Journal of Nursing Administration, 26*(4), 45–51.

Murray, M. E., & Henriques, J. B. (2003). An exploratory cost analysis of hospital-based concurrent review. *American Journal of Managed Care, 19*(7), 512–518.

National Center for Health Workforce Analysis. (2002). *What is behind HRSA's projected supply, demand, and shortage of registered nurses?* Rockville, MD: U.S. Department of Health and Human Services:. Retrieved November 28, 2008, from http://bhpr.hrsa.gov/healthworkforce/reports/behindrnprojections/4.htm#x23

Oakley, D., Murray, M. E., Murtland, T., Hayashi, R., Anderson, H. F., Mayes, F., et al. (1996). Comparisons of outcomes of maternity care by obstetricians and certified nurse midwives. *Obstetrics & Gynecology, 88*(5), 823–829.

Pappas, S. H. (2007). Describing costs related to nursing. *Journal of Nursing Administration, 17*(1), 32–40.

Poisal, J., Truffer, C., Smith, S., Sisko, A., Cowan, K., Keehan, S., et al., & the National Health Expenditures Accounts Projections Team. (2007). Health spending projections through 2016: Modest changes obscure Part D's impact. *Health AffairsWeb Exclusive.* Retrieved February 21, 2008, from http://content.healthaffairs.org.ezproxy.library.wisc.edu/cgi/content/full/26/2/w242

Swansburg, R. C., & Sowell, R. L. (1992). A model for costing and pricing nursing service. *Nursing Management, 23*(2), 33–36.

Yoder-Wise, P. (2007). Key forecasts shaping nursing's perfect storm. *Nursing Administration Quarterly, 31*(2), 115–119.

Chapter 33

Aiken, L., Clarke, S., Sloane, D., Sochalski, J., & Silber, J. (2002). Hospital nurse staffing and patient mortality, nurse burnout, and job dissatisfaction. *Journal of the American Medical Association, 288*, 1987–1993.

Albrecht, S. (1972). Reappraisal of conventional performance appraisal. *Journal of Nursing Administration, 2*(2), 29–35.

Arnold, E., & Pulich, M. (2003). Personality conflicts and objectivity in appraising performance. *Health Care Manager, 22*(3), 227–232.

Burns, N., & Grove, S. K. (2001). *The practice of nursing research: Conduct, critique & utilization* (4th ed.). Philadelphia: Saunders.

Cameron, K. S., & Quinn, R. E. (1999). *Diagnosing and changing organizational culture: Based on the competing values framework.* Reading, PA: Addison-Wesley.

Carroll, J. S., & Edmondson, A. C. (2002). Leading organizational learning in health care. *Quality and Safety in Health Care, 11*, 51–56.

Christensen, M. (1990). Peer auditing. *Nursing Management, 21*(1), 50–52.

Conlon, M. (2003). Appraisal: The catalyst of personal development. *British Medical Journal, 327*(7411), 389–391.

Detert, J. R., Schroeder, R. G., & Mauriel, J. J. (2000). A framework for linking culture and improvement initiatives in organizations. *Academy of Management Review, 25*(4), 850–863.

Donaldson, M. S., & Mohr, J. J. (2000). *Exploring innovation and quality improvement in health care microsystems: A cross-case analysis.* Washington, DC: Institute of Medicine, National Academies Press. Retrieved November 28, 2008, from www.nap.edu/openbook/NI000346/html/65.html

Duncan, D. (2007). The importance of managing performance processes well. *Kai Tiaki Nursing New Zealand, 13*(10), 25.

Frank, B. (1998). Performance management. In J. A. Dinenemann (Ed.), *Nursing administration: Managing patient care* (2nd ed., pp. 461–484). Stamford, CT: Appleton & Lange.

Gershon, R. R. M., Stone, P. W., Bakken, S., & Larson, E. (2004). Measurement of organizational culture and climate in health care. *Journal of Nursing Administration, 34*(1), 33–40.

Greguras, G. J., Robie, C., Schleicher, D. J., & Goff, M. (2003). A field study of the effects of rating purpose on the quality of multisource ratings. *Personnel Psychology, Inc., 56*, 1–21.

Hersey, P., Blanchard, K. H., & Johnson, D. E. (2008). *Management of organizational behavior: Leading human resources* (9th ed.). Upper Saddle River, NJ: Pearson Education.

Institute of Medicine (IOM). (2000). *To err is human: Building a safer system.* Washington, DC: National Academies Press.

Institute of Medicine (IOM). (2001). *Crossing the quality chasm: A new health system for the 21st century.* Washington, DC: National Academies Press.

Institute of Medicine (IOM). (2003). *Priority areas for national action: Transforming health care quality.* Washington, DC: National Academies Press.

Institute of Medicine (IOM). (2004). *Keeping patients safe: Transforming the work environment of nurses.* Washington, DC: National Academies Press.

Jawahar, M. (2006). Correlates of satisfaction with performance appraisal feedback. *Journal of Labor Relations, 27,* 213–234.

Letvak, S. (2003). The experiences of being an older staff nurse. *Western Journal of Nursing Research, 25*(1), 45–46.

McKirchy, K. (1998). *Powerful performance appraisals: How to set expectations and work together to improve.* Franklin, NJ: The Career Press.

Merriam-Webster's Collegiate Dictionary (10th ed.). (1997). Springfield, MA: Merriam-Webster.

Nauright, L. (1987). Toward a comprehensive personnel system: Performance appraisal—Part IV. *Nursing Management, 28*(2), 29–32.

Needleman, J., Buerhaus, P., Mattke, S., Stewart, M., & Zelevinsky, K. (2002). Nurse-staffing levels and the quality of care in hospitals. *The New England Journal of Medicine, 346,* 1715–1722.

Nemeth, L. (2005). *Implementing change in primary care practice.* Unpublished doctoral dissertation. Charleston, SC: Medical University of South Carolina.

Parse, R. R. (1997). Leadership: The essentials. *Nursing Science Quarterly, 10*(3), 109.

Parse, R. R. (2004). Power in position. *Nursing Science Quarterly, 17*(2), 101.

Reason, J. (2000). Human error: Models and management. *British Medical Journal, 320*(7237), 768–770.

Robinson, K., Eck, C., Keck, B., & Wells, N. (2003). The Vanderbilt Professional Nursing Practice Program—Part 1: Growing and supporting professional nursing practice. *Journal of Nursing Administration, 33*(9), 441–450.

Schein, E. H. (1992). *Organizational culture and leadership* (2nd ed.). San Francisco: Jossey-Bass.

Smith-Trudeau, P. (2008). Culturally sensitive performance appraisals that lead to reenergized managers and employees. *Vermont Nurse Connection,* November, December, January, 5.

Stetler, C. B. (2003). Role of the organization in translating research into evidence-based practice. *Outcomes Management, 7*(3), 97–103.

Stone, F. M. (1999). *Coaching, counseling & mentoring: How to choose & use the right technique to boost employee performance.* New York: AMACOM.

Studer, Q. (2003). *Hardwiring excellence.* Gulf Breeze, FL: Fire Starter Publishing.

The American Heritage Dictionary of the English Language. (2000). Boston: Houghton Mifflin. Retrieved November 28, 2008, from www.bartleby.com/61/11/C0801100.html

The Joint Commission (TJC). (2008). *Revised chapter program—OBS chapter: HR.* Oakbrook Terrace, IL: Author. Retrieved March 2, 2008, from www.jointcommission.org/NR/rdonlyres/86B6B609–3D33–4008–8A40–1D84AEE7D002/0/obs_sii_hr_revised_chapter.pdf

The Joint Commission (TJC). (2009). *National patient safety goals.* Oakbrook Terrace, IL: Author. Retrieved November 28, 2008, from www.jointcommission.org/GeneralPublic/NPSG/

Ward, D. (2003). Self-esteem and audit feedback. *Nursing Standard, 17*(37), 33–36.

Chapter 34

Anderson, C. (2002). Past victim, future victim? *Nursing Management, 33*(3), 26–31.

Beech, B., & Leather, P. (2005). Workplace violence in the health care sector: A review of staff training and integration of training evaluation models. *Aggression and Violent Behavior, 11,* 27–43.

Beugre, C. D. (2005). Understanding injustice-related aggression in organizations: A cognitive model. *International Journal of Human Resource Management, 16*(7), 1120–1136.

Botting, J. M. (2001). Picking up the pieces. *Security Management, 45*(1), 26–39.

Brown, H. (1998). Armed against terrorism. *Occupational Health & Safety, 67*(10), 172–176.

Bruser, S. (1998). Workplace violence: Getting hospitals focused on prevention. *The American Nurse, 30*(3). Retrieved November 28, 2008, from http://nursingworld.org/MainMenuCategories/ANAMarketplace/ANAPeriodicals/TAN/1998/MayJuneFeaturesViolence.aspx

Carroll, V., & Morin, K. (1998). Workplace violence affects one-third of nurses: Survey of nurses in seven SNAs reveals staff nurses most at risk. *American Nurse, 30*(5), 1. Retrieved November 28, 2008, from www.nursingworld.org/search.aspx?SearchMode=1&SearchPhrase=Workplace+violence+affects+one-third+of+nurses%3a+Survey+of+nurses+in+seven+SNAs+reveals+staff+nurses+most+at+risk&SearchWithin=2

Center for Violence Prevention and Control. (1996). *A guide to courses that include content pertinent to violence prevention and control.* Minneapolis, MN: University of Minnesota: Retrieved November 28, 2008, from www1.umn.edu/cvpc/pub_coursedir.html

Corbo, S. A., & Siewers, M. H. (2001). Hazardous to your health: Don't get burned when tempers ignite. *Nursing Management, 32*(3), 44C–44F.

Dietz, J., Robinson, S. L., Folger, R., Baron, R. A., & Schulz, M. (2003). The impact of community violence and an organization's procedural justice climate on workplace aggression. *Academy of Management Journal, 46*(3), 317–326.

Dolan, J. B. (2000). Workplace violence: The universe of legal issues. *Defense Counsel Journal, 67*(3), 332–341.

Edwards, R. (1999). Prevention of workplace violence. *Aspen's Advisor for Nurse Executives, 14*(8), 8–12.

Egger, E. (2000). Reasonable and appropriate action important in preventing violent crime. *Health Care Strategic Management, 18*(10), 13–14.

Elliot, P. P. (1997). Violence in health care. *Nursing Management, 28*(12), 38–41.

Gerberich, S. G., Church, T. R., McGovern, P. M., Hassen, H. E., Nachreizer, N. M., Geisser, M. S., et al. (2004). An epidemiological study of the magnitude and consequences of work related violence: The Minnesota Nurses' Study. *Occupational and Environmental Medicine, 61*, 495–503.

Ginn, G. O., & Henry, L. J. (2002). Addressing workplace violence from a health management perspective. *SAM Advanced Management Journal, 67*(4), 4–10.

Harulow, S. (2000). Ending the silence on violence. *Australian Nursing Journal, 7*(10), 26–29.

Henry, L. J., & Ginn, G. O. (2002). Violence prevention in health care organizations within a TQM framework. *Journal of Nursing Administration, 32*(9), 479–486.

Hoag-Apel, C. M. (1999). Smart safeguards for the ED. *Nursing Management, 30*(5), 31–33.

Hogh, A., & Viitasara, E. (2005). A systematic review of longitudinal studies of nonfatal workplace violence. *European Journal of Work and Organizational Psychology, 14*(3), 291–313.

Jossi, E. (1999). Defusing workplace violence. *Business & Health, 17*(2), 34–49.

Kreitzer, M. J., Wright, D., Hamlin, D., Towey, S., Marko, O., & Disch, J. (1997). Creating a healthy work environment in the midst of organizational change and transition. *Journal of Nursing Administration, 27*(6), 35–41.

Law, T. P., & Pettit, F. A. (2007). Insuring for workplace violence. *Risk Management, 54*(11), 14–18.

Litke, R. (1996). Defusing the workplace time bomb. *Journal of Property Management, 61*(4), 16–21.

Matchulat, J. J. (2007). Separating fact from fiction about workplace violence. *Employee Relations Law Journal, 33*(2), 41–22.

McKenna, B. G., Smith, N. A., Poole, S. J., & Coverdale, J. H. (2003). Horizontal violence: Experience of registered nurses in their first year of practice. *Journal of Advanced Nursing, 42*(1), 90–96.

McKoy, Y. L., & Smith, M. H. (2001). Legal considerations of workplace violence in healthcare environments. *Nursing Forum, 36*(1), 5–14.

McMillan, I. (1995). Losing control. *Nursing Times. 91*, 40–43.

McPhaul, K. M., & Lipscomb, J. A. (2004). Workplace violence in health care: Recognized but not regulated. *The Online Journal of Issues in Nursing, 9*(3). Retrieved November 28, 2008, from www.nursingworld.org/MainMenuCategories/ANAMarketplace/ANAPeriodicals/OJIN/TableofContents/Volume92004/No3Sept04/ViolenceinHealthCare.aspx

Murray, M. G., & Synder, J. C. (1991). When staff are assaulted. *Journal of Psychosocial Nursing and Mental Health Nursing, 29*(7), 24–29.

National Audit Office. (2003). *A safer place to work: Protecting NHS hospital and ambulance staff from violence and aggression*. London, UK: The Stationary Office.

National Institute for Occupational Safety and Health (NIOSH). (1996). *National Institute for Occupational Safety and Health, current intelligence bulletin 57—Violence in the workplace: Risk factors and strategies*. Washington, DC: NIOSH, Centers for Disease Control and Prevention, U.S. Department of Health and Human Services.

National Institute for Occupational Safety and Health (NIOSH). (2002). *Violence: Occupational hazards in hospitals*. Washington, DC: NIOSH, Centers for Disease Control and Prevention, U.S. Department of Health and Human Services. Retrieved November 28, 2008, from www.cdc.gov/niosh/docs/2002–101/

Occupational Safety and Health Administration (OSHA). (2004). *Guidelines for preventing workplace violence for health care and social service workers. OSHA publication 3148–01R 2004*. Washington, DC: OSHA, U.S. Department of Labor.

O'Leary-Kelly, A. M., Griffin, R. W., & Glew, D. J. (1996). Organization-motivated aggression: A research framework. *Academy of Management Review, 21*(1), 225–253.

Paetzold, R. L., O'Leary-Kelly, A. M., & Griffin, R. W. (2007). Workplace violence, employer liability, and implications for organizational research. *Journal of Management Inquiry, 16*(4), 362–370.

Rugala, E. R., & Isaacs, A. R. (Eds.). (2004). *Workplace violence: Issues in response*. Washington, DC: U.S. Department of Justice, Federal Bureau of Investigation (FBI). Retrieved November 28, 2008, from www.fbi.gov/publications/violence.pdf

Sheehan, J. P. (2000). Protect your staff from workplace violence. *Nursing Management, 31*(3), 24–25.

Smith, A. P. (2001). Removing the fluff: The quality in quality improvement. *Nursing Economic$, 19*(4), 183–185.

Smith-Pittman, M. H., & McKoy, Y. D. (1999). Workplace violence in healthcare environments. *Nursing Forum, 34*(3), 5–13.

Spector, P. E., Coulter, M. L., Stockwell, G., & Matz, M. W. (2007). Perceived violence climate: A new construct and its relationship to workplace physical violence and verbal aggression, and their potential consequences. *Work and Stress, 21*(2), 117–130.

Tzeng, H., & Ketefian, S. (2002). The relationship between nurses' job satisfaction and inpatient satisfaction: An exploratory study in a Taiwan teaching hospital. *Journal of Nursing Care Quality, 16*(2), 39–49.

Violence threatens the workplace. (1998). *The Internal Auditor, 55*(5), 13.

Wagner, C., Groenewegen, P. P., de Bakker, D. H., & van der Wal, G. (2001). Environmental and organizational determinants of quality management. *Quality Management in Health Care, 9*(4), 63–77.

Wheeler, H. (1998). Nurse occupational stress research 5: Sources and determinants of stress. *British Journal of Nursing, 7*, 40–43.

Chapter 35

Agency for Healthcare Research and Quality (AHRQ). (2005a). *Altered standards of care in mass casualty events: Bioterrorism and other public health emergencies.* AHRQ Publication No. 05–0043. Rockville, MD: Author. Retrieved May 26, 2009, from http://www.ahrq.gov/research/altstand/

Agency for Healthcare Research and Quality (AHRQ). (2005b). *Surge capacity and health system preparedness.* Rockville, MD: Author. Retrieved May 26, 2009, from http://www.ahrq.gov/news/ulp/btsurgemass/

Agency for Healthcare Research and Quality (AHRQ). (2007). *Mass medical care with scarce resources: A community planning guide.* AHRQ Publication No. 07–0001. Rockville, MD: Author. Retrieved May 26, 2009, from http://www.ahrq.gov/research/mce/

American-Firefighter.com. (2004). *Members from three incident management teams travel to Florida.* Retrieved November 29, 2008, from www.american-firefighter.com

American Nurses Association. (2007). *Adapting standards of care under altered conditions.* Center for Health Policy, Columbia University School of Nursing, Draft document for comment purposes only: September 2007.

Ashcroft, T. (2001). Braced for disaster. *Nursing Management, 32*(5), 49–52.

Christian, M. D., Hawryluck, L., Wax, R. S., Cook, T., Lazar, N. M., Herridge, M. S., et al. (2006). Development of a triage protocol for critical care during an influenza pandemic. *Canadian Medical Association Journal, 175*(11), 1377–1381.

Disaster Relief Library. (2004). *Disaster dictionary.* Atlanta: American Red Cross, CNN Interactive, and IBM.

Drenkard, K., Rigotti, G., Hanfling, D., Fahlgren, T., & LaFrancois, G. (2002). Health care system disaster preparedness. Part 1. Readiness planning. *Journal of Nursing Administration, 32*(9), 461–469.

Ehrat, K. (2001). Executive nurse career progression: Skills, wisdom and realities. *Nursing Administration Quarterly, 25*(4), 36–42.

English, J. F., Cundiff, M. Y., Malone, J. D., Pfeiffer, J. A., Bell, M., Steele, L., et al. (1999). *Bioterrorism readiness plan: A template for healthcare facilities.* Washington, DC: The Advisory Board Company. Retrieved November 29, 2008, from www.advisory.com

Fahlgren, T., & Drenkard, K. (2002). Health care system disaster preparedness. Part 2. Nursing executive role in leadership. *Journal of Nursing Administration, 32*(10), 531–537.

Hanfling, D. (2006). Equipment, supplies, and pharmaceuticals: How much might it cost to achieve basic surge capacity? *Academic Emergency Medicine, 13*(11), 1232–1237.

Hick, J. L., & O'Laughlin, D. T. (2006). Concept of operations for triage of mechanical ventilation in an epidemic. *Academic Emergency Medicine, 13*(2), 223–229.

Inova Health System. (2001a). *All-hazards disaster preparedness plan. Annex B.* Falls Church, VA: Inova Health System.

Inova Health System. (2001b). *All-hazards disaster preparedness plan. Annex C.* Falls Church, VA: Inova Health System.

Inova Health System. (2001c). *All-hazards disaster preparedness plan. Annex R.* Falls Church, VA: Inova Health System.

Kaji, A. H. (2004). *Hospital disaster preparedness in Los Angeles County.* Los Angeles: University of California Los Angeles. Retrieved November 29, 2008, from www.ph.ucla.edu/epi/layne/EPI226.html

Kraus, C. K., Levy, F., & Kelen, G. D. (2007). Lifeboat ethics: Considerations in the discharge of inpatients for the creation of hospital surge capacity. *Disaster Medicine and Public Health Preparedness, 1*(1), 51–56.

Lindholm, M., & Uden, G. (2001). Nurse managers' management, direction, and role over time. *Nursing Administration Quarterly, 25*(4), 14–29.

Macintyre, A. G., Christopher, G. W., & Eitzen, E. (2000). Weapons of mass destruction events with contaminated casualties: Effective planning for health care facilities. *Journal of the American Medication Association, 283*(2), 242–249.

McLaughlin, S. B. (2001). *Hazard vulnerability analysis tool.* Chicago: American Society for Healthcare Engineering.

Myers, F. E.III. (2001). Bioterrorism: Responding to militant microbes. *Nursing2001, Hospital Nursing, 31*(9), 32hnl–32hn4.

New York State Department of Health Task Force on Life and the Law. (2007). *Allocation of ventilators in an influenza pandemic.* Albany, NY: Author. Retrieved May 26, 2009, from http://www.health.state.ny.us/diseases/communicable/influenza/pandemic/ventilators/

Phillips, S. J., & Knebel, A. (2007). *Mass medical care with scarce resources, a community planning guide.* Prepared for Agency for Healthcare Research and Quality Contract No. 290–04–0010, February, 2007, AHRQ Publication No. 07–0001.

Pletz, B., Cheu, D., Russell, P., & Nave, E. (1998). *Hospital emergency incident command system update project: About the HEICS III project* (3rd ed., Vol. I). (Grant Contract #EMS-6040.) San Mateo, CA: San Mateo Health Services Agency, Emergency Medical Services.

Richter, P. (2004). *Hospital disaster preparedness: Meeting a requirement or preparing for the worst?* Chicago: American

Society for Healthcare Engineering of the American Hospital Association.

Testimony of Secretary Chertoff, U.S. Department of Homeland Security, before the U.S. House of Representatives Committee on Homeland Security. (2008). *FY 2009 Budget Request.* Cannon House Office Building. www.dhs.gov/xnews/testimony/testimony_1203008767192.shtm

The White House. (2002). *Homeland security presidential directive-3.* Washington, DC: The White House, President George W. Bush. Retrieved November 29, 2008, from www.whitehouse.gov/news/releases/2002/03/20020312–5.html

U.S. Department of Homeland Security. (2004). *Fact sheet: National incident management system NIMS.* Washington, DC: Author. Retrieved November 13, 2004, from www.dhs.gov/xnews/releases/press_release_0363.shtm

Vecchio, A. (2000). Plan for the worst before disaster strikes. *Health Management Technology, 21*(6), 28–30.

Wetter, D. C., Daniel, W. E., & Treser, C. D. (2001). Hospital preparedness for victims of chemical or biological terrorism. *American Journal of Public Health, 91*(5), 710–716.

Chapter 36

Abbott, P. A., & Lee, S. M. (2001). Informatics: A new dimension in nursing. *Imprint, 48*(3), 51–52.

American Nurses Association (ANA). (2007). *New criteria for recognition of terminologies supporting nursing practice.* Retrieved November 30, 2008, from www.nursingworld.org/DocumentVault/NursingPractice/DraftNursingTerminologiesRecognitionCriteria.aspx

Austin, C. (1979). *Information systems for hospital administration.* Ann Arbor, MI: Health Administration Press.

Bakken, S., Warren, J., Lundberg, C., Casey, A., Correia, C., Konicek, D., et al. (2001). *An evaluation of the utility of the CEN categorical structure for nursing diagnoses as a terminology model for integrating nursing diagnosis concepts into SNOMED.* Paper presented at the MEDINFO 2001, Amsterdam.

Ball, M. J. (2003). Hospital information systems: Perspectives on problems and prospects, 1979 and 2002. *International Journal of Medical Informatics, 69*, 83–89.

Ball, M. J., & Douglas, J. (1988). Integrating nursing and informatics. In M. J. Ball, K. J. Hannah, U. Jelger, & H. Peterson (Eds.), *Nursing informatics: Where caring and technology meet* (pp. 11–17). New York: Springer-Verlag.

Bates, D., Cullen, D., Laird, N., Petersen, L., Small, S., Servi, D., et al. (1995). Incidence of adverse drug events and potential adverse drug events: Implications for prevention. *The Journal of the American Medical Association, 274*(1), 29–34.

Blewitt, D. K., & Jones, K. R. (1996). Using elements of the nursing minimum data set for determining outcomes. *Journal of Nursing Administration, 26*(6), 48–56.

Brokel, J. (2007). Creating sustainability of clinical information systems. *Journal of Nursing Administration, 37*(1), 10–13.

Button, P., Androwich, I., Hibben, L., Kern, V., Madden, G., Marek, K., et al. (1998). Challenges and issues related to implementation of nursing vocabularies in computer-based systems. *Journal of the American Medical Informatics Association, 5*(4), 332–334.

Clark, J. L., & Lang, N. (1992). Nursing's next advance: An internal classification for nursing practice. *International Nursing Review, 39*(4), 109–111.

Coenen, A., Marin, H., Park, H., & Bakken, S. (2001). Collaborative efforts for representing nursing concepts in computer-based systems: International perspectives. *Journal of the American Medical Informatics Association, 8*(3), 202–211.

Coiera, E. (2000). When conversation is better than computation. *Journal of the American Informatics Association, 7*(3), 277–286.

DeJong, G. (2007). *Setting the stage: The case for another paradigm.* Council for the Advancement of Nursing Science Special Topics Conference, Washington, DC.

Delaney, C., & Huber, D. (2001). Clinical testing of a national standardized minimum data set designed to capture the management context of health care delivery. In *Proceedings of the AMIA Annual Symposium.* Washington, DC.

Donabedian, A. (1986). Criteria and standards for quality assessment and monitoring. *Quarterly Review Bulletin, 12*(3), 99–100.

Graves, J., & Corcoran, S. (1989). The study of nursing informatics. *Image: Journal of Nursing Scholarship, 21*(4), 227–231.

Hannah, K., Ball, M., & Edwards, M. (2006). *Introduction to nursing informatics.* New York: Springer.

Hardiker, N. (2003). Determining sources for nursing terminology systems. *Journal of Biomedical Informatics, 35*, 279–286.

Hardiker, N., & Rector, A. (2001). Structural validation of nursing technologies. *Journal of the American Medical Informatics Association, 8*(3), 212–221.

Huber, D., & Oermann, M. (1999). Do outcomes equal quality? *Outcomes Management for Nursing Practice, 3*(1), 1–3.

Huber, D., Schumacher, L., & Delaney, C. (1997). Nursing management minimum data set (NMMDS). *Journal of Nursing Administration, 27*(4), 42–48.

Huber, D. G., Delaney, C., Crossley, J., Mehmert, M., & Ellerbe, S. (1992). A nursing management minimum data set: Significance and development. *Journal of Nursing Administration, 22*(7–8), 35–40.

Ingenerf, J. (1995). *Taxonomic vocabularies in medicine: The intention of usage determines different established structures.* Paper presented at the MEDINFO 95. British Columbia: Vancouver.

Institute of Medicine. (2004). *Keeping patients safe.* Washington, DC: National Academies Press.

International Organization for Standardization (ISO). (2002). *Health informatics: Integration of a reference terminology model for nursing* (Committee Document No. ISO/TC 215/N 142). Geneva, Switzerland: Author.

Iowa Intervention Project. (1997). *Nursing outcomes classification (NOC)*. St. Louis: Mosby.

Jones, S., & Moss, J. (2006). Computerized provider order entry: Strategies for successful implementation. *Journal of Nursing Administration, 36*(3), 136–140.

Kennedy, R. (2003). The nursing shortage and the role of technology. *Nursing Outlook, 51*(Suppl.), 33–34.

Kimmel, K., & Sensmeier, J. (2002). *A technological approach to enhancing patient safety*. Chicago: HIMMS.

Kopp, B., Erstad, B., Allen, M., Theodorou, A., & Priestley, G. (2006). Medication errors and adverse drug events in an intensive care unit: Direct observation approach for detection. *Critical Care Medicine, 34*(2), 415–425.

Leape, L., Bates, D., Cullen, D., Cooper, J., Demonaco, H., Gallivan, T., et al. (1995). Systems analysis of adverse drug events. *Journal of the American Medical Association, 274*(1), 35–43.

Lorenzi, N., & Riley, R. (2003). Organizational issues = change. *International Journal of Medical Informatics, 69*, 197–203.

Maas, M., Johnson, M., & Moorhead, S. (1996). Classifying nursing-sensitive patient outcomes. *Image: Journal of Nursing Scholarship, 28*(4), 295–301.

Maas, M. L., Delaney, C., & Huber, D. (1999). Contextual variables and assessment of the outcome effects of nursing interventions. *Outcomes Management for Nursing Practice, 3*(1), 4–6.

Meadows, G. (2002). Nursing informatics: An evolving specialty. *Nursing Economic$, 20*(6), 300–301.

Mills, M., Romano, C., & Heller, B. (1996). *Information management in nursing and health care*. Philadelphia: Springhouse.

Moss, J. (2003). A method for evaluating nursing documentation. *Health IT Advisory Report, 4*(8), 14–17.

Moss, J., Andison, M., & Sobko, H. (2007). An analysis of narrative nursing documentation in an otherwise structured intensive care clinical information system. Chicago. *Proceedings of the American Medical Informatics Association Annual Symposium*, 543–547.

Moss, J., Coenen, A., & Mills, M. (2003). Evaluation of the draft international standard for a reference terminology model for nursing actions. *Journal of Biomedical Informatics, 36*(4–5), 271–278.

Moss, J., & Xiao, Y. (2004). Improving operating room coordination: Communication pattern assessment. *Journal of Nursing Administration, 34*(2), 93–100.

Moss, J., Xiao, Y., & Zubaidah, S. (2002). The operating room charge nurse: Coordinator and communicator. *Journal of the American Medical Informatics Association, 9*(Suppl. 6), 70–74.

O'Brien, K., & Anderson, J. (2007). *High quality, efficient care for Medicare beneficiaries—but at what cost?* Health Care Compliance Association. Retrieved February 2, 2008, from www.foley.com/files/tbl_s31Publications/FileUpload137/4556/Compliance_OBrienAnderson.pdf

Ornstein, C. (2003). *Hospital heeds doctors, suspends use of software*. Retrieved November 30, 2008, from www.latimes.com/news/printedition/california/la-me-cedars22jan22,0,15283.story

Petersen, L., Woodard, L., Urech, T., Daw, C., & Sookanan, S. (2006). Does pay-for-performance improve the quality of health care? *Annals of Internal Medicine, 145*(4), 265–272.

Phoenix Health Systems. (2004). *HHS fact sheet: Harnessing information technology to improve healthcare*. Montgomery Village, MD: Author. Retrieved May 31, 2004, from www.hhs.gov/news/press/2004pres/20040427a.html

Staggers, N., Bagley Thompson, C., & Snyder-Halpern, R. (2001). History and trends in clinical information systems in the United States. *Journal of Nursing Scholarship, 33*(1), 75–81.

Stenson, R. (2003). *Failure to check database, misunderstanding led to teen's death*. Oakland, CA: California Healthcare Foundation.

Stetson, P., McKnight, K., Bakken, S., Curran, C., Kubose, T., & Cimino, J. (2001). *Development of an ontology to model medical errors, information needs, and the clinical communication space*. Washington, DC: Paper presented at the AMIA Annual Symposium.

U.S. Department of Health and Human Services (USDHHS). (2004). *Secretary Thompson, seeking fastest possible results, names first health information technology coordinator*. Washington, DC: Author. Retrieved November 30, 2008, from www.dhhs.gov/news/press/2004pres/20040506.html

Vogelsmeier, A., Halbesleben, J., & Scott-Cawiezell, J. (2008). Technology implementation and workarounds in the nursing home. *Journal of the American Medical Informatics Association, 15*, 114–119.

Werley, H., & Lang, N. (Eds.). (1988). *Identification of the nursing minimum data set*. New York: Springer.

Winslow, E., Nestor, V., Davidoff, S., Thompson, P., & Borum, J. (1997). Legibility and completeness of physicians' handwritten medication orders. *Heart & Lung: The Journal of Acute & Critical Care, 26*(2), 158–164.

Chapter 37

Aiken, L., Havens, D., & Sloane, D. (2000). The Magnet nursing services recognition program: A comparison of two groups of Magnet hospitals. *American Journal of Nursing, 100*, 26–35.

American Nurses Credentialing Center (ANCC). (2009). *Magnet Recognition Program® manual: Recognizing nursing excellence*. Silver Spring, MD: Author: Retrieved May 26, 2009, from http://www.nursecredentialing.org/Magnet.aspx

Baptist Health Care. (2004). *Baptist Health Care: Mission, values, vision*. Pensacola, FL: Author. Retrieved November 30, 2008, from www.bhcexpansion.org/Values.aspx

Below, P. J., Morrisey, G. L., & Acomb, B. L. (1987). *The executive guide to strategic planning.* San Francisco: Jossey-Bass.

Collins, J. C., & Porràs, J. I. (1994). *Built to last: Successful habits of visionary companies.* New York: HarperBusiness.

Collins, J. C., & Porràs, J. I. (2004). *Built to last: Successful habits of visionary companies.* New York: HarperCollins.

Crossan, F. (2003). Strategic management and nurses: Building foundations. *Journal of Nursing Management, 11*(5), 331–335.

Fidellow, J. A., & Hogan, M. (1998). Strategic planning: Implementing a foundation. *Nursing Management, 29*(6), 34, 36.

Martin, M. (1998). Achieving the right balance with strategic planning. *Nursing Management, 29*(5), 30–31.

McClure, M. L., & Hinshaw, A. S. (2002). *Magnet hospitals revisited: Attraction and retention of professional nurses.* Silver Spring, MD: American Nurses Credentialing Center.

Peters, T. (1987). *Thriving on chaos.* New York: HarperCollins.

Puetz, B. E., & Shinn, L. J. (1997). *The nurse consultant's handbook.* New York: Springer.

Woods, S. L. (2001). Using evidence-based approaches to strategically respond to the nursing shortage. *Critical Care Nursing Clinics of North America, 13*(4), 511–519.

Chapter 38

Alward, R. R., & Camunas, C. (1991). *The nurse's guide to marketing.* Albany, NY: Delmar Publishers.

Andreasen, A. R., & Kotler, P. (2008). *Strategic marketing for nonprofit organizations.* Upper Saddle River, NJ: Pearson Prentice Hall.

Buresh, B., & Gordon, S. (2006). *From silence to voice: What nurses know and must communicate to the public* (2nd ed.). Ithaca, NY and London, UK: ILR Press.

Graham, P. (1993). Marketing's domain: A critical review of the development of the marketing concept. *Marketing Bulletin, 4,* 1–11.

Grant, R. M. (1991). *Contemporary strategy analysis* (3rd ed.). Malden, MA: Blackwell Publishers.

Harvard Business School Press. (2006). *Marketer's toolkit: The 10 strategies you need to succeed.* Boston, MA: Harvard Business School Publishing Corporation.

Harvey, J. W. (1998). Marketing in the new health care environment. In J. A. Dienemann (Ed.), *Nursing administration: Managing patient care* (2nd ed., pp. 185–206). Stamford, CT: Appleton & Lange.

Joint Commission on Accreditation of Healthcare Organizations (JCAHO). (2002). Oakbrook Terrace, IL: Author. Retrieved November 30, 2008, from www.jointcommission.org/NR/rdonlyres/5C138711-ED76–4D6F-909F-B06E0309F36D/0/health_care_at_the_crossroads.pdf

Kotler, P. (1999). *Kotler on marketing: How to create, win, and dominate markets.* New York: The Free Press.

Kotler, P. (2000). *Marketing management* (Millennium ed.). Upper Saddle River, NJ: Prentice-Hall.

Kotler, P. (2003). *Marketing insights from A to Z.* Hoboken, NJ: John Wiley & Sons.

Kotler, P., & Armstrong, G. (2008). *Principles of marketing* (12th ed.). Upper Saddle River, NJ: Pearson Prentice Hall.

Kotler, P., & Clarke, R. N. (1987). *Marketing for health care organizations.* Englewood Cliffs, NJ: Prentice-Hall.

Kramer, M., & Schmalenberg, C. (1988). Magnet hospitals: Institutions of excellence, Part 1. *Journal of Nursing Administration, 18*(1), 13–24.

Needleman, J., Buerhaus, P., Mattke, S., Stewart, M., & Zelevinsky, K. (2002). Nurse-staffing levels and the quality of care in hospitals. *The New England Journal of Medicine, 346*(22), 1715–1722.

Schnaars, S. P. (1991). *Marketing strategy: Customers and competition* (2nd ed.). New York: The Free Press.

Woods, D. (2002). Realizing your marketing influence. Part 1. Meeting patient needs through collaboration. *Journal of Nursing Administration, 32*(4), 189–195.

Woods, D., & Cardin, S. (2002). Realizing your marketing influence. Part 2. Marketing from the inside out. *Journal of Nursing Administration, 32*(6), 323–330.

Zander, K. (1992). Nursing care delivery methods and quality. *Series on Nursing Administration, 3,* 86–104.

Zell, A. J. (2002). *Change: An opportunity.* Portland, OR: Ambassador of Selling.

Index

Note: Page number followed by *f* indicates figures, *b* indicates boxes, and *t* indicates tables.

D

U

V